Textbook of Ear, Nose, Throat and Head & Neck Surgery

Clinical and Practical

Third Edition

P. Hazarika
MBBS, DLO, MS, FACS, FRCS (Edin), FIAO FUWAI, Fellow of UICC

Ex-Professor and Head, Department of ENT–Head & Neck Surgery
Kasturba Medical College, Manipal

D.R. Nayak
MBBS, MS, FICS, Fellow of UICC

Professor and Head, Department of ENT–Head & Neck Surgery
Kasturba Medical College, Manipal

R. Balakrishnan
MBBS, MS (ENT), DNB

Professor and Head of Unit II, Department of ENT–Head & Neck Surgery
Kasturba Medical College, Manipal

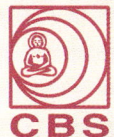

CBS Publishers & Distributors Pvt Ltd

New Delhi • Bengaluru • Chennai • Kochi • Mumbai • Pune
Hyderabad • Kolkata • Nagpur • Patna • Vijayawada

Textbook of Ear, Nose, Throat and Head & Neck Surgery
Clinical and Practical

Third Edition: 2013
Reprint: 2014
First Edition: 2007
Second Edition: 2009
Revised Second Edition: 2012
Copyright © Authors and Publishers

ISBN: 978-81-239-2316-1

Published by Satish Kumar Jain for
CBS Publishers & Distributors Pvt Ltd
4819/XI Prahlad Street, 24 Ansari Road, Daryaganj, New Delhi 110 002, India.
Ph: 23289259, 23266861, 23266867   Fax: 011-23243014   Website: www.cbspd.com
e-mail: delhi@cbspd.com; cbspubs@airtelmail.in.
Corporate Office: 204 FIE, Industrial Area, Patparganj, Delhi 110 092
Ph: 4934 4934   Fax: 4934 4935   e-mail: publishing@cbspd.com; publicity@cbspd.com

Branches

- **Bengaluru:** Seema House 2975, 17th Cross, K.R. Road,
  Banasankari 2nd Stage, Bengaluru 560 070, Karnataka
  Ph: +91-80-26771678/79   Fax: +91-80-26771680   e-mail: bangalore@cbspd.com
- **Chennai:** 20, West Park Road, Shenoy Nagar, Chennai 600 030, Tamil Nadu
  Ph: +91-44-26260666, 26208620   Fax: +91-44-42032115   e-mail: chennai@cbspd.com
- **Kochi:** 36/14 Kalluvilakam, Lissie Hospital Road, Kochi 682 018, Kerala
  Ph: +91-484-4059061-65   Fax: +91-484-4059065   e-mail: kochi@cbspd.com
- **Mumbai:** 83-C, Dr E Moses Road, Worli, Mumbai-400018, Maharashtra
  Ph: +91-22-24902340/41   Fax: +91-22-24902342   e-mail: mumbai@cbspd.com
- **Pune:** Bhuruk Prestige, Sr. No. 52/12/2+1+3/2 Narhe, Haveli
  (Near Katraj-Dehu Road Bypass), Pune 411 041, Maharashtra
  Ph: +91-20-64704058, 64704059, 32392277   Fax: +91-20-24300160   e-mail: pune@cbspd.com

Representatives

- **Hyderabad**   0-9885175004
- **Nagpur**   0-9021734563
- **Kolkata**   0-9831437309, 0-9051152362
- **Patna**   0-9334159340
- **Vijayawada**   0-9000660880

Printed at: HT Media Ltd., Noida

Foreword

Dr. P. Hazarika, Dr. D.R. Nayak and Dr. R. Balakrishnan should be congratulated for writing this book *Textbook of Ear, Nose, Throat and Head & Neck Surgery*. The authors are committed to providing a textbook that can be used by undergraduate students, residents and practising doctors in the Indian perspective.

This book will be rewarding to become a resource of information for the readers and help in generating the interest to pursue this field of speciality. The knowledge acquired from this book will definitely help in understanding the mechanism and management. The book contains 377 illustrations and line diagrams, 85 flowcharts, tables and 653 clinical operative photographs.

The authors have extensive training and experience in otolaryngology and are certainly well qualified to do this work.

I believe that this book will be an excellent contribution to otorhinolaryngology and head and neck surgery.

Prof. S.K. Kacker
MS, FRCS (London), FAMS
Otorhinolaryngologist (Ear, Nose and Throat Specialist)
Former Professor and Head, Department of ENT, and
Director
All India Institute of Medical Sciences,
New Delhi

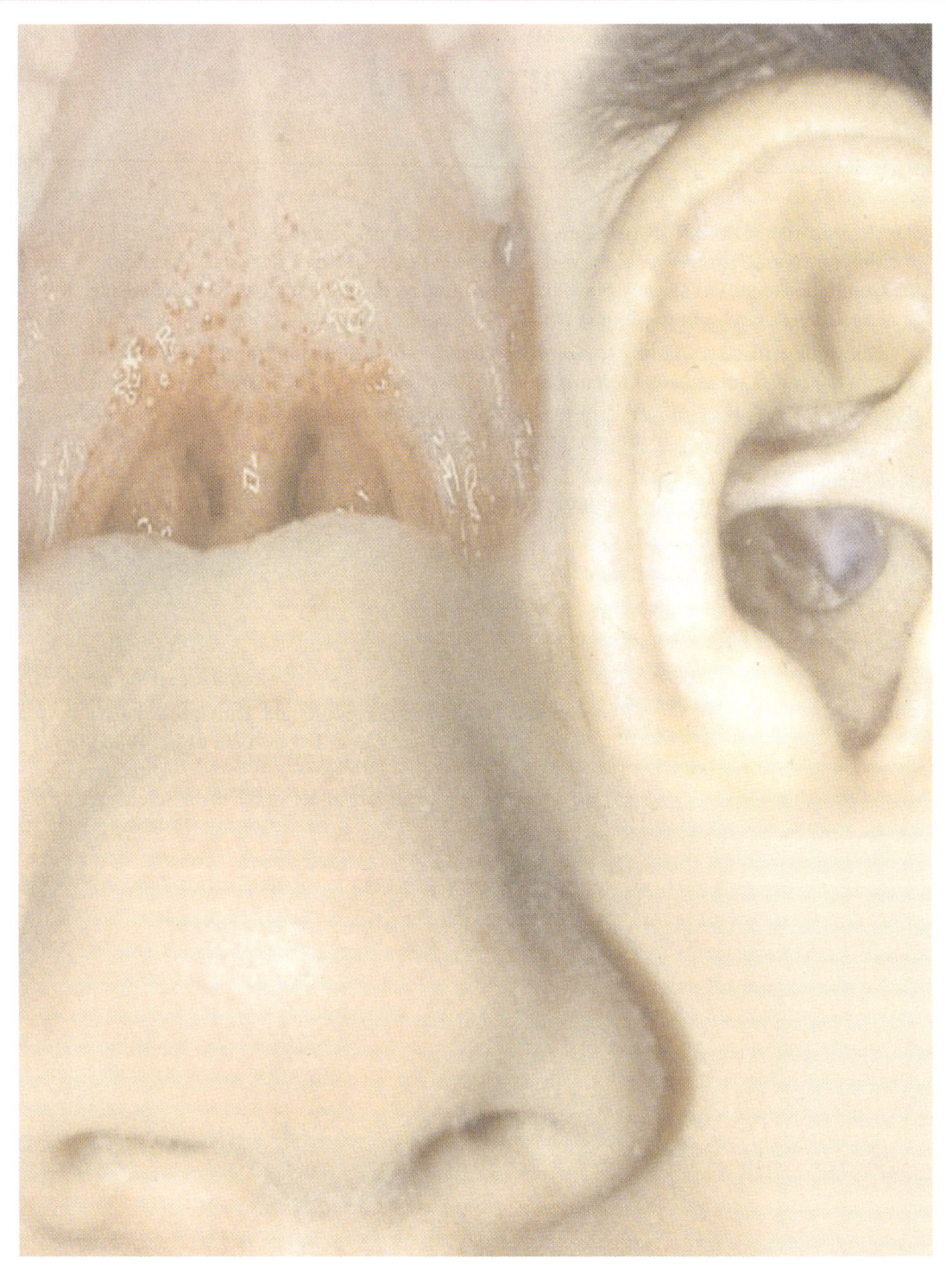

Preface to the Third Edition

It is our pleasure to bring out the third edition of this unique textbook after its first edition was published in 2007. The second edition was brought out in 2009 followed by the revised edition in 2012. We are thankful to all the readers including undergraduate and postgraduate students, teachers and practising doctors for accepting it as a standard textbook in ENT and encouraging us to come out with this new edition. This book has been thoroughly updated and revised in this edition. Replacement of drawings and pictures, especially in otology, and addition of a few relevant topics have been done as per the undergraduate requirement and suggestions received from various students and teachers.

We sincerely hope that the third edition of the book will be widely accepted and appreciated by the student community as well as teachers.

P. Hazarika

D. R. Nayak

R. Balakrishnan

"If you would not be forgotten
as soon as you are dead and rotten,
Either write something worth reading
or do things worth writing."

— Benjamin Franklin
US author, diplomat, inventor, physicist and politician (1706–1790)

— *Poor Richard's Almanack* (1738)

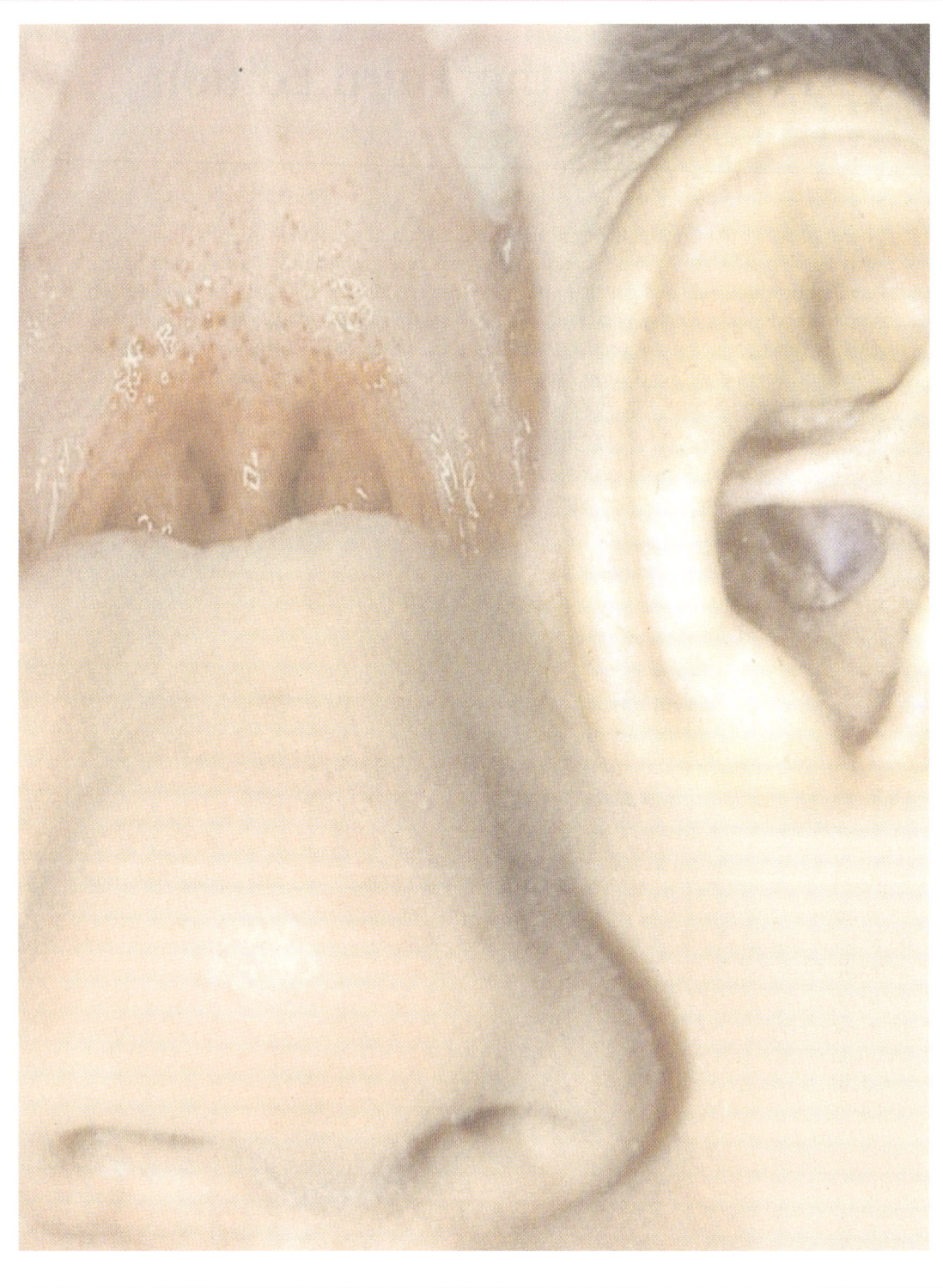

Preface to the First Edition

There are many undergraduate otolaryngology textbooks available, however, a textbook covering all the aspects of otolaryngology and head and neck surgery is a rarity in Indian perspective. The present multi-authored book covering the entire field of otolaryngology and head and neck surgery is very unique and informative from the MBBS student's viewpoint. It incorporates theoretical knowledge based on numerous developments in this speciality and also covers the clinical and practical aspects of the subject to help the students during their examinations.

The systematic organization of the chapters is necessary to retain a sensible balance while our knowledge has expanded in some areas more than the others. The chapters on recent advances, anesthesia and operative surgeries are incorporated to give a broad understanding and update in the knowledge of rapidly developing clinical otolaryngological practice.

Increased number of chapters with inclusion of clear and concise illustrations, clinical and operative methods and colour photographs of rare and interesting diseases, detailed description of the use of instruments has made this textbook very voluminous. The authors believe that this expansion is essential and necessary to inform the readers regarding the voluminous increase of knowledge in our speciality. The authors have confined themselves in their chapters to deal only with contemporary questions and problems and together synthesize the information on recent advances. Numerous books and journals have been referred before offering the critical evaluation of the recent advances.

The cover page of this book is designed by Urvashi Patankar from London, who is a known graphic designer and has done a very good job. The senior author is instrumental in persuading her to take up this work. Cover page has rightly represented area of skull base, broncho-oesophagology along with general otorhinolaryngology.

This book contains 377 illustrations and line diagrams, 85 flow charts and tables, and 653 number of clinical operative color photographs which makes the study of this book more interesting and enjoyable.

It will be very rewarding for the authors if this book becomes a resource of information for the readers and helps in generating the interest to pursue this field of speciality. The knowledge acquired from this book will definitely help in understanding the mechanism and management of the complication in the head and neck interface. This is critical to avoid diagnostic and surgical pitfalls while providing safe and effective care by practising otolaryngologist.

P. Hazarika
D. R. Nayak
R. Balakrishnan

Acknowledgements

It is after the completion of our work that we realize the immense necessity of writing this page, in an effort to acknowledge those who in all their possible ways have helped us in carrying out and completing this book. Of course, this small return in a few words is only a fraction of what we were given by them.

We take the privilege to express our profound sense of gratitude to late Prof. B.R. Das MBBS, DLO, FRCS (Edin), FRCS (Glas), Assam Medical College, who had a towering and divine influence in initiating this project of ours. We have the pleasure to place on record the concise and concrete suggestions as well as the goodwill offered to us by Prof. L.H. Hiranandani, Prof. K. Kameshwaran, Prof. A.L. Mukherjee, Prof. K.K. Ramlingam, Prof. R.C. Deka, Dr. Vishanathan and Dr. Mahadevaiah in response to a few of our queries in connection with this book. We owe a deep sense of gratitude to these great teachers of otorhinolaryngology of our times. Our special thanks to Prof. Santosh K. Kacker, former Professor of ENT and Director, All India Institute of Medical Sciences, New Delhi, for giving the Foreword.

We are grateful to our founder beloved President of MAHE, Dr. Ram Das M. Pai, Dr. Raj Warrior, Vice Chancellor of MAHE, and Dr. R.S.P. Rao, Dean of KMC, Manipal, who kindly permitted us to carry on the work on this book in this institution lacking which, we fear, it would not have been possible to bring this work to light.

It is worthwhile to express a word of appreciation to Dr. Suresh Pillai, Dr. Sherry Jacob, Dr. Kailesh Pujary, Dr. Parul Pujary, Dr. Asha Kumar, Dr. Jaspal Sahota, Dr. Sajeev George, Dr. S.A. Mallik, Dr. Vivek. C. Abraham, Dr. N.L.N. Reddy, Dr. A. Suneel, Dr. Navneet, Dr. Avneesh, Dr. Ajay Lavania, Dr. Raghavendra Rao, Dr. Ramananda Shetty, Dr. Rodney Rodrigues, Dr. Hemant, Dr. Harish Kundaje, Dr. Mahesh, Dr. Ranveer, Dr. Seema E.P., Dr. Pallavi, Dr. Sunil, Dr. Deepika, Dr. Sajilal, Dr. Aishwarya, Dr. Vijaya, Dr. Ramakrishna, Dr. Deepa, Dr. Archana, Dr. Jyothi, Dr. Gopi, Dr. Abhishek, Dr. Deichu and Dr. Navneet.

We do always have an indebted honor for Dr. Peddhibottala Kumararaja, Assistant Professor, Department of ENT, Medical College, Karimnagar, for his many-fold help in the initial stage of the work. We also deeply appreciate Dr. Rohit Singh, Assistant Professor of ENT, for his constant encouragement, and help at the crucial stage of the work particularly during proofreading and Dr. Prashant Prabhu for the timely correction of 2nd revised edition. We are also thankful to Dr. Manushrut, Pg. in ENT, for helping in addition of targeted Chemotherapy and IMRT.

We shall be failing in our duties if we do not offer our heartful gratitude to our parents late Mr. and Mrs. L.C. Hazarika; late Mrs. and Dr. B. Nayak; and Prof. K.R. Iyengar and Mrs. Lakshmi Iyengar. We are also thankful to our wives and children Mrs. Reema Hazarika, Dr. Manali Hazarika, Mrinmoy Hazarika, Mrs. Sujata D. Nayak, Shweta, Chinnu, Mrs. Sudha Balakrishna, Ananthu and Srividya for their constant encouragement and support.

Our secretary Mrs. Thulasi also deserves our thanks for help along with nonteaching staff of the department Mr. Seetharam, Mrs. Mangala, Mr. Bhaskar, Mr. Sudhakar, and Sister (Mrs.) Shanthi, Mrs. Malathi, Mrs. Mohini, Mrs. Usha, Mrs. Baby, Mrs. Vasanthi and Mrs. Bhavani.

Our special thanks to Mrs. Urvashi and Neil Patankar (London) for the preparation of an attractive cover page [first edition]. We shall be failing in our duties unless we offer our gratefulness to our patients who so optimistically offer themselves to our surgical efforts to cure such diseases.

Contents

Section 3: Pharynx and Esophagus

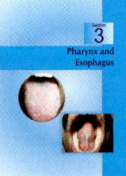

Section 4: Larynx and Trachea

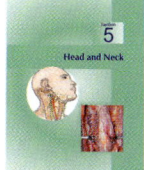

Section 5: Head and Neck

Section 6: Anesthesia in ENT: Head and Neck Surgery

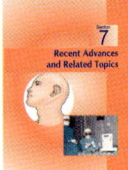

Section 7: Recent Advances and Related Topics

Section 8: Instruments and Radiology

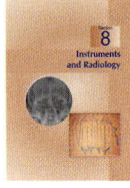

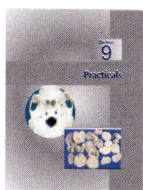

Section 9: Practicals

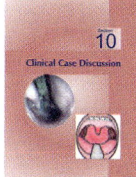

Section 10: Case Studies

Abbreviations Used

CSOM: Chronic suppurative otitis media
TTD : Tubo-tympanic disease
AAD : Attico-antral disease
URI : Upper respiratory infection
EAC : External auditory canal
MEM : Middle ear mucosa
HOM : Handle of malleus
TM   : Tympanic membrane
ETO : Eustachian tube orifice
ABL : Absolute bone conduction
N   : Normal
DNS : Deviated nasal septum
PND : Post nasal drip
WNL : Within normal limits
URTI : Upper respiratory tract infection
PPW : Posterior pharyngeal wall
PSQ : Posterosuperior quadrant
TMJ : Temporomandibular Joint
PNS : Paranasal sinus
ODH : Orodental hygiene
IT   : Inferior turbinate
IM   : Inferior meatus
MT   : Middle turbinate
MM   : Middle meatus
OP   : Organophosphorus

EAR

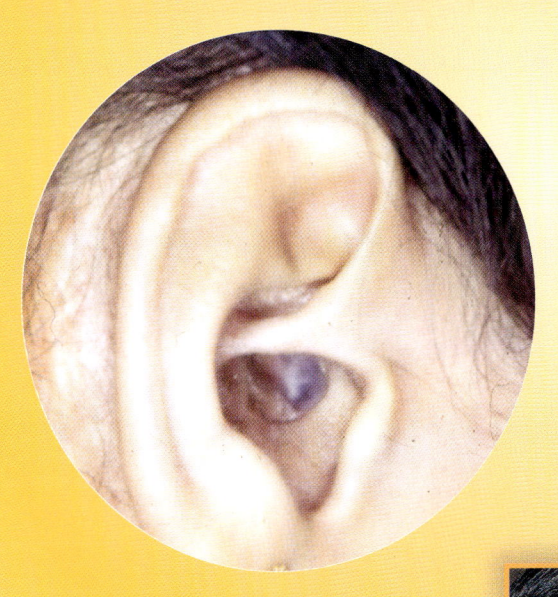

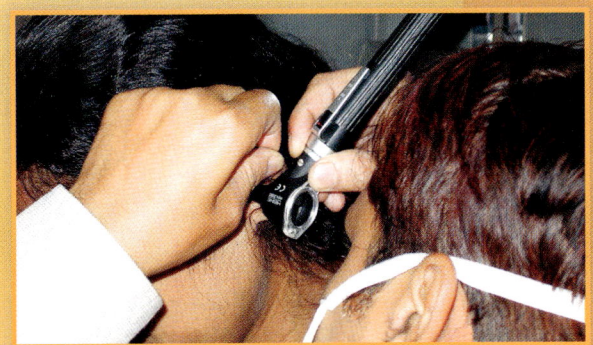

Embryology of the Ear

Ear has a very complex source of development. The sound conductive apparatus develops from the branchial apparatus whereas the sound perceptive apparatus develops from the ectodermal otocyst (pars otica). Because of this dual source of origin the developmental anomaly that produced commonly affects either the sound conductive system which includes anomaly of the external and/or the middle ear or the sound perceptive apparatus which includes the labyrinth. Both these anomalies rarely coexist because of different source of origin.

Development of the External Ear

This develops around the first branchial cleft.

The Pinna

Around 6th week of intrauterine life six hillocks or 'tubercles of His' appear around the first branchial cleft (Fig. 1.1). The first tubercle is derived from the first branchial arch and the rest from the 2nd branchial arch. Some authors believe that the first 3 tubercles develop from the first arch and the rest from the 2nd arch.

Structures derived from Various Hillocks

1. Tragus
2. Crus of the helix
3. Helix

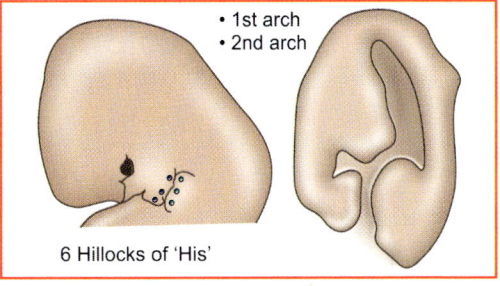

Fig. 1.1: Development of external ear from six hillocks

4. Antihelix
5. Scapha and the antitragus
6. Ear lobule

The ear takes definitive form by the end of third month of intrauterine life. Defective fusion of the tubercles gives rise to preauricular sinus and failure of the development of the hillocks causes anotia. Defective development of 4th tubercle can cause absence of antihelix leading to 'bat ear' deformity.

External Auditory Canal

This develops around the first branchial cleft as an invagination into a funnel-shaped pit to form a primary external auditory canal. Subsequent medial growth with a solid core of ectoderm leads to formation of a meatal plate called the secondary

3

external auditory canal. Between 8th and 10th week of IUL, the solid core of epithelium undergoes canalization forming the definitive external auditory canal.

Anomalies of the External Auditory Canal

1. Complete atresia
2. Shallow depression
3. Changes in the curvature of the canal
4. Stenosis

Development of Tympanomastoid Cavity and Eustachian Tube (Fig. 1.2)

Around 3rd week of IUL the first pharyngeal pouch develops which is phylogenetically the aquatic gill apparatus. This outpouching of the first pharyngeal pouch gives rise to two components namely:

1. The proximal narrow part which forms the eustachian tube.
2. The distal dilated part which gives rise to the developing middle ear cleft and is known as the tubotympanic recess. This forms the definitive tympanic cavity by progressively and systematically invaginating into the adjacent mesenchyme.

Towards the later part of the fetal life a diverticulum appears from the tubotympanic recess which subsequently forms the mastoid antrum. This antrum is about 3 mm thickness at birth and it increases 1 mm every year till it reaches the adult size of 15 mm thickness.

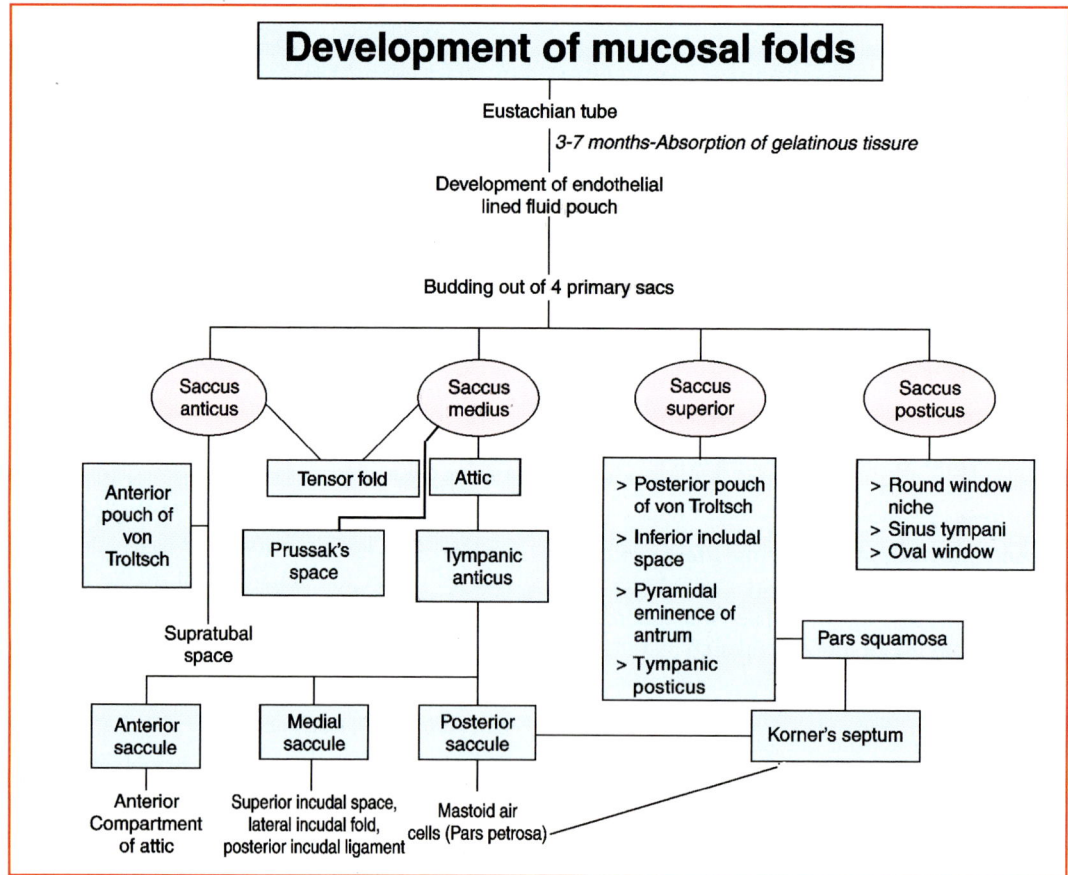

Fig. 1.2 Development of mucosal folds

Development of Ossicles

Anson in 1959 described the details of the development of the ossicles. The first arch cartilage (Meckel's cartilage) forms the head of the malleus and the body of the incus. The second arch forms the manubrium (handle) of the malleus and the long process of the incus and the crurae of the stapes. These sources of development confirm the various developmental anomalies involving the ossicles as encountered during surgery. The foot plate of the stapes develops from three sources namely:

1. The outer periosteal layer of the otic capsule.
2. Middle enchondral layer from the otic capsule.
3. Inner endosteal layer is same as the endosteum of the bony labyrinth and develops from the periotic mesoderm.

Development of Middle Ear Spaces and Folds

The envelopment of the ossicles by the mucous membrane lining of the tubotympanic recess occurs between 3–7 months of IUL. This mucous lining while encircling the ossicles form numerous folds and spaces as follows (shown in Figs 1.3, 1.4, 1.5a to d).

COMPARTMENT AND FOLDS OF THE TYMPANIC CAVITY (Figs 1.5a to d)

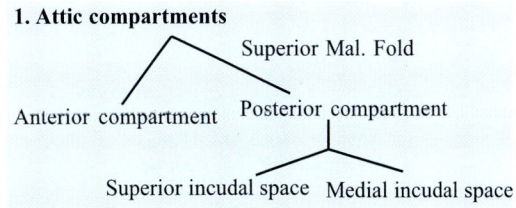

1. Attic compartments

- Anterior compartment
- Superior Mal. Fold
- Posterior compartment
  - Superior incudal space
  - Medial incudal space

2. Compartment of mesotympanum

Upper part of the mesotympanum is a reduplication of middle ear mucosa

Anterior malleolar fold	Posterior malleolar fold
• Neck of malleus to ant. margin of tympanic sulcus.	• Neck of malleus to post margin of tympanic sulcus.

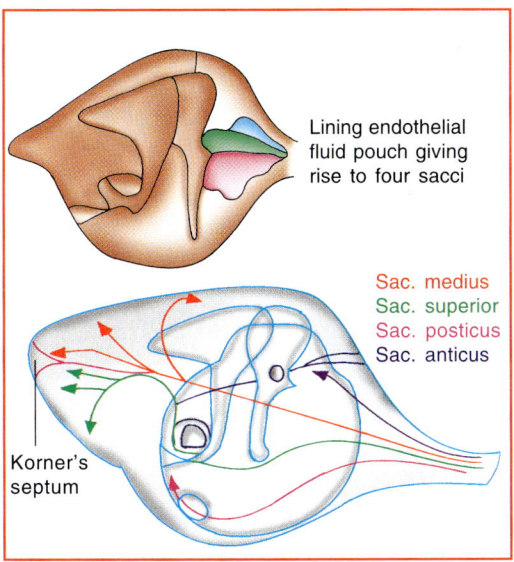

Lining endothelial fluid pouch giving rise to four sacci

Sac. medius
Sac. superior
Sac. posticus
Sac. anticus

Korner's septum

Fig. 1.3: Showing development of four primary sacs

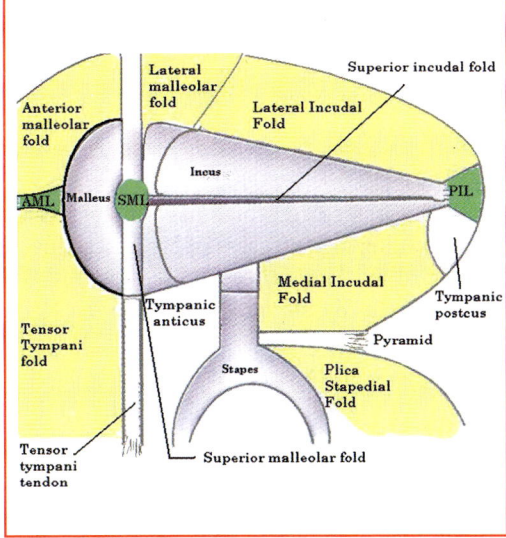

Fig. 1.4: Various middle ear folds and boundaries of tympanic anticus (TA)

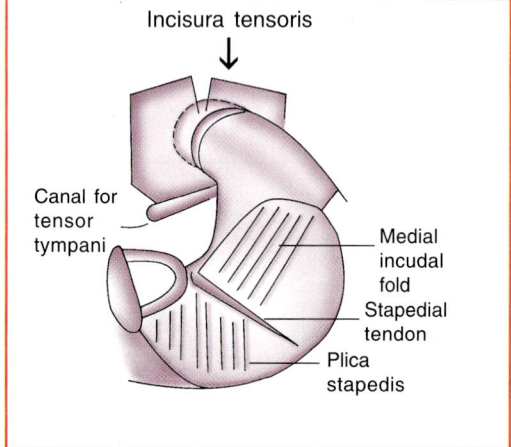

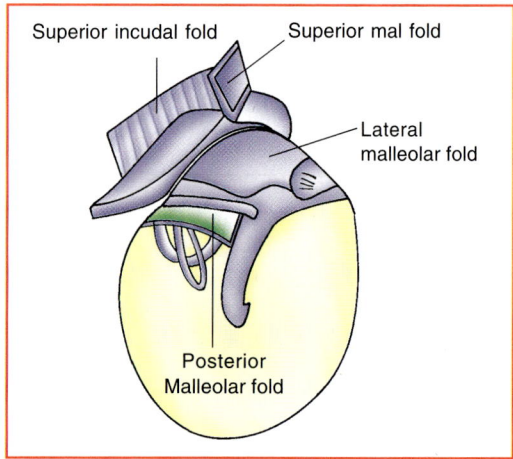

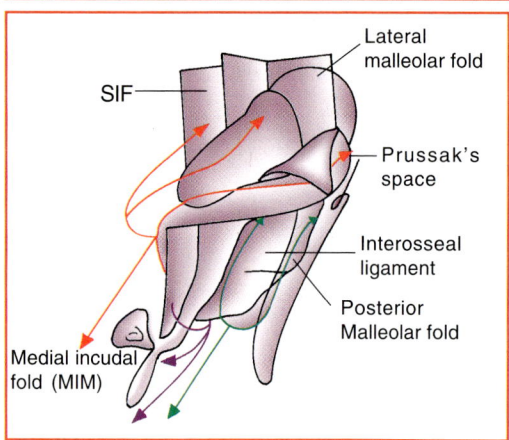

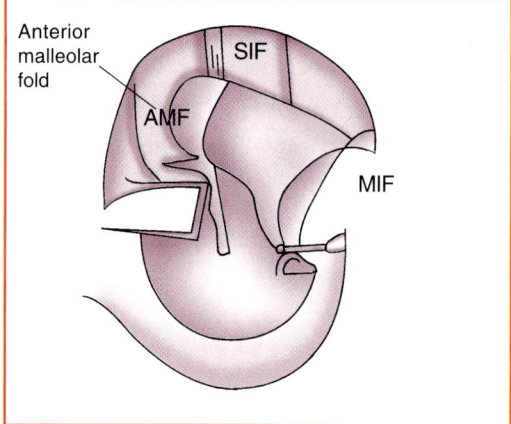

Figs 1.5a to d: Showing various mucosal folds that are developed during the process of development and the middle ear spaces that are formed from these folds

Prussak's Space (Figs 1.5c and 1.6)

It is a potential space which may be the first to involve during the extension of cholesteatoma, it is bounded by (Fig. 1.6)

- Laterally by shrapnell's membrane (Pars flacida)
- Medially by the neck of malleus
- Superiorly by fibers of lateral malleolar fold
- Inferiorly lateral process of malleus

Development of the Inner Ear

The inner ear develops from the otic capsule (pars otica). Initially a thickening appears in the ectoderm of the hindbrain known as otic placode.

It later invaginates forming otic cyst which is also known as otic capsule. Subsequent differentiation of this otic cyst leads to formation of membranous labyrinth. The mesoderm surrounding the otic capsule forms the bony labyrinth which attains the adult size at around 4th week of fetal life.

Pneumatization of mastoid: It is the process by which the aircell system extends as an outgrowth from the epithelial sac of the middle ear and antrum in conjuction with the enlargement of temporal bone which starts immediately after birth. Both genetic and acquired factors have been implicated to influence pneumatization process. The mastoid

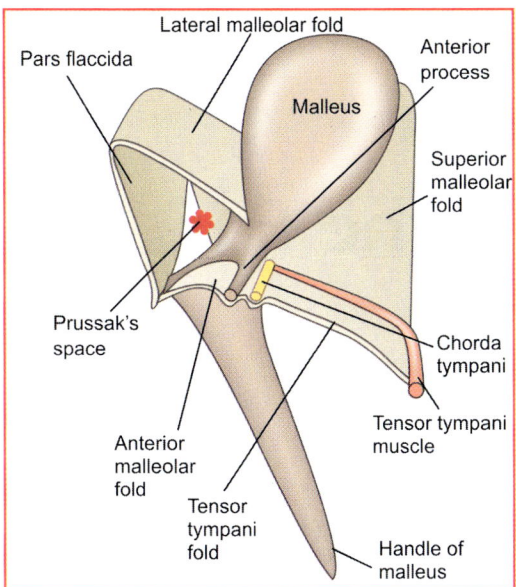

Fig.1.6: Boundaries of Prussak's space

process develops at the end of 1st year due to the contraction of the sternocleidomastoid muscles as the child tries to lift the head. In 80% of cases mastoid is fully pneumatized and in rest of the cases it may be partially pneumatized or sclerotic. Based on this the mastoid can be of three types:

1. Cellular (Well pneumatized)
2. Diploeic (Poorly pneumatized) few small-sized cellar
3. Sclerotic (Non-pneumatized) abscence of cells that are replaced with dense, compact bone. Sclerotic mastoid can be divided further into:
   - Primary sclerotic mastoid (not developed)
   - Secondary sclerotic mastoid (aquired).

Theories of faulty pneumatization:

1. Tumarkin theory: Poor ventilation of the middle ear cleft due to eustachian tube dysfunction leading to arrest of pneumatization.
2. Wittmaark theory: He proposed that otttis media in infancy and early childhood leads to poor ventilation of middle ear cleft causing arrest of pneumatization.
3. Diament was of the view that pneumatization of the mastoid bone is determined by hereditary factors.
4. Genetic factors were also implicated by Stern
5. Graham and Brackmen: The size of mastoid depends upon the final size of the skull in an individual as in acromegaly (large expansive mastoid) and in microcephaly (underdeveloped mastoid).

Classification of Mastoid Air Cell System

Allam (1969) classified the pneumatized spaces of the temporal bone into five different regions: middle ear region, mastoid region, perilabrynthine region, petrous apex region and accessory region (Fig. 2.19).

1. Middle ear region: Hypotympanic cells, etc.
2. Mastoid region
   - Central. Antum and Penantral cells
   - Peripheral. Tegnien cells, sinodural cells, pensinus cells, retrofacial cells and tip cells
3. *Perilabyrinthine region:* Supra and infralabyrinthine
4. Petrous apex region. Apical cells
5. Accessory region Zygomatic, squamous, occipital, styloid and pentubal cells

POINTS TO REMEMBER

1. The sound conducting apparatus develops from the branchial apparatus, whereas the sound perceptive apparatus from the ectodermal otocyst.
2. The pinna develops from the six hillocks around the 1st branchial cleft.
3. Defective fusion of tubercles gives rise to preauricular sinus.
4. The outpouching of the 1st pharyngeal pouch gives rise to a proximal narrow part that forms the eustachian tube and distal dilated part that forms the middle ear cavity.
5. Prussak's space is a potential space lateral to the sharpnell's membrane and medially by the neck muscles that can be involved during the extension of cholesteatoma.

2

Anatomy of the Ear

"Otology is almost unique even in the later part of the 20th century in not being able to explain at least a few of its diseases in biochemical terms"
— Ruben 1975.

Ear is divided into three parts (Fig. 2.1):
  1. External ear
  2. Middle ear
  3. Inner ear

EXTERNAL EAR

It consists of pinna and external auditory canal. Pinna develops from **six tubercles** around the **1st branchial cleft** whereas external auditory canal develops from the **1st branchial cleft.**

External auditory canal is the only cul-de-sac in the body lined by skin.

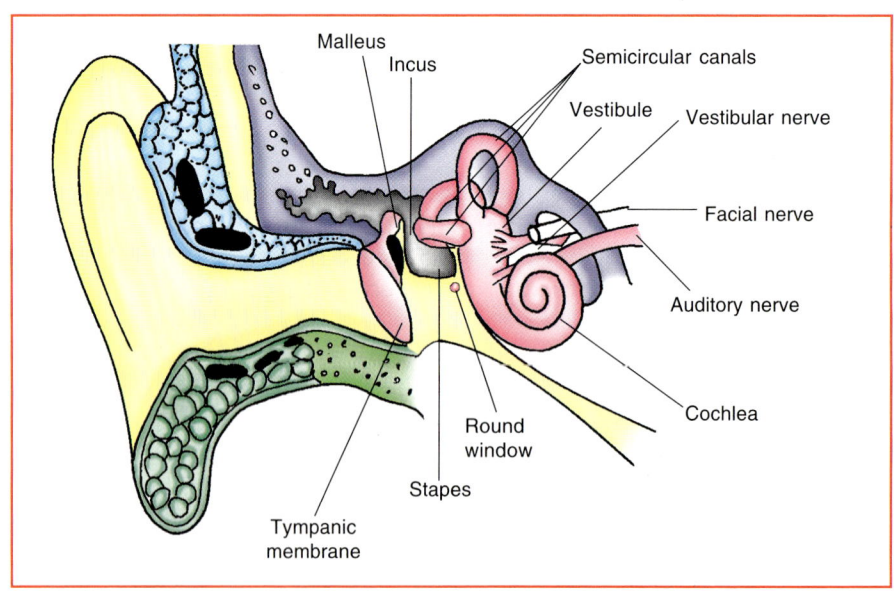

Fig. 2.1: Cross section of ear: External ear, middle ear and inner ear

Pinna (or auricle) is the prominent part of the external ear composed of **a single sheet of yellow elastic cartilage** covered by fat, subcutaneous tissue and skin. It has two surfaces—**medial (cranial) and lateral.** The lateral surface is concave with folds and hollows. The medial surface is convex. The most prominent outer fold is called **the helix** and the fold in front is the anti-helix. In front of the **anti-helix** is a hollow called concha which is divided by root of helix into Symba and cavum conchae.

Cavum conchae leads inwards to the external auditory canal. Anterior to the cavum conchae there is a small cartilaginous projection known as **tragus**. In the upper part of the cavum conchae, in front of the anti-helix, there is a triangular space known as **fossa triangularis.** There is also a boat shaped space in between the upper part of helix and anti-helix known as **scaphoid fossa** (Fig. 2.2).

The whole of the pinna is composed of a single sheet of cartilage except in the lobule and in the space between the cruss of the helix and tragus. This space is called **incisura terminalis** (Fig. 2.3). Since this area is devoid of cartilage, otologists can safely give an incision here for procedures in the ear to avoid postoperative perichondritis. The skin lining on the lateral or outer surface of the pinna is firmly adherent to the perichondrium of the cartilage with minimal or no subcutaneous tissue. Hence, the outer surface of the pinna is more prone to **frost bite**. In the cranial surface there is more subcutaneous tissue and the skin is loosely adherent to the underlying cartilage. Cysts like **sebaceous cyst** are commonly seen on this surface. The cartilage of the pinna **extends medially** to form the cartilaginous part of the external auditory canal.

External auditory meatus is **S-shaped** and approximately 2.5 cm in length. It has **two** parts - the outer one-third is **cartilaginous** and inner two third is **bony**. The cartilaginous part is a continuation of the auricular cartilage. It is firmly attached to the bony part by fibrous tissue. In infants, the cartilaginous meatus may remain collapsed because of the non development of the bony part. Hence, to examine the deeper part of the meatus in an infant, one has to pull the pinna outward, downward and backward.

It has two fissure the "**fissure of Santorini**" in the cartilaginous canal through which the parotid or superficial mastoid infections can appear in the meatus, or vice versa.

The external auditory canal is directed first inward, backward and upward and then goes forward, downward and medially. Isthmus is the

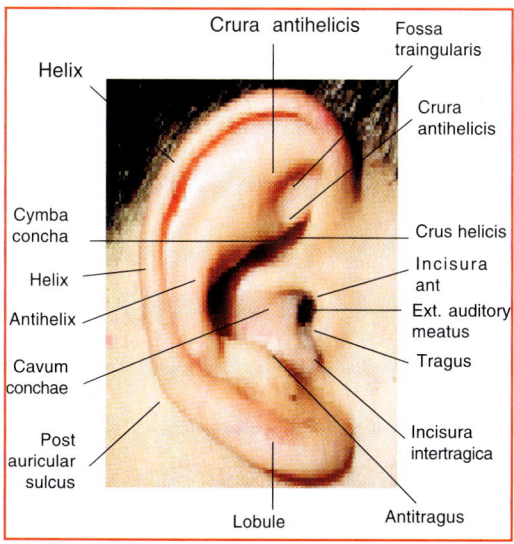

Fig 2.2: Parts of pinna

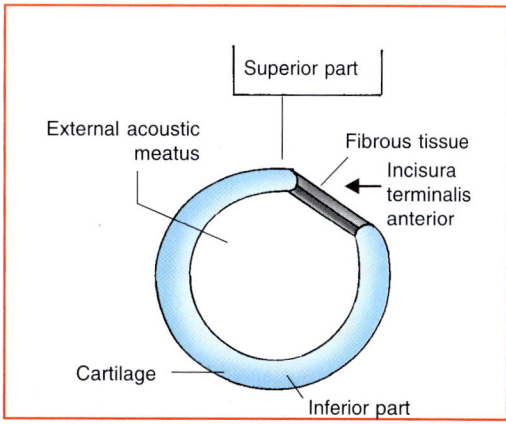

Fig. 2.3: Cross section of external auditory canal (Cartilaginous part)

narrowest part of the canal lying medial to the junction of bony and cartilaginous parts, nearly 5 mm lateral to the tympanic membrane. To examine the deeper part of the EAC in adult one has to pull the pinna upward, backward and laterally. The roof and posterior wall of the external auditory canal are **shorter** than the floor and anterior wall. Thus, the tympanic membrane fits obliquely in the deeper end of the canal.

The anterior wall goes sharply forward to the tympanic membrane to form a blind pouch known as the **anterior recess**. Examination of this area is likely to be missed on routine otoscopic examination unless one takes care. This may be a common site for **foreign body impaction lodgement**.

Skin of cartilaginous canal is loosely applied and contains hair follicles, ceruminous and sebaceous glands and these are absent in the skin of bony canal. Thus furunculosis occurs only in the outer cartilaginous canal and diffuse inflammation may occur in the bony canal.

The skin lining the tympanic membrane and bony canal has a self-cleansing property due to migration of the keratin layer of epithelium from drum towards the cartilaginous portion. Migration is rapid near the attachment of handle of malleus and slows as it reaches the canal. Loss of this property is seen in keratosis obturans.

Relation

It is closely related to the temporomandibular joint and parotid gland **anteriorly**. Mastoid antrum and mastoid air cells are the **posterior** relations.

Nerve Supply (Figs 2.4a and b)

Nerve supply of pinna

Greater auricular nerve is common to lower one-third of both the surfaces. Upper two-third of the medial surface is supplied by the lesser occipital nerve and the upper two-third of the lateral surface is supplied by the auriculotemporal nerve.

Nerve supply of external auditory canal

The anterior wall, floor and contiguous portion of the tympanic membrane are supplied by the auriculotemporal nerve. Rest of the canal and

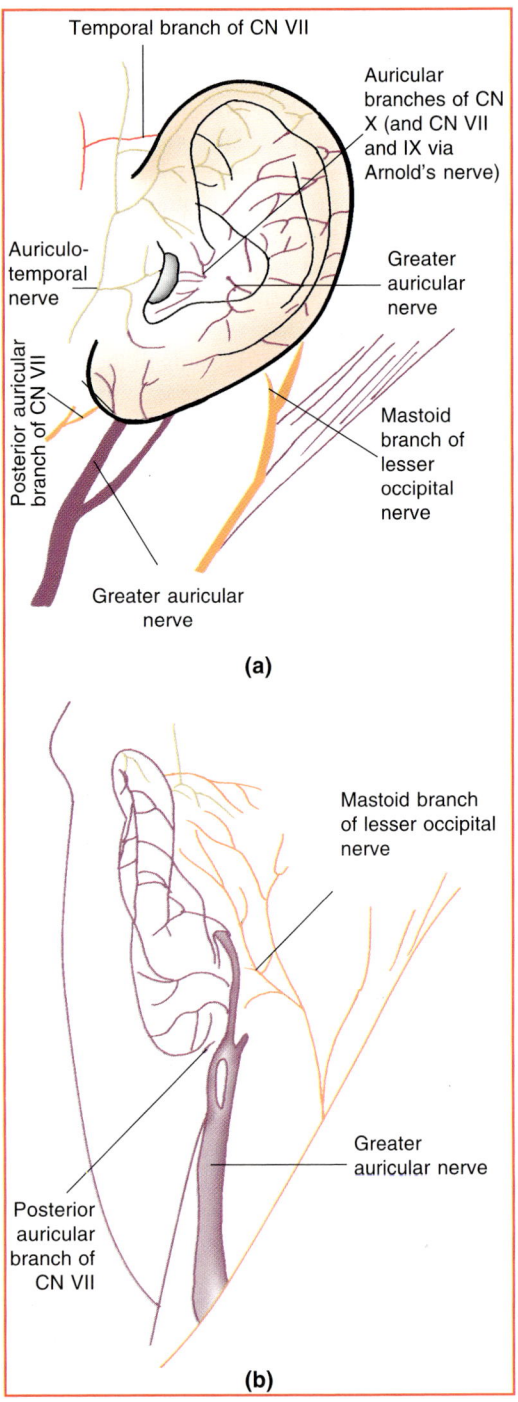

Figs 2.4a and b: Nerve supply of pinna

posterior part of the tympanic membrane are supplied by the tympanic branch of vagus, also known as **Arnold's nerve**. While cleaning the posterior meatal wall with a cotton swab, **cough is produced** which **reminds us of the presence of this vagal branch**. It is also thought that a twig from the facial nerve is incorporated with the tympanic branch of vagus and distributed along with it as evident in **herpes zoster infection**.

Blood supply is from the branches of the external carotid vessel.

Lymphatic Drainage (Fig. 2.5)

From the anterior wall it drains to the pre-auricular lymph nodes lying on the surface of the parotid gland in front of the tragus. The posterior wall drains to the post-auricular gland. The floor and lobule drains into retro-auricular gland.

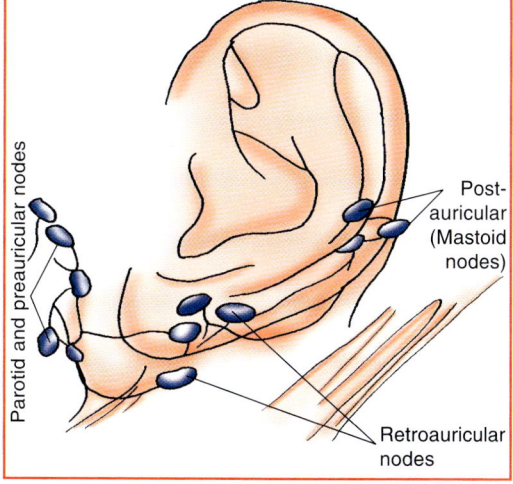

Fig. 2.5: Lymphatic drainage of pinna and external auditory canal

Tympanic Membrane (Ear drum; Drum Head) (Fig. 2.6)

It is a thin semitranslucent membrane pearly white in color, lying obliquely in the medial end of the external auditory canal, with the angle of 55°, forming the major part of the lateral wall of the

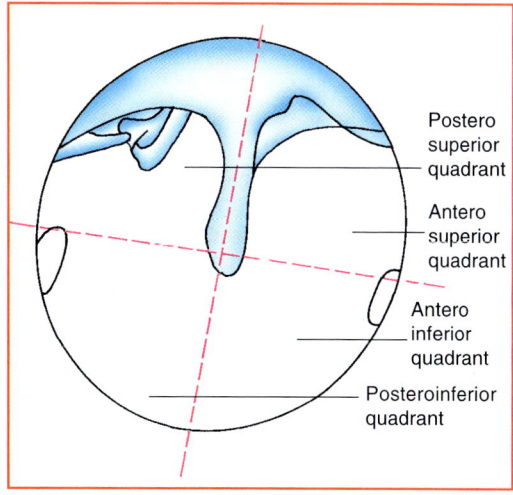

Fig. 2.6: Quadrants of right tympanic membrane

middle ear. Peripheral part of the tympanic membrane is thicker and rounded (except in the upper part) known as the annulus tympanicus. The annulus tympanicus is attached at its circumference to the tympanic sulcus. This tympanic sulcus ends in a notch known as the **Notch of Rivinus** in the upper part. There are two folds seen arising from the **Notch of Rivinus** to the lateral surface of malleus known as **anterior and posterior malleolar folds**.

Tympanic membrane consists of three layers except in the upper part

1. Outer cuticular or epithelial layer which is continuous with the skin of the external ear.
2. Middle fibrous layer has both circular and radial fibers. Radial fibers normally merge with the annulus tympanicus. This middle layer is missing in the upper part.
3. Inner mucosal layer which is continuous with the middle ear mucosa.

Tympanic membrane consists of two parts

1. **Pars tensa** is the larger part below the malleolar folds. It has all the three layers and is tense. The inner surface at the center is

attached to the handle of malleus. When light is reflected over the tympanic membrane, the anteroinferior part is the most illuminated part in the pars tensa.

2. **Pars flaccida (Shrapnell's membrane; attic)** is a triangular area above the malleolar folds which is thin and devoid of fibrous tissue and annulus. It fits into the **notch of Rivinus** (Fig. 2.7).

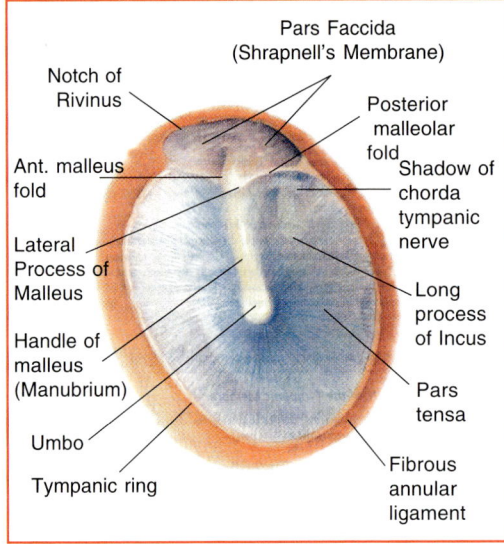

Fig. 2.7: Parts of left tympanic membrane

The ear drum measures approximately 10 mm in vertical diameter and 9.0 mm in horizontal diameter. It is oval in shape and placed obliquely at an angle of 55 degrees with the floor of the meatus. The inner surface is convex. The point of its greatest curvature is called **umbo** which corresponds to the tip of the handle of malleus on the inner surface (Fig. 2.8).

Blood Supply (Figs 2.9 a and b)

The outer surface of the tympanic membrane is supplied by manubrial artery whose origin is not known and also by the deep auricular branch of the maxillary artery.

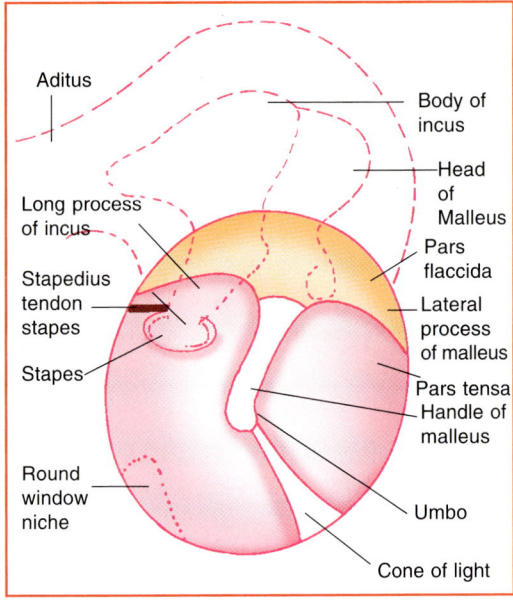

Fig. 2.8: Lateral wall of right tympanic cavity with its relation to the middle ear ossicles

The inner surface of the tympanic membrane is supplied by the following arteries

- Anterior tympanic branch of the maxillary artery.
- Posterior tympanic branch of stylomastoid artery.
- Inferior tympanic artery, a branch from the ascending pharyngeal artery.
- Arteria nutricia incudomallea, a twig from the middle meningeal artery.

Venous Drainage

The external jugular vein provides drainage for the outer surface. The inner surface is drained by the transverse sinus and the venous plexus located around the eustachian tube.

Nerve Supply

The outer surface is supplied by the auriculotemporal nerve in the anterior half and tympanic branch of vagus in the posterior half. Tympanic plexus supplies the inner surface.

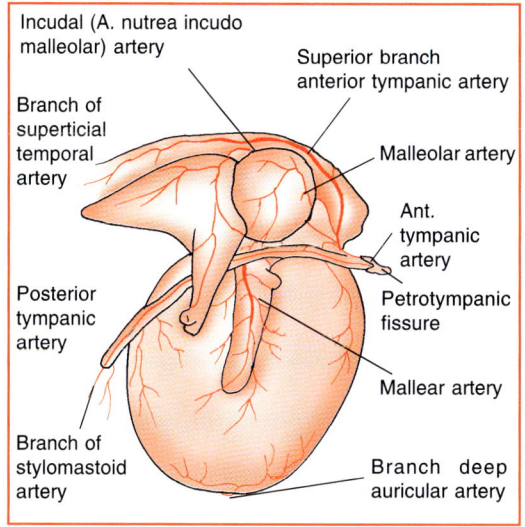

Fig. 2.9a: Blood supply of inner surface of tympanic membrane

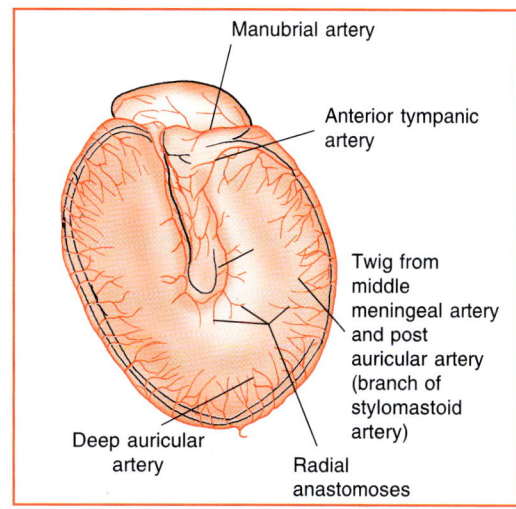

Fig. 2.9b: Blood supply of outer surface tympanic membrane

MIDDLE EAR CLEFT

Structures of Tympanic Cavity
(Figs 2.10 and 2.11)

The entire middle ear cleft is lined by columnar ciliated and pavement epithelium. It is an extension of the respiratory mucous membrane from nasopharynx. The middle ear cleft consists of:

1. Eustachian tube
2. Tympanic cavity
3. Mastoid antrum
4. Aditus ad antrum
5. Mastoid air cells.

EUSTACHIAN TUBE

Eustachian tube connects tympanic cavity to nasopharynx, it is approximately **3.6 cm long in average adult**. It is directed upward, backward from lower opening in the lateral wall of nasopharynx, towards the upper opening in anterior wall of tympanic cavity. Whereas it is directed downward, forward medially from the tympanic cavity. The nasopharyngeal opening lies behind posterior end of inferior turbinate. Tympanic opening is higher than the pharyngeal opening. *Tube is more horizontal and relatively wider, shorter in infants and young children.* The upper or posterolateral one-third is bony whereas lower or anteriomedial two third is cartilaginous. It is widest in entrance to tympanic cavity and narrow at its lower end, where tube is flattened at a diameter of 2 mm. Tubal tonsils are seen near the pharyngeal end of the tube which may at times cause eustachian tube obstruction because of hypertrophy.

There is also presence of fibrofatty tissue related to membranous part of cartilaginous tube specially in the region of nasopharynx which is known as **Ostmann's pad of fat.** This keeps the ET tube closed, thereby protecting the tube from **nasopharyngeal reflux**.

The fossa of Rosenmuller which lies behind the nasopharyngeal orifice is normally packed with small but well organized lymph nodes. It is the most common site for **nasopharyngeal malignancy.**

Blood Supply of Eustachian tube

Arterial supply: Ascending pharyngeal and middle meningeal artery and also from artery of pterygoid canal.

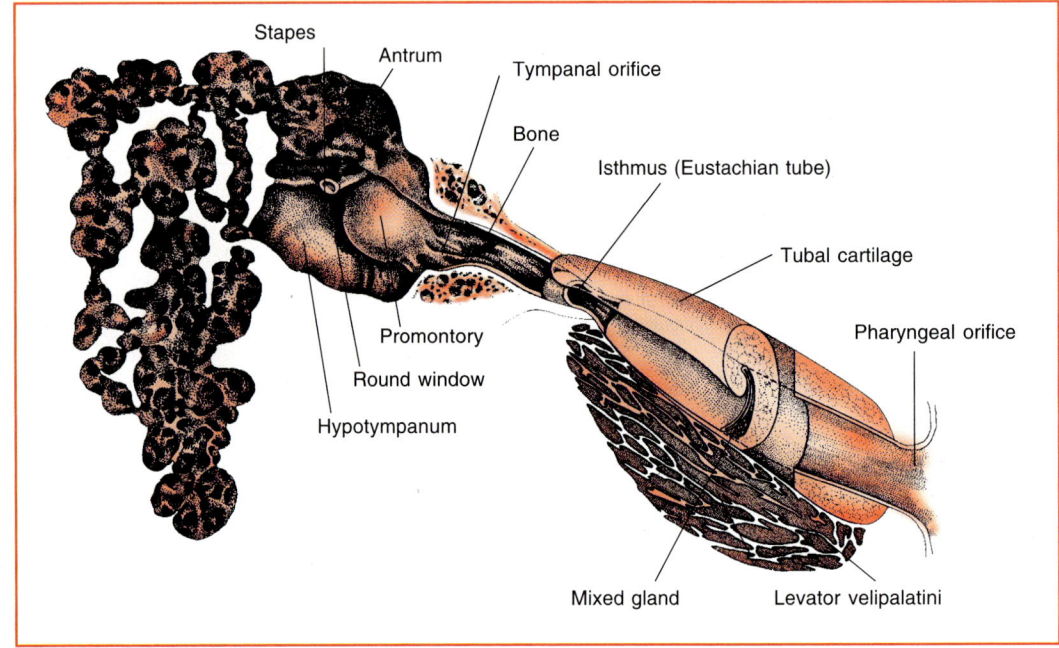

Stapes
Antrum
Tympanal orifice
Bone
Isthmus (Eustachian tube)
Tubal cartilage
Pharyngeal orifice
Promontory
Round window
Hypotympanum
Mixed gland
Levator velipalatini

Fig. 2.10: Diagrammatic representation of middle ear cleft

Venous Drainage: Pterygoid plexus.

Functions of Eustachian Tube

1. Ventilation of middle ear cleft—It plays a major role in equalizing middle ear pressure with atmospheric pressure.
2. Prevents reflux of nasopharyngeal secretion.
3. Clearance of middle ear secretions.

TYMPANIC CAVITY (the middle ear)

The tympanic cavity lies between the external and inner ear and shaped like a biconcave disc. The vertical and anteroposterior diameters are 15 mm, while the transverse diameter is 6 mm at the upper part, 2 mm at the center and 4 mm at the lower part (Fig. 2.12).

It is a six sided cavity with a roof, floor, anterior, posterior, medial and lateral walls. The tympanic cavity is divided into three parts:

- Epitympanum
- Mesotympanum
- Hypotympanum

Epitympanum (attic)

It is situated above the malleolar folds of the tympanic membrane. It contains the head of the malleus, incudomalleolar joint and body and short process of the incus. It connects the mastoid antrum via the aditus posterosuperiorly.

Mesotympanum

It is situated medial to the pars tensa of the tympanic membrane.

Hypotympanum

It is situated below the level of the tympanic membrane.

Anterior mesotympanum and hypotympanum are lined by columnar ciliated epithelium. The posterior mesotympanum, aditus and mastoid area are lined by pavement epithelium.

Lateral Wall

It is formed by the tympanic membrane and partly by a portion of squamous part of the temporal

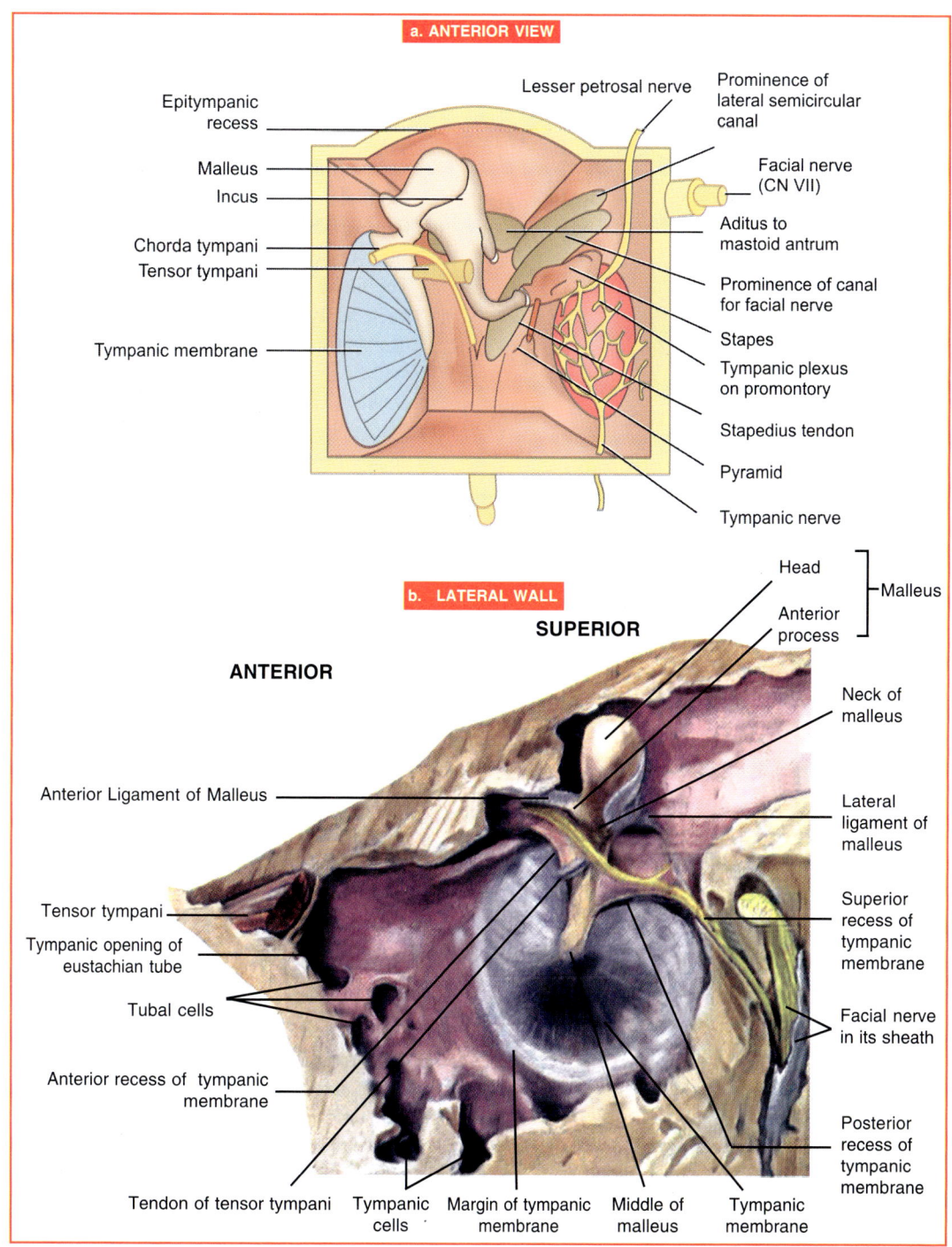

Figs 2.11a and b: (a) Three dimensional view of middle ear, (b) Lateral wall of middle ear

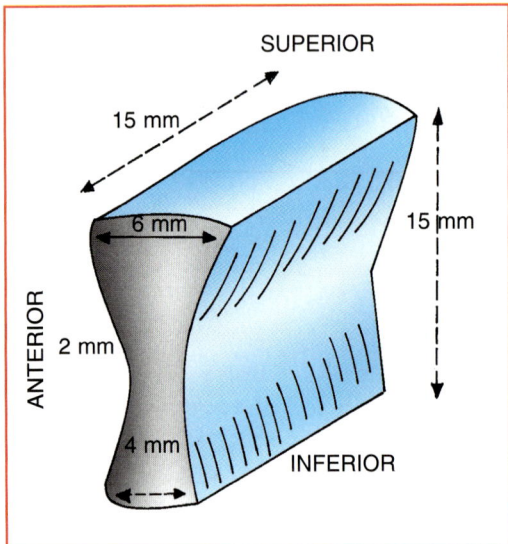

Fig. 2.12: Biconcave middle ear cavity

bone. This wall separates the middle ear from external ear.

Medial Wall (Fig. 2.13)

It separates the middle ear from the inner ear. It has several important structures:

(a) **Promontory** is the most prominent and bulging part of the medial wall formed by the basal turn of the cochlea.

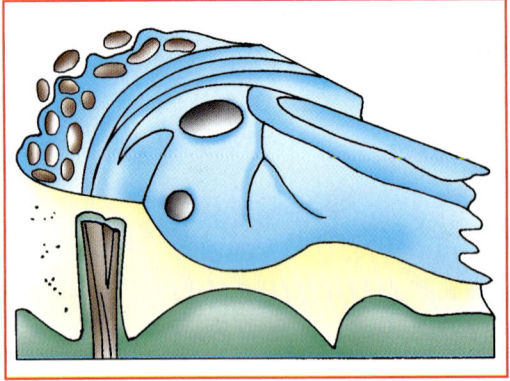

Fig. 2.13: Medial wall of middle ear

(b) **Bony Lateral Semicircular Canal** lies posterosuperior to the promontory above the oval window.

(c) **Oval Window (Fenestra vestibuli)** lies between the middle ear and the scala vestibuli of the cochlea. It is closed by the footplate of stapes and the annular ligament.

(d) **Round Window (Fenestra cochlea)** is situated below and behind the promontory. The niche of the round window is directed posteriorly. It is closed by the secondary tympanic membrane and separates the middle ear from the scala tympani of cochlea.

(e) **Facial Nerve** runs in the bony fallopian canal above the oval window.

Anterior Wall

Anterior wall separates middle ear cavity from internal carotid artery. There are various structures passing through the anterior wall to the tympanic cavity. They are as follows:

(a) Canal for chorda tympani nerve
(b) Canal for tensor tympani muscle
(c) Eustachian tube
(d) Anterior malleolar ligament
(e) Anterior tympanic artery

Posterior Wall

The upper part of the posterior wall shows the opening of aditus, which leads backwards from the posterior epitympanum to the mastoid antrum. Below the aditus there is a triangular bony projection known as processus pyramidalis through the apex of which is transmitted the stapedius tendon. The vertical portion of facial nerve courses down the posterior wall to its exit in the stylomastoid foramen.

- Facial recess (**Suprapyramidal recess**) and sinus tympani (**Infrapyramidal recess**) (Fig. 2.14).

  Two recesses extend posteriorly from the mesotympanum that are often impossible to

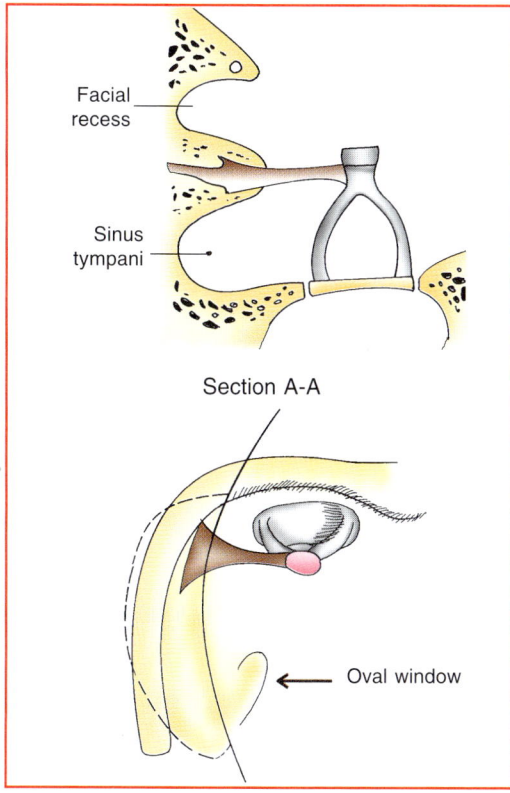

Facial recess

Sinus tympani

Section A-A

Oval window

Fig. 2.14: Diagrammatic representation of facial recess and sinus tympani

visualize directly. These spaces, the **facial recess** and **sinus tympani,** are the most common location for cholesteatoma persistence after ear surgery. The sinus tympani lies between the facial nerve and the medial wall of the mesotympanum and is very difficult to access surgically. The facial recess (suprapyramidal) is lateral to the facial nerve, bounded by the fossa incudis superiorly and the chorda tympani nerve inferiorly, posterosuperior meatal wall laterally and pyramid medially. It may be directly accessed via a posterior tympano- tomy approach, through the mastoid (posterior tympanotomy or facial recess approach).

- **Sinus tympani** (Infrapyramidal recess): The niche of two labyrinthine window communicate at the posterior extremity with the deep recess which is known as sinus tympani. Laterally it is separated from the facial recess by the pyramid.

Floor

It is formed by a thin plate of bone which separates the middle ear from the bulb of the internal jugular vein lodged in the jugular fossa. In the presence of a bony dehiscence in this area the jugular bulb may come into the middle ear to become a content of it.

Roof

The roof of the middle ear is separated from the middle cranial fossa by a thin plate of bone known as tegmen tympani and tegmen antri.

Ventilatory Anatomy

Normally the middle ear cleft is well ventilated. The air comes through the eustachian tube from the nasopharynx to the anterior mesotympanum. From here the air column goes up to the anterior epitympanum via the isthmus tympanic anticus and then goes backward to the posterior epitympanum. Part of this air passes through the aditus to ventilate the mastoid air cells and part of it comes down via isthmus tympanic posticus to ventilate the posterior mesotympanum. In a well pneumatized mastoid, ventilation of the posterior mesotympanum takes place also through the posterior wall. From the posterior mesotympanum, air percolates to the hypotympanum. Disorder of this ventilatory anatomy has a great bearing in the etiopathogenesis of various inflammatory diseases of the middle ear.

Contents of the Middle Ear
(Figs 2.15 and 2.16)

(a) Ossicles

Three tiny bones which conduct the sound from the ear drum to the oval window.

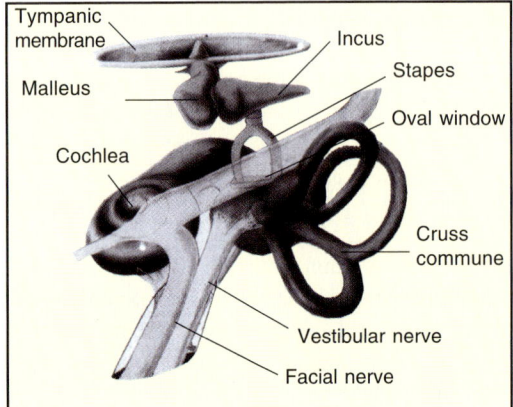

Fig. 2.15: Middle and inner ear with its nerve supply shown as single unit along with tympanic membrane and ossicular chain in relation to middle and inner ear

- **Malleus (hammer)** is the largest and lateral most ossicle measuring 8 mm in length. It has a head, neck, handle and anterior and lateral processes. The head is situated in the epitympanum. A lateral (short) process projects laterally from the neck while the handle is firmly fixed to the pars tensa of the ear drum.
- **Incus (anvil)** has a body, short process and long process. The body articulates with the head of malleus in the attic and the short process projects into the attic. The long process projects downwards behind the

handle of malleus, running parallel to it and articulates with the head of the stapes via the lenticular process.

- **Stapes (stirrup)** is the smallest ossicle measuring about 3.5 mm and consists of head, neck, footplate and anterior and posterior crura. The footplate of stapes is held to the oval window by the annular ligament.

(b) Muscles

- The tensor tympani and stapedius muscles decrease the movement of the ossicles.
- The tensor tympani is inserted to the neck of malleus. First arch muscle supplied by branch of mandibular nerve (V_3).
- The stapedius is inserted to the neck of the stapes. Second arch muscle supplied by branch of facial nerve, i.e. nerve to stapedius.

(c) Mucosal folds and ligaments—keep the ossicles in place.

(d) Nerves

- Chorda tympani is a branch of the facial nerve which carries the sense of taste. It enters the middle ear cavity from the posterior wall, runs forwards and lateral to the incus and medial to the malleus, escaping out through the anterior wall.
- The tympanic plexus lies on the promontory. It is formed by tympanic branch of glossopharyngeal nerve and sympathetic fibers from the plexus around the internal carotid artery. It also carries the secretomotor

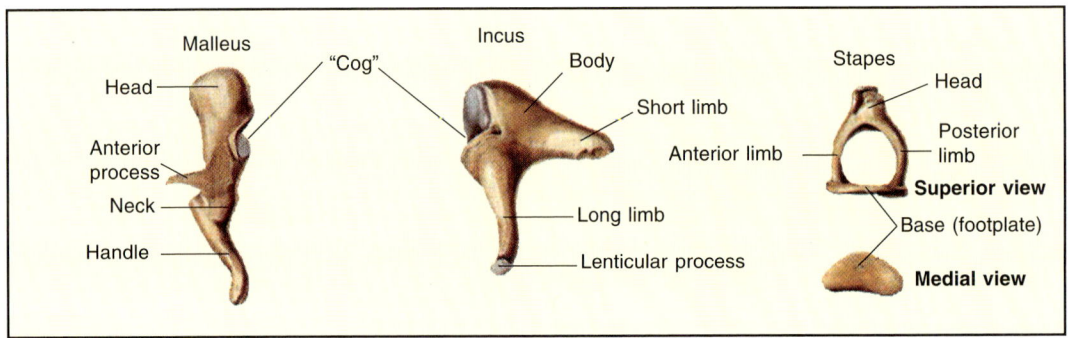

Fig. 2.16: Malleus, incus and stapes from left to right

to the parotid gland. Tympanic plexus innervates the medial surface of tympanic membrane, tympanic cavity, mastoid air cells and bony eustachian tube. Tympanic branch of glossopharyngeal nerve can be sectioned in middle ear for treating the **Frey's syndrome.**

(e) **Vessels:** Plexus of vessels of stylomastoid artery and from caroticotympanic artery.

Mastoid

The mastoid consists of **three parts**

1. **Aditus ad antrum** is a short canal connecting the epitympanum with the mastoid antrum. The short process of incus lies on its floor. The facial nerve runs in its canal in the floor, while the lateral semicircular canal lies in the medial wall. The bone lateral to the aditus appears like a bridge during ear operations (Fig. 2.17).

2. **Mastoid antrum** is the largest air cell in the mastoid bone. The antrum is an important landmark in the surgery of the mastoid bone, and is always present.

   - Anteriorly, the antrum receives the aditus. The facial nerve also lies anterior to the antrum.
   - Medially, it is related to the horizontal/ posterior semicircular canal.

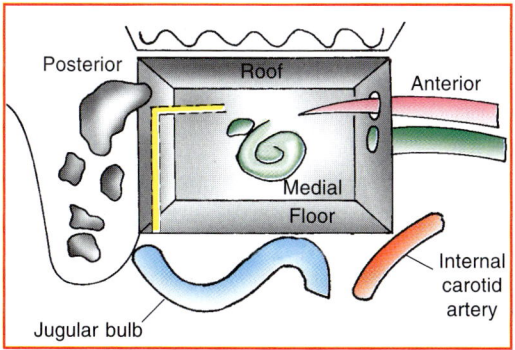

Fig. 2.17: Relation of mastoid with middle ear cavity

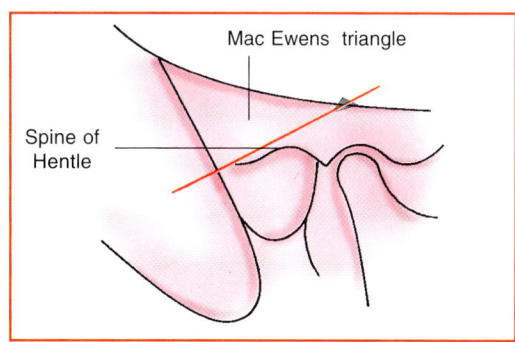

Fig. 2.18: Mac Ewens triangle

- Roof is formed by the tegmen antri.
- Lateral wall is formed by the cortex of the mastoid bone which lies medial to the suprameatal triangle. Its thickness can be upto 15 mm or 1.5 cm.

Mac Ewen's (Suprameatal) triangle (Fig. 2.18)—It forms bony surface marking of the antrum. It is bounded by temporal line of supramastoid crest and posterosuperior bony meatal wall and the line drawn connecting the suprameatal crest and the bony meatal wall.

Posteroinferiorly, the antrum communicates with numerous mastoid air cells.

Sinodural angle (Citelli's angle) Angle between tegmen antri and sigmoid sinus.

3. **Mastoid air cells** are variable in number, size and distribution. They communicate with the mastoid antrum.

   There are three types of mastoid process:

   (a) **Cellular,** with large and numerous air cells.

   (b) **Diploic,** with small and less numerous air cells.

   (c) **Sclerotic,** with air cells practically absent.

   - The cellular mastoid account in about 80% of subjects and is considered to be normal. The diploic and sclerotic types may be due to the blockage of the eustachian tube. The air cells are located mainly in petromastoid and squamous parts of the temporal bone. In a well developed mastoid they are grouped as follows (Fig. 2.19)

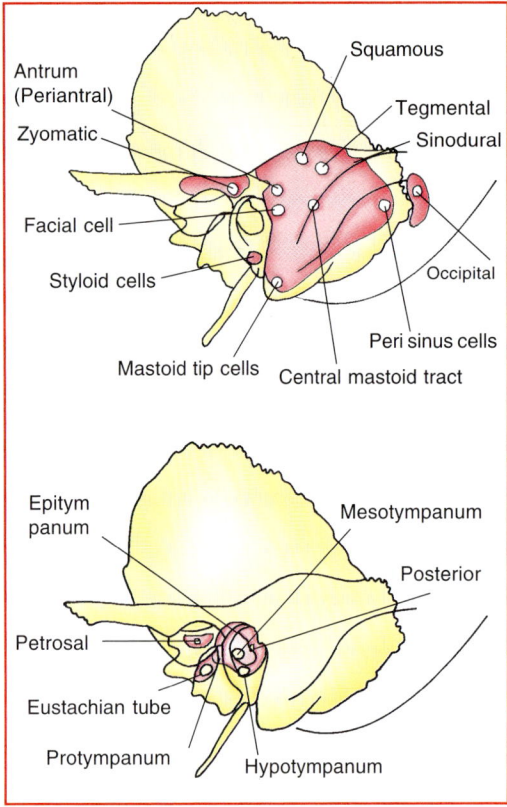

Fig. 2.19: Different group of mastoid air cells

- **Central group**
  Periantral cells
- **Peripheral group**
  Dural
  Perisinus
  Sinodural
  Tip
  Retrofacial
- **Labyrinthine group**
  Supra and infralabyrinthine cells
- **Petrous group: Apical cells**

- **Accessory group**
  Squamous
  Occipital
  Zygomatic
  Peri-tubal
  Styloid

Development of Mastoid

Mastoid develops from squamous and petrous bone. The persistent petrosquamosal lamina (bony plate)—the **Korner's Septum,** is surgically important as it may cause difficulty in locating the antrum. It divides mastoid air cells into medial and lateral group. Mastoid antrum lies medial to the septum which may be difficult to reach or may lead to incomplete removal of disease during mastoidectomy. So to reach antrum, Korner's septum has to be removed.

Development of mastoid process depends entirely on development of sternocleidomastoid muscle. Hence, its development does not begin until the end of first year of life, when the infants begin to hold their head erect. It does not form a definite elevation until the end of the second year and achieves its definite size only at puberty. So there is no actual mastoid process at birth and mastoid portion of temporal bone remains flat and stylomastoid foramen remains in surface of mastoid process. The facial nerve will be lying very superficial and may be injured in conventional postauricular mastoid incision. So to avoid injury to the nerve, postauricular incision has to be done more horizontally.

Relations of the Middle Ear Cleft (Fig. 2.20)

External ear lies lateral to the ear drum.

Temporal lobe of the brain and meninges are above the antrum, aditus and epitympanum. The tegmen plate separates the middle ear cleft from the structures in the middle cranial fossa.

Cerebellum is posteromedial to the mastoid air cells.

Inner ear is medial to the antrum, aditus and tympanum.

Horizontal semicircular canal is an important landmark which lies **posterosuperior to the facial nerve.**

Fifth and sixth cranial nerves lie close to the **apex** of the petrous pyramid.

Facial nerve—The horizontal part runs downward in the medial wall of the tympanum.

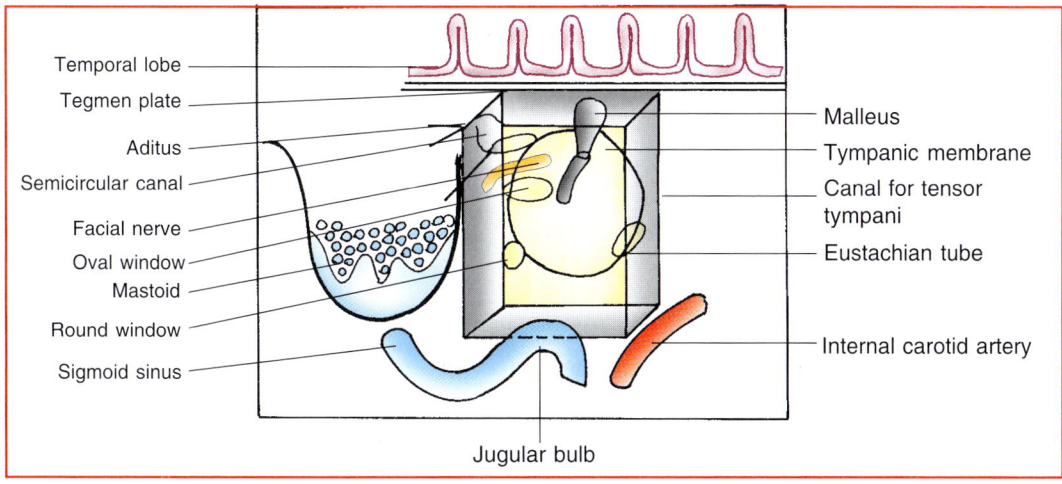

Fig. 2.20: Relation of middle ear cleft

The vertical part runs downward behind the tympanum and in front of the mastoid cells and emerges out through the stylomastoid foramen.

Lateral sinus is posterior to the mastoid cells.

Jugular bulb is in close contact with the floor of the tympanum.

Internal carotid artery is anterior to the tympanum.

Blood Supply (Fig. 2.21)

The blood supply of middle ear is from the branches of

- Middle meningeal artery
- Maxillary artery
- Ascending pharyngeal artery
- Stylomastoid branch of the posterior auricular artery.

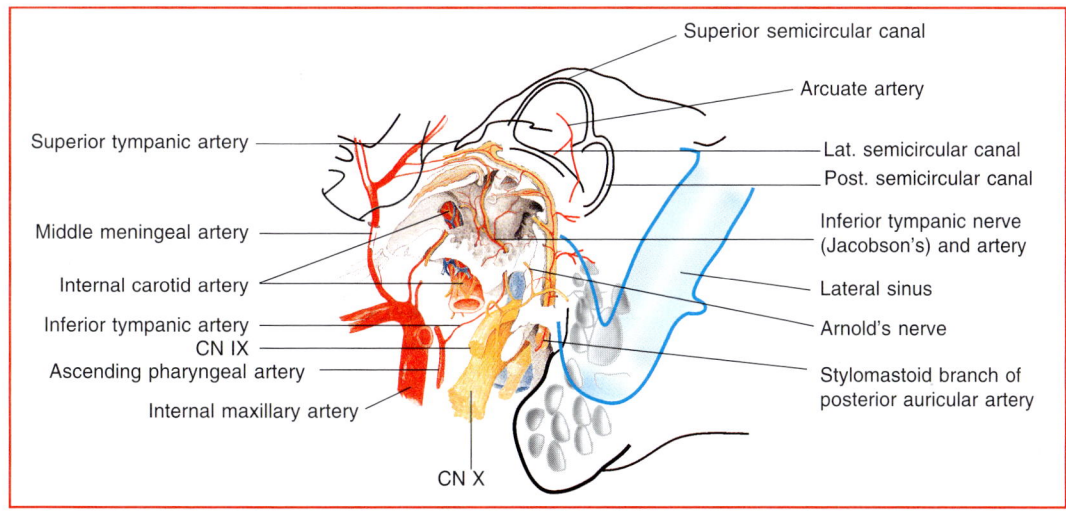

Fig. 2.21: Blood and nerve supply of middle ear

Nerve Supply (Fig. 2.21)

Sensory: Tympanic branch of the ninth cranial nerve **(Jacobson's nerve)** supplies through the tympanic plexus.

Motor: Tensor tympani muscle is supplied by the mandibular division of the trigeminal nerve and the stapedius muscle is supplied by the facial nerve.

Lyphatic Drainage

The lymphatics drain to the preauricular and the retropharyngeal lymph nodes.

INNER EAR

Development

It starts in the 3rd week of the intrauterine life and is completed by the 16th week of the intrauterine life.

Membranous labyrinth develops from the otic capsule. This differentiates into various structures, like sensory end organ of hearing and equilibrium.

Bony labyrinth develops from the otic capsule. This is a mesenchymal condensation surrounding the membranous labyrinth. Soon this is converted into cartilage. Between the cartilage and the labyrinth is loose periotic tissue. This tissue disappears around the utricle and saccule to form the vestibule. It also disappears around the semi-circular ducts to form the semicircular canals.

In the cochlea two spaces are formed on either side of the cochlear duct known as scala vestibuli and scala tympani.

Anatomy

The inner ear is well protected and lies inside the petrous temporal bone, between the medial wall of the middle ear and the internal auditory canal. It is composed of:

1. **The bony labyrinth** has a central part called bony vestibule which is connected anteriorly to the bony cochlea and posteriorly to the three bony semicircular canals (Fig. 2.22).

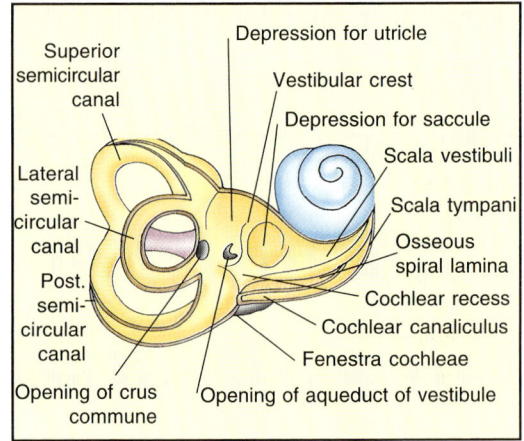

Fig. 2.22: Diagrammatic representation of bony labyrinth

2. **The membranous labyrinth** has the same named structures as the bony labyrinth which floats on the perilymph and itself has endolymph (Fig. 2.23).

Anatomy of the Bony Labyrinth (Fig. 2.22)

Divided into 3 parts:

(a) Bony vestibule
(b) Semicircular canals.
(c) Cochlea

(a) Bony Vestibule

Vestibule is the central part of the bony labyrinth and is compared to a standard aspirin tablet (5 mm). It lies between the medial wall of the middle ear and lateral to the internal acoustic meatus, anterior to the semicircular canal and posterior to the cochlea.

On the lateral wall of the vestibule there is a bean-shaped opening called **fenestra vestibulae (oval window)** occupied by the footplate of the stapes and surrounded by annular ligament. On the front half of the medial wall there is a marked depression called **spherical recess.** This is a space for saccule. This wall is perforated by minute holes called **maculae cribrosa media** for the passage of the inferior vestibular nerve filaments. Behind is another depression called the elliptical recess **containing utricle.** The two recesses are separated by a vestibular crest, the anterior end being the **vestibular pyramid.** Vestibular crest splits inferiorly to enclose the **cochlear recess** for cochlear nerve filaments. The pyramid and elliptical recess are perforated by small holes called **macula cribrosa superior** also called **Mike's dot,** (It is an important landmark in translabyrinthine approach) for nerves to utricle and ampulla of superior and lateral semicircular canals respectively. Below the elliptical recess, there is a diverticulum called **aqueduct of vestibule** plugged in life by the endo- lymphatic duct and one or two small veins.

(b) Semicircular Canals

They are three in number:

1. Superior
2. Posterior or vertical
3. Lateral semicircular canals.

Each occupies two-thirds of a circle and is unequal in length. The diameter is 0.8 mm. All three canals show dilatation at one end called **ampulla** containing vestibular sensory epithelium.

Superior semicircular canals length 15 to 20 mm **lies transverse to the bony axis of the petrous portion of temporal bone.** Anterolateral end is ampullated and opens in the upper lateral part of the vestibule. The other end fuses with the superior limb of the posterior vertical canal to form crus commune, 4 mm length, which opens in the medial part of the vestibule.

The lateral semicircular canal projects as a rounded bulge into aditus and antrum of the middle ear cleft. It is 12 to 15 mm long, lies at an angle of 30° to the horizontal plane. The ampullary end opens into the upper part of the vestibule, posterior end into the lower part below the orifice of the crus commune.

Posterior semicircular canal 18 to 22 mm long lies *parallel and very close to the posterior surface of the petrous portion of the temporal bone.* Lower ampullated limb opens into the lower part of the vestibule and the upper limb joins the crus commune. The angle formed by three semicircular canal is **solid angle**, whereas the triangle bounded by the bony labyrinth anteriorly, sigmoid sinus posteriorly and dura superiorly is known as **Trautman's triangle,** which is a weakest part.

(c) Cochlea

Cochlea resembles a common snail. It forms the anterior portion of the bony labyrinth.

It is 5 mm from base to apex and 9 mm around its base, length of the tube is 30 mm. It is a hollow tube having 2 and three-fourth turns around a conical central axis called **'modiolus'.** The base of modiolus is directive toward internal auditory meatus and is perforated for the passage of cochlear nerve. The apex lies medial to tensor tympani muscle (internal carotid artery). The osseous spiral lamina winds around modiolus and along the basilar membrane, it separates the scala media (cochlear duct) from scala tympani. Within this bony canal lies the membranous cochlear duct. There are **three longitudinal channels** within the cochlea: **scala vestibuli** above, **scala tympani** below and **scala media** in between. Scala vestibuli communicates with scala tympani at the apex of the cochlea called **helicotrema.**

Scala vestibuli is in continuity with the vestibule at the oval window closed by the stapes footplate. Scala tympani is separated from the tympanic cavity by the secondary tympani membrane at the fenestra cochlea. Central perforation leads to a foramen central in the body of modiolus, where nerves for the apex are accommodated. The nerve for the first turn and 3/4th of the cochlear tube pass through the **peripheral tractus**

spiralis foraminosa. At once the nerves pair off towards the margin of ganglion and from here nerves communicate via the osseous spiral lamina with **the organ of corti.**

Anatomy of the Membranous Labyrinth
(Figs 2.23 and 2.24)

The membranous labyrinth can be broadly divided into three parts based on physiology:

1. Membranous vestibular labyrinth
2. Membranous semicircular canal
3. Membranous cochlear labyrinth

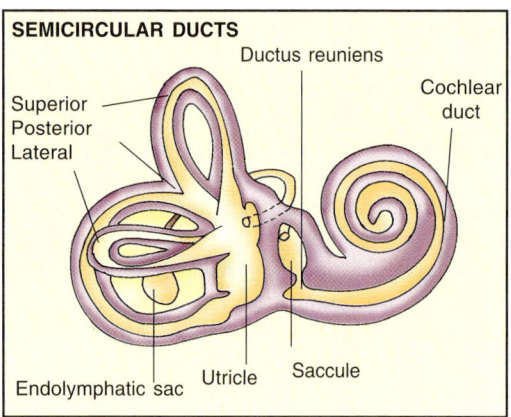

Fig. 2.23: Membranous labyrinth shown floating inside the bony labyrinth

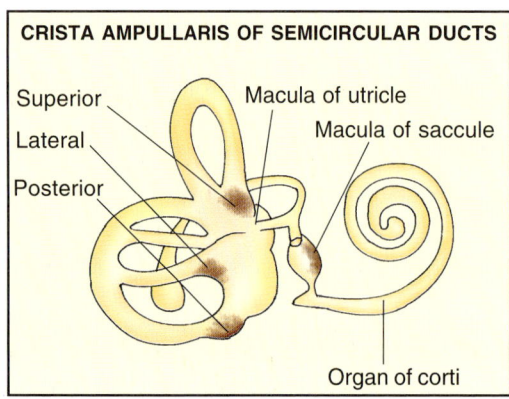

Fig. 2.24: Showing specialized epithelium in the membranous labyrinth

The membranous labyrinth contains endolymph and the specialized vestibular and cochlear receptors. It lies within the bony labyrinth, floating on the perilymph.

1. *Membranous Vestibular Labyrinth*

It consists of:
- Saccule
- Utricle
- The **endolymphatic duct** and sac.

Saccule is connected to the cochlear labyrinth by the **membranous cochlear reuniens.** Saccule and utricle are connected to each other indirectly by the endolymphatic duct. Saccule occupies the spherical recess in the bony vestibule and it contains specialized vestibular epithelium. Utricle is bigger in size than the saccule and occupies the elliptical recess of the bony vestibule.

The three semicircular canals open into the **posterior wall of the utricle by five openings.** Anteriorly, it connects to the saccule indirectly via the endolymphatic duct. It also contains specialized vestibular receptor organs.

Vestibular Receptor Organs

- Macula
- Cristae

Macula

Vestibular receptor organs of the saccule and utricle are called **macula.** Macula of the saccule lies vertically in the medial surface of the saccule, whereas in the utricle it lies horizontally. These specialized vestibular receptor organs are composed of **hair cells, supporting cells and gelatinous mass** (Fig. 2.25).

This gelatinous mass is composed of **mucopolysaccharides** thought to be secreted by the supporting cells. Macular gelatinous mass contains additional materials made up of calcium carbonate crystals known as **otolith or statoconia.** Hence, the gelatinous mass is sometimes known as **statoconial membrane.**

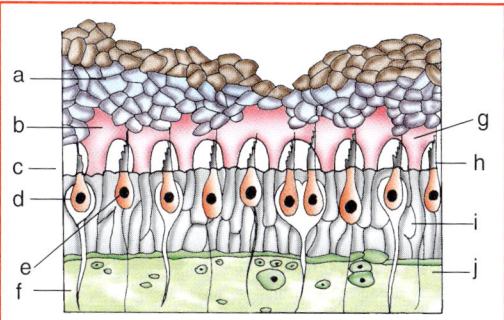

Fig. 2.25: Microscopic structure of Macula
a =Otoconia, b = Gelatinous layer, c = Reticular membrane, d =Hair cell type I, e = Hair cell type II, f = Nerve fibers, g = Subcupular meshwork, h =Subcupular space, i = Supporting cells, j = Basement membrane

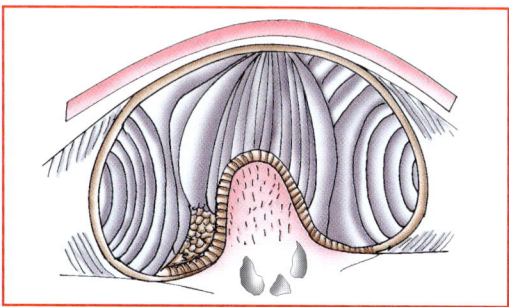

Fig. 2.26: Structure of ampullary end of semicircular duct over the crista lie sensory hair cells interspersed with supporting cells. Hair from sensory cells projects into the gelatinous substance of cupula

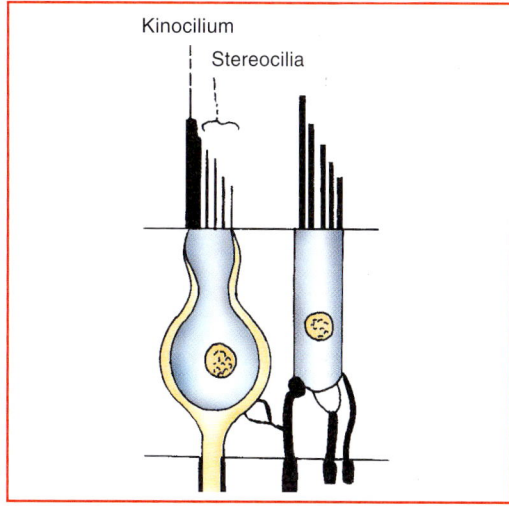

Fig. 2.27: Kinocillia and steriocillia type—1 (flask shaped cell) and type—2 (cylindrical cell)

2. *Membranous Semicircular Canal*

Cristae ampullaris: The membranous semicircular canal occupies the bony semicircular canals. It opens through the five openings into the posterior wall of the utricle (Fig. 2.24). One end of each semicircular canal gets dilated before entering the utricle. The dilated part is filled in the ampullary end of the bony semicircular canal. It accommodates the specialized vestibular epithelium known as **cristae.** This cristae also has hair cells, supporting cells and gelatinous mass (Fig. 2.26). The gelatinous mass in the cristae is dome shaped hence called **cupula**.

The hair cells are of two types (Fig. 2.27)

Type 1 are flask shaped with nerve chalice; Type 1 cells are predominantly seen in the summit of the cristae.

Type 2 are cylindrical with no nerve chalice. Type 2 cells are found more towards the periphery in the cristae.

The hair cells consist of one kinocilium which is tall and prominent; many small cilia (60–110) known as steriocilia which are smaller than the kinocilium. The kinocilium in the macula are not uniformly arranged. A curve line called **striola** divides each macula into medial and lateral halves.

3. *Membranous Cochlea*

Cochlear duct (scala media): It occupies mid portion of the cochlear canal and is triangular in cross section. Floor is formed by *basilar membrane*, roof by *Reissner's membrane* and lateral wall by *stria vascularis* and bony wall of cochlea. Basilar membrane supports *organ of corti*, containing the sound receptors.

The thin area of basilar membrane in its inner part is called ***Zona Arcuata,*** thicker outer part is ***Zona Pectinata.***

Organ of corti is spread like a ribbon along the entire basilar membrane. It consists of the ***tunnel of corti*** which is composed of two rows of rods of inner and outer hair cells. It forms a triangle with the basilar membrane and contains cortilymph. There is one row of hair cells on the inner whereas outer row has 3 or 4 rows of hair cells. Inner rods are 3500 and outer rods are 12000. Rods are expanded like a cap on top. Sensory cells arranged in two groups as inner and outer hair cells. In the fetus and newborn, there are 3500 inner hair cells and 13000 outer hair cells. As age advances there is generalized reduction in the number of hair cells. Hair cells are supported by pillar cells, Deiter's cells and Hensen's cells. The tips of the outer hair cells are attached to the undersurface of tectorial membrane (Figs 2.28 a and b).

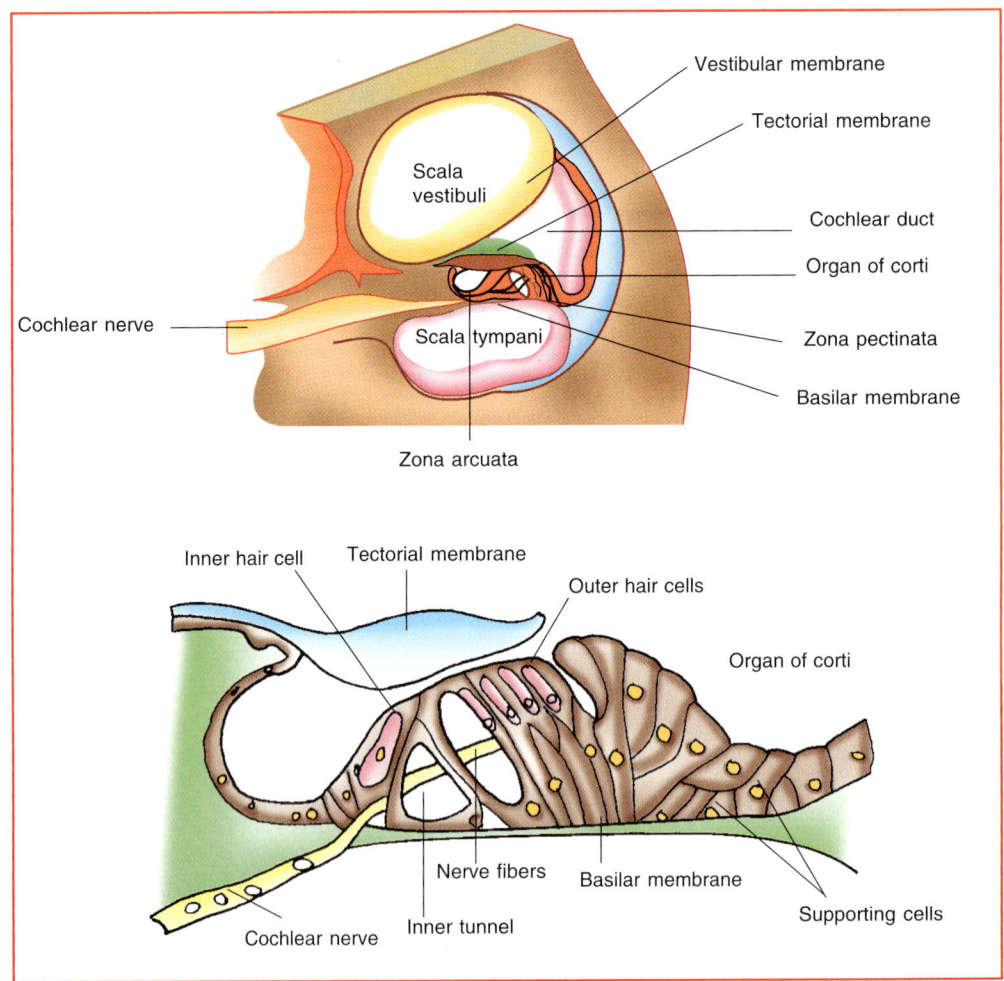

Figs 2.28a and b: (a) Structure of organ of corti (b) Diagrammatic microscopic view of organ of corti

Tectorial membrane: It consists of gelatinous matrix with delicate fibers, it overlies the organ of corti. The shearing force between the hair cells and tectorial membrane produces stimulus to hair cells.

Lateral wall 'stria vascularis': It is thought to play an active role in the maintenance of the ionic composition and electrical potential of the endolymph.

Roof formed by *Reissner's membrane.*

Blood Supply of Inner Ear (Fig. 2.29 and Flow chart 2.1)

Internal auditory artery arises from the anterior inferior cerebellar artery (AICA). It accompanies the facial and vestibulocochlear nerves in the internal acoustic meatus and usually divides into three branches to *supply the inner ear*:

- *Anterior vestibular artery* to supply the macula of utricle and crista of superior and lateral semicircular canals

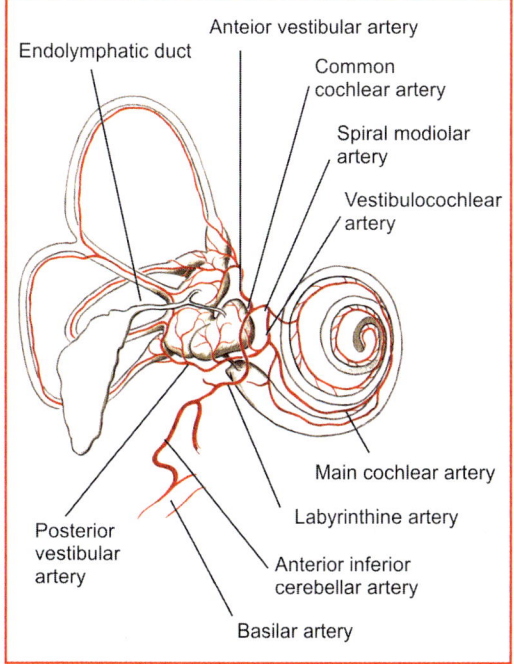

Fig. 2.29: Blood supply of inner ear

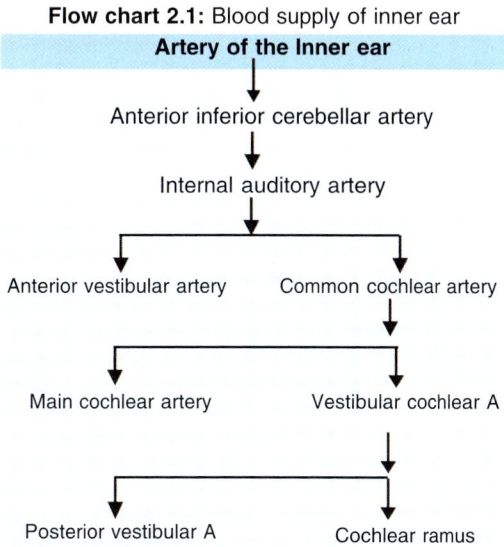

Flow chart 2.1: Blood supply of inner ear

- *Vestibulocochlear branch* to supply the posterior semicircular canal
- *Cochlear branch* to supply the cochlea.

AUDITORY PATHWAY

First order neurons are located in the spiral ganglion and are bipolar (Fig 2.30). Peripheral processes innervate the organ of Corti and central processes terminate in the dorsal and ventral cochlear nuclei (Fig. 2.31).

Second order neurons lie in the dorsal and ventral cochlear nuclei. Most of the axons cross over in the trapezoid body and terminate in the superior olivary nucleus. Many end in the trapezoid body or lateral lemniscus and some remain uncrossed.

Third order neurons lie in the superior olivary nucleus. The axons cross from lateral lemniscus and reach the inferior colliculus.

Fourth order neurons lie in the inferior colliculus. Their axons pass through the inferior brachium to reach the medial geniculate body (some fibers directly reach the medial geniculate body).

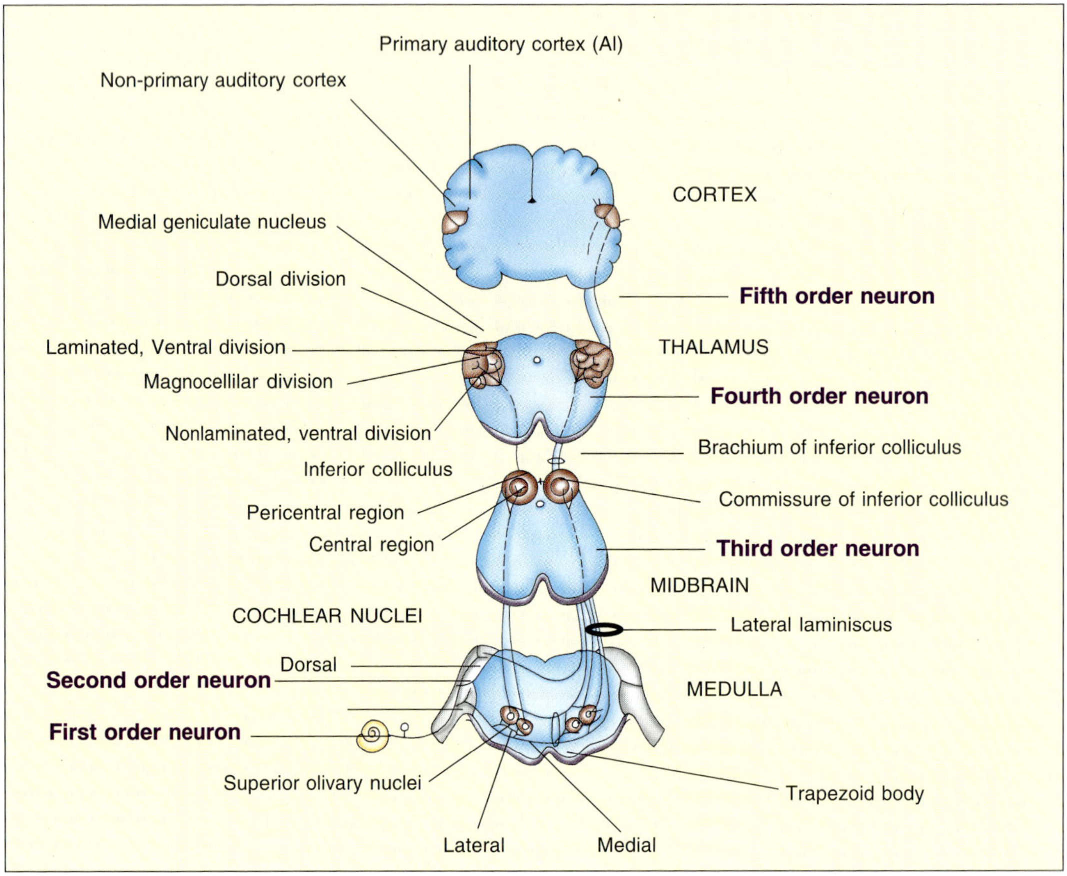

Fig. 2.30: The auditory pathway

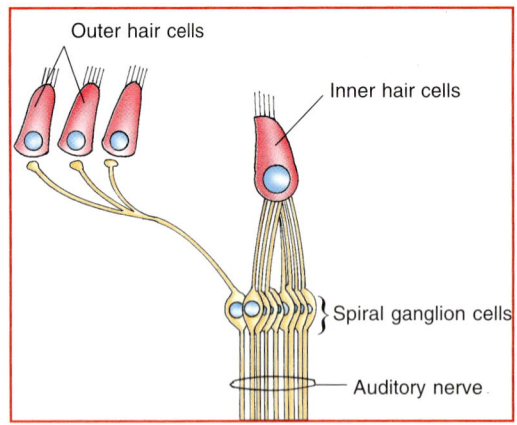

Fig. 2.31: First order neuron starting from hair cells to spiral ganglion cells and auditory nerve

Fifth order neurons lie in the medial geniculate body. Their axons form the auditory radiation which passes through the part of the internal capsule to reach the auditory area in the temporal lobe.

Vestibular Pathway (Fig. 2.32)

Vestibular receptors are the macula of the saccule and utricle and the cristae of the ampullae. They are innervated by the peripheral processes of bipolar neurons of the vestibular ganglion which is situated in the internal acoustic meatus. The central processes form the vestibular nerve which ends in the vestibular nuclei (Flow chart 2.2).

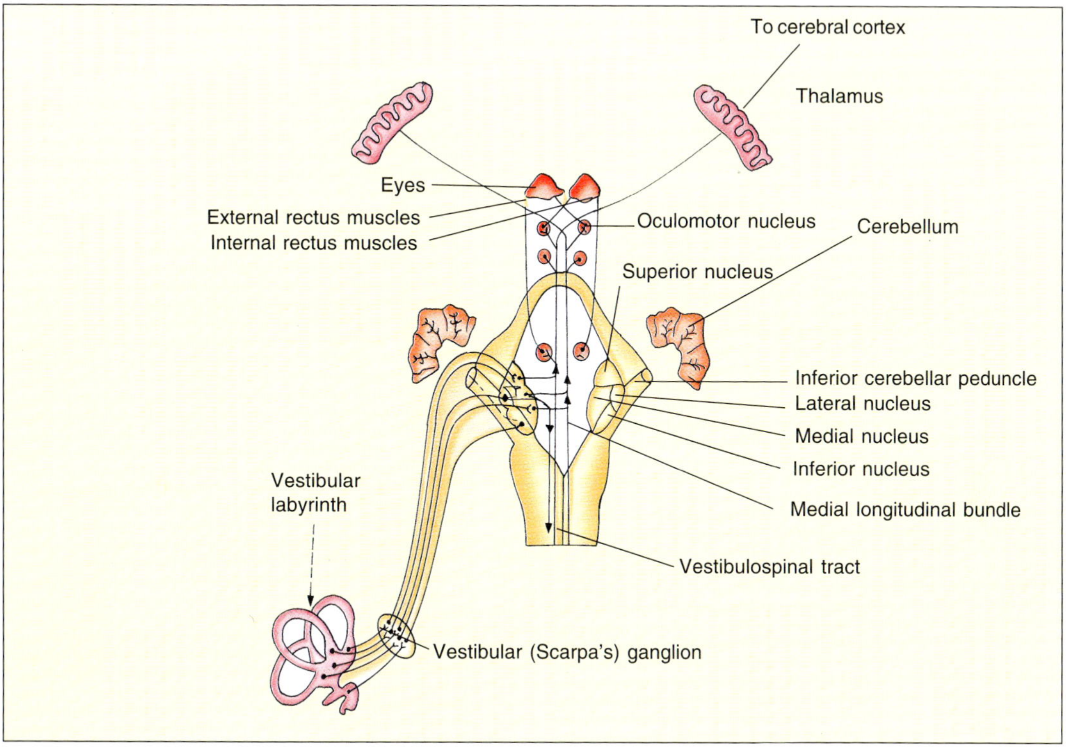

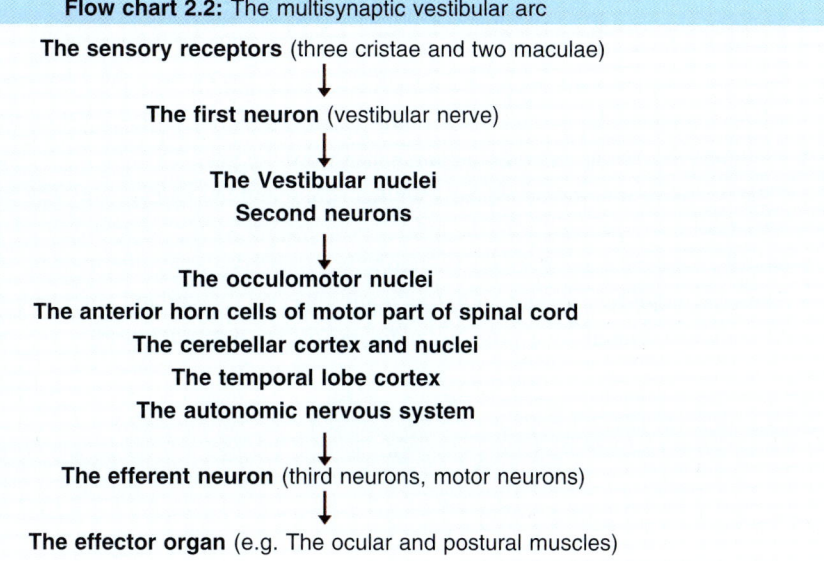

Fig. 2.32: The central connection of the vestibular nerve

Flow chart 2.2: The multisynaptic vestibular arc

The sensory receptors (three cristae and two maculae)

↓

The first neuron (vestibular nerve)

↓

The Vestibular nuclei
Second neurons

↓

The occulomotor nuclei
The anterior horn cells of motor part of spinal cord
The cerebellar cortex and nuclei
The temporal lobe cortex
The autonomic nervous system

↓

The efferent neuron (third neurons, motor neurons)

↓

The effector organ (e.g. The ocular and postural muscles)

Second order neurons lie in the vestibular nuclei. These send fibers to the following:

1. Archicerebellum through inferior cerebellar peduncle (vestibulo-cerebellar tract).

2. Motor nuclei of brain stem (chiefly 3, 4 and 6) through the medial bundle

3. The anterior horn cells of the spinal cord through the vestibulo-spinal tract. The impulses arising in the labyrinth can influence the movement of eyes, head, neck and trunk through the vestibular pathway.

Internal Auditory Canal (Fig. 2.33)

Internal auditory canal (IAC) is lined by dura. It is nearly 1 cm in length. It passes in the petrous temporal bone in lateral direction. The lateral end (fundus) of the canal is closed by cribriform plate having numerous apertures through which the auditory nerve, facial nerve, vestibular nerve, internal auditory artery and vein pass.

Fundus is divided by a vertical plate of bone which separate it from the inner ear. On the medial aspect, the plate is divided by transverse crest into smaller upper and larger lower area. Anteriorly

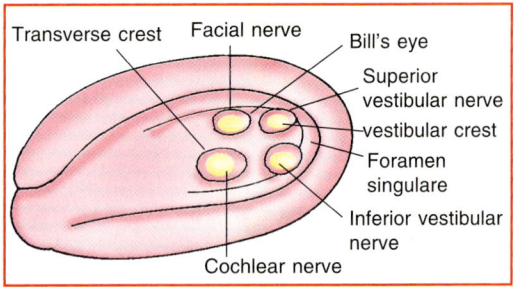

Fig. 2.33: Cross section of internal auditory canal

above the crest is opening of facial canal, behind this and separated from it by a vertical ridge called as BILL's BAR is the superior vestibular area. It shows a small depression containing numerous opening for the passage of filaments of vestibular nerve to utricle, saccule and superior, lateral semicircular canal. Below the transverse crest anteriorly lies the cochlear nerve. Inferior vestibular nerve lies behind cochlear nerve which carries fibers to the saccule. Foramen singulare lying behind and slightly below the inferior vestibular nerve through which singular nerve passes to supply posterior semicircular canal.

POINTS TO REMEMBER

1. Incisura terminalis in situated between the crus of helix and tragus, and is devoid of cartilage.
2. The skin on the outer surface of the pinna is firmly adherent to the perichondrium of the cartilage.
3. The malleolar folds separate the pars tensa from the pars flaccida.
4. The tympanic membrane is pearly white in color and lies at an angle of 55° with the floor of the meatus.
5. Middle ear cleft consists of eustachian tube, tympanic cavity and mastoid air cell system.
6. The eustachian tube is more horizontal and relatively wider and shorter in children.
7. Mac Ewen's triangle is a surgical landmark for the mastoid antrum.

Physiology of the Ear

3

When sound signal strikes the tympanic membrane, the vibration is transmitted to the stapes footplate through a chain of ossicles. The movements of the stapes causes pressure changes in the labyrinthine fluids which move the basilar membrane. This stimulates the hair cells of the organ of corti which acts as a transducer (Fig. 3.1).

MECHANISMS OF HEARING

Mechanisms of hearing (Flow chart 3.1) can be broadly divided into:
1. Mechanical conduction of sound.
2. Transduction of mechanical energy to electrical impulses.
3. Conduction of electrical impulses to brain.

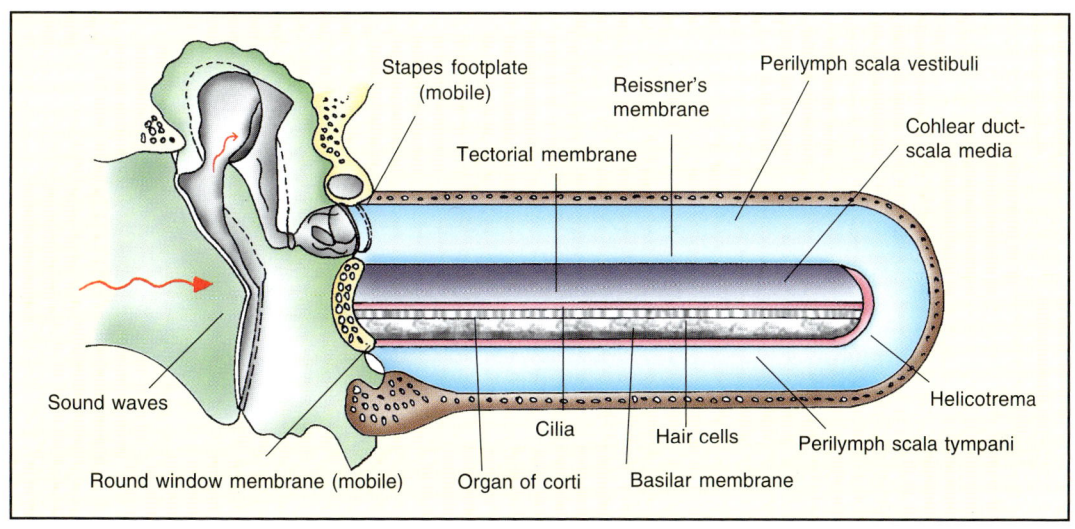

Fig. 3.1: Mechanism of hearing showing tympanocochlear relationship

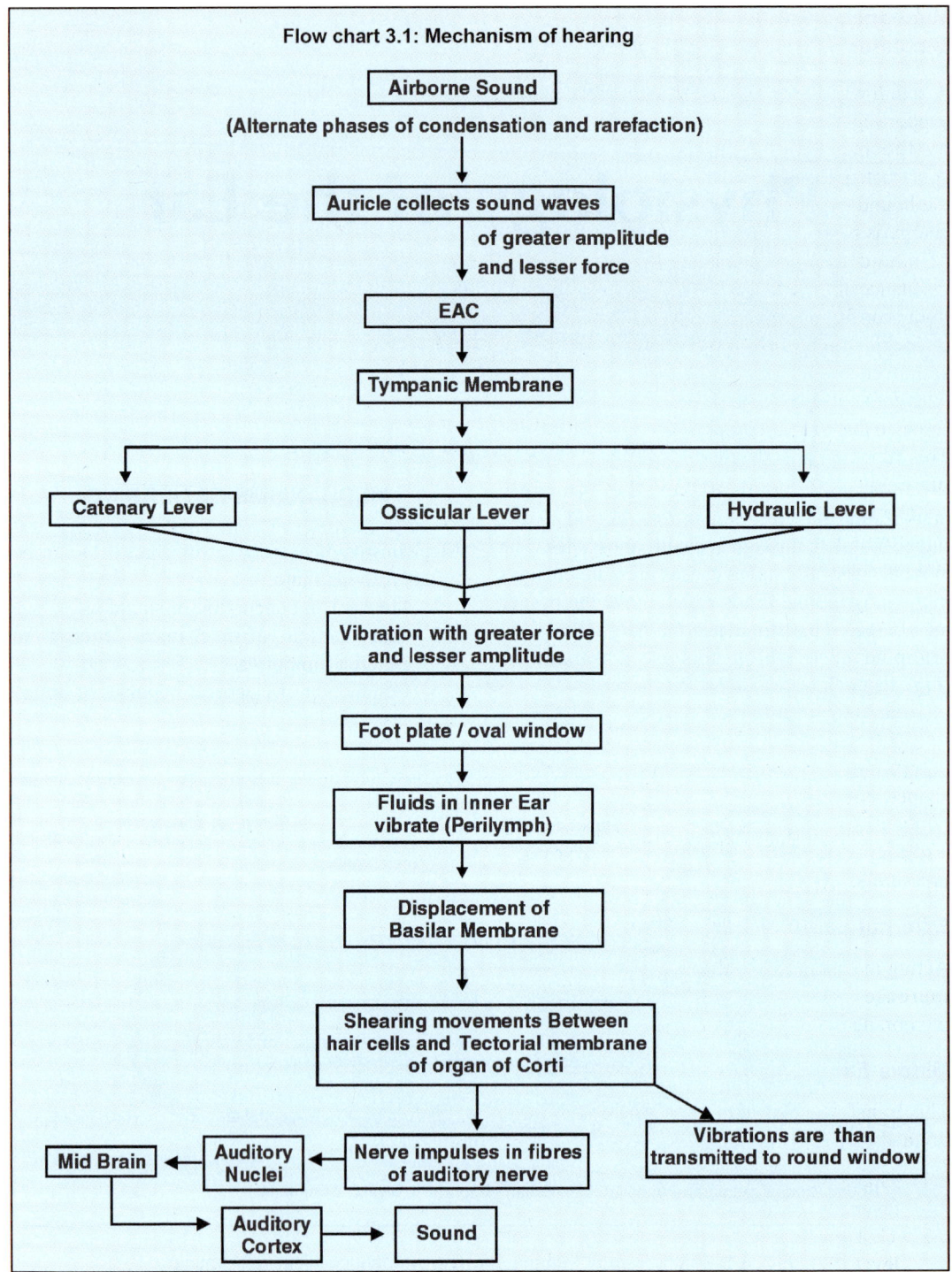

Flow chart 3.1: Mechanism of hearing

Mechanical Conduction of Sound (Acoustic Transformer)

A sound wave, on arriving at the boundary of its supporting medium, may be reflected or absorbed by the material of which the boundary is constructed. For example, if the medium is air and the boundary is water, 99.9 percent of the sound energy is reflected. The resistance to the passage of sound through a medium is its acoustic resistance or impedance. A similar situation exits in the ear when air conducted sound has to travel to cochlear fluids. So to compensate this loss of sound energy, nature has made middle ear to convert sound of greater amplitude, but lesser force, to that of lesser amplitude and greater force. This function of middle ear is called **impedance matching**.

The major contributors to the human acoustic transformer are the pinna, external auditory canal, and the middle ear sound conduction system.

Pinna

The pinna, because of their location and shape, serve to gather sound arriving from an arc of 135° relative to the direction of the head. This pattern rejects sound arriving from the ear and serves to determine the origin of the sound. The horn-shaped conchea then acts like a megaphone to concentrate the sound at the entrance of the auditory canal. This action increases sound pressure as much as 6 dB (2 times).

External Auditory Canal

Acting in concert with the effect of the pinna, can increase sound pressure at the tympanic membrane by 15 to 22 dB at 4000 Hz.

Middle Ear Transformer Mechanism

The transformer system of middle ear can be divided into three stages:

1. That provided by the eardrum (catenary lever.
2. That provided by the ossicles (**ossicular lever**).
3. Provided by the difference in surface area between the tympanic membrane and the stapes footplate (**hydraulic lever**).

1. *Catenary lever*
   Helmholtz was first to propose a concept of a catenary lever to the action of the tympanic membrane. A familiar example of this type of lever is a tennis net. The tighter a tennis net is stretched, the greater the force exerted on the posts holding it. Because the bony annulus is immobile, sound energy applied to the tympanic membrane is amplified at its central attachment, the malleus. It is estimated that even though the curvature of the tympanic membrane is variable, the catenary lever provides at least a two times (2x) gain in sound pressure at the malleus. Force exerted on the stretched curved fibers of the tympanic membrane are amplified at its point of attachment, the annular bone and the malleus handle. The annular bone is immobile, so that the malleus is the recipient of this magnified energy, directing it into the ossicular chain for transmission to the perilymphatic fluid.

2. *Ossicular lever*
   Handle of malleus is 1.3 times longer than long process of the incus, providing a mechanical advantage of 1.3. The catenary and ossicular levers, acting in concert provide an advantage of 2.3 (Fig. 3.2).

3. *Hydraulic lever*
   Helmholtz's third concept of impedance matching which is referred as **areal ratio**. The effective vibratory area of tympanic membrane is 55 mm sq. whereas foot plate area is 3.2 mm sq. Hence effective areal ratio is 14:1. This is a mechanical advantage provided by tympanic membrane. The product of areal ratio into lever ratio is known as transformer ratio. i.e., $14 \times 1.3 = 18:1$.

   Phase difference
   In normal ear, sound pressure waves never reach the oval window and round window

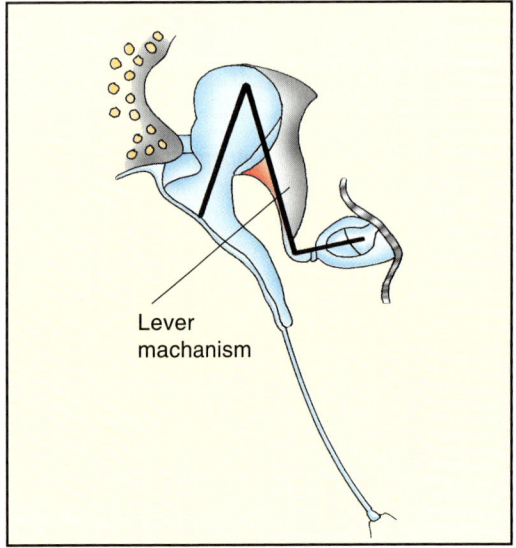

Fig. 3.2: Diagrammatic representation of Ossicular lever mechanism

in the same phase, due to presence of tympanic membrane, middle ear and air cushions. If air waves reach round window and the oval window at the same time it cancel the effect of sound waves leading to stasis of perilymph. This reciprocal action at oval window and round window is called as phase difference. Therefore, loss of this phase difference (due to large perforation) may lead to deafness. However in normal case sound wave reaches oval window earlier than round window which is also an added advantage of hearing.

Transduction Function of the Cochlea

What is Transduction?

It is the conversion of mechanical energy of movement of sound to electrical energy, which is followed by electrical event in the cochlear nerve. Many theories have been put forward while exploring the mehanics and mode of encoding in the cochlea which have been modified with the present day knowledge.

When the stapes is pressed onto the oval window, pressure is exerted to the perilymph in scala vestibuli which is transferred to the scala media. This causes downward movement of the basilar membrane exerting pressure in the scala tympani. This is transmitted in turn to the round window which bulges into the middle ear. When the stapes and oval window move out, there is an upward movement of the basilar membrane. The elastic tension built up in the basilar fibers initiates a wave which travels towards the helicotrema. This wave is comparable to the movement of a pressure wave along the arterial walls.

Each wave is weak at the onset but becomes stronger as it reaches its natural resonant frequency.

High frequency waves travel a short distance and die. Low frequency waves travel a long distance and die. This is because the energy in the wave is completely dissipated. The nature of interaction between the membrane and the fluids is complicated and many theories were put forward based on experimental findings and hypothesis.

Difference in chemistry of perilymph and endolymph is shown in Fig. 3.3 and Table 3.1.

- **Transduction by Hair Cells**

  Many theories were put forward regarding transduction by the hair cells. It is obvious now that auditory nerve endings are not only stimulated electrically but also by chemical transmitters.

  Major steps involved in transduction are:
  - The **Basilar Membrane** and the organ of Corti move up and down with sound stimulus. This causes a shearing action between the tectorial membrane and the reticular lamina causing the stereocilia to bend sideways.
  - This **bending of the hair** bundles opens the channel to allow K^+ to flow into the hair cell, resulting in depolarization.
  - **Depolarization** spreads to the lower part of the cell causing Ca^+ channels to open.

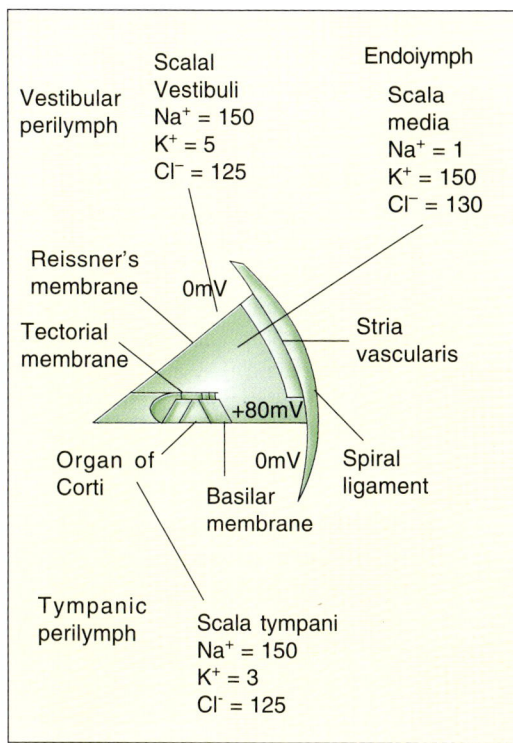

Fig. 3.3: Chemistry of cochlear fluid

Table 3.1: Chemistry of cochlear fluids	
Perilymph	*Endolymph*
1. Origin	
Maybe from CSF or an ultra filtrate of plasma from perilymphatic capillaries.	Secreted by stria vascularis
2. Site	
Scala tympani Scala vestibuli.	Scala media

Endolymph is sole source of oxygen supply for the organ of corti which itself has no blood supply.

- Ca$^+$ causes **transmitter vesicles** to fuse with the basal part of the cell membrane. This fusion releases transmitter substance.
- The **transmitter substance** i.e. amino acid glutamate diffuses across the synaptic cleft to initiate action potential in the auditory nerve fiber.

Electrical responses of cochlear hair cells

Using microelectrodes, four gross potentials have been extensively studied,

- **Endocochlear potential:** In relation to the perilymph, the endolymph in the scala media has a positive potential of +80mV and a high K$^+$ concentration. This is known as *endocochlear potential.* It is dependent on adequate O$_2$ and is produced by stria vascularis. When the K$^+$ is driven into the cell by this big potential gradient, large voltage is given triggering the natural impulses.

- **Cochlear microphonics:** Described by Wever and Bray are generated by the outer hair cells at the apical region. It produces the AC current wave form of stimulating sound and represents the K$^+$ flow through the outer hair cells. Cochlear microphonics is absent in any part of the cochlea where outer hair cells are damaged.

- **Summating potential:** It is a DC potential that follows the envelope of stimulating sound. Several origins have been cited; probably arising from inner hair cells with a small contribution from outer hair cells, this is a rectified derivative of sound signal.

- **Auditory nerve action potential:** It is neural discharge in the auditory nerve produced at the presence of stimulus. Each fiber has optimum stimulus frequency for which the threshold is lowest. Amplitude increases while latency decreases with intensity over 40 to 50 dB range.

Conduction of Electrical Impulses to the Brain

Hair cells peripheral, spiral ganglia central
↓
Cochlear nerve / **Auditory nerve**
↓
Ventral and dorsal **c**ochlear nucleus
↓
Superior olivary nucleus
↓
Lateral lemniscus
↓
Inferior colliculus
↓
Medial geniculate body
↓
Auditory cortex
Mnemonic - AC SLIM

Physiology of the cerebral cortex

Area of auditory pathway to the cerebral cortex is illustrated as primary auditory cortex excited by medial body.

Secondary auditory cortex excited secondarily by impulses from primary auditory cortex, thalamic area adjacent to medial body.

Sound frequency perception in the primary auditory cortex

Six different tonotopic maps have been found in both the primary and secondary auditory cortex. Low frequency sounds are located anteriorly and high frequency sounds posteriorly. One of the large maps in the primary auditory cortex discriminates the sound frequency, another map detects direction of sound.

Theories of Hearing

- **Helmhotz's place theory (1883):** postulated that the basilar membrane acts as a series of tuned resonators similar to a piano string. Each pitch would cause resonant vibration of the basilar membrane which is particular to its own place. Thus, the frequency was analyzed. High frequency waves excite the basal region and low frequency the apical region.

- **Rutherford's frequency/Telephone theory (1886):** Proposed that all frequencies activate the entire length of the basilar membrane along with the hair cells. He postulated that the frequency of the signal is represented by the rate of firing of the auditory nerve fibers. He believed that all vibrations are portrayed by the nerve impulses to the brain without complex vibrations in the cochlea.

- **Wever's volley resonance theory (1949):** Combines both the place and telephone theories postulating that:
  - High frequencies (5000 Hz) are perceived in the basal turn;
  - Low frequencies (1000 Hz) stimulate nerve action potential equal to frequency stimulation;
  - Intermediate frequencies (1000–5000 Hz) are represented in the nerve by asynchronous discharges which then combine actively to represent the frequency of stimulus.

- **Von Bekesy's travelling wave theory (1960)** This Wave begins from the base and moves towards the apex.
  Travelling wave is independent of frequency. The region of maximum displacement varies according to frequency. High pitched sounds cause a short travelling wave not beyond the basal turn. Low frequency stimuli cause maximum displacement near the apex. Middle frequency changes occur in between these two. It is now known that the basilar membrane is much more sharply tuned for frequency filtering. The basilar membrane becomes less selective in tuning at high

stimulating intensities due to non linearity of its response. The sharp tuning and non - linearity is due to an active mechanical amplifier which uses biological energy to boost the membrane vibration.

VESTIBULAR SYSTEM

It was Mach in 1875 who identified the role of the vestibular apparatus in the perception of motion. *This consists of functional subdivisions -*

Semicircular canals—Sense of head rotation.

Otolith organs—Stimulated by gravity and linear acceleration of the head.

Physiologically, the vestibular labyrinth transduces mechanical energy (linear and angular) into electrical activity (nerve action potential) which is interpreted by the brain to allow conscious awareness of the position and movement. Transduction and coding—common to both maculae and cristae.

Mechanical event is bending of hair cells. When the macula surface is tilted, otoliths slide down carrying gelatinous membrane and attached cilia. On head rotation, the endolymph pushes the cupula which carries cilia with it.

Bioelectric Events

There is a constant resting or tonic discharge in many of the afferent fibers from the receptors. Bending the cilia modulates the discharge. On bending of the stereocilia towards the kinocilium depolarization with increase in impulse frequency while bending away from the kinocilium causes hyperpolarization with decrease in impulse frequency. Thus, membrane deformation of hair shearing surface alters its electrical conductance.

Reflex Responses Distributes as Follows:

1. *Superior vestibular nucleus*: Receives impulses from cristae of semicircular canal and cerebellum.
2. *Lateral vestibular nucleus*: Receives impulses from macula of utricle and cerebellum.

3. *Medial vestibular nucleus* : Input from cristae and cerebellum.
4. Descending vestibular nucleus receives the impulses from macula of utricle and saccule.

Efferent Activity

Vestibular nuclei connect with **five main systems.**

1. Oculomotor nuclei (3,4,6) by way of MLF and multisynaptic connections in reticular formation.
2. Motor part of spinal cord by reticulospinal, vestibulospinal and inferior part of MLF.
3. Cerebellum.
4. Autonomic nervous system.
5. Cerebral cortex by multisynaptic pathways.

Functions of Vestibular Nuclei

1. *Superior nucleus:* Control of semicircular canal—ocular reflex.
2. *Lateral nucleus:* Vestibulospinal activity.
3. *Medial nucleus:* Co-ordinating eye, head and neck movements through medial longitudinal bundle.
4. *Descending nucleus:* Mainly to cerebellum and recticular formations.
5. *Subjective awareness* is by vestibulocortical projections.

Functions of Utricle and Saccule

Utricle and saccule respond to the slightest tilt and to fine acceleration of the head. Such a movement results in compensatory ocular reflexes where by the visual axis is fixed when the head is deviated slightly.

Macula of the saccule is at right angles to the macula of the utricle and may serve linear acceleration.

Functions of Semicircular Ducts

They respond to angular acceleration. The horizontal pair are for rotation about a vertical axis. Posterior and superior canals respond to tipping displacement of the head about a horizontal axis.

Movement of endolymph within the ducts stimulate cristae causing reflex nystagmus. The slow component is vestibular and the fast component cerebral. In clinical practice, nystagmus is named in the direction of the fast component.

Postural Reflexes

Labyrinthine reflexes maintains the posture.

1. **Static reflexes:** It is the postural reaction at rest. Together with reflexes from muscles, joints and others. They include the following labyrinthine (utricular) reflexes:
   - Tonic labyrinthine reflexes–with effect on the limbs, neck, trunk and eyes.
   - Labyrinthine righting reflexes
   Restore the body to normal position when it is brought to rest in abnormal position.
2. **Kinetic reflexes:** Postural reactions of the body during movement.
   - Angular as in movement of rotation in any plane.
   - Progressive as in movement in a straight line.

In general, kinetic reflexes bring the body into normal stance while it is maintained by activation of various static reflexes.

Vestibular Physiology

Saccule and utricle are known as **static labyrinth** whereas semicircular canals are known as **dynamic labyrinth** because it is associated with kinetic balance.

Saccular macula responds to the tilting movement of the head, i.e. if the head is tilted to the right side, the right saccular macula will get stimulated whereas the left saccular macula will remain static. The utricular macula responds to forward and backward movement of the head. The cristae of the semicircular canals responds to turning of the head, i.e. angular acceleration.

The **bending of hair cells towards the kinocilium causes depolarization** with increase in impulse frequency, whereas bending towards the steriola will produce less stimulation due to hyperpolarization. The hair cells of the utricle and saccule are divided by an arbitrary line called **striola.** The bending of utricular hair cells away from striola causes hyperstimulation due to depolarization whereas the bending of saccular hair cells towards the striola causes decrease stimulation (Fig. 3.4).

Bending of hair cells of the cristae towards utricle (ampullofugal) movement in the lateral semicircular canal causes hypostimulation. However, some authors believe that the ampullofugal movement in the lateral semicircular canal causes hyperstimulation whereas **ampullopetal movement** in the vertical semicircular canal causes less stimulation.

Fibers, both afferent and efferent, form a plexus of unmyelinated fibers from which myelinated fibers arise and go to the bipolar cells in Scarpa's ganglion of the internal auditory canal.

Otolith Physiology

Otoliths are stretch receptors. When a tangential force, regardless of its origin is applied over the macula, the otoconia slide over the surface of the sensory epithelium stimulating the hair cells. The position of otoliths changes whenever the head position is changed or during head displacement with a component of linear acceleration.

The Dynamics of the otoliths is comparable to those of a low pass filter i.e., displacement due to linear acceleration is greater for lower frequencies, including stimulation with constant acceleration, than for higher frequencies.

The nerve fibers innervating the macular organs are sensitive to changes in position of the head. *Each fiber has a preferred direction of tilt to which it responds maximally.* Thus the movements of head are appreciated along a vector in a three dimensional space. The mechanical deformation of the hair bearing surface alters its electrical conductance. The endolymph has a +40mV potential compared to the -50mV in the substance of sensory epithelium. Electrical modulation of the resting discharge

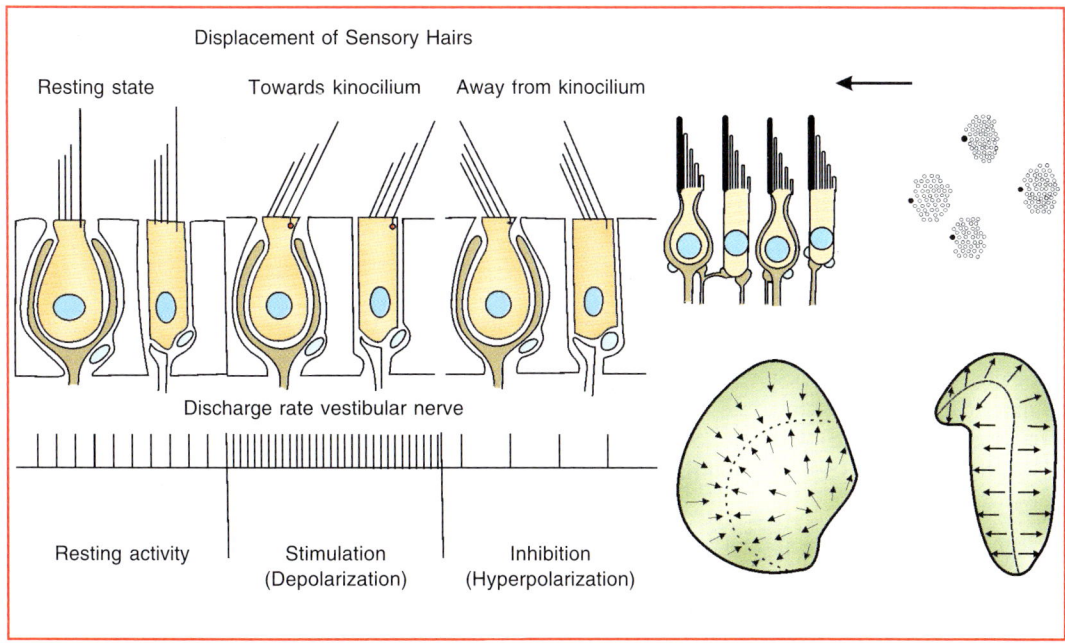

Fig. 3.4: Showing relation between hair cell orientation and pattern of stimulation of the innervating nerve fibers

arises when electrical current leaks from the top of the cell membrane.

Saccules are affected by lateral tilt of the head. When head is tilted to right, macula of right saccule hangs downwards - pulls on its macula and maximal stimulation is produced. Whereas the macula of the left saccule points upwards, rests on its macula producing minimal stimulation.

Ventral/dorsal deflection of the head affects macula of utricle when the head is straight, macula of the utricle points upwards producing minimal stimulation. Forward or backward bending makes the macula pendant, pulling on the macula producing maximal stimulation.

A tilt of as little as 2.5° stimulates the appropriate macula. The frequency of the impulse generated by the hair cells is directly related to the strength of the stimulation. They show little adaptation.

Mode of Action of Semicircular Canals

Effective stimulus to each semicircular canal is rotation of head in the plane of its canal.

When the head starts to rotate, *e.g.*: to the right, the endolymph in the semicircular canals, which lie at right angles to the axis of rotation tends to lag behind the movement and it moves to the left initially.

With regard to the flow of the endolymph, the left ampulla is **Leading** and the right one **Trailing.**

Rotation to right—endolymph moves to left.

After the initial inertia is overcome, endolymph no longer lags behind the movement of head. It flows in the same direction.

Cupula swings back because of its elasticity, to its normal position, as long as the movement exists in the same velocity and direction and resting discharge is resumed. When the movement ceases, the endolymph tends to continue to rotate and cupula is displaced in the opposite direction and hair cells are bent in that direction. Swinging in a particular direction in any canal increases the stimulus while in the opposite direction decreases the stimuli. Thus in any movement there is an increase in frequency of impulse in one ampula and decrease in its opposite side/ampulla.

This combination of increased and decreased stimuli form the basis of interpretation of the direction of the movement. Accordingly in the above example—when the movement ceases, since the chain of events occur in a way opposite to that at the start, a subjective impression of motion in the reversed direction occurs. Finally the cupula regains the resting potential and sense of movement ceases.

The various impulses produced by the hair cells are transmitted to the vestibular nucleus via vestibular fibers. The vestibular system has diffuse connections with central nervous system like with ocular nuclei complex, anterior horn cells of spinal cord, cerebellum, higher centers in the brain.

Ewalds Law

The vestibular physiology was well clarified by Ewald's experiments. He came out with three major observations.

1. Head and eye movement always occur in the plane of the canal being stimulated and in the direction of the endolymph flow.
2. In the horizontal canal, ampullopetal endolymph flow causes a greater response than ampullofugal flow.
3. In the vertical canals ampullofugal flow causes greater response than ampullopetal flow.

Vestibular Tract

Some salient features and **points to ponder.**
1. Vestibular nuclear complex occupies the dorsolateral region of the rostral medulla and caudal pons.

2. Vestibular nuclear complex-Afferent-efferent connections.
3. Reflex responses:

Stimulation of the vestibular sensory epithelium causes Two reflex responses.

1. **Vestibulo-ocular reflex** a means by which humans stabilize gaze so that image can be fixed on the fovea of the retina during head movement.
2. **Vestibulospinal reflex** to maintain the normal posture of the head, trunk and limbs.

Vestibulo-ocular Reflex

Utriculopetal stimulus in one labyrinth is matched by an equal but opposite, utriculofugal displacement in the functionally paired canal of the other ear. Accordingly the lateral canals form one pair while the posterior canal pair with the opposite side superior canal.

Taking as an example – utriculopetal deviation of the cupula of the right horizontal canal, occurs with an utriculofugal movement of the cupula of the left horizontal canal. This results in an increase in the firing rate of the right afferent nerve and an equal but opposite response in the left afferent nerve. The right afferent information exerts an excitatory influence on the agonist muscles and an inhibitory influence on the antagonist muscles. The left afferent information reduces the excitatory influence on the antagonist muscles and disinhibits the agonist muscles. This results in contraction of the left lateral rectus and the right medial rectus muscles producing deviation of the eyes to the left.

If the stimulus is large, such that the compensatory movement cannot be obtained within the confines of the orbit, a fast movement in the opposite direction occurs. This fast movement is central, initiated and mediated by the reticular formation, cutting off the incoming flow from the vestibular nucleus and reticular activating neurons directing the ocular muscle nuclei to return the eyeballs to the point of gaze at which the slow component began.

The combination of this alternating slow and fast movements in opposite directions is called **nystagmus.**

Three controlled oculomotor systems are of clinical importance with reference to the vestibular ocular reflex.

1. **The saccadic system:** Generates rapid eye movement to correct errors in the direction of gaze and bring the desired object of fixation to the fovea in the shortest possible time. It is produced voluntarily or reflexly.

2. **Smooth pursuit system:** Low velocity accurate tracking eye movement enabling a moving target to be stabilized on the fovea. It is most efficient in low velocity targets and cannot occur in the absence of a target.

3. **Optokinetic nystagmus:** It is the reflex oscillation of the eyes induced by movements of large areas of target, *e.g.* jerking movements of the eyes of a passenger travelling in a train as he views the passing landscape. There are two types of optokinetic reflex: (a) Pursuit and (b) Non-Pursuit. Pursuit optokinetic reflex is normal and requires foveal vision while non-pursuit depends on the peripheral retina and occurs abnormally with central scotoma.

Vestibulo-spinal Reflexes

The vestibular system influences posture and orientation through neck, axial and limb motor neurons. The basic resting activity of the vestibular labyrinth which discharges impulses at a steady rate is responsible for maintaining normal tone.

Stimulation of the semicircular canal causes deviation of the head which tends to restore it to its former position.

Backward rotation of the head stimulates the posterior vertical canal and inhibits the anterior ones. This activates muscles which tends to tilt the head forwards.

Similarly, limb and trunk muscles respond to head movements with contractions appropriate to prevent falling and to maintain balance and restore normal posture. The control of posture is by way of the myotactic reflex. The lateral vestibulo-spinal, medial vestibulo-spinal and reticulo-spinal tracts are the three major pathways by which the vestibular information influences spinal anterior horn cells.

The immediate responses to stimulation are generated by the semicircular canals but after correction of the initial movement, macular stimuli maintain the necessary muscle tone.

POINTS TO REMEMBER

1. Middle ear acts as an acoustic amplifier (transformer) to compensate for the loss of sound energy due to the impendence offered by the cochlear fluid (Impendence matching).

2. The receptor organ of hearing is organ of corti.

3. Membranous cochlea (scala media) is filled with endolymph and is rich in potassium.

4. Endolymph is actively secreted by the stria vascularis.

5. Wever's volley theory states that high frequencies are perceived in the basal place mechanism turn and low frequency by telephone mechanism (rate of firing)

6. Utricle and saccul respond to linear acceleration and the semicircular canal responds to angular acceleration.

4

History Taking and Clinical Examination

History taking and careful clinical examination is very much essential to establish a proper diagnosis. No amount of present day sophisticated investigations can replace thorough history taking and careful clinical examination.

History taking for ear diseases can be described under the following headings:

- Chief complaints
- History of presenting symptoms
- Past history
- Family history
- Personal history
- Treatment history
- General examination
- Local examination
- Systemic examination
- Provisional diagnosis
- Differential diagnosis.

Chief Complaints

Common Symptoms of Ear Diseases

- Discharge
- Hearing impairment
- Otalgia (pain in the ear)
- Tinnitus

- Vertigo
- Itching
- Blocked sensation
- Feeling of fullness
- Autophonia
- Neuro-otological symptoms like:
  (a) Fever
  (b) Headache
  (c) Stiffness of neck
  (d) Facial nerve palsy
  (e) Vomiting
  (f) Diplopia
  (g) Cervicofacial pain
- Swelling and deformity.

HISTORY OF PRESENTING ILLNESS

All the above mentioned symptoms have to be analyzed under the following heading. Pertinent questions have to be asked, to know how did the disease start and what is the duration? How has it progressed up to this moment? Whether onset is sudden or gradual? All these questions should be asked strictly and impartially, without the influence of a preconceived idea which may tend to mislead the patient from the beginning. These questions lead to a thorough investigation of the patient's hereditary and medical history.

Discharge from the Ear

Onset

Sudden : ASOM
Gradual : CSOM

Duration

Long duration	:	Chronic suppurative otitis media, Eczematous otitis externa
Short duration	:	Acute suppurative otitis media, Ruptured furunculosis
Intermittent	:	Tubotympanic type of chronic suppurative otitis media

Type of Discharge

Watery discharge	:	CSF otorrhea, otitis externa (eczematous)
Serosanguinous	:	Fungal infection, diffuse otitis externa
Mucoidal	:	CSOM tubotympanic type, fungal infection, granular myringitis
Mucopurulent	:	CSOM (tubotympanic), secondary infection in CSOM, tuberculous otitis media (painless otorrhea)
Purulent	:	Furunculosis, mastoiditis, Malignant otitis externa, Atticoantral type of CSOM.
Blood stained	:	CSOM with granulation, malignant otitis externa, glomus tumor, etc.

Consistency of the Discharge

Viscid and tenacious discharge in tubotympanic disease.

Odor

Odorless: Allergic otitis externa, CSOM (tubotympanic).
Foul smelling (Fishy smell): Atticoantral disease.

Quantity

Profuse	Tubotympanic,
Scanty	Atticoantral.

Associated Conditions

- Discharge increases with cold, head bath, pharyngitis and tonsillitis, enlarged adenoids seen in tubotympanic type of CSOM.

Hearing Impairment (Deafness)

Onset

- *Sudden:* Impacted wax, vascular or viral deafness, acoustic trauma
- *Gradual:* Presbyacusis, acoustic neuroma, otosclerosis, noise induced hearing loss
- *Unilateral*: CSOM, mumps, Herpes Zoster oticus, acoustic neuroma, etc.
- *Bilateral:* Presbyacusis, Meniere's disease, otosclerosis, noise induced hearing loss
- *Progressive*: Meniere's disease, presbyacusis, otosclerosis, acoustic neuroma, tympanosclerosis
- *Fluctuating:* Meniere's disease, perilymph leak.

Autophony (Hearing his own voice louder in the ear) Secretory otitis media.

Paracusis willis

- Hearing better in noisy place-otosclerosis, whereas hearing better in a quiet place - suffering from SN loss.

Diplacusis

- Differences in the pitch of the tone in different ear is found in Meniere's disease.

Recruitment

- A relatively small increase in intensity of the auditory stimulus may cause frank discomfort to the listener as seen in cochlear pathology.

Otalgia (Pain in the Ear)

Pain in the ear may be because of the local and referred causes. Whenever the patient complains of pain the following questions should be asked in the history of presenting symptoms.

Onset

- *Sudden: e.g.* furunculosis, acute otitis media, trauma like otitic barotrauma

- *Gradual:* otitis externa secondary to CSOM, malignancy, malignant otitis externa

Duration

- *Short duration:* ASOM, perichondritis of ear pinna
- *Long duration*: Malignancy

Nature of the Pain

- *Dull :* eczematous otitis externa, secretory otitis media, impacted wax
- *Sharp:* furunculosis, otitic barotrauma
- *Throbbing pain:* ASOM

Relieving Factors

- Pain relieves with discharge from the ear- acute suppurative otitis media (ASOM)

Aggravating Factors

- Pain increasing on swallowing—ASOM.
- Pain increasing on yawning and chewing- furunculosis arising from anterior canal wall
- Pain increasing on pulling the pinna and pressing the tragus—otitis externa.

Radiating Pain

Furuncle arising from anterior wall, pain radiates to preauricular region and posterior wall to the mastoid region.

Referred Pain (Otalgia)

- Referred pain to the ear is because of nerve supply from 5th, 9th and 10th cranial nerves and $C_{2,3}$ to the ear.

Referred pain via 5th nerve

- *Dental:* Caries tooth, impacted molar, malocclusion
- *Oral cavity:* Benign or malignant ulcerative lesion
- Temporomandibular joint disorders like Costen syndrome, T.M joint arthritis.

Referred pain via 9th nerve

- Base of tongue malignancy
- Oropharynx—Acute tonsillitis, peritonsillar abscess, benign or malignant ulcers of the soft palate or tonsils.
- Elongated styloid process also known as Eagles syndrome.

Referred pain via 10th nerve

- Ulcerative lesions of vallecula, epiglottis, larynx or laryngopharynx.

Referred pain via C2, C3

- Cervical spondylosis, caries spine.

Symptoms associated with Otalgia

- Tinnitus—Acoustic neuroma
- Itching—Otomycosis

Tinnitus

It is the name given to the symptom of noises in the head or ear. It is very common and sometimes may be the only symptom. It may be regarded as a sign of irritation to the cochlea or central auditory pathway. Tinnitus should be clinically evaluated as follows:

Duration of Tinnitus

- *Short:* Middle ear pathology.
- *Long:* Meniere's disease, acoustic neuroma, palatal myoclonus, glomus jugulare, patent cochlear duct, ototoxicity.

Types of Tinnitus

- Subjective type
- Objective type

Subjective type: Sounds like ringing, whistling or roaring is heard by the patient without the presence of such a sound. This can also be psychogenic and functional in origin, apart from diseases like Meniere's, ototoxicity, etc.

Objective type: This is heard not only by the patient but also by the examiner, e.g. palatal myoclonus, patulous eustachian tube, vascular bruit, arteriovenous malformation, etc.

Nature

- *Continuous:* Otosclerosis, acoustic neuroma, acute noise trauma.
- *Intermittent and fluctuant:* Meniere's disease.
- *Pulsatile:* Glomus tumors, strychnine poisoning.
- *Relieving factors:* By putting pressure at the side of the neck in vascular causes.
- *Aggravating factors:* By smoking—cochlear pathology, ototoxicity. Yawning and blowing–eustachian dysfunction.

Vertigo

Sensation of rotation of surrounding environment with respect to person. **Vertigo without loss of consciousness** is mainly of peripheral origin—BPPV, labrynthitis. Vertigo with loss of hearing is seen in Meniere's disease, acoustic neuroma, bacterial labrynthitis. **Vertigo with loss of consciousness** is mainly because of central pathology.

Past History

History of similar illness in the past. Past history of drug intake, especially in sensorineural hearing loss and bronchial asthma. Following are the commonly associated past illnesses that can cause ear diseases.

- Diabetes mellitus
- Allergy and bronchial asthma
- Hypertension
- Tuberculosis
- Syphilis
- Childhood diseases
- Radiation
- Bleeding condition
- Connective tissue disorder
- Hyperthyroidism

Family History

History of consanguineous marriage causes high incidence of deaf-mutism and other congenital disorders. Otosclerosis runs in the family.

Personal History

- Occupation
- Diet
- Personal hygiene
- Smoking and alcohol
- Loss of weight
- Pan chewing

Treatment History

Any past medication and surgery should be enquired for better planning of the treatment.

CLINICAL EXAMINATION

Clinical Examination of the Ear

Equipment for Ear Examination

Both indirect and direct light sources are used
1. Bull's eye lamp—indirect light source.
2. Head mirror.
3. Head light—direct light source.
4. Ear specula of various sizes—The largest speculum which can be conveniently inserted into the ear canal should be used.
5. Siegel's pneumatic speculum.
6. Tuning fork—256, 512, 1024 Hz are preferred to assess the speech frequency.
7. Jobson Horne probe can be used as a cotton wool carrier to clean the discharge from the external auditory canal before examining the tympanic membrane.
8. Tilley's or Hartmann's forceps.
9. Eustachian tube catheters.
10. Otoscope—It gives a magnified view of the part to be examined.
11. Suction apparatus—This is one of the important equipment in ENT and is used to remove the secretions from the external ear and helps in proper examination.
12. Microscope—Either attached with ENT equipment unit or separate entity.
13. Otoendoscope.

In examining the ear with a forehead mirror good illumination is necessary. Any fairly powerful lamp such as Bull's eye lamp will be sufficient. Daylight will suffice for the examination of the external auditory meatus, but is less satisfactory for the drum head. The source of light is arranged on the left side of the patient slightly above the level of his ear. The patient is seated sideways to the surgeon who sits opposite the ear to be examined and reflects light onto it.

Examination of the External Ear

Inspection

Pre auricular region and pinna: Look for swelling, scar, sinus and other skin changes. The pinna should be inspected for congenital and acquired abnormalities.

Palpation: It should be done in a systematic manner like the following:

Superficial palpation: By means of digital palpation both the soft tissues and the cartilaginous framework are explored.

- **Soft tissue:** Mobility of the tissue on the cartilage is absent in malignant or cicatricial lesions.
  Any thickening or swelling in the pinna can be due to hematoma, tumors and gumma- tous lesion.
  Cartilaginous framework: It should be palpated to find out any deficiency or loss of cartilage—whether cartilage is completely developed or not and whether cartilage alone or soft tissue is also involved.

Deep Palpation

Eliciting the tragal tenderness: Using the tip of index finger on tragus in the pretragal region a fair degree of pressure is exerted. In case of acute inflammation of external ear as in otitis externa, furunculosis, etc. it causes severe pain.

Traction of pinna: When pinna is pulled upwards, backwards and outwards should not cause pain in normal cases unless the patient has otitis externa.

Examination of Postauricular Region

Inspection

Examination should be done to rule out the following conditions like postoperative scar, dermatitis, erysipelas, etc.

- **Change in general contour of mastoid:** Examiner should stand behind the patient to see the change in mastoid configuration on both sides.

Palpation

1. **Skin (superficial palpation):** Normal skin over postauricular region is mobile.
   - Temperature of the skin will increase in mastoiditis and abscess.
   - Contour and boundaries of the swelling if any should be noted.
   - Tenderness (Deep palpation): Mastoid tenderness should be elicited by pressing with the tip of forefinger or thumb in three different areas of mastoid namely Mac Ewan's triangle (cymba concha), midpoint of the posterior border of mastoid and tip of the mastoid. Both Mac Ewan's triangle and mid point of posterior border of mastoid are very important points to elicit mastoid tenderness in mastoiditis.

Examination of Neck

Examination of neck may be of vital importance in case of Bezolds abscess, Citelli's abscess where pus from the mastoid may track inferiorly along the sternocleidomastoid or may track anteriorly along the digastric tendon into the submaxillary triangle respectively. In case of internal jugular vein thrombosis internal jugular vein may be palpated as a hard cord anterior and deep to the sternocleidomastoid.

Examination of External Auditory Canal

This may be direct (Fig. 4.1) or by using instruments. Popularly used instrument is aural speculum (Fig. 4.2).

1. Direct Examination

External auditory canal has a S shaped curvature which consists of bone and cartilage which require special retraction and manipulation to make

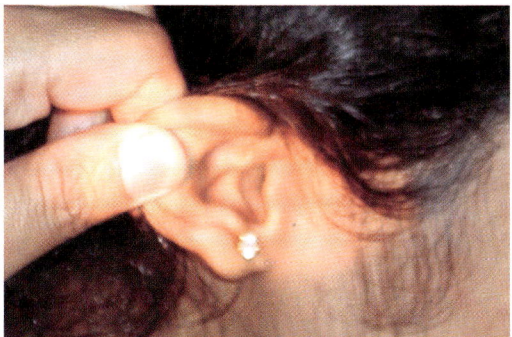

Fig. 4.1: Direct examination

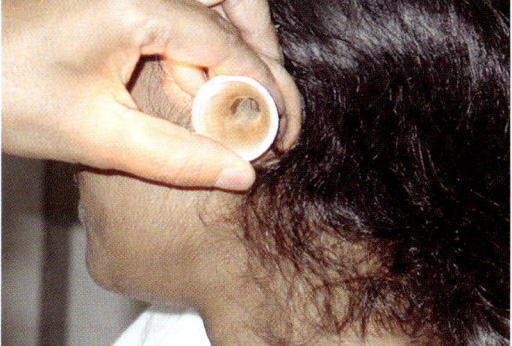

Fig. 4.2: Aural examination

to inspect the ear drum without the use of a ear speculum. The following points to be examined during this procedure.

External auditory canal—may show the following abnormalities:

- **Narrow canal** (Fig. 4.3)
  (i) Congenital- atresia
  (ii) Acquired - scar following trauma, burns, bony tumor like osteomas, etc.
- **Wide canal:** Patients in whom tympano-mastoidectomy is done, syphilis, oto-sclerosis (Fig. 4.4).

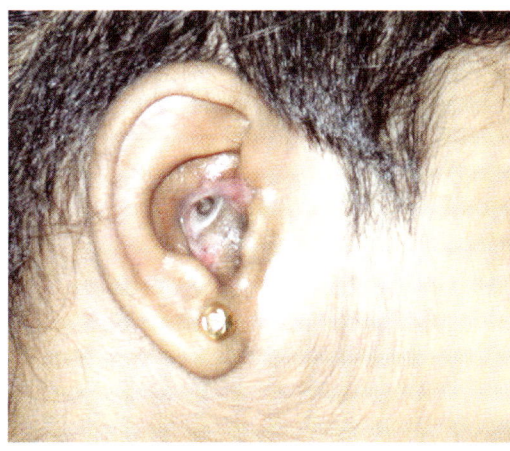

Fig. 4.3: Narrow external auditory canal

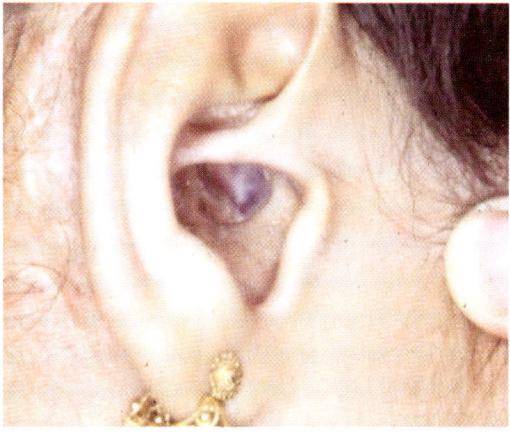

Fig. 4.4: Post-mastoidectomy wide external auditory canal

the ear canal straight for examination purposes. For direct examination patient is seated sideways in such a way that examiner faces the ear to be examined with a good source of light and direct this light on to the auditory meatus. On completion of the above examination, patients head is tilted slightly opposite from the ear being examined.

The pinna is held between thumb and index finger of left hand when examining right ear and of the right hand when examining the left ear and ear is pulled upwards, backwards, outwards in adults, downwards and laterally in infants and young children. The other three fingers are placed on the temporal region serving as fulcrum. This manipulation will straighten the ear canal to a certain extent and provide a better view in preliminary examination.

In case where canal is wide and follows a straight line, this examination permits examiner

- **Foreign body:** Vegetative and non-vegetative.
- **Impacted wax:** Hard blackish mass occluding whole of the external auditory canal.
- **Tumor:** Both benign and malignant.
- **Discharge:** Profuse and thin discharge usually from middle ear pathology, whereas slight and thick discharge from the external auditory canal.

2. Aural Speculum Examination
(Instrument examination)

For this examination a proper and adequate size aural speculum preferably black coated is selected and introduced into the external auditory canal. Aural speculum will help examination of deep meatus and tympanic membrane. Most commonly used speculum is Toynbees and Gruver's speculum.

Aim of this speculum is to straighten the canal and it should be long enough to reach the deepest obstacle which is at the junction of the bony and cartilaginous canal. Specula are circular with diameters varying between 2 and 7 mm. The speculum used should correspond to the size and permeability of the canal. In rare cases, it may be necessary to fall back upon **forced dilatation** of the canal to examine the drum. In such cases a dilating speculum can be used the best being Moores instrument. The dilation is extremely painful and **should be performed under general anesthesia.** When greater precision and details are required a special speculum like **seigel's pneumatic speculum** or an **endoscopic speculum** or **otoendoscope** or **otoscope** can be used (Fig. 4.5).

Technique of speculum examination: Patient is placed as per direct examination when the examiner focuses the light from his head mirror or head light on to the auditory meatus. The pinna is held between the middle and ring fingers of the left hand and pull upwards and backwards. The speculum is held in the right hand and gently introduced into the canal. Once speculum has been introduced it is held in place by the thumb and

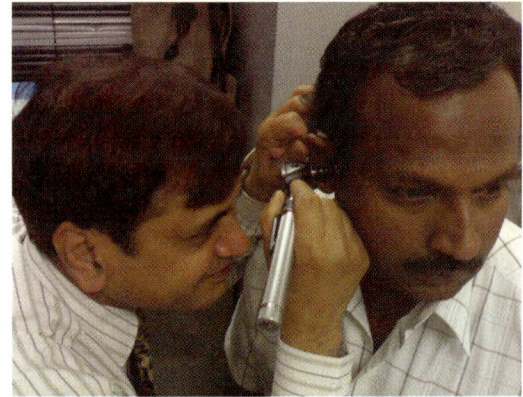

Fig. 4.5: Otoscopic examination

index finger of the left hand in order to free the right hand for cleaning and probing. The speculum should be introduced with the **utmost gentleness** with a slow rotatory movement to facilitate its passage. One should not be surprised when the patient coughs while introducing the speculum which is due to irritation of auricular branch of vagus nerve.

3. Palpation of the External Auditory Canal

This examination is made directly with finger or with instruments.

- **Finger Palpation:** Direct digital palpation is done by inserting the tip of the index finger

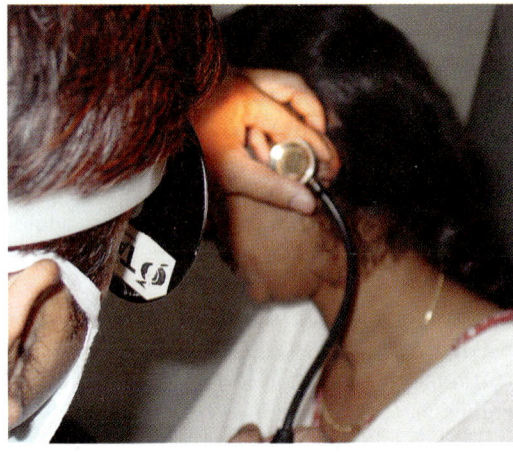

Fig. 4.6: Seigel's pneumatic speculum examination

into the canal. By this the consistency of the lesion is felt and also the condition of condyle of mandible can be felt.

- **Instrumental:** The probe or stylet which is angulated is preferred and introduced through the speculum which will prevent obstruction of examiner's vision. It helps to determine the consistency, shape and direction of a fistula.

4. Otomicroscopic examination (EUM) is of more precise diagnostic method. When canal is obstructed by secretion or foreign body it is necessary to clean the canal as completely as possible either by dry mopping or suction cleaning under microscopic vision.

Examination of the Tympanic Membrane

To make an effective examination of tympanic membrane it is first necessary to be properly oriented with the normal anatomy of the tympanic membrane. To achieve this, the examiner should first examine the upper part of the drum and look in front of its upper pole for a small yellowish prominence. This is the short or lateral process of malleus. This landmark is particularly important since it is almost always present even when the rest of malleus has disappeared.

From this Prominence
(Short or Lateral Process) Originate

1. Anteriorly, a horizontal line, often scarcely perceptible extending to the periphery of the drum, this is the anterior malleolar fold.
2. Posteriorly, a small similar line, but a little longer, this is the posterior fold, or posterior malleolar fold.
3. Inferiorly and posteriorly a whitish bony landmark is seen at an angle of 45° called handle of malleus and its tip is called the umbo. The convexity of the umbo will be directed medially towards middle ear.
4. A light reflex can be observed, triangular in shape which is placed anteriorly and inferiorly called **Cone of light**. The cone

of light is always projecting anteroinferiorly in normal tympanic membrane because the tympanic membrane is placed obliquely in the deep part of the external auditory canal.

It is customary to divide the drum topographically into four sectors or quadrants. This is done by drawing an imaginary line horizontally touching the tip of the umbo, and a second line vertically along the long axis of the handle of malleus. The quadrants are known as:

- Anterosuperior quadrant
- Posterosuperior quadrant
- Anteroinferior quadrant
- Posteroinferior quadrant.

After orientation is achieved the tympanic membrane should be examined in relation to:

I. Color.
II. Position.
III. Mobility.
IV. Changes in surface.

I. Color

Normal drum appears greyish white. If this color is changed some pathological condition should exists as follows.

- ***Congested drum:*** Indicates an inflammation, *e.g.* acute otitis media, myringitis bullosa, active otosclerosis, glomus jugularis, excessively crying child, etc. Congestion with yellowish tint is sometimes the sign of an acute suppurative otitis media. In stage of suppuration the congestion may be diffuse or localized. Localized in the handle of the malleus in acute otitis media or in subacute otitis media. Generalized congestion in acute simple or necrotising otitis media.

- ***Dark grey slate color:*** This color is an indication of tubal occlusion. This type of drum does not light up well (Dull appearance).

- ***A dull white***, thickened, cotton-like drum, is found in certain types of sclerosis (senile) or following scarring and changes after otitis media popularly called as chalky white patch or tympanosclerotic patch.

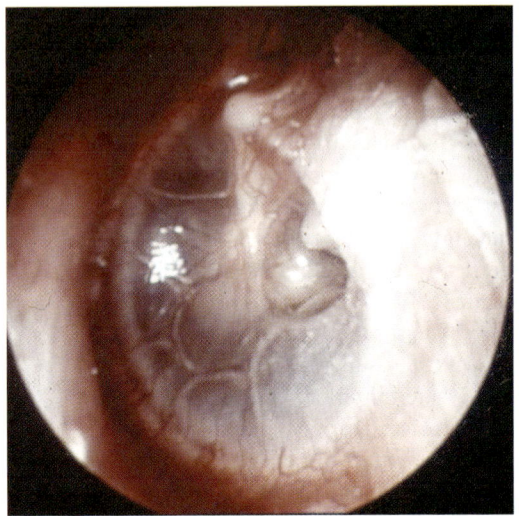

Fig. 4.7: Secretory otitis media

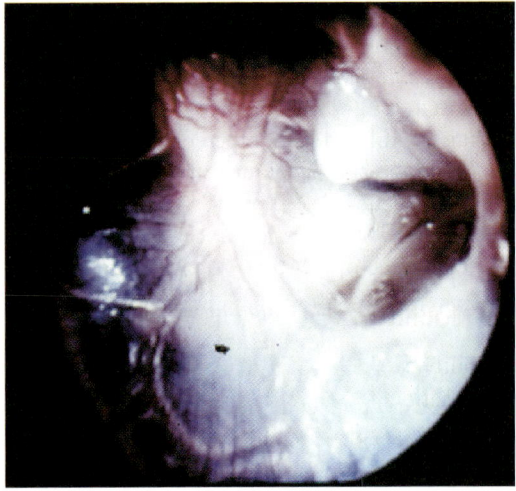

Fig. 4.8: Retracted drum

- *A dull* lusterless occasionally bulging tympanic membrane is seen in secretory otitis media or glue ear (Fig. 4.7).

- *A slight* vasodilatation of blood vessels caused by the irritation of the canal, or probing with a stylet, should not be confused with a pathological condition. Such congestion may be especially pronounced along the handle of malleus.

- *A blue drum* is sometimes found when infection is entirely absent. It is seen in transudative type of otitis media, glomus juglare, high jugular bulb, cholesterol granuloma and Van der Hoeve syndrome.

- *A dark blue* drum is seen in case of hemotympanum following head injury.

II. Position

Normally, the drum inclines downwards and medially. The upper portion is much more closer to the examining eye than it's lower portion. The drum may change position so that it protrudes outwards towards the examiner or it may be pulled inwards towards the tympanic cavity. The following are the commonly known abnormal position:

Bulging drum: Apparent increase in length of the handle of malleus, decrease in the short process and absence of the cone of light. The bulge may be due to blood (trauma, hemorrhagic otitis media), pus (purulent otitis media), air following tubal insufflation or tumors.

Retracted drum (Fig. 4.8): Apparent shortening of the handle of malleus, exaggeration of the prominence of the short process and anterior and posterior malleolar folds and distortion of the cone of light reflex. **It may be due to insufficient tubotympanic aeration (eustachian tube dysfunction)** or adherence of the drum to the medial wall of the middle ear cavity (atelectatic drum). The retracted tympanic membrane have been classified into four grades depending on the amount of **retraction of pars tensa (Sade's classification)**.

Grade 1 : Mild retraction not touching the long process of incus.

Grade 2 : Retracted drum touching the long process of incus.

Grade 3 : Retracted drum touching the promontory.

Grade 4 : Drum plastered to the promontory.

Retraction of Pars flaccida has been classified into four grades according to **Tos's classification**:

Grade 1 : Mild attic retraction, without touching the neck of malleus

Grade 2 : Attic retraction touching neck of malleus.

Grade 3 : Limited outer attic wall erosion with extent beyond osseous malleus.

Grade 4 : Severe outer attic wall erosion.

III. Mobility

Mobility can be examined with the aid of seigle's pneumatic speculum or by valsalva maneuver. During compression the triangular light reflex changes shape and the handle of malleus moves. If it does not change or move there is evidence of more or less complete loss of mobility of the tympanic membrane.

The mobility is decreased or absent in:
- Adhesive otitis media which may be due to adhesion and scars following necrotising otitis media.
- Ankylosis of the ossicular chain.
- Eustachian tube dysfunction.

Other methods of testing the mobility is by increasing the air pressure inside the middle ear cavity by insufflation of the eustachian tube while at the same time examining the drum through an otoscope which is called as **Toynbee's maneuver.** The tympanic membrane also seen moving along with breathing in case of **patulous eustachian tube** called as hyper mobile tympanic membrane.

IV. Changes in the Surface

In pathological conditions the following changes can occur on the surface of the membrane calcareous deposits (tympanosclerotic patch), scars or thinned out membrane, bullas and perforation.

(a) **Calcareous deposits:** These look like white plaques of varying sizes and shapes, resembling small pieces of plaster of paris on the drum.

(b) **Bulla:** Bullas vary in number and are seen by the examiner as grey, reddish or bluish in color, resembling small pearls attached to the surface of the drum.

The location of a perforation is extremely variable. Determination of the exact location is most essential for diagnostic therapeutic and prognostic accuracy. The perforation may be central, attic or marginal.

MIDDLE EAR

Direct examination of the middle ear is not possible under normal conditions. Only a small area can be observed through the perforated or thin drum, i.e. a part of the incus, a shadow of the round window niche and in case the drum is extremely thin the chorda tympani nerve is seen.

In case of large central perforation labyrinthine wall, promontory and ossicle may be seen. The stapes may also be seen in posterosuperior perforations.

Changes in the tympanic membrane may give us an indication as to the condition of the middle ear cavity and its contents. All these parts may however be hidden by granulations or polyp arising from the middle ear.

Instrumental Examination

A blunt probe or stylet is used to test the softness of the granulation tissue, point of origin of the polyp, resistance of the promontory, denuded bone in an osteitic area and orifice of a fistula.

Eustachian Tube

It is a communication canal between the middle ear and the pharynx. It maintains the equilibrium between the pressure of the middle ear and the atmosphere. Any obstruction whether partly or complete causes a reabsorption of air from the middle ear with consequent retraction of the drum as a result of a higher atmospheric pressure. Due to its deep-seated anatomical location, the eustachian tube can only be examined indirectly with the help of several instruments and various methods. To test eustachian tube patency it is necessary to insufflate air into the eustachian tube by various methods such as:

- Valsalva maneuver
- Toynbee maneuver
- Politzerization
- Catheterization
- Frenzel's maneuver (nasopharyngeal pressure test).

Tuning Fork Tests

The commonly performed tests are Rinne, Weber and absolute bone conduction tests. The commonly used tuning fork (Fig. 4.9) tests are of the frequencies of 256, 512 1024. The details of the technique have been described under the chapter of hearing evaluation.

Fistula Test

It is done by applying intermittent pressure over the tragus, or by seigelization with an pneumatic speculum. Ask the patient to look straight ahead, and check for nystagmus directed towards the opposite side. The patient may complain of vertigo. (Details are given in examination of the labyrinthine function).

Facial Nerve

It is important to differentiate between upper motor neuron palsy and lower motor neuron palsy by asking the patient to show various facial expressions like:

- Frowning (wrinkling of the forehead)
- Movement of the eyelids (closing of the eyes)
- Smiling or showing the teeth (angle of the mouth).
- Loss of nasolabial fold.

Examination of the Eye

Inspection of the eye may reveal features such as hypertelorism or coloboma associated with congenital hearing disorder syndrome. The presence of blue sclera (osteogenesis imperfecta) and interstitial keratitis (congenital syphilis, Cogan's disease) should be noted.

On fundoscopy, papilloedema may be seen in space occupying lesions such as cerebellopontine angle tumors, temporal lobe abscess, otitic hydrocephalus. Eye movements for nystagmus should be observed. The absence of corneal reflex is usually a late sign of acoustic neuroma.

Examination of Other Cranial Nerves

Paralysis of the VI nerve may be associated with lesions in the petrous apex, e.g. (Gradenigo's syndrome). The involvement of last four cranial nerves are frequently associated with stage 3 malignant otitis externa and advanced glomus jugulare tumor. Loss of corneal reflex is seen in acoustic neuroma.

Examination of the Nose and Throat

A full examination of the nose and throat must always be carried out to rule out rhinitis, sinusitis, pharyngitis, tonsillitis, nasopharyngitis, etc.

Functional Examination of Hearing

Plethora of clinical tests of hearing were introduced in the 19th century and, although, the majority have been superseded by more sensitive and reliable audiometric tests, some knowledge of these clinical tests is of value.

Clinical tests of auditory function may be divided into four types:

1. **Finger friction test:** Rubbing or snapping of the forefinger and thumb is a test

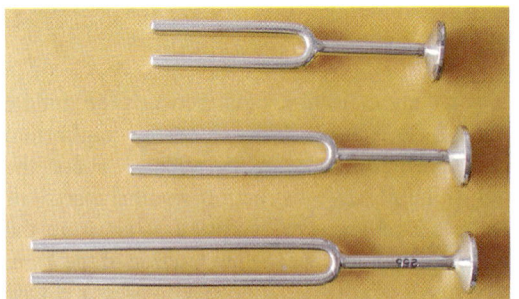

Fig. 4.9: Gardiner browns tuning fork

commonly employed by neurologists, for screening for both threshold of hearing deficits and sound localization.

2. **Lever pocket watch test:** With the introduction of the Quartz watch, lever pocket watch tests, have become obsolete, although for many years they were a valuable tool in audiometric screening in the absence of more sophisticated equipment.

3. **Speech test:** Speech test can be done in any of the following ways. However, free field speech test is most popular. These are
   (a) Freefield speech test by whisper, conversation
   (b) Recorded voice test
   (c) Speech audiometry.
   (d) Monitored speech through a closed circuit. In this the patient must be 20 feet from the examiner.

Requirements for Speech Test
- Testing room should be reasonably quiet.
- The eye must be shielded to prevent lip reading.
- The ear under test is directed towards the examiner.
- The non-test ear is blocked by assistant's index finger on tragus.
- Speech test material should be spondee and phonetically balanced, example: "Black Bird", "night tight", etc.
- Whisper test should be done with whisper with residual air after an ordinary expiration.
- Speech materials if audible at a distance of 20 feet is considered to be normal.
- Despite these precautions, great care must be exercised in using clinical speech tests to assess auditory thresholds.
- Clinical tests of auditory function may enable the clinician to distinguish a conductive from sensorineural loss or in identifying the presence of a feigned hearing loss. It is basically a qualitative test but the quantity of deafness can also be assessed by an experienced otologist.

4. **Tuning fork tests:** The most clinical information may be obtained using tuning forks that vibrate naturally at 256, 512, 1024 and 2048 Hz. These are the frequencies commonly used in clinical practice.

The following precaution should be taken:
1. The test should be performed in a quiet room.
2. The prong should be struck sharply against some resistance, e.g. Elastic object like, hard rubber, thenar eminence, femoral condyle.
3. The prong should be **struck at a point about one-third of its length from the free end**, thus keeping overtones to a minimum and producing a pure tone. The following tuning fork tests are commonly used in practice.
   - **Rinne's test**
   - **Weber's test**
   - **Absolute bone conduction test (Modified Schwabach's test).**

Rinne's Test

In this test the vibrating tuning fork is kept over the mastoid and when the patient indicates that the sound has stopped, the tuning fork is placed 2.5 cm in front of the external auditory canal (Fig. 4.10). Rinne is said to be positive if the patient still hears the sound and negative if the sound is not heard. Alternatively, the vibrating tuning fork is placed in front of the external canal and on the mastoid intermittently and the patient is asked to indicate with which the hearing is better.

In cases with severe unilateral sensorineural deafness, the vibrating tuning fork may be heard when placed on the ipsilateral mastoid but not in front of the ear. This is due to trans- mission of the vibrations to the healthy ear and is referred to as a **'false Rinne negative'** and it may be differentiated from a true negative by masking the non test ear with Barany's noise box. The rinne is positive in patient with normal hearing.

Weber's Test

This test is performed in conjunction with the Rinne test and is of particular value in cases

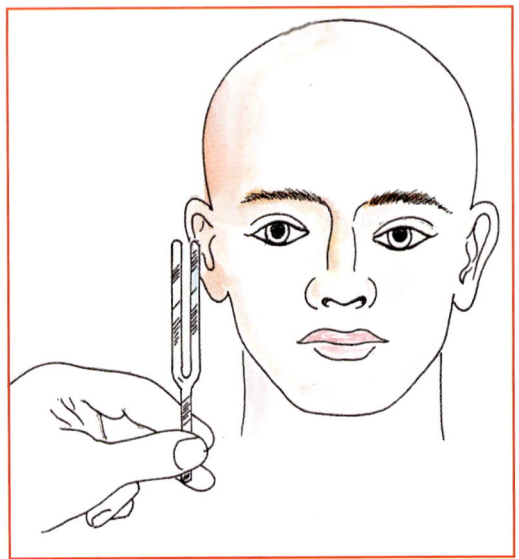

Fig. 4.10: Rinne's tests

of unilateral hearing loss. In this test the vibrating tuning fork is placed in the middle of the forehead or on the vertex. Then the patient is asked in which ear the sound is heard better. Normally it is heard equally in both ears. In conductive deafness it is heard louder in the worse ear and in Sensorineural deafness it is heard louder in the better ear. This is called as lateralization. In conductive loss lateralization of sound to the bad ear is either due to loss of ambient noise or **failure to dissipate sound** because of the ossicular discontinuity.

Absolute Bone Conduction or Modified Schwabach's Test

It is done to investigate a possible decrease in bone conduction. To conduct this test the examiner himself should have normal hearing or normal cochlear reserve. In this test the patients bone conduction is compared with that of the examiners.

The patient external auditory canal is blocked by pressing over tragus while putting the buzzing tuning fork on the mastoid bone. When the patient no longer hears any sound, the same tuning fork to be shifted to the examiner's mastoid of the same ear to compare.

In conductive hearing loss both the patients and examiner hears the fork for the same duration, whereas in sensorineural deafness patient hears the tuning fork for shorter duration which is interpreted as ABC down or short. **The result of the ABC is interpreted as normal or short.**

Schwabach's Test

This test is similar to ABC except that the ear canal is not occluded. In conductive hearing loss, the Schwabach is lengthened where as for normal hearing the sensorineural hearing loss it is normal and reduced respectively

Gelle's Test

This test constitutes an excellent method of determining the functioning of the ossicular chain and especially the stapes.

The air pressure in the external auditory meatus is altered using a Seigle's speculum. In the normal individual or those with a sensorineural loss increasing the meatal pressure results in a decreased sensation of loudness from a bone conducted stimulus.

No alteration of bone conduction thresholds indicates fixation of the stapes in case of otosclerosis.

Bing Test

This test is based on the principle that, when a vibrating tuning fork is placed on the cranium and it ceases to be heard (primary perception) in the normal ear, and when the external auditory canal is plugged hears it again (secondary perception). Increased loudness for bone conducted stimuli (less than 2 KHz), occurs in the normal patients or those with a sensorineural loss when the external meatus is occluded (presence of secondary perception). There is no change when a conductive deafness is present.

Tuning Fork Test for Malingering or Non-organic Deafness

1. *Stenger's test:* The principle of this test is that if two equal and identical sounds strike normal ears, the individual receives the impression in one ear only, i.e. the one nearest to the sound. The patient is blindfolded and the examiner holds two similar tuning forks (512) struck with moderate intensity and held at 25 cms from each ear. Malingeer will say that he hears in the normal ear only. The fork on the deaf side is advanced by 3 inches towards the ear. Patient who is maligering deafness will deny hearing the sound at all.

2. *Chimani Moos test:* A modification of the Weber test to detect non-organic hearing loss. If a tuning fork is placed on the forehead the malingerer states that he hears the sound in his good ear (simulating a sensorineural deafness). If the meatus of the good ear is occluded, the truly deaf patient still hears the sound in the occluded ear but the malingerer may deny that he hears the tuning fork at all.

Others tests being: Teal test and Lombard test.

POINTS TO REMEMBER

1. Tragal tenderness can be elicitated in case of furunculosis of external ear.
2. The site for eliciting the mastoid tenderness are over the cymba concha, midpoint of posterior border of the mastoid and tip of the mastoid.
3. False negative Rinne is seen in severe sensorineural hearing loss.
4. Tuning fork tests are done for subjective assessment of hearing.
5. Gelle's test is an excellent method of determining the functioning of the ossicular chain and especially the stapes.
6. Toynbee's maneuver is done to test the mobility of the tympanic membrane.
7. Hyper mobile tympanic membrane can be seen in patulous eustachian tube.

Audiology and Assessment of Hearing

TYPES OF AUDIOMETRY

Subjective Audiometry

1. Pure tone audiometry

It includes measurement of hearing acuity by using pure tones (Single frequency sound) to estimate the air conduction and bone conduction thresholds of hearing for various frequencies. The primary purpose of pure-tone audiometry tests is to determine the type, degree, and configuration of hearing loss. The following measurement is done.

- *Air conduction threshold:* Minimum perceivable intensity of sound presented adjacent to pinna-conduction through external and middle ear.
- *Bone conduction threshold:* Minimum perceivable intensity of sound presented on the mastoid process directly stimulates the inner ear.

Pure-tone thresholds indicate the softest sound audible to an individual at least 50% of the time and the hearing level are measured in decibels. Frequency is measured in hertz, which are cycles per second. Usually frequencies of 250-8000 Hz are used in testing as this range represents most of the speech spectrum. The hearing sensitivity is plotted on an audiogram, which is a graph displaying intensity as a function of frequency.

Advantages

- Tests various frequencies
- Both qualitative and quantitative (type and severity of hearing loss)
- Documentation
- Compare serial audiograms/pre and post treatment audiograms
- May give clue to diagnosis

Disadvantages

- Subjective test
- Patient should understand instructions—cannot be done in children and psychiatric patients.
- Not accurate for medico-legal purposes if malingering suspected.
- Masking to be done to avoid involvement of non-test ear in the test.

Features of Conductive Deafness

- Normal BC thresholds
- Increased AC thresholds
- Air-Bone (AB) gap
- Usually lower tones affected
- Loss usually < 60–70 dB
- Carhart's notch is present in otosclerosis.

Features of Sensorineural Deafness

- Both air and bone conduction thresholds are raised—No AB gap
- Dip at 4K in noise induced hearing loss
- Bilateral sloping (decending) curve in presbyacusis

Degree of hearing loss
- Normal hearing (0–25 dB)
- Mild hearing loss (26–40 dB)
- Moderate hearing loss (41–55 dB)
- Moderate-severe hearing loss (56–70 dB)
- Severe hearing loss (71–90 dB)
- Profound hearing loss (> 90 dB).

Pure tone audiometry (PTA) will give a graphical representation of different hearing loss. Both quantity and quality can be studied (Fig. 5.1a and b).

Pure tone audiometry showing profound bilateral sensorineural hearing loss in a congenitally deaf child (Fig. 5.2a).

Pure tone audiometry showing bilateral (Fig. 5.2b) and unilateral conductive (Fig. 5.2c) hearing loss secondary to middle ear pathology.

Pure tone audiometry showing bilateral acoustic dip at 4 kHz in the bone conduction thresholds suggestive of noise-induced hearing loss (Fig.5.2d).

Pure tone audiometry showing unilateral sensorineural deafness with positive **glycerol test** suggestive of Meniere's disease (Fig. 5.2e).

Pure tone audiometry showing low frequency conductive hearing loss suggestive of bilateral secretory otitis media (Fig. 5.2f).

2. Speech audiometry: It is used to analyze graphically the percentage of words heard correctly by the subject.

***Normal ears:* 100% discrimination score is usually achieved by 60 dB intensity levels.**

Conductive deafness: 100% discrimination score or near is usually reached but at higher intensity level. (Pure tone audiometry (PTA) test).

Sensory or cochlear deafness: Often patients are unable to reach high scores (*e.g.* 50–70% max.) before discrimination deteriorates.

3. Bekesy self-recording audiometer based on Sweep and fixed frequency testing can be done as follows (Fig. 5.3a to 5.3d).

Type I	:	Normal ears and conductive hearing loss
Type II	:	Sensory deafness
Type III	:	Neural deafness.
Type IV	:	Common in neural than in sensory deafness.
Type V	:	Non-organic hearing loss- malingering

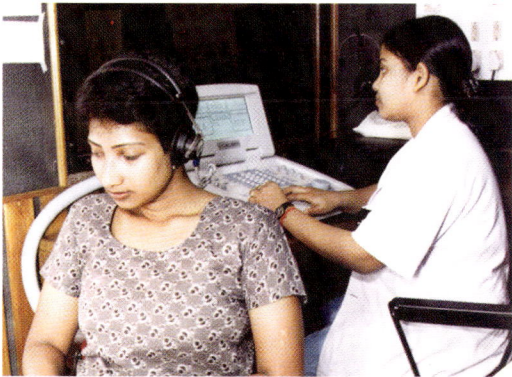

Fig. 5.1a: Pure tone audiometry in progress (air conduction)

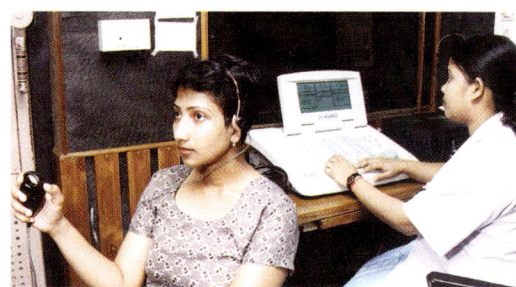

Fig. 5.1b: Pure tone audiometry in progress (bone conduction)

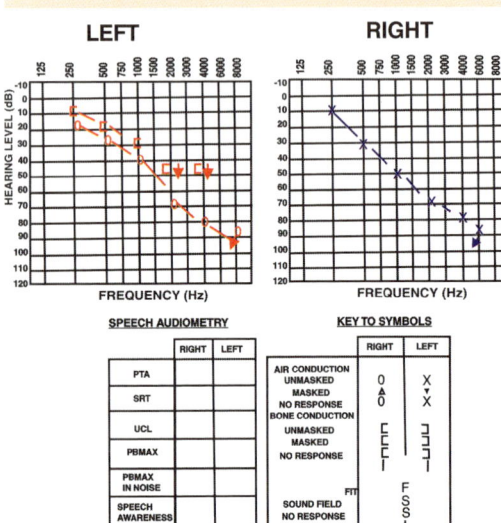

Fig. 5.2a: Pure tone audiometry showing high frequency sensorineural hearing loss

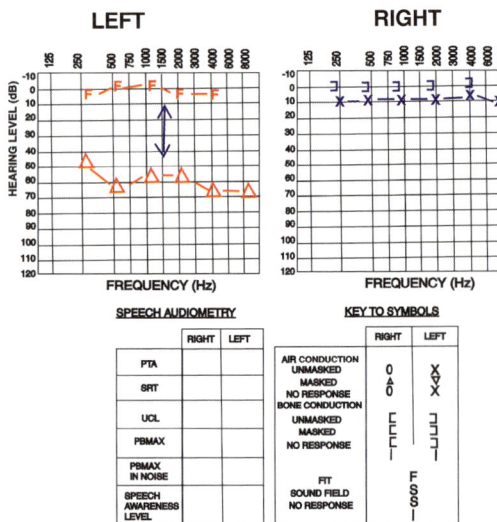

Fig. 5.2c: Pure tone audiometry showing unilateral conductive hearing loss secondary to middle ear pathology

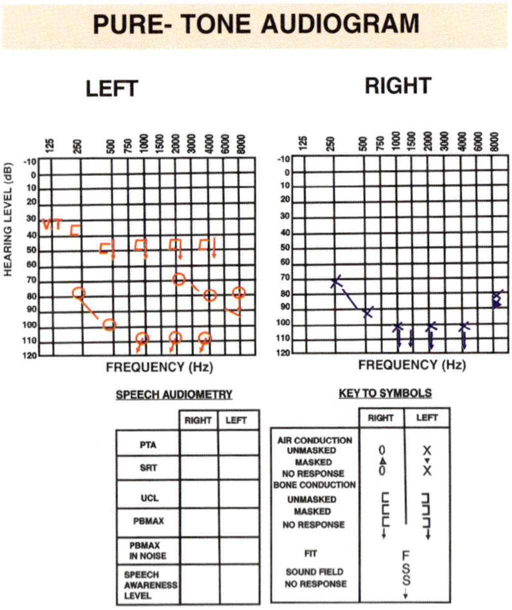

PURE- TONE AUDIOGRAM

LEFT   **RIGHT**

Fig. 5.2b: Pure tone audiometry showing profound bilateral sensorineural hearing loss in a congenitally deaf child

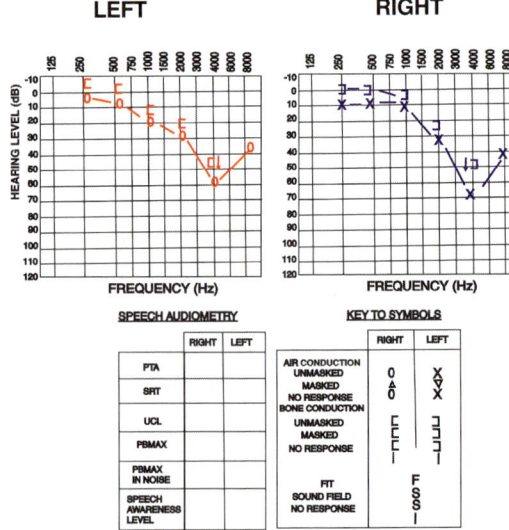

Fig.5.2d: Pure tone audiometry showing bilateral acoustic dip at 4 KHz in the bone conduction thresholds suggestive of noise-induced hearing loss

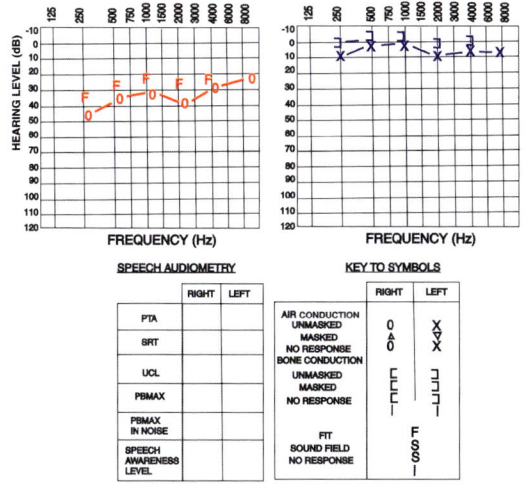

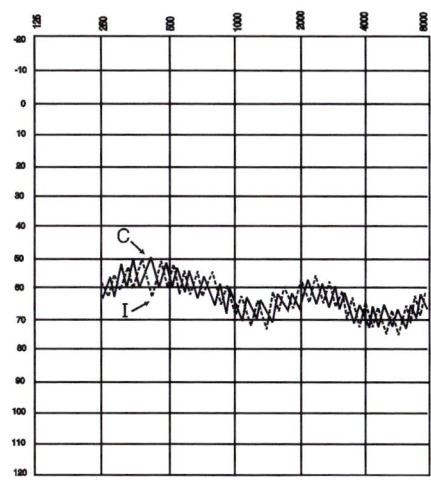

Fig. 5.3a: Type I—Tracing overlap one another found in normal and middle ear pathology

Fig. 5.2e: Pure tone audiometry showing unilateral sensorineural deafness with positive glycerol test suggestive of Meniere's disease

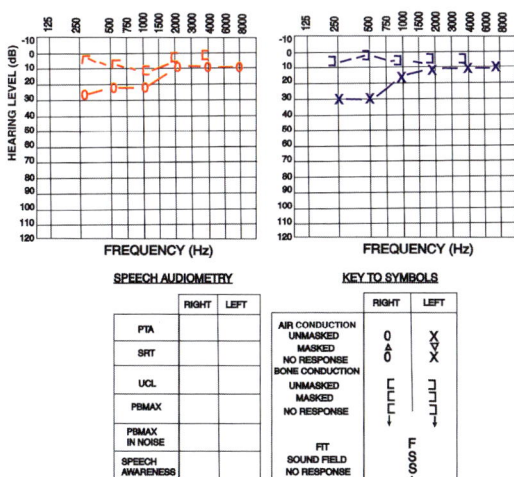

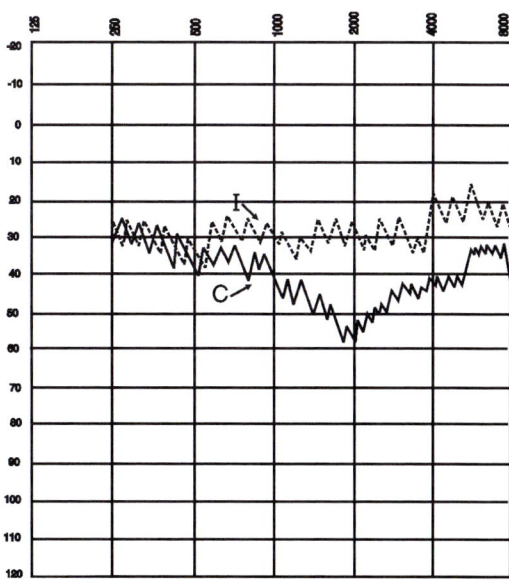

Fig. 5.2f: Pure tone audiometry showing low frequency conductive hearing loss suggestive of bilateral secretory otitis media

Fig. 5.3b: Type II—Seen in cochlear pathology. Tracing overlap at low frequency and separates between 500-1000 Hz.

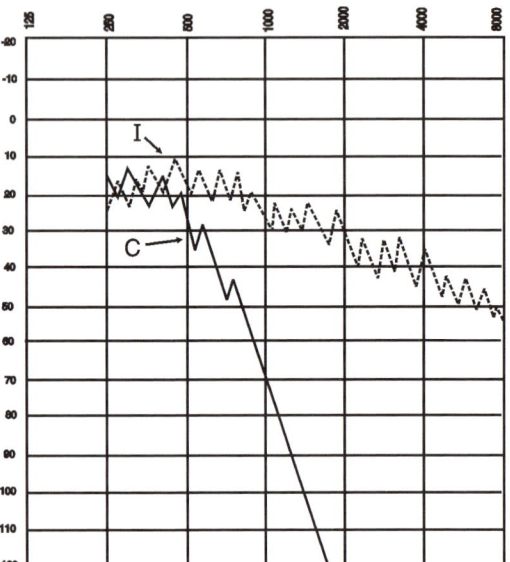

Fig. 5.3c: Type III - Continuous tracing falls abruptly away from the interrupted tracing. Mostly found in disorders of 8th cranial nerves

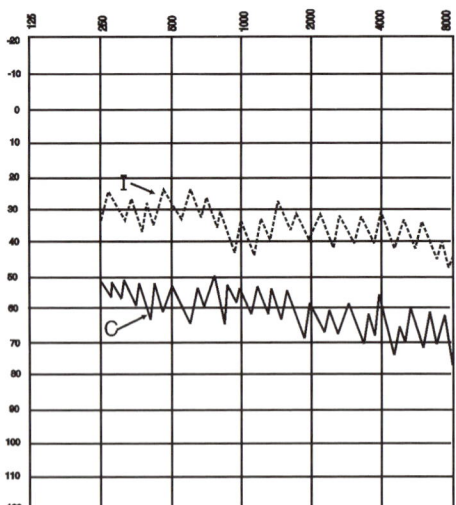

Fig. 5.3d: Type IV - Continuous tracing runs below the interrupted tracing of all frequencies seen in some accoustic nerve disorder

Objective Audiometry

1. Impedance audiometry tympanometry: The term impedance means resistance to flow of energy. The details are given in the next chapter (Fig. 5.4a to 5.4d).

2. Brain stem evoked response audiometry (Fig. 5.5): Measurement of the tiny physiological electrical events occurring in response to sound stimulation. Brain stem response stimuli in the form of clicks, these electrical potentials are picked up from the vertex by surface electrodes (the details are given in the next chapter).

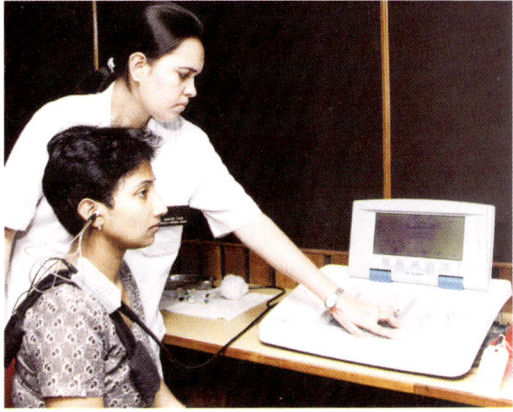

Fig. 5.4a: Impedance audiometry in progress

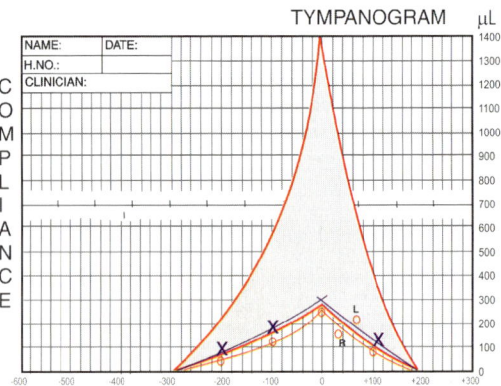

Fig. 5.4b: 'As' type of curve with low compliance seen in otosclerosis

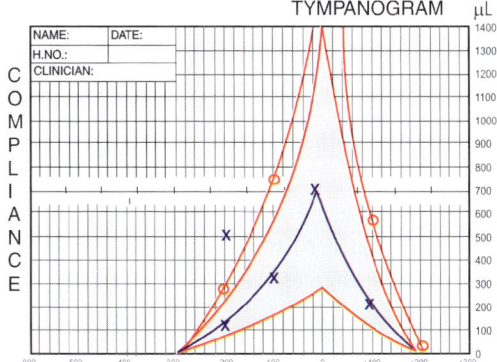

Fig. 5.4c: 'Ad' type of curve with increase compliance seen in ossicular discontinuity

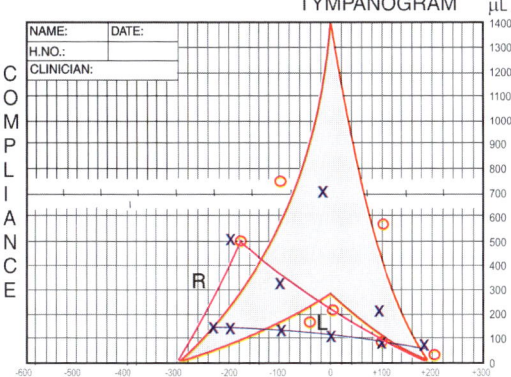

Fig. 5.4d: Right type C curve due to negative middle ear pressure left side B type curve (flat) suggestive of fluid in the middle ear

3. Otoacoustic Emissions (Fig. 5.6)

Hearing tests in infants and children

Following are the methods to determine the hearing loss in children.

- Reflex test: At birth Moro's or startle reflex.
- At 3 months: Blinking or frowning.
- At 5 months: Eyes turn towards a sound source.
- At 6 months: The head turns towards a sound source.

Behavioral Test

1. From 7 to 18 months, distraction test is used.
2. At 18 months - 2 years, co-operation of the child is sought to sound hence called co-operation test.
3. Between 2 and 5 years- Performance test the child may be asked verbally to perform tasks.

Subjective Audiometry for Children

- Peep show audiometry.
- Conditioned audiometry.

Objective Audiometry for Children

- Impedance audiometry
- Brainstorm evoked response audiometry
  These tests can be done in infants under general anesthesia.

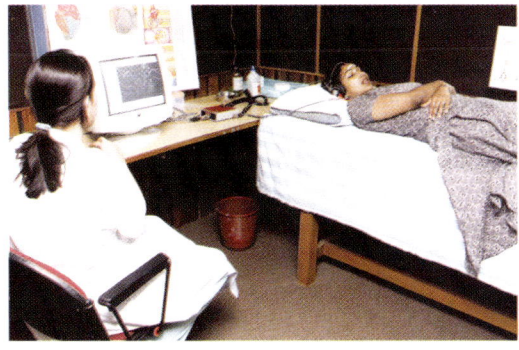

Fig. 5.5: Showing BERA in progress

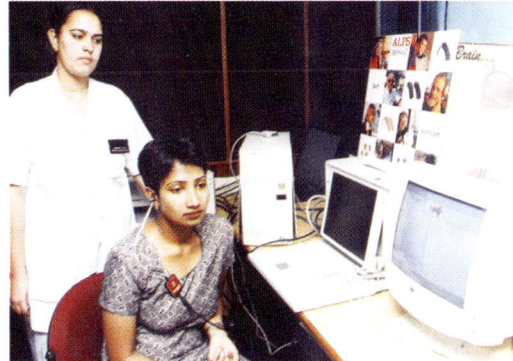

Fig. 5.6: Showing otoacoustic emissions test in progress

IMPEDANCE AUDIOMETRY AND ITS CLINICAL APPLICATIONS

It is one of the main objective audiometric tests. The introduction, principles and inference are given below.

Acoustic impedance means resistance to flow of acoustic energy. This is expressed in ohms.

Three factors impede the flow of sound:
1. Stiffness provided by the tympanic membrane, ossicles and inner ear fluid on the foot plate of stapes.
2. Mass provided mainly by the ossicles.
3. Friction or resistance by the ligaments in the middle ear. Admittance is the reciprocal of impedance. It refers to how much sound energy enters the ear. Admittance is expressed in milli ohms.

Impedance

It can also be expressed by the terms compliance or accommodation, expressed in cubic centimeter of air. It is also known as resistance.

The acoustic impedance is determined mainly by the stiffness of the middle ear system. Mass and friction have negligible effect. Therefore, by allowing a low frequency sound to enter the ear and noting the amount of sound energy that passes into the inner ear and the amount reflected back, one can determine the stiffness of the middle ear system. In brief, since a stiff system offers more impedance, less sound is conducted through it and, therefore, less admittance; while in a flaccid system, the impedance is less and admittance is more. Maximum admittance occurs when the pressure in the external auditory canal and in the middle ear are equal.

Aim of impedance: To assess the middle ear function, i.e. to determine whether the middle ear system is stiff or lax.

Apparatus 1: Ear Probe—probe tip containing three tubes:
- Tube used to deliver probe tone generated by a 220 Hz oscillator driving a miniature receiver.
- Microphone to pick up energy in the canal which is reflected back depending on the impedance.
- Manometer to increase or decrease the pressure in the external canal using an air pump.

Apparatus 2: In the opposite ear conventional ear phone connected to a suitable sound source which delivers signals used to measure threshold for acoustic reflex.

Patient Preparation
1. Wax in the external ear should be removed.
2. Otoscopy to assess the tympanic membrane.
3. Sedation in case of a child.
4. To choose a proper ear tip the external canal has to be assessed by the audiologist. The patient has to be instructed not to move, to avoid deep respiration and to avoid talking and swallowing.

Procedure
1. Probe to be applied to the ear.
2. Increase the pressure to + 200 mm of H_2O.
   - Reduce the pressure serially to 100, 50, 0 upto–400 mm of H_2O to test the compliance at various pressures.
   - Draw a graph with pressure on the X-axis and compliance on the Y-axis. This is the pressure versus compliance function curve described by Terkildsen.
   - The normal middle ear pressure is ± 25 mm of H_2O but for practical purposes ± 100 mm of H_2O is taken as normal.

Inference

Static compliance is the difference between maximum compliance and the compliance at + 200 mm of H_2O. Normal range is 0.3–1.7 cc (Brevs). If it is more than 1.7 cc it suggests a highly loose ossicular system. Less than 0.3 cc means a stiff ossicular system. A positive middle ear pressure is rarely encountered :
- In early stages of acute otitis media,
- After blowing the nose, and
- While crying.

Types of Tympanograms and their Significance

Jerger described A, As, Ad, B and C types of tympanograms (Fig. 5.4b to 5.4d).

Type A : The peak is near 0 pressure and is seen in normal ears.

Type As: The peak is at 0 but the amplitude of the peak is low. This is due to an increased stiffness of the system and is seen in (a) Otosclerosis, (b) Tympanosclerosis, (c) thick graft in myringoplasty.

Type Ad: The peak is around 0 but the peak amplitude is abnormally high. This means that the system is more compliant than normal and is seen in (a) ossicular discontinuity (if air-bone gap is >60 dB), (b) Flaccid tympanic membrane and (c) Monomeric tympanic membrane.

Type B: It is a flat curve denoting that pressure changes do not have much effect on the compliance. The possible causes from the external canal inwards are:

1. Impacted wax
2. Foreign body
3. Secretory otitis media
4. Adhesive otitis media
5. Perforated TM
6. Patent grommet

If the compliance is more than 2.5 cc. with type B curve, it indicates perforation with eustachian tube block. Here the volume of the middle ear cavity is also included to give this high value. This can be used to check the patency of the grommet also.

Type C: In this, the peak is shifted to the negative side. Two types of curves are got:

- Sharp pointed curve
- Humped curve

Humped curve indicates collection of fluid in early stages and reduced mobility. It is seen in:

Type A: Middle ear negative pressure

Type B: Early secretory otitis media

Type C: Eustachian tube dysfunction

Liden et al have described a type D and a type E curve.

Type D: A notched graph, seen in scarred tympanic membrane and in flaccid tympanic membrane.

Type E : An undulating graph, seen when a high frequency sound is applied (8000Hz). This is due to an increased mass factor seen in thick grafts after myringoplasty or in any other condition causing increase in mass.

Eustachian Tube Test

The needle of the meter moves with respiration if the eustachian tube is patulous. In tympanic membrane perforation with a patent eustachian tube, no tracing is possible as an air tight seal is not obtainable. A pin hole perforation can be indirectly diagnosed.

Acoustic Reflex

It is the contraction of the stapedius muscle causing a change in impedance. The minimum sound intensity required to produce stapedial reflex is called stapedial reflex threshold (SRT). Reflexes are bilateral and can be measured on the ipsilateral and contralateral side. For ipsilateral the reflex is measured in the ear in which the tone is given while for contralateral the reflex is tested in the ear opposite to which the tone is given.

Normally, the reflex occurs about 70–90 dB above the patients threshold, *e.g.* if the threshold is 10 dB, 80–100 dB will be the SRT.

Possible Findings

1. In conductive deafness, the reflex will be absent or unobtainable because 70-90 dB above SL is not possible in an ordinary audiometer.

2. In sensory neural deafness, the reflex will be absent or present depending on the degree of deafness i.e. absent in severe deafness and present in mild to moderate deafness.

3. In cochlear pathology, the reflex occurs in less than 70dB above SL due to recruitment.

4. In retrocochlear pathology, the relax is obtained at a higher intensity or is absent due to tone decay.

5. In facial nerve paralysis, if the lesion is proximal to the stapedius muscle there will be no reflex.
6. Abnormalities of the stapedius muscle can cause absent ipsilateral reflex.
7. In damage to the brain stem at the pons, the ipsilateral reflex is present but the contralateral relax is absent on both sides.
8. Lesions in the higher areas of the auditory cortex usually produce no abnormalities in either ipsilateral or contralateral reflex because they are above the auditory reflex area.
9. To find out the pure tone threshold in a deaf mute child which helps in selecting a hearing aid.
10. In otosclerosis to select the ear for surgery. The ear with the better static compliance value is easy to operate and the results will be better. If the maximum compliance is less than 0.3 cc, usually a type III or type IV footplate is encountered.

Advantages
   (a) Purely objective test.
   (b) Non-invasive.
   (b) Assess middle ear function accurately.
   (d) Possible to test children and uncooperative patients.
   (e) Malingering can be detected.

Recruitment

It is a phenomenon wherein the growth of loudness of sound of increasing intensity is greater than in normal ear. This condition occurs in sensorineural deafness and is associated with disease of the cochlea. Quiet sounds cannot be heard by the patients but loud sounds are heard as greater intensity than normal producing discomfort.

Two mechanisms of recruitment have been suggested:
   • The sensation of loudness is determined by number of cochlear nerve fibers which are activated by stimulating sound. Recruitment depends on the fact that each cochlear nerve makes contact with several hair cells.

If a sound of weak intensity is applied to the deafened ear, the stimulation of the remaining outer hair cells is only sufficient to activate a few of the nerve fibers which innervate them. Therefore the sensation of loudn- ess experienced by the deafened ear is less than normal. If a sound of strong intensity is applied, the stimulation of inner ear cells is able to saturate a large number of nerve fibers. The sensation of loudness experienced by the deafened ear will now equal that of normal ear.
   • At very high intensities, the deafened ear may hear the sound louder than the normal ear (over recruitment).

This can result in loss of speech discrimination and intolerance of loud sounds especially when hearing aid is worn.

Clinically if recruitment is present then the site of disorder is cochlear rather than retrocochlear.

Tests for Recruitment

1. Alternative binaural loudness balance test (ABLB).
2. Loudness discomfort level.
3. Stapedial reflex threshold measurements.

Alternative Binaural Loudness Balance Test (ABLB): It is used to detect recruitment in unilateral cases. A tone of 1000 Hz is played alternatively to normal and affected ear. The test is started 20 dB above the threshold of deaf ear and then repeated at every 20 dB rise until the loudness is matched. In cochlear lesions, partial complete or over recruitment may be seen.

Speech Audiometry (Fig. 5.7): This measures the patient's ability to understand speech. A series of words from a tape recorder is presented via headphones to the patient. The words range from 500 to 2000 Hz and the intensity is varied. The results are charted by recording the total percentage of words correctly repeated by patient at each intensity.

A—Hearing is normal that means all the words will be understood.

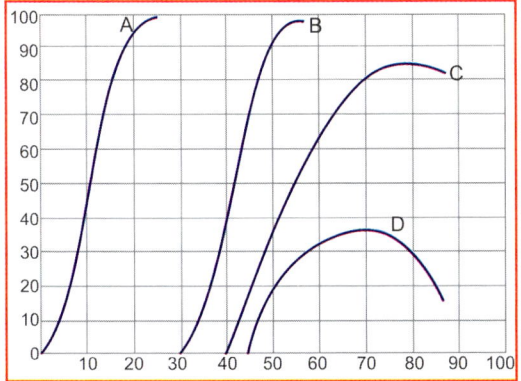

Fig. 5.7: Speech audiometry

A – Normal
B – Conductive deafness
C – Sensorineural deafness poor
  discrimination (Cochlear)
D – Sensorineural deafness – severe
  loss of discrimination (Retrocochlear)

B—Conductive deafness: All the words will be understood but they will need to be played louder than the normal subject.

C and D: There is a loss of ability to discriminate speech. This is seen in sensorineural deafness.

Speech Reception Threshold (SRT): It is intensity at which the patient can repeat 50% of the spondee words. Normal SRT is within 10 dB of the average of pure tone threshold of three speech frequencies (500, 1000, 2000 Hz). An SRT better than pure tone average by more than 10 dB suggest functional hearing loss.

Speech audiometry is valuable method of assessing the actual disability produced by deafness and it can be used to predict the usefulness of a hearing aid or the benefit which might be obtained by an operation. It is also useful in helping to localize a lesion causing sensorineural deafness.

In cochlear deafness the ability to discriminate speech is relatively well maintained. But in retrocochlear deafness caused by disease involving the acoustic nerve or brain stem there is often a severe loss of ability to hear speech which is far worse than PTA would incite.

Tone Decay Test

It is a measure of nerve fatigue and is used to detect retrocochlear lesion.

This test may be performed with standard audiometry and is believed to be useful in distinguishing lesions from cochlea from those in other areas of auditory pathway.

Threshold is established for a selected frequency (say 1000 Hz) and the tone allowed to persist unchanged in intensity until the patient indicates it can no longer be heard. The intensity is then raised again until it is heard and until it decays, and so on, intensity being charted against time. Normally the threshold tone is perceived for longer than half a minute, and should not 'decay' during this time by more than 5 dB.

Normal person can hear a tone continuously for 60 seconds. In nerve fatigue he stops hearing earlier.

BRAIN STEM EVOKED RESPONSE AUDIOGRAM (ERA; BERA)

The measurement of the tiny physiological electric events occurring in response to sound stimulation are assessed by this audiometry. Details about the principle and technique are as follows:

SYNONYMS

BSERA	–	Brain stem Evoked Response Audiogram
ABR	–	Auditory Brain stem Response
BEP	–	Brain stem Evoked Potential
AER	–	Auditory Evoked Response.

Introduction

Jewitt (in 1970) should be credited to be the first person to introduce BERA. It is a non-invasive, objective audiological investigation and has become the single most reliable indication of a retrocochlear pathology specially acoustic neuroma.

Principle

Sound waves entering cochlea—transduced to electrical potentials—transmitted via VIII nerve - through known relay station—brain stem.

These electrical responses are picked up by surface electrodes and represented graphically. Each wave in the graph is thought to be generated by major processing centers of the auditory system.

Procedure

- One ear should be tested at a time.
- Stimulations like clicks, filtered clicks tone bursts and tone pips are used. Patient is comfortably seated in a recliner and is placed in an acoustically isolated and electrically shielded room. Patient may be awake and adequately relaxed or sleeping (to reduce myogenic potentials).
- Tho following three surface electrodes are used:
    i. Active electrode kept on the vertex.
    ii. Reference electrode kept on earlobe/ mastoid of tested ear.
    iii. Ground electrode kept on earlobe/ mastoid of opposite ear.

An earphone is kept on the tested ear and a series of 1000 to 1200 clicks are given at a rate of 5–50/sec. The neurogenic potentials elicited are recorded for the first 10 millisecond. This is the time taken for the electrical responses to be carried to the brain stem alone.

The graph represents 5 waves, i.e. from I to V. Each wave is known to arise from known centers in the auditory pathway. Thus we have:
- Wave I—VIII nerve.
- Wave II—Cochlear nuclei.
- Wave III—Superior olivary complex.
- Wave IV—Lateral lemniscus.
- Wave V—Inferior colliculus.

Interpretation of the graph is done in terms of:
1. Absolute latency delay.
2. Interwove latency delay (I to III, III to V & I to V).
3. Latency/Intensity function.
4. Absence of expected waves.
5. Deformities of waves.
6. Wave amplitude.
7. Threshold of wave V.

Of all these parameters, latency of wave V appears to be the most consistent abnormality and least affected when intensity increases.

Latency of each wave decreases with increase in intensity, but the interwove relationship remains normal.

Upper Limits of Normal Values

Latency of wave V	- 5.9 m.s.
I - V interval	- 4.4 m.s.
I - V interaural difference	- 0.29 m.s.

Advantages

- It can be used in infants and children.
- It can be used in cases of mentally handicapped like cerebral palsy, mental retardation and aphasia.
- It can be used in unconscious patients.
- It can be used as a test to identify malingering.
- It can be used to assess early neurological lesions like multiple sclerosis, demyelinating disease, etc.
- ***The biggest advantage is in the diagnosis of acoustic neuroma.***

Disadvantages

- No standardization exists at present for BERA.
- Wave V is not recorded if hearing level is 75 dB at 3KHz.
- Normally, latency of wave V increases in old age, conductive hearing loss and pure sensorineural hearing loss.
- Wave I is not easily identifiable in BERA.

Oto Acoustic Emission

It has been found that the normal cochlea generates a sound—believed to be due to biological activities of outer hair cells. This sound can be picked up, recorded and measured by placing a microphone receiver in the deep external meatus. This is called as **oto acoustic emission**.

They are of two types: Spontaneous OAE and Evoked OAE

- **Spontaneous oto acoustic emissions** are generated spontaneously and they do not require stimulation and generally found in 50% of normal hearing subjects and has no diagnostic importance.
- **Evoked otoacoustic emissions (EOAE)** has to be evoked by presenting a sound stimulus to the ear.

    The EOAEs are measurable in essentially all normal hearing persons irrespective of age and very reliable response can be obtained objectively.

    EOAEs are usually elicited by presenting clicks at intervals of 20 mili seconds and

response is obtained as a series of waves having latency of 5 to 15 seconds after on-set of the stimulus.

If a recordable EOAE is obtained, it indicates that the subject has a normal middle ear and cochlear mechanism.

If EOAE is absent, it indicates that there is probably some problem in middle ear or cochlea which needs to be further evaluated.

Indication

1. Very useful objective screening of hearing in neonates
2. Detection of early cochlear damage due to ototoxicity and noise trauma

All these audiological investigations help in differentiating cochlear from retrocochlear lesions (Table 5.1).

Table 5.1: Difference between cochlear and retrocochlear lesion

	Normal	**Cochlear**	**Retrocochlear**
PTA	Normal	Sensorineural hearing loss	Sensorineural hearing loss
Speech discrimination score	90–100%	Below 90%	Very poor
Roll over phase	Absent	Absent	Present
Recruitment	Absent	Present	Absent
SISI score	low (0–15%)	Over 70%	0–20%
Threshold tone decay test	0–15db	Less than 25 db	Above
Stapedial reflex	Normal	Normal	Abnormal
BERA	Normal	Normal	Delayed or absent
(Interval between Wave I and V)			

POINTS TO REMEMBER

1. Pure tone audiometry can be used to study the qualitative and quantitative analysis of hearing loss with a graphical representation.
2. Speech audiometry is use to analyze graphically the percentage of words heard correctly by the subject.
3. Brainstem evoked response audiometry (BERA) is used for measurement of the tiny physiological electrical events occurring in response to the sound stimulus
4. Impendance audiometry is use to assess the middle ear function i.e. to know if the middle ear system is stuff or lax.
5. Recruitment is a phenomenon wherein the growth of loudness of sound of increasing intensity is greater than in normal ear.

6

Hearing Loss

Hearing loss is defined as impairment of hearing and its severity may vary from mild to moderate or profound.

Hearing loss is characterized by

- Type of loss (conductive, sensory, neural)
- Location of the problem (external ear, middle ear, cochlea, auditory nerve, central)
- Mode of onset (sudden/insidious)
- Rate of progression
- Degree of loss (mild, moderate, severe)

- The condition that causes it (etiology)
- Bilateral or unilateral.

Classification (Flow chart 6.1)

1. Congenital
2. Acquired.

CONGENITAL HEARING LOSS

Many hereditary conditions produce hearing loss at birth or later in life due to secondary

Flow chart 6.1: Classification of hearing loss

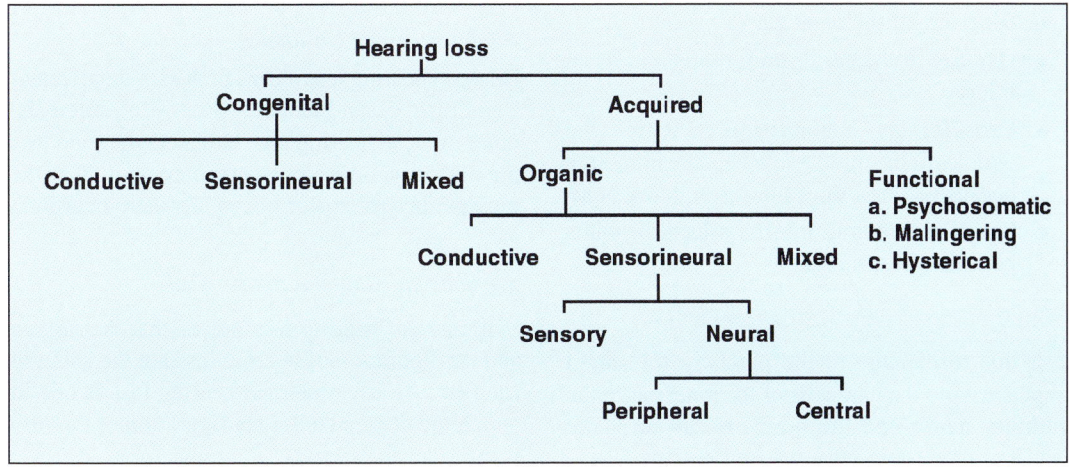

degeneration of the inner ear structures. These usually occur as recessive conditions that often skip generations within a family (discussed later in detail under **Childhood deafness**).

Hereditary Causes
1. Waardenburg's syndrome affected people often have eyes of different color, a white forelock, widest eyes and progressive hearing loss.
2. Usher's syndrome (retinitis pigmentosa)
3. Alport's syndrome (deafness and kidney disease).

Other Causes
- Congenital cholesteatoma
- Fixation of malleus
- Meatal atresia
- Fixation of stapes footplate
- Ossicular discontinuity.

ACQUIRED HEARING LOSS

Conductive Hearing Loss (CHL)

It is caused by anything that interferes with the transmission of sound from the outer to the inner ear. Possible causes include:
- Middle ear infections (Otitis media)
- Collection of fluid in the middle ear (glue ear in children)
- Blockage of the outer ear (by wax)
- Damage to the ear drum by infection or an injury
- Otosclerosis, a condition in which the ossicles of the middle ear become immobile because of growth of the surrounding bone
- Rarely, rheumatoid arthritis affects the joints between the ossicles.

Sensorineural Hearing Loss (SNHL)

It is due to damage to the pathway for sound impulses from the hair cells of the inner ear to the auditory nerve and the brain. It can be acute (sudden) or chronic sensorineural hearing loss.

1. Sensory Deafness
- Age related hearing loss - the decline in hearing that many people experience as they grow older
- Acoustic trauma (injury caused by loud noise) to the hair cells
- Viral infections of the inner ear (may be caused by viruses such as mumps or measles
- Meniere's disease (abnormal pressure in the inner ear)
- Certain drugs, such as aspirin, quinine and aminoglycoside antibiotics, which can affect the hair cells.

2. Neural Deafness
- Acoustic neuroma, a benign (non-cancerous) tumour affecting the auditory nerve
- Viral infections of the auditory nerve (such as mumps and rubella)
- Infection or inflammation of the brain covering, *e.g.* meningitis
- Multiple sclerosis
- A brain tumor
- Stroke.

The difference between conductive and sensorineural hearing loss and their management has been depicted in Table 6.1

Bilateral versus Unilateral

Bilateral hearing loss means both ears are affected. E.g: Presbycusis, Meniere's disease, otosclerosis, noise induced hearing loss. Unilateral hearing loss means only one ear is affected, e.g. CSOM mumps, herpes zoster oticus, acoustic neuroma, etc.

Symmetrical versus Asymmetrical

Symmetrical hearing loss means that the degree and configuration of hearing loss are the same in each ear. An asymmetrical hearing loss is one in which the degree and/or configuration of the loss is different for each ear.

Table 6.1: Differences between CHL and SNHL

	CHL	SNHL
A. Cause	Interferes with transmission of sound from outer, middle ear to the inner ear	Damage to the pathway for sound impulses from the hair cells of inner ear to auditory nerve and brain.
B. Tunning fork test		
1. Rinne test	Negative (BC>AC)	Positive (AC>BC)
2. Weber test	Lateralized to poorer ear	Lateralized to better ear
3. Absolute bone conduction test	Normal	Reduced
C. Audiometry		
1. Threshold elevated	AC only	Both AC and BC
2. Hearing loss severity	< 60dB	May exceed > 60dB
3. Speech discrimination	Good	Poor
4. Air bone gap	Present	No AB gap
5. Frequency involved usually	Involves low frequency	Involves high frequency
D. Management	Medical or surgical	Usually medical (hearing aids, rehabilitative procedures, etc.)
	(a) Removal of obstructive pathology in external / middle ear (e.g. Wax foreign body, benign tumors of external ear or fluid in middle ear).	(a) Treating the underlying cause, e.g. Hormonal replacement therapy in hypothyroidism
		(b) Surgical sealing of the fistula in case of perilymph fistula, etc.
	(b) Stapedectomy in otosclerosis	(c) Cochlear implant
	(c) Tympanoplasty	
	(d) Hearing aids	

Progressive Versus Sudden Hearing Loss

Progressive hearing loss is a hearing loss that becomes increasingly worse over time, e.g: Meniere's disease, presbyacusis, otosclerosis, acoustic neuroma, tympanosclerosis. A sudden hearing loss is one that has an acute or rapid onset and therefore occurs quickly, requiring immediate medical attention to determine its cause and treatment. Sudden hearing loss is usually the vascular, viral, bacterial labyrinthitis.

Fluctuating versus Stable Hearing Loss

Fluctuating hearing loss is typically a symptom of conductive hearing loss caused by ear infection and middle ear fluid. This also occurs in other conditions such as Meniere's disease, perilymph leak, etc.

Degree of Hearing Loss

Social classification

Normal	0–20 dB
Mild	20–40 dB
Moderate	40–60 dB
Severe	60–80 dB
Profound	>80 dB

Goodman's classification

Normal	0–15 dB
Minimal	15–25 dB
Mild	25–40 dB
Moderate	40–55 dB
Moderately severe	55–70 dB
Severe	70–85 dB
Profound	> 85 dB

Functional Hearing Loss (Non-organic)

This term broadly includes inability to hear because of psychological causes with no underlying organic lesions. This deafness can be either of conscious or unconscious origin.

1. *Feigned deafness or malingering:* Conscious origin, in order to gain a definite advantage
2. *Hysterical:* Unconscious origin, organ of hearing is normal
3. *Psychosomatic:* Unconscious origin, but there may be an organic change in auditory apparatus resulting from mental causes.

The patient may present with
   a. Total hearing loss in both ears
   b. Total loss in one ear
   c. Exaggerated loss in one or both ears.

Approach towards patients with functional deafness

1. High index of suspicion
2. Patients gain confidence
3. Patient can be blindfolded for tuning fork and voice test
4. Inconsistent results on repeat pure tone and speech audiometry test
5. Absence of shadow curve while testing bone conduction.

6. **Stenger's test:** It is performed with two matched tuning forks and depends on the principle that two tones of equal frequency and tonal quality cannot be heard at the same time if one is louder than other. The subject is introduced with two tuning forks of equal frequency at a same distance from each ear. The patient will claim to hear in the normal ear. Now bring the tuning fork on the side of feigned deafness nearer, while keeping the tuning fork on the normal side at the same distance. The malingerer will deny hearing even though tuning fork on normal side is at the same place where it was heard earlier. This test is more precisely carried out with two audiometers.

7. **Chimani-Moos test:** A 512 tuning fork when placed on vertex will be heard in deaf ear in conductive deafness and in the better ear in perceptive deafness. The malingerer will usually claim to hear in so called good ear, there by representing perceptive deafness. Now if good ear is occluded he should still hear the fork better in the good ear, but in case of malingering he will more likely to claim to hear nothing.

8. **Erhard's Test:** Erhard's loud voice test exposes feigned unilateral hearing loss.

9. **Lombard's Test:** Is done using Barany noise box over normal ear with true hearing voice markedly raised.

10. Delayed side tone test is done using delayed speech feedback mechanism.

11. **Acoustic reflex threshold:** Discussed under impedence audiometry.

12. **Electric response audiometry:** Discussed under BERA.

SOCIAL AND MEDICOLEGAL ASPECTS OF DEAFNESS

Hearing loss mainly refers to the impairment of hearing where as deafness is the term which includes little or no hearing.

Deafness can be defined as those in whom the sense of hearing is nonfunctional for ordinary purposes of life. It includes patients with hearing loss of more than 90 dB in the better ear or total loss of hearing in both ears.

Classification of Deafness

1. Clinical
2. Educational
3. Sociological

1. Clinical classification (Table 6.2)

2. Educational classification

The Ministry of Education recognizes three grades of deafness according to classroom capacities and makes provision for the deaf children. They are as follows.

- **Grade I:** Those who can obtain proper benefit from education provided in ordinary school.
- **Grade II:** Those who require special educational arrangements but do not need educational methods used for deaf children.
- **Grade III:** Educational methods are required for deaf children without naturally acquired speech or language.

3. Sociological classification

In favor of employment in public bodies various companies have their own classifications (e.g. Table 6.3).

1. How do we calculate degree of handicap?
Various systems have been adopted to find the degree of handicap. Few examples are given in the Flow chart 6.2.

Flow chart 6.2: Calculation of binaural (Bilateral) handicap

Calculate average of pure tone audiometric thresholds at hearing frequencies of 500, 1000, 2000 Hz (A) for worse ear

↓

Deduce 25 dB from it
(i.e. A -25 dB)

↓

Multiply it by 1.5, i.e.
(A - 25 dB) x 1.5
(This is percentage of hearing impairment)
in worse ear %

↓

Calculate hearing impairment for other ear also in the similar way

↓

% handicap = $\frac{(\text{better ear \% x 5}) + \text{worse ear \%}}{6}$

2. Degree of handicap in presbyacusis correction is made by deduction of 0.5% per annum for each ear of age after 64.

OTHER FORMS OF HEARING LOSS

(a) Noise trauma
(b) Ototoxicity
(c) Presbyacusis
(d) Sudden sensory neural hearing loss
(e) Inflammations of labyrinth
(f) Familial progressive sensorineural hearing loss.

Table 6.2: Clinical classification of deafness

Classification	Social difficulty	Clinic voice test	Pure tone audiogram
Normal hearing	None	18ft or more	No loss over 10dB
Mild deafness	Long distance speech	Not over 12ft	10-30 dB loss
Moderate deafness	Short distance speech	Not over 3 ft	Upto 60 dB loss
Severe deafness	All unamplified voices	Raised voice at meatus	Over 60 dB loss
Total profound deafness	Voices never heard	Nil	Over 90 dB loss

Table 6.3: Recommendation about the categories and the tests required
(Dept. of Personnel, Govt. of India)

Category	dB level	Speech discrimination	% of impairment
I. Mild hearing impairment	26 to 40 dB in better ear	80 to 100% in better ear	Less than 40%
II. Moderate hearing	41 to 55 dB in better ear	50 to 80% in better ear	40 to 50%
III. Severe hearing impairment	56 to 70 dB hearing impairment in better ear	40 to 50%	50 to 75%
IV. a) Total deafness	No hearing	No discrimination	100%
b) Near total deafness	91 dB and above in better ear	No discrimination	100%
c) Profound hearing impairment	71 to 90 dB	Less than 40% in better ear	75 to 100%

Facilities to be offered to the disabled

Category I : No special benefits

Category II : Considered for hearing aids at free or concessional costs only.

Category III : Hearing aids, free of cost or at concessional rates. Job reservation - benefit of special employment exchange. Scholarships at school.

Catergory IV : Hearing aids, facilities of reservation - special employment exchange. Special facilities in school like scholarships. Hearing aids - exemption from 3 language formula.

NOISE INDUCED HEARING LOSS

Environmental noise is a common and preventable cause of hearing loss. These transient noise can be either impulse noise that results from an explosion or impact noise that results from collision. Flow chart 6.3 depicts various type of noise trauma.

Etiology (Flow chart 6.3)

1. One- time exposure to loud sound (Acoustic trauma).

Flow chart 6.3: Noise induced hearing loss (NIHL)

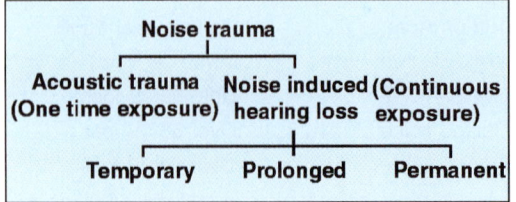

2. Repeated exposure to sounds at various loudness levels over an extended period of time. Sound of less than 80 decibels, even after long exposure, are unlikely to cause hearing loss.

Effects of Noise Trauma

(a) Functional
(b) Structural changes in cochlea

Factors affecting the damage caused by Noise trauma are

1. Frequency of noise
2. Intensity and duration of noise
3. Continuous / Interrupted noise
4. Susceptibility of individual
5. Pre-existing ear disease

Pathophysiology of Noise Trauma

1. Temporary threshold shift

- First change of hazardous noise is temporary shift of threshold level.

- Characterized by 4 kHz dip
- Accompanied with tinnitus
- Recovers after sometime
- Cause for temporary shift has been postulated as: (a) The depletion of the metabolic enzymes (b) Diminished oxygen tension, which leads to reversible alterations in the sensory cells.

2. **Permanent Threshold Shift**
   - Develops as the result of longer and continuous exposure to the damaging noise.
   - 4 kHz notch widens at higher frequencies followed by lower frequencies.
   - Develops as a result of irreversible morphological changes in the hair cells.

Why 4 kHz dip?

(a) Anatomical location of 4 kHz area of the basilar membrane corresponds to that area of basal turn (of cochlea) where it is firmly attached and therefore more prone for torsion and pressure changes in the perilymph.

(b) More prone for vascular injuries in this area.

(c) Reflex contraction of intratympanic muscles in response to loud sounds shift the sound towards higher frequencies.

(d) Due to increase resonance of external auditory, meatus, there is increase in amplitude of sound waves in this frequency level.

Structural changes in cochlear components following exposure to loud sound

Loud sound
↓
Outer hair cells involved
↓
Supporting hair cells
↓
Inner hair cells/ Basilar membrane
↓
Cochlear neurons atrophy
↓
Few cases degeneration of organ of corti.

Predisposing Factors of NIHL

Individuals of all ages, including children, adolescents, young adults and older people can develop NIHL. Exposure occurs in the workplace, in recreational settings and at home. Noisy recreational activities include target shooting and hunting, snow mobiling, riding go-carts, woodworking and other noisy hobbies and playing with power horn, cap, guns and model airplanes. Various famous terminologies have been used for occupational noise induced hearing loss. E.g. Copper smith's deafness, Black smith's deafness, Boilermaker's deafness, etc. Harmful noises at home include vacuum cleaners, garbage disposals, gas powered lawn movers, leaf blowers and shop tools.

Symptoms

1. Sounds may become distorted or muffled and it may be difficult for the person to understand speech. The individual may not be aware of the loss, but it can be detected with a hearing test.

2. Associated tinnitus.

Signs: Audiogram shows typical notch at 4 kHz for both air and bone conduction (Fig. 6.1) in early stages. In advanced stage the AC and BC thresholds are raised even for other frequencies.

Treatment

NIHL is preventable. All individuals should understand the hazards of noise and how to practice good health in everyday life.

- Know which noises can cause damage (those above 90 decibels) (Table 6.4).
- Wear earplugs or other hearing protective devices when involved in loud activity (special earplugs and earmuffs are available at hardware stores and sporting good stores).

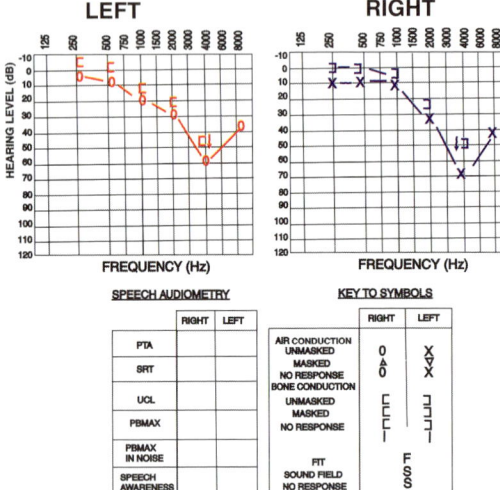

Fig. 6.1: Pure tone audiometry showing bilateral acoustic dip at 4 kHz in the bone conduction thresholds suggestive of noise-induced hearing loss

Table 6.4: Permissible exposure for continuous noise or a number of short term exposures [Govt. of India, Ministry of labor, model rules under factories act- 1948 (corrected up to 31.3.87)]

Noise level (dBA)	Permitted daily exposure (hours)
90	8.0
92	6.0
95	4.0
97	3.0
100	2.0
102	11/2
105	1.0
110	1/2
115	1/4

- Be alert to hazardous noise in the environment.
- Advice children who are too young to protect themselves.

- Make family, friends and colleagues aware of the hazards of noise.
- Have a medical examination by an otolaryngologist and a hearing test by an audiologist to identify and measure hearing loss and to rehabilitate persons with hearing impairment (Table 6.3).

OTOTOXICITY

Definition

Ototoxicity can be defined as a capacity of a drug or chemical to damage the inner ear structure or derange its function. Damage may occur in the auditory or vestibular portion or in both parts of the inner ear.

It is quite clear that several classes of drug regularly damage the inner ear, where as some occasionally do and others might certainly cause harm.

The following **classification** of different groups of drugs are followed by many otologists:

1. **Drugs that are certainly ototoxic**
   - Aminoglycoside antibiotics
   - Cisplatin
   - Salicylates
   - Quinine
   - Diuretics like fursemide, bumetide
2. **Drugs that certainly cause a hearing loss**
   - Macrolide antibiotics
3. **Drugs that may alter hearing and balance**
   - Glycopeptide antibiotic (vancomycin)
4. **Centrally acting agents**
   - Imipramine
   - 5 Hydroxy tryptamine
   - Carbamazepine

Pharmacokinetics of Aminoglycosides
(Figs 6.2a and b)

Since aminoglycosides are commonly used drugs it has been mentioned in detail. Pharmacokinetic reactions are different with different drugs. The half life of aminoglycosides in perilymph and endolymph appears much greater than in the

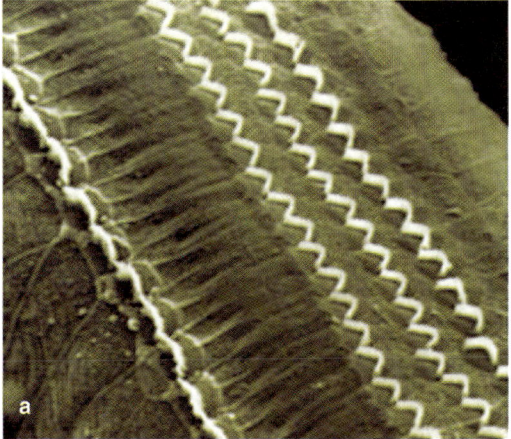

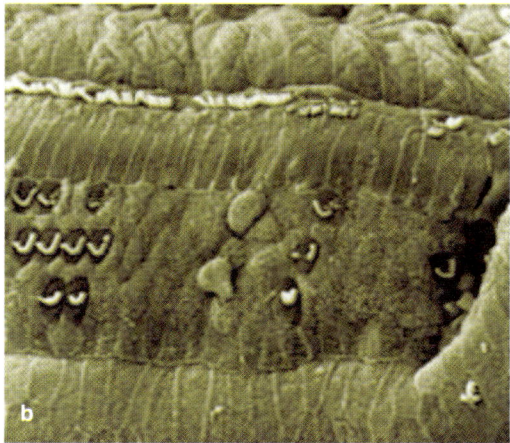

Figs 6.2a and b: (a) Showing outer and inner normal hair cells. (b) Showing the damaged hair cells due to aminoglycosides toxicity

Clinical Features

Clinical features are same for all the types of ototoxic drugs, however its severity, timing and duration of the effect may vary from drugs to drugs.

1. **Tinnitus:** It is most often the first warning symptom. It is usually high pitched and continuous when it starts and may be unilateral or bilateral.
2. **Hearing loss:** There may be different pattern of hearing loss with different ototoxic agent. There is often a delay in the onset of hearing loss when the aminoglycosides are the culprit.
3. **Balance disturbances (Disequilibrium):** Most of the patients are severely unsteady, bedridden in the worst cases, as there are altered labyrinthine responses to head movement. No nystagmus is observable. The caloric and rotational tests show a bilateral loss of labyrinthine function. This is known as **bobbing oscillopsia**. Patient may also experience vertigo and a sense of continuous rotation after turning the head or turning over in the bed.

But true rotatory vertigo is rare. Vestibulo-toxicity of the aminoglycosides may not become apparent immediately since the patients are often ill and confined to bed. Even on mobilization their unsteadiness may be ascribed to the debility of the illness.

Investigations
1. Monitoring of drug concentration in body
2. Pure tone audiometry
3. Caloric test
4. Electrocochleography
5. Otoacoustic emission
6. BERA.

Management of Ototoxicity

1. Early recognition and discontinuation of the drug.
2. Hearing aid should be prescribed if there is severe hearing loss.

blood. This high concentration of amino-glycosides in the endolymph is blamed to be the cause of ototoxic actions. Other non-amino-glycoside antibiotics may not affect the inner ear when given in the systemic form but the local application has definite harmful effect on the inner ear.

The aminoglycoside may generate tinnitus by altering hair cell function whereas salicylates may alter the afferent or efferent pathway directly. The loop diuretics may alter the activities of the striavascularis.

3. Tinnitus should be treated with mild hypnotics or by tinnitus maskers.
4. Disequilibrium should be treated with reassurance and regular physiotherapy including vestibular exercises, wearing of soft, thick padded shoes, avoidance of walking in darkness and unnecessary head movement.

PRESBYACUSIS

Definition

Presbyacusis is defined as a sensorineural hearing loss associated with increase in chronological age but patient may or may not be aware of the hearing loss in the initial stage.

Predisposing Factors

- **Aging** effect on the hearing nerve can be started earlier than usual cases in the following conditions:
  - People working in **noisy environment.**
  - **Ototoxicity.**
  - **Diabetes** and other generalized systemic and metabolic disorders.

Pathology

Histopathologically four distinct types have been described according to the area of degeneration.

1. **Neural presbyacusis:** Early degeneration affect the dendritic process (cochlear neuron) of osseous spiral lamina. In severe cases there will be loss of ganglion cell and afferent axon.
2. **Sensory presbyacusis:** There is loss of inner and outer hair cell in the basal turn. Secondary cochlear neural degeneration is common. Audiometric studies show high frequency losses with good discrimination score.
3. **Metabolic presbyacusis:** This is associated with degenerative changes of stria vascularis

of middle and apical turn of cochlea. Pathological changes consists of degeneration of all the three layers of stria vascularis most prominently in the apical region of the cochlea. Audiometry shows flat SN hearing loss with good speech discrimination score.
4. **Mechanical presbyacusis:** Commonly associated with degeneration of the spiral ligament rupture and thickening of the basilar membrane. Audiometry shows descending type (sloping type) of curve.

Clinical Features

1. **Deafness:** This will be bilateral symmetrical and gradual in onset and progressive in nature. Patient will find it difficult to understand in a noisy environment and discrimination will be very low.
2. **Tinnitus:** Tinnitus may be accompanied with high frequency sensorineural hearing loss in the initial stage.
3. **Vertigo:** This is seen in 30% of cases. Whether it is of labyrinthine origin is not certain. Elderly people may also have vertiginous symptoms due to brainstem and central vascular changes.
4. **Distortion of speech:** It may occur in one or both ears, may be sometimes annoying for music lovers.
5. **Recruitment may be positive:** Recruitment means loud or high intensity sound causing discomfort in hearing.

Investigations

1. **Tuning Fork test**
   - Rinne is positive but short.
   - Weber is lateralized to the better ear.
   - ABC is reduced.
2. **Audiogram**
   In early cases high frequency sensorineural hearing loss will be present. In late cases the low frequency is also involved (Fig. 6.3).

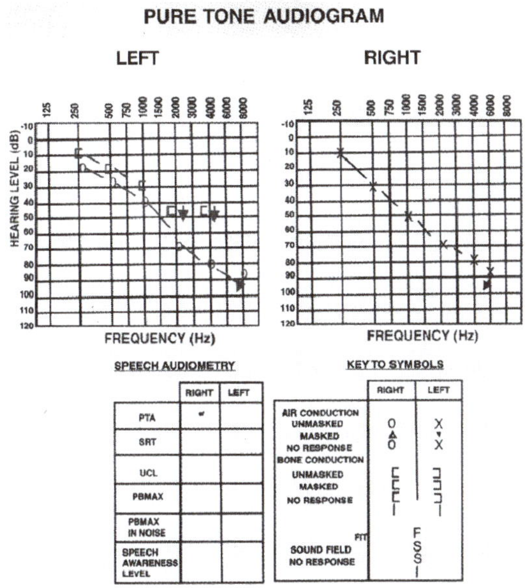

PURE TONE AUDIOGRAM

Fig. 6.3: Pure tone audiometry showing high frequency sensorineural hearing loss

Differential Diagnosis

1. *Cochlear otosclerosis:* Sensorineural hearing loss in advanced **otosclerosis** will show normal bone conduction in lower tone in contrast to marked air conduction loss. In presbycusis the air and bone gap are approximately equal. The paracusis Willis will often present in otosclerosis.
2. *Meniere's disease:* Hearing loss will be fluctuating in character. Glycerol test will be positive.
3. *Acoustic trauma:* The audiogram will show sudden dip at 4KHz. History of noise trauma may be present.

Treatment

1. *Prophylaxis*
   - Avoidance of noise.
   - Avoidance of high fat diet.
   - Avoidance of cold, excessive smoking and stress.
2. *Psychological Support*
   Information and explanation regarding the disease process and its effect in the body is very important and helpful for the patient.
3. *Hearing Aids*
   Discussed later in this chapter.
4. *Drugs*
   No specific drugs are available to improve the hearing. However B1, B6, B12 and iron may be tried in long term basis to prevent deterioration of hearing.

Prognosis

Prognosis depends on the type of hearing loss. Gradually increasing deafness is very common type which will not lead to complete deafness. When the deafness is sudden, catastrophic and very severe, the rehabilitation with hearing aid may be difficult.

SUDDEN SENSORINEURAL HEARING LOSS

It can be defined as a deterioration of more than 35 dB in atleast three adjacent frequencies occurring with in 3 days; with allowance for a long period of onset if the loss is more severe. Loss can be partial or complete. Usually it is unilateral and may be accompanied by tinnitus or vertigo.

Causes

- Trauma and labyrinthine membrane rupture
- Postoperative (perilymph fistula)
- Infections: Bacterial/Viral
- Vascular lesions like hemorrhage, arterial occlusions or vasospasm in diseases like diabetes, polycythemia or sickle cell trait
- Acoustic neuroma
- Immune complex diseases
- Cochlear otosclerosis
- Endolymphatic hydrops
- Multiple sclerosis
- Psychogenic deafness, etc.

Investigations

1. Careful history and examination

2. Auditory function test
3. Radiological examination of temporal bone to rule out acoustic neuroma
4. Serial viral antibody studies for VDRL, FTA
5. Blood glucose level for diabetes
6. ESR and circulating immune complexes to rule out autoimmune pathology.

Treatment

The effective management depends on
- Investigations to establish diagnosis
- Empirical medication
- Specific treatment for underlying cause
- Psychological rehabilitation
  1. Bed rest (in head raised position)
  2. Sedation to relieve anxiety and associated giddiness
  3. Steroid therapy: Prednisone, 10 days course of 15 mg TID per oral. After 10 days dose it is tapered off.
  4. Inhalation of carbogen (5% CO_2 + 95% O_2). It increases cochlear blood flow.
  5. Vasodilator drugs i.v. histamine acid phosphate in first 3 days has been reported to be effective (contraindicated in patients with peptic ulcers or allergic diseases.
  6. Low molecular weight dextran. Contra-indicated in cardiac failure and bleeding disorders.
  7. Hyperbaric oxygen therapy
  8. Antiviral agents (acyclovir) have been tried in patients with suspected viral etiology.

Prognosis

Depends on:
- Onset
- Duration
- Severity.

25–50% of patients may recover spontaneously. Recovery may be total or partial. Younger patients and those with moderate losses have better prognosis.

CHILDHOOD DEAFNESS AND DEAF MUTISM

The childhood deafness presents a special problem to the otolaryngologist because of difficulties in detecting the deafness before one year of age causing rehabilitation problems. To avoid the permanent effect upon language development, the hearing loss in the childhood must be detected and treated promptly before the critical period of language acquisition has passed, i.e. before the age of six months, rehabilitation for the speech should be started.

Childhood deafness associated with other impairments and disabilities make the rehabilitation programme much more difficult. The management of hearing impairment in children is most effective if undertaken by a consultant led multidisciplinary team including otolaryngologist, audiologist, pediatrics, genetics, plastic surgeon, speech therapist, psychiatrist, social worker, educationist and voluntary body.

Assessment, diagnosis and management of hearing impaired child is best undertaken in a child friendly environment.

Causes of Hearing Impairment in Children

Causes can be divided broadly into two headings:
  1. Congenital hearing impairment.
  2. Acquired hearing impairment.

1. Congenital Hearing Impairment
  a. Genetic
  b. Non-genetic

(a) Genetic Causes

Genetics can involve either the conductive apparatus or sensorineural apparatus or both.

Conductive Apparatus Anomalies
  1. Pointed pinna
  2. Lop ear

3. Exostosis
4. Microtia
5. Absence of pinna
6. Atresia of external auditory canal with or without ossicular fixation or malformation, i.e.
   - Treacher Collins syndrome
   - Klippel-Fiel syndrome
   - Alport's syndrome
   - Goldenhar syndrome
   - Mohr's syndrome
7. Conductive anomalies associated with pigmented disorders.
   - Fornis syndrome
8. Associated with eye disorders.
   - Crypt ophthalmus
   - Duane's syndrome
9. Associated with renal disorders.
   - Nephrosis
   - Renal-genital syndrome
   - Taylor's syndrome

Sensorineural System Malformation

Common malformations are either aplasia or heredodegeneration.
- Michael's syndrome (complete lack of development of inner ear)
- Mondini's syndrome (Incomplete development of bony and membranous labyrinth)
- Scheibe's syndrome (Cochleosaccular aplasia with normal bony labyrinth)
- Bing- Siebenmann syndrome (malformation of membranous labyrinth with a normal osseous labyrinth)

(b) Non-genetic Causes

Intrauterine
- Environmental hazards
- Diabetes
- Toxemia
- Ototoxic drugs
- Teratogenic chemicals
- Infections
- Rubella
- Cytomegalovirus
- Measles
- Chicken pox
- Herpes
- Toxoplasma
- Syphilis
- Provirus
- HIV

Perinatal
- Low birth weight
- Hyperbilirubinemia
- Anoxia

Neonatal Infections
- Meningitis
- Encephalitis
- Septicemia

Developmental
- Delayed auditory maturation

2. Acquired Hearing Impairment

- **Infection**
  - Viral
  - Meningococcal
  - Chronic suppurative otitis media

- **Trauma**
  - Acoustic trauma
  - Iatrogenic
- **Perilymph leak**
- **Endolymphatic hydrops**
- **Ototoxic drugs.**

Evaluation of Hearing Loss in Children

Evaluation of deafness in children from birth to five years of age presents a special problem in terms of assessment and rehabilitation. Evaluation of hearing in this category of patients is very challenging as well as frustrating. Child with significant hearing loss will have a serious communication handicap leading to deaf mutism. Delays in identification of the hearing loss causes irretrievable loss of time for rehabilitation.

Measurement of hearing in children is in real terms the evaluation of a child's behavioural responses in a controlled setting to the presentation of various acoustic stimuli. Children with sensorineural hearing loss have delayed speech and language and may also have a coexisting aphasia or dyspraxia unrelated to the hearing impairment.

The two main tenets of hearing evaluation in deaf mute are as follows:
1. No child is too young for hearing loss.
2. The earlier the identification of hearing loss the better the prognosis for hearing evaluation.

The following are hearing test batteries used to evaluate the hearing in children.

1. *Reflex tests for the first 6 months*
   - At birth Moro and oropalpebral or startle reflex.
   - At 3rd month: Blinking and frowning to sounds.
   - At 5th month: Eyes turn towards the sound source.
   - At 6th month: The head turns towards the sound source.

2. *Behavioural tests*
   - **Distraction Test:** (7th to 18th month) - In this test the children are in a state of attention, while a tester makes a sound to the side and out of site of children. The child will respond positively to the sound. The sound should be produced at minimal sound intensity level, and presented at each side at a distance of 1 meter. The tests are made of low pitch sound like voice and low pitched rattle and high pitch sound and high pitch rattle. Rhythmic repetition of letter S or rustle of tissue paper.
   - **Cooperation Test:** 18th months–2 years —Cooperation of a child is sought to sound. The child should be given few toys to play with, and when the child is busy playing with the toys, very quietly at a distance of one meter from each ear. Simple sentences like put the

dolly in the pram, put the doggy in the buff, show me your hair, etc. should be asked.

3. *Performance test*
   - 2–5 yrs - child may be asked verbally to perform task. In this test child makes a learned response to a given sound. In this test manipulation toys can be given, which can produce different sounds. Sounds should be made at a distance of 2 meters and child can be taught to respond and repeat the sound.

4. *Objective tests*
   - Impedance audiometry.
   - BERA.

Treatment

The treatment of the deaf child with delayed speech is a multidisciplinary approach. The speciality consists of:
1. Otolaryngologist
2. Audiologist
3. Speech therapist
4. Pediatricians
5. Child psychologist
6. Specially trained teachers
7. Social workers
8. Engineers.

1. **Counselling of the parents:** After the diagnosis of deaf mutism the parents should be counselled to accept the child and treat him at par with normal child. Over indulgence and also negligence on the part of the parents care may severely interfere with the growth as well as the speech development of a child. The parents should realize that, they are not the only parents in this world to have a deaf child.

2. **Fitting of a bilateral hearing aid:**
   - Preferably body worn are best for the child. While wearing the hearing aid, the child should be encouraged to listen to

the sound and to pay attention to the speaker's facial and lip movement while speaking. This can be learned initially from the speech pathologist/audiologist and must be taken up subsequently in the natural environment of the home by the parents.

- Bonc anchoring hearing aid (BAHA) have been advised for children with atresia, microtia and having recurrent ear discharge.
- Hand wire system and induction loop system are used for group reading. This is best done in a specially designed room where amplifier is connected to one or more microphone or induction loop wired in a room and connected to an amplifier to create an electromagnetic field to facilitate group hearing.

3. **Communication Methodology:** The two major methods in the education of deaf are:

   (a) *Oral approach*: This encourages to develop vocabulary after training and it is more preferred.

   (b) *Manual approach*: Here deaf people communicate with sign language.

4. **Cochlear Implant:** In profoundly deaf child with developed cochlea is giving very good results, if it is done between 2 to 4 years.

5. **Educational placement of the deaf child:** Selection of the school for the deaf children should be done by the specially trained teacher, child psychologist and social workers in consultation with the parents.

Usually the schools has been classified as:

1. Special school for the deaf children where mostly sign languages are taught.

2. Special class for deaf in normal school, where special instruments for amplification are used in group or individual form where a specially trained teacher will teach.

3. The normal school—Here the children with moderate deafness with hearing aid are selected.

HEARING AIDS

Hearing aid is a device where a sound will be amplified by electrical or mechanical means. The hearing aids are mostly electrical and transistorized. Following are the basic components of a hearing aid.

Microphone

Microphone collects the sound and transforms it into electrical energy. The microphone is usually magnetic type. The microphone again consist of a diaphragm which will convert sound energy into mechanical energy.

Amplifier

The function of amplifier is to increase the electrical voltage which is received from the microphone. This increases in voltage is mostly done by the implanted transmitter into the amplifier.

Receiver

The receiver will transfer the electrical energy back into sound wave which have much greater amplitude than those which fell upon the microphone. Most receivers are **air conduction** type. Also there are receiver of **bone conduction type.** These are magnetic receiver in which diaphragm is connected to a vibrator.

It is placed behind the ear against the mastoid bone and sets of vibration in the skull when they are transmitted to the bony labyrinth and the fluid in the cochlea.

Batteries

Batteries are used to supply the power.

Features of Hearing Aid

1. On and off switch.

2. Volume control.

3. Tone control: It is fitted to and aid to modify the frequency characteristic of the amplifier.

4. In the normal position, the normal frequency response of the instrument is produced. In high position, only the higher frequency will be amplified without interfering low and mid frequencies. If the position is marked low, amplification of the upper frequency is reduced.

Telephonic Device

Telephone conversation is made possible through the hearing aid by placing a special device like induction coil.

Types of Hearing Aids (Figs 6.4 to 6.7)
1. Body worn hearing aids are usually prescribed for individual with profound hearing loss of mixed type.
2. Postaural hearing aid.
3. Ear canal hearing aid.
4. Spectacle type hearing aid.
5. Implantable hearing aid.
6. Bone anchored hearing aid.
7. Digitally programmable and remote control hearing aid.

Indications

1. Hearing aid can be prescribed to all types of deafness which cannot be cured by medicine or surgery.
2. People who are reluctant for surgery.
3. Contraindication for surgery.

Selection of a Hearing Aid

It is the duty of the otologist and audiologist to find out the proper indication and selection of cases to get the maximum benefit from the hearing aid. Most of the selection are done from the type of audiogram (PTA and Speech audiometry). Many of the patients with sensorineural hearing loss do not find the hearing aid convenient and cannot tolerate because of the poor speech discrimination score. To avoid this, patient can be prescribed for **digitally programmed remote control hearing aid** to minimize the tolerance.

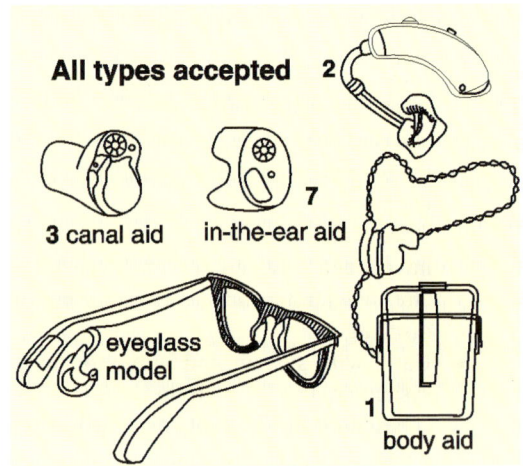

Fig. 6.4: Different types of hearing aids

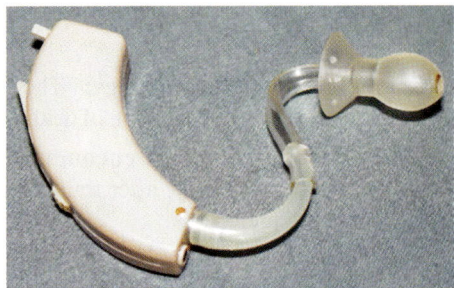

Fig. 6.5: Postaural hearing aid (Behind the Ear BTE)

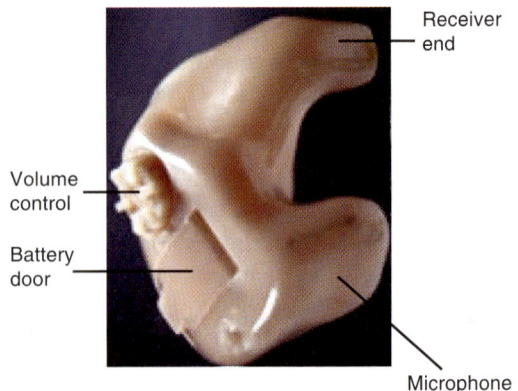

Fig. 6.6: Ear hearing aid

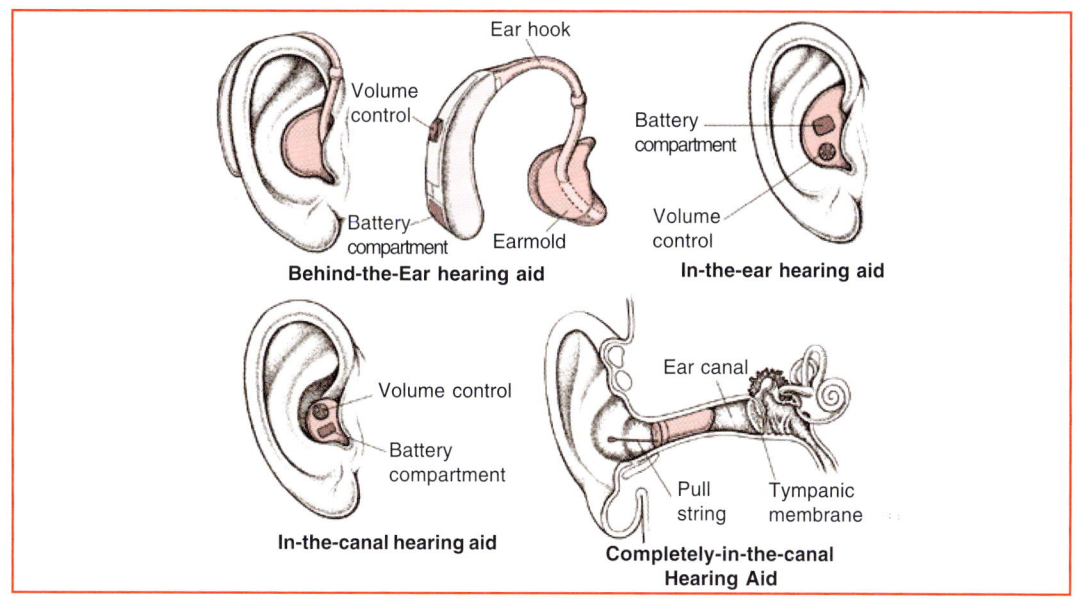

Fig. 6.7: Hearing aid in situ

IMPLANTABLE HEARING DEVICES

Several types of devices can be considered for implantable hearing devices. These include

- Bone-anchored hearing devices
- Middle ear implant
- Cochlear implants
- Auditory brainstem implants

Bone-anchored Hearing Devices (BAHA)

The BAHA device is a percutaneous implantable device primarily used for conductive hearing loss, or more recently, for single-sided sensorineural hearing loss. The original device was designed to treat conductive or mixed losses and has become popular for hearing rehabilitation in patients with congenital ear malformations or refractory chronic ear disease. An osseointegrated titanium fixture with a percutaneous abutment is implanted in the postauricular area (Fig. 6.8). An external sound processor is attached to the abutment at will. A microphone in the processor, which vibrates the bone in the skull by means of the fixture, picks up sound. The sound is transmitted directly to the inner ear on the side with conductive hearing loss, bypassing the middle ear. The BAHA device can be placed bilaterally in patients with bilateral disorders to allow for sound localization and to improve speech recognition in noise (Fig. 6.8).

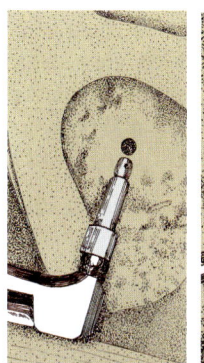
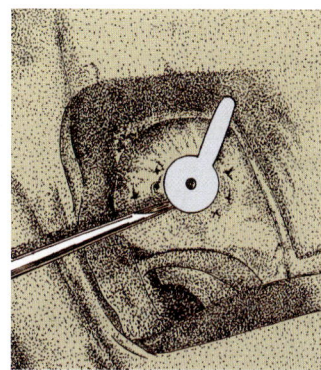

Fig. 6.8: Implanting the titanium fixture of bone anchored hearing aid (BAHA)

Middle Ear Implant

The Middle Ear Transducer (MET) was first introduced as a semi-implantable device but was recently made totally implantable. Fully implanted MET ossicular stimulator (FIMOS), it is fully implantable electro mechanical device which is intended to benefit the patient suffering from moderate to severe sensorineural hearing loss. This device resides completely beneath the skin without any visibility in the ear canal and thus eliminating the need of any external device or processor. It eliminates the disadvantages of conventional hearing aids. The added advantage of this device is that the wearer will use this device throughout the day during all normal activities including showering and swimming (Fig. 6.9).

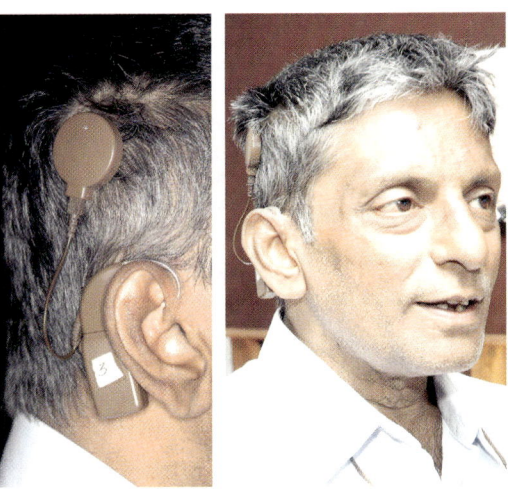

Fig. 6.10: Showing cochlear implant advanced bionics Hi Resolution 90 K (clarion)

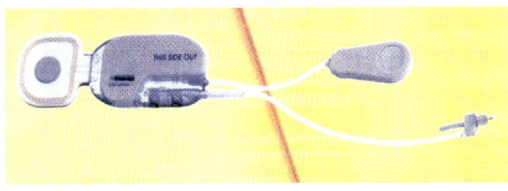

Fig. 6.9: Fully implanted MET ossicular stimulator

Cochlear Implant

Definition

Cochlear implant is an electrical device, which is used in profoundly deaf patients to electrically stimulate the cochlear nerve. There are single channel and multichannel cochlear implants. Multiple electrode system is regarded to be better as it gives multichannel stimulation which provides more speech understanding.

Principle of Cochlear Implant

Cochlear implants have basically an **external and an internal part. The external part consists of a** microphone, a speech processor and a transmitter coil. **The internal part** consists of a receiver stimulator and electrode array (Fig. 6.10).

1. The external transmitter coil will be held in position by the magnet of the receiver stimulator.
2. The microphone transmits sound into a voltage waveform. This voltage is applied to a speech processor which may be body worn or behind the ear via a small cable.
3. The speech processor, filters the speech wave form into frequency bands. The output of the filters are referred to a map of the patients electric current threshold and comfortable listening level for the individual electrode. Thus, a code is produced for the stimulus parameter. This code together with the power is transmitted to the implanted receiver stimulator by the external transmitter.
4. This receiver stimulator of internal part directs the current pulses to the appropriate electrodes array lying close to the auditory fibers which lies close within the basal turn of the cochlea. The current excites the auditory population of the auditory nerve fibers to stimulate the pattern of the auditory nerve activity in response to sound, thereby

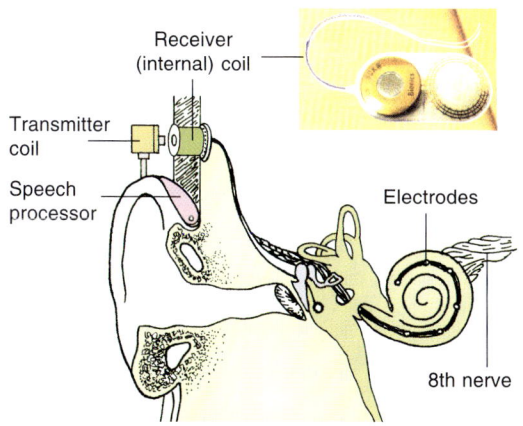

Fig. 6.11: Multichannel cochlear implant

providing meaningful representation of speech and environmental sound specifically by a multichannel cochlear implant (Figs 6.11 and 6.13).

Patient Selection

1. Congenital deafness.
2. Acquired profoundly deaf patient with above 80dB loss in postlingual deafness.
3. Acquired profoundly deaf child with normal cochlear development. Implant between 2 to 4 years of age gives best result.
4. Postlingual profound deafness caused by meningitis is not a good candidate for cochlear implant. Meningitis initiates new bone formation leading to cochlear obliteration making insertion of the electrode difficult.

Investigations

1. Audiological investigations
   - Pure tone audiometry.
   - Speech audiometry.
   - Aided audiometry.
   - BERA is specially needed for children.
   - Promontory stimulation test is more important in children to anticipate post implant results.
   - Neurocochleography.
   - Otacoustic emission audiometry.
2. Speech evaluation.
3. Radiological investigations to know the size and shape of the cochlea : CT scan and MRI of temporal bone - axial and coronal.
4. Surgical fitness.

Steps of Surgical Procedure (Figs 6.12a and b)

1. Wide postauricular flap is used for safe placement of the implant over the mastoid bone. Incision is small in minimally ***invasive cochlear impart.***
2. Making of the bed in the temporo-occipital bone for receiver stimulation.
3. Posterior typanotomy approach to visualize the round window.
4. Widening of the round window opening (Cochleostomy).
5. Insertion of electrode array through the cochleostomy into the basal turn of the cochlea.
6. Closure of the cochleostomy with fibrofatty tissue to prevent CSF leak.
7. Placement and stabilization of receiver stimulator.
8. Closure of incision in layers.
9. Postoperative care.
10. Suture removal after 10 to 12 days.
11. Switch on mapping after 2 months.

Rehabilitation

It is done by the audiologist, speech therapist, psychiatrist, engineers, family member, social worker and teachers, etc (Fig. 6.13). Difference between hearing aid and cochlear implant is described in Table 6.5.

Auditory Brainstem Implants

Auditory brainstem implants (ABIs) were designed to be used in neurofibromatosis type 2 (NF-2) in which tumors involving complexes of both cranial nerve VII and VIII render the patient anacusic. These devices, which bypass the cochlea

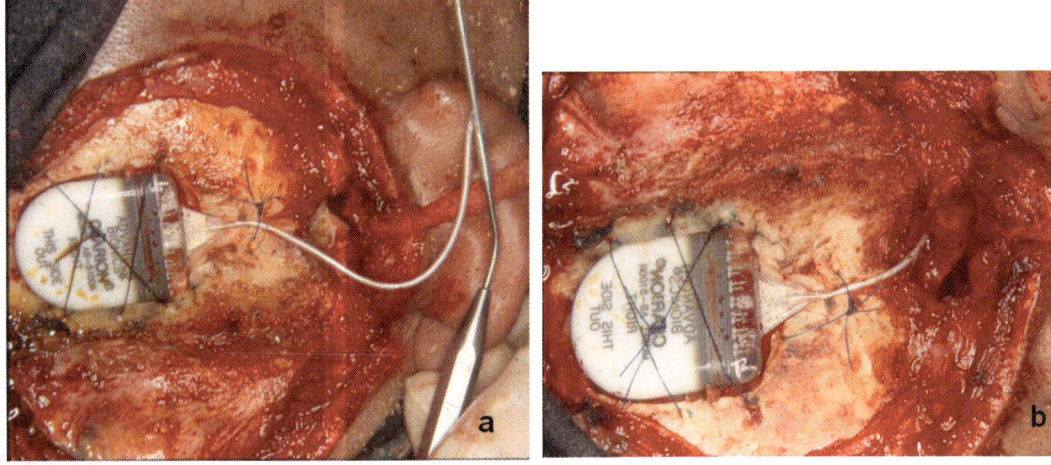

Figs 6.12a and b: (a) Showing Placement and stabilization of receiver stimulator before inserting the electrode through cochleostomy, (b) after insertion of electrode through the cochleostomy.

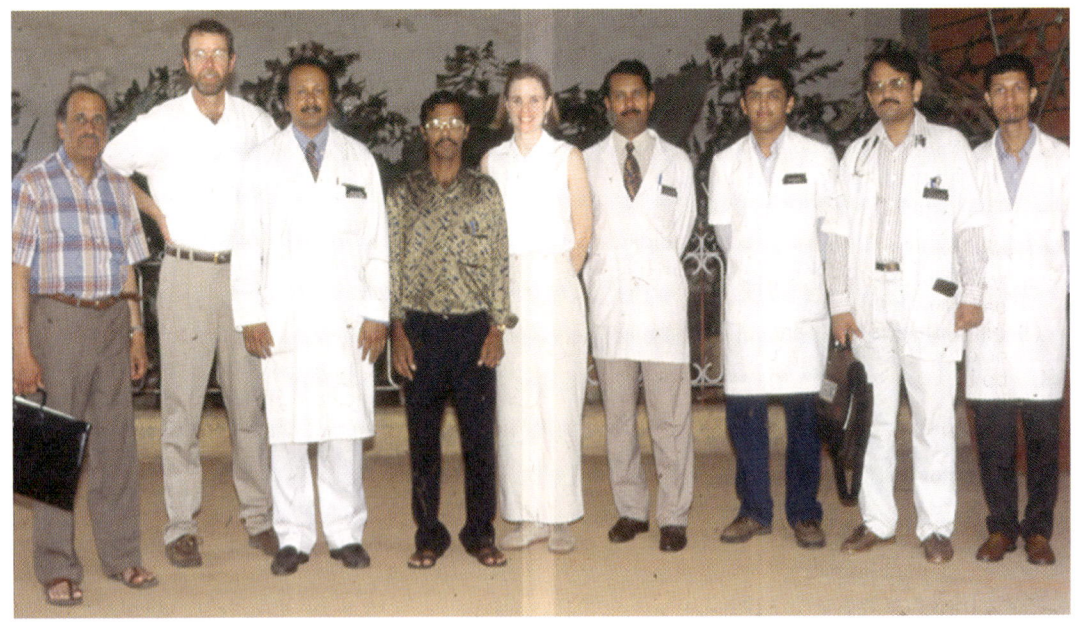

Fig. 6.13: First Manipal cochlear implant group with patient in 1994 headed by the senior author (Third from the left)

Table 6.5: Difference between Hearing aids and Cochlear implants

Hearing Aid	Cochlear implant
Concept : Amplify sounds reaching the ear	Direct stimulation of spiral ganglion of auditory nerve
Indications : SNHL Deaf child CHL, when surgery is not feasible due to various reasons	Profound sensory neural hearing loss

Components: • Microphone
• Amplifier
• Receiver (Earphones)
	(a) External part
	    - Microphone
	    - speech processor
	    - Transmitter coil
	(b) Internal part
	    - Receiver stimulator
	    - Electrode array

Types: (a) Non electrical
        Electrical
(b) Air conduction type (MC)
        Bone conduction type
(c) Implantable hearing aids
	Depending on number of electrodes and channels
	(i) Nucleus 24' 'contour'
	(ii) Clarion C-11
	(iii) MED-EL combi 40+

Advantages
(i) Cost effective as compared to cochlear implant
(ii) Good patient compliance
(iii) Used in patients where surgery is not feasible
(iv) Done on OPD basis
	(i) Better efficacy in postlingual deaf cases
	(ii) Better results in children in prelingual deafness
	Observed in terms of
	    - Speech intelligibility scores
	    - Language development rate expressive skills
	(iii) More useful for patients having profound SNHL

Disadvantages (i) May cause intolerable destortion of sound in patients with SNHL (ii) Difficult to use in patients with discharging ear or otitis external (Bone conduction type can be used in these cases)	(i) Cost factor (ii) Can not be used in psychologically imbalanced individuals (iii) Involves surgical procedure (technically dificult) (iv) Long postoperative rehabilitation programmes (v) Longer programmes hospital stay
Complications : 1. Recurrent infections of external auditory canal and middle ear	1. Facial nerve palsy 2. Wound infection /dehiscence 3. Device failure (early/late) 4. CSF leak (rare) 5. Post op vertigo 6. Post op meningitis (rare) 7. Extrusion/ Exposure of device (rare)

and cochlear nerve, are implanted into the lateral recess of the fourth ventricle adjacent to the cochlear nucleus to provide the patient with auditory perception. These devices are usually implanted after the tumor is resected, during the same operation.

Dr. William House and William Hitselberger implanted the first ABIs in 1979. The latest ABI incorporates a digital speech. The device is indicated in patients with NF-2 aged 12 years or older. Implantation may occur during tumor removal on the first or second side or as a separate procedure. The patient should be medically and psychologically suitable, and no audiologic criteria are applied.

ABIs have been used with varying success in patients born with cochlear nerve aplasia, those with traumatic cochlear-nerve avulsion, and those in whom cochlear implantation is unsuccessful (for salvage treatment).

POINTS TO REMEMBER

1. Stenger's test and chimani-moos test are done to detect functional deafness (malingering).
2. Environmental noise is a common and preventable cause of hearing loss.
3. Acoustic trauma is caused by single exposure to very loud and high intensity noise.
4. Noise induced hearing loss is caused by repeated exposure to sound at various loudness levels (above 90 db)
5. Acoustic dip at 4 KHz in the bone conduction threshold of pure tone audiometry is suggestive of noise induced hearing loss.

Functional Examination of Vestibular System

7

Spontaneous Nystagmus

Nystagmus should be assessed by asking the patient to sit in front of the examiner. The examiner keeps moving the fingers 45 cm from the patients eyes and moves it right, left up and down taking care not to move more than 30 degrees from the central position to avoid gaze nystagmus. Presence of spontaneous nystagmus indicates an organic lesion which may be peripheral (lesion at the labyrinth or 8th nerve) or central (lesion at vestibular nuclei, brain stem or cerebellum). Peripheral vestibular nystagmus is horizontal rotatory and have both fast and slow components. Peripheral nystagmus is fatiguable but reproducible.

Corneal Reflex

Small cotton wool is taken in the examiner's hand and the patient is asked to look forward and straight when the examiner will touch the sclera first and then the cornea. In normal on touching the cornea the patients eyes should blink on both the sides. Blinking will be absent in case of loss of corneal reflex signifying cerebelopontine angle pathology.

Fistula Test

This may be elicited by pressing the tragus or **by** using sieges pneumatic speculum. The interpretations of the fistula test are as follows:

Positive fistula test means that patient will complain of vertigo while performing the test and nystagmus will be directed towards opposite side.

Inference

(a) Positive fistula test implies that there is a fistula connecting middle and inner ear. Commonest site of fistula formation is lateral semicircular canal.

(b) Negative fistula test in presence of a fistula may be there when the labyrinth is dead or the fistula is covered by granulation tissue or cholesteatomal mass (False negative fistula sign).

(c) Fistula test positive without a fistula in case of early congenital syphilis where the annular ligament is lax and mobile known as **Hennebert's sign**. Also the same is reported in presence of Menniere's disease. When giddiness is produced more by loud noise rather than pressure it is known as **Tullio phenomenon,** which is seen in association with labyrinthine fistula and following fenestration surgery.

Postural Tests

Romberg's Test

Patient is asked to stand with feet together and arms by the side with eyes open first, then with

91

eyes closed. In peripheral lesion patient sways to the side of the lesion but in central lesion patient shows instability.

Sharpened Romberg's Test

If the above Romberg's test is normal, the patient is asked to stand with one heel of one foot in front of the toes of the other with arms folded across the chest, inability to perform this indicates vestibular impairment.

Gait Test

The patient is asked to walk along a straight line to a fixed target with eyes open and then closed. In case of peripheral lesion patient deviates to the affected side.

Unterberger's Test

Patient is asked to stand with hands out stretched and closed eyes. He will be asked to march on the spot inside a circle. Patient having unilateral paralytic labyrinthitis will deviate towards that side. In presence of active irritative lesion, the balance disturbances is so significant that the patient will not be able to perform the test for three seconds.

Positional Test (Hall Pike Test)

It is done when patient complains of vertigo during change of head posture. Patient sits on the edge of the couch, examiner holds the patient's head and turns 45 degrees to the right and then places him to supine position, and then bring the head down 20 degree below horizontal plane and patient's eyes are observed for nystagmus.

The test is repeated on the left side. The nystagmus is checked for latency, duration, direction and fatiguability.

Caloric Test (Fig. 7.1a)

Caloric test is a very commonly done vestibular test; patient will be put in a couch with head end elevated to 45 degrees and each ear will be irrigated with hot and cold water to stimulate the vestibular labyrinth.

Principle

Water at 30 or 44 degrees centigrade is run into the ear under certain standard conditions. Nystagmus is produced in the normal person with a healthy labyrinth. Hot water heats the fluid in the duct, the specific gravity of the fluid falls and the fluid rises, i.e. moves towards the ampulla. This causes nystagmus with quick component to the stimulated side. When cold water or air is used it produces nystagmus in the opposite direction.

The normal duration of the nystagmus is 3 to 4 minutes and this test is interpreted as follows:

(a) **Canal paresis** is present if the duration of nystagmus is reduced equally for both hot and cold tests. The condition may be unilateral or bilateral. If there is no nystagmoid response with cold and hot water then it signifies a dead labyrinth (Fig. 7.1b).

(b) **Directional preponderance:** There is preponderance of nystagmus is one particular direction to both cold and hot water. This feature is seen in both central and peripheral lesions and require additional investigations like BERA and CT/MRI scan to differentiate (Fig. 7.1b)

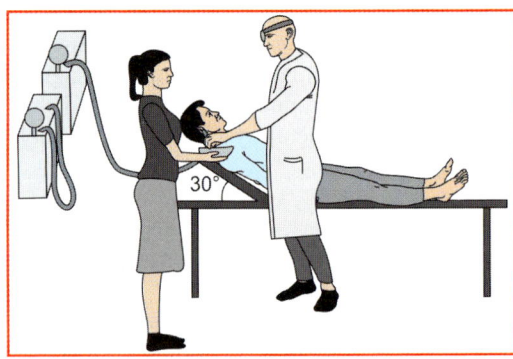

Fig. 7.1a: Caloric test

Cold Tap Water Test (Modified Kobrak Test)

It is done with patients head tilted to 60 degrees backward to place the horizontal canal in vertical position. 5 ml. of ice water is taken in a syringe to irrigate the external auditory canal and then the nystagmus is seen towards the opposite side. If

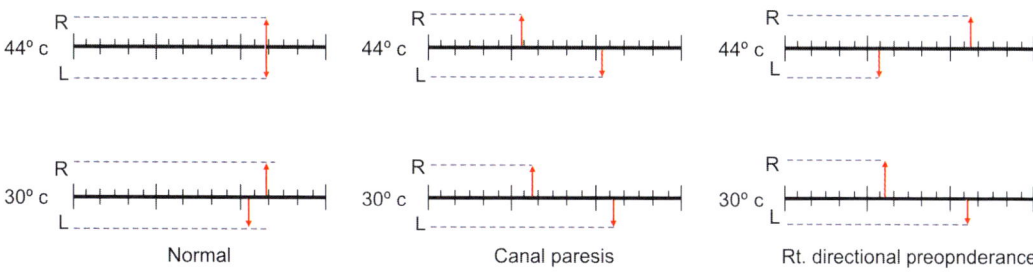

| Normal | Canal paresis | Rt. directional preopnderance |

Fig. 7.1b

no nystagmus is elicited, upto 40 ml. of ice water can be used for irrigation increasing by 10 ml. each time, if no response is elicited then it indicates a dead labyrinth.

Cold Air Test (Dundas Grant's Test)

This test is done in middle ear pathology or mastoidectomy cavity.

Rotation test

Stimulation of semicircular canal is done by rotatory movement that causes displacement of endolymph with the corresponding stimulation of nerve endings.

Cupulometry

This is a form of rotational test in which subjective vertigo and objective nystagmus following gentle rotational stimuli are recorded electrically.

Electronystagmography

It is now accepted as routine investigation in vertiginous patients. This is based on principle of corneoretinal potential to answer the following questions:

1. Abnormality in vestibular system or not?
2. Peripheral or central vestibular system problem?
3. If peripheral, which side is involved?
4. If central, what region is likely to be involved?
5. Is lesion static, progressive or recovering?

Advantages

1. To record nystagmus with the subject's eyes closed by attaching electrodes (Fig. 7.2).
2. Small amplitude nystagmus, not visible to the eye, can be identified and distinguished from other non-nystagmic eye movements.
3. Can be used to do electro-oculography.
4. It allows the accurate measurement of various nystagmus like slow phase velocity, amplitude, frequency, duration, fast phase velocity, total numbers of beats, latency, etc.

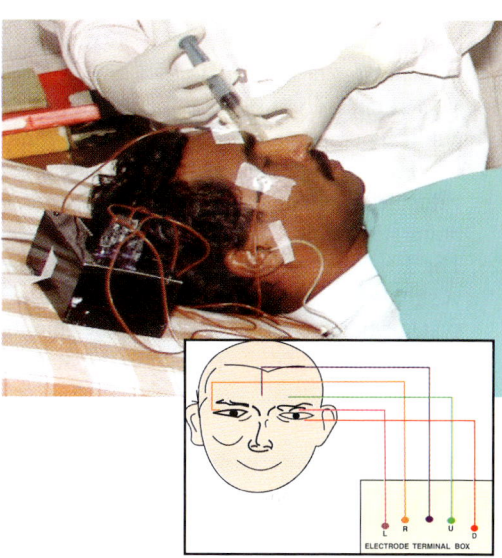

Fig. 7.2: Attachment of electrodes in 2+1 ENG channel

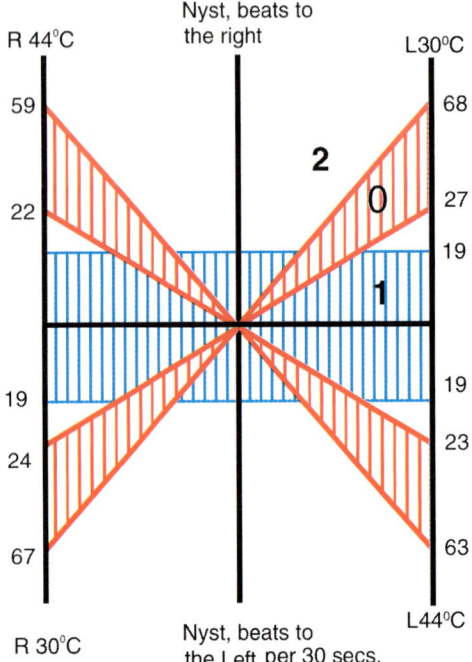

Fig. 7.3: Claussen butterfly chart
Normal - 0, Hypoactive - 1, Hyperactive - 2

5. It facilitates proper documentation and provides an accurate record, a documentary evidence for medicolegal cases.
6. It facilitates vivid picture for teaching and publication and an easier patient follow-up.
7. ENG studies the vestibular reflex which gives valuable information about the integrity of the brain stem.
8. The ENG test assesses the integrity of the vestibulo-oculo reflex system and the related systems like the saccadic system, the smooth pursuit system and the optokinetic system.

Disadvantages

1. No characteristic wave configuration or abnormalities from which one can directly pinpoint the nature and site of the lesion.
2. It cannot record nystagmus in certain kind of nystagmus where corneoretinal potential is absent and in cases of purely rotational nystagmus.
3. The ENG test does not assess the functional integrity of the vestibulospinal reflex system.

THE ELECTRONYSTAGMOGRAPH MACHINE

Types

- For routine clinical ENG it is preferable to use a machine with an AC amplifier. A DC amplifier is ideal for recording the true steady position of the eyes in the entire duration of the eye deviation. DC technique has a major drawback of drift of baseline which may be confused with the tracing produced by deviation of the eyes. An AC amplifier avoids this problem but true position of eyes in sustained position cannot be recorded.
- This machine can be a **multichannel** or a **single channel** apparatus.
- **Computerized ENG** is now a new additional armamentarium to neurootologist. The main advantage being reduced time spent and accurate interpretation of the ENG recording.
- **Telemetric ENG** allows a time and place independent recording of nystagmus by the patient himself at the time of the attack, it can also be used in the clinic for online computerized ENG recording.

Methodology

Various tests done during ENG procedure are:
1. Calibration
2. Spontaneous nystagmus test
3. Gaze test
4. Optokinetic nystagmus test
5. Positional test
6. Paroxysmal nystagmus test
7. Caloric test

FOLLOWING ARE FEW SAMPLE ENG GRAPHS IN NORMAL AND DISEASED PATIENTS
(ENG graphs in normal and diseased patients Figs 7.4 to 7.12)

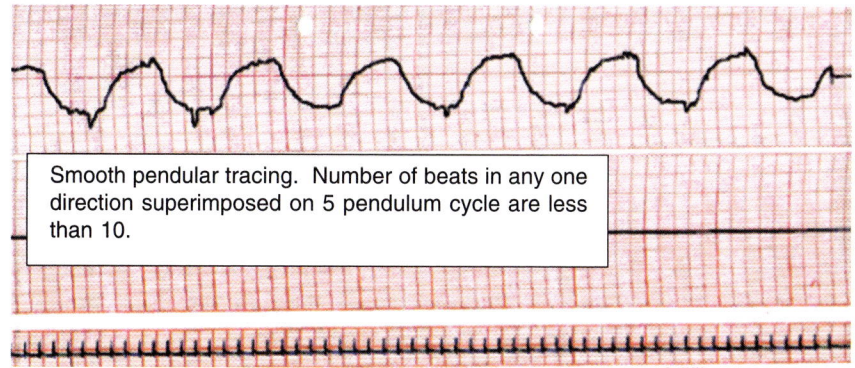

Smooth pendular tracing. Number of beats in any one direction superimposed on 5 pendulum cycle are less than 10.

Fig. 7.4: Pendular tracing of normal patient

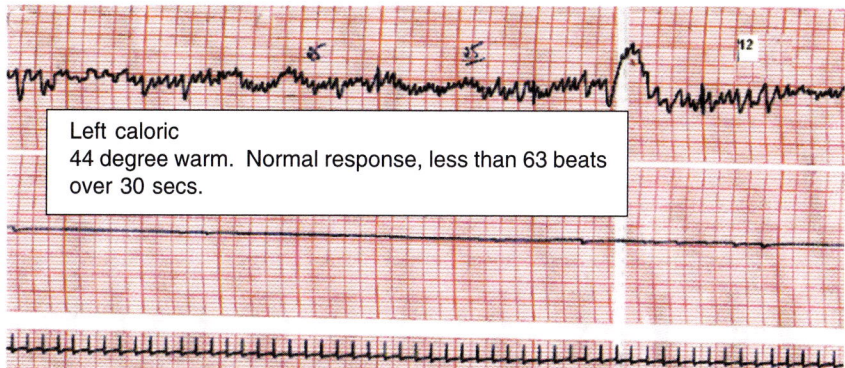

Left caloric
44 degree warm. Normal response, less than 63 beats over 30 secs.

Fig. 7.5: Caloric test showing normal left warm response

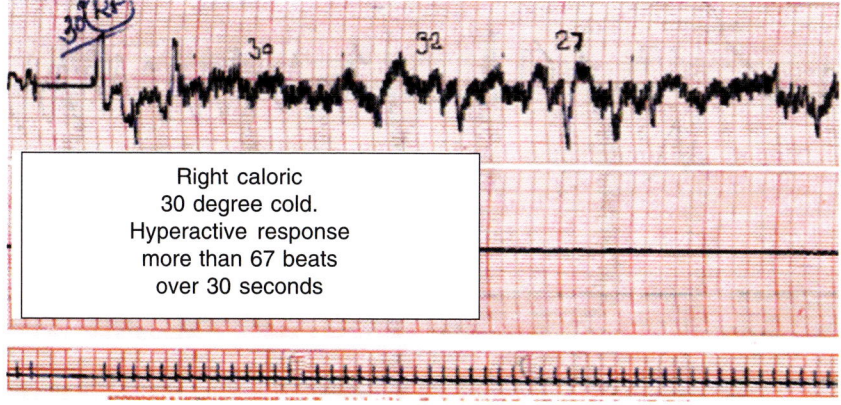

Right caloric
30 degree cold.
Hyperactive response
more than 67 beats
over 30 seconds

Fig. 7.6: Caloric test showing right cold hyperactive response

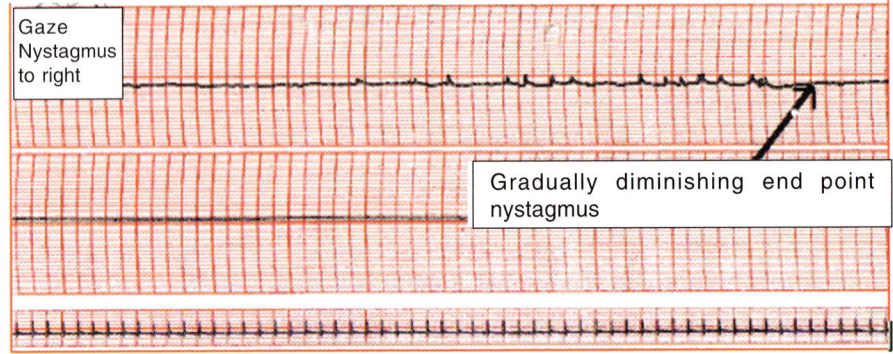

Fig. 7.7: ENG tracing showing gaze nystagmus to right, gradually diminishing: Physiological end point nystagmus

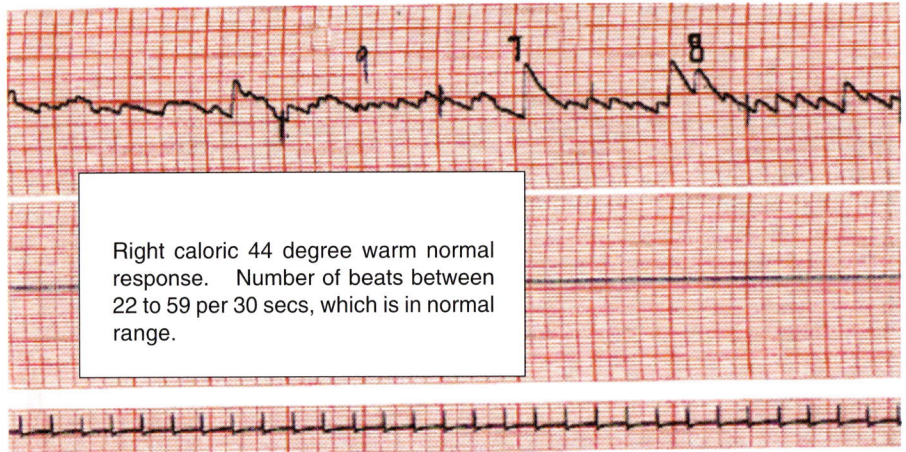

Fig. 7.8: A 32 year old female presented with giddiness, history of menorrhagia. O/E Pallor positive. Caloric test showed normal ENG tracing

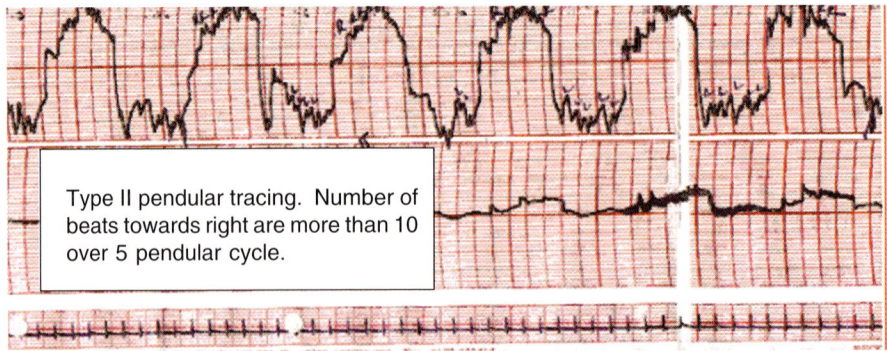

Fig. 7.9: A 65 year old male, vertigo 2 year duration, on labyrinthine sedatives

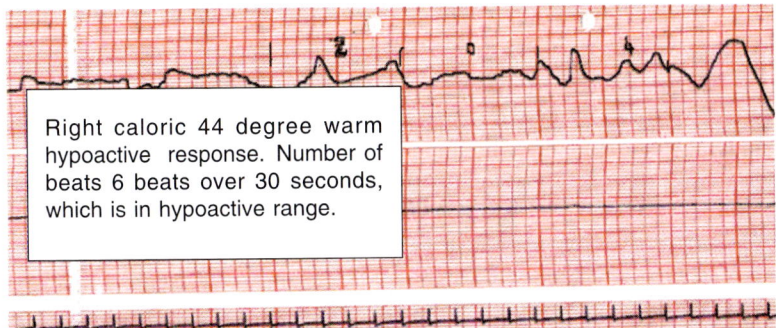

Right caloric 44 degree warm hypoactive response. Number of beats 6 beats over 30 seconds, which is in hypoactive range.

Fig. 7.10: A 52 year old male, vertigo 3 year duration associated with vomiting, caloric test showed right peripheral lesion, PTA showed features of menniere's. CT Scan was normal. Patient was subjected to intratympanic gentamycin therapy

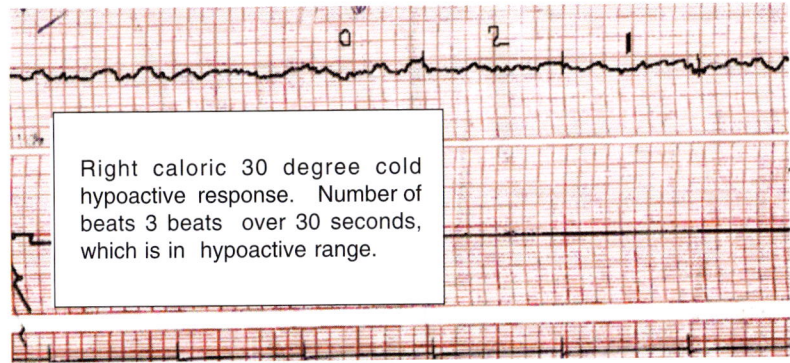

Right caloric 30 degree cold hypoactive response. Number of beats 3 beats over 30 seconds, which is in hypoactive range.

Fig. 7.11: A 42 year old male, post-trauma (right side head), presented with vertigo positional variation to right, O/E Positional test positive to right, Caloric test showed right peripheral vestibular lesion, features suggestive of BPPV. CT head normal. Patient was put on adaptation exercises

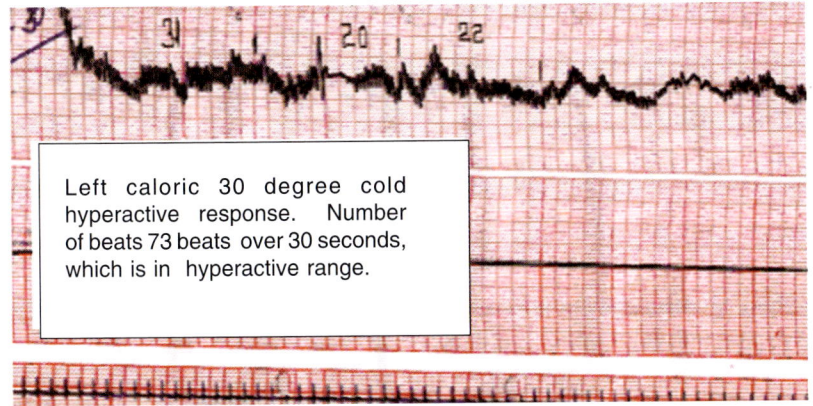

Left caloric 30 degree cold hyperactive response. Number of beats 73 beats over 30 seconds, which is in hyperactive range.

Fig. 7.12: A 38 year old male, presented with post-myringoplasty (left sided) vertigo. Caloric test showed left peripheral vestibular lesion

8

Vertigo

Vertigo is not a disease in itself but rather a symptom that can have any number of causes.

Definition

A feeling "in which the external world seems to revolve around the individual or in which the individual seems to revolve in space".

Incidence

5% of patients visiting the general practitioner are suffering from vertigo, whereas 10% of patients visiting the otorhinolaryngologist have vertiginous symptom.

Nomenclature

Paroxysmal vertigo: Sudden attack comes on quickly, lasts for a short time.

The single attack: Sudden intense attack fading away slowly.

Chronic vertigo: Usually not severe, may have long history.

Positional vertigo: Momentary vertigo occurs following sudden movements of head in certain positions.

Dizzy spells: Lasting a few seconds occurring irregularly.

What causes vertigo?

Contradictory information from

1. Vestibular system
2. Visual system
3. Proprioceptive system (muscles, joints)

Causes of Vertigo (Flow chart 8.1)

The causes of vertigo can be classified as follows:

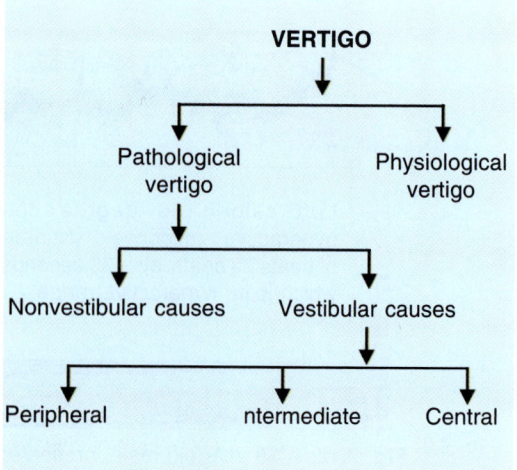

Flow chart 8.1: Causes of vertigo

Physiological Causes

1. Mismatch among three stabilizing sensory systems, as in motion sickness, height vertigo, visual vertigo (motion pictures).
2. The vestibular system is subjected to unfamiliar head movements to which it has never adapted, as in sea sickness.
3. Unusual head and neck positions.

Pathological Causes

1. Vestibular Causes *(Fig. 8.1)*

(a) Peripheral causes: arises in vestibule

- Benign paroxysmal positional vertigo (BPPV)
- Meniere's disease
- Labyrinthitis
- Head injuries and surgical trauma
- Pressure vertigo

(b) Intermediate causes: arises in nerve

- Vestibular neuronitis
- Acoustic neuroma
- Drugs

(c) Central causes: arises in vestibuli nuclei

- Vertibrobasilar insufficiency (VBI)
- Arteriosclerosis
- Cervical spondylosis
- Whiplash injury
- Acoustic neuroma

2. Nonvestibular causes

- Ocular vertigo
- Anemia
- Cardiovascular (orthostatic hypotension)
- Cerebrovascular disorders
- Psychogenic
- Brain tumors
- Epilepsy
- Head injury
- Multiple sclerosis
- Hypoglycemia
- Migraine

NYSTAGMUS

"Involuntary rhythmical oscillation of the eyes".

Nystagmus is defined as involuntary eye movements usually triggered by inner ear stimulation (Flow chart 8.2). It usually begins as a slow pursuit movement followed by a fast, rapid resetting phase. Nystagmus is named by the direction of the fast phase. Thus, nystagmus may be termed right beating, left beating, (collectively horizontal), up-beating or down-beating (vertical) or direction changing.

It can occur physiologically from vestibular or optokinetic stimulation or pathologically from various diseases (central or peripheral—Tables 8.1a and 8.1b).

Nystagmus has a slow phase and a fast phase *By convention nystagmus is named after fast phase* (Fig. 8.2).

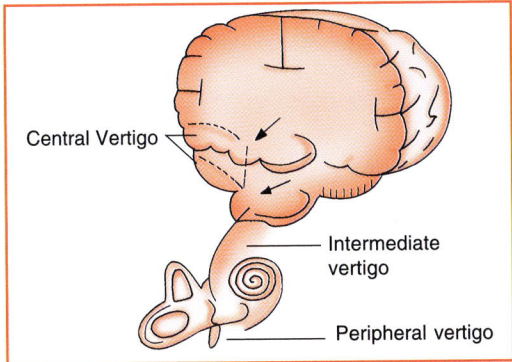

Fig. 8.1: Diagrammatic representation of sites of the lesion in case of vertigo

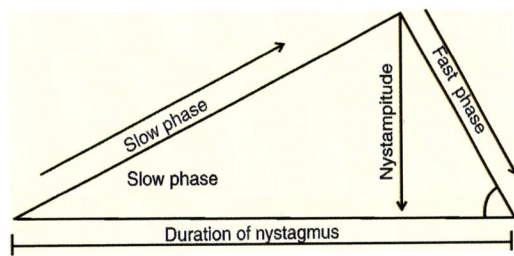

Fig. 8.2: Showing a nystagmus beat with its slow and fast components

Table 8.1a: Differences between central and peripheral vertigo

Sign/Symptoms	Peripheral	Central
Direction of associated nystagmus	Unidirectional : fast phase opposite lesion	Unidirectional/bidirectional
Purely horizontal nystagmus without torsional component	Common	Uncommon
Vertical or purely torsional nystagmus	Never present	May be present
Visual fixation	Inhibits nystagmus and vertigo	No inhibition
Severity of vertigo	Marked	Often mild
Direction of spin	Towards fast phase	Variable
Direction of fall	Towards slow phase	Variable
Duration of symptoms	Finite (min, days, weeks) but recurrent	May be chronic
Tinnitus and/or deafness	Often present	Usually absent
Associated abnormalities	None	Extremely common
Common causes	Infection, Meniere's, neuronitis, ischemia, trauma, toxin	Vascular, demyelinating, neoplasm

Table 8.1b: Dix—Hallpike maneuver (Positional test)

Features	Peripheral positional vertigo	Central Positional vertigo
Latency	3–40 sec	None, immediate vertigo and nystagmus
Fatiguability	Yes	No
Habituation	Yes	No
Intensity of vertigo	Severe	Mild
Reproducibility	Non reproducible	Reproducible
Direction of the nystagmus	Towards undermost ear and enhanced by removing ocular fixation	Variable
Incidence	Common	Rare

Flow chart 8.2: Mechanism of origin of nystagmus

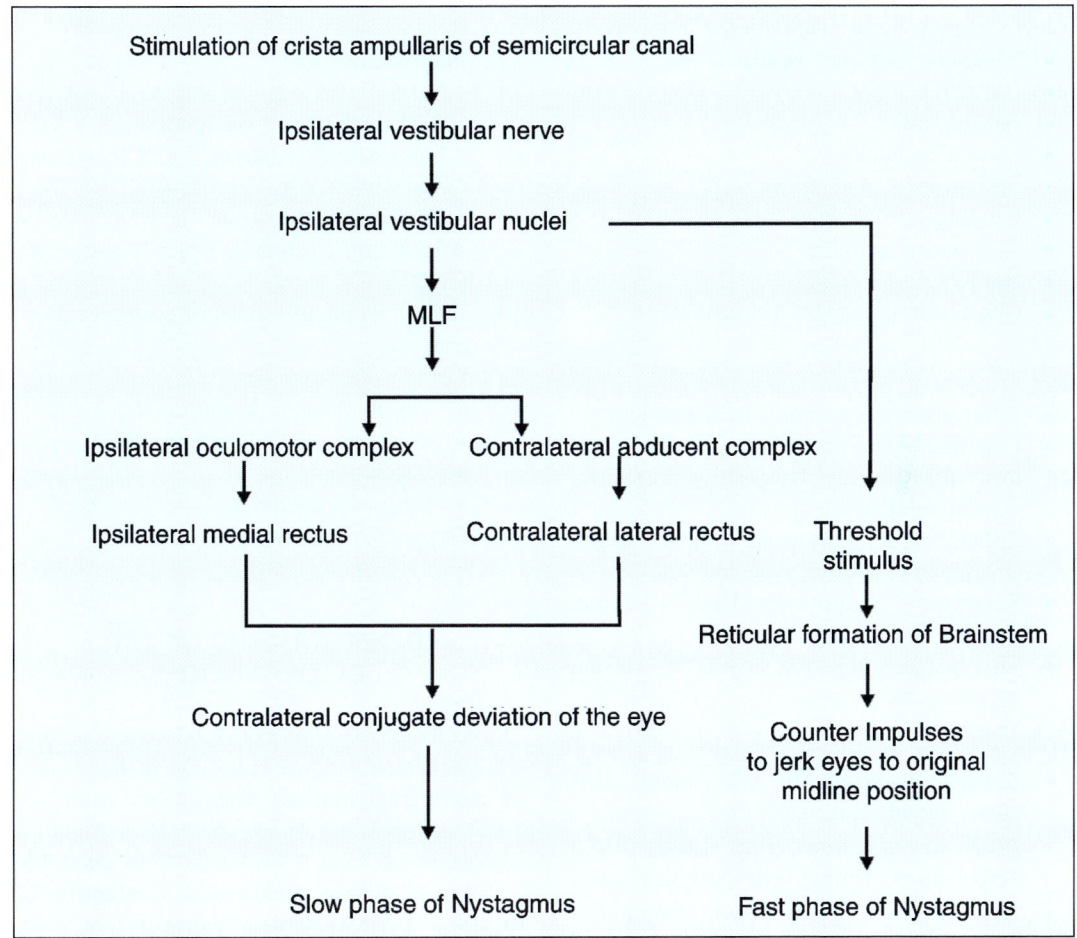

Nystagmus is of Two Types

(a) Spontaneous nystagmus

- When looking straight ahead
- When focusing on fixed spot
- When looking side ways
- When following a moving object

(b) Induced nystagmus

- When head is in a particular position
- While focussing position of head
- While turning the head

Alexander's Law for Peripheral Nystagmus

- **1st Degree:** Present only when patient looks in the direction of fast phase of nystagmus

- **2nd degree:** Present when patient looks straight ahead.

- **3rd degree:** Present even when patient looks in the direction of slow phase. Above degrees indicate the untenary of nystagmus.

When to Seek Medical Help?

When vertigo is associated with the following:
- Severe or 'different' headache
- Blurred vision
- Hearing loss
- Speech problems
- Weakness in a leg or arm
- Fainting
- Problems in walking
- Numbness or tingling
- Chest pain or changes in heart rate

Important Points in History Taking

- Description of symptoms by the patient
- Classification of vertigo attacks (which type, how debilitating, frequency, duration, vegetative symptoms)
- Influencing circumstances (injuries, drugs, stress, eating pattern, systemic illnesses)
- Secondary symptoms like diabetes, hypotension
- Tinnitus, hearing loss, headache, nausea/ vomiting, etc.

Examination
- ***General examination:*** Temperature, B.P. pulse, blood tests, etc.
- ***ENT examination:*** Ear drum, EAC, nasopharynx. Tuning fork tests, fistula test
- ***Neurological examination:*** Cerebellar dysfunction, corneal reflex and special test.
- Hearing test (SISI tone decay, BERA, otoacoustic reflex).
- ***Balance tests:*** Romberg test, Unterberger test, Babinski-Weill test, Barany Pointing test.
- Eye movement tests. Nystagmus tests; Caloric test (modified Kobrak test, Fitzgerald—Hallpike test, cold air caloric test), electronystagmography, optokinetic test.
- Positional tests (Hallpike maneuvre).
- CT Scan, MRI (as and when required) (Table 8.2).

Management of Vertigo

1. Reassurance/psychological support
2. Pharmacotherapy
   - Vasodilators, e.g.: Betahistine
   - Antiemetics, e.g.: Domperidone
   - Labyrinthine sedatives, e.g.: Cinnarizine
   - Anxiolytics, e.g.: Alprazolam
   - Diuretics, antioxidant
3. Adaptation exercises, Epley's maneuver (BPPV).
4. Intratympanic injections of gentamycin
5. Surgery.
   Conservation procedure
   - Endolymphatic decompression
   - Selective vestibular neurectomy
   - Sacculotomy
   - Codi tack operation
   Destructive procedure
   - Labyrinthectomy

UNDERSTANDING OF THE DIZZY PATIENT

The vestibular labyrinth has a basic resting activity and discharges at a steady rate even in the absence of an external stimulus. These as we know, are equal but opposite. Approach to the vertiginous patients is shown in Table 8.2 and Flow chart 8.3.

When a sudden pathological diminution of function of one vestibular system occurs, there exists a major imbalance. The involved side is no longer able to deliver its equal and opposite fund of information to the brain. The sequelae of this imbalance is a manifestation of a relative hyper-function of the intact side, leading to uncontrolled and prolonged vestibular reflexes. This disparate message arrives at the cerebral cortex and is interpreted in the light of past experience as a con-dition of constant motion. This misinterpretation is a rotatory sensation when the whole end organ is involved because the six semicircular canals predominate over the four otolith organs. Thus, vertigo results, i.e. sensation of a rotatory nature, pitching, yawning or rolling character but always rotational in nature.

Table 8.2: Key items in the history of dizzy patients

Disorders	Onset	Symptoms	Precipitating factors
Vestibular neuritis	Acute dizziness	Vertigo, dysequilibrium N/V, oscillopsia	Spontaneous exacerbated by head movements
Labyrinthitis	Acute dizziness	Vertigo, dysequilibrium N/V, oscillopsia, hearing loss and tinnitus	Spontaneous exacerbated by head movements
Wallenberg's syndrome (dorsal medullary infarct)	Acute dizziness	Vertigo, dysequilibrium N/V, tilt, laterpulsion, ataxia, crossed sensory loss, oscillopsia	Spontaneous exacerbated by head movements
Bilateral vestibular dificit or > 3 days from a unilateral vestibular defect	Chronic dizziness	Dizzy, dysequilibrium occasionally oscillopsia	Induced by head movements, walking exacerbated when walking in the dark or on uneven surfaces
Mal de debarquement	Chronic dizziness	Rocking or swaying as if on a boat	Spontaneous while lying or sitting Rarely occurs while in motion
Oscillopsia	Chronic dizziness	Subjective illusion of visual motion	Spontaneous with eyes open
Anxiety / Depression	Chronic dizziness	Lightheaded, floating or rocking	Induced by eye movements with head still
Benign paroxysmal positional vertigo	Spells : seconds	Vertigo, lightheaded, nausea	Positional: lying down, sitting up or turning over in bed, bending forward
Orthostatic hypotension	Spells : seconds	Lightheaded	Positional : Standing up
Transient ischemic attacks	Spells : minutes	Vertigo, lightheaded dysequilibrium	Spontaneous
Migraine	Spells : minutes	Vertigo, dizziness motion sickness	Usually movements induced
Panic attack	Spells : minutes	Dizzy, nausea diaphoresis, fear palpitations, paresthesis	Spontaneous or situational

Contd..,

Contd..,

Disorders	Onset	Symptoms	Precipitating factors
Motion sickness	Spells : hours	Nausea, diaphoresis dizzy	Movement induced, usually, visual-vestibular mismatch
Meniere's disease	Spells : hours	Vertigo dysequilibrium, ear fullness, hearing loss and tinnitus	Spontaneous, exacerbated by head movements

Abbreviation : N/V - Nausea or vomiting

Flow chart 8.3: Approach to a vertiginous patient

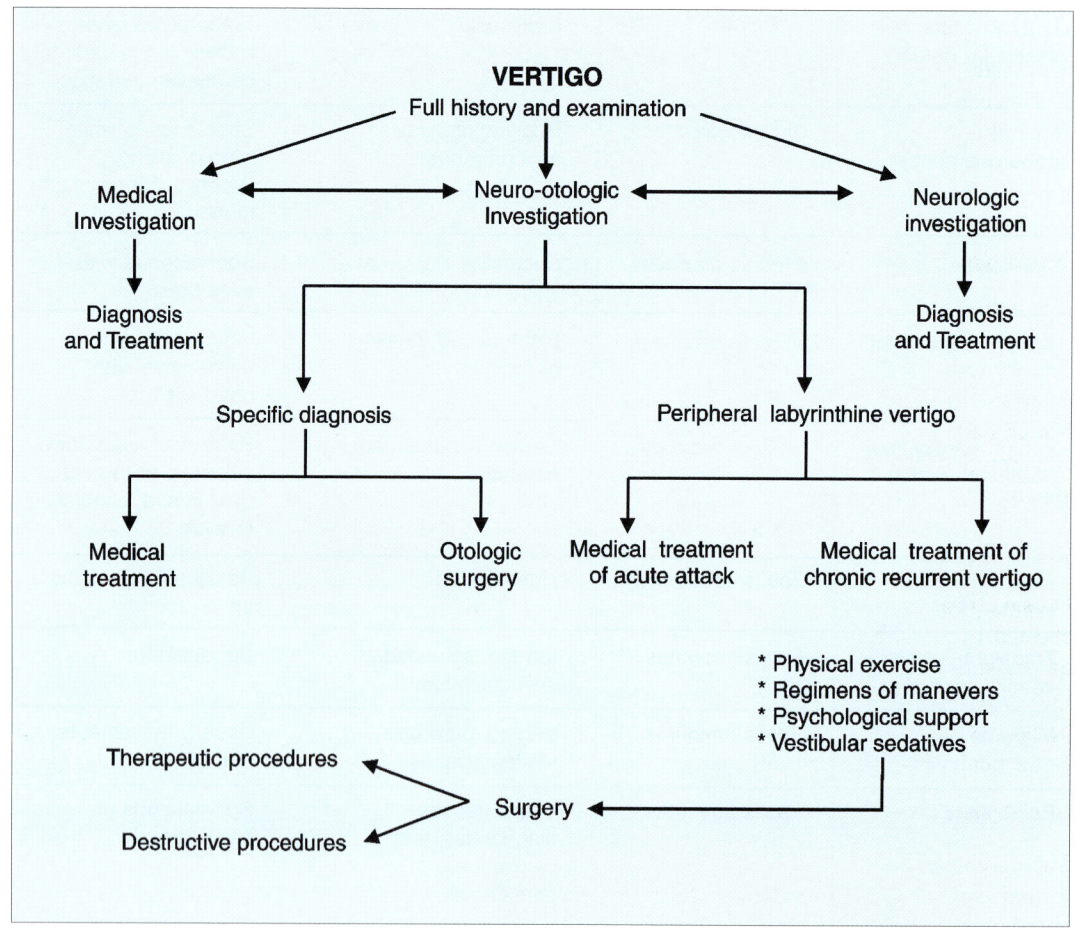

Eyes

The visual (slight) system makes us aware of our surroundings and the position of our bodies in relation to our surroundings. Any imbalance in the vestibular system leads to mismatch of information to the cerebellum. This imbalance in discharges arrives at the eye muscle nuclei and the reticular formation which is misinterpreted. The eye muscle nuclei deviate eyes in the direction of last gaze, to retain orientation.

This is how the slow component of the nystagmus is born. Subsequently, inhibitory neurons in the reticular formation cut off the incoming flow from vestibular nuclei and at the same time reticular activating neurons direct the ocular muscle nuclei to return the eyeballs to the point of gaze at which the slow component began to deviate.

This compensatory or recovery phase is faster and is known as the quick component of the nystagmus. The reticular activating neurons enters into a refractive period after firing and the vestibular nuclei inflow resumes. The chain of events repeat again.

Spinal Cord

The same imbalanced information goes to the anterior horn cells of the spinal cord and instructs postural and locomotor muscles to meet the new situation that has come. Leading to staggering to ataxia.

Vagal Stimulation

Dorsal efferent nucleus of the vagus nerve is also cheated by this imbalanced impulse. Cessation of peristalsis occurs in a mild form. If the imbalance is massive and continuous, reverse peristalsis occurs resulting in nausea and vomiting as the nucleus is heavily stimulated.

Physiology of Repair and Compensation

The cerebellum in a matter of minutes, causes virtual shut down of electrical activity of the vestibular system, by virtue of its profound inhibitory influence on the vestibular activity (Cerebellar lamp). Though, imbalance of a greater magnitude is not eliminated, it serves to eliminate imbalance of a lower magnitude. This is because only those incoming via medial nuclei are clamped, impulses coming fibers via fibers from other nuclei are not affected by the cerebellar clamp.

Restoration of equilibrium brings about resolution of uncontrolled reflexes, i.e.

1. Restoration of health to the diseased system.
2. Central suppression of the intact side by invocation of inhibitory tracts in the central nervous system.
3. Generation of a new electrical activity in the under discharging system, to balance the normal but now relatively hyperactive.

Benign Paroxysmal Positional Vertigo

Benign paroxysmal positional vertigo (BPPV) is probably the most common cause of vertigo. BPPV was first described by Barany in 1921.

BPPV is defined as an abnormal sensation of motion that is elicited by certain critical provocative positions. The provocative positions usually trigger specific eye movements (i.e., nystagmus). The character and direction of the nystagmus are specific to the part of the inner ear affected and the pathophysiology.

Pathophysiologic Mechanisms
(Fig. 8.3)

1. Canalithiasis
2. Cupulolithiasis
1. **Canalithiasis** (literally, 'canal rocks') is defined as the condition in which otoconial debris are floating freely in the canal portion of the semicircular canals (SCCs).
2. **Cupulolithiasis** (literally, 'cupula rocks') refers to condition where otoconial debris are adhered to the cupula of the crista ampullaris. That is they reside in the ampulla of the SCCs and are not free floating.

Classic BPPV (canalithiasis) is the most common variety of BPPV. It involves the posterior SCC. It is due to the most dependent portion of the posterior semicircular canal.

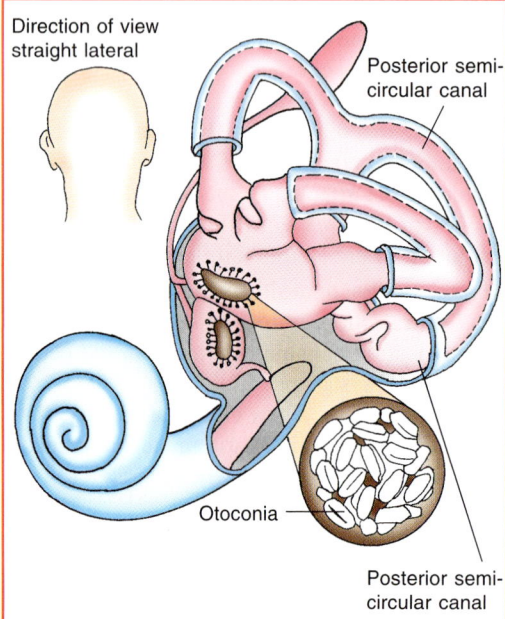

Fig. 8.3: Pathogenesis of BPPV showing displaced otoconia

The **pathognomonic** nystagmus pattern of BPPV consists of:

1. The nystagmus is rotational and geotropic.
2. There is a latency of onset, usually around 1 to 5 seconds.
3. The duration of nystagmus is short, usually 20 to 30 seconds, and always less than 1 minute.
4. The nystagmus is associated with vertigo, which follows the same time course as the nystagmus.
5. The nystagmus is fatiguable, that is, it becomes progressively weaker and disappears with repeated testing.
6. The nystagmus is reversible with return of the head to the upright position.

Incidence

Sex: Womens are more commonly affected.
Age: BPPV seems to have a predilection for the older population (average age, 51 to 57.2 yrs). It is rarely observed in individuals younger than 35 years without a history of antecedent head trauma.

Predisposing factors
- Acute alcoholism
- Major surgery
- CNS disease

Causes
- Idiopathic
- Trauma
- Miscellaneous

Associated Factors

- Cervical vertigo
- Ear diseases like
  - Otitis media
  - Vestibular neuritis
  - Sudden SNHL
  - Meniere's disease
  - Otosclerosis
  - Acoustic neuroma
- Vertibrobasilar insufficiency
- CNS disease

Differential Diagnosis

- Perilymphatic fistula
- Drug or alcohol intoxication
- Meniere's disease
- Neurovascular compression
- Psychogenic vertigo.

Symptomology

- The onset of BPPV is typically sudden. Many patients wake up with the condition, noticing the vertigo while trying to sit up suddenly. Thereafter, propensity for positional vertigo may extend for days to weeks, occasionally for months or years. In many, the symptoms periodically resolve and then recur.

- People who have BPPV do not usually feel dizzy all the time. Severe dizziness occurs as attacks triggered by head movements. At rest between episodes, patients usually have few or no symptoms.

- Classic BPPV is usually triggered by the sudden action of moving from the erect position to the supine position while angling the head 45 degree toward the side of the affected ear.
- When BPPV is triggered, patients feel as though they are suddenly thrown into a rolling spin, toppling toward the side of the affected ear. Symptoms start very violently and usually dissipate within 20 or 30 seconds. This sensation is triggered again upon sitting erect; however, the direction of the nystagmus is reversed.

Sign

- The physical examination findings in patients affected by BPPV are generally unremarkable. All neurotologic examination findings except those from the Dix-Hallpike maneuver may be normal.

- The Dix-Hallpike maneuver is the standard clinical test for BPPV. The finding of classic rotatory nystagmus with latency and limited duration is considered pathognomonic. A negative test result is meaningless except to indicate that active canalithiasis is not present at that moment. (Refer to Chapter Functional Examination of Vestibular System) - Fig. 8.4.

Investigations

Since the Dix-Hallpike maneuver is pathognomonic, laboratory tests are not needed to make the diagnosis of BPPV. However, since a high association with inner ear disease exists, laboratory workup may be needed to delineate these other pathologies.

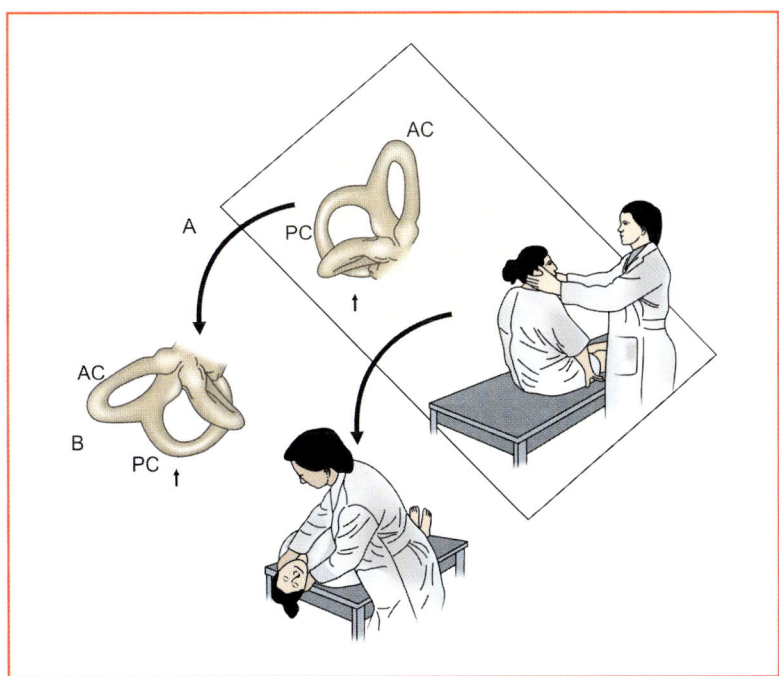

Fig. 8.4: Position of the semicircular canal Dix-Halpike test BPPV. Shows the movement of debris in right posterior SCC during the rest and after performing the test

- Imaging studies are not needed in the workup of a patient in whom BPPV is suspected.
- Electronystagmography
- Torsional eye movement cannot be demonstrated directly, but occasionally electronystagmography (ENG) is helpful in detecting the presence and timing of nystagmus.
- Caloric test results can be normal or hypofunctional.
- BPPV can originate in an ear with an absent caloric response because the **nervous and vascular supply to the horizontal canal is separate from that of the PSCs.**
- *Audiogram*: The result of an audiogram may be normal.
- *Posturography*: Posturography results are often abnormal but follow no predictable or diagnostic pattern.

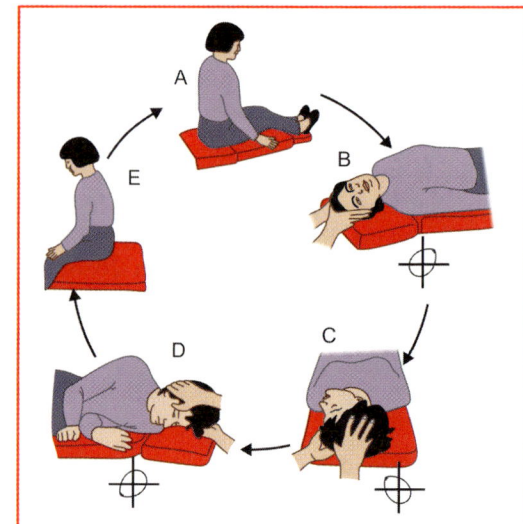

Fig. 8.5: Steps of Epley's maneuver

Treatment

Medical Care: Treatment options include:

- Watchful waiting
- Vestibulosuppressant medication
- **Vestibular rehabilitation:** Vestibular rehabilitation is a noninvasive therapy that can have success after lengthy periods. Patients can be instructed in Cawthorne exercises that seem to help by dispersing particles.
- **Canalith repositioning, (CRP):** Epley maneuver (for canalithiasis) and Semont maneuver (for cupulolithiasis).

Epley Maneuver (Fig. 8.5)

The patient sits on the examination table, with eyes open and head turned 45 degrees to the right.

A. The physician supports the patient's head as the patient lies back quickly from a sitting to supine position, ending with the head hanging 20 degrees off the end of the examination table.

B. The physician turns the patient's head 90 degrees to the left side. The patient remains in this position for 30 seconds.

C. The physician turns the patient's head an additional 90 degrees to the left while the patient rotates his or her body 90 degrees in the same direction. The patient remains in this position for 30 seconds.

D. The patient sits up on the left side of the examination table.

E. The procedure may be repeated on either side until the patient experiences relief of symptoms.

Surgical Care

- Surgery is usually reserved for those in whom CRP fails
- Labyrinthectomy
- Posterior canal occlusion
- Singular neurectomy
- Vestibular nerve section
- Transtympanic aminoglycoside application.

VESTIBULAR NEURONITIS

It is characterized by the sudden onset of vertigo, nausea and vomiting without deafness and tinnitus as a result of labyrinthine stimulation by various factors like:

1. Virus
2. Age—adolescent groups are more affected
3. Sex—equally seen in both sexes
4. Idiopathic.

Pathophysiology

It is an inflammatory process in the vestibular nerve which is self limiting.

Clinical Features

- **Vertigo:** Persistent and frequent in the beginning and becomes paroxysmal and less frequent, lasts maximum for 3 weeks and usually does not recur.
- **Nausea and vomiting** due to vestibular disturbances.
- **Normal hearing** as cochlea is spared
- **Nystagmus:** Spontaneous nystagmus of horizontal type is present.

Investigations

- Audiometry
- Caloric test shows canal paresis and directional preponderance
- Electronystagmography

Treatment

- Bed rest and reassurance
- Labyrinthine sedatives
- Prochlorperazine maleate
- Promethazene
- Theodine
- Cinnarizine, betahistine

POINTS TO REMEMBER

1. The vestibular nystagmus is always fine, horizontal and has both slow and fast component and does not last for more than 6 weeks.
2. The direction of nystagmus is determined by fast component.
3. Tullio phenomenon is associated with giddiness in response to loud noise and may be seen following fenestration surgery.
4. Canal paresis is present if the duration of nystagmus is reduced equally for both hot and cold tests.
5. Vestibular neuronitis occur as a sudden onset of vertigo, nausea, vomiting without deafness and tinnitus.
6. Epley's maneuver is used to treat BPPV.

9

Tinnitus

Tinnitus is the perception of sound in the head or the ears. The term tinnitus is derived from the Latin word *tinnier,* meaning to ring. Estimates of patients with tinnitus range from 10 to 15% of the population (30–40 million people). Of patients presenting with ear-related symptoms, 85% report experiencing tinnitus as well. Both adults and children report experiencing tinnitus.

CLASSIFICATION

Tinnitus should be clinically classified as follows (Flow chart 9.1):

Duration of Tinnitus

- *Short:* Middle ear pathology.
- *Long:* Meniere's disease, acoustic neuroma, palatal myoclonus, glomus jugular, patent cochlear duct, ototoxicity.

Types of Tinnitus

- Subjective type
- Objective type.

Subjective Type

Sounds like ringing, whistling or roaring is heard by the patient without the presence of such a sound. This can also be psychogenic and functional in origin, apart from diseases like Meniere's, ototoxicity, etc.

Objective Tinnitus

This is heard not only by the patient but also by the examiner, *e.g.* palatal myoclonus, patulous eustachian tube, vascular bruit, arteriovenous malformation, etc.

Nature

- *Continuous:* Otosclerosis, acoustic neuroma, acute noise trauma.
- *Intermittent and fluctuant:* Meniere's disease
- *Pulsatile:* Glomus tumors, strychnine poisoning.
- *Relieving factors:* By putting pressure at the side of the neck in vascular causes.
- *Aggravating factors: By smoking*—cochlear pathology, ototoxicity. *Yawning and blowing-*eustachian dysfunction.

Evaluation

Tinnitus is not a disease in itself but rather a reflection of underlying disease so it must be evaluated properly.
1. History taking
2. Clinical examination

Flow chart 9.1: Classification of tinnitus

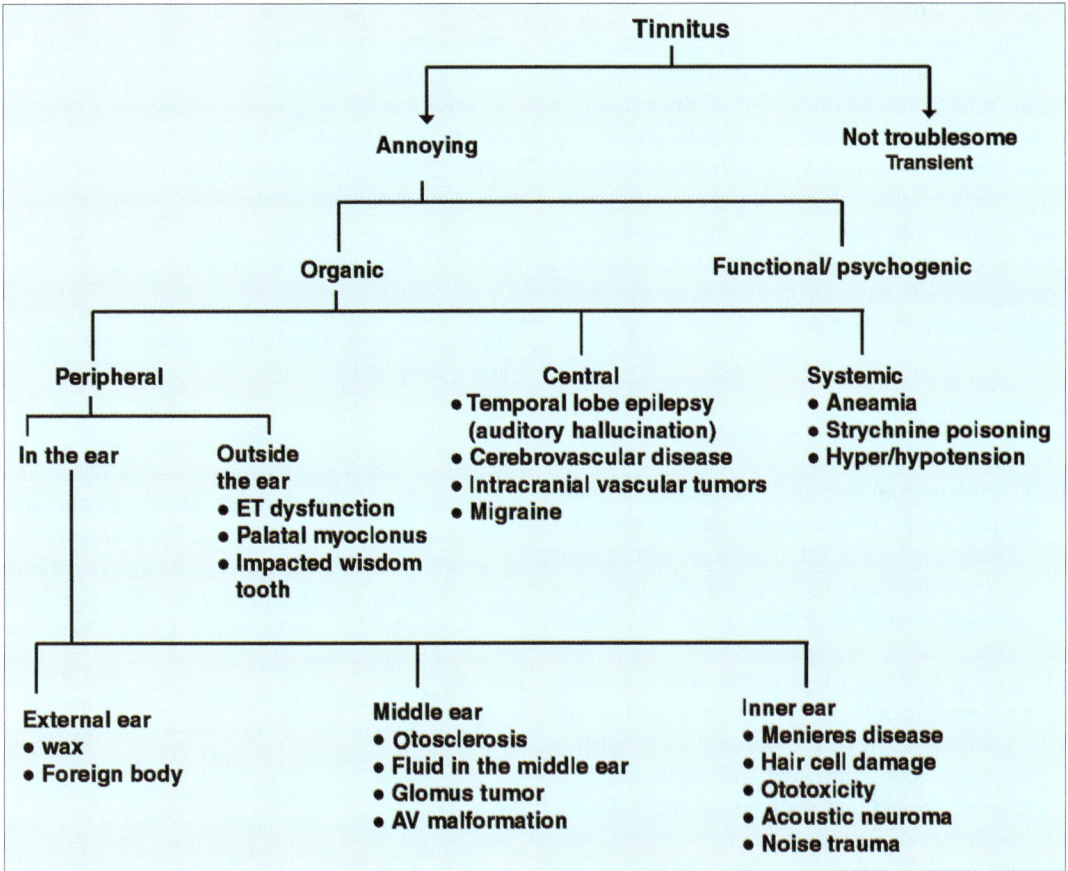

3. Audiometric testing
4. Radiological investigations
5. Laboratory studies

History Taking

The evaluation of a patient with tinnitus should start with a carefully taken history.

a. The patient's description of the tinnitus is very important, it can provide key information during the initial evaluation.
   - The quality of the sound, especially whether it is pulsatile or non pulsatile
   - The perceived location
   - The pitch
   - The loudness
   - Constant or episodic
   - Onset
   - Alleviating/aggravating factors
b. History of infection
c. History of trauma, noise exposure, medication usage
d. Medical history—Diabetes, hypertension
e. Associated hearing loss/vertigo, pain
f. Family history of hearing loss

Many drugs have been linked to tinnitus. Although almost any medication can be a possible cause of tinnitus the most frequently implicated drugs are the anti-inflammatories, antibiotics, and antidepressants. Both aspirin and quinine are associated with tinnitus. This tinnitus is high frequency, tonal in nature, and accompanied by a temporary threshold shift.

The tinnitus is reversible with cessation of the medication. Aminoglycoside antibiotics are also often implicated as the cause of drug-induced tinnitus. Other medications include loop diuretics and chemotherapeutic agents such as cisplatin and vincristine. Any of the heterocyclic anti-depressants (i.e. amitriptyline, imipramine) can cause tinnitus. This is interesting because antidepressants have also been investigated for the treatment of tinnitus.

Clinical Examination

a. Complete head and neck exam
b. General physical exam
c. Otomicroscopy to look for a middle ear mass or motion of the tympanic membrane with respiration. A glomus tympanicum can be seen as a reddish mass in the middle ear or a dehiscent jugular bulb may be seen as a bluish mass.
d. With a history of pulsatile tinnitus, the physician should search for an audible bruit by auscultating the external canal with a Toynbee tube, and over the orbit, mastoid process, skull, and neck using the bell and diaphragm of a stethoscope.

The heart should be auscultated for murmurs. The patient should perform light exercise to see if this increases the pulsatile tinnitus. Tinnitus of arterial origin will often worsen with exercise. Venous induced tinnitus may decrease with light pressure on the neck, turn-ing the head, or with the Valsalva maneuver.

Audiometry Testing

a. Pure tone audiometry
b. Speech discrimination
c. Tympanometry
d. Acoustic reflex measurements.

Radiological Investigations

Weissman and Hirsch recently reviewed the imaging of tinnitus. *They recommend contrast-enhanced computed tomography of the temporal bones and skull base as the first line study for evaluating pulsatile tinnitus.* The diagnosis of glomus tympanicum tumors is made on the bone algorithm scans which best shows the extent of the mass. It is usually not possible to see enhancement of a small tumor confined to the middle ear on a CT study.

Laboratory Studies

Hematocrit, fluorescent treponemal antibody absorption tests, blood chemistry, thyroid studies, and a lipid battery.

Treatment

Multiple etiologies and poorly understood mechanisms of tinnitus have led to the attempt at multiple treatment modalities. These include:

- **Diet modification and habituation:** Avoidance of stimulants such as coffee, tea, chocolate, cola, and other caffeine containing medications as well as smoking cessation may help some patients.
- **Medications:** Many medications have been researched for the treatment of tinnitus, including lidocaine, tocainide, carba-mazepine, benzodiazepines, tricyclic antidepressants, and ginko biloba. Lidocaine administered intravenously has been shown to improve tinnitus but is impractical to use clinically.
- **Masking:** Hearing aids, maskers, or combinations of the two may help some patients. If the patient has some hearing loss, amplification of background noise by a hearing aid can decrease tinnitus. A masker produces sound to mask the tinnitus and decrease the annoyance to the patient. There are combination of hearing aids/maskers which can be used. They are called as *tinnitus instruments*.
- **Electrical stimulation:** Electrical stimu-lation of the cochlea has been studied for the treatment of tinnitus. Transcutaneous, round window, and promontory stimulation

of the cochlea have shown some benefit. Direct currents may produce permanent damage and cannot be used clinically.

- **Acupuncture:** Hypnosis has been tried with no concluding evidence of improvement.
- **Recently** tinnitus retraining therapy has been tried with promising results. It consists of one to one directive counselling and sound therapy.

- **Surgery:** Surgical treatment of tinnitus is used in the treatment of arteriovenous malformations, vascular tumors, oto-sclerosis, and acoustic neuroma.
- Some patients need only reassurance that the tinnitus is not a sign of a serious medical disease. Patients should be instructed to avoid medications, which are known to cause tinnitus such as aspirin and NSAIDs.

POINTS TO REMEMBER

1. Tinnitus is the perception of sound in the ear, head and can be subjective or objective.
2. Tinnitus is not a disease in itself but rather a reflection of underlying disease, which should be evaluated.

10

Otalgia

Otalgia (Pain in the ear)

Pain in the ear may be because of the local and referred causes. Whenever the patient complains of pain the following questions should be asked in the history of presenting symptoms.

Onset
- *Sudden:* e.g. Furunculosis, acute otitis media, trauma like otitic barotrauma
- *Gradual:* Otitis externa secondary to CSOM, malignancy, malignant otitis externa.

Duration
- *Short duration:* ASOM, perichondritis of ear pinna
- *Long duration:* Malignancy

Nature of the Pain
- *Dull:* eczematous otitis externa, secretory otitis media, impacted wax
- *Sharp:* furunculosis, otitic barotrauma
- *Throbbing pain:* ASOM

Relieving Factors

- Pain relieves with discharge from the ear - acute suppurative otitis media (ASOM)

Aggravating Factors

- Pain increasing on swallowing—ASOM
- Pain increasing on yawning and chewing - furunculosis arising from anterior canal wall

- Pain increasing on pulling the pinna and pressing the tragus—otitis externa.

Radiating Pain

Furuncle arising from anterior wall, pain radiates to preauricular region and posterior wall to the mastoid region.

Referred Pain (Referred Otalgia)

- Referred pain to the ear is because of nerve supply from 5th, 9th and 10th cranial nerves and C2, 3, to the ear (Fig. 10.1).

Referred Pain via 5th Nerve

- Dental—Caries tooth, impacted molar, malocclusion
- Oral cavity—Benign or malignant ulcerative lesion
- Temporomandibular joint disorders like Costen syndrome, TM joint arthritis

Referred Pain via 9th Nerve

- Base of tongue malignancy
- Oropharynx—Acute Tonsillitis, peritonsillar abscess, benign or malignant ulcers of the soft palate or tonsils.
- Elongated styloid process also known as Eagle's syndrome.

Referred Pain via 10th Nerve

- Ulcerative lesions of vallecula, epiglottis, larynx or laryngopharynx

Referred Pain Via C2, C3

- Cervical spondylosis, caries spine

Symptoms Associated with Otalgia Like

- Tinnitus—Acoustic neuroma
- Itching—Otomycosis.

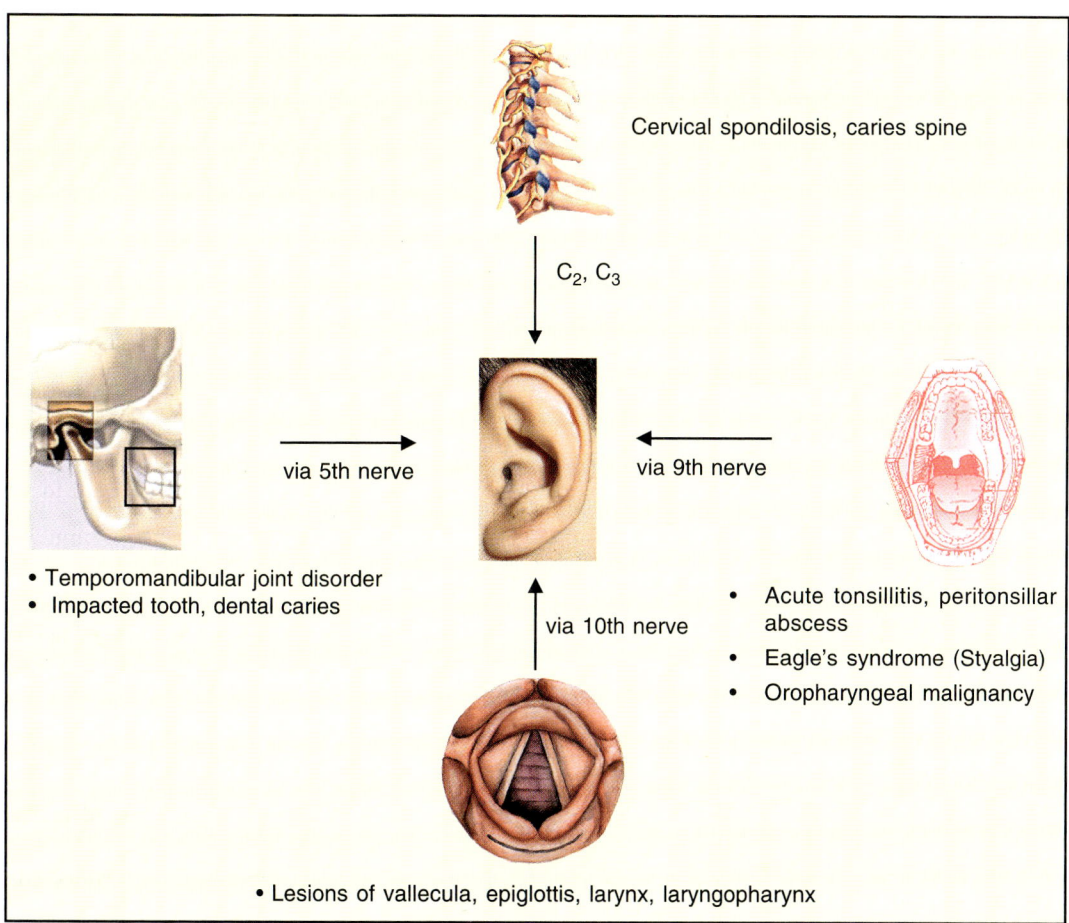

Cervical spondilosis, caries spine

C_2, C_3

via 5th nerve

via 9th nerve

- Temporomandibular joint disorder
- Impacted tooth, dental caries

via 10th nerve

- Acute tonsillitis, peritonsillar abscess
- Eagle's syndrome (Styalgia)
- Oropharyngeal malignancy

- Lesions of vallecula, epiglottis, larynx, laryngopharynx

Fig. 10.1: Diagrammatic representation of referred pain to the ear

---

POINTS TO REMEMBER

1. Referred otalgia: Pain perceived in the ear through radiation from areas with source of nerve supply like traumatic, inflammatory and neoplastic conditions of larynx, pharnx, oral cavity and cervical spine.
2. Persistent ear pain can be associated with T.M. Joint dysfunction and should be evaluated.

Disorders of Eustachian Tube

EUSTACHIAN TUBE DYSFUNCTION

Normal Eustachian tube function is essential for the well-being of the middle ear cleft as it maintains the equilibrium between middle ear pressure and the atmosphere (Anatomical details and functions have been described in Chapter Anatomy of the Ear). Any obstruction whether partly or complete causes a resorption of air from the middle ear with consequent retraction of the drum as a result of a higher atmospheric pressure. Eustachian tube dysfunction is characterized by a middle ear pressure of less than 100 mm H_2O. The patient will notice this as a mild hearing loss and feeling of pressure in the ear. If the process continues and the tube does not reopen then a serous exudates occurs which is associated with a more severe hearing loss, discomfort in the ear, occasionally tinnitus and in some patient dizziness. Throat infections may be transmitted by the tube to the middle ear causing otitis media. This is more common in children because their tube is shorter and straighter and has an exuberance of lymphoid tissues in throat. The difference between adult and infant Eustachian tube is given in Table 11.1.

Flow chart 11.1: Disorders of Eustachian tube

Disorders of Eustachian tube	
Mechanical	**Functional**
• Nasal allergy	• Patulous eustachian tube (seen in old, debilitated patients)
• Chronic infections of sinuses	
• Adenoids, nasopharyngeal tumors	• Down's syndrome
• Cleft palate	• Congenital anamolies
• DNS	

Eustachian tube obstruction can be either anatomical, functional or both (Flow chart 11.1).

Mechanical obstruction may be due to:

1. Nasal allergy
2. Chronic infection in the nose and sinuses
3. Adenoids, nasopharyngeal tumors
4. Cleft palate
5. DNS

Functional obstruction is caused by collapse of the tube due to poor function of tensor veli palatine muscle, e.g. in children with Down's syndrome.

Investigations

Eustachian tube patency can be tested by various methods like
- Valsalva maneuver
- Toynbee maneuver
- Politerization
- Catheterization
- Frenzel's maneuver (nasopharyngeal pressure test)
- Radiology
  - E.T. salphingography
  - CT Scan
  - X-ray submento-vertical view.

Treatment

This is directed at eliminating infection in the nose and sinuses combined with the patient attempting the Valsalva maneuver. Local and systemic decongestants, local steroid spray like fluticasone, budesonide, local antihistamines like azelastine, systemic antihistamines like l-cetrizine, ebastine, loratidine are used to treat any allergic element.

PATULOUS EUSTACHIAN TUBE

It may occur in elderly patients, particularly those with debilitating disease and marked weight loss.

Congenital anomaly may account for a small number of cases. Patients suffering from this condition complain of the loudness of their own voice (autophony) while their hearing is reduced for other voices and sounds. They may be aware of their own breath sound and the patient's breathing can be heard through an auscultation tube inserted into external auditory meatus.

An unduly open or patulous Eustachian tube is sometimes associated with atrophic changes in the mucous membrane of the nose and pharynx. The mucosa of the whole tube may be affected or changes may be limited to the pharyngeal opening. On examination, the characteristic sign is the inward and outward movements of the tympanic membrane while breathing.

Treatment is usually unnecessary and patient may be reassured. Some patients get symptomatic relief after insertion of grommet in the drumhead. If the symptoms are distressing to the patient it is worth injecting a little Teflon paste into the anterior part of the Eustachian cushion or by nasal endoscopic correction.

ACUTE TUBAL CATARRH

This usually occurs after an upper respiratory tract infection, particularly sinusitis or influenza. The epithelial lining of the tube becomes congested and edematous resulting in tubal blockage without involving middle ear.

Patient complains of blockage of ear. On swallowing, feeling of blockage is temporally relieved. There may be occasional earache. The nasal and pharyngeal symptoms are those of an upper respiratory tract infection.

On examination, there is usually nasal obstruction with a mucopurulent nasal discharge. Tympanic membrane is retracted but its color is normal with a few dilated surface vessels. The condition usually resolves as the upper respiratory tract symptoms disappear. Treatment comprises rest in ventilated room, nasal decongestants and anti-histaminic and local steroid spray.

Table 11.1: Differences between adult and infant eustachian tube

	Infant	Adult
Length	13–18 mm	36 mm
Placement	More horizontal and less angulated shorter, wider and straighter	Forms an angle of approximately 45° with horizontal and is more angulated
Bony portion	Longer and wider	Approximately one third of the total length of tube so comparatively shorter than infants
Cartilaginous portion	Flaccid, retrograde reflux of nasopharyngeal secretions can occur thereby making middle ear more prone for infection	Rigid and remains closed thereby protecting middle ear from the reflux
Ostmann's pad of fat	Less in volume	Large and helps to keep the tube closed
Density of elastin	Less dense, so tube does not close efficiently	Comparatively more which helps the tube to close by recoil action of the cartilage
Ventilatory function	Not well developed	Well developed

CHRONIC TUBAL CATARRH

It presents with chronic tubal obstruction without any active disease in the tympanic cavity. Predisposing factors are adenoiditis, nasal allergy, allergic fungal sinusitis and chronic infection in the nose and paranasal sinuses.

The presenting symptom is intermittent deafness with discomfort. Otoscopy shows retracted tympanic membrane which does not move on Valsalva's maneuver. Tuning fork and audiogram show mild to moderate conductive deafness.

Infection or allergy of nose and paranasal sinuses is to be controlled. Nasal decongestants and anti-histamines are prescribed. Politzerisation or Eustachian catheterization is done after nose is free of infection. Myringotomy with grommet insertion may be needed for middle ear aeration. Adenoidectomy is done in children to prevent recurrence.

POINTS TO REMEMBER

1. The length of adult Eustachian tube is 36 mm.
2. In infants the Eustachian tube is more shorter, wider and horizontal and therefore Eustachian tube dysfunction and middle ear infection are common.
3. Functional obstruction of the Eustachian tube is associated with Down's syndrome due to poor function of tensor velipalati.
4. Autophony (loudness of one's own voice) is associated with patulous Eustachian tube.

Diseases of the External Ear

12

CONGENITAL ANOMALIES OF THE EXTERNAL EAR

Abnormalities of the Auricle

1. **Minor variations of the auricle**
   - Darwin's tubercle
   - Bat ear (antihelix poorly formed)
   - Wildermuth's ear (helix under developed and antihelix is prominent)
   - Mozart's ear (helix and antihelix are found fused together)
   - Pre-auricular appendage
   - Pre-auricular pit or sinus

2. **True deformities**
   - Macrotia
   - Microtia
   - Microtia with syndrome
     - Treacher Collins syndrome
     - Pierre Robin syndrome
     - Potter's syndrome
   - LADD syndrome
   - Anotia with or without atresia of the external auditory canal.

3. **Congenital fistula**

4. **Congenital tumor**
   Cavernous hemangioma

Abnormalities of the External Meatus

- Atresia
- Atresia without microtia
- Atresia with microtia (Fig. 12.1)
- Abnormal middle ear with atresia
- Atresia with inner ear affected

Etiology

- Fetal alcohol syndrome
- Drugs like thalidomide, warfarin, hydantoin, methotrexate
- Radiation to maternal pelvis
- Virus rubella

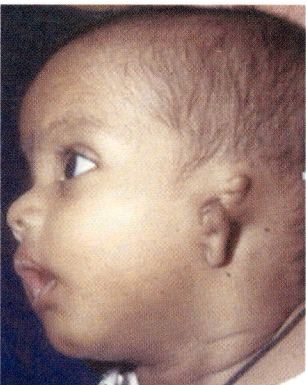

Fig. 12.1: Atresia with microtia

Treatment

- Surgical correction/ otoplasty procedures should be planned for true deformity before school going age.
- Darwin's tubercle and Bat ear can be corrected surgically with less morbidity.
- Prosthetic ear can also be used before surgical correction of microtia.
- Hearing aid and speech therapy for bilateral atresia till the date of surgery.
  - Bilateral body worn or behind the ear hearing aid.
  - BAHA (bone anchoring hearing aid) becoming popular but expensive indicated for severe conductive loss (Fig. 12.2).

SWELLING AND DEFORMITY OF THE EAR AND PINNA

1. **Preauricular region**
   - Preauricular cyst
   - Preauricular lymphadenopathy
   - Preauricular sinus.
   - Collaural fistula.
2. **Pinna**
   - **Congenital**
     - Cavernous hemangioma
     - Arteriovenous malformation (Figs 12.3a and 12.3b)
   - **Cyst**
     - Pseudocyst of pinna

- **Benign tumors**
  - Papilloma
  - Cutaneous horn
  - Keloid
  - Neurofibroma
  - Keratocanthoma
- **Malignant**
  - Squamous cell carcinoma
  - Basal cell carcinoma
  - Melanoma
- **Inflammatory conditions**
  - Chondrodermititis nodularis
  - Chronica helicis
  - Hematoma auris
  - Perichondritis
3. **Postauricular**
   - **Cyst**
     - Sebaceous cyst
     - Pseudocyst pinna
   - **Fistula and sinus**
   - **Mastoid abscess**

Treatment: Treatment of inflammatory condition, deformity and tumors are discussed separately in other chapter.

INJURY TO THE AURICLE / PINNA

Etiology

1. Trauma
   - Household accidents
   - Road traffic injury.

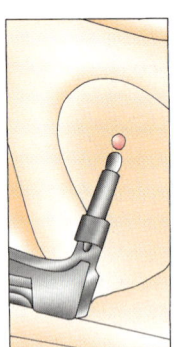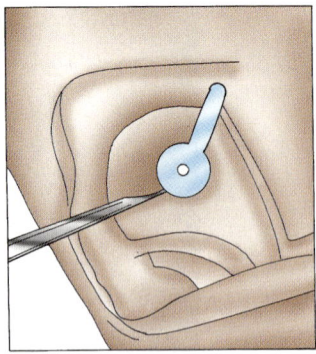

Fig. 12.2: Bone anchoring hearing aid after making drill hole in mastoid

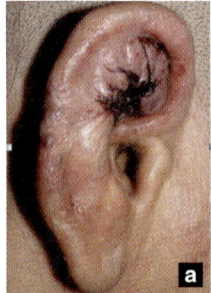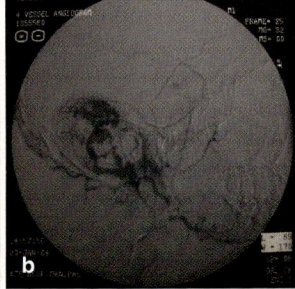

Figs 12.3a and b: (a) Arteriovenous malformation (b) Angiogram of the same patient showing tortuous supply from post-auricular artery

2. Occupational hazards
   - Burns
   - War injury
   - **Frost bite:** Exposure to extreme cold causes formation of ice crystals and obstruction to the vessels in the exposed area often pinna. Pinna becomes red initially and blue or white later depending on duration of exposure. Complete or partial loss of pinna can occur except the ear lobule.
     Treatment
     Rewarming, debridement if gangrenous, analgesics, antibiotic, toxoid.
3. Sports injuries as in boxing, wrestling, football.

Classification

1. **Injury without loss of tissue** (Fig. 12.4)
   - Small bruises
   - Lacerations
   - Hematoma (extravasation of blood between the perichondrium and cartilage).
2. **Injury with tissue loss:** Avulsion of pinna.

Clinical Examination

1. On inspection there is a fresh wound on the pinna.
2. Skin is stretched over a doughy swelling.

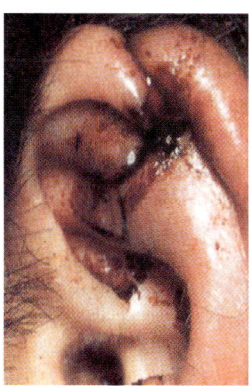 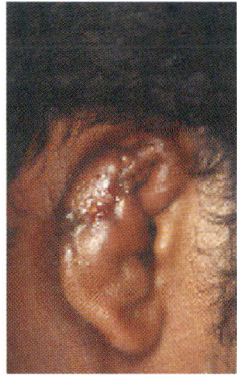

Fig. 12.4: Injury without tissue loss

3. Swelling may be localized or diffuse depending on the amount of collection.

Treatment

- The main objective of treatment is to avoid deformity.
- Tetanus toxoid should be given as prophylactic measure.
- No active treatment is required for a small bruise. Sometimes pressure bandage with 24% strong lead subacetate may be required.
- An antibiotic course should be started. Penicillin or a broad spectrum antibiotic may be given as prophylactic measure.
- In case of hematoma auris, aspiration of blood under strict aseptic conditions may be done.
- Incision and drainage-Incision is made parallel to the helix for cosmetic acceptibility. A pressure bandage is put.

Suturing can be done if Required

- Injury with loss of tissue requires adequate treatment.
- Wound debridement is done to normalise the tissue.
- Perichondritis should be prevented at all cost by using proper antibiotics and wound care.
- Repair with free and pedicled flap or prosthetic reconstruction may be required for major injuries like avulsion of pinna.

PERICHONDRITIS

Definition

Inflammation of the perichondrium with collection of pus between the perichondrium and cartilage.

Pathology (Flow chart 12.1)

Infection is essentially by pseudomonas or *staphylococcus aureus*. Occasionally, untreated or infected hematoma auris may lead to perichondritis. The cartilage gets it's vascular supply from the perichondrium. When there is collection of serous fluid or pus between the perichondrium and cartilage because of trauma or inflammation, the perichondrium will be **lifted away from the cartilage.** This will cut off the blood supply to the cartilage causing avascular necrosis. Extensive damage of the cartilage will lead to a deformity of the pinna known as **cauliflower deformity.**

Flow chart 12.1: Pathology

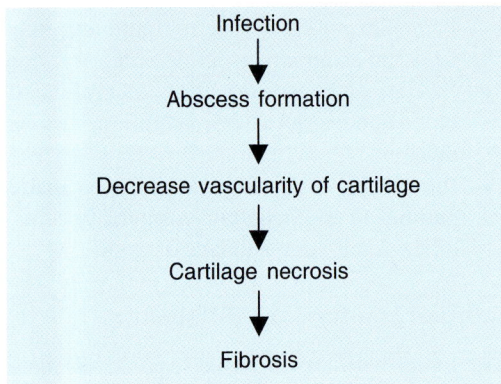

Infection

↓

Abscess formation

↓

Decrease vascularity of cartilage

↓

Cartilage necrosis

↓

Fibrosis

Deformed Pinna (Cauliflower ear)

Etiology

1. **Accidental injury** at home, road traffic injury. Hematoma auris can lead to perichondritis.
2. **Surgery** like mastoidectomy, meatoplasty, in the presence of otitis externa, endaural incision in the presence of infection.
3. **Spread from the superficial wound infection** from surrounding areas, as in infected preauricular sinus, parotid fistula, may lead to perichondritis (Fig. 12.5).

Symptoms

1. Feeling of burning sensation and warm feeling in the ear.
2. Stiff and painful movement of the ear.
3. Swelling:

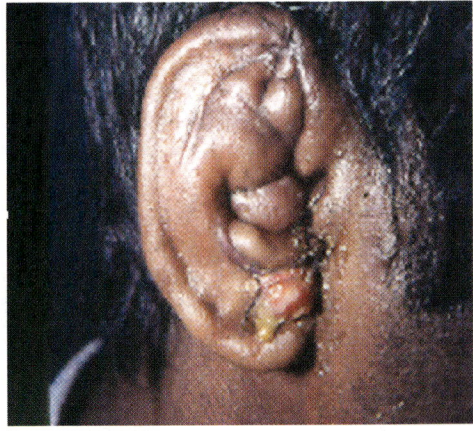

Fig. 12.5: Perichondritis (cauliflower ear)

- Localised
- Diffuse/multiple cystic

4. Deformity leading to cauliflower ear.
5. Pinna may be prominent.
6. Fever, bodyache.

Signs

1. Tenderness
2. Fluctuation in the presence of pus.

Treatment

- Prevention of perichondritis and hematoma auris is the principle.
- Lacerated wounds need regular antiseptic dressing.
- Antibiotics should be given based on culture and sensitivity of a swab taken from the affected area. Broad spectrum antibiotics should be started awaiting the results. The drug is continued if the symptoms improve within 48 hour.
- Local application of aluminium acetate.
- Aspiration under strict aseptic conditions.
- Incision and drainage and insertion of a drainage tube having multiple openings.
- Application of 20% silver nitrate/absolute phenol at the site, for cauterization of granulation tissue.
- Pressure bandage.

WAX/CERUMEN

Definition

It is a mixture of ceruminous and sebaceous gland secretions mixed with desquamated epithelium in the external auditory canal.

It is brownish or yellowish in color due to oxidative causes.

Ceruminous glands secrete watery fluid whereas sebaceous gland has a fatty secretion. It may become black or greyish when mixed with desquamated keratinized epithelium. Excretion of wax from the external auditory canal is helped by movement of the jaw while eating and talking.

Functions

1. Anti-bacterial action.
2. Traps dust and foreign body.

Causes of Excessive Wax Collection

1. Excessive formation.
2. Excessive desquamation of the canal wall.
3. Less oily sebaceous secretion.
4. Presence of stiff hair.
5. Presence of a narrow canal.
6. Presence of exostosis.
7. Excessive obliquity of the canal.
8. Occupational factors - seen among miners.
9. Living in a hot and dry climate.
10. More in apprehensive patients.

Diagnosis

Done by otoscopic examination.

Symptoms

1. Deafness—present when the canal is completely occluded and occasionally, it is sudden in onset. It is of conductive type.
2. Irritation and itching.
3. Otalgia when there is associated otitis externa.

4. Tinnitus and vertigo.
5. Cough reflex—initiated through tympanic branch of vagus.

Treatment

- Syringing for soft wax.
- Waxolytic agents for impacted wax to soften the wax. It can then be removed by syringing / suctioning.
- Use a hook or forceps—Hooking for firm wax. Before hooking, a small tunnel has to be made in the posterosuperior part between the canal and the wax (Fig. 12.6a to c).

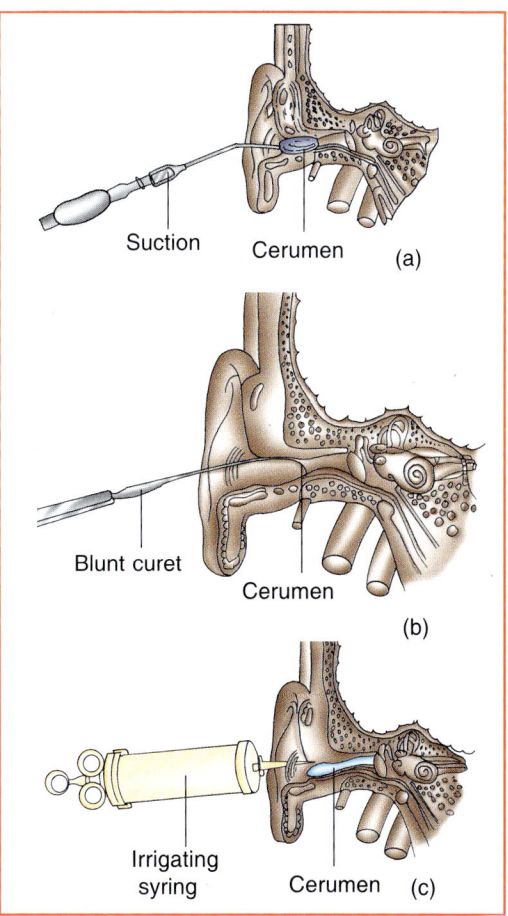

Figs 12.6a to c: (a) Wax removal by suction, (b) cleaning by hooking, (c) Syringing

KERATOSIS OBTURANS

Definition

It is a firm mass consisting of wax, desquamated keratinised epithelium and cholesterol in the external canal simulating a cholesteatoma mass. It is associated with osteitis, granulation tissue formation in the deep bony canal.

Etiology

1. Unknown.
2. Hyperemia of the canal skin.
3. Irritability of the epidermis.
   The mass is closely attached to the meatal wall and pressure effect causes erosion of the bone and widening of the bony meatus. This makes removal of the mass difficult.

Clinical Features

1. Pain—severe
2. Deafness—conductive type.
3. Tympanic membrane usually not involved.
4. Ocassionally associated with bronchiectasis and sinusitis in young adults.
5. Granulation tissue obscuring the view of the blackish mass is seen on examination of the ear.
6. Tinnitus
7. Discharge from the ear.
8. Facial nerve palsy of LMN type may occasionally occur.

Treatment

- General anesthesia is often necessary for removal of the mass.
- Use of waxolytic agents like 2% sodium bicarbonate solution to help soften the wax and facilitate removal.
- Sometimes an endaural approach may be required for removal of the mass.

Prevention

- Routine check up by an experienced otologist.
- Frequent cleaning of the external auditory canal.

FOREIGN BODY OF THE EAR

Classification (Flow chart 12.2)

Flow chart 12.2: Types of foreign bodies in the ear

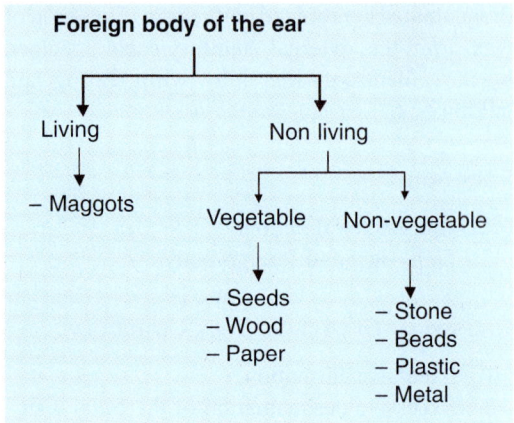

Incidence

1. Common in children.
2. Pateints with schizophrenia.
3. In persons who are bored.

Symptoms

Depends on the type of foreign body. In case of living foreign body the complaints are of pain, crawling/irritable sensation and / or noise in the ear. Vegetable foreign bodies in the ear present with irritation and deafness.

Treatment

Animate - living
- Immobilization of maggots with maggot oil/chloroform/ethyl chloride and remove with the help of forceps or hook.

Animate—nonliving (Fig. 12.7)
- Remove with currete and hook

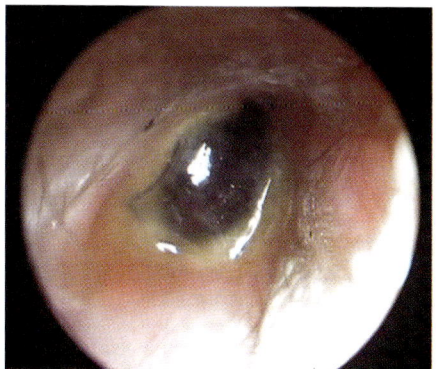

Fig. 12.7: Showing a dead insect in the external auditory canal

Inanimate—organic
- Absolute alcohol to be instilled if impacted and then remove it with hook or forceps. ***Syringing should not be tried as organic foreign bodies are hygroscopic.***

Inanimate—inorganic
- Syringing or hook or forceps can be used. Impacted inanimate foreign body may require endaural approach for removal if it cannot be removed with curet and hook due to inadequate exposure (Fig. 12.9).

Syringing

- How do you do syringing?
  It is done with an aural syringe.
- What solution do you use?
  Normal saline or any other solution at body temperature.
- Why cold water is not used?
  Cold water causes giddiness by initiating caloric response.
- Why hot water is not used?
  It causes burns and also stimulates the vestibular apparatus.

Contraindications

1. If there is history of previous ear discharge which means that the patient had a pre-existing perforation of the tympanic membrane.
2. If there is any history of head injury which may cause a fracture line connecting the middle ear and intracranial fossa.
3. Living vegetable foreign body.

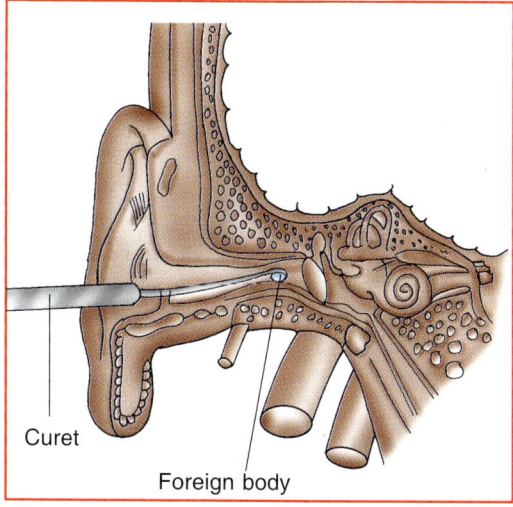

Fig. 12.8: Removal of foreign body by blunt curet

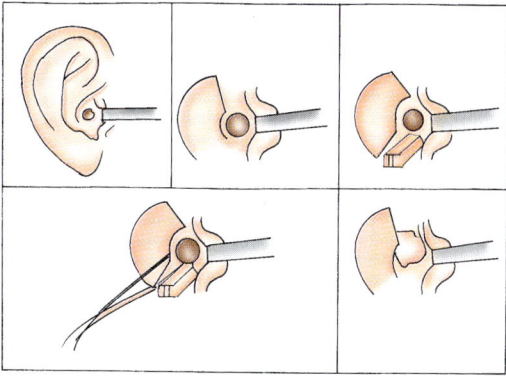

Fig. 12.9: Endaural incision showing the removal of severely impacted foreign body

Complications

1. Traumatic tympanic membrane perforation.
2. Vaso-vagal attack.
3. Further impaction of the foreign body.
4. Labyrinthine stimulation causing vertigo.

NON-INFLAMMATORY LESIONS OF THE EXTERNAL EAR

Auricle may be inflicted by a variety of lesions that are not primarily inflammatory in nature although they can get infected secondarily. The lesions in the auricle are very often overlooked in the routine clinical examination.

The Preauricular Tag and Accessory Auricle

They are small nodular masses found anterior to the tragus. When these masses are composed of skin and fat only, they are called skin tags. When it contains cartilage in addition to fat and skin, it is called **accessory auricle.** They are usually bilateral.

Treatment

It consists of simple excision purely based on cosmetic reason. However, position of the facial nerve should be kept in mind to avoid injury during surgery.

PREAURICULAR PIT

Pits are skin lined depression that are found on or just anterior to the anterior crus of helix. They are usually bilateral and develop from abnormalities of fusion of 'hillocks of His' during auricular development. It occasionally consists of small amount of cheesy keratin debris. If infected it may lead to pain, swelling associated with purulent discharge.

Treatment

1. Antibiotic

2. Complete excision of the pit may be required along with removal of part of the helical cartilage.

Preauricular Sinus/Fistula
(Figs 12.10a and b)

It is deeper. It is lined by squamous or columnar epithelium extending medially to end blindly. It may open into the external auditory canal, parotid

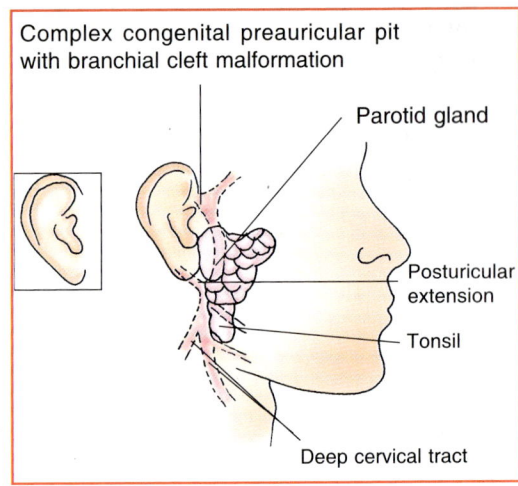

Complex congenital preauricular pit with branchial cleft malformation

Parotid gland

Posturicular extension

Tonsil

Deep cervical tract

Fig. 12.10a: Different sites of opening of the preauricular sinus

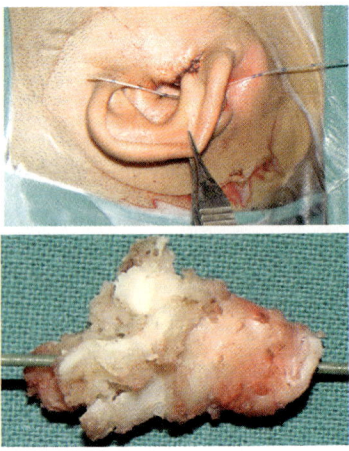

Fig. 12.10b: Collaural fistula and tract after complete excision

gland or in the region of the neck as collaural fistula.

Symptoms

Recurrent attacks of pain, swelling and discharge.

Investigations

Sinogram or fistulogram should be done whenever possible to know the extent of the tract.

Treatment

Complete surgical excision of the tract is necessary to prevent recurrence.

Cutaneous Cyst

They are usually congenital in origin, arise from the epidermis or the root of the hair follicle. Cutaneous cysts are seen more commonly in the postauricular skin. These cysts are normally insidious in onset, soft to firm in consistency and non-tender, slow growing. It may be inflamed if it is ruptured or may get infected. Infected cysts are red, tender and may discharge if the cyst ruptures (Fig.12.11).

Treatment

1. Antibiotics if infected.
2. Complete surgical excision.

Winkler's Nodule (Chondrodermatitis Nodularis Chronica Helices) (Fig. 12.12)

It is a benign lesion occuring in the rim of the helix commonly seen among the elderly people. Exposure to sunlight is blamed. Sunlight breaks the elastin fibers and trauma initiates chronic inflammation that extends down to the perichondrium.

Secondary epithelial changes develops leading to transdermal elimination of degenerated connective tissue.

On examination: The lesion is red nodular usually with a central depression or crater which is tender. The fundus of the crater is the cartilage or the perichondrium accounting for the tenderness. Tenderness is the distinguishing feature to rule out senile keratosis, keratocanthoma, cutaneous horns and carcinoma.

Treatment

Medical Treatment
Topical steroids and adhesive bandage to minimize the contact of the nodule while sleeping

Surgical Treatment
Full thickness excision of the nodule. The cartilage defect may be closed by the local advancement flaps.

Gouty Tophi of the Auricle (Fig. 12.13)

It is normally seen in the patient suffering from hyperuricemia. The uric acid crystals form a

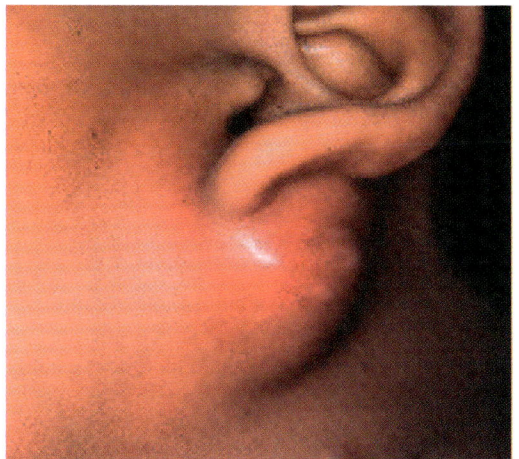

Fig. 12.11: Infected cutaneous cyst

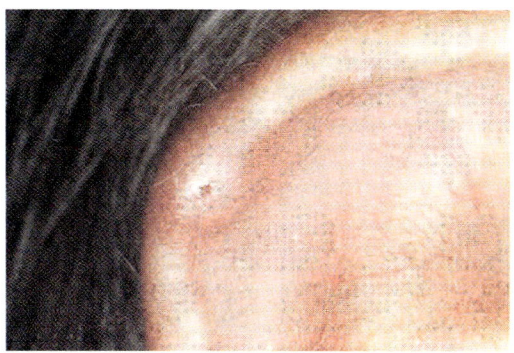

Fig. 12.12: Winkler's nodule

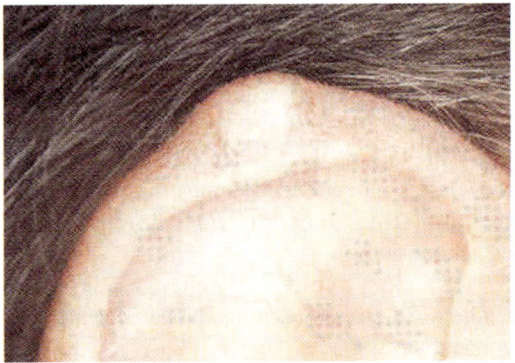

Fig. 12.13: Gouty tophi

subcutaneous nodule **most commonly on the helix.**

Nodule appears yellowish or salmon pink and is hard and gritty to touch. There is always erythemia and tenderness of the overlying skin.

Treatment

1. Dietary control of serum uric acid level.
2. Colchicine or Allopurinol drug to reduce the uric acid level.
3. Anti-inflammatory drugs like aspirin.

Hypertrophic Scars and Keloids
(Fig. 12.14)

Hypertrophied scars remain confined to the original site of injury. Histologically it consists of mature collagen. Whereas keloids often invade the adjacent untraumatized tissue causing various great cosmetic and functional deformity.

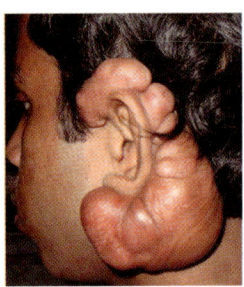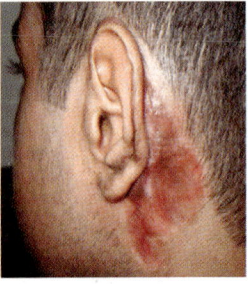

Fig. 12.14: Post-auricular keloid (preoperative and postoperative)

Histologically hypertrophic scar consists of mature collagen. Keloid contain mature collagen and thick acellular eosinophillic bundle of collagen with nodular or concentric arrangement. Collagen synthesis in keloids is 3 times greater than in hypertrophic scars and 20 times greater than in normal scars. Keloids are more seen in dark skin individuals and commonly seen in the lobule of the ear.

Treatment

1. Small keloid are best left alone with the advice of not to use ear rings in any form.
2. Topical injection of steroid with triamcinalone acetate is very effective in fresh keloid.
3. Full excision of the keloid with preservation of adjacent skin.
4. Area is closed with minimum trauma using fine non-absorbable sutures. Postoperatively the area is infiltrated with triamcinalone and hyaluronidase.
5. Use of gamma interferon injection of 5 million units in 1 ml for 1 week after excision of keloid, prevents its for their growth.
6. Laser assisted excision -KTP -532 laser, ND YAG, CO_2 laser are used for excision of keloid.
7. Silicone gel sheets and silicone occlusive dressings have been used with varied success in the treatment of keloids after surgical excision The sheets can be worn for as long as 24 h/d for up to 1 year. Good results have been seen after laser excision.

Solitary Fibromyositis

Solitary Adult Myofibroma

Myofibroma presents as small, solitary or multiple (myofibromatosis) dermal, subcutaneous or sometimes deep intramuscular nodules, usually seen in children.

Occurence of this lesion in the pinna in adult is very rare and is first reported by Balakrishnan and Pujary et al (1999).

Nodule is tender and skin over the nodule will be stretched and shiny and fixed to underlying cartilage.

Histopathological examination revealed a picture of myofibroma with hemangiopericytoma like pattern and haphazardly arranged fascicles of long spindle shaped cells with elongated nuclei around dilated vascular spaces.

Treatment

It consists of wide excision with reconstruction if necessary. Margin of the excised mass should be free of the disease.

INFLAMMATORY CONDITIONS OF EXTERNAL EAR

OTITIS EXTERNA

Definition

It is an acute inflammation of the skin lining the external auditory canal.

Classification

There are three classifications as follows:

A. **1. Localized**
- Circumscribed, e.g. furunculosis
- Diffuse, e.g. cellulitis

2. Generalized: Inflammation is not only in the external auditory canal but also in the pinna and skin of the surrounding structures.

B. **1. Infective**
- Bacterial—Furunculosis
- Viral—Herpes zoster/simplex
- Fungal—Otomycosis.

2. Reactive
- Eczema.
- Neurodermatitis
- Seborrheic dermatitis
- Psoriasis

Reactive due to exposure to allergens or contact with toxic agents.

C. **Malignant Otitis Externa**
Severe form of otitis externa associated with temporal bone osteonecrosis which is very painful and may involve the cranial nerves like facial, glossopharyngeal, vagus and hypoglossal nerves with resultant paralysis. It is seen in elderly diabetic patients.

FURUNCULOSIS

Definition

It is inflammation of the hair follicles commonly by *Staphylococcus aureus*. It is usually seen in the outer or cartilaginous part of the external auditory meatus. Furunculosis may occur as a single lesion or it may spread to the surrounding structures causing cellulitis (subcutaneous spread).

Etiology

1. **Predisposing Factors**
   1. Scratching the ear canal with dirty fingers or contaminated sticks.
   2. Trauma to the skin of the ear canal.
   3. Use of dirty and contaminated hearing aid, ear mould, stethoscope.
   4. Allergy
   5. Hereditary
   6. Immunocompromised patients, e.g. diabetics.
   7. Depression.
2. **Exciting Factors**
   1. *Staphylococcus aureus.*
   2. Gram negative organisms like pseudomonas and proteus

Symptoms

1. Pain—acute, excrutiating. If furuncle is arising from the anterior canal wall pain is aggravated while chewing.
2. Deafness—conductive deafness if there is complete occlusion of external auditory canal by the furuncle.
3. Discharge—purulent discharge from the ear if the furuncle bursts.

Signs

1. Prominence of pinna if the furuncle is associated with cellulitis. In this case pus will be trickling down from the ear.
2. Tenderness is present while moving the pinna or pressing on the tragus.

3. Ear canal may be stenosed. Furuncle may be seen.
4. Tympanic membrane appears normal on otoscopic examination

Differential Diagnosis (Table 12.1)

1. Acute mastoiditis
2. Subperiosteal mastoid abscess
3. Diffuse otitis externa

Treatment

- 10% Icthymol with glycerin pack. Glycerin is hygroscopic and therefore, helps to reduce the swelling and pain. Icthymol is a local irritant which increases the vascularity of the area and has bacteriostatic action also. Packing should be done two or three times daily.
- Antibiotics
- Analgesic
- Incision and drainage
- Prevent recurrence

Diffuse otitis externa (swimmers ear)

It is a diffuse form of inflammation of the external ear involving the entire bony meatus and can also extend to the cartilaginous part that can be presented in the acute or chronic stage.

Etiology: Maceration, scratching, clumsy instrumentation

Causative agent: *Pseudomonas, Proteus, Staph. aureus*, etc.

Pathology: In acute stage there is hyperaemia and infiltration of inflammatory cells into the epithelial and subepithelial layer. Cellulitis can develop in severe cases including involvement of periauricular soft tissue. Desquamation of meatal skin produces cheesy debris. In chronic stage meatal skin becomes thickened and hypertrophied, due to infiltration of lymphocytes and fibroblasts leading to meatal stenosis.

Clinical features: Pain in the ear is the most predominant feature in the acute stage than in chronic. Itching and purulent discharge are often present in both groups. Deafness is present if canal is completely occluded with discharge.

On examination: Pain on gentle or genle traction of the pinna may be present. Ear canal may be associated with serous discharge that may turn out to be purulent. If the condition is not treated or resolved within 4 weeks it leads to chronic stage with thickening of meatal skin and later stenosis.

Treatment: Aural toilet is very important that includes meticulous cleaning of the external ear under microscope and application of topical antibiotics with steroid ear drops. Systemic antibiotic may be given in severe cases taking care of the causative agent. In chronic cases alluminium acetate soaked wick can be applied to achieve a dry ear early.

OTOMYCOSIS

Definition

It is fungal infection affecting the external ear (Fig. 12.15). The incidence of fungal infection is high in

Table 12.1: Differences of Furunculosis and Mastoiditis

Furunculosis	Mastoiditis
1. No history of middle ear infection	History of middle ear infection
2. Tragal tenderness present	Mastoid tenderness present
3. Discharge is purulent **never** mucoid, moderate in amount	Discharge is mucoid to mucopurulent, profuse and pulsatile
4. Enlargement of preauricular and postauricular lymph node	No enlargement of pre and postauricular nodes
5. Conductive deafness mild due to occlusion of meatus	Conductive hearing loss is moderate to moderately severe
6. Normal tympanic membrane	Perforation and congestion of tympanic membrane
7. Swelling is confined to the cartilaginous part	Sagging of posterosuperior bony meatal wall
8. X-ray mastoid shows clear air cells	X-ray mastoid shows clouding of air cells

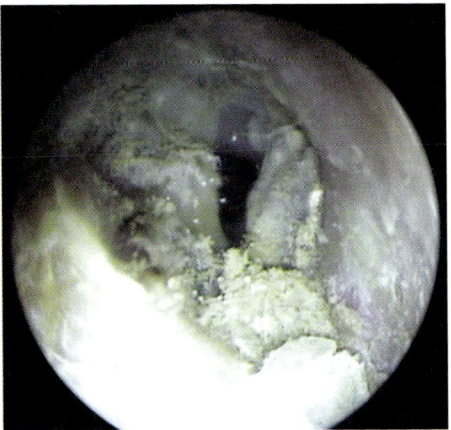

Fig. 12.15: Otomycosis in the external auditory canal

tropical and subtropical countries. Diabetes and other immunocompromised states predispose to otomycosis. *Aspergillus niger* is the commonest fungus to cause otomycosis The other fungi encountered are *Candida albicans* and *Aspergillus fumigatus*.

Organisms of Otomycosis

- *Aspergillus niger*: Black-headed filamentous growth.
- *Aspergillus fumigatus*: Green/brown.
- Candida albicans: White and creamy.
- Dermatophytes
- Actinomycosis

Symptoms

1. Irritation of the external canal. This is the **most common** symptom when infected with *Aspergillus niger*.
2. Pain predominant symptom in case of *Aspergillus flavus* infection. Also, pain may be caused by mixcd infection with fungi and bacteria.
3. Deafness—uncommon, but may be present if there is complete occlusion of the canal by the fungal mass.
4. Itching-more common in *Aspergillus niger.*
5. Discharge—sometimes minimal mucoidal discharge may be seen in the ear canal which is the byproduct of the fungal infection.

Signs

1. Pinna usually, is normal but in extensive cases skin may be infected and blebs may be seen.
2. External ear canal may be congested, ulcerated and the fungal mass will be seen.
3. Tympanic membrane may be congested occasionally but is otherwise normal.

Fungal mass is seen in three forms:

1. Dry, whitish/brownish sheets.
2. Wet and darkish white, resembling *wet blotting paper.*
3. Wet and blackish or brownish.

Investigations

1. Ear swab for culture and sensitivity and fungal smear.
2. Blood sugar estimation to rule out diabetes in severe and recurrent cases.

Treatment

1. Thorough cleaning of the fungal flakes from the external ear canal by syringing or suction cleaning.
2. Painting of the canal with either 2% salicylic acid or 1% gentian violet.
3. Anti-fungal ear drops, e.g. Nystatin.
4. Prevention of recurrent infection by keeping the ear dry.
5. Treatment of the underlying cause like diabetes.

MALIGNANT OTITIS EXTERNA

Definition

It is a severe progrcssive infection starting in the external auditory meatus, progresses rapidly involving the temporal bone and adjacent soft tissue. It is commonly seen in elderly, diabetic patients and other immunocompromised conditions.

Etiology

Causative factor: *Pseudomonas aeruginosa.* Predisposing factors are as follows:

1. Uncontrolled diabetes above 55 years of age.
2. Immunocompromised patients—AIDS, etc.
3. Malnutrition
4. Anemia (children)
5. Organ transplant recipient.

Pathogenesis

The infection starts as a cellulitis of the external auditory meatus, which is insiduous in onset. The infection spreads rapidly to the adjacent soft tissue, tympanomastoid suture, fissures of Santorini followed by cellulitis of the skull base. Infection also spreads along the vascular channel within the tympanic and petrous bone. This infective process produces a number of exotoxins and enzymes including an elastase which digests vessel wall. Some enzymes will have collagenase effect.

Involvement of the mastoid causes spread to the lateral, superior and inferior petrosal sinus producing osteomyelitis of the petrous apex, floor of the middle cranial fossa and basisphenoid. The 9th, 10th, 11th and 12th cranial nerves may also get involved in late cases. Contralateral involvement of the petrous apex and basisphenoid have also been seen in few cases. Infection leads to granuloma formation.

Clinical Features

Symptoms

- Pain—severe continuous pain in the external and deep meatus.
- Discharge—mucopurulent in the initial stage, purulent and blood stained in the late stages.
- Deafness—sensorineural hearing loss.
- Facial nerve palsy—lower motor neuron type.

Signs

- Pinna will be doughy on palpation.
- Tenderness on pulling the pinna.
- Mastoid tenderness in late cases.

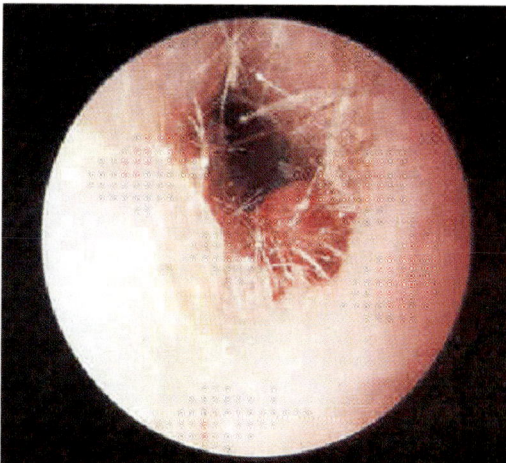

Fig.12.16: Granulation in floor of EAC in malignant otitis externa

Otoscopic Examination (Fig.12.16)

1. External auditory canal (EAC) is narrow and discharge is present.
2. Granulation tissue in the deep meatus is the hallmark finding.
3. Sagging of the posterior meatal wall.
4. Tympanic membrane is normal in early cases.
5. May show bulge, congestion and granulation if middle ear is involved.
6. Signs of multiple cranial nerve paralysis in late cases.

Investigations

- Ear swab for culture and sensitivity test.
- Blood examination—complete blood picture
- Fasting blood sugar, erythrocyte sedimentation rate.
- Renal function tests and liver function tests are important because the patient has to be treated with antibiotics for longer duration
- CT scan /MRI with gallium contrast will show evidence of temporal bone involvement and extent of the disease.
- Isotope bone scan - demonstrates increased uptake in the region of skull base in active

cases (traditionally was diagnosed by technetium -99).

- A greater degree of diagnostic accuracy by single photon emission tomograph (SPECT) with two radionuclide tracer.

Treatment

- Antipseudomonal antibiotics are to be selected after culture and sensitivity tests. Antibiotics are usually given for a period of three months. Commonly recommended antibiotics are gentamycin/tobramycin, ticarcillin, etc. Maintainence dose of antibiotics is important to prevent relapse.
- Control of diabetes—insulin and other anti-diabetic therapy.
- Surgical treatment mainly consists of drainage of the subperiosteal abscess and removal of necrotic sequestrated bone
- Laser therapy-Author's personal experience of use of KTP -532 laser in excision of granulation is very satisfactory. So author recommends the laser surgery to prevent recurrence of granulation tissue
- Prognosis is usually bad.

Herpes Zoster Oticus (Ramsay Hunt's Syndrome)

Herpes zoster oticus may present clinically as an isolated herpetiform eruption of the external ear. It is, therefore, convenient to consider the disease, although primarily neurological, under otitis externa due to a virus infection.

Herpes zoster, considered in general, arises from inflammation of one or more posterior sensory root ganglia or their cranial analogs, and has been called posterior polimyelitis.

Organism

- *H. simplex*
- *H. zoster*

Features of H. zoster

- Site of affection: Geniculate ganglion of the facial nerve.

- May also involve the IX and X cranial nerves.
- Attacks are more common in adults than in children.

Sign and Symptoms

- Severe otalgia
- Sometimes disturbance of hearing and balance
- Vesicular eruptions on external auditory canal or pinna of the affected ear (The vesicles) are in the epidermis and are associated with a swelling of prickle cells called balloon cells.
- Facial nerve palsy (LMN type)

Hunt divided the syndrome into three clinical groups they are:

1. Herpes auricularis
2. Herpes auricularis with facial palsy
3. Herpes auricularis with facial palsy and auditory symptoms.

Treatment

1. Symptomatic treatment
2. Oral acyclovir—800 mg 5X/Day (To be started within 72 hours of the onset of rash).

TUMORS OF THE EXTERNAL AUDITORY CANAL

OSTEOMA AND EXOSTOSIS

Definition (Fig.12.17)

They are bony tumors that may occur in the deeper portion of the external auditory canal.

There are two types:

1. Multiple of ivory bone origin (exostosis)
2. Solitary of cancellous bone origin (osteoma).

Exostosis is more common than osteoma and can arise from any wall of the external auditory canal whereas solitary osteoma arise from the posterior wall by a narrow base and appear as a smooth rounded body which may be completely filling the canal.

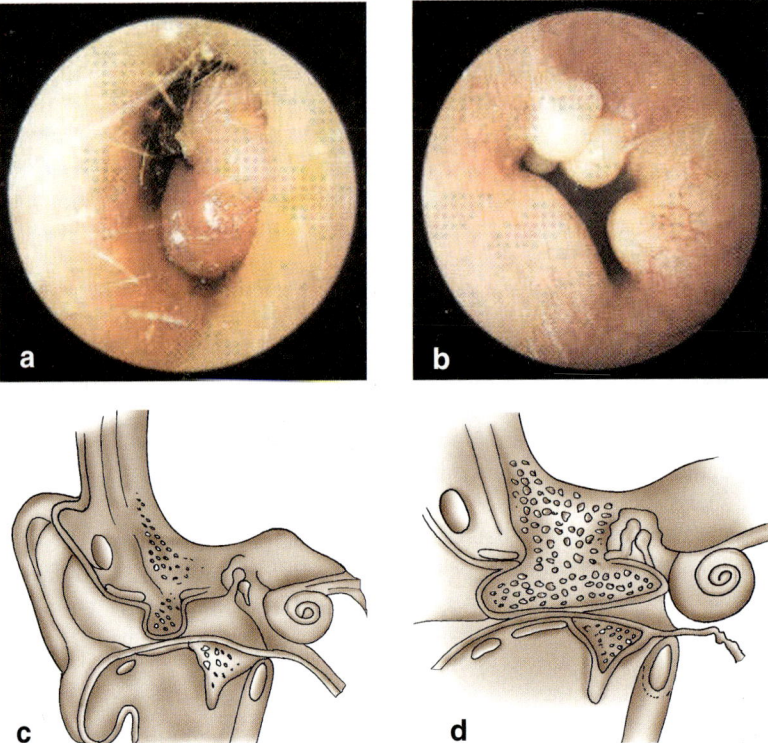

Figs 12.17a to d: (a) Solitary osteoma (b) Multiple osteoma, (c and d) Diagrammatic representation of osteoma arising from bony canal wall

Etiology

- **Swimming:** Repeated entry of cold water into the external auditory canal in swimming and diving is regarded as a primary cause for exotosis formation.
- **Otitis** externa of long duration may also initiate formation of osteoma.
- **Chronic suppurative otitis media:** The discharge may stimulate the skin of the canal leading to osteoma formation.

Symptoms

1. Usually asymptomatic and diagnosed as an incidental finding.
2. Irritation and itching because of the wax collection.
3. Blocked sensation in the ear.

4. Deafness—if the osteoma is large enough to block the canal.
5. Pain is usually associated with otitis externa.

Signs

1. On examination, a hard mass in the deeper part of the external auditory canal is seen. It may be covered by impacted wax.
2. Tympanic membrane is not seen if the osteoma is occluding the canal.
3. Excessive accumulation of wax may be seen due to defective cleansing mechanism of the ear.

Treatment

- Asymptomatic—no treatment.
- Symptomatic multiple osteoma—excised with a microdrill.

- Solitary osteoma—Chiselled with an osteotome along with canal skin.
- Skin grafting—If there is extensive loss of canal skin during surgery.

MALIGNANT TUMORS

Common tumors of the pinna and external auditory canal are:
- Squamous cell carcinoma
- Adenocarcinoma
- Melanoma
- Basal cell carcinoma
- Sebaceous cell carcinoma

Etiology

Mostly unknown
The known causative factors are:
1. Chronic inflammation in the form of otitis externa.
2. Radiation
3. Carcinogens within cerumen. Alpha toxin B is a potent hepatic carcinogen which can occasionally be a transient contaminant of the ear canal.

Squamous Cell Carcinoma

It is commonly seen in the bony external auditory canal and presents with blood stained ear discharge with an ulcerating mass in the external auditory meatus. It may spread to middle ear and other part of temporal bone, parotid gland and skull base. In advanced cases can produce pain and facial nerve paralysis.

Investigations

- Punch biopsy to confirm the diagnosis.
- CT scan
- Audiometry.

Treatment (Figs 12.18a to c) and (Figs 12.19a to d)
1. Radiotherapy for early malignancy.
2. Surgery
   - Lateral temporal bone resection/sleeve excision of external auditory canal—In early case
   - Wide excision—Partial temporal bone excision which includes the tympanic bone, temporomandibular joint and parotid gland.
3. Chemotherapy - Results are not satisfactory.

Adenocarcinoma (Fig. 12.20a)

This may appear as a papillary or cystic growth in the external auditory canal. It causes obstruction of the external auditory canal. Pain is mostly seen in adenoid cystic carcinoma. It has a long natural history.

Treatment (Fig. 12.20b)
1. Wide excision of the external auditory canal and surrounding bone.

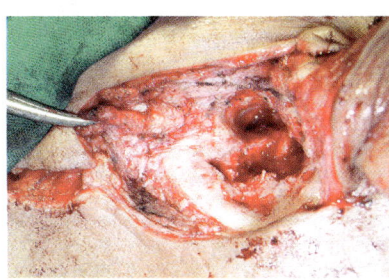 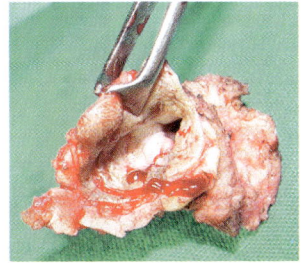 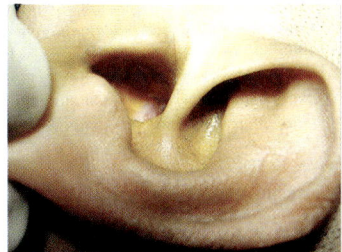

Fig.12.18a: Intraoperative photograph of sleeve excision   **Fig. 12.18b:** Specimen of sleeve excision   **Fig. 12.18c:** External auditory canal after sleeve resection

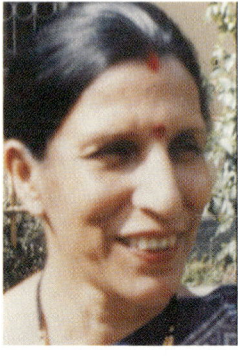

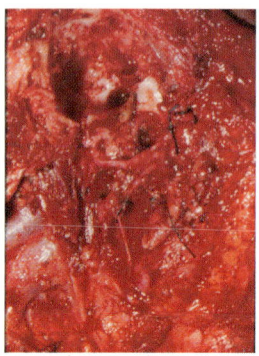

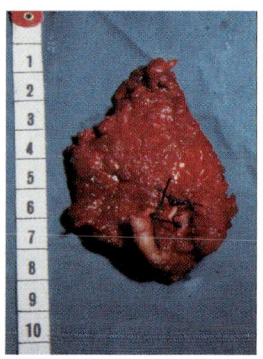

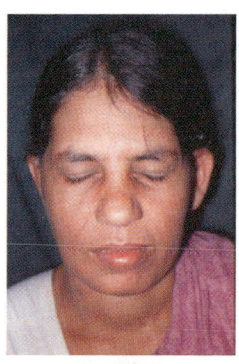

Fig. 12.19a: Post sleeve excision photograph showing no facial palsy

Fig.12.19b: Partial temporal resection with preservation of facial nerve

Fig.12.19c: Specimen of partial temporal bone resection

Fig. 12.19d: Post operative partial temporal resection having no facial palsy

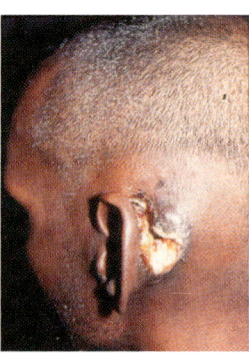

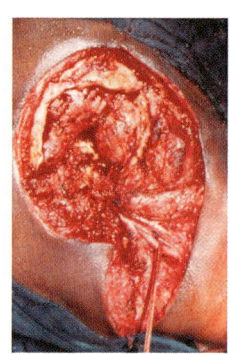

Figs 12.20a and b: (a) Preoperative picture of adenocarcinoma (b) Intraoperative photograph of subtotal petrosectomy with exposing dura middle and posterior cranial fossa

2. Extended radical mastoidectomy, excision of dura
3. Total petrosectomy in extensive cases.

Malignant Melanoma

It is rare, mostly seen in the pinna. It appears as a black mole. Usually it is a very aggressive tumor. Spontaneous regression has been reported in rare cases.

Investigations—Biopsy.

Biopsy

Treatment

1. Surgical excision
2. Radiotherapy
3. Chemotherapy

Basal Cell Carcinoma
(Figs 12.21a and b)

It usually presents in the pinna as a small non healing ulcerative growth. It is commonly seen in tropical climates.

Biopsy is confirmatory.

Treatment

Surgical excision and reconstruction.

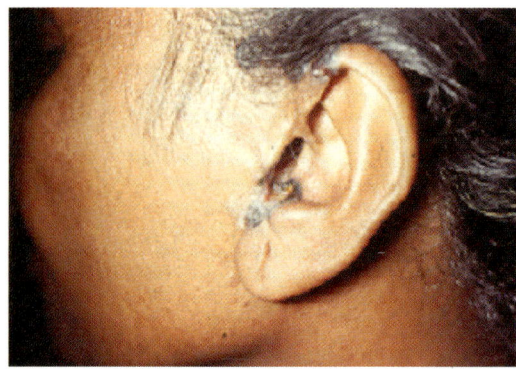

Fig. 12.21a: Basel cell carcinoma

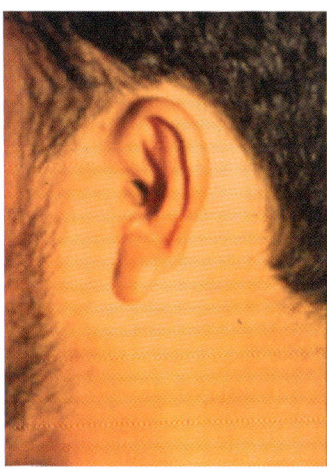

Fig. 12.21b: Postoperative photograph of surgical exicision and reconstruction

Sebaceous Cell Carcinoma

This is an extremely rare tumor that can occur in any part of the body. It is commonly seen in the head and neck region mainly in the concha of the ear and nose. Tumor is confirmed by biopsy.

Treatment
Excision.

INFLAMMATORY DISEASES OF THE TYMPANIC MEMBRANE

MYRINGITIS BULLOSA HEMORRHAGICA

Definition

It is a painful inflammatory condition of the tympanic membrane characterised by the formation of blisters of various sizes on the tympanic membrane and deep ear canal.

Etiology

Exact cause is not known. Possible organisms are:
1. Viruses
2. Mycoplasma
3. Bacteria

Clinical Features

Symptoms
- Pain - sudden in onset, severe in nature and seasonal.
- Fullness of the ear.
- Blood stained discharge, not foul smelling.
- Mild conductive hearing loss may be present.

Signs
Otoscopic examination—presence of blisters or bullae on the tympanic membrane and deep external auditory canal (Fig. 12.22).

Bullae may be filled with serous or hemorrhagic fluid. This involves both the tympanic membranes.

Treatment
- Analgesics
- Topical antibiotic and steroid ear drops.
- Systemic antibiotics if associated with bacterial infection.

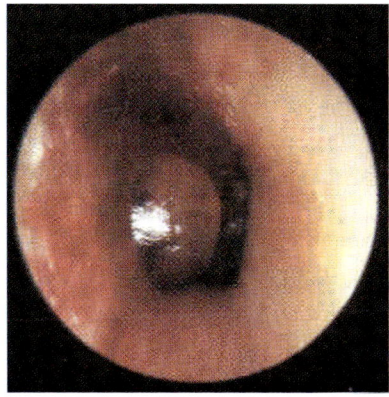

Fig. 12.22: Otoscopic view of blisters of the tympanic membrane in case of myringitis bullosa

GRANULAR MYRINGITIS

Definition

This is an inflammatory process of the tympanic membrane characterised by the appearance of patchy granulations over the surface of the tympanic membrane.

Causative factors—not known.

1. Tubal dysfunction producing negative pressure in the middle ear is blamed.
2. Fungal infection—possibility of fungal infection has to be ruled out.

Clinical Features

Symptoms

1. Mild pain.
2. Ear discharge—mostly mucoidal and tenacious.

Signs

- Presence of granulation tissue on the tymapanic membrane which may be localised to any quadrant of the tympanic membrane but most frequently to the posterosuperior and central part.

Treatment

1. Antibiotic ear drops after culture.
2. Silver nitrate cautery of the granulation tissue in multiple sittings

TRAUMATIC PERFORATION OF THE TYMPANIC MEMBRANE

Etiology

1. Faulty technique of cleaning the ear
2. While removing a foreign body from the ear
3. Forceful syringing
4. Increase in air pressure while slapping
5. Travelling in an non-pressurised air craft
6. Blast
7. Sudden fluid compression while diving
8. Forceful blowing of the nose
9. Associated with head injury

Symptoms

1. Pain in the ear
2. Discharge - mainly blood stained.
3. Deafness - usually conductive type.
4. Tinnitus.
5. Vertigo.

Signs

1. Fresh bleeding or blood clot is seen in the external auditory canal.
2. Tympanic membrane perforation seen is mostly central and the margins of the perforation are irregular and congested (Fig. 12.23).
3. Tuning fork tests and audiometry will show a conductive deafness.

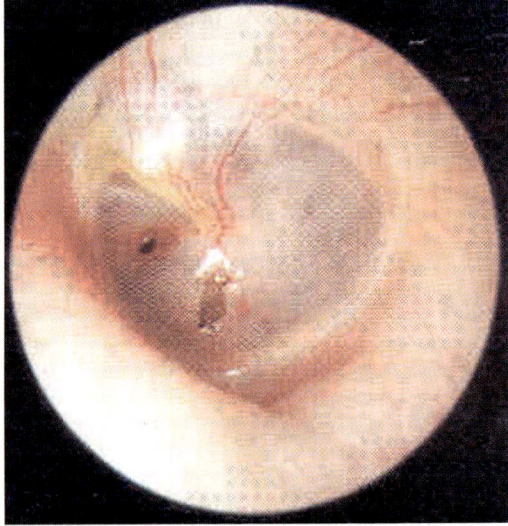

Fig. 12.23: Otoscopic view of tympanic membrane after blast injury

Treatment

- External auditory canal in the affected side should be plugged with a cotton ball.
- No ear drops should be instilled.

- No attempt should be made to clean the ear.
- Antibiotics, anti-inflammatory, analgesics and nasal decongestants should be prescribed.
- If infected, should be treated as chronic suppurative otitis media.
- If perforation persists inspite of the above conservative treatment, margins of the perforation can be cauterized with trichloroacetic acid and silver nitrate. If it still persists, the perforation is closed by myringoplasty or tympanoplasty.

Eczematous otitis externa: It is an allergic dermatitis of external ear that may accompany typical atopic eczema or other primary skin conditions.

Associated conditions: Atopic Triad (Family History)
- Eczematous Dermatitis (Atopic Dermatitis)
- Allergic Rhinitis
- Asthma

Provocative factors: Emotional stress, excessive sweating, food allergy, low humid conditions leading to dryness of the skin.

Pathology:

Acute stage: Irritation, redness, edema, are common. Vesication, weeping and crust formation can be seen in severe cases.

Chronic stage: The skin becomes hypertrophied due to secondary infection leading to scaling and fissure and finally stenosis of the external auditory canal.

Clinical feature: Itching and swelling associated with discharge is the main presenting feature. Deafness is present if the meatus is completely excluded.

On examination: External auditory canal may be swollen and red associated with ulcerations, fissuring, scaling in the acute stage and thickening, narrowing and stenosis in the chronic stage.

Treatment:

Acute stage
- Application of hydrocortisone ointment
- Systemic antihistaminics

Chronic stage
- Packing the canal with aluminum acetate wick
- Steroid ear drops can prevent itching
- Surgical: Canal plasty, treatment of atopy

Seborrhoeic otitis externa: It is a greasy, scaling and crusting condition of external auditory canal.

Etiology
- Not fully understood
- Associated with seborrhoeic dermatitis (dandruff) of scalp
- Superimposed infection
- Malassezia furfur, a lipophilic yeast, thought to play a role in the development of this condition.

Clinical Features

Greasy yellow scales line, the external auditory canal that commonly affects postauricular sulcus and lobule itching and scratching leads to secondary infection and discharge

Treatment: Shampoo: Selenium sulphide
- Salicylic acid and sulphur 2% aq. cream
- AURAL TOILET
- Secondary infection must be controlled before the basic treatment.

POINTS TO REMEMBER

1. Perichondritis of the pinna can give rise to cauliflower deformity, if associated with extensive cartilage necrosis.

2. Syringing should not be tried in case of organic foreign bodies as they are hygroscopic.

3. Malignant otitis externa is a very severe form of condition that is associated with osteonecrosis of the temporal bone and can give rise to life-threatening complications. This condition is seen in diabetes melitus and other immunocompromise condition.

13

Temporal Bone Fracture

The temporal bone is the most complex bone in the human body. It houses many vital structures, including the cochlear and vestibular end organs and the facial nerve, carotid artery and jugular vein. Involvement of none or all of these structures in temporal bone fractures is possible.

Etiology

- Head injuries, physical assaults, falls, road traffic accidents, gunshot wounds.
- Males aged 21 to 30 years comprise the most commonly involved group.

Classification

Fractures of the temporal bone are commonly classified based on the relationship of the fracture line to the long axis of the temporal bone (Fig. 13.1).

A. **Longitudinal fractures** are the most common accounting for 70 to 90% of the temporal bone fractures. This fracture extends along the length of the temporal bone.

B. **Transverse fractures** extend directly across the petrous bone and make up about 10 to 30% of temporal bone fractures.

C. **Mixed fractures** display some characteristics of each of the above.

Longitudinal Fractures

Longitudinal fractures comprise 70 to 90% of all temporal bone fractures.

Mechanism of Injury

They are caused by a lateral force over the mastoid or squamous bone.

Extent

The fracture line parallels the long axis of the petrous pyramid. It starts in the pars squamosa, extends through the posterosuperior bony external

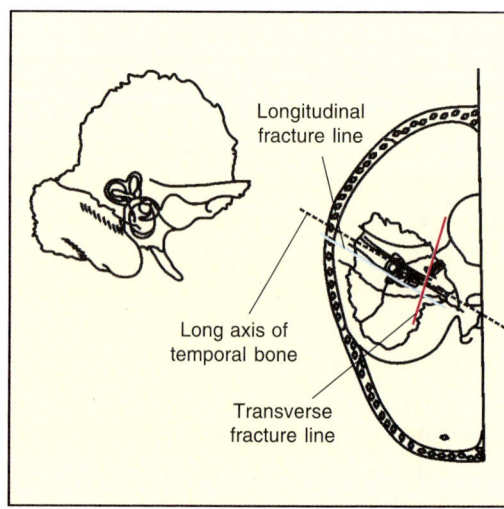

Fig. 13.1: Temporal bone fracture

canal, continues across the roof of the middle ear space anterior to the labyrinth, and ends in the middle cranial fossa near the foramen spinosum.

Oblique fractures produce a similar fracture line in the middle cranial fossa but differ externally. Oblique fractures cross the petrotympanic fissure and longitudinal fractures are contained within it. They are grouped with longitudinal fractures.

Signs and Symptoms

1. Bleeding into the ear canal from skin and tympanic membrane laceration.

2. Ossicular chain disruption producing conductive hearing loss, sensorineural hearing loss may occur as a result of concussive damage.

3. *Facial nerve paralysis (10–20%):* The injury site is usually the horizontal segment distal to the geniculate ganglion. This results from edema, intraneural hemorrhage, bony fragment impingement and dehiscence of the nerve.

4. Cerebrospinal fluid (CSF) otorhinorrhea is common but usually temporary.

5. Bilateral fractures are present in 29% of all fractures.

Transverse Fractures

Transverse fractures comprise 10 to 30% of all temporal bone fractures.

Mechanism of Injury

They are usually caused by a frontal or parietal blow but may result from an occipital blow.

Extent

The fracture line runs perpendicular to the long axis of the petrous pyramid and starts in the middle cranial fossa, crosses the petrous pyramid transversely, and ends at the foramen magnum. It may extend through the internal auditory canal and injure the nerves directly. Cochlear and vestibular structures are usually destroyed.

Signs and Symptoms

1. Profound sensorineural hearing loss rarely, a mixed hearing loss may occur.

2. Severe ablative vertigo. The vertigo persists until compensation occurs. Nystagmus is common.

3. *Facial nerve paralysis (50%):* The injury site is anywhere from the internal auditory canal to the horizontal segment proximal to the geniculate ganglion. Pneumolabyrinth may be a sign. Medial fractures can occur without otic capsule involvement (true skull base fractures).

4. Hemotympanum

5. The battle sign (ecchymosis of the post-auricular skin) may be noted in either type of fracture.

Histopathologically, hair cell loss, ganglion cell loss, and supporting cell loss occur. Rarely, labyrinthitis ossificans occurs from trauma or subsequent infection. This must be kept in mind when considering the placement of cochlear implants after temporal bone fracture.

Penetrating Wounds

Stab wounds and gunshot wounds are the most common penetrating wounds. Gunshot wounds medial to the geniculate ganglion are usually fatal. The otic capsule may act as a missile deflector, protecting the brain.

Associated injuries of cranial nerves (other than the seventh), intracerebral damage and arterial or venous injury can occur. These are the most severe of the temporal bone injuries.

Gunshot wounds to the temporal bone often result in profound sensorineural hearing loss, facial nerve disruption and CSF leak.

Differences between longitudinal and transverse fractures are given in Table 13.1.

Examination

A complete neuro-otologic examination, as well as a complete nose and throat examination is mandatory.

	Transverse fracture	Longitudinal fracture
Table 13.1: Differences between longitudinal and transverse fractures		
Incidence	10 to 30%	70 to 90%
Mechanism of injury	Frontal or parietal blow	Lateral force over the mastoid or squamous bone
Fracture line	Runs perpendicular to the long axis of the petrous pyramid	Parallel to the long axis of petrous pyramid
Cochlear and vestibular structure	Involved	(Tympanic membrane, perforation, ossicular chain disruption)
Type of hearing loss	Sensorineural	Conductive loss
CSF otorhinorrhea	Rare	Common
Vertigo	Severe	Minimal
Hemotympanum	Common	Rare(bleeding from ear)
Facial nerve paralysis	50%	<20%

1. Look for the impact site on the skull.
2. Taking aseptic precautions, examine the external canal for blood or CSF. Lacerations, step deformities and tympanic membrane lacerations/perforations. Check for hemotympanum.

   Do not lavage the ear canal and do not use packing in the canal unless bleeding is difficult to control, because either may introduce infection to the cochlea and labyrinth, as well as to the brain and meninges.
3. If the patient's condition permits, test the hearing with tuning forks. Complete audiometric testing can be performed later.
4. Examine the eyes for nystagmus. Severe nystagmus (ablative) often occurs in patients with transverse fractures. If the patient is conscious, determine if he or she has vertigo.
5. Examine the mandible and mid face for fractures.
6. Examine the facial nerve. Checking for paralysis (and determining whether it is of immediate or delayed onset) is crucial. This may be difficult to determine if the patient is intubated or comatose or if muscle relaxants have been administered. Painful stimuli may elicit a grimace response, even in comatose patients.

Investigation

High-resolution CT scanning of the temporal bones is useful in injuries complicated by CSF leak or facial paralysis and is typically ordered as axial and coronal images, with 1 - mm slices and magnified views of the temporal bones.

Complications and its Management

These patients may have multiple trauma injuries; therefore, stabilization of the patient must be accomplished first. The cervical spine should be evaluated before manipulation of the head.

1. **Hearing Loss**

   Conductive hearing loss is frequently observed with longitudinal fractures and is caused by hemotympanum, tympanic membrane perforation partial or complete ossicular chain disruption. Ossicular chain dislocation is more common than ossicular chain fracture. Tympanic membrane perforations and hemotympanum usually resolve in 3 to 4 weeks.

   Axial and coronal high-resolution CT scans are helpful for diagnosis of ossicular chain dislocation.

   Incudostapedial joint separation: The incudostapedial joint is the most common site of traumatic separation because the incus has weak attachments to the malleus and the stapes. The malleus is anchored by the tensor tympani muscle and its tendon, and the stapes is anchored by the stapedius muscle and its tendon. They contract during trauma and pull the incus medially. This movement is accentuated by the trauma, causing medial dislocation of the incus.

Most nondisruptive conductive hearing losses resolve spontaneously. If conductive hearing loss is present at greater than 30 dB after 3 months, consider surgical exploration.

Sensorineural hearing loss: Severe-to-profound sensorineural hearing loss most commonly occurs in patients who have transverse fractures with otic capsule involvement. Partial sensorineural loss is also possible. Mild high-frequency loss (5 KHz notch) may occur in longitudinal fractures from cochlear concussion. When vertigo is present with fluctuating or progressive hearing loss, traumatic endolymphatic hydrops or perilymphatic fistula is the diagnosis.

Mixed hearing loss: Mixed conductive and sensorineural hearing loss may be difficult to detect in the presence of severe sensorineural hearing loss. Surgical correction is considered when gain from correction of the conductive component is expected.

2. Vertigo

Causes:

- Transverse temporal bone fractures usually cause damage to the cochlea and semicircular canals; subsequent vertigo is usually severe and ablative.
- Post-traumatic benign paroxysmal positional vertigo is common.
- Perilymphatic fistula may also cause paroxysmal vertigo. Onset of fistula and its symptoms may be delayed. This diagnosis is considered when fluctuating

hearing loss and vertigo are present in the immediate post-traumatic period. Medical treatment initially consists of bed rest, head elevation, and stool softeners. Surgical exploration may be indicated in persistent perilymphatic fistulas.

- *Traumatic endolymphatic hydrops:* Vertigo usually resolves over 3 to 6 months; however, may persist in elderly patients. Vestibular rehabilitation or canal repositioning may be of value in BPPV.

3. Cerebrospinal Fluid Fistula

CSF fistula may occur as a result of dural tear in all types of temporal bone fractures. The leak almost always stops within 4 to 6 weeks.

Presentation

A. Otorrhea, through a canal laceration or tympanic membrane laceration, is usually the presenting symptom.
B. CSF can also be observed in the middle ear behind an intact tympanic membrane after the blood resorbs.
C. Rhinorrhea may be the only symptom.

The most common sites of fistula are the tegmen tympani, internal auditory canal and posterior mastoid air cells.

Investigations

1. Testing the fluid for glucose is helpful but lacks specificity.
2. Beta 2 transferrin assay is the most accurate diagnostic test for CSF.
3. The halo test using a filter paper may be helpful (separates CSF from blood).
4. High-resolution CT scans and CT cisternography in localizing the site of CSF leak. If the bony defect is not identified, metrizamide myelography is usually the next diagnostic procedure of choice.

Treatment

- CSF leaks tend to close spontaneously with elevation of the head, bed rest, stool softeners, cessation of sneezing and nose blowing.

- Intermittent lumbar punctures or indwelling lumbar drains.
- Acetazolamide or other dehydrating agents may be used.
- The use of antibiotics in the presence of CSF fistula is controversial.
- Surgical exploration may be indicated in persistent perilymphatic fistulas.

4. **Meningitis**

The risk of meningitis is very low in patients with leaks lasting less than 7 days. Incidence increases to 33 to 54% in leaks lasting greater than 7 days. The risk of meningitis increases in patients who have temporal bone fractures with CSF fistula, open lacerations, and co-existing infections.

5. **Facial nerve paralysis**

In longitudinal fractures

The most common site of facial nerve involvement is the horizontal segment of the intratympanic portion distal to geniculate ganglion (compression and ischemia are usually the cause). Onset may be immediate or delayed and partial or complete.

In transverse fractures

The usual location of injury is anywhere from the internal auditory meatus to the horizontal segment proximal to the geniculate ganglion (the nerve is avulsed or severed by the comminuted bone fragments). Facial nerve paralysis is usually immediate in onset and complete.

Management

1. Delayed—onset paralysis: Almost always recovers.

2. Immediate paralysis of a partial nature also almost always recovers; these patients should be treated conservatively.

3. Immediate complete paralysis usually means a severed nerve. Recovery rates are lower for immediate - onset paralysis. Facial nerve decompression may be done in immediate onset paralysis.

6. **Rare complications**

Abducent nerve paralysis usually occurs in the area of the Meckel's cave and the Dorello canal. Recovery within 6 months is usual. Alternate eye patching may be the only treatment necessary.

Trigeminal nerve damage usually occurs in the area of the Meckel cave; treatment is conservative. Mastication muscles may be involved.

Sigmoid sinus thrombosis occurs but is rare. The Griesinger sign (mastoid emissary vein thrombosis due to thrombus extension) may be noted.

Treatment may require exploration of the sinus and ligation of the jugular veins in the neck.

Post-traumatic cholesteatoma is a late complication of temporal bone fracture and is caused by skin entrapment in the cranial vault or temporal bone. Treatment is surgical.

Sympathetic cochleolabyrinthitis is a rare complication of temporal bone fracture. The condition is very significant because of the potential for hearing loss in the only ear with hearing. Treatment includes immuno-suppression.

POINTS TO REMEMBER

1. Longitudinal fracture comprise 70 to 90% of all temporal bone fractures.
2. In transverse fracture, facial nerve paralysis is usually immediate in onset and complete.
3. Longitudinal fracture is commonly associated with conductive hearing loss where as transverse fracture is associated with sensorineural hearing loss.

14

Diseases of the Middle Ear

OTITIS MEDIA

Definition

It is the inflammation of the mucous membrane of the middle ear cleft.

Classification

1. Acute otitis media
   - Non suppurative (inlcuding Barotrauma)
   - Suppurative
2. Chronic otitis media
   - Non-suppurative
     - Otitis media with effusion
     - Adhesive otitis media.
     - Tympanosclerosis
   - Suppurative
3. Specific type of otitis media (tuberculosis syphilis, diphtheria).

NON-SUPPURATIVE OTITIS MEDIA

Otitis media with efffusion:
Synonyms: Secretory otitis media, Glue ear, Serous otitis media, Seromucinous otitis media.

Definition

It is the accumulation of non-inflammatory exudate in the middle ear cavity following a series of pathological changes in the mucous membrane of the middle ear. Commonly seen in children.

Etiology (Fig. 14.1)

The exact etiology is not known.

1. **Tubal occlusion:** In children, enlargement of the adenoids and any infection in the nose or throat can give rise to tubal occlusion. Tubal occlusion will produce negative pressure in the middle ear cavity causing tympanic membrane retraction. Also, the middle ear mucosa will absorb the air from the middle ear producing more negative pressure. These are the key factors in

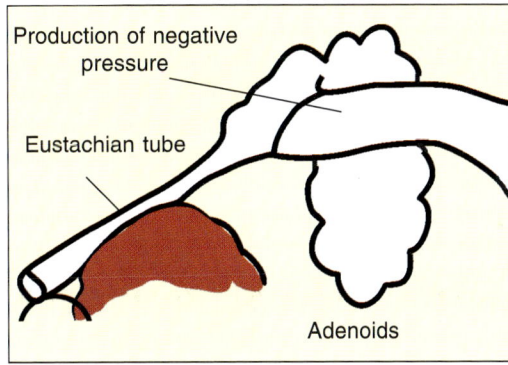

Fig. 14.1: Production of negative pressure in middle ear due to occlusion of ET by adenoid hypertrophy

145

producing changes leading to the formation of sterile effusion in the middle ear cavity. Exudate may be of varying consistency from thick tenacious mucous to thin serous. In children it is very viscid, tenacious and mucoid, hence called *glue ear.*

2. **Allergy**: Can cause mucosal edema of the Eustachian tube orifice.

3. **Hypogammaglobulinemia:** Predisposes to inflammatory response because of low immune status.

Pathogenesis (Fig. 14.2)

Symptoms (Often asymptomatic)

1. Blocking sensation of the ears.
2. Deafness - conductive type. It is usually bilateral in children and unilateral in adults.
3. The child's performance in school will be low.

4. Wooly feeling in the ear.
5. Autophony.

Associated symptoms

- Nasal discharge.
- Nasal obstruction.

Signs

1. Tympanic membrane appears dull and lusterless but may occasionally appear congested in the initial stage.
2. Retraction of the tympanic membrane.
3. Evidence of fluid in the middle ear in which the fluid level may be seen as an air bubble (Fig. 14.3).
4. Mobility of the tympanic membrane is decreased.
5. *Tuning fork tests* : Rinne test - negative on the affected side. Weber test - lateralised to the affected side. Absolute bone conduction -normal.

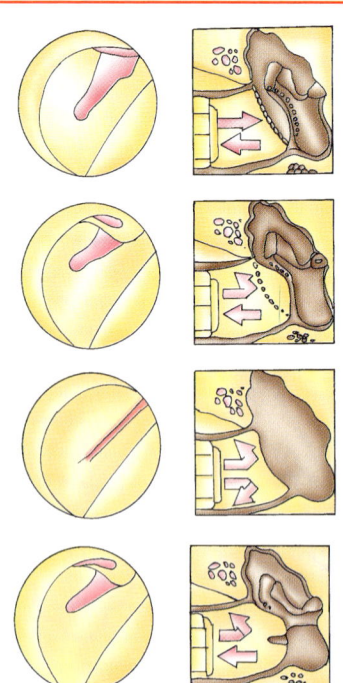

Normal
Position- neutral
Color - normal
Translucency- translucent
Mobility- moves briskly with slight positive and negative pressure

Negative Middle Ear Pressure
Position- retracted
Color - normal
Translucency - translucent
Mobility - moves only with applied negative pressure

Acute otitis media
Position- full to bulging
Color - red (can be pink, white or yellow)
Translucency - opaque
Mobility - poor when both positive and negative pressures are applied.

Fluid level
Position- retracted
Color - yellow or amber
Translucency - translucent
Mobility - restricted, fluid and bubble seen with applied pressure.

Fig.14.2: Diagrammatic representation of secretory otitis media

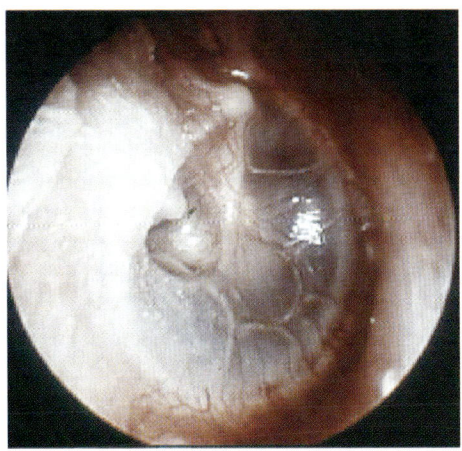

Fig. 14.3: Fluid level and air bubble

Investigations

1. Plain X-rays

- Water's view of paranasal sinus to rule out nasal and sinus infection.

- Lateral view of nasopharynx to rule out hypertrophied adenoids.

2. Audiometry

(a) Pure tone audiometry—conductive deafness, commonly in the low frequencies because of increase of mass factor in the middle ear (Fig. 14.4).

(b) Impedance audiometry will show a flat curve with a shift in compliance to the negative side (Fig. 14.5).

Treatment

1. Prevention of the secretory otitis media.
2. Removal of the possible cause, e.g. adenoidectomy.
3. Anti-allergy treatment—antihistamines, desensitization.
4. Advise the child to sit in the front row in school.
5. Myringotomy with grommet insertion. (Fig. 14.6)

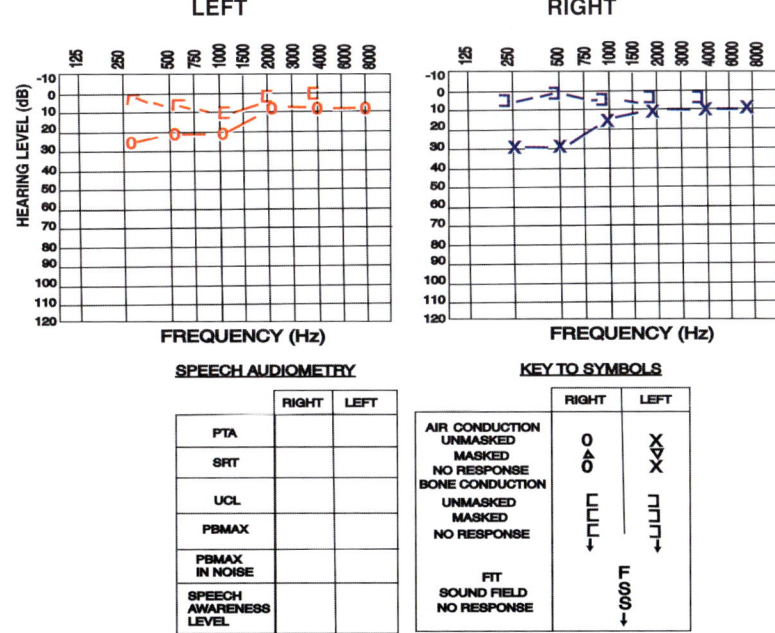

Fig. 14.4: Pure tone audiometry showing low frequency conductive hearing loss

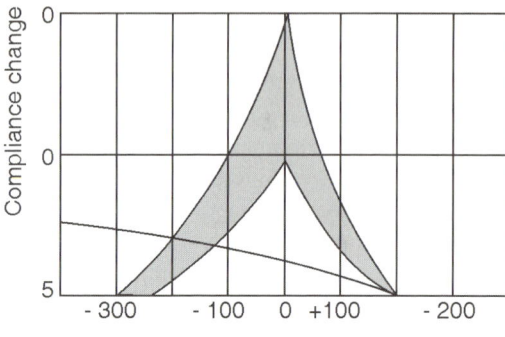

Fig. 14.5: Impedance audiometry will show a flat curve with a shift in compliance to the negative side

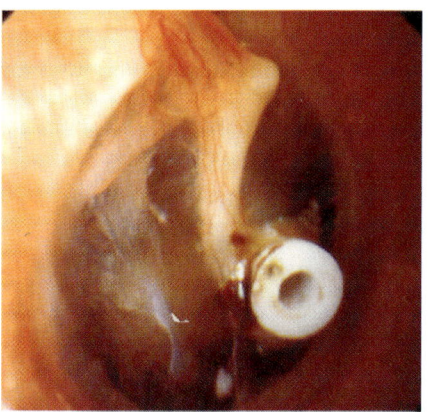

Fig. 14.6: Grommet in situ in right TM in antero inferior quadrant

OTITIC BAROTRAUMA

It is the term applied to the damage that results from failure of the Eustachian tube to equalize air pressure on either side of the tympanic membrane, occurs most commonly during descent from high altitude in an aircraft or descent in under water diving. The eustachian tube functions as, one way valve that allows air to flow passively from the middle ear to the nasopharynx. It must be opened actively by muscle contraction during swallowing to permit the passage of air in the reverse direction.

During the aircraft descent the increased atmospheric pressure pushes the tympanic membrane medially and pain is experienced. The Eustachian tube must be opened actively by swallowing or by valsalva to facilitate the entry of air in to the middle ear. Occasionally an excessive air pressure difference may force the soft tissue near the ET opening into the lumen thus resulting in a locked Eustachian tube (ET). This happens when there is

- Air travel while there is a functional problem with ET tube, e.g.: URTI.
- Sleep during descent of an aircraft from high altitude.
- In-flight, alcohol leading to sleep thus causing Eustachian tube muscle relaxation.
- Patient undergoing hyperbaric O_2 therapy in decompression chamber.

Symptoms

1. Pain
2. Hearing loss
3. Tinnitus
4. Sensation of wooliness in ear.
5. Swishing sensation in ear on movement.

Signs

1. Erythema of tympanic membrane.
2. Solitary or multiple interstitial hemorrhages on tympanic membrane.
3. Linear streaking in the pars flaccida and along the sides of handle of malleus.
4. A golden yellow serous exudates or a frank hemotympanum.
5. In severe cases rupture of tympanic membrane or round window can occur in which case patient will have vertigo or fluctuating sensory neural hearing loss.

Treatment

1. Prevention is by
   - Avoiding air travel during URTI
   - Topical nasal decongestants such as oxymetzoline or Xylometazoline HCl

0.1% or oral systemic decongestants with regular valsalva maneuver during aircraft descent.
  • Avoidance of alcohol on the journey.
2. The effusion of barotrauma tends to resolve spontaneously in 6 weeks usually.
3. Topical and systemic decongestants.
4. Myringotomy and ventilation tube insertion.

ACUTE SUPPURATIVE OTITIS MEDIA

It is also known as acute otitis media; ASOM.

Definition

It is an acute suppurative inflammation of the periosteal layer of the middle ear cleft by suppurative organisms.

Incidence

It is commonly seen in children but adults may also get affected.

Etiology

Routes of Infection
1. Infection through the Eustachian tube to the middle ear, following chronic tonsillitis, chronic rhinitis, chronic sinusitis and adenoiditis may give rise to ASOM.
2. Traumatic perforation—infection may come through the perforation.
3. Hematological—blood borne infection is very rare.

Common Organisms
  • Streptococcus
  • Pneumococcus
  • *H. influenza*
  • *Moraxella catarrhalis*
  • Pseudomonas

Clinical Features

(Signs and symptoms are described in stages).

  • Stage I - Stage of hyperemia.
  • Stage II - Stage of exudation.
  • Stage III - Stage of suppuration.
  • Stage IV - Stage of coalescent mastoiditis.
  • Stage V - Stage of complications.
  • Stage VI - Stage of resolution.

Stage I—Stage of Hyperemia

Pathology

In this stage, the mucosa in the middle ear and the Eustachian tube will get congested because of invasion by microorganisms. The hyperemia may extend to the antrum and mastoid region.

Symptoms
1. Earache—mild to moderate.
2. Obstruction or fullness of the ear.
3. Fever
4. Deafness—mild conductive type.
5. Associated symptoms like running nose, nasal obstruction.

Signs
1. Tympanic membrane—congested.
2. Landmarks of the tympanic membrane may be distorted associated with dilated radial blood vessels (cart wheel appearance).
3. Nasal mucosa congestion or mucopurulent discharge on rhinoscopy.

Treatment
1. Antibiotics
2. Analgesics and antipyretics
3. Decongestants
4. Nasal drops
5. Menthol or Tincture benzoin steam inhalation.

Stage II—Stage of Exudation (Fig. 14.7)

Pathology

In addition to hyperaemia, there will be collection of the exudate in the middle ear cavity.

Symptoms
1. Pain will increase.

2. Blocking sensation of the ear will increase.
3. Deafness increases.

Signs

1. Tympanic membrane—thick, congested, loss of landmarks; bulging.
2. X-ray mastoid - haziness, cloudy.

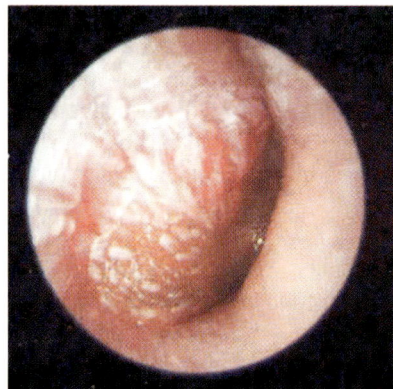

Fig. 14.7: Stage of exudation producing bulge in tympanic membrane

Treatment

1. Antibiotics
2. Myringotomy

Stage III—Stage of Suppuration

Pathology

The collected exudate in the middle ear will increase producing tension on the tympanic membrane. This in time will produce pressure necrosis in the pars tensa of the tympanic membrane leading to a small central perforation. Thus, the ear starts draining. The discharge may be blood stained initially, then serosanguinous and later the discharge may be mucopurulent. In this stage, the mucoperiosteum of the middle ear cleft will be thickened by the neoformation of many capillaries in the young fibrous tissue infiltrated with lymphocytes, plasma cells and polymorphs.

Symptoms

1. Pain is less, because of discharge. There will be a feeling of well being.

2. Discharge—blood stained, serosanguinous, mucopurulent.

Signs

1. Tympanic membrane will show small central perforation.
2. Pulsatile discharge present through the perforation is called *Light house sign*.
3. X-ray mastoid is cloudy, but the walls of the mastoid air cells are intact.

Treatment

1. Aural toilet—dry mopping or suction cleaning.
2. Broad spectrum antibiotic ear drops like gentamicin, neosporin.

Stage IV—Coalescent Mastoiditis/ Surgical Mastoiditis

There will be reinfection in the middle ear seen usually after a period of two weeks after the previous stage. This reinfection will produce a series of pathological changes in the middle ear cleft.

Pathology (Flow chart 14.1)

Symptoms

1. Earache increases after a period of two weeks of remission.
2. Fever.
3. Discharge from the ear, most often mucopurulent.
4. Deafness will increase.

Signs

1. Thickening of periosteum over the mastoid, so mastoid becomes smooth (ironed out mastoid) is the first sign of acute mastoiditis.
2. Mastoid tenderness can be elicited.
3. Discharge is copious and continuous. It reappears immediatly after wiping, called "reservoir" sign.
4. Tympanic membrane—central perforation with polypoidal middle ear mucosa.

Flow chart 14.1: Pathogenesis of coalescent mastoiditis

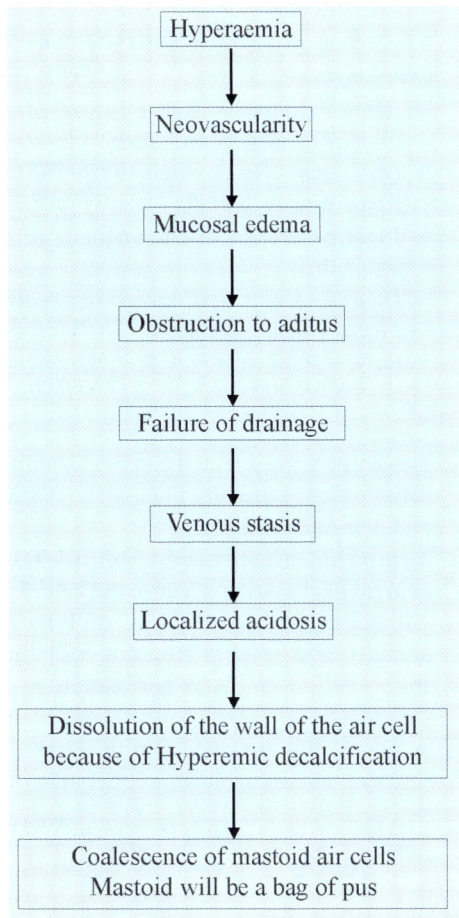

5. Sagging of the posterior superior meatal wall is the cardinal sign.
6. ESR will be high.
7. X-ray mastoid will show clouding of air cells

Treatment

- Surgical—Cortical mastoidectomy and drainage of the pus.

Stage V—Stage of Complications

Untreated cases can lead to many complications which can be divided into two groups— intracranial and extracranial (discussed in chapter 15).

Pathology

Complications may occur either by erosion of bone or by hyperemic decalcification (or) thromboembolic phenomena.

Symptoms and signs will depend on the type of complication and have been described separately else where.

Treatment

Depends on the type of complication.

Stage VI—Stage of Resolution

Pathology

As resistance of the host overtakes the virulence of the organism or because of proper antibiotic therapy, the acute infection begins to subside.

The first evidence of resolution will be dimmunition or cessation of ear discharge. Later on, the pathological process will resolve and the ear comes back to normal. It is rare for an acute infection like suppurative otitis media to leave any permanent residue.

ACUTE NECROTIZING OTITIS MEDIA

Acute necrotizing otitis media is a special form of acute suppurative otitis media that occurs mostly in infants and young children, suffering from scarlet fever, measles, pneumonia, influenza or some other systemic illness.

There is an early necrosis and distruction of most of the tympanic membrane, with its annulus, mucosa of the promontory, ossicular chain and even mastoid air cells. The infecting organism is mostly beta hemolytic streptococcus.

Tympanic membrane usually shows a total perforation with foul smelling purulent discharge. Necrotic ossicles may be seen.

Healing is followed by fibrosis or ingrowth of squamous epithelium leading to secondary acquired cholesteatoma.

Early institution of intravenous antibiotics therapy is indicated. Cortical mastoidectomy may be needed if the condition gets complicated by acute mastoiditis.

CHRONIC SUPPURATIVE OTITIS MEDIA

Definition

It is defined as chronic inflammation of muco-periosteal lining of the middle ear cleft.

Classification

1. Tubotympanic type otitis media (safe type)
   - *Inactive (mucosal):* Permanent perforation without discharge
   - *Active (mucosal) COM:* Permanent perforation with discharge
   - *Healed:* Tympanosclerosis; healed perforation
2. Atticoantral type otitis media (dangerous type)
   - *Inactive (squamous):* Retraction with no cholesteatoma
   - *Active (squamous):* Retraction pocket with cholesteatoma
   - Secondary acquired cholesteatoma.

TUBOTYMPANIC TYPE

Etiology

1. **Predisposing factors**
   - Inadequate/improper treatment of ASOM.
   - Infection from surrounding areas like nose, nasopharynx and oropharynx.
   - Some diseases like tuberculosis are chronic from the beginning.
   - Pneumatization of mastoid—sclerotic mastoids are more prone for CSOM.
2. **Exciting factors**
   - Gram negative organisms *like Pseudo-monas, proteus, E. coli*
   - Streptococcus.
   - Staphylococcus.

Symptoms

1. **Discharge:** Profuse, intermittent, predo-minantly mucoid occassionally muco-purulent, non foul smelling, whitish/yellowish and tenacious. It increases with attacks of cold.

   Depending on the discharge it is divided into *four stages:*
   - *Active*—Actively discharging ear at the time of clinical examination.
   - *Quiescent*—No ear discharge for less than 3 to 6 months period.
   - *Inactive*—No ear discharge for more than 6 months.
   - *Healed*—Central peroration has healed.
2. Deafness—Mild conductive
3. Earache—If associated with otitis externa.

Signs

1. Discharge is present in the external auditory canal which is usually mucoidal, tenacious and non-foul smelling.
2. **Tympanic membrane** (Fig. 14.8)—A **central perforation** occur in the pars tensa without any involvement of the tympanic annulus. Size of the perforation will range from small to very large perforation in the pars tensa.
   - Small, pinpoint perforation (less than 25%) is seen in acute suppurative otitis

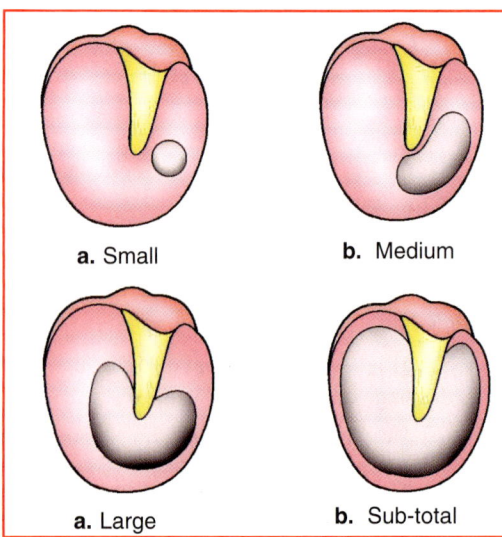

a. Small   b. Medium

a. Large   b. Sub-total

Fig. 14.8: Types of central perforation

media and also in trauma. If it is difficult to detect a small perforation the following tests can be done, i.e.

(a) **Bonsin's test:** It consists of painting the drum with 1 in 20% solution of silver nitrate causing the perforation to stand out as a black spot against a white background.

(b) If asked to do forced valsalva, air leakage can be heard.

(c) However if a drop of sterile water or antibiotic ear drops is given in the ear and patient is asked to do valsalva, air bubbles can be seen.

- **Medium size (25–50%)** involves more than one but less than two quadrants of the tympanic membrane.
- **Large perforation (50–75%).** A subtotal perforation involves all the 4 quadrants of tympanic membrane except the annulus.
- Complete or total perforation when there is loss of substance involving the entire tympanic membrane including the annulus found in atticoantral disease.

Middle ear can be easily visualized through a large perforation. In case of suppuration, medial wall is covered by thick red granular and sometimes polypoidx`x al mucous membrane.

Other Structures that can be identified are as follows (Fig. 14.9):

- Promontory
- Oval window
- Round window niche
- Eustachian tube orifice

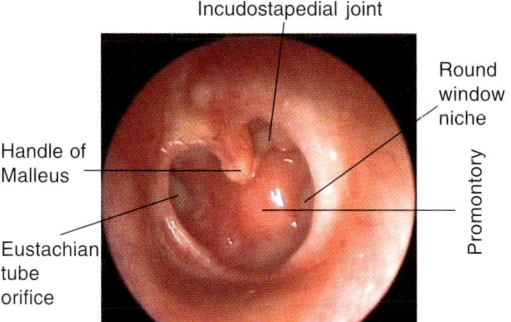

Fig. 14.9: Showing sub-total central perforation

- Parts of ossicular chain
- Stapedius tendon.

3. Tuning fork tests
Rinne—negative.
Weber—lateralized to the affected side.
ABC—normal.

Investigations

- **Culture and sensitivity** of the discharge in case of active stage.
- **Examination under microscope**
  1. To see the margin of the perforation.
  2. To rule out any ingrowing epithelium.
  3. To see granulation tissue and polyp.
  4. To see any evidence of cholesteatoma.
  5. For precise collection of swab from middle ear.
  6. To rule out any hidden pin hole perforation.
  7. To see status of middle ear mucosa.
  8. To see the status of ossicular chain if possible.
- **Pure tone audiogram:** Mild conductive loss between 20 to 30 dB.

  Patch test: This test is performed as a out patient procedure (Flow chart 14.2). The material used in patch test can be thin paper commonly taken from cigarette foil and which is cut into size of perforation. Before patching, a pure tone audiogram is taken. Then perforation is closed with the same cut thin paper. Patching of perforation is always better if paper is soaked in vaseline. A repeat audiogram is done after patching.

  Interpretation of patch test are
  1. Improved hearing means intact ossicular chain.
  2. Decreased hearing means ossicular fixity or discontinuity.
  3. No improvement means in technical fault or improper patching.
- **X-ray of mastoids:** To rule out mastoiditis
- **X-ray of paranasal sinuses:** To rule out sinusitis
- **X-ray soft tissue neck lateral view:** To rule out adenoid enlargement.
- **Diagnostic nasal endoscopy**

Flow chart 14.2: Showing procedure of patch test

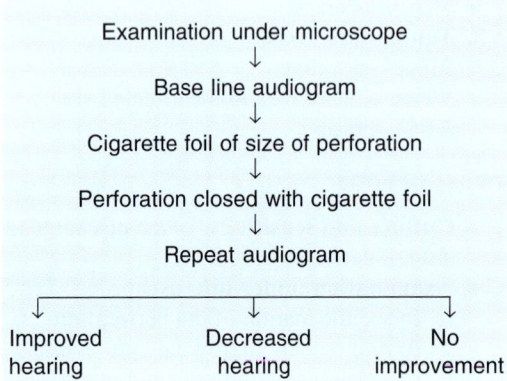

Examination under microscope
↓
Base line audiogram
↓
Cigarette foil of size of perforation
↓
Perforation closed with cigarette foil
↓
Repeat audiogram

| Improved hearing | Decreased hearing | No improvement |

Treatment

Medical Management

- Aural toilet by (a) dry mopping, (b) wet mopping or (c) suction cleaning. Wet mopping is discouraged nowadays. Suction cleaning is the best method but may not be possible in children.
- Antibiotic ear drops after culture and sensitivity report.

Surgical management of tubotympanic disease
- **Removal of septic foci**, e.g. Tonsillectomy, adenoidectomy, sinus wash.
- **Myringoplasty** if hearing loss is below 40 dB, **tympanoplasty** if above 40 dB.
- If X-ray mastoid shows mastoiditis, do cortical mastoidectomy.

Preoperative Advice

- Avoid entry of water into the ear by plugging with a cotton ball or by using an ear plug and by avoiding swimming.
- Common cold should be treated immediately.

ATTICO-ANTRAL OR DANGEROUSTYPE

It is usually associated with cholesteatoma formation.

Cholesteatoma is defined as a sac in the middle ear, which is lined by keratinizing stratified squamous epithelium containing desquamated epithelium as keratin debris. It is also described as skin in the wrong place. This structure has a capacity for progressive and independent growth at the expense of underlying bone and has tendency to reccur, unless removed completely.

- The mechanism of bony erosion of cholesteatoma are not completely understood. Various factors are mentioned below (Flow chart 14.3):
  1. Earlier it was thought the physical pressure of cholesteatoma causes bony erosion.
  2. At the cellular level the chief factor in bony erosion is activation of osteoclasts.
  3. It is believed that release of inflammatory mediators such as the cytokinin, interleukin 1 alpha, from macrophages and epidermal keratinocytes are being important in osteoclast activation. Other humoral factors that have been suggested are prostaglandin, Cathepsin D and parathyroid hormone like protein.

- In addition to bone destruction **new bone formation** can occur in cholesteatoma mostly seen in attic and mastoid antrum (Flow chart 14.3).

Flow chart 14.3: Showing mechanism of bony erosion in cholesteatoma

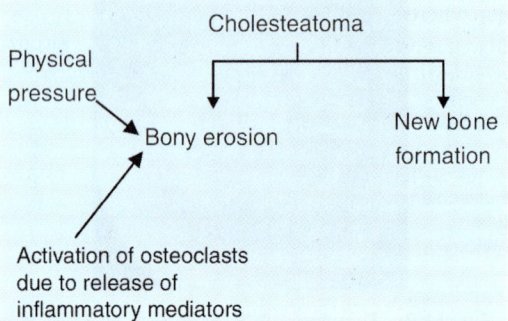

Cholesteatoma

Physical pressure → Bony erosion

New bone formation

Activation of osteoclasts due to release of inflammatory mediators

Flow chart 14.4: Classification of cholesteatoma

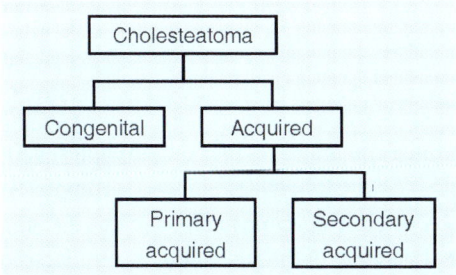

Classification of Cholesteatoma
(Flow chart 14.4)

Congenital Cholesteatoma

It arises from embryonic epidermal cell rests in the middle ear cleft or temporal bone. It may occur at

- Middle ear
- Petrous apex (or)
- Cerebellopontine angle.

A middle ear congenital cholesteatoma usually presents as a white mass behind an intact tympanic membrane. It may also spontaneously rupture through the tympanic membrane.

Levenson criteria for diagnosis

- A white mass behind normal tympanic membrane
- Normal pars flaccida and pars tensa
- No prior history of otorrhea
- No prior history of otological procedure
- Canal atresia and intramembraneous and giant cholesteatoma

Primary acquired cholesteatoma occurs in the ear where there is no previous history of ear discharge from the ear or tympanic membrane perforation.

Secondary acquired cholesteatoma always occurs in an already diseased ear where there is a pre-existing tympanic membrane perforation.

Etiopathology

The exact etiopathology is unknown but various theories have been put forward for the formation of cholesteatoma. Cholesteatoma is a white, pultaceous mass having bone eroding capacity either by expansion or by liberation of some chemical enzyme .

Theories

1. **Retraction pocket theory (Primary acquired cholesteatoma)** (Fig. 14.10a)
   Eustachian tube obstruction will produce negative pressure in the middle ear cavity as a result there will be formation of a retraction pocket at the attic region which will hamper the normal migratory action of the epithelium of the external auditory meatus. This will produce accumulation of the desquamated epithelium in the attic and pressure necrosis of the tympanic membrane forming cholesteatoma of the middle ear. This theory holds good in explaining the primary acquired cholesteatoma. There are other theories of genesis of primary cholesteatoma which is shown in flow chart 14.5.
2. **Theory of migration** (Fig. 14.10b)
   Skin of the external auditory meatus will migrate to the middle ear cavity through the tympanic membrane perforation leading to secondary acquired cholesteatoma formation in the middle ear.
3. **Metaplasia theory** (Fig. 14.10c)
   Because of recurrent/chronic infection normal columnar epithelium turns into squamous epithelium by metaplasia.
4. **Implantation theory**
   At the time of middle ear surgery squamous epithelium may get implanted.

Other Theories of Epithelial Abnormality

- Invasive hyperplasia of basal layer of meatal skin adjoining of the upper margin of tympanic membrane has been postulated in this theory. Papillary invasion with central cornification enters the epitympanum without tympanic membrane perforation. This speaks in favor of primary acquired cholesteatoma (Fig. 14.10d).

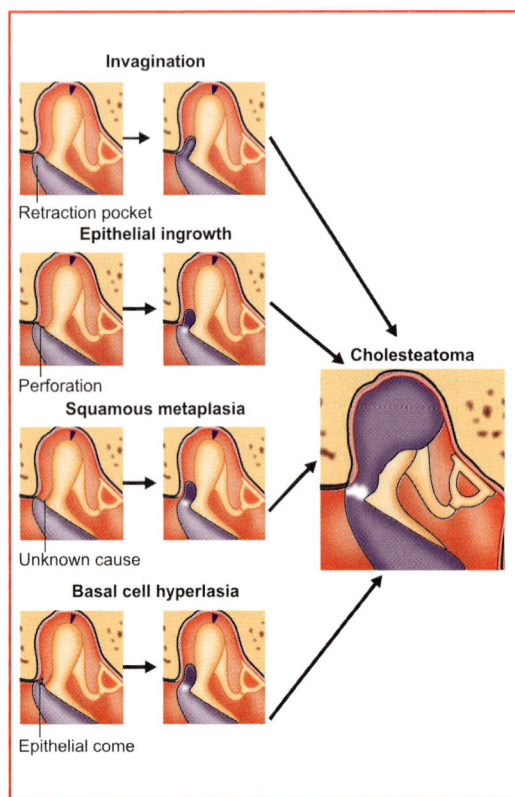

Fig. 14.10: Theories of pathogenesis of aural cholesteatoma

- Invasive hyperkeratosis and acanthosis of deep meatal skin has also been postulated.

Typical Growth Pattern of Cholesteatoma

The most common sites of acquired cholesteatoma listed by their frequency.

- Posterior epitympanum
- Posterior mesotympanum
- Anterior epitympanum

It is not unusual for multiple cholesteatoma sac to occur in the same ear involving two or even all three of these typical routes. While great majority of cholesteatoma follow one or more of this common pathway, others assume unusual patterns presumably because of anatomic variation of middle ear fold and the ligaments which channel the cholesteatoma growth.

Pars Tensa Cholesteatoma

Ossicular chains are involved at a relatively early stage. Long process of incus and stapes suprastructure are the common ossicles. This causes moderate to severe conductive deafness. Occasionally the hearing is well preserved by

Flow chart 14.5: Pathogenesis of primary acquired cholesteatoma

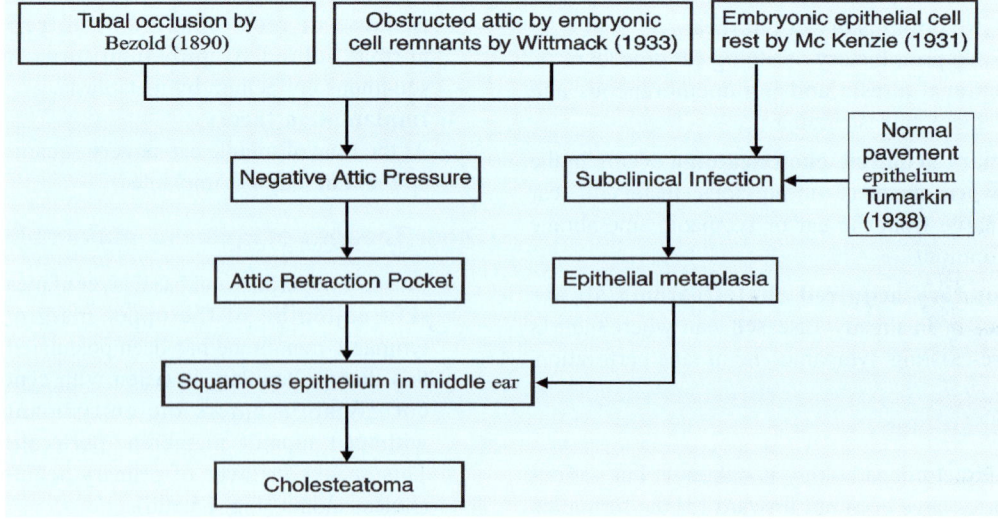

- A retraction on to the stapes head or
- Bridging of ossicular chain defect by cholesteatoma **(cholesteatoma hearers).**

Pars Flaccida Cholesteatoma (Fig. 14.11)

Pars flacida cholesteatoma is frequently with ostitiis, granulation tissue and erosion of outer attic wall or scutum. As the cholesteatoma expands the ossicular head of malleus and incus becomes surrounded by squamous epithelium. The involvement of the ossicular chain occurs relatively late in disease process. It is not uncommon to encounter large pars flaccida cholesteatoma with an intact ossicular chain and relatively a minor degree of conductive deafness. Further progression of disease occurs anteriorly in to the anterior epitympanum and posteriorly into the mastoid antrum and its air cell system.

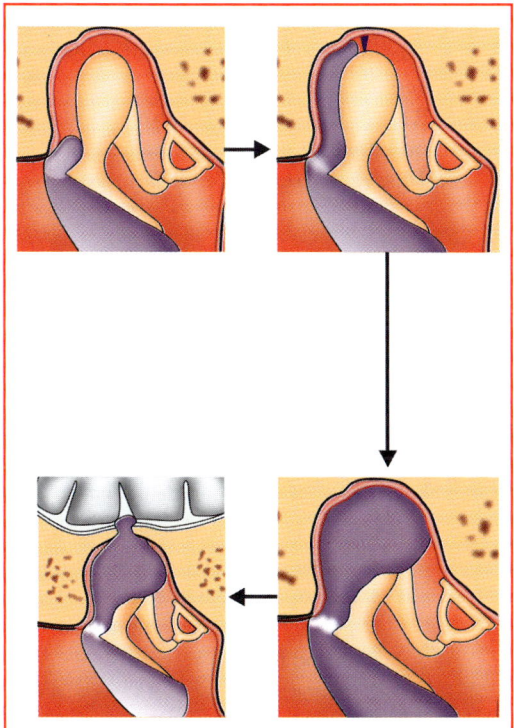

Fig. 14.11: Growth pattern of pars flaccida cholesteatoma

Clinical Features

Symptoms

- **Ear discharge:** It is foul smelling scanty predominantly purulent, occasionally blood stained and has no relation with upper respiratory tract infection.
- **Deafness:** Progressive conductive deafness
- **Itching and pain in the ear:** May be caused by otitis externa or may be an early symptoms of complication.
- **Tinnitus and giddiness:** May be early symptoms of complication.

Sign

Otoscopic examination reveals

1. Foul Smelling discharge in the external auditory canal.
2. Granulation tissue in posterosuperior part of deep meatus.
3. Tympanic membrane shows attic, marginal or total perforation (Figs14.12 and 14.13a and b).
4. Occasionally granulation tissue or polyp may be seen coming out of perforation.
5. Whitish cholesteatoma flakes can be seen through perforation.
6. Mastoid tenderness present.
7. Tunning fork shows the rinne negative, weber lateralized to the affected side, ABC normal.

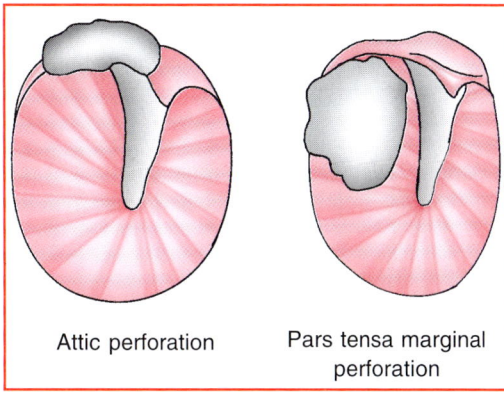

Attic perforation   Pars tensa marginal perforation

Fig. 14.12: Attic and marginal perforation

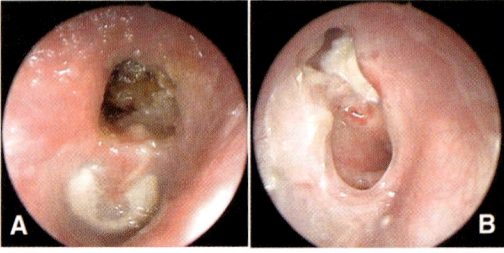

Figs 14.13a and b: (a) Perforation in the pars flaccida (b) Showing double pathology involving both pars tensa and pars flaccida (total perforation)

Differences between tubotympanic and attico antral disease is given in Table 14.1.

Investigations

(a) Examination under microscope
(b) Culture sensitivity from ear discharge
(c) Rigid oto-endoscopy—to see the facial recess and sinus tympani if possible
(d) Audiogram (PTA)
(e) Imaging
 1. **X-ray Mastoid (Schullers and law's view):** To see the bony erosion , to see the anatomy of mastoid, occasionally to diagnose cholesteatoma which gives the cotton wool appearance.

Differential diagnosis of cavity in the mastoid -
 • Mega antrum
 • Post mastoidectomy cavity
 • Cholesteatoma
 • Eosinophilic granuloma

 • Tuberculosis
 • Multiple myeloma
 • Large emissary vein
 • Large facial neuroma
 • Cholesterol granuloma
 • Carcinoma
2. **CT scan:** Features seen in high resolution are the following:
 • Blunting of the scutum is the earliest sign.
 • Erosion and destruction of lateral attic wall (normal **figure of eight** pattern is lost)
 • Widening of aditus
 • Displacement and destruction of ossicles
 • Labyrinthine fistula formation.
 • Erosion into the facial canal
 • Dehiscence of the tegmen tympani and sinus plate
 • Destruction of mastoid or natural mastoidectomy
 • Erosion of posterior and roof of external auditory canal
3. **MRI:** MRI provides complimentary information by allowing characterization of soft tissue masses.

Management

Aims and Objective

1. Primary objective is to make the ear safe and dry

Table 14.1: Differences between tubotympanic and atticoantral disease

	TTD	*AAD*
Parts involved	Anteroinferior	Posterosuperior
Discharge	Mucoid, profuse, non foul smelling	Mucopurulent to purulent scanty, foul smelling, often blood stained
Perforation	Central type	Marginal type, involving the attic
Polyp	Usually pale	Pink and fleshy
Granulation tissue	Rare	Common
Cholesteatoma	Absent	Present
Complications	Rare	Common
Audiogram	Mild- moderate conductive hearing loss	Conductive or mixed hearing loss

2. To restore or to improve the hearing
3. To maintain the normal anatomical appearance of ear by avoiding open mastoid cavity

Surgical Management

Surgical management is the main line of treatment in atticoantral disease. Conservative or medical line of management has no role in making the ear safe. Surgical management can be broadly divided in two groups which consist of:

1. **Canal wall down mastoidectomy**
2. **Canal wall up mastoidectomy**

   Canal wall down mastoidectomy consist of **radical or modified radical** mastoidectomy. These procedure ensures safety and dry ear but functional improvement may not be achieved .

Canal wall up mastoidectomy is also known as **combined approach tympanoplasty** where functional improvement can be achieved but not the safety.

Medical Management

In patient who are medically unfit for surgery or in some patients with **cholesteatoma in only hearing ear**, conservative medical management is only therapeutic option with topical antibiotic and steroid.

However ideal medical treatment would be topical agent which has the potential for either eliminating the squamous epithelium or reducing its activity in order to curtail the production of desquamated debris. Study have shown that **5 - Flurouracil** has some useful activity in this aspect. Initial studies in which 5 flurouracil was applied to the cyst wall of early cholesteatoma, relapsing cholesteatoma and in large discharging cavity showed inhibition of keratin formation and otorrhea (Flow chart 14.6).

Adhesive Otitis Media

Adhesive otitis media has been defined as a long standing adhesive process as a result of inflammation (Fig. 14.14 and Flow chart 14.6). An inflammatory reaction may subside, allowing the tissue to attain its normal character. Sometimes there is inflammation terminating with formation of scar tissue. Fibroblast lay down new fibrous tissue which becomes more dense. Avascular fibrosis is specially found to occur if mucous membrane has been converted into granulation tissue by chronic infection. The tympanic membrane becomes adherent to the medial wall of the middle ear. It can also present as adhesions, fibrosis of tympanic membrane, **ankylosis** of the ossicular chain, **tympanosclerosis**, i.e. hyaline

Flow Chart 14.6: Management of AAD

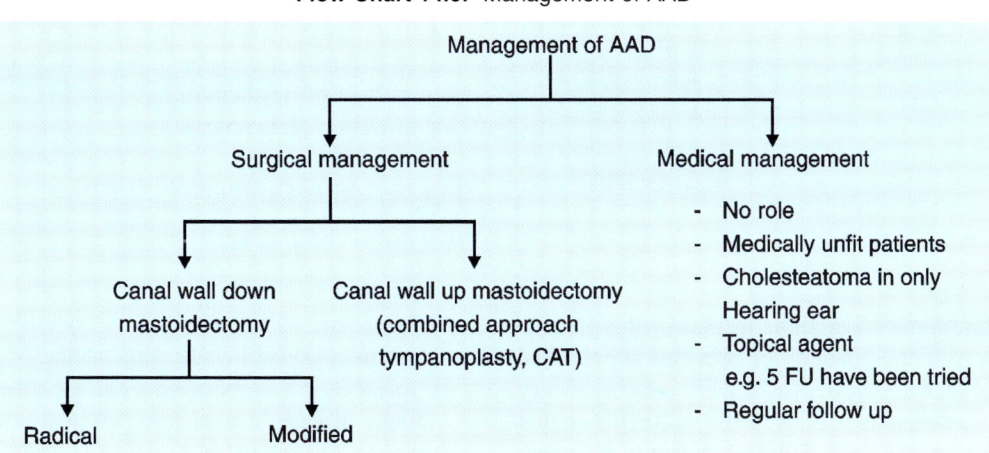

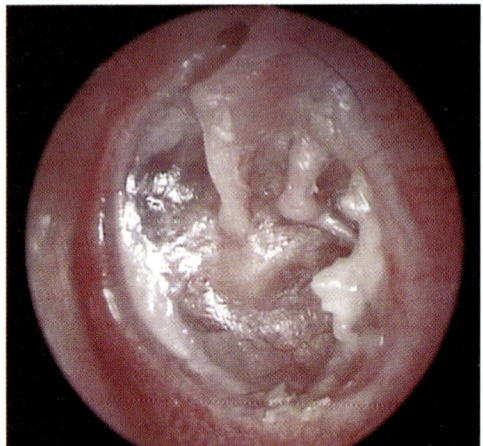

Fig.14.14 Adhesive otitis media

degeneration of collagen and calcium deposits in the submucosal layer (Flow chart 14.7).

Flow Chart 14.7: Post-inflammatory pathological changes

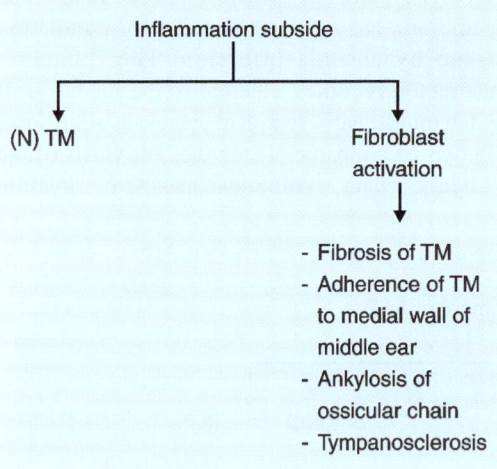

Etiology

Inflammatory reaction: In half of the patients there is usually history of previous suppurative otitis media. In other cases there may be history of-non suppurative otitis media with effusion that passed unnoticed. **Tough adhesions between**

portion of **ossicular chains and** medial wall of middle ear or **Tympanosclerotic patch**, incudomalleal joint fusion or tympanosclerosis of round window niche can occur. Classification of adhesive otitis media and retraction is given under atelectasis (Page 163).

Symptoms

1. *Deafness*: The symptom that brings patient to otologist is deafness. Conductive loss not often exceeding 50dB.
2. *Tinnitus*: Not uncommon
3. Paracusis willis is rare

Signs

1. Retracted and lusterless tympanic membrane draping the middle ear structures.
2. Absent or restricted mobility of TM on siegelization.
3. Eustachian tube catheterization shows abnormal inflation or complete obstruction.

Treatment

- Surgical measures will aim at remobilization of sound pressure transformer system, which is a elusive technical goal as the division of adhesion can be followed by further adhesion due to surgical trauma.
- Stapedectomy may have a theoretical application.
- Exploratory tympanotomy only as a means of offering a chance of natural hearing mechanism restoration.
- Provision of hearing aid.

Chronic Otitis Media with Effusion

It occurs as a sequel to

- Acute otitis media
- In patients who have had no documented recent episode of acute otitis media.
- Associated factors considered are allergy, sinus disease, nasopharyngeal obstruction due to adenoid or neoplasm.

Treatment

1. Use of corticosteroids in the form of nasal spray or systematically is thought to useful in clearing the middle ear fluid.
2. 21–30 day course of full antibiotic therapy is recommended as viable bacteria have been demonstrated in the middle ear fluid.
3. Myringotomy and insertion of ventilation tube along with treatment of the primary condition (like adenoidectomy).
4. *H. influenza* type B vaccine in which the capsular polysaccharide is conjugated with a protein heptovalent pneumococcal conjugate vaccine is under trial in prevention of AOM.

SPECIFIC TYPES OF OTITIS MEDIA

Tuberculous Otitis Media

Etiology

1. Infection is secondary to pulmonary tuberculosis in most of the cases. It infects the middle ear via tube by coughing up sputum laiden with tubercle bacilli.
2. Less commonly it may be acquired by contact with infected sputum or by drinking milk from infected cow.
3. It may be blood borne from tuberculous focus in other parts.

Pathology

Disease is insidious in onset with involvement of tympanic cavity resulting in thickening, extensive edema and infiltration of the mucosa of tympanic cavity by giant cells. Spontaneous multiple perforations and thin scanty odorless discharge occurs. Extensive granulation tissue in the middle ear and mastoid can lead to early facial nerve palsy.

Symptoms

1. *Ear discharge*: Painless, serosanguinous discharge occasionally blood stained.

2. *Hearing loss*: Early and severe hearing loss out of proportion to the symptoms
3. *Facial paralysis*: High incidence of facial paralysis seen. It may be the presenting symptom in children.

Signs

1. Multiple perforations with extensive granulation tissue in the middle ear.
2. Enlarged pre -auricular lymph node.

Diagnosis

1. Culture of the ear discharge,
2. *Biopsy*: Demonstration of the acid fast bacilli from the granulation,
3. *Chest X-ray*: To rule out pulmonary tuberculosis,

Treatment

1. Systemic antitubercular therapy of the primary focus.
2. Local treatment in the form of aural toilet.
3. *Surgical treatment*: Mastoidectomy indicated if complication is involved. Medical treatment preceeds any surgical treatment as surgical treatment may fail in absence of systemic therapy

Syphilitic Otitis Media

Rare condition where the spirocheates reach the middle ear through eustachian tube from the lesions that are present in the nose or nasopharynx. Bone necrosis and sequestrum formation are common leading to foul smelling discharge.

Sensory neural hearing loss, tinnitus and vertigo occurs due to spircheatal invasion of the sensory end organs and nerves.

Diptheritic Otitis Media

May accompany diptheritic croup and nasopharyngitis. Dipheritic membrane may form in the middle ear. Complication occur frequently leading to destruction of tympanic membrane, ossicles and infection of contiguous structures leading to necrosis of mastoid, temporal bone and the mastoid.

TYMPANOSCLEROSIS

Definition

It is an abnormal condition of the middle ear characterized by hyaline degeneration of the fibrous layer of the tympanic membrane and the middle ear mucosa.

Etiology

1. It is an irreversible condition from an imperfect healing process in response to inflammation of middle ear space.
2. Patient with previous grommet tube insertion has 59% chance of TS patch.
3. Patient with only myringotomy has 13% chance of TS patch formation.
4. Autoimmune cause.

Pathogenesis (Flow chart 14.8)

It appears histologically as a hyalinization of the subepithelial connective tissue of the tympanic membrane and middle ear. In most instances hyalinization is associated with calcification.

- When tympanosclerosis plaque occur within tympanic membrane, they are limited to lamina propria and it causes only very minimal conductive hearing loss.
- Middle ear tympanosclerosis can cause ossicular fixation and result in more severe degree of conductive hearing loss.

Types of Tympanosclerosis

1. ***Sclerosing mucositis:*** It is more superficial and amenable to total surgical removal.
2. ***Osteoclastic mucoperiostitis:*** An invasive form which often defies complete removal.

Treatment

1. Operation for the removal of a large plaque in the membrane and middle ear extension.

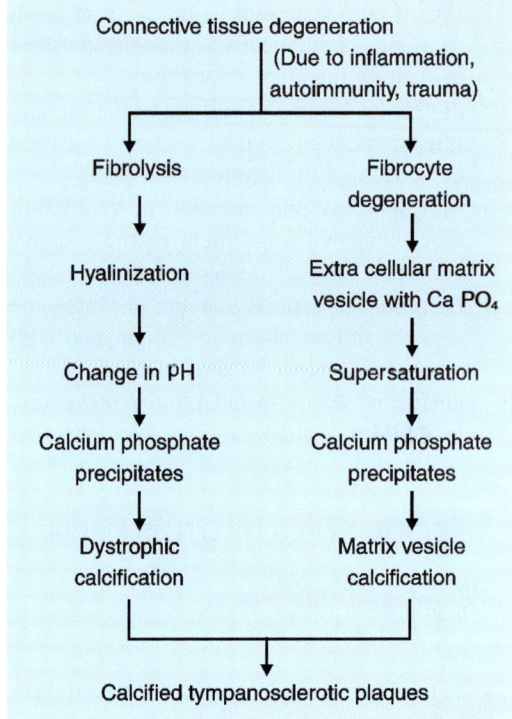

Flow chart 14.8: Pathogenesis of tympanosclerosis

This should only be undertaken if there is patent eustachian tube.

2. Ideally the ossicles should be remobilized and adhesions should be divided especially of incudomalleolar joint.
3. If the drum head adheres to the ossicles and promontory the membrane should be separated.
4. Tympanosclerosis at round window and stapes head is a contraindication to surgery and these patients should be subjected to hearing aid trial.

Atelectasis

The middle ear atelectasis signifies collapse of the tympanic membrane so that it becomes displaced inwards towards the promontory. The condition occurs in association with eustachian tube malfunction which leads to inadequate ventilation of middle ear cleft. Thus it is closely related to chronic secretary otitis media.

Retraction of Pars Tensa (Sade's Classification)

Grade 1: Mild retraction not touching the long process of incus

Grade 2: Retracted drum touching the long process of incus

Grade3: Retracted drum touching the promontory

Grade 4: Drum plastered to the promontory

Retraction of Pars Flaccida (Tos's Classification)

Grade 1: Mild attic retraction, not touching neck or malleus

Grade 2: Attic retraction touching neck or malleus.

Grade 3: Limited outer attic wall erosion

Grade 4: Severe outer attic wall erosion

Treatment

Restoration of the middle ear ventilation forms the basis of treatment and every effort should be made to treat the cause of Eustachian tube dysfunction in nose or nasopharynx as outlined in secretory otitis media.

For Pars Tensa Retraction

For grade 1 and 2 myringotomy and grommet insertion.

For grade 3 and 4
a. Hearing aid trail
b. Tympanoplasty with cartilage or sialastic interposition to attain adequate middle ear space.

For Pars Flaccida Retraction

Grade 1 and 2 - Repeated suction and cleaning. Regular follow up.

Grade 3 and 4 - Canal wall down mastoidectomy.

POINTS TO REMEMBER

1. Acute necrotizing otitis is a special form of suppurative otitis media where early destruction and necrosis of tympanic membrane occurs. The condition is commonly caused by virulent form of β-hemolytic streptococcus.

2. Tubotympanic type of chronic suppurative otitis media is always associated with intermittent profuse non foul smelling mucopurulent discharge.

3. Atticoantral type of chronic suppurative otitis media is always associated with continuous purulent, scanty fowl smelling discharge.

4. Tympanosclerosis is a condition associated with hyalinization of the subepithelial tissue of tympanic membrane and middle ear. Middle ear tympanosclerosis can cause ossicular fixation leading to severe conductive hearing loss.

15

Complications of Suppurative Otitis Media

There is decline in the incidence of complication due to early diagnosis and also due to availability of good antibiotics.

Complications of CSOM/ASOM
(Fig. 15.1)

I. *Extracranial*
1. Mastoiditis and mastoid abscess
2. Facial nerve paralysis
3. Labyrinthitis
4. Petrositis
5. Otogenic tetanus

II. *Intracranial*
1. Extradural abscess
2. Subdural abscess
3. Brain abscess
4. Lateral sinus thrombosis
5. Otitic hydrocephalus
6. Meningitis

Mode of Spread of Infection (Fig. 15.2)

1. Bone erosion (cholesteatoma)
2. Thrombophlebitis

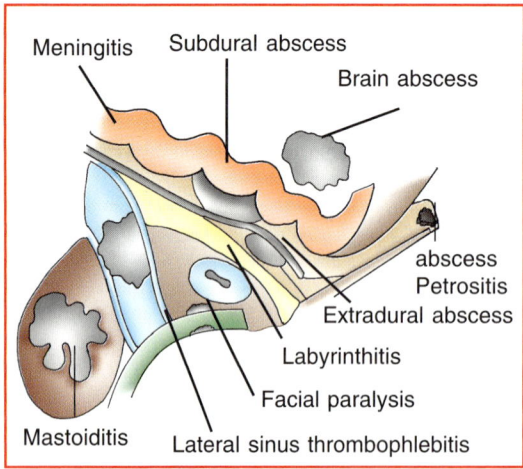

Fig. 15.1: Complications of SOM

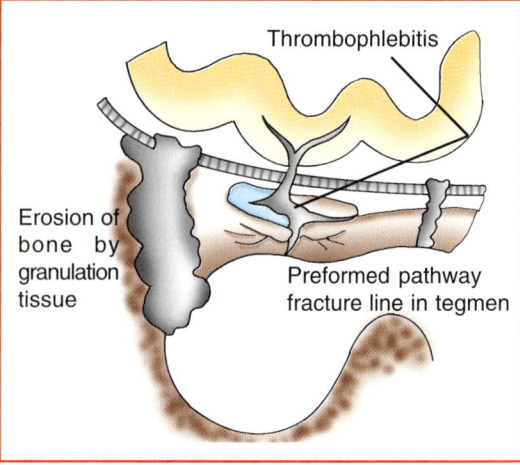

Fig. 15.2: Mode of spread of infection

3. Periphlebitis
4. Preformed pathways—Oval window, round window.

Spread through different walls of the middle ear (Flow chart 15.1)

1. **Through the posterior wall**
   - Acute mastoiditis in cellular mastoid.
   - Facial nerve palsy in sclerotic or acellular mastoid.
   - Lateral sinus thrombosis.
   - Trautman's triangle—cerebellar abscess.
   - Through solid angle—superior petrosal sinus thrombosis.

2. **Through the medial wall**
   - Labyrinthitis

3. **Through the roof**
   - Extradural abscess
   - Subdural abscess
   - Temporal and cerebellar abscess
   - Meningitis
   - Brain abscess

4. **Through the floor**
   - Thrombosis of the jugular bulb

Signs and symptoms of impending complications in CSOM are

1. Persistent pain and headache on the affected side.
2. High temperature with chills and rigors.
3. Giddiness either persistent or recurrent.
4. Twitching of the facial muscles on the affected side.
5. Positive fistula test.

EXTRACRANIAL COMPLICATIONS

ACUTE MASTOIDITIS

Definition

An acute inflammation of the middle ear cleft involving the mastoid air cell system associated with destruction of intercelluar septae due to hyperaemic decalcification.

Etiology

Organisms

- Streptococcus
- Staphylococcus

Flow chart 15.1: Spread of infection through different walls of the middle ear

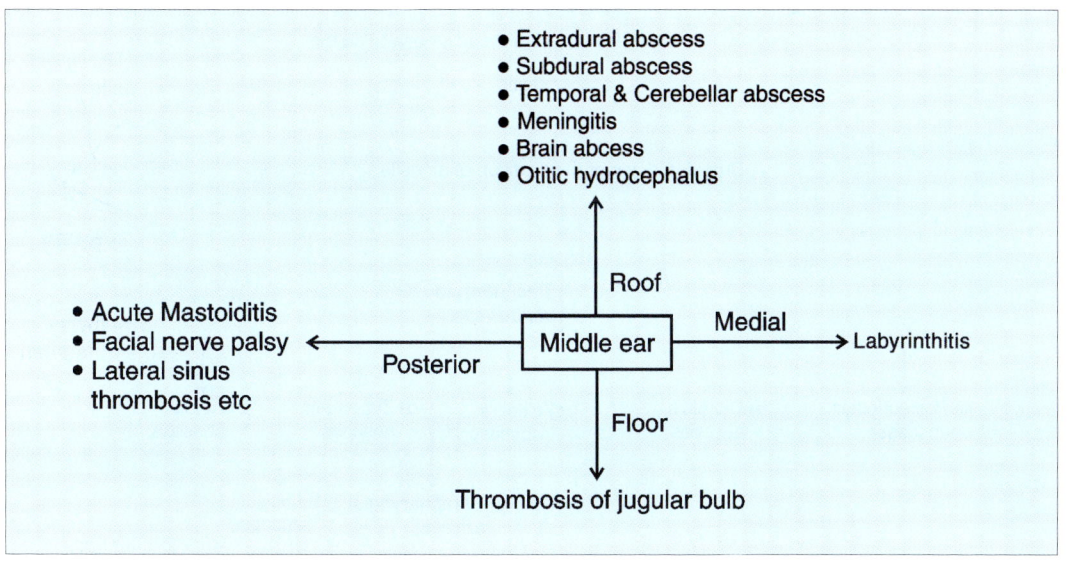

- Pneumococcus
- Hemophilus influenza
- Pseudomonas

Spread

- Infection spreads from the middle ear cavity through the aditus to the mastoid air cells.
- Blood borne infection.
- Trauma especially penetrating injury.

Pathology (Flow chart 15.2)

When acute infection reaches the mastoid air cells, there will be congestion and edema of the mucous membrane of the air cells associated with osteitis resulting in collection of purulent exudate in the air cells. Pressure of the purulent exudate will produce venous stasis leading to local acidosis. This results in breaking down of the partition of the air cells and abscess formation due to hyperemic decalcification. These abscesses coalesce and cause gradual erosion of the bone. If there is erosion of the cortex of the mastoid, the abscess may get collected beneath the periosteum producing a subperiosteal mastoid abscess. Later on, it may pass out through the skin producing a postauricular fistula. The pus can tract down to various sites to produce the following abscesses.

1. **Postauricular abscess:** The postauricular collection of pus beneath the periosteum

Flow chart 15.2: Showing pathophysiological progression of acute mastoid air cell disease

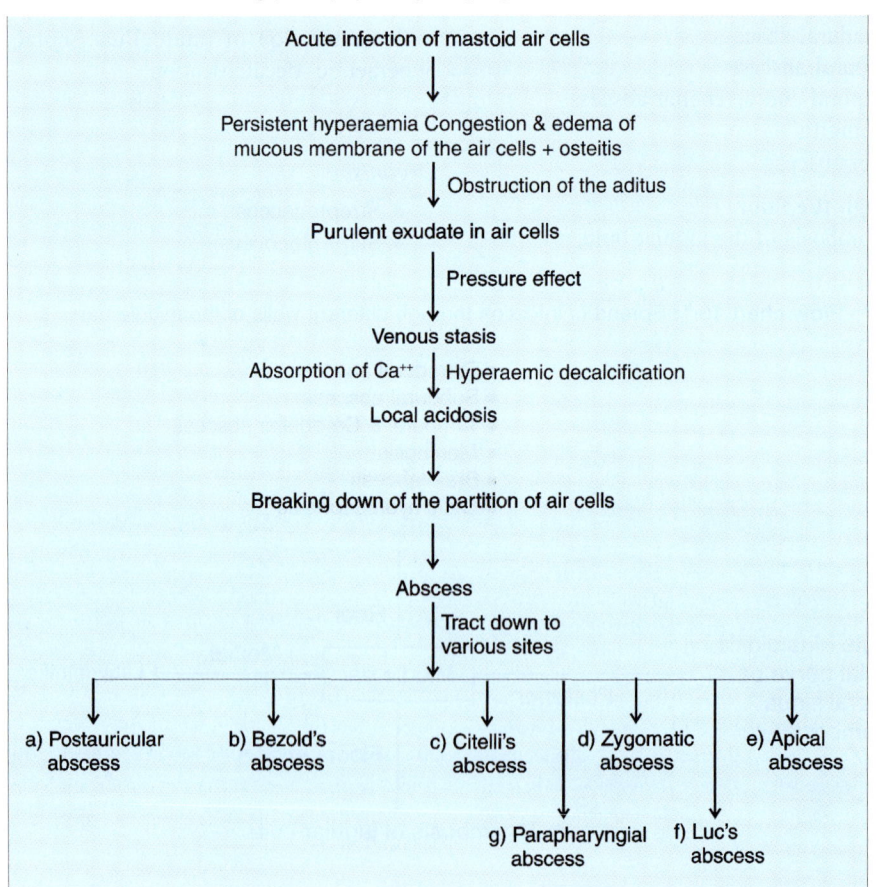

behind the pinna. Here the auricle is displaced forwards and outwards a fluctuant mass can be palpated behind the ear.

2. **Bezold's abscess:** Results from the perforation and necrosis of the mastoid tip. Pus will collect under the anterior border of the sternocleidomastoid muscle. This pus may also extend along the digastric into the submandibular triangle when it is called Citelli's abscess.

3. **Zygomatic abscess:** Abscess extends anteriorly to the zygomatic process producing facial and eyelid swelling.

4. **Apical abscess:** Abscess extends upto the petrous apex producing Gradenigo's syndrome. It consists of diplopia, cervicofacial pain, deafness and ear discharge.

5. **Pharyngeal abscess:** This occurs along the peritubal cells in the cortex.

6. **Luc's abscess:** It is an abscess in the deep external auditory canal as a result of pus breaking through the bony canal wall.

Clinical Aspects

Symptoms

1. Pain and swelling in the mastoid region.
2. Fever
3. Deafness—conductive type
4. Discharge—mucopurulent.

Signs

1. Thickening of the periosteum of the posterior auricular region.
2. Tenderness over the mastoid antrum, mastoid tip and posterior border of mastoid.
3. Postauricular swelling—tender, fluctuating, warm and congested.
4. Discharge—profuse, purulent and foul smelling. **Mastoid reservoir sign** may be positive. In mastoid reservoir sign there will be immediate filling of deep external auditory meatus with pus immediately after cleaning or mopping of pus.

5. Tympanic membrane shows a perforation which may be central or marginal.
6. Sagging of the posterosuperior meatal wall.
7. Profound conductive deafness.
8. Tuning fork tests
   • Rinne's test—negative
   • Weber's test—lateralized to the diseased side
   • ABC test—normal

Investigations

1. Complete blood picture shows— Leucocytosis.
2. Culture and sensitivity of the discharge.
3. PTA - conductive deafness.
4. X-ray mastoid—cavity or cloudiness.
5. CT Scan.

Differential Diagnosis

1. Furunculosis with cellulitis.
2. Sebaceous cyst.
3. Postauricular lymphadenitis.

Treatment

Aim

• Resolution of the infection.
• Prevention of intracranial infection.
   1. Antibiotics in the early stage of mastoiditis.
   2. Incision and drainage of the abscess.
   3. Simple mastoidectomy if the disease is localized in the mastoid region only.

Masked Mastoditis

Masked mastoiditis is a type of acute mastoiditis where partial treatment with antibiotics leads to failure of resolution with a low grade granular osteitis developing in the mastoid bone.

This condition may cause headache, earache and general malaise, but more often it is silent disease. Its danger lies int he fact that it can have the same consequences as acute coalescent mastoiditis, i.e. abscess formation including extra and intracranial complication as a result of necrosis of the mastoid bone.

The symptoms are less severe in comparison to acute coalescent mastoiditis. The discharge from the ear is mucopurulent but moderate in amount. Ear ache is less severe or may be completely absent. Deafness is present and is conductive in type unless the labyrinth is involved.

The signs are similar to that of acute coalescent mastoiditis although the inflammatory response may be less.

Management: The investigations are the treatment are same as acute coalescent mastoiditis.

LABYRINTHITIS

Definition

It is the inflammation of the labyrinth as an extension of otitis media and purulent meningitis.

Etiology

1. **Trauma:** Fracture of the skull, surgical trauma like mastoidectomy or stapedectomy in the presence of suppurative infection.
2. **Bacterial infection** of the middle ear through the round or oval window.
3. **Meningitis:** Bacterial meningitis may lead to retrograde spread of infection to the membranous labyrinth or extension of infection along the fluid pathway that connects the subarachnoid space and peri-lymphatic space of the cochlea, i.e. through the cochlear aqueduct.

Classification

Labyrinthitis may be classified as follows:

1. Circumscribed labyrinthitis
2. Diffuse serous labyrinthitis
3. Diffuse suppurative labyrinthitis
   - Acute suppurative labyrinthitis
   - Chronic or fibro-osseous labyrinthitis.

Circumscribed Labyrinthitis

It is a localized perilabyrinthitis following inflammatory condition where the pathological fistula formation occurs mainly into the lateral semicircular canal.

Causes

1. Cholesteatoma—one of the most common causes.
2. Congenital syphilis.
3. Granulomatous disease.
4. Temporal bone tumors.
5. Chronic otitis media (Acute exacerbation)
6. Pneumococcal type 3 infection of the middle ear and mastoid, i.e. acute coalescent mastoiditis.

Pathology

Any part of the middle ear cavity can be involved but most commonly seen in the lateral semi-circular canal. Fistula usually erodes the bony labyrinth but also can extend into the membranous labyrinth in few cases.

In late cases the pathological processes are much more likely to become diffuse. There will be primary breakdown of middle ear mucosa followed by resorption of a portion of the labyrinthine capsule. Bone resorption begins along the vascular channel.

Symptoms

1. Recurrent attacks of dizziness and nausea aggravated by movements of the head and body which lasts about a week.
2. Temperature and hearing are within normal limits or there may be mild conductive loss.

Signs

1. Spontaneous nystagmus towards the diseased ear is present during the attacks.
2. Fistula sign will be positive.

Investigations

1. CT scan of the temporal bone.
2. Audiogram.

Treatment

Medical treatment: Antibiotics preferably in the acute stage along with labyrinthine sedatives.

Surgical treatment: Mastoidectomy and closure of fistula in otitis media.

Diffuse Serous Labyrinthitis

It is a diffuse intralabyrinthine non-suppurative inflammatory condition.

Causes

1. Secondary to pre-existing circumscribed labyrinthitis.
2. Chronic suppurative otitis media - untreated.
3. Mastoidectomy operation in the presence of circumscribed labyrinthitis.
4. Trauma.
5. Surgery of the inner ear.

Pathology

The essential pathology is that of nonpurulent inflammation of the labyrinth with cellular infiltration of serous or serofibrinous exudate. This usually occurs as a result of chemical changes in the perilymphatic space caused by a toxic or suppurative process which impinges on the membrane barrier of the labyrinth such as round window causing the bony fistula.

Symptoms

1. Vertigo—Spontaneous and rotational.
2. Sensorineural hearing loss—Acute onset but temporary.
3. Temperature—Normal.

Signs

1. Nystagmus—usually to the side of the disease.

2. Fistula sign is positive if secondary to circumscribed labyrinthitis.

Differential Diagnosis

1. Suppurative labyrinthitis—sensorineural hearing loss is present which is total and permanent. In serous labyrinthitis hearing loss is temporary.

Treatment

Medical

- Absolute bed rest
- Antibiotics
- Labyrinthine sedative

Surgical

This is contraindicated in the early stage. Surgery may be required later where antibiotics fail to control the infection and in cases of cholesteatoma.

Diffuse Suppurative Labyrinthitis

It is a diffuse purulent peri- and endo-lymphatic condition.

Causes

1. Chronic suppurative otitis media.
2. Subdural abscess or meningitis.

Pathology

Acute stage consists of an infiltration of the labyrinth with polymorphonuclear leukocytes combined with destruction of the soft tissue structures. Osseous labyrinth may become necrosed in parts. Granulation tissue formation which may form a wall around the necrotic bone forming one or more sequestra. Paralysis of facial nerve may occur and infection may extend into the intracranial structures if it is virulent.

The chronic stage follows 2 to 3 weeks after the onset of acute suppurative labyrinthitis. The granulation tissue gradually changes to fibrous tissue associated with calcification and new bone formation. The new bone formation may partly or completely fill the labyrinthine spaces from 6 months to several years in about 50% of cases.

Symptoms

1. Onset is acute in acute suppurative type.
2. Nausea
3. Vomiting
4. Vertigo
5. Ataxia
6. Deafness—profound sensorineural type.

In chronic variety, the above symptoms are insidious in onset due to compensatory action of the opposite labyrinth. The temperature is normal.

Posture of the patient: In acute stage patient will be curled up in the bed lying to the side of the healthy ear down most and affected ear upper most to get rid of the vertigo.

Signs

1. *Nystagmus*: horizontal or rotatory type.
2. *Fistula sign*: negative because of the dead labyrinth.

Investigations

1. *Caloric test*: Canal paresis.
2. *Audiogram*: Profound sensorineural hearing loss.
3. CT scan
4. CSF examination to rule out meningitis.

Treatment

Medical: Absolute bed rest, labyrinthine sedative and antibiotics.

Surgical: Mastoidectomy with labyrinthectomy may be necessary in patient with threatening intracranial complications.

PETROSITIS

Definition

Petrositis is the infection of the petrous apex leading to the coalescence of petrous apex air cell with formation of empyema. It is very often secondary to otitis media, occurs less commonly than the mastoiditis.

Clinical Features

1. Onset may be acute or chronic.
2. Three D's:
   - Diplopia
   - Discharge (foul smelling)
   - Deafness
3. Cervicofacial neuralgia
4. ***Gradenigo's syndrome*** consists of otorrhea, retro-orbital pain (V nerve involvement) lateral rectus palsy (VI nerve palsy).
5. Associated symptoms of headache, fever and vomiting.

Investigations

1. Plain X-Ray (Towne's and Stenver's view)
2. CT-Scan/MRI to compare the pneumatization of both the sides.

Treatment

1. *Medial management:* In case of acute petrositis.
   - I/V chloramphenicol with flucloxacillin
2. *Surgical management:* Mainly designed for chronic cases. Preferred surgeries consists of:
   1. Simple mastoidectomy and exploration of tract to the apex.
   2. *Eagleton's approach* provides wide exposure of the dura of middle fossa.
   3. *Almoor's anterior approach:* The petrous apex is approach through a triangle bounded by tegmen tympani above,

carotid artery anteriorly and cochlea posteriorly.

4. *Ramadiers-Lamperts approach:* The petrous apex explored through the posterior wall of the bony carotid canal.

5. *Frenckner's operation:* Petrous apex approached through under the arch of superior semicircular canal.

INTRACRANIAL COMPLICATION

LATERAL SINUS THROMBOSIS

Definition

It is defined as the inflammation of the lateral or sigmoid sinus with the formation of thrombosis inside the lumen of the sinus.

Commonest Organisms

1. Streptococcus
2. Pneumococcus type 3

Route of Infection

1. **Bony destruction or erosion:** Chronic inflammation of the middle ear (choles-teatoma) spreads to the mastoid which will erode the bony wall of the lateral sinus by means of osteitis. The infecting organism will come in touch with the wall of the sigmoid sinus which will initiate the thrombus formation.

2. **Progressive thrombophlebitis:** Infection without thrombus formation. The infecting organism may transverse to the sinus through it's tributaries without eroding the bony wall of the sinus.

3. **Preformed pathway:** Infection may travel through the preformed pathway to the sinus.

Pathology

When the virulence of the organism is high and resistance of the host is low, the infective organism will cause the inflammatory changes in the wall of the sigmoid sinus. This in turn will initiate thrombus formation inside the lumen of the sigmoid sinus to seal and localize the infection. The thrombus may keep accumulating inside the lumen and go as far down upto the internal, jugular vein or it may go up to the confluence of the sinuses.

Symptoms

1. Fever resembles malarial fever. It is a high swinging type fever accompanied by chills and rigors. In between the attacks the patient will have a sense of well being. This fever is also known as **picket fence fever.**
2. Headache due to perisinus abscess or raised ICT
3. Projectile vomiting and neck rigidity i.e. is the patient has an emaciated look due to the progressive anemia.
4. Ear discharge.
5. Deafness.
6. Ophthalmoplegia.
7. Blindness.

Signs

1. **Tenderness** can be elicited over the mastoid which may also be there along the anterior border of the sternocleidomastoid. On palpation, there is a cord like feeling along the anterior border of the sterno-cleidomastoid.
2. **Gresinger's sign:** Inflamed swelling and edema in the middle of the posterior border of the mastoid.
3. **Tobey - Ayer test** is positive i.e. on putting pressure on the neck there will be fluctuation of reading seen in the barometer connected to the lumbar puncture site for collection of CSF in a normal individual but the same is absent in lateral sinus thrombosis (Fig. 15.3).
4. **Crowe-Beck test:** Pressure on the jugular vein of healthy side produces engorgement of the retinal veins and supra orbital veins. Engorgement relieves on release of pressure.
5. **Progressive anemia.**

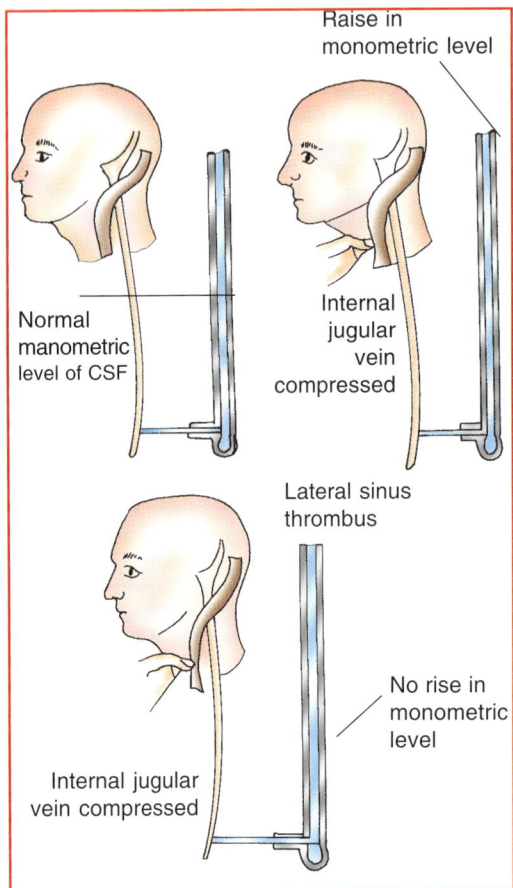

Fig. 15.3: Digrammatic representation of Tobey-Ayer test

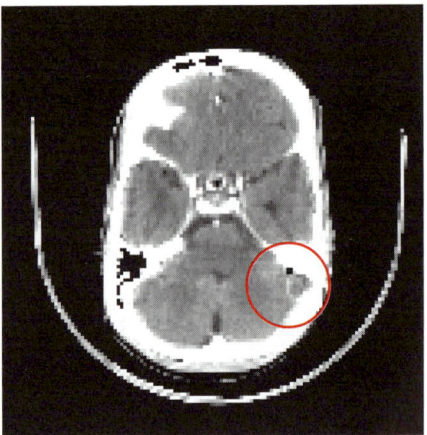

Fig. 15.4: CT scan axial cut showing delta sign

Treatment

1. Antibiotics to be selected after blood culture; adequate dose should be given.
2. Surgical: If no improvement of the symptoms after the first 48 hours after starting antibiotics, then radical mastoidectomy is done followed by removal of the thrombus or ligation of the sigmoid sinus.
3. Anticoagulants like heparin or dicumarol may be given.

A. Extradural Abscess

Extradural abscess is formed by direct extension following bone erosion. The abscess is situated between eroded inner cortex and duramater (Fig. 15.5). It is one of the most common intracranial complications. The size and rate of enlargement depends on the exact location of the abscess.

Common sites

1. Around the lateral sinus.
2. Opposite the middle cranial fossa by destroying the tegmen plate and more anteriorly to the petrous apex by destroying the petrous pyramid, opposite the posterior cranial fossa by destroying the bone in the **Trautmann's triangle.**

Investigations

- Hemoglobin—low.
- Blood culture and sensitivity.
- Peripheral smear to rule out malarial infection.
- Fundoscopy to rule out papilloedema.
- X-ray mastoid—erosion.
- CT scan can show the sinus thrombosis. Delta sign (enhancement of sinus walls but not the contents, filling defect) may be seen positive in the axial cuts (Fig.15.4)
- MRI with contrast will show the thrombus.

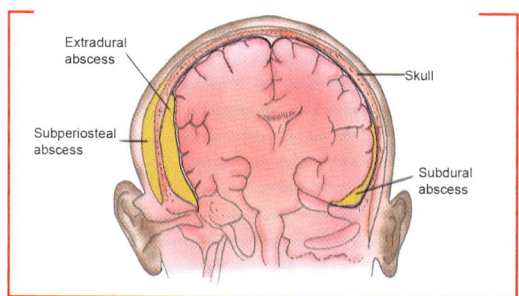

Fig. 15.5: Extradural abscess, subdural abscess, and subperiosteal abscess

Pathology

This abscess is well encapsulated. The spread of infection from the petrous apex can cause a middle fossa extradural abscess, medial to the arcuate eminence, precipitating the **Gradenigo's syndrome**.

A posterior fossa abscess occurs in close association with the lateral sinus and is frequently associated with the lateral sinus thrombophlebitis. The spread of the posterior fossa abscess is limited medially by the internal auditory meatus.

Clinical Features

The clinical pattern depends on the site of the abscess, it's duration and the rate of it's development. Most of the time, it is an incidental finding. However, the following symptoms in a chronically discharging ear should be suspected.
1. **Earache:** Steady, throbbing and boring.
2. **Discharge:** Profuse, creamy and sometimes pulsatile. Rate of discharge and degree of pulsation of the discharge may sometime increase by compression of the internal jugular vein.
3. **Headache**.

Investigation

CT Scan.

Treatment

1. Antibiotics.
2. **Surgical:** Radical or modified radical mastoidectomy with wide removal of the bone around the abscess.

B. Subdural Abscess

It is an abscess in which pus is collected between duramater and arachnoid. Multiple abscesses may occur in the subdural space.

Pathology

The rate of spread of abscess probably determines the clinical and pathological pattern. The dura is very resistant to infection. The granulation tissue is usually formed on its inner surface to localize the inflammatory reaction. The granulation tissue may eventually be converted to fibrous tissue. Eventual necrosis of dura may lead to infection of the subdural compartment. The abscesses are initially seropurulent and later become frankly purulent and extends over the surface of the cerebellar hemisphere. Continuing granulation tissue invasion will localize the developing abscess. The abscess may remain near the site of invasion or may extend widely with the production of the pus which will act like a space occupying lesion. Adjacent cortical vein will show thrombophlebitis producing multiple small abscess.

Clinical Features

1. Progressively severe malaise, fever, headache.
2. Patient becomes toxic.
3. Focal epileptic fits.
4. Behavioral changes in rapid succession i.e. confusion, stupor, etc.
5. Neck rigidity.

Investigations

- CSF study:
  - Increased CSF pressure.
  - Polymorphs 500 to 800
  - Glucose normal.
  - No microorganism on culture.
- CT scan.
- Fundoscopy—papilloedema.

Treatment

- Antibiotics.
- Drainage through multiple burr holes followed by modified radical mastoidectomy.

C. Brain Abscess

It is a circumscribed collection of inflammatory product involving both the cerebellar and temporal lobe. Temporal lobe abscesses are more commonly encountered. Development of otogenic brain abscess occurs within a period of 1 to 2 weeks.

Pathology

The infective organism will produce a local pachymeningitis which may be followed by thrombophlebitis penetrating the cerebral cortex of the temporal lobe or the cerebellum. Infection may also extend along periarteriolar **Virchow-Robin** space into cerebral white matter. The cerebellar abscess are frequently preceded by lateral sinus thrombophlebitis. They usually lie within the lateral lobe of the cerebellum. The formation of abscess usually undergo the following stages.

1. **Stage of encephalitis,** i.e. micro-organism migrate along the perivascular sheath of pial vessels into the substance of the brain causing focal necrosis and liquefaction with a surrounding zone of intense edema.

2. **Stage of localization:** There is formation of a capsule of inflammatory tissue and fibrosis.

3. **Stage of enlargement:** Abscess begin to enlarge after varying period.

4. **Stage of rupture:** Temporal lobe abscess may rupture into the lateral ventricle or onto the surface of the brain to develop meningitis.

   Cerebellar abscess may rupture into the fourth ventricle which may produce herniation into the foramen magnum.

Clinical Features

It is divided under two headings.

1. **Symptoms and signs of raised intracranial pressure**
   - Headache-usually on the side of the lesion.
   - Malaise.
   - Nausea and projectile vomiting.
   - Fever—low grade and later hypothermia
   - Apathy and drowsiness.
   - Delirium and convulsion.
   - Pulse rate may vary - slow if pressure is more.
   - Papilloedema.

2. **Localizing symptoms and signs**
   Temporal lobe abscess
   1. Dysphagia
   2. Homonymous upper quadrantic hemianopia due to involvement of lower fibers of optic radiation.
   3. Jacksonian convulsion.
   4. Paralysis—contralateral face and arms.
   5. Hallucination of smell and taste.
   6. Nominal aphasia in case of left temporal abscess difficulty in naming known objects.
   7. Contralateral extension plantar reflex.

Cerebellar Abscess

1. Headache —suboccipital and tend to radiate down the neck.
2. Neck stiffness.
3. Weakness and loss of tone on the affected side (Head may be tilted towards the side of the lesion).
4. Vertigo.
5. Nystagmus.
6. Ataxia—tendency to fall to the same side.
7. Past pointing—finger to nose and heel to shin tests are impaired on the side of the abscess.
8. Paralysis of 6th and 7th cranial nerve occasionally.
9. Pupillary paralysis, hemiplegia, status epilepticus, bradycardia, hypotension,

irregular and slow respiration occur in the end of the manifestation stage, when the patient will die.

Investigations

1. CT scan or MRI.
2. *CSF analysis*: Lumbar puncture at times may be dangerous.

Treatment

1. Antibiotics.
2. Drainage of the brain abscess by multiple burr holes followed by mastoidectomy (modified or radical).
3. Lateral sinus thrombophlebitis to be treated.

Otitic Hydrocephalus

Definition

This is a condition characterised by increased I.C. pressure syndrome probably secondary to the bilateral sinus thrombophlebitis but without enlargement of the ventricles.

Clinical Features

- Onset may be gradual, may be weeks or years after the ear infection.

Symptoms

1. Headache
2. Drowsiness
3. Blurred vision, nausea and vomiting with occasional diplopia

Signs

Papilloedema, nystagmus, CSF pressure exceeds 300 mm of water.

Differential Diagnosis

Brain abscess.

Investigations

CT and MRI shows normal site ventricles.

Treatment

1. Steroids
2. Diuretics
3. Antibiotic therapy
4. Repeated lumbar puncture
5. Long term lumbo peritoneal shunting may be required.

Meningitis

This complication occurs as a result of spread of infection through the tegmen plate due to preformed pathway or erosion of bone by cholesteatoma. The other route of spread are sinus plate, labyrinth following suppurative labyrinthitis.

The clinical features include headache, vomiting and high grade fever associated with neck stiffness and positive Kernig's sign. In severe cases drowsiness, delirium and papilloedema can occur.

Treatment

High dose of broad spectrum antibiotics and mastoidectomy.

POINTS TO REMEMBER

1. Complication of suppurative otitis occurs following spread of infection through (a) Bony erosion (b) Thrombophlebitis (c) Preformed pathways (d) Periphlebitis.
2. Picket fence fever is a characteristic feature of lateral sinus thrombophlebitis.
3. Gresinger's sign is positive in lateral sinus thrombophlebitis.
4. Fistula sign is positive in circumscribed labyrinthitis, which is commonly associated with a fistula in the lateral semicircular canal.
5. Gradenigo's syndrome consists of otorrhea, retro-orbital pain and lateral rectus paralysis.
6. Cerebellar abscess are frequently preceded by lateral sinus thrombophlebitis.

16

Otosclerosis

Definition

It is a common hereditary disease of localized bone derived from the otic capsule. Here, the normal laminar bone is removed by osteoclasts and replaced by unorganized bone of greater thickness, vascularity and cellularity (spongy interwoven cancellous bone).

The inner ear develops from the otic capsule. It has 14 or more ossification centers and normal laminar bone formed by this process will have three layers:

1. Periosteal layer
2. Enchondral layer
3. Endosteal layer

It will also have residual cartilage. They are known as fissula ante fenestrum and fossula post fenestrum which are situated in front and behind the oval window respectively. Otosclerotic focus occurs mainly in the region of the fissula ante fenestrum.

Types of Otosclerosis

See Flow chart 16.1 for various types of otosclerosis.

Etiology

The exact etiology is not known
- Hereditary—because it runs in the family

Flow chart 16.1: Types of otosclerosis

Types of otosclerosis		
Stapedeal otosclerosis	Cochlear	Histological type
• Anterior focus	• Round window area or other areas of the otic capsules is involved	• Lesion detected only on post-mortem
• Posterior focus		
• Lobster—claw type		
• Biscuit type		
• Circumferential type (Footplate and the Stapedial crura cannot be identified)		

- Autosomal dominant
- Racial-common in Caucasian
- Hormonal - otosclerotic activity is more during pregnancy and puberty.
- Age group 15 to 45 years.
- Male : Female = 1:2

Pathogenesis

Otosclerosis is a localized irregularly progressive disease involving primarily the otic and labyrinthine capsules of the temporal bone. It is characterized by the replacement of normal enchondral bone by spongy vascular bone. The sites of predilection are characterized by the presence of embryonic fibrocartilage, namely the fissula ante fenestrum and fossula post fenestrum just anterior and posterior to the stapes footplate.

The first indication of disease is enlargement of the perivascular space. Bone is absorbed by osteoclastic activity and new bone is deposited by osteocytes. The osteocytes are found in the advancing edge of the lesion which extends to the otic capsule by finger-like projections. These lesions contain vascular spaces in the center. The result is disorganized bone rich in osteocytes with enlarged marrow spaces rich with blood vessels and connective tissue with multinucleated giant cell osteoclasts in the center absorbing the disorganized bone. This process of resorption and replacement of bone occurs ultimately leading to the deposition of lamellar bone.

As the otosclerotic focus gradually replaces periosteal layer of the otic and labyrinthine capsules and approaches the middle ear surface the overlying mucoperiosteum increases in thickness and becomes vascular due to neovascularization and vascular shunting. It is seen as a reddish hue through the translucent ear drum.

As the disease advances the focus from the predicted site involves the oval window causing fixation of the stapes. Gradually the whole of the footplate is involved and in very advanced cases the otosclerotic focus involves both the oval and round window including the cochlear bony labyrinth and the term **malignant otosclerosis** is used.

Sometimes the otosclerotic focus involves the bony labyrinth of the cochlea without associated stapes fixation and the term cochlear otosclerosis is used.

Histopathology of Otosclerosis

Otosclerotic lesion may be characterized histologically as **active** and **inactive** depending on their stage of bone remodeling and growth tendency. Active lesions are recognized by their spongy structure, immature osseous tissue with numerous dilated vascular channels with osteoclastic giant

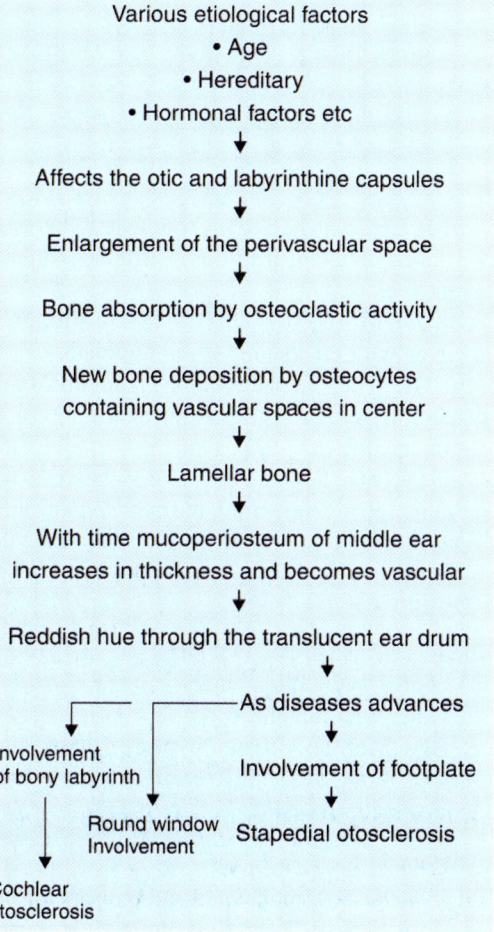

cells. Inactive lesions represent end stages of otosclerotic bone transformation process characterized by solid, compact, lamellar, mosaic-like tissue containing tiny marrow spaces and small infrequent blood vessels.

Schuknecht and Barber used the following criteria as indicative of histologic activity in an otosclerotic focus:

1. Area of nonosseous tissue showing increased vascularity and cellularity.
2. Evidence of osteoclastic bone resorption or osteoblastic new bone formation.
3. Increased vascularity and fibrous thickening of overlying mucosa.
4. Affinity of the osseous tissue for acidophilic stains.

Using these criteria there was a direct correlation of the size of the lesion and the histologic activity.

Depending on the amount of otosclerotic bone deposition in the region of the footplate of stapes, they are divided into (Fig. 16.1).

Type I: Less than half of the footplate is involved and normal thin bluish appearance of the footplate is retained.

Type II: More than half of the footplate is involved with thickening of the footplate.

Type III: Whole of the footplate is involved and appears thickened. The margin of the footplate can be identified.

Type IV: Otosclerotic bone is deposited in the entire footplate obliterating the oval and/or round window.

Histologically

The foci demonstrates two phases:

1. Early spongiotic phase
2. Late sclerotic phase

Blue Mantles: Area of hypercellularity with areas of blood vessels. Remodelled bone with blood vessels around it.

Symptoms

1. **Voice** is low modulated and the patients are soft spoken. Because bone conduction is

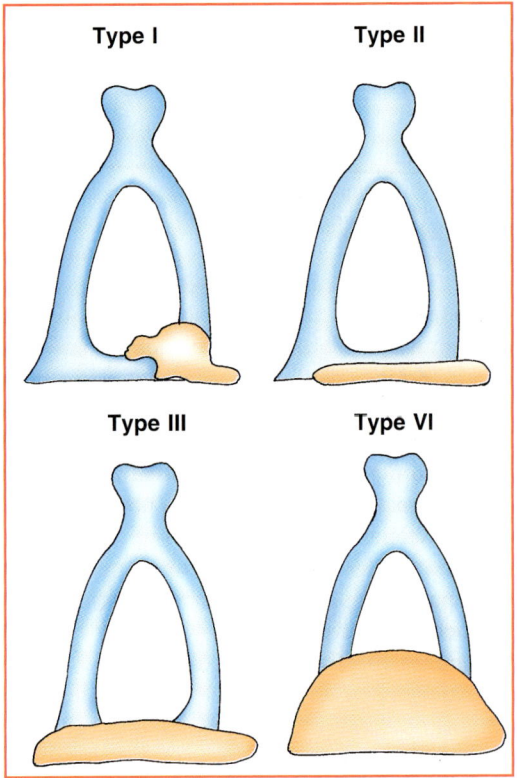

Fig. 16.1: Types of footplate

more and patient hears their own voice louder.

2. **Deafness:** Mainly conductive, sensorineural or mixed in cochlear type. **Paracusis Willisii**, i.e. the patient will hear better in noisy surroundings as in a restaurant (as people tend to speak in a louder voice against a background noise).

3. **Tinnitus:** Patient complain of associated noise and is more commonly with cochlear otosclerosis and active disease

4. **Vertigo:** Persistent and frequent in the beginning and becomes paroxysmal and less frequent, lasts maximum for 3 weeks and usually does not recur.

5. **Bezold's triad:** Absolute negative rinne, raised lower tone limit, prolonged bone conduction.

Signs

1. Otoscopy—the external auditory canal is wider than normal but the tympanic membrane is usually normal. In active otosclerosis, a congested area may be seen in the tympanic membrane which is known as **flamingo pink blush or Schwartz sign.**
2. Tuning fork tests.
   - (a) Rinne's test—negative
   - (b) Weber's test—lateralized to the affected side.
   - (c) Absolute bone conduction—normal.
   - (d) Gelle's test—positive in case of fixed stapes footplate.
3. Audiogram will show an air bone gap. In few patients one may find a notch or dip at 2000Hz in the bone conduction curve known as **Carhart's notch. Cookie Bite pattern** is seen in mixed hearing loss as in cochlear otosclerosis. Carhart notch is a mechanical artifact, not a true representation of cochlear reserve. Notch is commonly attributed to:
   - (a) Loss of inertial component of bone conduction by stapes fixation.
   - (b) Fixation of stapes disrupts normal ossicular resonance, happening at about 2000 Hz.
   - (c) Relative perilymph immobility due to stapes fixation disturbs the normal compressional mode of bone conduction.
4. Impedance will show low compliance.
5. CT scan of temporal bone 20 degree coronal section. Loss of definition of margins of oval window to narrowing and finally complete obliteration of the oval window opening and niche. Cochlear otospongiosis shows **double ring effect** due to spongiosis within the thickened capsule.

Differential Diagnosis

1. Ossicular discontinuity behind an intact drum.
2. Congenital fixation of ossicles, mainly the stapes footplate.
3. Secretory otitis media.
4. Fixed malleus syndrome
5. Tympanosclerosis.

Treatment

Medical

There is no medical treatment of otosclerosis, however sodium fluoride has been tried to hasten the maturity of active focus and arrest further cochlear loss. Sodium fluoride can be given especially in cochlear otosclerosis given in 50mg b.i.d divided doses for one to two years.

Surgical

Various surgical procedures have been developed for the treatment of otosclerosis which include:

1. Stapedectomy.
2. Small fenestra stapedectomy.
3. Stapedotomy (Fig. 16.2).

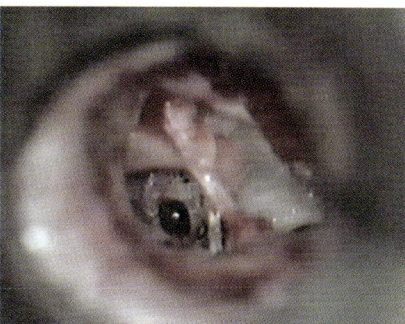

Fig. 16.2a: Otosclerotic foci in stapes footplate

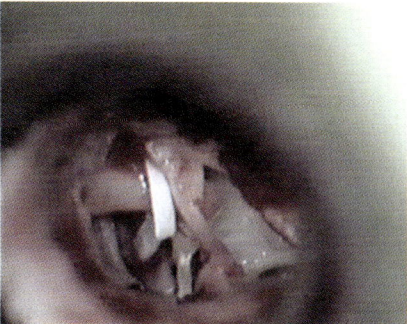

Fig. 16.2b: Teflon piston placed after stapedotomy

4. Stapedotomy with stapedius tendon preservation.
5. Vein-graft Teflon interposition operation.
6. Laser stapedotomy.

Indications for Surgery

- Bone conduction of 0 to 25db and air conduction of 45 to 65 db.
- Air bone gap should be at least 15 db.
- Speech discrimination score of 60% or more.

Contraindication

- Age >70 years
- Children less than preadolescent age group.
- Conductive losses from other causes like tympanoslcerosis.
- Otitis media
- Only hearing ear
- Pregnancy
- Stapedial/cochlear otosclerosis with poor air bone gap
- Vertigo and clinical evidence of secondary labyrinthine hydrops.
- Sportsmen.

POINTS TO REMEMBER

1. Otosclerosis is a disease of the otic capsule, where normal endochondral bone is replaced by spongy vascular bone formation leading to ankylosis of the footplate of the stapes.
2. Schwartz size is positive in active otosclerosis.
3. Paracusis willisii is a feature seen in otosclerotic patient, where, the patient can hear better in a noisy surrounding.

17

Facial Nerve and its Disorders

Anatomy of the Facial Nerve

Facial nerve is a mixed nerve having motor, sensory and secretomotor fibers.

- **Sensory and secretomotor** fibers are carried by nervus intermedius of Wrisberg and relayed into the tractus solitarius and superior salivary nucleus in the medulla and pons respectively. The sensory root (nervus intermedius of Wrisberg) has afferent fibers conveying taste sensation from the anterior two-third of tongue, and efferent fibers which are secretomotor to the lacrimal gland, and submandibular and sublingual salivary glands.
- The nucleus for the **motor fibers** lies on the pons. It supplies the muscles of facial expression.

Nerve has basically two parts

1. Supranuclear part
2. Infranuclear part.
   - Intratemporal part
   - Extratemporal part.

However, for the purpose of topographical analysis, the intratemporal part has been further divided into nuclear, suprageniculate, geniculate, suprastapedial, infrastapedial, infrachordal and extracranial. The composition of this nerve in each of these segments are different and therefore produces different symptoms and signs. By employing special tests, the level of lesion can be detected.

Supranuclear Part (Fig. 17.1)

The supranuclear part has fibers from both the cerebral cortex and supplies the muscles of the upper part of the face. Motor fibers from its nucleus in the pons hooks around the 6th cranial nerve and comes out into the cerebellopontine angle through the lower border of the pons. The efferent secretomotor fibers arise from the superior salivary nucleus and join the course of the facial nerve in the cerebellopontine angle to supply the lacrimal, submandibular and sublingual salivary glands and also the glands of the nasal and palatine mucosa. Taste fibers from the anterior 2/3rd of the tongue are carried by the chorda tympany nerve in the main nerve trunk to travel upto the cerebellopontine angle where it gets separated to join the nucleus of the tractus solitarius in the medulla. The somatic afferent fibres from the posterosuperior part of the tympanic membrane, external auditory canal and concha also run in the main nerve trunk.

Intratemporal Part (Flow chart 17.1)

The facial nerve passes through the internal auditory canal along with the vestibulocochlear

Flow chart 17.1: Intratemporal part

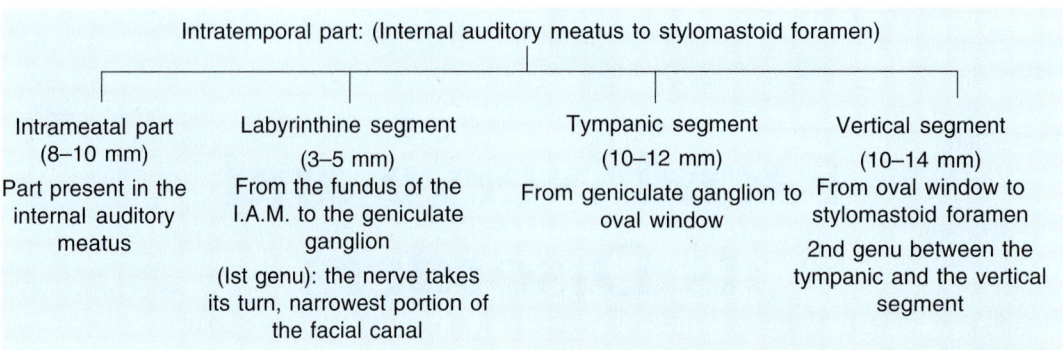

Intratemporal part: (Internal auditory meatus to stylomastoid foramen)			
Intrameatal part (8–10 mm) Part present in the internal auditory meatus	**Labyrinthine segment** (3–5 mm) From the fundus of the I.A.M. to the geniculate ganglion (Ist genu): the nerve takes its turn, narrowest portion of the facial canal	**Tympanic segment** (10–12 mm) From geniculate ganglion to oval window	**Vertical segment** (10–14 mm) From oval window to stylomastoid foramen 2nd genu between the tympanic and the vertical segment

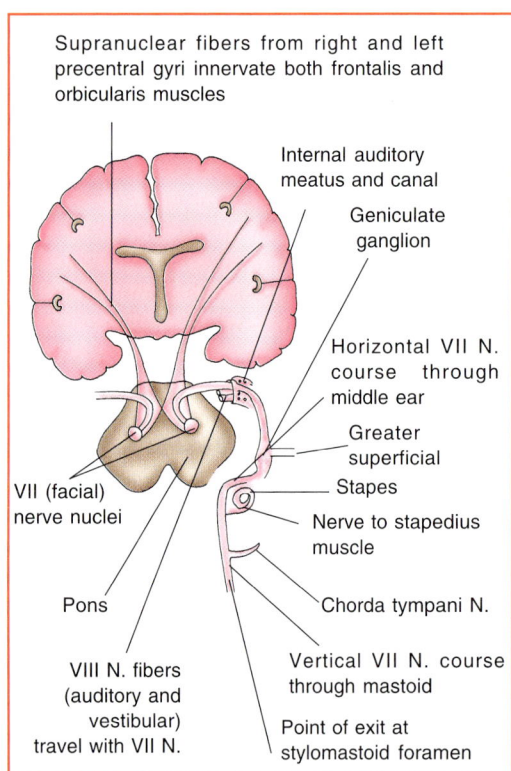

Fig.17.1: Course of the facial nerve (supranuclear and infranuclear) and its branches

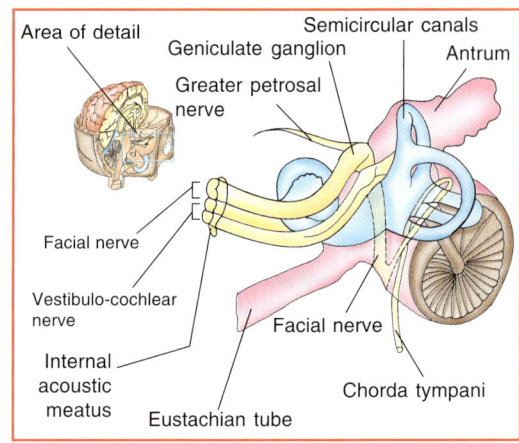

Fig. 17.2: Intratemporal course of facial nerve

The nerve turns backward and lying within the bony fallopian canal, it runs above the oval window (horizontal portion). It then turns downwards (vertical portion) in the posterior wall of the middle ear and emerges out via the stylomastoid foramen.

The intratemporal part is of immense surgical importance to the otolaryngologist.

Branches

1. **In the geniculate ganglion:** Greater superficial petrosal nerve carries preganglionic parasympathetic or secretomotor fibers. Also carries the taste sensation from the soft palate.

nerve and the internal auditory artery. It enters the middle ear behind the processus cochleariformis. At this site of bending the geniculate ganglion is situated (Figs 17.1 and 17.2).

2. **Within the canal:** Nerve to stapedius muscle, chorda tympany nerve.
3. **At the stylomastoid foramen:** Muscular branches to postauricular muscle, posterior belly of digastric and stylohyoid muscle.
4. **Terminal branches (face):** Temporal, zygomatic, buccal, marginal mandibular and cervical branches to supply the muscles of facial expression (Figs 17.3 and 17.4).

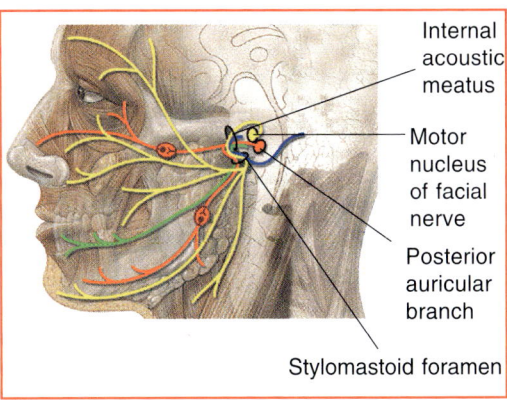

Fig. 17.4: Facial nerve supplying muscle of facial expression

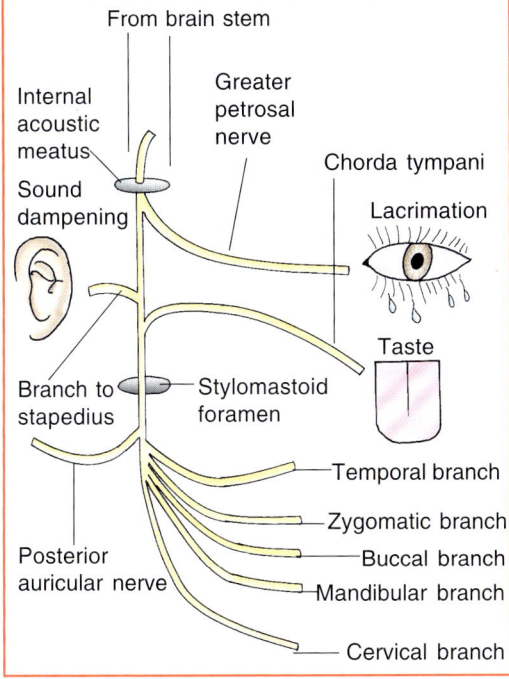

Fig. 17.3: Branches of facial nerve

Etiology of Facial Nerve Paralysis

A. Intracranial infranuclear lesions

1. Vascular thrombosis
2. Tumors
3. Multiple sclerosis
4. Poliomyelitis
5. Acoustic neuroma
6. Cysts
7. Primary cholesteatoma
8. Basal meningitis
9. Infective polyneuritis
10. Trauma
11. Head injuries

B. Intratemporal lesions
- **Congenital**
  1. Melkersson Rosenthal syndrome
  2. Mobius syndrome

- **Acquired**
1. Idiopathic—Bell's palsy
2. Trauma :
   - Temporal bone fracture
   - Post—surgical, e.g.: Mastoidectomy, stapedectomy.
3. Infective
   - Bacterial—otitis media
   - Viral—Herpes zoster oticus.
   - Tuberculous mastoiditis.
   - Malignant otitis externa.
4. Tumors:
   - Facial nerve neuroma.
   - Intracanalicular acoustic neuroma.
   - Glomus jugular.
   - Malignant tumors of middle ear and mastoid.

C. Infratemporal lesions
1. Trauma
   - Birth trauma

- Surgical trauma
  - Parotidectomy
  - Postauricular incision in children.
  - Surgery of temporomandibular joint.
2. Tumors
   - Malignant tumors of parotid gland.
   - Facial nerve neuroma.
   - Metastatic lymph nodes.

D. Miscellaneous causes

1. Temporary paralysis following local anesthesia infiltration.
2. Lead poisoning
3. Sarcoidosis
4. Polyneuritis
5. Poliomyelitis
6. Diphtheria
7. Syphilis
8. Glandular fever

Pathophysiology of Facial Nerve Paralysis

Sunderland has described the pathophysiological events associated with all types of disorders that afflict the facial nerve in five grades.

Grade 1. Neuropraxia—compression of axoplasm. Nerve is viable and returns to normal function when block is corrected.

Grade 2. Axonotemesis—compression persists with increase in intraneural pressure.

Grade 3. Neurotemesis—loss of myelin tube.

Grade 4. Partial transection—loss of myelin tube and disruption of perineurium.

Grade 5. Complete transection—loss of myelin tube, disruption of perineurium and disruption of epineurium.

- The first three grades of injury can occur with viral inflammatory immune disorder such as Bell's palsy and herpes zoster.
- Injuries of first and second grade have an excellent recovery usually occurs between one week to two months.

- Third grade injury recovery is moderate to poor in 2–4 months.
- Fourth and fifth grades injuries occur when there is disruption of nerve during surgery, temporal bone fracture, rapidly growing benign and malignant tumors.
- Fourth grade may very rarely recover where movement is barely perceptible from 4 to 18 months.
- Fifth grade injury will never recover.

Tests for Topographical Diagnosis

1. Schirmer tear testing for lacrimation.
2. Tests of stapedial reflex by impedance audiometry.
3. Tests for taste by
   - Electrogustometry
   - Application of chemical solutions on the tongue.
4. Tests for salivation—the volume of saliva is measured after sucking a fresh lemon for 60 seconds.

Electrodiagnosis

- Threshold excitability tests.
- Conduction velocity tests.
- Electromyography
- Estimation of voluntary motor unit potential.
  - Fibrillation action potential.
  - Polyphasic potential.

Radiological Tests

CT scan and MRI with contrast.

Sequelae of Degeneration

In case of facial nerve injury above grade III, produces the following abnormalities:

1. **Facial asymmetry** due to loss of motor power or contracture.
2. **Synkinesis** in which voluntary movement of one part of the face results in inadvertent movement of another, e.g. smiling may be associated with involuntary eye closure or

sweating over preauricular area while chewing (**Frey's syndrome**) because of the cross innervation of motor fibers.

3. **Crocodile tears** - Lacrimation during eating.
4. **Mass movement** resulting from lack of insulation of electrical impulses by the myelin sheath.
5. **Clonic facial spasm (Tics)**
6. **Ocular disturbances.**

General Management of Facial Nerve Paralysis

1. **Restoration of the continuity of the facial nerve.**
   - Facial nerve decompression.
   - Rerouting.
   - End to end anastomosis.
   - Cable grafting of the nerve with post auricular or sural nerve.
   - Dott's operation (intracranial facial nerve repair).
   - Faciohypoglossal anastomosis.

2. **Surgical rehabilitation**
   - Tympanic neurectomy in case of crocodile tears.
   - Muscle transplantation to prevent contracture and fibrosis of muscle by sling operation.
   - Selective facial nerve avulsion for facial nerve spasm.
   - Injection of botulinum to the muscle for facial spasm.
   - Prosthetic rehabilitation.
   - Tarsorraphy or gold implant for lid loading to manage eye closure.

3. **Electrical stimulation**
   - Galvanic stimulation to prevent fibrosis and contracture of paralyzed muscles.
4. **Physiotherapy:** Massage of the paralyzed facial muscles from down above. Circular massage should be avoided to prevent tear of muscle fibers.

Idiopathic Facial Paralysis (Bell's palsy)

It is the most common type of facial paralysis. The etiology of which is still obscure. The following theories have been put forth as the etiological factors:

1. **Ischemic theory :** Spasm occurring in the arterioles of the vasa nervosum causes ischemia of nerve and subsequent edema and compression of the nerve in the fallopian canal producing ischemic paralysis.
2. **Viral theory:** The viral theory is attractive because it explains the acuteness of the paralysis and self limiting course of Bell's palsy. It is also known that the facial paralysis is commonly affected by viral infections like Herpes zoster, poliomyelitis and infectious mononucleosis which proves that facial nerve is very prone for viral infection. Herpes simplex virus (HSV-1) has also been known to cause facial paralysis.
3. **Autoimmune theory:** This theory has not been well accepted by majority of the otologists but can be a cause in isolated cases.

Clinical Features

1. Loss of voluntary movement of facial expression on the side of the lesion.
2. Paralysis is of lower motor neuron type, i.e. all the muscles of facial expression on the affected side are paralyzed. The presence of muscle paralysis can be recorded by asking the patient the following questions:
   - *To close the eyes*: The patient will not be able to close the eye on the affected side. The eyeball will roll up on every attempt of closure (**Bell's phenomenon**) (Fig. 17.5a).
   - To show the teeth, to whistle and to blow the cheek. Facial asymmetry can be noted (Fig. 17.5b).
   - *To look upwards*: Absence of wrinkling of the forehead on the affected side which

is pathognomonic of lower motor neuron type of paralysis (Fig. 17.5c).

3. **Dryness** of the eye on the affected side in some cases. **This symptom has a bad prognostic value.**

4. Loss of sense of taste—**this also has bad prognostic value.**

5. Intolerance to loud noise (hyperacusis) due to paralysis of stapedius muscle.

6. Epiphora.

7. Pain is usually retroauricular but sometimes radiates to the face, pharynx and arm.

8. Decreased hearing.

Natural history of idiopathic paralysis

Idiopathic paralysis may be of two types:
1. Partial paralysis
2. Total paralysis

Partial paralysis: In this type there is no nerve degeneration and complete recovery is seen within 3 weeks. A small percentage of cases may go for complete paralysis.

Total paralysis: Vast majority of these cases recover. In very small number of cases, they go for total degeneration in which case, the recovery is never complete. **The total paralysis accompanied by severe pain in elderly people with loss of taste and lacrimation will have grave prognosis.**

Diagnosis

1. *From the history*: Acute onset.

2. *Clinical findings*: The facial paralysis is always isolated and peripheral in origin. Systemic disease is not evident.

Tests for topographical diagnosis as mentioned earlier to know the level of lesion.

Management

Management is very important and falls under two headings:
1. Treatment to minimize the denervation.
2. Treatment to maintain the muscle tone during the period of paralysis.

Treatment to minimize the denervation

Medical Management

1. **Corticosteroid therapy:** Considered to be an excellent treatment. Prednisolone - 1mg/kg/body wt./day in divided doses for first five days. If the paralysis remain incomplete the dose is to be tapered in the next 5 days. If the paralysis remain complete same dose of steroid is to be continued for a total period of 15 days and tapered to zero in the next 5 days. Prednisolone is discontinued after 21st day even though return of facial nerve function cannot be expected until 3 to 6 weeks.

2. **Acyclovir:** Acyclovir and prednisolone are the treatment of choice for Bell's palsy and herpes zoster palsy. This combination gives an excellent final outcome of recovery.

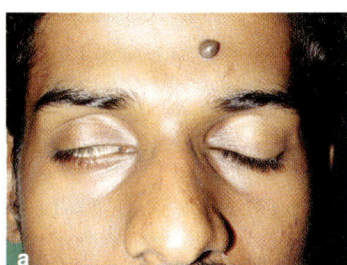 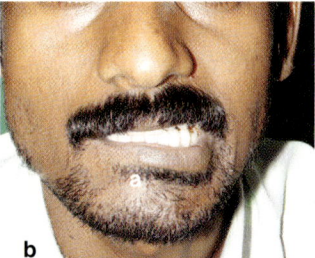 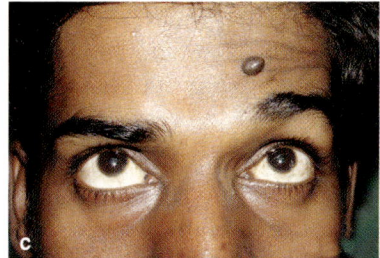

Figs 17.5a to c: Clinical pictures of Bells Palsy: (a) Incomplete closure of eye , (b) Facial assymetry, (c) Absence of wrinkling of the forehead on the affected side

Acyclovir can be given intravenously or orally.

Oral dose: 800 mg every 5 hrs.

Intravenous dose: 200 mg every 5 hrs for 10 days.

3. **Vasodilator therapy:** Nicotinic acid.
4. **Stennert's protocol:** This is a new line of management with the following drugs
   - Low molecular dextran IV infusion 1000cc /day for 3 days over a 16 hour period reduced to 500 cc over 8 hours for 10 days.
   - Hydrocortisone 200 mg /day for 2 days if the wt is below 70 kg; 250 mg/day for 2 days if wt is more than 70 kg reduce to 50 mg /day for 10 days and stop steroid therapy between 11 to 12th day.
   - Pentoxyphilline 10 mg/day added to the infusion (to any 1 pint of low molecular weight dextran)
   - Acyclovir 200 to 400 mg 5 times daily for 10 days.

Surgical Management

Surgery in case of Bell's palsy is done only in case of associated **BAD syndrome.**

B—Absence of Bell's phenomena
A—Anesthesia of cornea
D—Dry eyes.

Facial Nerve Decompression

It is still a controversial line of treatment regarding the time of surgery. It is suggested that the electroneurography and the clinical course of the paralysis are the best guidelines for selecting patients for facial nerve decompression. When electroneuronography demonstrates 70 to 90% degeneration within two weeks after onset- urgent surgical decompression will prevent the complete degeneration. Surgery after 2 weeks is not advised because active viral disease has abated and early regeneration stage is beginning. Decompression should be limited to the meatal and labyrinthine segment through a **middle cranial fossa approach.** The Transmastoid approach is no more popular nowadays.

Treatment to maintain muscle tone

1. Reassurance
2. Care of the eye
3. Care of the facial nerve
4. Prosthetic rehabilitation.

POINTS TO REMEMBER

1. Facial nerve is a mixed nerve having motor, sensory and secretomotor fibers.
2. Nervus intermedius of Wrisberg carries sensory and secretomotor fiber.
3. The supranuclear part has fibers from both the cerebral cortex and supplies the muscle of the upper part of the face.
4. Sunderland has described the pathophysiological events associated with disorders of facial nerve in five grades, i.e. (a) Neuropraxia, (b) Axonotemesis, (c) Neurotemesis, (d) Parital transection, (e) Complete transection.
5. Bell's palsy (Idiopathic facial paralysis) is the most common type of facial paralysis. Acyclovir and prednisolone are the treatment of choice for Bell's palsy.

18

Tumors of
the Middle Ear

GLOMUS TUMORS

Glomus tumors also known as chemodectomas or non-chromaffin paragangliomas, arise from the glomus bodies distributed along the parasympathetic nerve in the skull base, thorax and in the neck. However, the term glomus tumor is much more popular than the other terminologies.

The term **glomus tympanicum** is used for tumors arising from the middle ear promontory whereas the term **Glomus jugulare** tumor is used for tumor arising from the jugular foramen regardless of their extent. When they arise high in the neck extending towards the jugular foramen they are termed as **glomus vagale**.

When they arise in the carotid bulb, they are termed as **carotid body tumors** (Fig. 18.1).

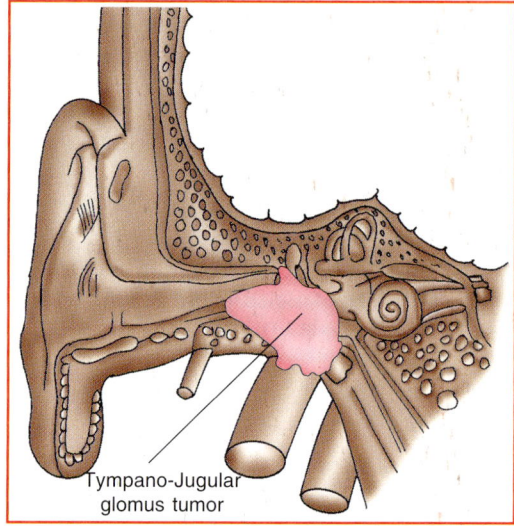

Tympano-Jugular glomus tumor

Fig. 18.1: Glomus tumor arising from jugular bulb

Pathology

Glomus tumors are the most common benign tumors that arise within the temporal bone. These tumours are hypervascular and they arise from the glomus bodies. The glomus bodies are found within the adventitia of the jugular bulb, in the course of the glossopharyngeal and vagus nerves including the tympanic canaliculus, retrofacial air cells, promontory and geniculate ganglion.

The clinical behavior of this tumor is very variable, it may present as a simple swelling in some cases whereas marked bone erosion, expansion with cranial nerve paralysis may be seen in other cases. The main blood supply to the glomus tumour is the ascending pharyngeal artery.

All these tumors secrete catecholamines, although few exhibit clinically evident hypersecretion, of nonadrenaline, adrenaline, dopamine, serotonin, vasoactive amines, glucagons, polycytokines, etc. have been described. A few patients may undergo malignant changes and metastasis.

Microscopically, glomus tumor resembles glomus bodies with rich supply of vascular spaces lined by epitheloid cells. Tumors that metastasize are usually more pleomorphic.

Clinical Features

Incidence

- Middle age group
- Females are commonly affected
- Female: male ratio of 3:1.
  Familial with autosomal dominant hereditary patterns and can be sporadic also.

Symptoms

- Hearing loss
- Pulsatile tinnitus
- Blocking and fullness of the ear in early cases
- Bleeding or blood stained discharge
- Otalgia
- Cranial nerve palsies—facial paralysis and may include 6th, 9th, 10th, 11th and 12th cranial nerve weakness producing symptoms like diplopia, hoarseness, aspiration and inability to lift the shoulder.

Signs (Fig. 18.2)

- A reddish-blue retrotympanic mass may be seen known as **rising sun** behind the drum.
- Bleeding and polypoidal mass is seen when there is invasion of the tympanic membrane.

- **Brown's sign** is positive, i.e. a smooth dark red middle ear mass that blanches in response to the applied pneumatic pressure via the otoscopic or seigelization.

Differential diagnosis of a reddish blue mass behind the tympanic membrane:

- Glomus tympanicum
- High jugular bulb
- Aberrant carotid artery
- Aneurysm of carotid artery
- Cholesterol granuloma
- Metastatic disease

Classification

Fisch (1979)

Type A—Tumor localized to the middle ear cavity.
Type B—Tympanomastoid tumors with no destruction of bone in the infralabyrinthine compartment in the temporal bone.
Type C—Tumors invading the bone of the infralabyrinthine compartment.
Type D—Tumors with intracranial extension.

Investigations (Fig. 18.3)

1. Audiogram is initially conductive but later profound sensorineural hearing loss in most of the cases occurs.

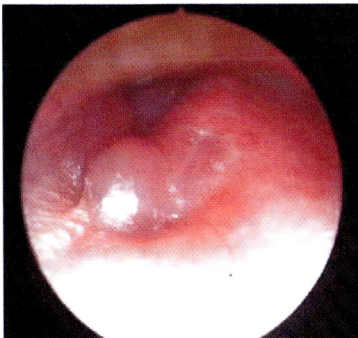

Fig. 18.2: Showing the rising sun appearance of glomus tumor

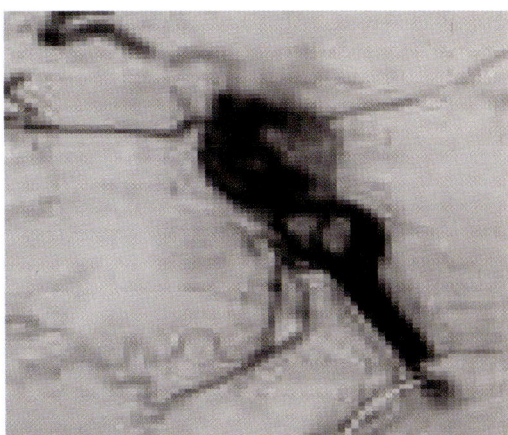

Fig. 18.3: Angiogram showing highly vascular glomus tumor

2 MRI with gadolinium contrast will show tumor extension, T1 weighted image have **salt and pepper** appearance.

3. CT scan may also be done, lateral tomography shows absence of normal crest of bone between the carotid canal and jugular foramen characteristic of glomus jugulare tumour, known as **Phelp's sign**.

4. Digital subtraction angiography helps to know the feeding arteries for preoperative embolization and to know the cerebral cross circulation.

5. 24 hour urine vanillylmandelic acid levels prior to surgery is required because some of the glomus tumors secrete catecholamines which can cause increase in blood pressure.

Treatment (Flow chart 18.1)

1. Surgery
   - Transmastoid excision of type A and B.
   - Lateral skull base surgery with infratemporal fossa extension for type C and type D.
2. Preoperative embolization before 48 hours of surgery can reduce intraoperative bleeding.
3. Radiotherapy and chemotherapy for unresectable tumors with intracranial extension.
4. KTP 532 laser and bipolar assisted excision of glomus tympanicum (Senior author has used this technique in his patients with very good results).

MALIGNANT TUMORS OF THE MIDDLE EAR

The squamous cell carcinoma is the commonest malignant tumor where as adenocarcinoma is rare.

Etiology
1. Unknown
2. Long-standing, neglected CSOM.

Spread
1. **Laterally:** External auditory canal and parotid gland.
2. **Upward:** Middle cranial fossa.
3. **Backwards:** Mastoid.
4. **Downwards**: Jugular fossa.
5. **Inwards**: Inner ear and C.P. angle and petrosphenoid angle.
6. **Forward**: Eustachian tube to the naso-pharynx.

Lymphatic drainage
Commonly retropharyngeal nodes.

Incidence
- Rarely seen
- Common in 6th decade
- Equal sex ratio

Flow chart 18.1: Management of glomus tumor

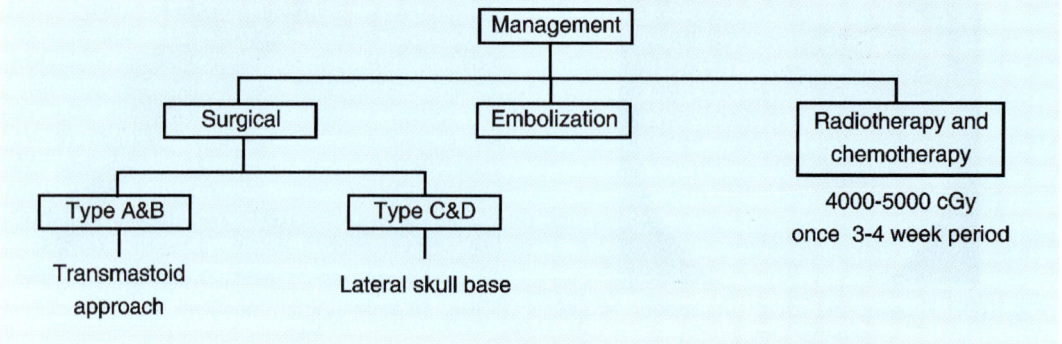

Symptoms

1. Blood stained ear discharge
2. Otalgia
3. Deafness

Signs

1. Granulations and polyp seen in the external auditory canal.
2. Evidence of lower cranial nerve palsy including the facial nerve in late cases.

Investigations

1. CT- Scan/ MRI
2. Biopsy

Treatment

1. Radiotherapy in early cases.
2. Surgery in the form of radical mastoidectomy/subtotal petrosectomy/total petrosectomy. Followed by postoperative radiotherapy.
3. Chemotherapy.

POINTS TO REMEMBER

1. Glomus tumors are known as chemodectomas.
2. Glomus tumor arising from the jugular foramen is called glomus jugular and those arising from the promontory of the middle ear are called glomus tympanicum.
3. Glomus tumors are the most common benign tumors that arise within the temporal bone.
4. It presents with pulsatile tinnitus.
5. Browne sign refers to blanching of a smooth dark redish middle ear mass on increasing the external ear pressure by seigelization.
6. Squamous cell carcinoma is the most common malignant tumor of the middle ear.

19

Diseases of the Inner Ear

MENIERE'S DISEASE

First described by Prosper Meniere. It is also known as *endolymphatic hydrops* and is characterized by episodic vertigo, fluctuant deafness and tinnitus. It is often associated with nausea and vomiting. It is also described as *labyrinthine hydrops* because of inner ear disease. The peak incidence is between 40–60 years of age. In 47% of cases bilateral involvement is seen.

Etiology

The exact etiology is not known. A number of factors have been blamed for are
1. Genetic: Present in certain major histo-compatibility patient.
2. Allergy: Presence of IgG, IgA and secondary component in the cells of the sac stroma.
2. Hormonal
3. Vasomotor instability and ischemia
4. Viral inoculation.
5. Autoimmune: Immunologically induced inflammation.
6. Psychosomatic

Etiology of Secondary Endolymphatic Hydrops

Secondary endolymphatic hydrops known to be secondary to otic capsule disease, like congenital or acquired syphilis, otosclerosis, Paget's disease and post-stapedectomy cases.

Atypical Meniere's Disease is a term which has been suggested to describe patients who complain of some but not all of the classical symptoms of the triad.

Variants of Meniere's Disease

(a) *Lermoyez syndrome*: Sudden sensorineural hearing loss which improves during or immediately after the attack of vertigo (Tinnitus, hearing loss vertigo).
(b) *Tumarkin's otolithic catastrophe*: Abrupt falling attacks of brief duration without loss of consciousness.

Pathophysiology (Flow chart 19.1)

The basic pathology in Meniere's disease is increased accumulation of fluid in the endolymphatic system causing engorgement (Figs 19.1 and 19.2) due to:
1. Excessive endolymph production in the stria vascularis.
2. Decreased absorption of endolymph in the endolymphatic sac.

Histopathologically

Damages are seen mainly in the inner ear. There will be dilatation of the cochlear duct, saccule

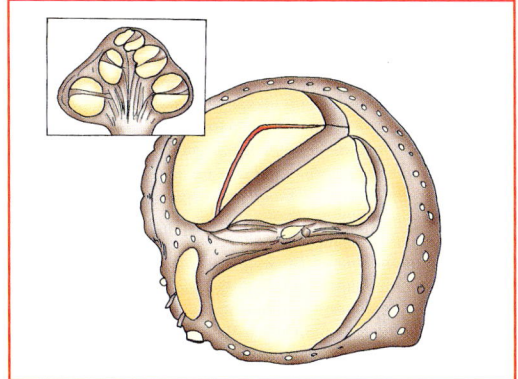

Fig.19.1: Bulging of Reissner's membrane

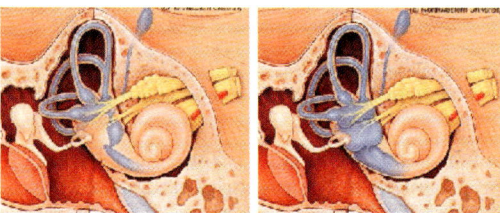

Fig.19.2: Normal and engorged membranous labyrinth

Flow chart 19.1: Pathophysiology of Meniere's Disease

Prodromal stage of gradual distension of endolymphatic system

↓

Distension progresses leading to thinning and atrophy of Reissner's membrane and saccular wall

↓

Rupture and sudden release of large volume of endolymph in small perilymph space

↓

Sensory and neural structure exposed to K^+ rich endolymph

↓

Sudden hearing loss and vertigo

↓

When perilymphatic compartment is restored to normal, symptoms subside

↓

Aided by the collapse, the rupture heals and the process is repeated.

and utricle. The Reissner's membrane bulges into scalavestibuli. There will be herniation of Reissner's membrane and later rupture of Reissner's membrane leads to leakage of K+ rich endolymph into perilymphatic space causing 8th nerve depolarization causing reduced vestibular neuronal outflow. Healing of the membrane improves auditory and vestibular function.

Incidence

- Seen equally in both sexes and family history is positive in 10–20% of cases
- Peak age incidence is to 40–60 years.
- Commonly unilateral but can affect both ears eventually in some cases.

Clinical Features

Symptoms

1. Vertigo (96%)

- Episodic, sudden onset
- Lasts for 24 minutes to 24 hours
- Rotatory in nature
- Associated with nausea, vomiting and diarrhea.
- No loss of consciousness
- Associated with nystagmus
- Patient gives history as if feeling on a *ship at the mercy of stormy sea.*

 Tullio's phenomenon: Subjective imbalance and nystagmus observed in response to loud sound, low frequency, noise exposure.

2. Hearing loss (88%)

- Fluctuant and progressive
- Initially low frequency loss and later high frequency loss
- Sensory neural hearing loss
- Dysacousis
- Diplacusis—difference in presentation of pitch between the two ears.

3. **Tinnitus**—associated low pitch noise (roaring sound) in the ear which comes in bouts.
4. **Feeling of aural fullness**
   Pattern of attack:
   vertigo⟶ deafness ⟶ tinnitus

Signs

1. Otoscopic examination - Normal.
2. Nystagmus is seen during the attacks. Nystagmus is horizontal rotatory having a fast and slow component. In between the attacks the nystagmus will be absent.
3. Tuning fork test indicates sensory neural hearing loss. Rinne test is positive, absolute bone conduction is reduced in the affected ear and weber is lateralized to the better ear.

Investigations

- **Pure tone audiometry:** There is sensorineural hearing loss. In early stages, lower frequencies are affected and the curve is of rising type. When higher frequencies are involved curve becomes **tent** shape (falling type) and later flat.
- **Speech audiogram:** It is to distinguish between cochlear and retrocochlear lesions. In Meniere's disease:
  a. Recruitment is positive
  b. SISI (Short increment sensitivity test) score is better than 70% in two thirds of patients.
  c. Tone decay test - There is no tone decay.
- **Electrocochleography** shows the changes that are characteristic of, and probably diagnostic of endolymphatic hydrops. There is a broadening of the SP/AP wave form, due to a relative enhancement of the summating potential (SP). The normal SP/AP ratio is around **20%.** In an ear with hydrops, the ratio is often as high as **30%.**

- **Vestibular function test**
  - *Caloric test:* These are abnormal in about three-quarters of patients. The commonest pattern is a **canal paresis**, but a directional preponderance towards the normal ear, or a combination of reduced

canal sensitivity and directional preponderance may be found.
- *Electronystagmography:* It is now accepted as routine investigation in vertiginous patients. This is based on principle of corneoretinal potential to answer the following questions:
  1. Abnormality in vestibular system or not?
  2. Peripheral or central vestibular system problem?
  3. If peripheral, which side is involved?
  4. If central, what region is likely to be involved?
  5. Is lesion static, progressive or recovering?
- *Glycerol test:* This glycerol dehydration test is performed by administering glycerol, flavored with orange juice or lime, by mouth in a dose of 1.5ml/kg. A pure tone audiogram, and electrocochleography are carried out before ingestion of the dose, and again 1½ to 2 hours later. Plasma osmolality should also be measured, since there can be no effect on the cochlea unless that rises by more than 10 mOsm/kg., and 15% improvement in PTA is significant and decrease in SP/AP ratio is seen.
- **Brainstem evoked response audiometry:** Measurement of the tiny physiological electrical events occurring in response to sound stimulation. Brain stem response stimuli in the form of clicks, these electrical potentials are picked up from the vertex by surface electrodes.
- *CT scan or MRI to rule out cerebellopontine angle pathology.*

Differential Diagnosis

1. Vestibular neuronitis
2. Benign paroxysmal positional vertigo
3. Cervical spondylosis
4. Acoustic tumors
5. Vertebrobasilar insufficiency
6. Labyrinthitis

7. Perilymph fistula
8. Migraine induced vertigo.

Treatment

The treatment of Meniere's disease or endolymphatic hydrops remains an enigma because the precise etiology of the disease is unknown.

General Measures

1. **Reassurance:** To relieve the patient's anxiety and explaining the nature of disease specially in acute attack.
2. Avoidance of smoking
3. Low salt diet
4. **Decrease intake of alcohol, coffee and tea.**

Medical Management

1. **Vestibular sedatives:** Drugs of the phenothiazine group with antihistamine properties are strong vestibular suppressants. They include *cinnarizine* and *procholorperazine.* Antihistamine such as promethazine (Phenergan) are also useful vestibular sedatives.
2. **Diuretics and dietary salt restriction:** Diuretics Thiazide triamterene can alter the fluid balance in the inner ear leading to a decrease in endolymph and resolution of the hydrops.
3. **Carbonic anhydrase inhibitors**
4. **Vasodilators** are used based on the hypothesis that ischemia of the stria vascularis causes Meniere's. The rationale is to improve the metabolic function of a diseased ear. IV histamine, isosorbide dinitrate, cinnarizine (a calcium antagonist), and betahistine (an oral histamine analog) have been used with purported success. Betahistine produces vasodilation of the capillaries, arterioles, and arterial-venous arcades in the stria vascularis and spiral ligament and lower endolymphatic pressure

5. **Clinical evidence of Meniere's disease** were found to have autoantibodies. This antibody treatment with immunosuppressive agents has gained favor. Systemic and intratympanic glucocorticoids, cyclophosphamide, and methotrexate have all been used by clinicians but this treatment is controversial.

Surgery to Medical Failures

1. **Chemical labyrinthectomy** has recently become popular in the treatment of patients with disabling vertigo that is persistent and refractory to medical management.
   - **Intramuscular streptomycin**
   - **Intratympanic gentamicin** (Fig. 19.3) allows treatment of unilateral Meniere's disease without producing systemic toxicity or effects on the opposite ear. The round window membrane serves as the primary route of entry into the inner ear with the annular ligament of the stapes serving as a secondary route. The solution may be used as a stock solution of 40 mg/cc at a pH of 5.4 or buffered to a pH of 6.4 by sterile 8.4% sodium bicarbonate to improve patient comfort. With the patient supine and the head turned away from the treatment ear the tympanic membrane is anesthetized with application of absolute phenol with swab stick. About 0.5 cc of solution is injected into the middle ear with 25 gauge needle over the round window niche in the posteroinferior quadrant of tympanic

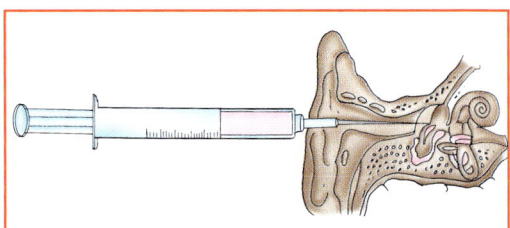

Fig. 19.3: Intratympanic gentamicin injection in low dose

membrane. The patient remains in this position for 30 minutes and is instructed not to swallow. We routinely schedule the injections weekly until effective treatment has occurred.

- **Gentamycin inner ear perfusion**—Low dose 10 mg per ml gentamicin infusion at 5 micro liter per hour for 10 days, through a microcatheter placed in round window niche. It is reported that vertigo is controlled in 95% while preserving hearing in 77%.

2. **Conservative operative procedures**
   - Endolymphatic sac decompression
   - Cochleostomy (cochlear endolymphatic shunt)
   - Cochlear dialysis
   - Sacculotomy (Fick's operation)
   - Grommet insertion
   - Cervical sympathectomy

3. **Surgery reducing vestibular activity without damaging the cochlea**
   - Vestibular nerve section
   - Ultrasonic destruction of vestibular labyrinth

4. **Destructive surgery**
   - Labyrinthectomy
   - Laser destruction of inner ear.

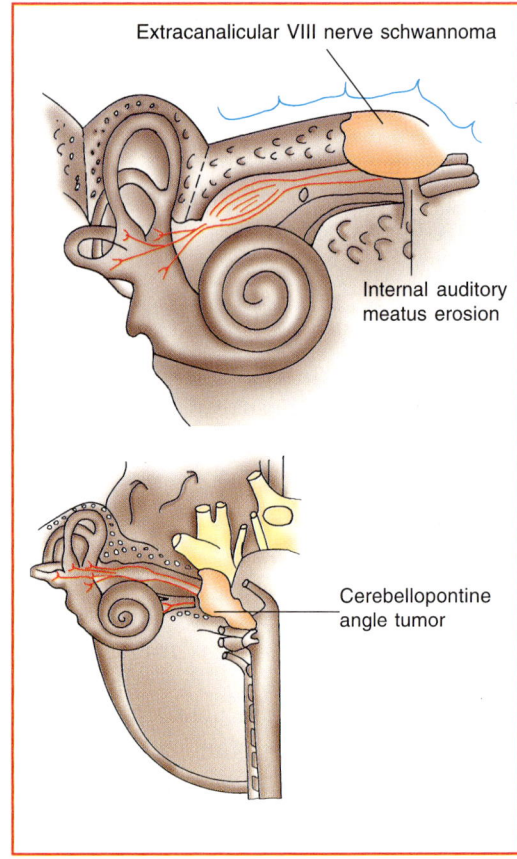

Fig. 19.4: Site of origin of acoustic tumor

ACOUSTIC NEUROMA

It is a benign Schwannoma of the 8th cranial nerve and is also known as neurilemmoma or neurinoma. It forms 8 to 10% of all intracranial tumors and 90% of all cerebellopontine angle lesions (Fig 19.4).

Pathology

It is a circumscribed encapsulated benign tumor. Malignant transformation is very rare. The shape and appearance varies according to the consistency in size of the tumor. Small tumors are generally pink or yellow and rubbery in consistency, whereas large tumors are more yellow, mottled and cystic in consistency.

Histopathologically, it is composed of Antoni A fibers which are compact and cellular and Antoni B fibers which are loosely packed and cellular.

Site of Origin

Arise from the vestibular nerve and more commonly from superior vestibular nerve. It arises from the Schwano-glial junction near the Scarpa's ganglion in the internal auditory meatus. This zone is termed as the *Obersteiner-Redlich zone*. There is abundance of Schwann cells in this region and hence it's origin from this area is more common. **It is necessary to know the growth pattern of the tumor because it determines** the chronology of symptoms. The growth patterns are :

- *Slow growth*: 0.02 cm per year
- *Medium growth*: 0.20 cm per year
- *Fast growth*: 1.00 cm per year

The tumor originates in the internal auditory meatus and gradually grows out into the cerebellopontine angle cistern, enlarges there, compresses the nerve and brain stem with increase in intracranial pressure, followed by death if untreated.

Clinicopathological Classification
(Flow chart 19.2)

Stage I (Otological Stage): Includes all intrameatal lesions, extrameatal tumors upto 2 cms, cause unilateral hearing loss with tinnitus.

Stage II (Trigeminal nerve involvement) Tumors more than 2 cms causes compression of trigeminal nerve leading to decrease corneal reflex.

StageIII (Brain stem and cerebellar compression): Ataxia, direction changing nystagmus (Brun's nystagmus) and involvement of lower cranial nerves (IX, X and XI).

Stage IV (Increase intercranial pressure): Papilloedema, headache and vomiting.

Stage V (Terminal stage): Failure of vital centers in brain stem causes coma and death.

Symptoms

- **Hearing loss:** Gradual, unilateral sensorineural hearing loss or asymptomatic sensorineural hearing loss, associated with impairment of speech discrimination out of proportion to the pure tone loss (67% of cases). Atypically, there may be sudden hearing loss in 26% of cases and normal hearing in 1 to 5% of cases.
- **Tinnitus (18%):** It is high pitched and continuous on the affected side. It coincides

Flow chart 19.2: Progression of Disease

Tumors from internal auditory
↓
Pressure effects on cochlear / facial nerve
↓
Erosion of walls of IAM
↓
Expansion in medial direction
↓
CP angle
↓
Tumor more than 2 cms
↓
Pressure effect on V, VI, IX, X and XII cranial nerves
↓
Brain stem cerebellar involvement
↓
Increase intracranial pressure
↓
Terminal stage

with the hearing loss for which the patient may not bother about the symptom. Unilateral tinnitus even if not accompanied by hearing loss should be investigated for acoustic neuroma.

- **Vertigo (18%):** Abrupt in onset, occurs early, lasts for days or weeks. It spontaneously resolves. It increases with head movement and exertion. Vertigo is seen more commonly and frequently in smaller tumors.
- **Cerebellar dysfunction (48%):** Ataxia or dysequilibrium which is continuous and unremitting, with tendency to fall towards the side of the tumor.
- **Trigeminal nerve dysfunction:** Numbness in the teeth, hypesthesia of the midfacial region. Atypically, trigeminal neuralgia.

- **Headache:** Occurs in the early and late part of the disease. Headache is seen in the fronto-occipital region of the ipsilateral side worse in the morning or precipitated by head movement and exertion.
- **Symptoms of raised intracranial pressure:** Commonly seen in large tumors. Vomiting, decreased visual acuity, diplopia, anosmia, etc.
- **Facial nerve palsy:** Occurs late and in large tumours.

On Examination

1. *Otoscopy*: Loss of touch sensation in the posterior superior meatal wall in some cases, known as *House and Hitselberger's sign.*
2. *Nystagmus*: Horizontal, rotatory.
3. *Loss of corneal reflex* (Fig.19.5)
4. Romberg's sign positive, i.e. tendency to fall to the affected side.
5. Past pointing is positive in very big tumors.

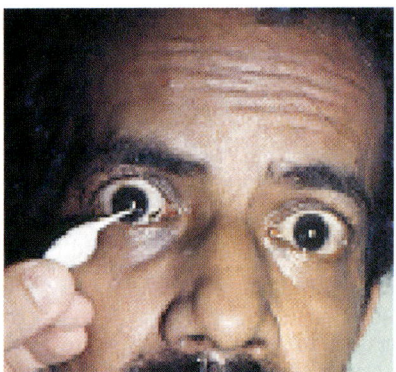

Fig. 19.5: Corneal reflex being done

Tuning Fork Tests

- Rinne's positive
- Weber is lateralized to the healthy side
- Absolute bone conduction is decreased

Investigations

1. Pure tone audiometry - high tone loss.
2. Speech reception threshold - 46 dB.

3. Speech discrimination score - very low, average 53%.
4. Recruitment and tone decay positive.
5. Acoustic reflex delay present.
6. Electrocochleography - Broadening of the AP and SP wave forms. Large cochlear microphony. Presence of action potential at stimulus intensity less than threshold and inaudible to the patient.
7. BERA: Most reliable audiological evaluation. Interval between wave 3 and wave 5 greater than 2 milliseconds for large tumors. Absence of the 5th wave is also seen in large tumors. Intra-aural latency differences more than 0.2 milliseconds suggests an acoustic neuroma.
8. Caloric test—Canal paresis in 90% of cases.
9. Electronystagmography—Direction changing nystagmus is seen once cerebellar connections are involved called as *Brun's nystagmus.*
10. Radiological evaluation—CT scan with contrast and MRI with *gadolinium* are the best radiological investigations to detect acoustic neuromas (Fig. 19.6).

Differential Diagnosis

1. Congenital cholesteatoma

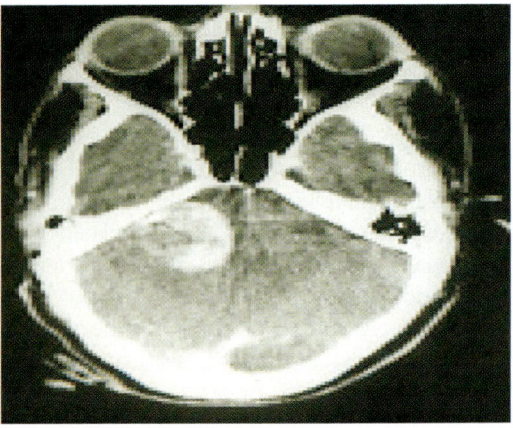

Fig. 19.6: CT scan showing left side acoustic tumor

Table 19.1: Advantages and disadvantages of surgical approaches to acoustic neuroma

Approach	Indications	Advantages	Disadvantages
Translabyrinthine	• Ideal for medium and large ANS because hearing preservation unlikely with tumors > 2 cm • Small ANS without serviceable hearing • Approach for facial nerve decompression and vestibular neurecetomy in the absense of serviceable hearing • Suitable approach for any tumor requiring exposure to CPA	• Highest rate of preserved facial nerve function (98.5% anatomic; 75% H-B I-IV) • Wide exposure to CPA • Facial nerve identified at CP angle and fundus • Immediate facial nerve repair possible • LImited cerebellar retraction • Low recurrence rate (0.4%)	• Total hearing loss • Short term vertigo if patient poorly compensated preoperatively • CSF leak 4 to 14%
Combined translabrynthine and transotic approach (Fisch approach)	Ideal for large tumor more than 3 cms without serviceable hearing	Wide exposure to CP angle and IAM	Total hearing loss
Restrosigmoid	ANS with serviceable hearing and minimal involvement of the IAC (especially smaller lesions) Meningiomas with limited IAC if serviceable hearing	Wide exposure Hearing preservation possible (35-65%) Facial nerve preservation possible 58-93%	Fundus not visualized Cerebellar retraction Postoperative headaches in 10% - postulated as intradural bone dust or adherence of nuchal muscles to dura Air embolism possible CSF leak 11–15% Recurrence 1–3%
Middle fossa	Intracanalicular ANS with minimal CPA involvement (<1cm) Tumors > 1cm is relative contraindication	Hearing preservation possible (up to 71%) Excellent facial nerve preservation (92%)	Not recommended in patients > 65 years old because dura is more adherent and fragile Temporal lobe retraction Must work around facial nerve to access tumor CSF leak 10%

2. Meningioma
3. Facial nerve Schwannoma
4. Arachnoid cyst

Treatment

Non-surgical

- Conservative observation in elderly patients with small tumors.
- *Stereotactic radiosurgery or Gamma knife:* Modern radiation protocols are stereotactic or gama-knife schema, with radiation doses of 1200 to 1400 rad most commonly employed. This causes arrest of growth of the tumor and also reduction in size. It is mainly used in
  - Patients who refuses surgery
  - Residual tumor
  - Contraindication to surgery

Complications includes trigeminal neuropathy, hearing loss, facial paresis.

- Chemotherapy
- Radiotherapy

Surgical

- Surgical approaches depends upon size and status of hearing shown in Table 19.1.

POINTS TO REMEMBER

1. Meniere's disease is a condition associated with formation of endolymphatic hydrops and is characterized by episodic vertigo, fluctuant deafness and tinnitus.
2. Tullio's phenomenon is associated with subjective imbalance and nystagmus in response to loud noise.
3. Acoustic neuroma is a benign schwannoma of the 8th cranial nerve that occurs in the cerebello-pontine angle. It arises from the Schwanno-glial junction and commonly from superior vestibular nerve.
4. Intratympanic gentamycin allows treatment of unilateral Meniere's disease without producing systemic toxicity or effects on the opposite ear.

Common Otologic Surgeries

20

COMMON OTOLOGIC SURGERIES

- Myringotomy and grommet insertion
- Myringoplasty
- Tympanoplasty
- Cortical mastoidectomy
- Modified radical mastoidectomy
- Radical mastoidectomy
- Stapedectomy

MYRINGOTOMY AND GROMMET INSERTION

"Myringotomy" is the incision of the tympanic membrane in order to drain suppurative or non suppurative effusion of the middle ear or to provide aeration in case of a malfunctioning eustachian tube. This procedure may be combined with the insertion of a ventilation tube or Grommet which keeps the opening patent.

Functions of Tympanostomy Tubes

- Eustachian tube bypass
- Support function of aeration and drainage.

Disadvantages of Tympanostomy Tubes

- Promote otitis media in children
- Contamination from EAC
- Does not serve barrier protection.

"However, studies have proved beyond doubt that tympanostomy tube placement greatly reduce rate of otitis media when the right tube is placed for right indications and for right period of time".

Indications for Myringotomy

- Relief of severe otalgia at the onset of illness or persistent signs and symptoms of acute middle ear infections.
- Presence or suspicion of suppurative complications of otitis media such as facial nerve paralysis or mastoiditis.
- Suspected cases of middle ear effusion.
- Hemotympanum.

Indications for Myringotomy and Grommet Insertion

1. Otitis media with effusion (OME)
2. Persistent retraction of tympanic membrane.
3. Radiation-induced secretory otitis media.
4. Patulous eustachian tube.
5. Treatment of Meniere's disease for intra-tympanic instillation of gentamicin or dexamethasone.
6. Salivary gland/choriostoma of the middle ear.
7. Hyperbaric oxygen therapy.

Anesthesia

- Routinely done under general anesthesia (GA) in all young children and large percentage of older children.
- Local anaesthesia (LA) is used in:
  - Cooperative child
  - Favourable ear canal anatomy.

Topical anesthetic drugs used include phenol, lidocaine.

Tube Selection

- Short term (6 months to one year) Shepherd Grommet style
- Permanent—T Tubes.

Technique

- Circumferential incision in posteroinferior quadrant for myringotomy in acute suppurative otitis media (Figs 20.1 and 20.2).
- Radial incision in anteroinferior quadrant is used for Grommet insertion.
- Middle ear effusion aspirated
- Insertion of tympanostomy tube (Figs 20.3 and 20.4).

- PSQ incision to be avoided for fear of:
  - Ossicular injury
  - Retraction pocket.

Postoperative Care

- Antibiotic ear drops in case of infection
- Avoid swimming
- Use ear plugs
- Regular OPD visits for follow-up of hearing assessment.
- Antihistamine and nasal decongestant and steroid like fluticasone, beclomethasone nasal spray.
- Mucolytic agents like ambroxol and bromhexine.

Complications

- Anesthetic complications.
- Operative complications like ossicular injury, bleeding due to high jugular bulb.
- Otorrhea
  - Can occur in some cases if the cause is not adequately treated or due to poor aural hygiene. Nasopharyngeal cancer can cause similar problem even after its treatment

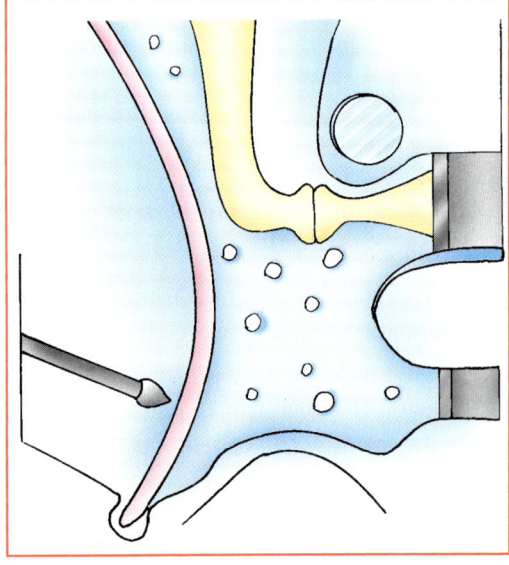

Fig. 20.1: Incising tympanic membrane

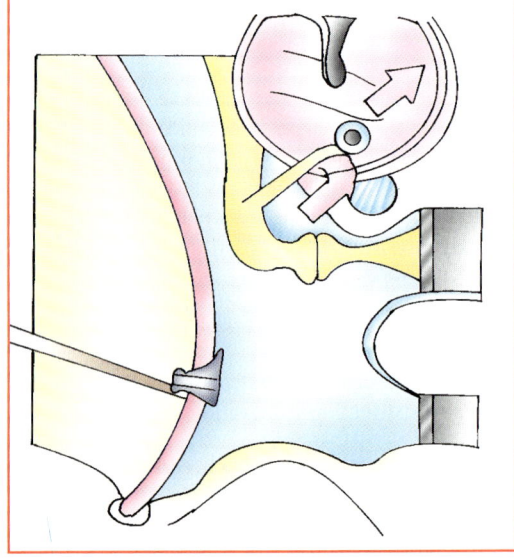

Fig. 20.2: Grommet in situ

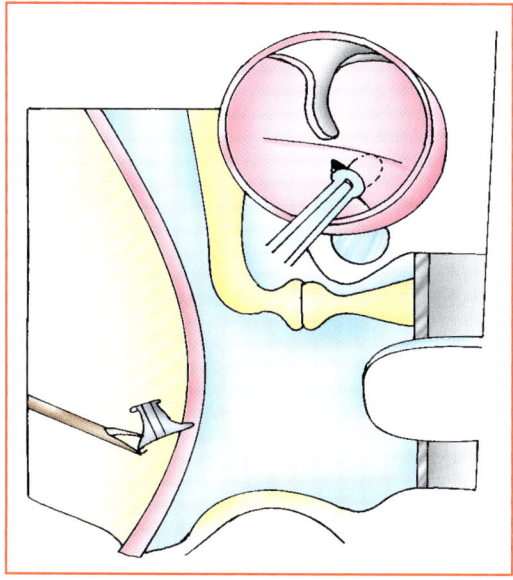

Fig. 20.3: Grommet being inserted

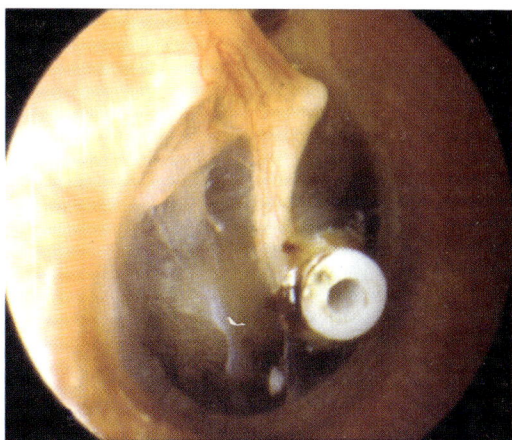

Fig. 20.4: Grommet in situ in the antero-inferior quadrant

- More common in children < 2 years, during upper respiratory tract infections (URTI)
- Early and late types
- Bacteriology in cases of suspected pseudomonas infection
- Myringosclerosis
- TM perforation
  - Smaller flanged Grommet (1-3%)
  - Stiff larger flanged T-tubes (30%)
  - Shorter flanged T-tubes (10%)
- Tympanostomy tube lost in middle ear
- Early extrusion
- Plugging of tube
  - With dried blood
  - Mucus
  - Granulation tissue.
- Tympanic membrane atrophy, retraction and atelectasis and cholesteatoma formation.

Laser Myringotomy

- Using CO_2 or KTP-532
- Used in highly vascular TM with decreased risk of bleeding and eschar blockage of ventilation tube.

MYRINGOPLASTY

Definition

Myringoplasty is a surgical procedure performed to repair or reconstruct the tympanic membrane with a suitable graft material.

It does not include removal of disease or reconstruction of ossicular chain.

Objectives of Myringoplasty

- To make the ear dry and trouble-free
- To improve hearing
- To enable proper hearing aid usage

Contraindication for Myringoplasty

- Acute URTI, Otitis externa
- Children below 12 years
- Only hearing ear with severe sensorineural hearing loss (SNHL) of opposite side
- Perceptive deafness more than 30 dB
- Marked loss of speech discrimination
- Uncontrolled systemic diseases like hypertension, diabetes mellitus, etc.
- Pregnancy

Prerequisites for Myringoplasty

- Ear should be dry at least for 3 months
- Healthy middle ear mucosa
- Patent eustachian tube
- There should be no focus of infection in nose, PNS and nasopharynx.
- Good cochlear reserve.

Graft Materials

1. Biological
2. Non-biological

Biological

Types	Sources
1. Autograft	Same person
2. Isograft	Genetically identical twin
3. Homograft (allogenous)	Another person (same species)
4. Heterograft (Xenograft)	Animals (another species) e.g calf fetal serosa, bovine jugular vein

Advantages of Autograft

- No immunological reaction
- Inexpensive
- No risk of HIV or other infections

Types of Autografts

1. Temporalis fascia (Ortegren -1958-59, Heermann -1961)
2. Tragal perichondrium (Goodhill et al -1964)
3. Conchal perichondrium
4. Tragal/conchal cartilage
5. Periosteum (Bocca et al -1956)
6. Vein (Shea -1960)
7. Fatty tissue from ear lobule (Ringenberg - 1962)
8. Subcutaneous tissue (Sale - 1969)
9. Fascia lata (Zollner -1956)
10. External auditory canal skin
11. Heterotopic skin (WullStein and Zollner 1950) - Split thickness and Full thickness
12. Dura (Homograft)

Advantages of Temporalis Fascia

- Location of donor site
- Easy to harvest
- Close histological and segmental kinship
- Low BMR—requires less nutrition—high survival
- No size limitation
- The only suitable autologous membrane for reconstruction of tympanic cavity and ear canal.
- It can be used as onlay / intermediate / underlay grafting.
- It can be used as more than one piece, overlapping the other.
- It can be used in sandwich techniques as one of the grafts with canal skin on the fascia.

Temporalis Fascia is An Extension of Deep Fascia of Neck

- It covers temporalis muscle and adjacent periosteum.
- It consists of two layers.
- Superficial layer of loose areolar tissue.
- Deep layer (lamina profunda) is aponeurotic and strong.

Aim of Myringoplasty

- Permanent closure of perforation with production of dry trouble free ear.
- To improve hearing function by restoration of hydraulic ratio and protection of round window.
- To restore a smooth continuous migratory tract to external auditory canal (EAC).

Classification of Myringoplasty Techniques

Myringoplasty techniques are classified into:

- Onlay
- Underlay techniques, based on the following.
  - Placement of graft in relation to lamina propria of drum remnants and fibrous annulus.
  - Underlay below (medial to) the annulus
  - Ovelay over (lateral to) the annulus

Onlay Technique

Steps of Onlay Technique

- Infiltration of postauricular area and ear canal with 2% lignocaine with 1:100000 adrenaline
- Postauricular ***Wilde's incision*** (Fig. 20.5b).
- Temporalis fascia graft harvestation
- Elevation of periosteal flap with anterior retraction of pinna
- De-epithelization of perforation margins
- **Vascular strip elevation** (Postcanal wall skin - Fig. 20.5a and b) and removal of anterior canal skin as free graft (Fig. 20.5c).
- Graft placement on fibrotympanic annulus and/ or tucking under the handle of Malleus (Fig. 20.5d).
- Replacement of free meatal skin graft and vascular strip (Fig. 20.5e).
- Packing of canal with gelfoam and umbilical tape
- Skin closure in two layers and mastoid dressing.

Advantages of Onlay

- Anterior recess can be visualized.
- Anterior over hang can be drilled out.
- Take up rate should be high as graft bed is broad.
- Middle ear space is not reduced.

Disadvantages of Onlay

- Poor exposure of vital areas of tympanic cavity.
- Delayed healing.
- Epithelial pearls from remnants of drum epithelium.
- **Blunting** of anterior meatal recess due to
  - Accumulation and organization of blood deep to graft.
  - Inadequate removal of anterior canal over hang.
  - Lateral healing of graft.
- Lateral displacement of graft.
- Inclusion or residual **cholesteatoma**.
- Retraction pocket due to E.T. dysfunction.

Underlay Technique

Technique of Underlay Myringoplasty

- After 4 quadrant infiltration of local anesthetic, **aural and end aural speculum** is introduced.
- Margins of tympanic membrane perforation are freshened.

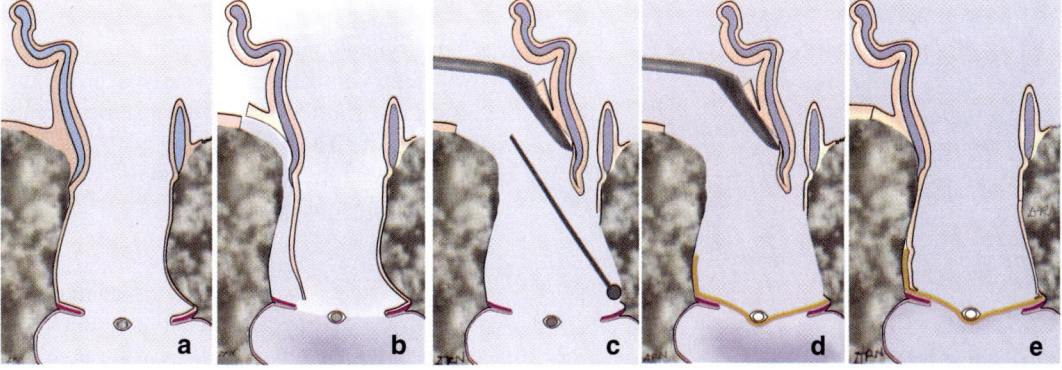

Figs 20.5a to e: Onlay technique of myringoplasty: (a) Perforation of the tympanic membrane, (b) Postauricular incision given and posterior canal wall skin (vascular strip) being raised and exposing posterior tympanic annulus, (c) Anterior canal skin being elevated and removed along with removal of skin over the entire annulus, (d) Graft placed over fibrotympanic annulus, (e) Placement of anterior canal wall skin and repostion of vascular strip over the graft

- A circumferential incision is given on the posterior meatal wall from 6 to 12 clock position, 3 to 4 mm lateral to annulus.
- Two lateral radial incisions given at 6 and 12 clock positions along tympanomastoid and tympanosquamous suturelines. This flap is elevated with a flap elevator and preserved (Figs 20.6a and b).
- Postauricular skin and periosteal incision given preferably just posterior to postaural groove. Same incision is extended upwards to procure the temporalis fascia graft.
- Anterior canal wall retractor is placed for reflecting the lateral posterior meatal wall.
- Tympanomeatal flap will be elevated and along with the annulus, taking care not to injure chorda tympani, long process of incus, handle of malleus. This elevation of meatal wall may requires 2 medial radial skin incisions.
- Temporalis fascial graft is placed lateral to the handle of malleus covering the perforation. This requires support of graft by pieces of dry gelfoam.
- Tympanomeatal flap will be replaced on the graft. Gelfoam is packed in deep meatus. Lateral posterior meatal wall flap is replaced, canal is then packed with gel-foam and medicated ribbon gauge.

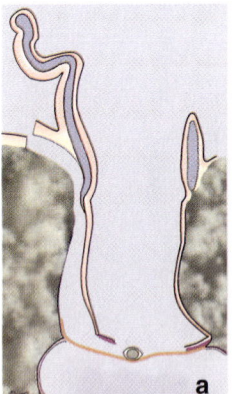 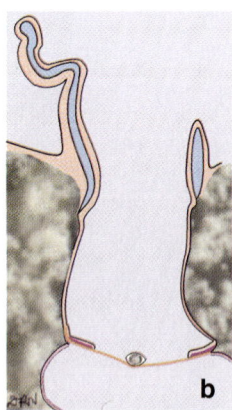

a   b

Figs 20.6a and b: (a) Graft placed under tympanic annulus after raising tympanomeatal flap (b) Graft placed under tympanic annulus and tympanomeatal flap repositioned

- Postauricular wound is closed in layers. Mastoid bandage is applied.

Advantages

- Simple and easy to perform, when perforation is small.
- Avoids extensive dissection of anterior meatal skin, thus preventing blunting of anterior recess.
- Ensures healing of drum at correct level relative to fibrous annulus and osseous remnant.

Disadvantages

- Reduction of middle ear space.
- Limited bed of raw area for graft reception.
- Difficult graft placement if perforation extends more anteriorly.
- Three layer formation of TM is unlikely.
- Anterior reperforation.
- Anterior tympanomeatal cholesteatoma.
- Blunting of anterior tympanomeatal angle can occur if anterior tympanic annulus has been separated from sulcus.

TYMPANOPLASTY

Definition

The term tympanoplasty was first used in 1953 by Wullstein. This refers to any surgical procedure involving reconstruction of tympanic membrane/ossicular chain. The term myringoplasty is inter changeable with the term tympanoplasty without ossicular reconstruction.

Physiologic Considerations

As sound waves travel from air to water/fluid medium 99% of energy is reflected at the air-water interface. This might be true in the case of ear also, if there was no middle ear ossicular chain. This prevents most of the sound energy being reflected. This transformer function of middle ear is accomplished primarily by the **'Hydraulic**

OPERATIVE STEPS OF UNDERLAY MYRINGOPLASTY

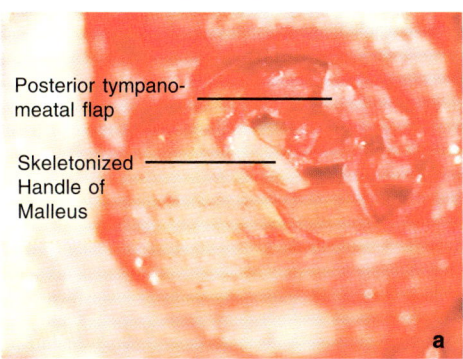

Posterior tympano-
meatal flap

Skeletonized
Handle of
Malleus

Fig. 20.7a: Posterior tympanomeatal flap raised and retracted anteriorly with exposure of middle ear

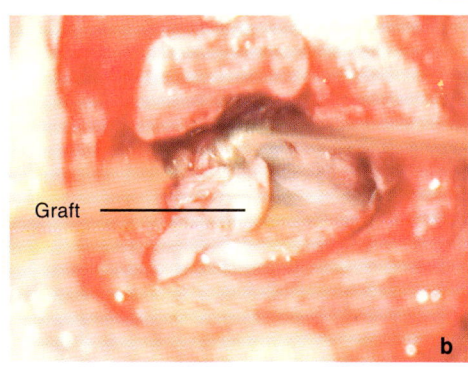

Graft

Fig. 20.7b: Graft being placed under the tympanom- eatal flap and over middle ear cavity

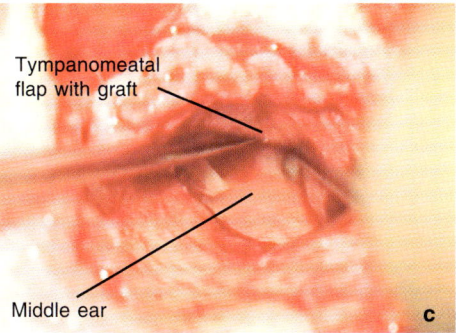

Tympanomeatal
flap with graft

Middle ear

Fig. 20.7c: Tympanomeatal flap along with graft retracted anteriorly exposing middle ear for placing gel foam

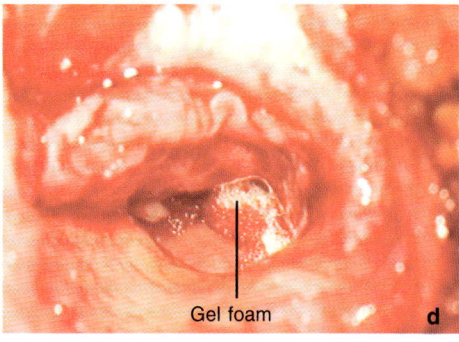

Gel foam

Fig. 20.7d: Gel foam being placed in middle ear

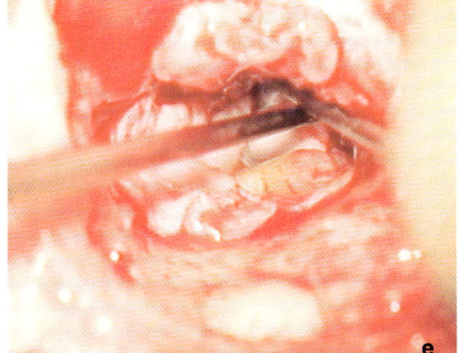

Fig. 20.7e: Tympanomeatal flap along with graft repositioned after placing gel foam in middle ear

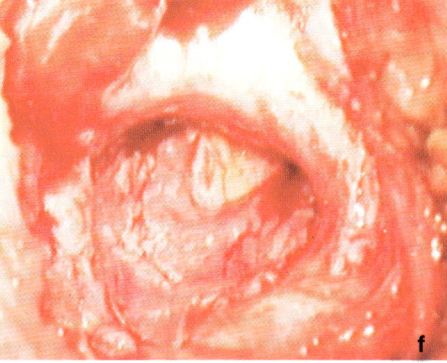

Fig. 20.7f: Graft in final position under the tympanic annulus

Effect', which is the ratio between the area of tympanic membrane and the stapes footplate (17:1). The 17 to 1 hydraulic ratio times the 1.3 lever ratio yields a total increase of pressure level at the oval window 22 times. This is termed as sound pressure transformer ratio of normal human ear. The 22 times increase of pressure equals 26.8 dB. The "round window" function as a relief door which moves to and fro with the vibratory movement of cochlear fluid column (Fig. 20.8).

A perforation of Tympanic membrane removes the sound protection from the round window with a tendency for sound to reach both windows at nearly the same moment and thus cochlear fluid movement will be less.

A small perforation, for example, which still isolates round window from direct sound stimulation results in less than 30 dB conductive deficit. But a large perforation with no round window protection disrupts the hydraulic effect, and a conductive deficit more than 30 dB is produced. In a total perforation there is loss of 40 to 45 dB and in ossicular discontinuity or fixation behind an intact drum, more than 60 dB loss occurs.

The frequencies involved in the hearing loss are influenced by the perforation. In a small perforation low frequency loss occurs.

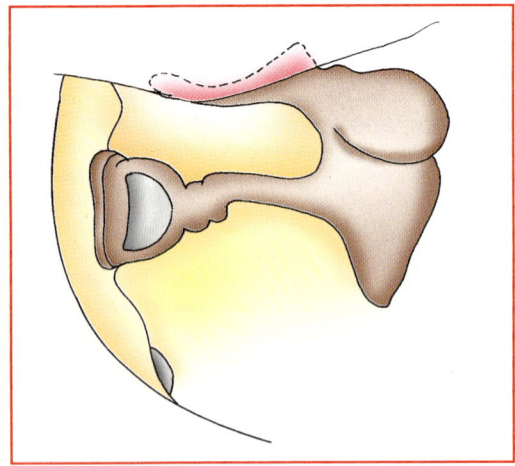

Fig. 20.8: Shows the position of ossicles

Tympanoplasty-Classification

Zollner and Wullstein's Classification (1953)

Type I: Perforated tympanic membrane with normal ossicular chain. The procedure includes inspection of the middle ear cleft with closure of the perforation (Fig.20.9a).

Type II: Sound transmission through a functioning but deformed ossicular chain *e.g.*, erosion of the malleus. Type II is modified to include any reformed mechanism joining the tympanic membrane with stapes footplate which retains a lever advantage. Thus there is Type IIa which is the original Type II reconstruction. Type IIb is malleus stapes assembly or malleus footplate assembly. Type IIc is a new reconstruction independent of the malleus (Fig. 20.9b).

Type III: Destruction of the tympanic membrane and ossicular chain but intact and mobile stapes. Tympanic membrane graft is kept in contact with the stapes head. It also gives sound protection to the round window - Fig. 20.9c. (Columella Tympanoplasty Sheehy 1987).

Type IV: Head, neck and crura of the stapes are missing, only a mobile footplate remains. Sound protection of the round-window, is given by putting a graft from ET to round-window, where mobile foot plate of the stapes is left exposed - Fig. 20.9d (Oval window or cavum minor tympanoplasty. Sheehy 1987).

Type V: Here the footplate is fixed. Fenestra is made to the horizontal semicircular canal. A graft seals off the middle ear to give sound protection to the round window (Fig. 20.9e).

Type VI (Gracice Ibanez): Sono inversion : Here the round window is left exposed to the direct impact of sound waves. Mobile footplate is protected by a small tympanic air space in continuity with the eustachian tube.

Austin's Classification of Anatomical Defects in Ossicular Chain (1971)

Isolated loss of malleus handle (29% of ossicular defects) and isolated loss of stapes superstructure.

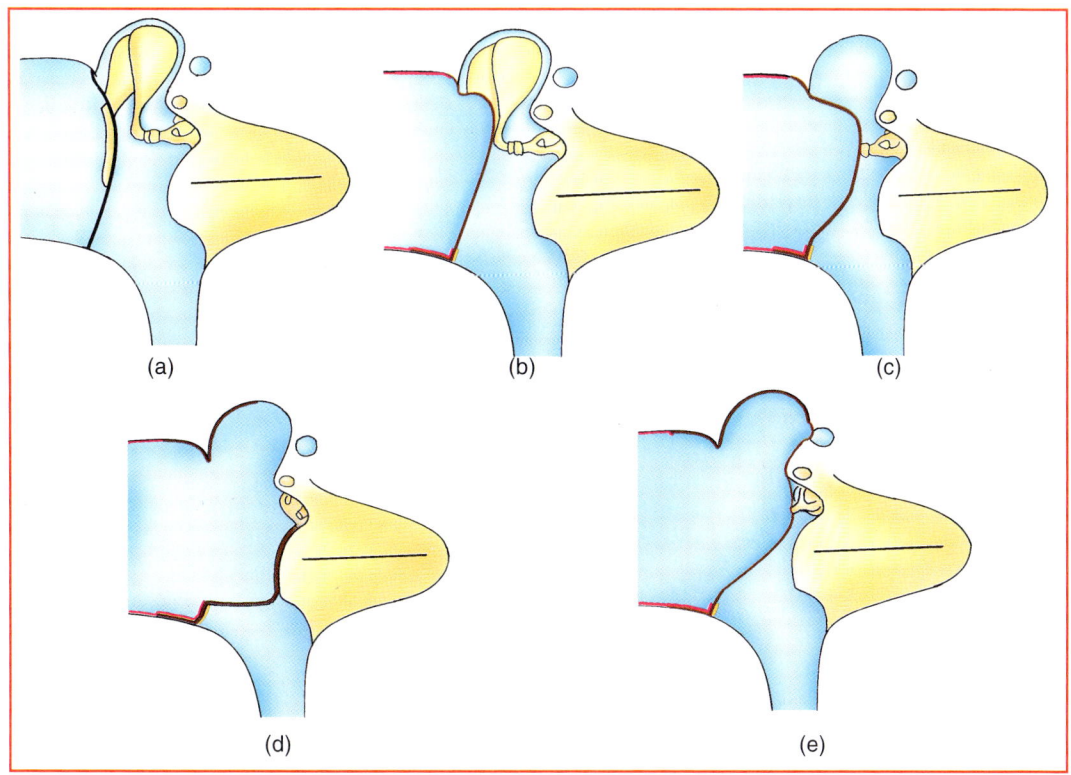

Figs 20.9a to e: Tympanoplasty types: (a) Type I - Graft placed over intact ossicular chain, (b) Type II - Graft placed over the incus in case of eroded malleus, (c) Type III - Graft placed over the stapes superstructure in case of eroded malleus and incus, (d) Type IV - Graft placed over mobile stapes foot plate when superstructure of stapes is eroded, (e) Type V - Graft placed over the fenestera made in horizontal semi circular canal in case of fixed stapes foot plate

1.7% of ossicular defects were not classified because of their rarity.

Incus absent in all cases and tympanic membrane repair required in all cases.

Type a: Malleus handle and stapes superstructure present requiring reconstruction of the tympanic membrane and ossicular chain from the handle of the malleus to stapes superstructure.

Type b: Handle of malleus absent, stapes superstructure present requiring reconstruction of the tympanic membrane, handle of malleus and incus.

Type c: Handle of malleus present. Stapes superstructure absent, requiring reconstruction of the tympanic membrane and reconstruction of the ossicular chain from the handle of malleus to stapes footplate.

Type d: Handle of malleus absent, stapes superstructure absent requiring reconstruction of the tympanic membrane and handle of malleus, incus and stapes superstructure.

Combined Approach Tympanoplasty (CAT) Synonyms : Canal up Mastoidectomy

Operative Procedure

Steps

1. Postauricular incision
2. Exposure of Mac Ewen's triangle

3. Forward elevation of posterior superior meatal wall
4. Cortical mastoidectomy with extension into attic
5. Identification of chordofacial angle - Short process of incus (Fossa incudes) superiorly, medially vertical portion of facial nerve, laterally post-superior meatal wall, inferiorly chorda tympani nerve.
6. Exposure of the chordofacial angle (Posterior tympanotomy) with the help of fine diamond end cutting burr.
7. Extension of the lower border of the exposed chordofacial angle to the hypotympanum visualize if necessary.
8. Ossicles and ossicular defect can be visualized adequately when various types of tympanoplasty as given below can be performed.
9. Various types of ossiculoplasties can also be performed in canal wall down mastoidectomy.

CORTICAL MASTOIDECTOMY

This is a transcortical opening of the mastoid air cell and the antrum. It is the initial stage of any transmastoid surgery of the middle ear, inner ear, facial nerve, endolymphatic sac, labyrinth, internal auditory canal and various procedures on the skull base for removing skull base tumors.

Other Terminologies for this Procedure

1. *Simple mastoidectomy*: Removal of diseases mucosa and bone along with incision and drainage gave its name simple mastoidectomy.
2. Schwartz mastoidectomy
3. Conservative mastoidectomy
4. Complete mastoidectomy

Incisions

1. Postauricular incision of Wilde (Sir William Wilde in 1853 introduced this).

2. End aural incision of Lempert (1st employed by Kessel in 1885. In 1929, Lempert advocated extracartilaginous endaural incisions).

Postauricular Incision

- Most widely used for mastoid access
- Gives best exposure
- Used in well pneumatized mastoids
- 8 to 10 mm behind postauricular crease
- Useful for Palva method of creating subcutaneous flap for mastoid obliteration.
- Heal rapidly, flap infection rare
- Unsightly scarring rare, cosmetically acceptable.
- Preservation of the size and anatomy of external auditory meatus.
- When placed more posteriorly provides wider exposure necessary for translabyrinthine, retro labyrinthine, retrosigmoid approaches to CP angle.
- Should not be placed directly on postauricular crease because cleaning becomes difficult.
- Under 2 years of age, incision should be horizontal just above the auricle (because antrum lies above and behind the meatus) and inferior portion of the incision must be more posteriorly placed.
- *Modification:* A secondary horizontal incision at right angle to the middle of the first incision can be given in extensive pneumatization extending posteriorly and superiorly to the lateral sinus.

End Aural Incision

- For temporal bones with restricted pneumatization.
- Poor exposure of posterior and inferior air cell tracts facial recess and eustachian tube.
- Limited access to labyrinth, jugular bulb and facial nerve.
- **Lempert 1:** Canal incision medial to bony cartilaginous junction extending along entire posterior half of the canal.

- **Lempert 2:** Superior incision extending from Lempert-1 incision laterally between tragus and root of helix at the meatus of ear canal.

Indications

1. ASOM not responding to antibiotic therapy and proceeding to coalescent mastoiditis.
2. Acute mastoiditis with impending or coexisting complications [subperiosteal abscess, zygomatic, Bezold's, Citelli's, meatal abscess (Luc's abscess), sagging of posterosuperior canal wall, positive reservoir sign, i.e. meatus fills immediately with pus after it has been mopped out].
3. Masked or latent mastoiditis
4. Prior to tympanoplasty
5. CSOM with mastoiditis where non-surgical management fails.
6. Refractory secretory otitis media.
7. Persistent profuse otorrhea
8. Exposure of otic capsule for cochlear implantation.
9. Exposure of mastoid segment of facial nerve.
10. Exposure of mastoid region in CAT to delinate vertical portion of facial nerve and to provide access for opening the posterior tympanotomy into middle ear.
11. Saccus decompression surgery for the safest and widest access to the posterior fossa dura.
12. Trans-labyrinthine operations to provide exposure of bony labyrinth needed for its exenteration to allow access to the internal auditory meatus.
13. Retro-labyrinthine approach to the vestibular nerve.
14. Exposure of sigmoid sinus for obliteration before petrosectomy.
15. Mastoid trauma
16. Exploratory cortical mastoidectomy

Contraindications

- No absolute contraindications
- Uncontrolled systemic diseases.

Anesthesia

General anesthesia is usually selected, IV thiopental for adults and inhalation of non explosive gas for children. If GA is not indicated, local anesthesia may be secured.

Position of Patient

Supine position with head turned towards the opposite side.

Foot end of the table should be lowered by 20 degree. Head lowered to the horizontal to dispose the plane of the middle fossa dura as near to vertical as possible.

Local infiltration with 2% xylocaine with 1 in 2 lakh adrenaline given behind the auricle over the mastoid process to block branches of greater auricular nerve supplying the auricle and meatus.

- Infiltration at the bony cartilaginous junction to block tympanic branch of auriculotemporal supplying anterior meatal wall.
- Auricular branch of vagus supplying the anterior surface of the mastoid and skin of the floor of the meatus.
- Auricular branch of the auricular temporal supplying the upper part of auricle and skin above the meatus and incisura terminalis.

Parts Cleaned and Draped

Postauricular incision put and deepened through subcutaneous tissue and muscle. Periosteum incised in T or Y or U-shaped manner elevated with farabeut's mastoid periosteal elevator. Spine of Henle, MacEwen's triangle and the posterior bony margin of the meatus visualized.

Mollisons self-retaining retractor is inserted to hold the soft tissues away from the underlying exposed bone.

The mastoid cortex is removed over MacEwen's triangle which is a rough guide to the position of the underlying mastoid antrum, using a drill fitted with large cutting burr driven by an electric motor. The antrum will be encountered at a depth of about 1.5cm in the adult. Antrum lies just above and behind the posterosuperior osseous meatal wall.

While searching for the antrum, surgeon should beware of:

1. Injuring a forward lying sigmoid sinus.
2. Injuring a low middle fossa dura
3. Injuring the pyramidal segment of the facial nerve
4. A false antrum—the result of a well developed Korner's septum.

After identification of the antrum, patency to attic is confirmed by saline irrigation or gently probing anteriorly with a Dundas Grant probe or cell seeker, which will slip into the aditus. Care should be taken to avoid displacement of the short process of the incus. Hard white bony horizontal semicircular canal is a recognizable landmark in the floor of the antrum.

Opening to the antrum is enlarged by removal of cells superiorly and posteriorly with a large curette or burr. From the antrum, various cell tracts are followed to their termination. Saline irrigation and suctioning done during drilling.

1. The vertical tract of cells from the antrum to the tip of the mastoid process is removed, establishes the initial groove. Position of the vertical portion of the facial nerve should be taken care of.
2. The sheet of cells that covers the sigmoid sinus is followed backward from the initial groove until the sinus plate is well defined and meets the outer cortex posteriorly, indicating the posterior limit of pneumatization.
   - Injury to the mastoid emissary vein should be avoided.
   - In front of the bulge of the sigmoid sinus plate, removal of cells will uncover the bone of **Trautmann's triangle**, protecting the dura of the posterior cranial fossa and leading anteriorly and medially to the so called **solid angle**, where the dense bone of the otic capsule protects the posterior semi circular canal.
   - Whenever this operation is performed for suppurative mastoiditis, the bone over the sigmoid sinus should be removed

sufficiently to allow insertion of a fine needle into that vessel to confirm that there is no thrombophlebitis within.

3. Cells at the tip of the mastoid process are cleaned out and the lateral wall of the tip is removed and within the mastoid digastric ridge is defined. Care should be taken of the facial nerve which lies at the anterior end of this ridge.

   Removal of the mastoid tip is advocated to allow soft tissue to fall in and partly obliterate the remaining cavity.

4. Cells that extend towards the jugular bulb medial to the digastric ridge between it and the sigmoid sinus are carefully excavated with large burr.
5. The sheet of cells against the tegmen plate is removed until the plate is defined and meets the cortex of the squama superiorly indicating the limit of pneumatization in superior direction.
6. The sinodural angle is cleaned out until the tegmen plate meets the sigmoid sinus plate at a sharp angle.
7. Remove cells extending forward into the posterior root of the zygomatic process without opening the epitympanum.
8. Clean out all small pneumatic cells medial to the antrum down to the hard bony posterior and superior semicircular canals. Define the posterior end of the bony horizontal semicircular canal by avoiding injury to or dislocation of the incus.

The landmarks for the vertical portion of the facial nerve may be located as the posterior end of the bony horizontal semicircular canal, digastric ridge tympanomastoid suture in the posterior bony meatal wall. Remove the remaining cells along the posterior bony meatal wall after defining the course of the facial nerve.

In the completed simple mastoid cavity, (Figs 20.10 and 20.11) the osseous superior and posterior meatal wall has been left standing, the tegmen and sinus plates are defined but intact, the cell tracts have been followed to their terminations from the antrum inferiorly to the tip,

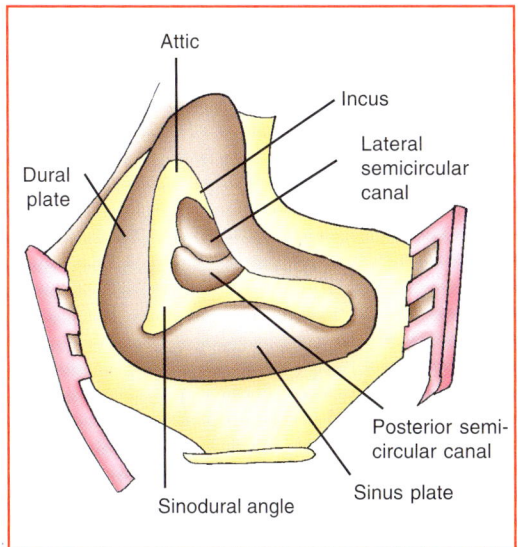

Fig. 20.10: Completed cortical mastoidectomy

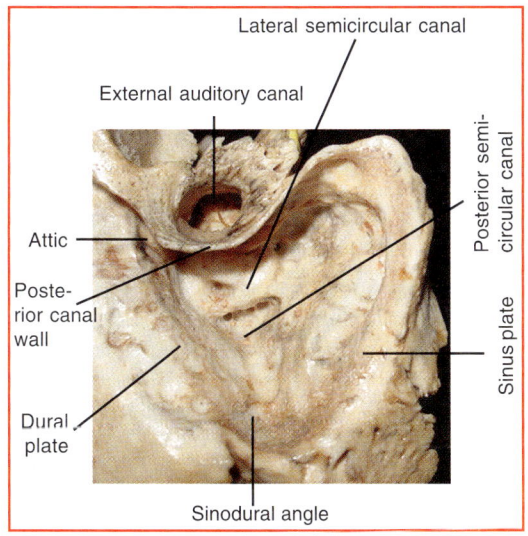

Fig. 20.11: Completed cortical mastoidectomy cavity in a dry temporal bone

superior and posterior osseous semicircular canals.

Overhanging cortex is removed with burr. Sinus plate or tegmen plate softened by disease should be elevated carefully from the underlying sigmoid sinus or dura and removed in small bites with a small curette until firm healthy bone and healthy sinus or dura without granulations are encountered .

Unnecessary exposure of sinus or dura should be avoided because it lays open fresh tissue to the **infection.**

Suture of the Wound

Complete mastoidectomy on a well localized coalescent mastoiditis no longer needs to be packed and left open. A drain or a ventilation tube leading to the antrum is sutured to the skin through a separate skin incision.

With antibiotic coverage, the wound may be sutured without any drainage.

Cavity debrided of any loose fragments of bone with warm sterile saline irrigation for hemostasis and removal of any remaining particles of bone. The skin and periosteum are approximate by interrupted sutures.

A mastoid dressing is applied.

Postoperative Care

- Appropriate antibiotics, anti-inflammatory, analgesic, decongestant can be continued.
- Keep the operated ear up.
- Facial movements checked once the patient is conscious.
- Look for nystagmus, vomiting, vertigo, Weber's test.
- The patient can be ambulatory on the day of surgery.

If needed, ventilation tube can be placed for ventilation, drainage of the cavity and is also useful for instilling antibiotic drops. Tube can be removed when no secretion is aspirated or when it is greater than 0.5 ml. Keep the ear dry for 3 weeks.

posteriorly to the junction of sinus plate and cortex, superiorly to the junction of tegmen plate and cortex, anteriorly to the limit of pneumatization in the posterior root of zygoma, medially to the

Mastoid dressing can be removed on fifth or sixth day along with sutures.

Accidents during Surgery/Postoperative Complications

1. *Facial nerve injury:* Heat generated by diamond burr can cause nerve injury. This is minimized by use of constant suction and irrigation during dissection with diamond burr. Facial nerve can be traumatized during surgery.
2. *Sigmoid sinus injury:* Injury to the sigmoid sinus, the superior petrosal sinus, jugular bulb, mastoid emissary vein result in profuse bleeding which can be controlled by occlusion with gloved finger or gauze pad, packing with gel foam, surgical, bone wax, absorbable collagen, temporalis fascia graft.
3. Sigmoid sinus injury can lead to air embolism.
4. Injury to the dura with the escape of CSF
5. *Dislocation or removal of the incus:* Dislocation or removal of the incus results in severe permanent conductive hearing loss. This can be managed by tympanoplasty operation later on.
6. Persistence of discharge from the ear or mastoid process
7. Postoperative hematoma—leading to devitalization of wound edges.
8. Traumatic high tone loss for 4 to 8 KHz.
9. Meatal stenosis
10. Bony fixation of malleus and incus.

MODIFIED RADICAL MASTOIDECTOMY

Modified radical mastoidectomy (MRM) or canal wall down mastoidectomy is a surgical procedure where the disease process is eradicated from the middle ear cleft; followed by converting the mastoid cavity, middle ear and external auditory canal into a single, smooth, self cleansing cavity exteriorized through external auditory canal (EAC) leaving behind healthy tissues whenever possible for the future reconstruction of sound conducting mechanism.

Objectives of MRM

- Safe ear
- Dry ear
- Preservation and reconstruction of sound conducting mechanism

Indications for MRM

1. Cholesteatoma with recurrent ear discharge with sufficient cochlear reserve for future tympanoplasty mastoidotympanoplasty (Figs 20.12 and 20.13).
2. In atticoantral disease (AAD), where combined approach tympanoplasty :
   (a) Is difficult as in small sclerotic mastoids.
   (b) Cannot be done due to inexperience of the surgeon.
   (c) Should not be done in patient not willing to come for regular follow-up.
3. Disease in the only hearing ear.
4. Unconstructable posterior canal wall.
5. Labyrinthine fistula.
6. CSOM associated with severe complications.

Contraindications

1. Benign type of chronic otorrhea with a central perforation and without cholesteatoma.
2. Acute otitis media with coalescent mastoiditis.
3. Persistent secretary otitis media or chronic allergic otitis media.
4. Tubercular otitis media.

Approaches

Endaural Approach

a. More direct access to EAC and middle ear.
b. More accurate cutting of skin flaps.
c. Better assessment of accessibility and shape of cavity with respect to EAC after operation.
d. Cosmetic scar.

Postaural Approach

a. Wider exposure of mastoid cortex.

b. Easier access to posterior fossa dura, sigmoid sinus and Trautman's triangle

c. Greater sensory disturbance of pinna (rarely permanent).

Advantages of Canal Wall Down Mastoidectomy include:

1. Residual cholesteatoma is visible on follow up.
2. Recurrent cholesteatoma is rare.
3. Complete exteriorization of facial recess.
4. Second stage is rarely required.

Disadvantages include:

1. Mastoid cavity problems.
2. Shallow middle ear, which is difficult to reconstruct.
3. Position of pinna may be altered.
4. Postoperative vertigo due to caloric stimulation of lateral semicircular canal.

Preparation in Surgery

Patient

The hair is shaved 2 to 3 cm above and behind the ear. The skin is cleaned and sterile drape is applied. The mattress is taped securely to the operating table to prevent slipping when the table is tipped from side to side or into the Trendelenburg position. The patient is placed with his/her head at the end of table. The patient's head and shoulder should be as near the surgeon's side of the table as possible. The table is usually placed in a few degree of Trendelenburg position and rolled slightly towards the surgeon.

Anesthesia

Surgery can be performed under both LA as well as GA, but in children and for surgeries, which require more than 1.5 hrs, GA is preferred.

Local infiltration is given in postauricular area with 2 to 3 ml. of 2% xylocaine with adrenaline (if not contraindicated), 5 to 10 minutes before incision is made. Four-quadrant infiltration is given at the bony-cartilaginous junction of the posterior, superior, inferior and anterior canal walls.

Surgical Steps

Retroauricular skin incision is carried out along the hair-line and extends inferiorly over the mastoid tip into a crease of skin. The skin incision must be posterior enough to avoid lying over the exenterated mastoid bone.

The soft tissues are elevated for **exposure of mastoid.** The Periosteum covering the mastoid is incised and elevated. Landmarks seen on the Mastoid cortex are:

• External auditory meatus
• Suprameatal **spine of Henle**
• Suprameatal **triangle of MacEwen** defined by supramastoid crest (Posterior prolongation of upper border of root of zygoma) superiorly, posterosuperior margin of bony EAC anteriorly and a vertical tangential line drawn through the posterior margin of the EAC posteriorly.
• Temporal line.

Preservation of Posterior canal skin is done by elevating the posterior and superior canal wall skin along with posterior annulus and reflecting it anteriorly to prevent any injury from burrs.

Complete **cortical mastoidectomy** is performed. The landmarks seen after cortical mastoidectomy include:

• Dural (Middle Cranial fossa) plate.
• Sigmoid sinus plate.
• Sinodural angle plate.
• Thinned bony posterior canal wall.
• Bony lateral semicircular canal at the floor of antrum.
• Mastoid tip air cells.
• External genu of facial nerve.
• Fossa incudis.

Atticotomy (Epitympanotomy) is done by removing the triangular area of bone bounded superiorly along the suprameatal crest, inferiorly a line along the posterosuperior canal wall with apex pointing towards the zygoma (Fig. 20.12a).

The depth at which outer attic wall is reached is just lateral to the notch of Rivinus. The bony removal is carried out anteriorly to expose the short process of incus. Further anteriorly the incudomaleolar joint and head of malleus are seen. The dissection stops at the anterior wall of epitympanum. The malleus head and incus are removed if cholesteatoma matrix envelops them or goes medial to them. The malleus head is removed with a malleus nipper even if it is healthy, if wide clearance from the walls of the epitympanum is not obtained; otherwise the result is bony ankylosis (Fig. 20.12b).

Medial wall of Attic is divided by genu of facial nerve into **supralabyrinthine recess** (posteriorly) and **supratubal recess** (anteriorly). These spaces are adequately exenterated and exteriorized.

Facial bridge is that portion of posterosuperior bony meatal wall that bridges over the notch of Rivinus and overlies the ossicles. This is removed with cutting burr initially and diamond burr later, always working outwards and away from fallopian canal (Fig. 20.12c).

Anterior buttress is the projection of bone at the junction of anterior bony meatal wall and epitympanic tegmen. The drilling is done at anterior buttress, just lateral to the malleus head. Once this bone is removed, there will be a smooth curve from the middle fossa tegmen to epitympanic tegmen to the anterior wall of external auditory canal.

Posterior buttress is the projection of bone at the junction of posterior wall and the floor of the meatus, lateral to the facial nerve. Its removal causes the floor of EAC to slope off gently into the mastoid tip.

Facial ridge is that part of posterior bony meatal wall which houses the posterior bend and vertical segment of facial nerve. The tympanic fallopian canal is identified at the inferior edge of the lateral semicircular canal. The level of mastoid segment of facial nerve is determined by a line drawn from tympanic facial nerve (2nd genu) to stylomastoid foramen.

Lowering the facial ridge is performed with diamond burrs and suction irrigation. One should always work away from facial nerve. The bone is lowered up to the level of lateral semicircular canal in the vertical plane and floor of EAC (ideally up to the digastric ridge) in horizontal plane (Figs 20.12a to f). Lowering the facial ridge exposes the upper part of facial recess, pyramid, stapes and chorda tympani nerve (Fig. 20.12 d).

Extension of the squamous epithelium into facial recess or sinus tympani is considered as one of the most important factors for residual cholesteatoma. Cholesteatoma sac can be removed by careful dissection. Buckingham mirror or an angled endoscope can be used for better visualization.

Removal of cholesteatoma from oval window niche is done after completion of bone work to avoid prolonged exposure of inner ear.

Removal of cholesteatoma matrix from **round window membrane** should be made under direct vision. This requires removal of the upper edge of the round window niche with a diamond burr until the round window membrane is exposed.

Tympanoplasty

Tympanoplasty can be done in the same sitting or it can be done as a staged tympanoplasty. Various studies show better results with staged tympanoplasty. The indications for staged tympanoplasty include (Figs 20.12e and f):

Mucosal Factors

- Large area of diseased mucosa in the middle ear cleft.
- Large area of absent mucosa in the middle ear cavity.
- Absent mucosa over the promontory.

Ossicular Chain Factors

- Stapes foot plate fixation.
- Stapes suprastructure absent.
- Absent malleus handle with total TM perforation.

In all these cases, the graft tends to lateralise

Residual Cholesteatoma Factors

1. If cholesteatoma is seen in places where it is difficult to remove.

OPERATIVE STEPS OF MRM WITH TYMPANOPLASTY

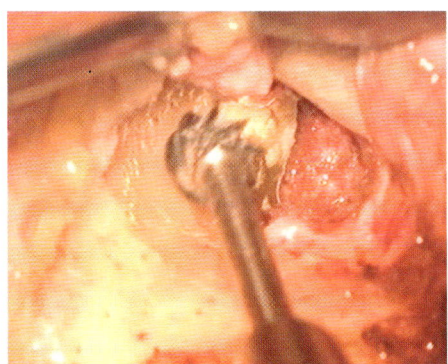

Fig. 20.12a: Atticotomy being done with the cutting burr

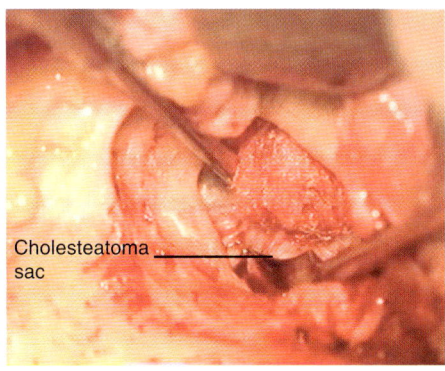

Fig. 20.12b: Cholesteatoma sac being removed from attic region

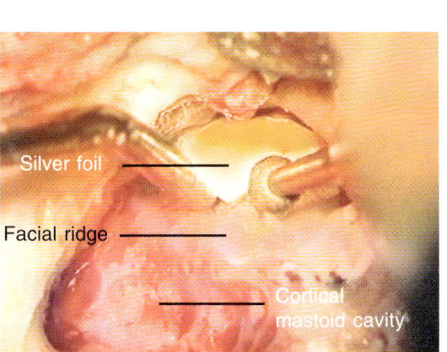

Fig. 20.12c: Middle ear cavity covered with the silver foil to protect middle ear remnant and facial rigde is lowered by diamond burr

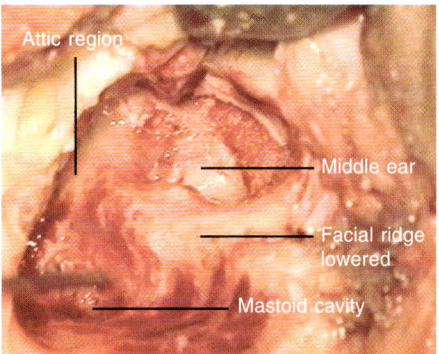

Fig. 20.12d: Mastoid cavity, middle ear, external auditory canal made into a single cavity

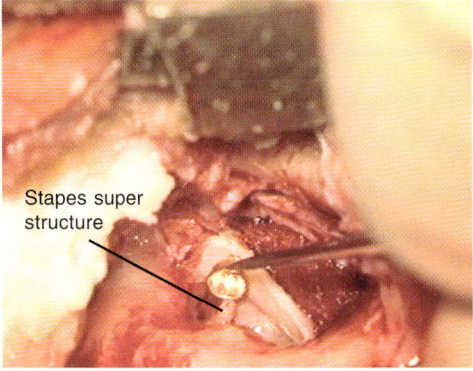

Fig. 20.12e: Gold prosthesis with the cartilage being kept over stapes for tympanoplasty

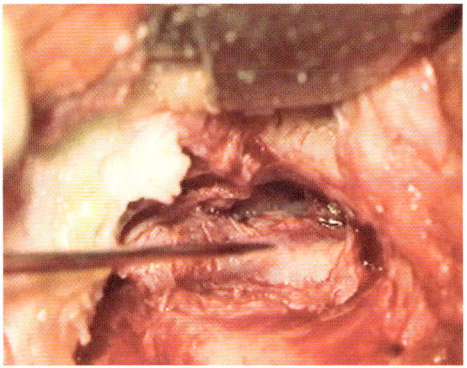

Fig. 20.12f: The graft placed above the gold prosthesis and the middle ear

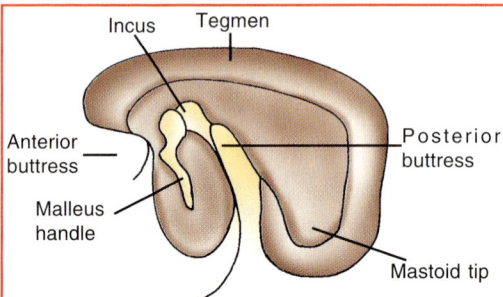

Labels: Incus, Tegmen, Anterior buttress, Malleus handle, Posterior buttress, Mastoid tip

Fig. 20.13: After removal of anterior butters of facial bridge

2. Presence of acute infection during surgery, which makes it difficult to differentiate between granulation tissue and cholesteatoma matrix.
3. Excessive bleeding in epitympanum during surgery (chances of residual cholesteatoma are high).

Objectives of Staging

• Obtain a disease free ear.
• Obtain better and permanent hearing results.
• Stabilization of TM.
  – Regrowth of middle ear mucosal lining.
  – Evaluation of Eustachian Tube function.

Timing of second stage of Tympanoplasty

• *For mucosal and ossicular chain factors*: 6 to 9 months.
• *For residual cholesteatoma factors*: 1 to 2 years.
  In staged tympanoplasty the first stage controls the irreversible diseased tissue of the ear after which reformation of tympanum takes place through regrowth of the mucosa over an inert mould placed in the middle ear, *e.g.* parrafin, teflon, sialastic and dental compound, etc. In second stage the mould is removed and sound conduction mechanism is reconstructed.

Conchomeatoplasty

Meatoplasty is the next step of the procedure. The idea of meatoplasty is to allow better aeration of the mastoid cavity and easy visualization of the entire cavity to facilitate postoperative care and self cleaning. Different techniques used for conchomeatoplasty include:

Korner's Technique

Wide posteriorly placed cartilagenous canal skin flap is elevated. Auricle is reflected anteriorly and the pedicle is delivered into the mastoid operative site. Conchal cartilage and soft tissue are removed. The flap is returned to its anatomical position having been thinned out permitting a wider meatal opening.

Sieberman's Technique

An inverted Y shaped incision is made in posterior skin. The flaps are pulled into operative side. Conchal cartilage and soft tissue are removed and the skin is placed down with three corner sutures.

Other techniques include

• Fisch's technique
• Yanagisawa's technique
• Panse and Portman's technique

Postoperative care

• To keep the ear dry.
• To avoid blowing of nose.
  Patient is reviewed after one month and asked regarding ear discharge, decreased hearing, giddiness.

Otoscopy is done to see

• Size of cavity
• Epithelial lining
• Discharge
• Granulations
• Lowering of facial ridge
• Adequacy of meatoplasty
• Graft status
  Pure tone audiogram is performed.

Complications of MRM

Intraoperative

1. Injury to:

- Dura mater
- Sigmoid sinus
- Facial nerve
- Labyrinth—Total hearing loss

2. Bleeding from the dura, sinodural angle, sigmoid sinus, middle ear and facial nerve. Bleeding may be the first indication that dura lies just below the drill.

Postoperative

1. Recurrent and residual cholesteatoma.
2. Persistent otorrhea—Regular cleaning at intervals of 6 to 12 months and necessary medication.
3. Inadequate epithelization of cavity.
4. Granulations in mastoid cavity
   - Thin layer—Apply 2 % gentian violet paint.
   - Large buds—$AgNO_3$ cautery and antibiotic steroid ear drops.
5. *Mucous or chocolate cyst*: Collection of serum in a mucosal lined pocket beneath the epithelium lining of a healed cavity.
6. Perichondritis.

Late

1. Stenosis of the mastoid cavity due to neo-osteogenesis.
2. Meatal stenosis and closure.
3. Mastoidocutaneous fistula.
4. Postauricular depression.
5. Graft failure.

Management of Complications

1. Bleeding

Bleeding may be the indication of dura underlying the drill. A change in the sound or feel of the drill also indicates the presence of underlying dura. Bleeding in sinodural angle may be controlled by bone wax. Larger defects can be covered with temporalis fascia graft.

Bleeding of sigmoid sinus is controlled by immediate digital pressure followed by application of bone wax. At the end of procedure bone wax is removed and defect is covered with fascia.

Diamond burr moving parallel to the nerve controls bleeding around the intact facial nerve canal. Cautery is to be avoided.

Bleeding in middle ear is controlled with cotton ball soaked in adrenaline and lignocaine or ferracrylum (Sepgard gel).

2. Facial nerve injury

Safest way to avoid injury is to identify the nerve.

The 4 common sites of injury are:
- First genu and geniculate ganglion
- Horizontal segment (tympanic portion)
- Second genu (pyramidal portion)
- Near the stylomastoid foramen

Following otologic surgery if patient awakens with facial paralysis, several steps must be taken. When local anesthesia has been applied, wait for 4 hours to allow its affect to subside. If the paralysis persists fallopian canal must be immediately explored. Traumatic injury to the facial nerve often requires repair of the nerve. Three major sensory nerves used in facial nerve grafting are ***greater auricular, lateral femoral cutaneous nerve and sural nerve.***

3. Labyrinthine injury

Injury to lateral semicircular canal can occur while drilling the dural plate.

Bone dust is placed over the defect and facial covering is placed over it.

4. Management of Mucous/chocolate Cyst

Simple puncture to evacuate the Mucoid brownish serum reduces the cyst but does not prevent its recurrence. If the cyst is sufficiently troublesome, it should be exposed and its mucoperiosteal lining should be removed.

5. Management of recurrent and residual cholesteatoma

Because such recurrences (residues) of cholesteatomas are easily seen, they are easily uncapped and do not carry the risk of complications. Management includes incision of the sac and evacuation of contents or cutting the margins of the Sac (marsupialization).

6. Management of stenosed mastoid cavity

The cavity is drilled again and then obliterated to keep it at level with external auditory canal.

7. Management of meatal stenosis

Much more commonly seen with endaural incision.

- *Moderate stenosis:* A vertical incision is made and conchal cartilage wedges are removed.
- *Almost complete stenosis:* Elliptical incision is made along with a perpendicular limb conchal cartilage wedges are removed.

8. Management of mastoidocutaneous fistula and postauricular depression

The retracted scar is excised full thickness in an ellipse. Subcutaneous tissue flap is designed posterior to the excised scar with an inferiorly based pedicle. The postauricular skin is undermined and the subcutaneous tissue flap is advanced anteriorly into the defect caused by the excision of the scar.

Discharging Mastoid Cavity

The causes include:
1. Inadequate conchomeatoplasty (Most important reason)
2. Too large cavity
3. Residual disease in
   a. Sinus tympani
   b. Facial recess
   c. Root of zygoma
   d. Mastoid tip
   e. Retrofacial region
   f. Sinodural angle
   g. Perisinus cells (Retrosigmoid cells)
   h. Retrolabyrinthine and supralabyrinthine cells
4. Recurrent disease
5. Inadequate lowering of facial ridge
6. Inadequate removal of anterior and posterior buttresses

7. Lining of the cavity by secretary respiratory epithelium
8. Exposed ETO with TM perforation
9. Deep cavity at mastoid tip
10. Nasal allergy
11. Brain abscess/extradural abscess draining in to mastoid cavity
12. CSF otorrhea.

RADICAL MASTOIDECTOMY

Definition

It is an operation performed to eradicate middle ear and mastoid disease in which, mastoid antrum, tympanum and external auditory canal are converted into a common cavity exteriorized through the external auditory meatus (this operation involves removal of all the structures excepting the footplate of stapes and does not involve any reconstructing or grafting procedure).

James L. Sheehy

Radical mastoidectomy is not very popular in modern days because of the non-feasibility of future reconstruction of the middle ear.

Indication for Radical Mastoidectomy

1. Unresectable cholesteatoma extending to eustachian tube.
2. Promontory cochlear fistula due to cholesteatoma.
3. Chronic perilabyrinthine osteitis or cholesteatoma that cannot be removed and must be cleaned and inspected periodically (Shambaugh).
4. Carcinoma of external auditory meatus and middle ear.
5. Childhood necrotizing acute otitis media leading on to secondary acquired cholesteatoma.

Steps of Radical Mastoidectomy

1. Exposure of the mastoid area.
2. Identification of mastoid antrum and completion of basic mastoidectomy (Schwartz or cortical mastoidectomy).

3. *Atticotomy:* Outer attic wall is removed and atticotomy is completed, using a small cutting burr, as described earlier under MRM.

4. *Canal wall down:* This is done as in case of the modified radical mastoidectomy taking care that the facial ridge is adequately lowered along the line of the facial canal. Lowering of the facial ridge is done by working along the axis of the facial canal (vertical segment) until the pyramidal process is exposed. All the disease along the facial recess area can be cleared once this step is completed. Meticulous clearance of cholesteatoma/disease from the sinus tympani may require removal of pyramid and bone anterior to the facial nerve, using fine diamond burr (Figs 20.14 to 20.18).

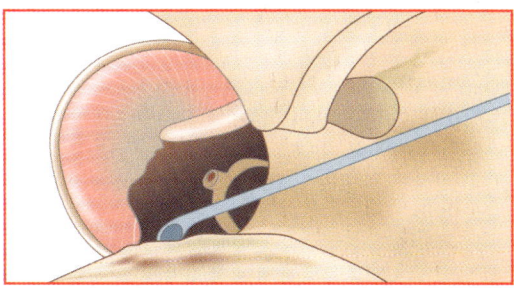

Fig. 20.16: Curette removes diseased tissue from facial recess

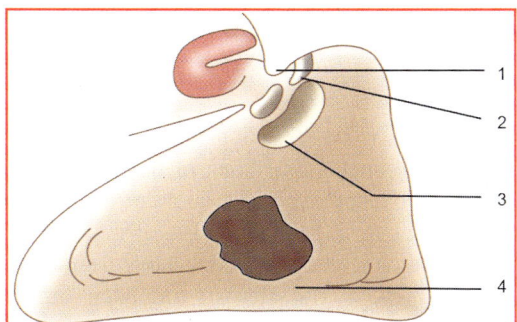

Fig. 20.14: After mastoidectomy (1) Anterior buttress (2) Incus (3) Lateral semicircular canal (4) Sigmoid sinus

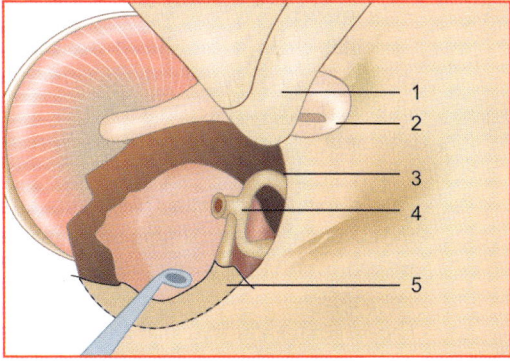

Fig. 20.17: Showing removal of posterior buttress (1) Anterior buttress (2) Malleus head (3) Chorda tympani (cut) (4) Stapes (5) bPyramidal process

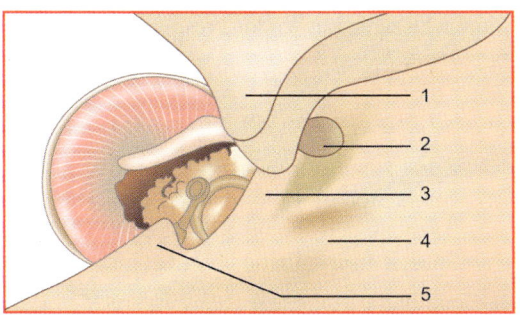

Fig. 20.15: Canal wall being lowered (1) Anterior buttress (2) Malleus (3) Facial canal (4) Horizontal semicircular canal (5) Posterior buttress

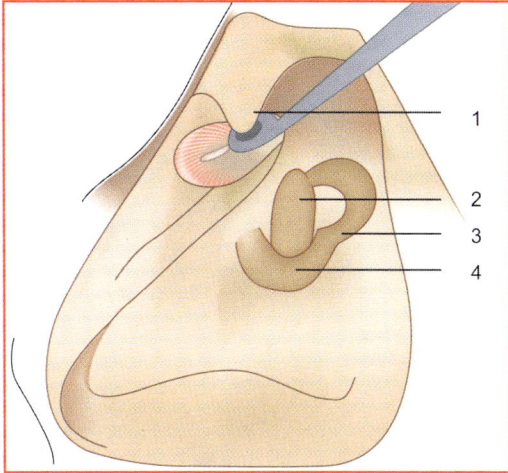

Fig. 20.18: Removal of anterior buttress (1) Anterior buttress (2) Lateral semicircular canal (3) Superior semicircular canal (4) Posterior semicircular

5. *Removal of middle ear contents:* This step marks the essential difference between radical mastoidectomy and modified radical mastoidectomy (in which healthy middle ear contents are preserved) (Fig. 20.19).

Under magnification, following steps are done:

i. The incudostapedial joint is seperated.

ii. The tensor tympani muscle is cut just medial to malleus and it is pulled out from its canal.

iii. The cochleariform process is fractured and removed.

iv. Ossicular chain is mobilized from attic space and they are removed using an alligator forceps. The stapes footplate is retained, if possible with its super-structure.

v. The tympanic membrane (with annulus) and all mucoperiosteal lining of the cavity are removed using a microelevator and cup forceps.

vi. The external auditory canal and the floor of hypotympanum is made level by

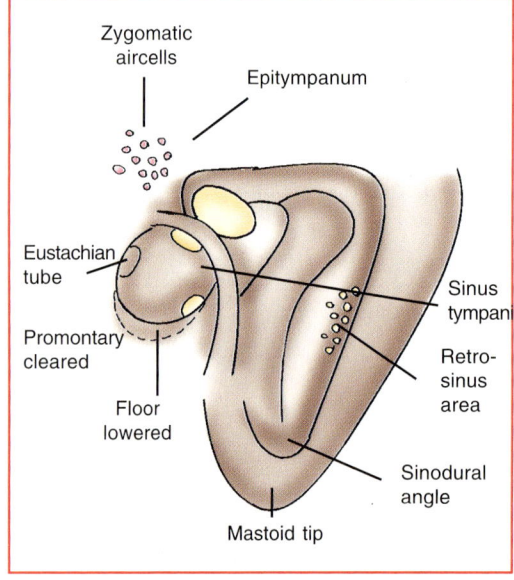

Fig. 20.19: Schematic diagram shows structures removed in radical mastoidectomy

removing the inferior bony annulus.

vii. Mucosa over the eustachian tubal orifices is curetted out and an attempt is made to seal the opening of eustachian tube by septal cartilage, ossicles, bone chips, muscle or fascia. This is to prevent future ingrowth of mucosa to middle ear space.

6. Polishing (smoothening) of the cavity. A large polishing burr is usually used for this purpose. This is done to avoid any pockets retaining pus or debris.

7. Soft tissue meatoplasty/cavity obliteration.

8. Wounds closure in layers.

Causes of cavity problems: Same as for MRM.

Complications: Same as of MRM.

STAPEDECTOMY

Introduction

Otosclerosis is a disease of the otic capsule where the normal enchondral bone of the footplate is replaced by spongy vascular bone formation causing ankylosis of the footplate of stapes to the oval window leading to a conductive deafness.

Treatment of otosclerosis has been largely restricted to surgical efforts. Various surgical procedures have been performed in the past like mobilization of stapes, stapes extraction, fenestration, stapedectomy, etc. Recently small fenestra stapedectomy, stapedotomy, stapedo-tomy with stapedius tendon preservation is gaining popularity.

Indications for Surgery

1. Bone conduction of 0 to 25 dB and air conduction of 45 to 65 dB.

2. Air bone gap should at least be 15 dB.

3. Speech discrimination score of 60% or more.

Contraindications as listed by Morrison in 1967 are:

1. General systemic illness like diabetes and bleeding disorders where the patient is unfit

for surgery or when patient's life expectancy is limited.

2. Old age above 70 years.
3. Surgery is not advocated in children below pre-adolescent age group.
4. Conductive losses from other causes like tympanosclerosis, etc. - These cases are highly prone to develop sensorineural hearing loss.
5. Stapes surgery should not be done until the tympanic defect is corrected as in otitis media.
6. Very early otosclerosis with minimal conductive hearing loss is not required to undergo surgery.
7. Only hearing ear with previous history of failure of surgery with associated sensorineural hearing loss in the other ear unless the hearing aid does not give relief.
8. In unilateral hearing loss where other ear is normal, surgery may not be necessary unless patient finds loss of binaural hearing as a great handicap.
9. Stapedial and cochlear otosclerosis with poor air-bone gap.
10. Presence of vertigo and clinical evidence of secondary labyrinthine hydrops especially fluctuating hearing loss. These patients have a high risk of developing a dead ear due to distended saccule.
11. Revision stapedectomy with adhesive changes is dangerous in which case surgery should be done in expert hand.
12. Second ear stapedectomy is still controversial due to risk of delayed or immediate senso-rineural hearing loss, vestibular damage, technical difficulties in the first ear surgery and abnormalities in caloric response.
13. In a young adult with rapidly spreading stapedial and cochlear otosclerosis and a positive Schwartze sign, surgery should be delayed till the activity is controlled by sodium fluoride.
14. Pregnancy is a definite contraindication and should be deferred for 12 months after parturition.
15. In those whose occupation includes considerable physical strain as in sportsmen, pilots there is increased risk of perilymph fistula.
16. In cases of bilateral otosclerosis it is better to operate in the worst ear.

John J. Shea is the originator of stapedectomy operation.

Special problems during stapedectomy

1. Abnormalities of the facial nerve.
2. Persistent stapedial artery.
3. Floating footplate
4. Biscuit footplate is a thickened footplate with well-defined margins produced by a primary focus in footplate.
5. Depressed footplate, submerged footplate
6. Damage to the chorda tympani nerve
7. Obliterative otosclerosis
8. Tympanic membrane tear
9. Fixed malleus
10. Round window closure
11. Fracture of long process of incus
12. Perilymph gusher

The operation

It depends on six basic steps:

1. Obtaining the tissue graft- temporalis fascia, perichondrium, vein, fat, clotted blood, etc.
2. Exposure of the oval window
3. Removal of stapes suprastructure
4. Footplate removal and creation of fenestra.
5. Tissue seal of the fenestra.
6. Prosthesis placement.

Details of surgical procedure for small fenestra stapedotomy/laser stapedotomy

1. Preparation of the canal wall.
2. Infiltration with Xylocaine and adrenaline at 4 points with help of endaural speculum
3. Magnification of 6X used and the middle ear entered through permeatal tympanotomy.
4. Tympanomeatal flap created by an incision from the 6 o'clock position 2 mm away from tympanic annulus outwards into the meatus

to meet another incision from 12 o'clock position immediately above the short process of malleus curving outwards and then downwards, 6mm away from the annulus at the 9 o'clock or 3 o'clock position in either ear (Fig. 20.20).

5. Elevation of flap using flap elevator (Fig. 20.21).

6. Fibrous annulus is identified with a sickle knife or a right angled probe and reflected out of the bony sulcus beginning at the posterosuperior angle and with the help of a microelevator from the rest of the sulcus. If a posterosuperior bony overhang overlying the oval window is present it should be removed by using a cutting burr or with the help of Lempert or House fine mastoid curette. (Figs 20.22 and 20.23)

7. Exposure and preservation of the chorda tympani nerve should always be attempted which is reflected anteriorly. If the chorda tympani creates surgical difficulties and inadequate exposure of the suprastructure of stapes then it may be divided (Fig. 20.24).

8. The lenticular process, the suprastructure of stapes, stapedius tendon and the footplate can now be visualized adequately (Fig. 20.25).

9. Ideally a control opening is made with the help of a straight pick or laser (KTP-532 is the commonly used one) in the posterior part of the footplate before the posterior crura is removed which may be done with the help of a crurotomy knife or microscissors or by using a cutting burr or laser that can easily be vaporized (Fig. 20.26).

10. Then, the opening is tailor-made to desired size depending on the size of the piston (common sizes available are 4 mm, 6 mm, 8 mm) with the help of hand burr or laser (rosette. formation) and diamond burr to take out the charred tissue after use of laser. If laser is being used, the facial nerve area is well covered with saline soaked gelfoam to prevent thermal injury due to laser.

11. Finally, the anterior crus is removed in similar fashion.

12. Temporalis fascia or vein grafted harvested earlier can be used to seal the opening site before piston is placed. Some people do not use vein or fascial graft. Instead, they place some gelfoam or fat/fascia around the piston.

13. Thus the lenticular process and the incudostapedial joint along with the stapedius tendon is preserved retaining its function.

14. Piston is then put in place into the opening site and the hook is anchored onto the lenticular process of incus. (Fig. 20.27)

15. Tympanomeatal flap is replaced and the external auditory canal is packed with gelfoam.

16. Mastoid dressing is applied.

Types of Prosthesis

Several types of prosthesis are used during stapes surgery like:

1. Robinson type with a metal stem designed to fit under the lenticular process, advantage being it is easy to insert and does not require trimming.

2. Causse type prosthesis made of Teflon designed to attach to the long process of incus. Can be used with small fenestra stapedotomy or total footplate removal.

3. Fisch/ Mc Gee type consists of a malleable ribbon like crook connected to a metal or Teflon stem. Its advantage is that it is easy to attach and crimp in position. It is ideal for small fenestra stapedotomy.

4. House type wire prosthesis is made of a thin metal wire used for total footplate removal. It is much more difficult to attach compared to the other prosthesis.

5. Velagrakis et al (1999) described a prosthesis which consists of a platinum ribbon and Teflon shaft. Its advantages are maximum visualization of the surgical field thereby allowing easy placement of the prosthesis.

6. Tange-RA et al (1998) advocated the use of Gold prosthesis.

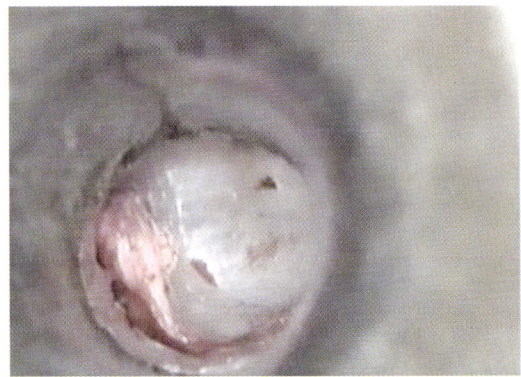

Fig. 20.20: Incision for tympanomeatal flap elevation

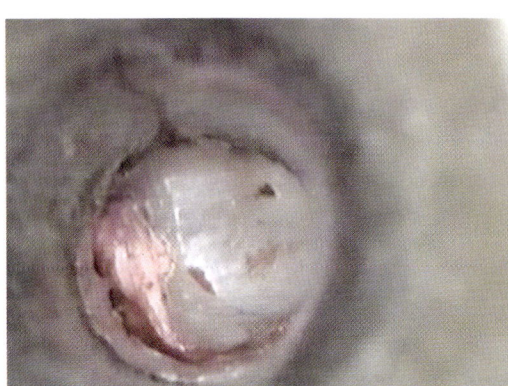

Fig. 20.21: Elevation of flap using flap elevator

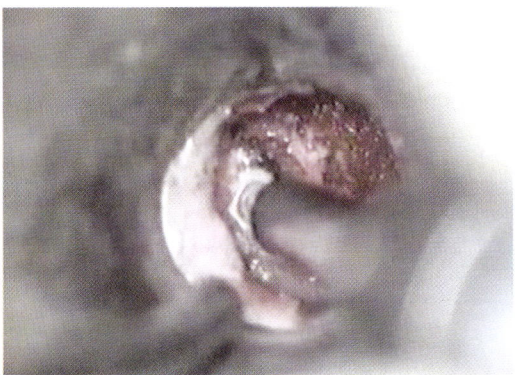

Fig. 20.22: Removal of PS Bony overhang with microdrill

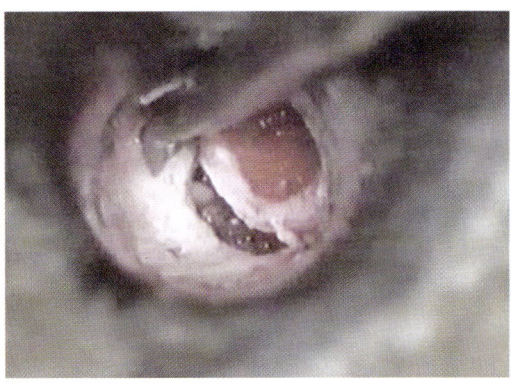

Fig. 20.23: Close up view

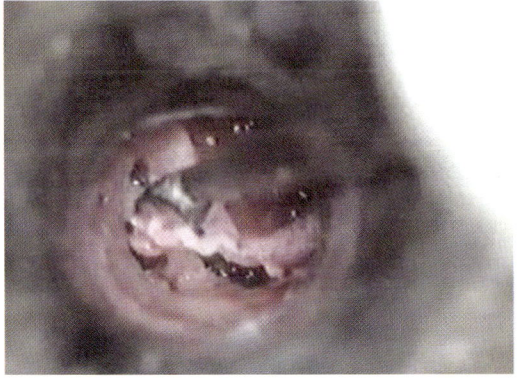

Fig. 20.24: Chorda tympani preserved

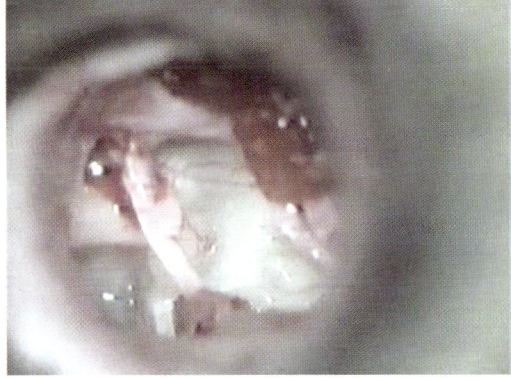

Fig. 20.25: Visualization of middle ear structures

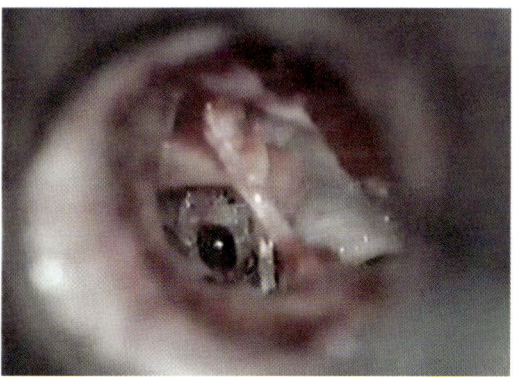

Fig. 20.26: Stapedectomy done

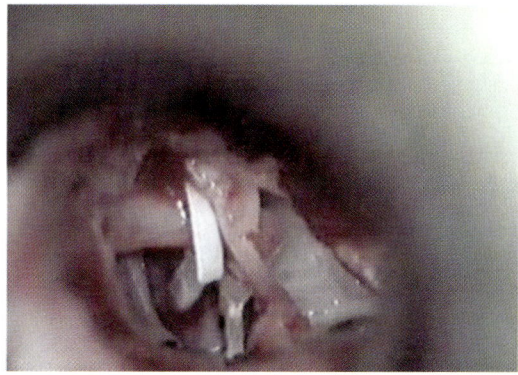

Fig. 20.27: Teflon piston fixed into long process of incus to fenestra of footplate

Postoperative Complications

1. Perilymph fistula
2. Acoustic trauma
3. Excessive movement of stapes
4. Rupture of membraneous inner ear
5. Delayed or immediate sensorineural hearing loss
6. Rapid loss of perilymph
7. Presence of blood in vestibule
8. Facial palsy
9. Injury to chorda tympani nerve
10. Reparative granuloma
11. Cerebrospinal fluid leak described by Causse and Causse in 0.3% due to widening of the cochlear aqueduct or a defect in the internal auditory canal.

Nose and Paranasal Sinus

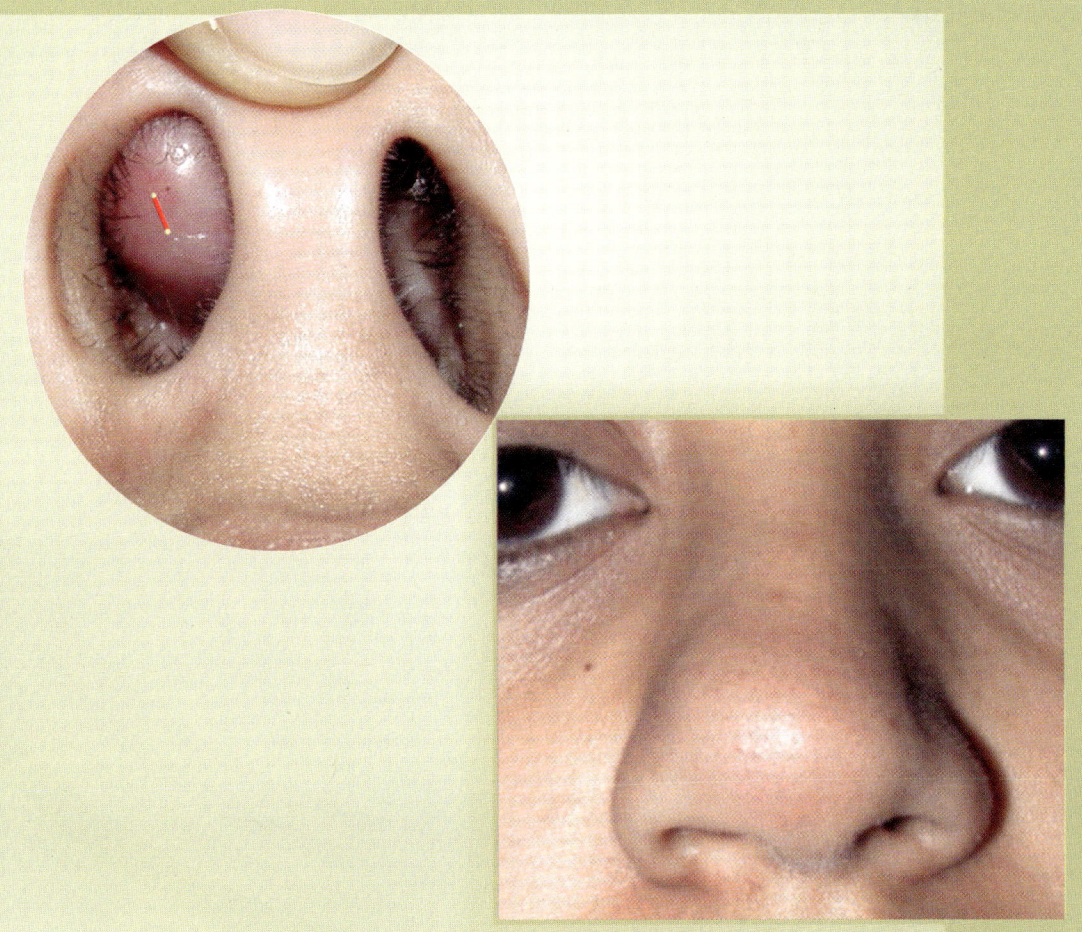

21

Anatomy of the Nose and PNS

NOSE AND PARANASAL SINUS

Nose is one of the most delicate organs in the body. The external nose serves the cosmetic function by enhancing the personality and the beauty of an individual. The nasal cavities act as the gateway to the respiratory tract, where it filters and conditions the inspired air in its respiratory zone. The olfactory zone serves the function of smell in humans, but is less effective in comparison to animals like the dog. The nasal mucosa serves many defensive functions like humidification and temperature regulation of inspired air, muco ciliary clearance and nasal reflexes. It also adds resonance to the voice.

The paranasal sinuses act as a constant source of sterile mucous blanket to replace the contaminated secretions in the nasal cavity through mucociliary clearance.

Anatomy of the Nose and Paranasal Sinuses

External nose
The external nose is a pyramidal structure and its skeletal framework is made up of bone and cartilages which maintain its shape. The upper angle of the nose where it is continuous with the forehead is called the **root** of the nose. The base of the nose is directed downwards. The base is triangular in shape and has two openings called the **anterior nares** or nostrils. The two nares are separated by the **columella**. These nares lead to the skin lined part of the nasal cavities called the **vestibule** of the nose. The free angle of the nose below forms its apex and is called the tip of the nose. It is connected to the root of the nose by the dorsum. The upper part of the dorsum is called the bridge.

Skeletal Framework of External Nose

It consists of bony and cartilaginous supportive framework (Fig. 21.1).

Bony part consists of the following
  1. Paired nasal bone

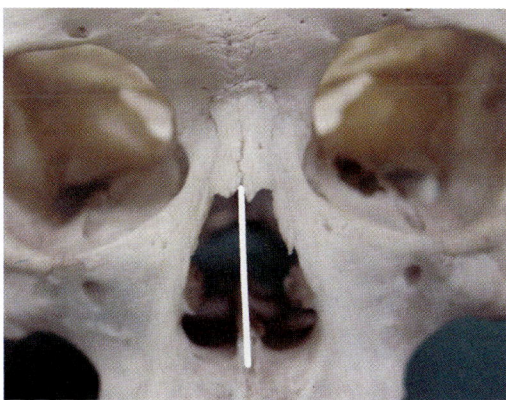

Fig. 21.1: Bony framework of face shows pyriform aperture and white line shows position of septum

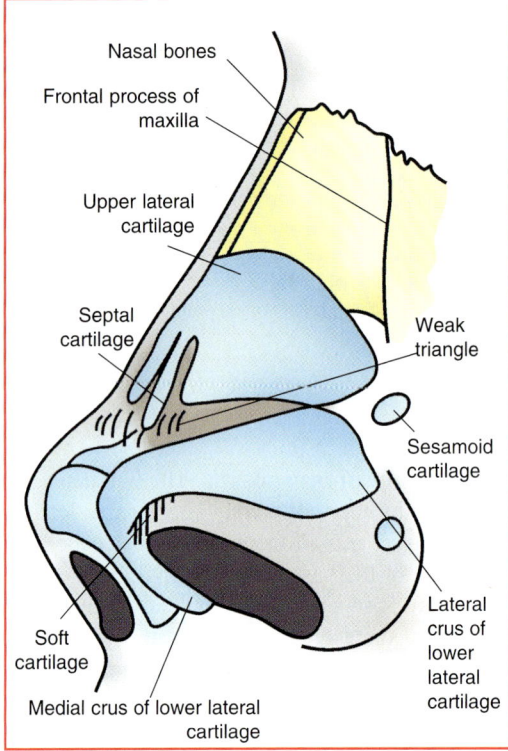

Fig. 21.2: Skeletal framewok of external nose showing its different parts

2. Paired frontal process of the maxilla
3. Nasal process of the frontal bone (Fig. 21.2)

The nasal bone articulates with the nasal process of the frontal bone superiorly, frontal process of the maxilla laterally, inferiorly with the upper lateral cartilage and medially with nasal bone of the other side. The junction between the two nasal bones forms the bridge of the nose. The nasal bone ossifies in a membrane from one center overlying the anterior part of the cartilaginous nasal capsule.

Cartilaginous part is made up of the following cartilages

1. Paired upper lateral cartilage
2. Paired lower lateral cartilage (alar cartilages)
3. Sesamoid cartilage
4. Anterior part of the septal cartilage

The upper lateral cartilage: It is triangular in shape and is attached above with the frontal process of maxilla and inferior margin of nasal bone. Medially it is continuous with the septal cartilage and is in fact a triangular flat expansion of the septal cartilage forming the middle third of the nose.

The lower lateral cartilage or the alar cartilage forms the lower third of the nose and is responsible for maintaining the projection and shape of the tip. It consists of slender medial crus and wider lateral crus. The two medial crurae support the columella. Each lateral crus forms the ala of the nose. The projection between the medial and lateral crurae of the cartilage supports the tip of the nose.

The minor **sesamoid cartilages** are present between the upper and lower nasal cartilages.

The **nasal cartilages** are made up of hyaline cartilages. Nasal bones and cartilages are connected to each other by periosteum and perichondrium, which is continuous. The upper and lower lateral cartilages prevent collapse of the vestibule during inspiration.

The skin covers the skeletal framework of the external nose, which is continuous with the skin of the columella and vestibule of the nose.

Nasal Cavity

The nasal cavity is divided into right and left nasal cavities by the nasal septum. Each nasal cavity has medial and lateral walls, a roof and a floor. The anterior most part of the nasal cavities lined by the skin is called the vestibule of the nose. Rest of the nasal cavities is lined by the respiratory epithelium below and olfactory epithelium above.

Vestibule

It is the entrance of the nasal cavity from the nostrils and is lined by skin containing hair follicles. It forms part of the dangerous area of face because of the presence of the retrograde venous drainage through ophthalmic veins (without valves), which can lead to complications like cavernous sinus thrombosis. The vestibule is demarcated from the nasal mucosa by the limen nasi, which corresponds to the superior margin of the lower lateral cartilage.

Columella

It is the part between the two nasal vestibules and forms the caudal end of the nasal septum. It is formed by the medial crurae of the two lower lateral cartilages. The lower lateral cartilages and the caudal end of the septum support the tip of the nose. Injury of any form to either caudal septum or lower lateral cartilages will change the shape of the tip.

Framework of the Nasal Cavity

In an articulated skull, the following bone/ cartilages bind each nasal cavity:

1. **The floor is formed by the**
   (a) Palatine process of the maxilla.
   (b) Horizontal process of the palatine bone.
2. **The roof consists of**
   (a) Cribriform plate of the ethmoid.
   (b) Nasal process of the frontal bone.
   (c) Body of the sphenoid.
3. **The medial wall is formed by**
   (a) Cartilaginous nasal septum
   (b) Bony nasal septum
   (c) Membranous columella

4. **Lateral wall consists of**
   (a) Medial wall of the maxilla.
   (b) Inferior concha
   (c) Middle and superior concha of the ethmoid bone (Fig. 21.3).

Medial Wall (Nasal Septum)

This is formed by bony and cartilaginous framework and is lined by the mucoperiosteum and the mucoperichondrium respectively. This forms the bulk of the nasal septum. The small caudal part is membranous (columella) and is lined by skin.

Following structures forms the **bony nasal septum** (Fig. 21.4).

Major contribution from

- Perpendicular plate of ethmoid
- Vomer
- Palatine crest
- Maxillary crest

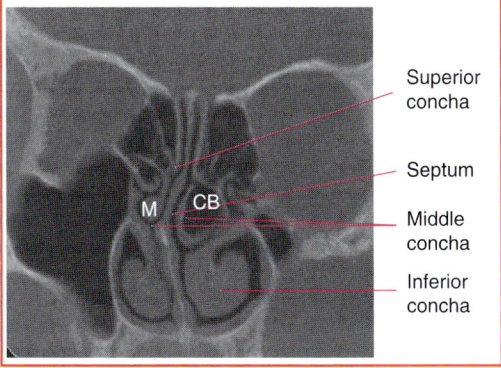

Fig. 21.3: CT scan of the nose and paranasal sinuses (M: Middle turbinate, CB: Concha bullosa)

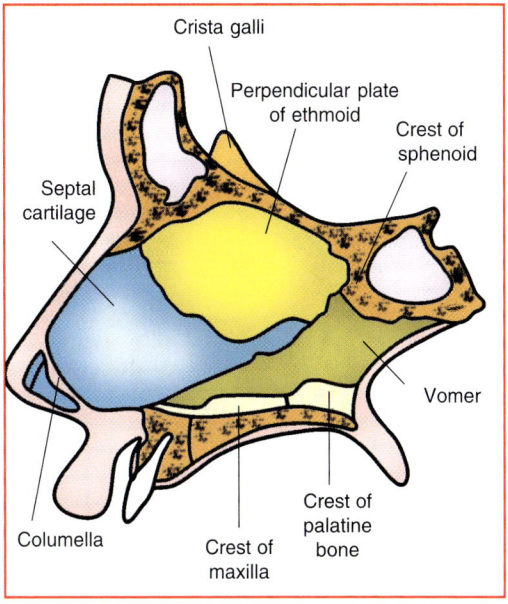

Fig. 21.4: Parts of the nasal septum

Small contribution from

- Nasal spine of the frontal bone
- Rostrum of the sphenoid
- Anterior nasal spine of the maxilla

The cartilaginous part of the nasal septum is formed by quadrangular cartilage with a contribution from upper and lower lateral cartilages.

Membranous columella: It is the membranous part of the septum between the medial crus of the lower lateral cartilage and the quadrangular cartilage. It is lined by skin.

Lateral Wall of the Nasal Cavity

Lateral wall is irregular and formed by the various bones and covered mainly by ciliated columnar epithelium. It is the main area of drainage for sinus secretions. Any change in its morphology or physiology may be a major cause of various sinus diseases.

The lateral wall is formed by the following bones

- Medial wall of the maxilla.
- Lateral mass of the ethmoid and lacrimal bone.

- Ascending process of the maxilla.
- Perpendicular part of the palatine bone.
- Medial pterygoid process of the sphenoid.

The features of the lateral wall (Figs 21.5a and b)

The lateral wall of the nasal cavity has three scroll shaped horizontal elevations called turbinates, i.e. superior, middle and inferior turbinates. Beneath and lateral to the turbinates are the three meatus, i.e. superior, middle and inferior meatus.

Superior Turbinate

It is part of the ethmoid bone. In some cases a small ridge may be seen above the superior turbinate called the supreme concha. The medial surface of the superior turbinate, corresponding part of the nasal septum and the area above it are lined by olfactory epithelium.

Middle Turbinate

It is formed by the middle concha, which is part of the ethmoidal bone. It has basal lamina, which passes laterally to join the lamina papyracea, and an ascending limb, which joins the cribriform

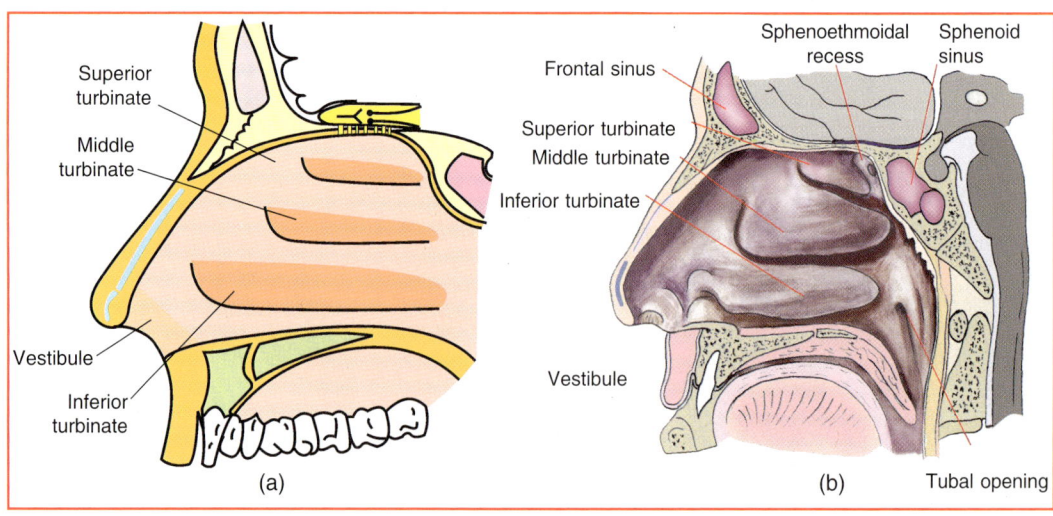

Figs 21.5a and b: (a) The lateral nasal wall. (b) Various structures in the lateral wall of the nasal cavity

plate. Fracture of the middle turbinate may cause avulsion of cribriform plate and CSF rhinorrhea and/or loss of sense of smell. This turbinate can be pneumatized by the ethmoidal air cell system and is called *Concha bullosa* (CB) (Fig. 21.3). Occasionally the turbinate may be *paradoxically curved* causing narrowing of the middle meatus. The posterior end of the middle turbinate points to the opening of the sphenopalatine foramen which actually represents a gap in the fusion between the sphenoid, palatine and ethmoid bones. It is covered by respiratory epithelium and its submucosa has limited cavernous venous plexus (erectile tissue).

Inferior Turbinate

It is composed of inferior concha, which is a separate bone. It is covered by respiratory epithelium and its subepithelium contains a rich cavernous venous plexus (erectile tissue).

Superior Meatus

It lies beneath the superior concha and has one or two openings for the posterior ethmoidal air cells.

Just above and posterior to the superior turbinate is a shallow depression called sphenoethmoidal recess. The sphenoid sinus drains into this recess.

Middle Meatus (Fig. 21.6)

It is one of the most important areas of the nose, from the surgeon's point of view. It is the most complex of the three meatus and it lies deep to the middle concha. The forward continuation of the middle meatus is called *atrium* of the nasal cavity. A curved ridge above the atrium is called the *agger nasi* and it may get pneumatized from the ethmoid and is known as *agger nasi air cell*. Just beneath the attachment of the middle turbinate, is a small thin plate of bone covered by mucoperiosteum, which is attached to the lamina papyracea superiorly and to the inferior concha inferiorly. This sickle shaped thin bone is called the *uncinate process*. Posterosuperior to the *uncinate process*, a rounded prominence is seen called the *bulla ethmoidalis*. It represents the middle ethmoidal air cells and is separated from the posterior ethmoid cells by *basal lamina* as discussed earlier. Between the uncinate process

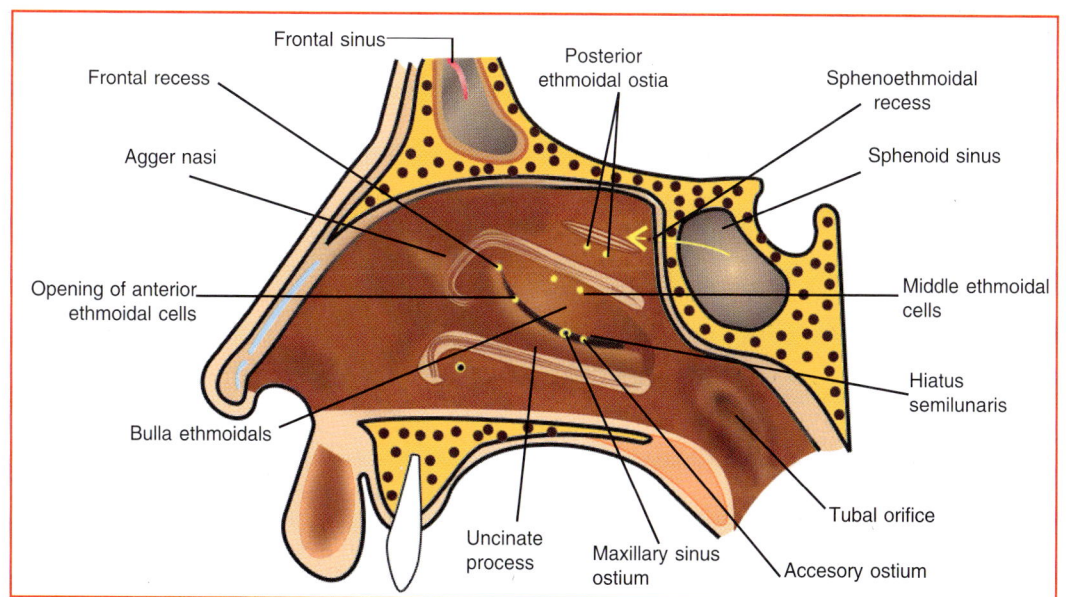

Fig. 21.6: Structure in the lateral wall of the nose after the turbinates are cut

and the bulla ethmoidalis, a slit-like semilunar shaped opening is present and is called *hiatus semilunaris*. This leads to a narrow three-dimensional space between the uncinate process and the bulla ethmoidalis laterally and middle turbinate medially and is called the ethmoidal *infundibulum*. Anterosuperiorly, the frontal sinus drains into the infundibulum through the frontal recess or through the anterior ethmoidal air cells. Few openings are seen on the surface of the bulla, which drains the anterior and middle ethmoid air cells. The natural ostium of the maxillary sinus opens into the hiatus and is located between the anteroinferior part of the bulla and the uncinate process. These important structures within the middle meatus as described above constitute the *ostiomeatal complex*.

Ostiomeatal Complex (Fig. 21.7)

This is defined as a micro architectural drainage pathway for anterior group of major paranasal sinuses and consists of a narrow cleft of ethmoidal infundibulum, between the uncinate process and bulla ethmoidalis. This cleft comprises of the ostium of the maxillary sinus and the frontal recess. Anatomical and pathological abnormalities in this region lead to persistent infection and disease within the major sinuses.

Roof of the Nose

This is formed by the cribriform plate of ethmoid and is considered part of the olfactory area *(dangerous area of the nasal cavity)*.

Olfactory area (dangerous area of nose): It is bounded laterally by the superior turbinate, medially by the corresponding part of the septum and superiorly by the cribriform plate. It is called as the dangerous area of the nasal cavity because the olfactory nerve fibers (Fig. 21.8) from this area pass through the cribriform plate into the anterior cranial fossa and can carry infection intracranially at the time of surgery/ trauma and also can be associated with CSF rhinorrhea.

The olfactory region of each of the two nasal passages in humans is a small area of about 2.5 square centimeters containing in total approximately 50 million primary sensory receptor cells. Olfactory region is lined by brownish epithelium and consists of three types of cells. They are:

1. Olfactory - bipolar receptor cells
2. Supporting cells consisting of microvilli
3. Basal cells - contain yellow pigment.

These cells are derived from the stem cells which have a unique capability to regenerate (Fig. 21.9).

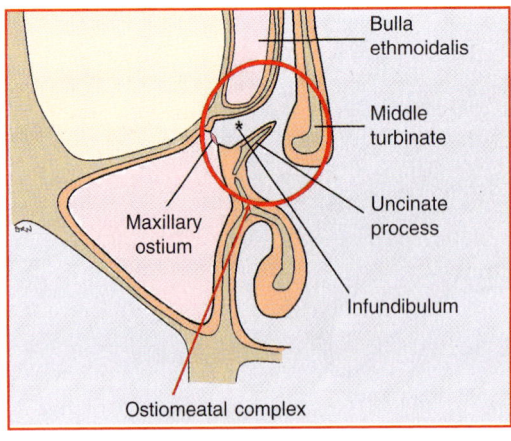

Fig. 21.7: Ostiomeatal complex

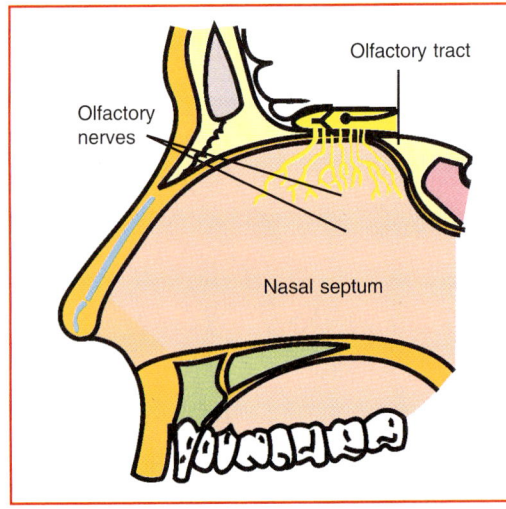

Fig. 21.8: Area supplied by the olfactory nerve

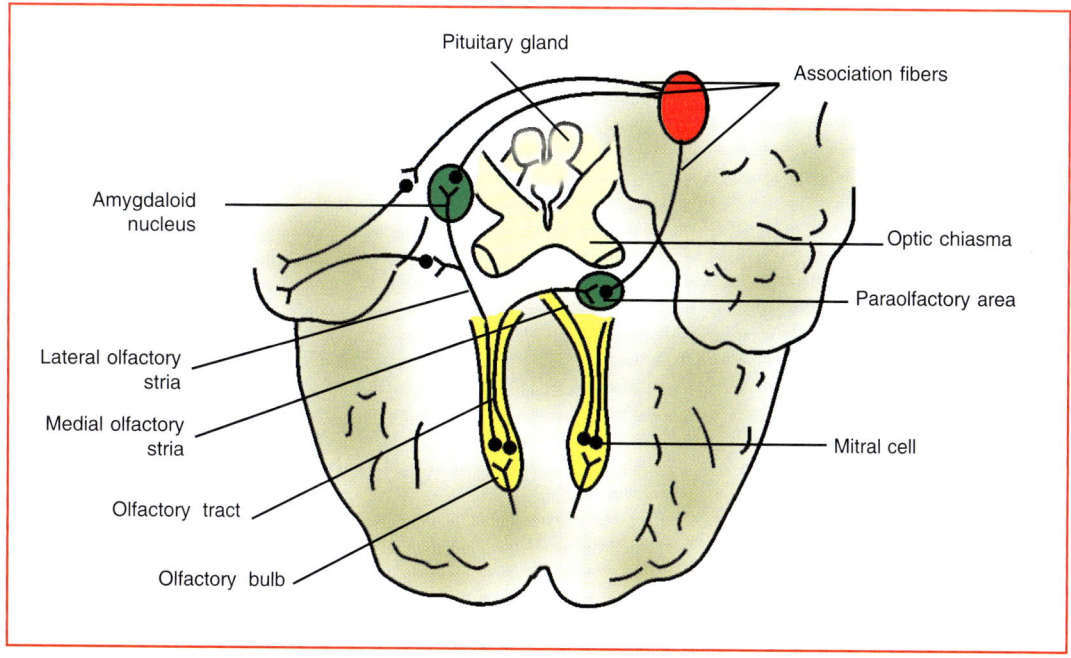

Fig. 21.9: Olfactory pathway

Blood Supply of Nasal Cavity
(Figs 21.10a and b)

Arterial supply

Derived from both internal and external carotid artery.

  1. **Derivatives of external carotid artery**
     1. Sphenopalatine artery
     2. Greater palatine artery
     3. Superior labial artery
  2. **Derivatives of internal carotid artery**
     1. Anterior ethmoidal artery
     2. Posterior ethmoidal artery

Blood Supply of the Lateral Wall of The Nose

Arterial

Sphenopalatine artery supplies all the turbinates and meatus. Anterior ethmoidal artery supplies the roof and lateral wall of nose. The superior labial supplies the alae nasi.

Venous

Cavernous plexus beneath the middle meatus.
  • Sphenopalatine and anterior facial vein
  • Ophthalmic vein
  • Veins on the orbital surface of the anterior cranial fossa
  • Superior sagittal sinus.

Blood Supply of the Nasal Septum

It is divided into anterosuperior, anteroinferior and posterosuperior.

The anterior ethmoidal artery supplies the anterosuperior part.

The anteroinferior part is supplied by

  • Long sphenopalatine artery, a branch of the internal maxillary artery. It is the main arterial supply to the septum. Also called **the artery of epistaxis**.
  • Anterior ethmoidal artery
  • Terminal branches of the greater palatine

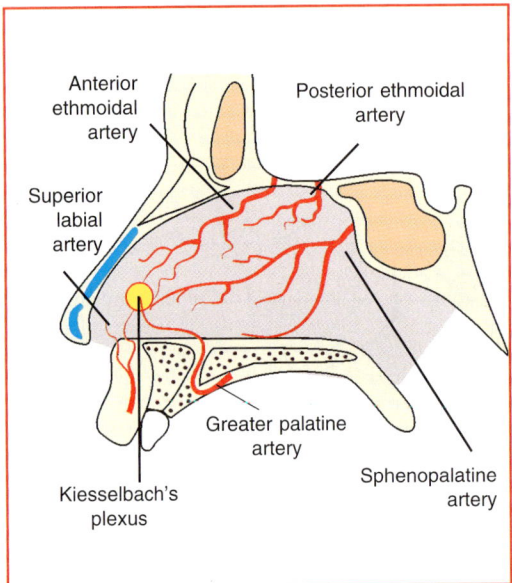

Fig. 21.10a: Blood supply of septum and showing Kiesselbach's plexus

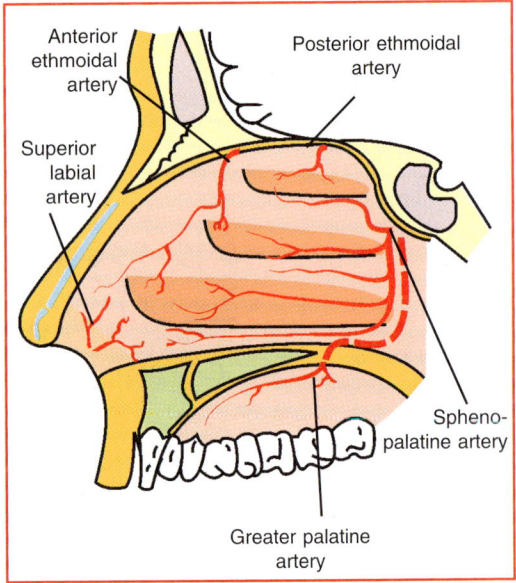

Fig. 21.10b: Blood supply of lateral wall of nasal cavity

- Septal branches of the superior labial (branch of facial artery) supply the tip of the septum.

All these arteries form an anastomotic plexus in the anteroinferior part of the nasal septum, known as *Kiesselbach's plexus* or *Little's area.* This is a frequent site for bleeding.

Venous arrangement of the Mucous Membrane of The Nose (Fig. 21.11)

Arterioles lying in the deeper part of the subepithelium forms the subepithelial periglandular capillaries which drains into the venous sinusoids and finally into the venous plexus. The entire vascular arrangement is controlled by autonomic nerve supply and is called erectile tissue.

Erectile tissue (subepithelial venous plexus)

It is seen in the inferior turbinate and posterior part of the middle turbinate and corresponding part of the nasal septum.

Autonomic Control (Figs 21.12a and b)

It maintains the congestion and the decongestion of the turbinates and regulates the airflow within the nasal cavity.

Sympathetic: Through the deep petrosal nerve
Parasympathetic: Through the greater petrosal nerve.

The deep petrosal nerve joins the superficial petrosal nerve to form the nerve of the pterygoid canal (vidian nerve). The sympathetic fibers through the nerve are derived from caroticotympanic plexus through the deep petrosal nerve.

Paranasal Sinuses (Fig. 21.13)

They are air filled spaces in the skull bones and are lined by mucosa, which drains into the nasal cavity by the mucociliary drainage.

They are eight in number, four on each side, namely the frontal, ethmoidal, maxillary and sphenoidal sinuses.

Functionally there are two groups.

1. *Anterior group:* These drain into the middle meatus.

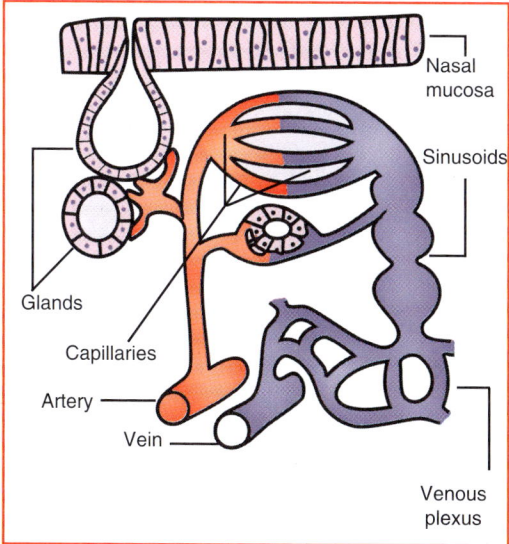

Fig. 21.11: Arrangement of subepithelial venous plexus

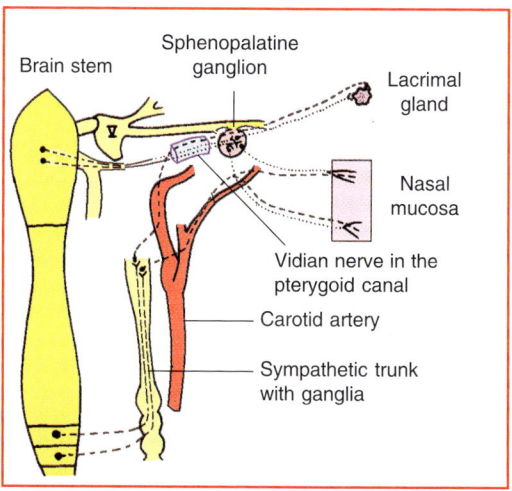

Fig. 21.12a: Autonomic supply of the nose

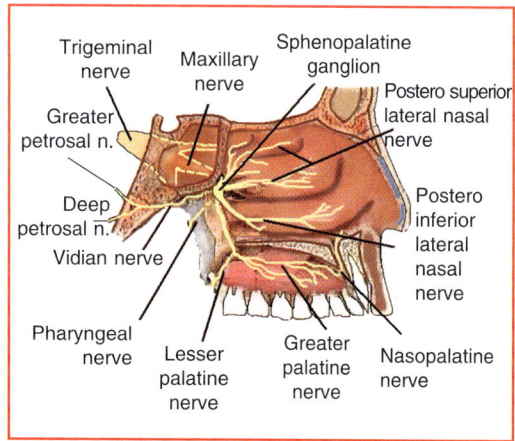

Fig. 21.12b: Nerve supply of the lateral wall of the nose

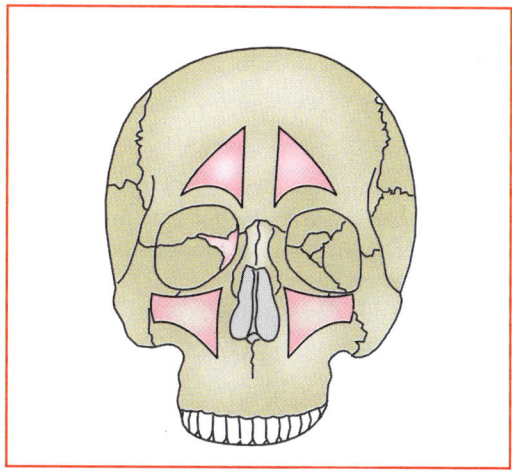

Fig. 21.13: Paranasal sinuses

(a) Frontal sinus
(b) Maxillary sinus
(c) Anterior ethmoidal sinus
(d) Middle ethmoidal sinus

2. *Posterior group:* These drain into the superior meatus/ sphenoethmoidal recess.

(a) Posterior ethmoidal sinus
(b) Sphenoid sinus

Maxillary Sinus (Antrum of Highmore) (Fig. 21.14)

This is a three sided pyramidal structure. In an adult its capacity is approximately 15 ml.

Base (medial wall) corresponds to the lateral wall of nasal cavity in relation to the middle and inferior turbinates. The ostium of the maxillary

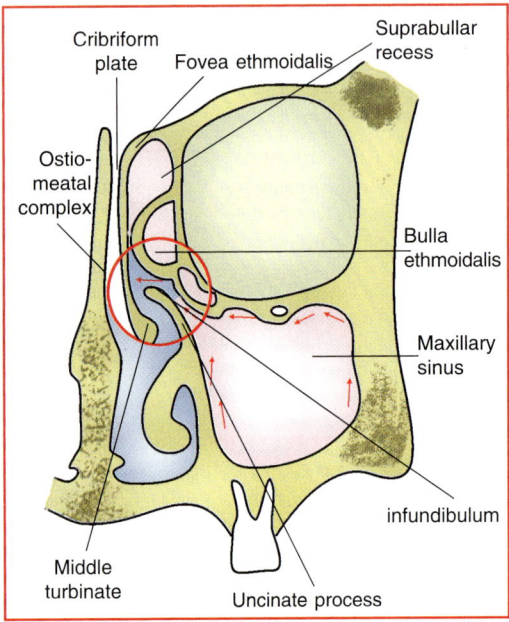

Cribriform plate

Fovea ethmoidalis

Suprabullar recess

Ostio-meatal complex

Bulla ethmoidalis

Maxillary sinus

infundibulum

Middle turbinate

Uncinate process

Fig. 21.14: Maxillary sinus

sinus opens in the medial wall and opens into the middle meatus between the uncinate process and the bulla ethmoidalis as described under lateral wall of the nasal cavity.

Apex is directed towards zygomatic process.

The three walls of this pyramid are:

(a) **Anterolateral wall** covered by the periosteum, soft tissue and skin of the cheek. It is relatively thinner in the canine fossa and is present lateral to the canine eminence. This site is used for approaching the maxillary sinus in *Caldwell-Luc operation*. This wall has an opening called infraorbital foramen, which is situated about one cm below the infraorbital margin. Infraorbital nerve and vessels emerges through this foramen.

(b) **Superior wall** (roof of antrum) is formed by orbital plate. This is covered by the orbital periosteum. At its midpoint in its inferior aspect is a groove, through which the infraorbital nerve and vessels pass before emerging out of the infraorbital foramen.

(c) **Posterior wall** is formed by a thin plate of bone and is related to pterygopalatine fossa, which consists of third part of internal maxillary artery, vidian nerve and the sphenopalatine ganglion. Posteromedially the bone is attached to pterygoid plates with a dehiscence called the sphenopalatine foramen. This opens into the lateral wall of the nose just behind the posterior end of the middle turbinate. This transmits the sphenopalatine vessels and the nerves.

Floor is formed by alveolar and palatine process of the maxilla. It lies at or above the floor of the nasal cavity in a child while it lies at a lower level in an adult.

Frontal Sinus (Figs 21.15 and 21.16)

It is pyramidal in shape and its volume, size and shape is variable. It can also be rudimentary. The two frontal sinuses are often asymmetrical in shape. Bony septa may partially subdivide it into one or more compartments. Its average capacity is about 7 ml in adults. It is not present at birth and it usually develops after the age of about five years as an extension of the anterior ethmoidal air cell.

Position it is situated between the inner and outer table of the frontal bone. It occupies variable amount of frontal bone.

Floor is formed by orbital roof. As it is relatively thin, it is used as a surgical approach.

Medially it is separated from the other frontal sinus by a thin interfrontal septum.

Posterior wall is related to anterior cranial fossa.

Anterior wall is covered by periosteum and skin of the forehead.

Ethmoidal Sinuses

It is well developed in children and it occupies the medial wall of the orbit and upper third of the lateral wall of the nose. It consists of 7 to 15 cells on each side and is divided into two groups based on their drainage. The ethmoidal air cells are small and do not have regular disposition, symmetry or fixed number.

Anterior group consists of anterior and middle ethmoidal air cells and drain into the middle meatus. It is separated from the posterior group by a thin bone arising from the middle turbinate called **basal lamina**.

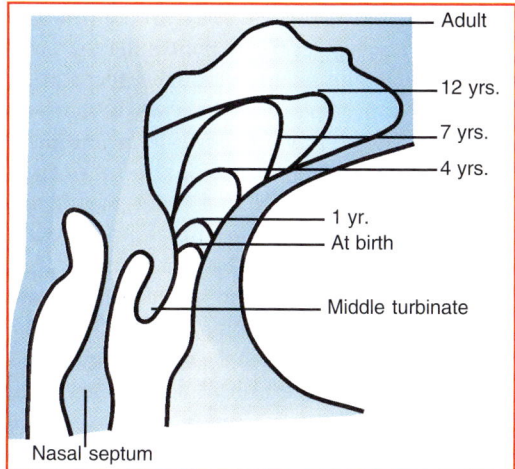

Fig. 21.15: Development of frontal sinus with age

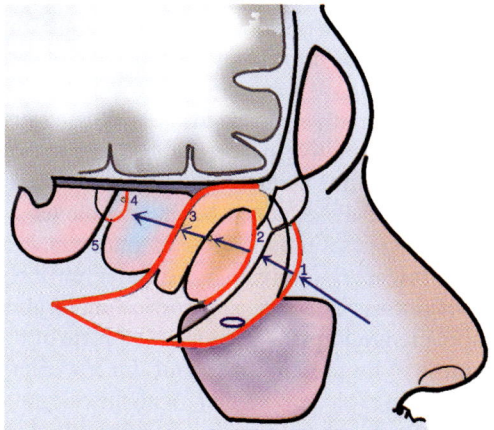

Fig. 21.16: Various lamellae from anterior to posterior dividing the sphenoethmoids: (1) uncinate, (2) bulla ethmoidalis, (3) basal lamella, (4) lamellae additional, (5) anterior wall of sphenoid

Posterior ethmoid drains into the superior meatus (Figs 21.16 and 21.6).

Superior wall of ethmoid labyrinth: The ethmoidal roof is formed by **fovea ethmoidalis** and is related to the anterior cranial fossa. The fovea slopes medially and downward. Its medial part is thinner and may be easily injured. The fovea is at a higher level than the cribriform plate, especially in its lateral part.

Lateral: It is formed by a papery thin bone called the **lamina papyrecea.** Here it is related to orbit and the lacrimal sac.

Posteriolaterally it is related to the sphenoid sinus. The posterior ethmoid cells may extend lateral to the sphenoid sinus where it is related to the optic nerve. These cells are called the **Onodi cells.**

Medially the ethmoid labyrinth is related to nasal cavity. The uncinate process and the bulla ethmoidalis are part of the ethmoid labyrinth. A semi-lunar opening between these two, drains the infundibulum of the 'ostiomeatal complex', which is described under the lateral wall of the nasal cavity.

Sphenoidal Sinuses

This is situated in the body of sphenoid. The sinuses of the two sides are divided by an asymmetrically placed median intersphenoidal septum. The sphenoid sinus drains into the sphenoethmoidal recess. It is related to a number of important structures because of its situation in the skull. The distance between sphenoid ostium to the anterior nasal spine is 7 cm.

Relations (Fig. 21.17)

Superiorly

1. Pituitary gland bulges into the sphenoid sinus posterosuperiorly. This is often used as a surgical approach (trans-sphenoidal hypophysectomy).
2. Optic chiasma
3. Olfactory tract
4. Frontal lobe of the brain.

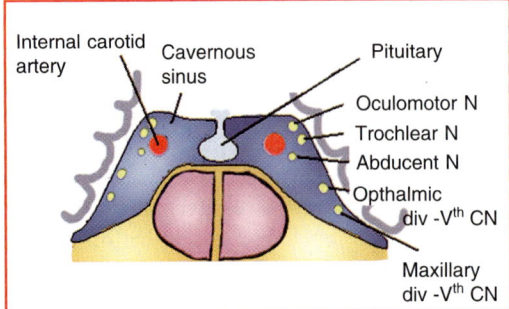

Fig. 21.17: Sphenoid sinus and its relations

Anteriorly

1. Sphenopalatine foramen
2. Sphenoidal crest
3. Nasal cavity.

Inferiorly

1. Nasopharynx and choanae
2. Vidian nerve is situated inferolaterally and its position helps in vidan neurectomy.

Posteriorly

1. Basilar artery
2. Brain stem

Laterally

1. Cavernous sinus and its contents (III, IV, V and VI cranial nerves)
2. Internal carotid artery.

Blood Supply of the Paranasal Sinuses

Infraorbital and superior dental arteries derived from the internal maxillary artery supply maxillary sinus.

Branches of the anterior and posterior ethmoidal artery supply ethmoidal sinus and frontal sinus.

Sphenoid sinus is supplied by pharyngeal branch of the internal maxillary artery.

Development of the Nose and Paranasal Sinuses (Figs 21.18a and b)

Nose develops from a number of mesenchymal processes surrounding the primitive stomodeum.

The **frontonasal process** arises between the central aspect of the forebrain and the epithelial roof of the mouth. A highly specialized ectodermal tissue called **olfactory placode** develops during the fifth week of intrauterine life, on each side of ventral surface of the frontonasal elevation. This divides it into **median and lateral nasal processes.** The **olfactory placode** sinks in to form the olfactory pit.

The extension of the mesenchyma from the median process gives rise to premaxillary process of the developing mouth. This subsequently also forms the upper lip and medial crus of the lower lateral cartilage. In the mean time anterior mesenchymal process, the **maxillary process** develops from the dorsal end of the mandibular arch and this fuses with the lateral nasal process the two being separated by the nasomaxillary groove. Ectoderm along the boundaries of these two process remains, giving rise to the **naso-lacrimal ridge** from which the **nasolacrimal duct** arises later. The **lateral nasal process** forms the **nasal bones**, the upper lateral cartilages and the lateral crus of the lower lateral cartilages. The median maxillary process fuses with the median nasal elevation leading to the formation of the **primitive external nares.** From this a deepening pit in the mesenchyma produces the nasal cavity. The primitive nose and mouth are separated by the **bucconasal membrane,** which disappears later to facilitate communication posteriorly through a primitive choana. This is situated just behind the primitive palate. Failure to canalize leads to **choanal atresia.** Initially the external nares are widely separated but later come closer as the frontonasal process reduces gradually. The **primitive nasal septum** is initially entirely cartilaginous. The superior portion undergoes ossification to form the perpendicular plate of the ethmoid. The premaxillary and the maxillary process establish the continuity with the primitive nasal septum thus defining the two primitive nasal cavities. On each side of the anterior nasal septum, an invagination of the ectoderm represents the *vomero-nasal organ*. The vomer ossifies in the connective tissue covering the residual posterior inferior cartilage from two centers, which unite below the cartilage creating a deep groove in which the quadrilateral cartilage lodges. As the growth continues the bony lamellae fuse and the cartilage gets absorbed. At puberty the lamellae are almost completely united with the everted alae. An anterior groove remains suggestive of the vomer's bi-lamellar origin. On the lateral wall of the nose a series of elevation appears within the nasal cavity at 6th week of intrauterine life, which ultimately forms the turbinates.

Development of Paranasal Sinuses

The *primordial of the sinuses* arises rather late during the prenatal period. The frontal sinus is the last to develop. In the first and second month of intrauterine life, the main features of the nasal cavities are defined. The *paranasal sinuses arise as localized epithelial invaginations* or recesses of the nasal mucosa, after the second month. These recesses become the ostia of the various sinuses.

The maxillary sinus and sphenoidal sinus arise as mucosal recesses during the third prenatal month. The invagination developing from the hiatus semilunaris forms the future maxillary sinus. The ethmoidal cells originate during the 5th and 6th months of the intrauterine life from the middle and superior meatus into anterior and posterior groups respectively.

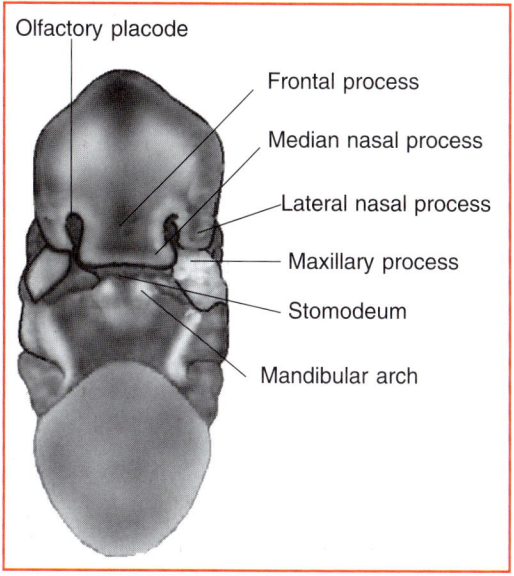

Olfactory placode
Frontal process
Median nasal process
Lateral nasal process
Maxillary process
Stomodeum
Mandibular arch

Fig. 21.18a: Development of various arches and developing nose

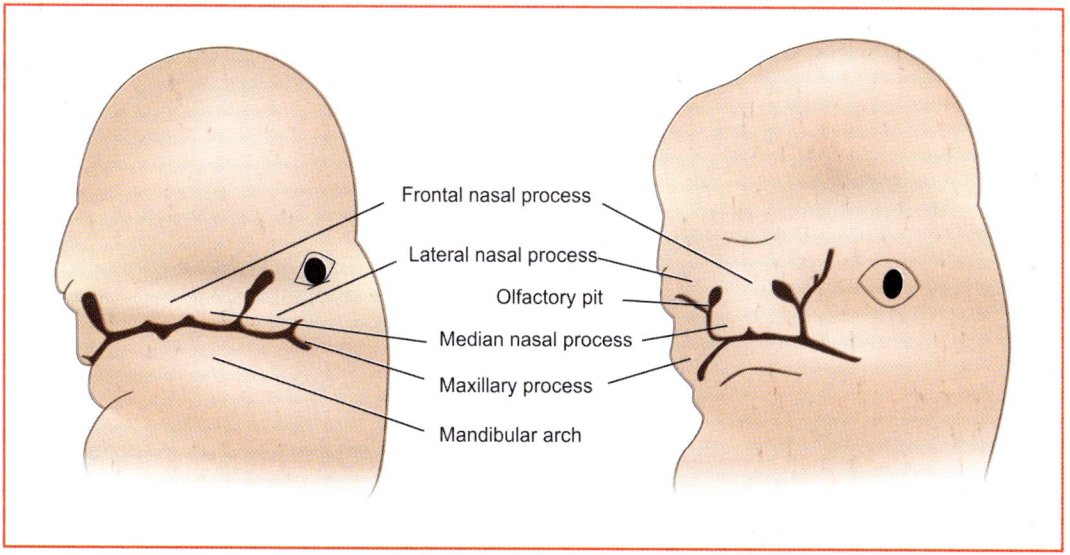

Frontal nasal process
Lateral nasal process
Olfactory pit
Median nasal process
Maxillary process
Mandibular arch

Fig. 21.18b: Development of nose

POINTS TO REMEMBER

1. The nasal cavity acts as the gateway to the respiratory tract, where it filters and conditions the inspired air into its respiratory zone.
2. The olfactory zone serves the function of smell in humans, but is less effective in comparison to animals like dog, etc.
3. The external nose is supported by bony and cartilaginous framework.
4. The ostiomeatal complex consists of a narrow cleft between uncinate process and bulla ethmoidalis and comprising of ethmoidal infundibulum, maxillary ostium and frontal recess.
5. The olfactory area is considered as the dangerous area of nose as the infection from this area can be carried through the cribriform plate to the anterior cranial fossa.

Physiology of the Nose and Paranasal Sinuses

22

Functions of The Nasal Cavity

1. Nasal respiration
2. Protection of the lower respiratory tract
   (a) Filtration
   (b) Air-conditioning of inspired air (temperature and humidity regulation)
   (c) Mucociliary function
   (d) Sneeze reflex
3. Vocal resonance
4. Olfaction
5. Outlet to the lacrimal secretions

Nasal Respiration (Figs 22.1a and b)

The contribution of the nose to the airflow in the respiratory tract is of considerable importance. 50 percent of the total resistance is contributed by the nasal cavities. Man is an obligatory nasal breather for the first six months of life. 85 percent of the adults are nose breathers and only resort to an oral or oronasal route under demanding situations such as exercise or in pathological conditions. It has been estimated that an adult inspires up to 10,000 liters of air daily (Kerr, 1997).

Nasal airway resistance: The nasal vestibule is the first component of nasal resistance. The nasal vestibule is composed of compliant walls that are liable to collapse from the negative pressures

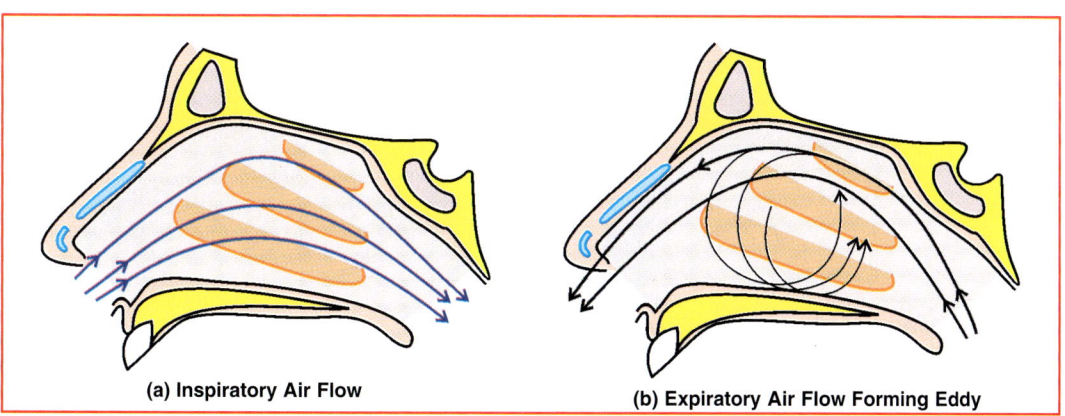

(a) **Inspiratory Air Flow** (b) **Expiratory Air Flow Forming Eddy**

Figs 22.1a and b: Inspiratory and expiratory phases of nasal airflow generated during inspiration (kerr, 1997). The vestibule has been termed the external nasal valve. It contributes to one third of the nasal airway resistance. The valve region is formed slightly posterior to the posterior edge of the lower lateral cartilage and the nasal septum contributes most of the remaining two third of the resistance (Fig. 22.2).

Inferior and middle turbinates contain erectile tissue, the anterior end of which has a major effect on nasal resistance and functions as an internal nasal valve.

Inspiratory air currents pass vertically up through the anterior nares at a rate of 2 to 3 m/s. The flow converges to a laminar pattern at a velocity of 12 to 18 m/s at the narrowest point i.e. the nasal valve after which the flow becomes horizontal. Laminar flow is important for cleaning and conditioning of the air. Most of the air conditioning occurs along the middle meatus and the floor of the nose, but eddying occurs in olfactory area.

Expiratory air currents are most turbulent, with air flowing through the nasal cavity, sweeping inspired air out of the olfactory region. The expiratory flow produces eddies in the region of the middle meatus. The sinuses are ventilated only in the expiratory phase by air that has been pretreated by the respiratory mucosa and are relatively sterile. The uncinate process probably protects the sinuses by diverting the inspired air that is rich in allergens and bacteria - *(Nayak et al 2001)* (Figs 22.3a and b).

Changes in the nasal resistance are primarily the result of a vascular response and erectile tissue controlled by autonomic nervous system, mainly the sympathetic system. This determines the state of engorgement of the erectile tissue.

Factors Affecting the Nasal Resistance

(a) *Age:* Maximum resistance is found in infancy and it reduces as the age advances
(b) *Nasal cycle*: A physiological cycle of spontaneous reciprocating nasal

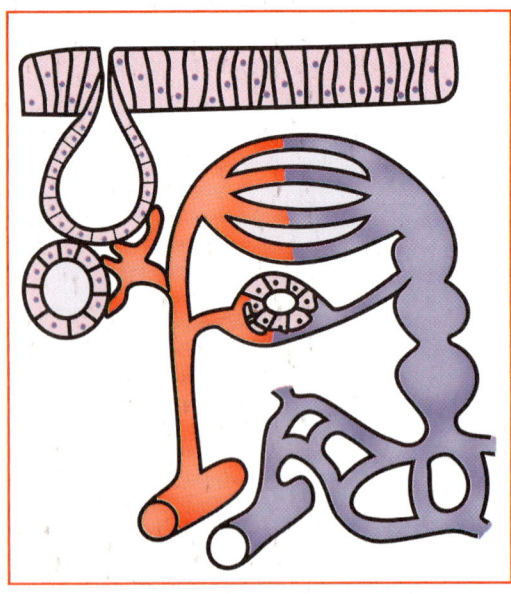

Fig. 22.2: Erectile tissue in the subepithelium of the turbinates

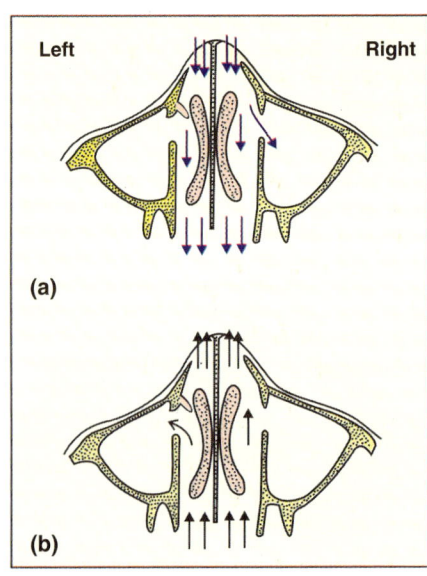

Figs 22.3a and b: Normal air flow during inspiration and expiration on the left side and the effect of uncinate process removal on ventilation of sinus in the right side

congestion and decongestion alternating between the two nasal cavities.

This was first described by Kayser in 1895 and is probably controlled by respiratory areas in the brain stem closely associated with respiratory activity. The duration of the cycle varies from 2 to 7 hrs. It is absent in laryngectomies and tracheostomized patients.

(c) *Exercise:* With increase in exercise the nasal resistance decreases probably due to increase in the sympathetic activity on the erectile tissue.

(d) *Respiration:* Resistance is slightly lower during inspiration compared to that during expiration. Hyperventilation results in vasodilatation and a rise in resistance.

(e) *Posture:* Change of posture leads to change in nasal resistance due to alteration in jugular venous pressure.

(f) *Nasal reflexes:* Like sneezing can influence the nasal resistance. Sneezing results from a number of mild mechanical and chemical stimuli to the nasal mucosa and is associated with increased secretion and congestion. The trigeminal nerve, respiratory muscles and the autonomic nervous system usually mediate this.

(g) *Skin and air temperature:* Atmospheric air can affect the skin temperature, which reflexly alters the nasal mucosal blood flow as part of the thermoregulatory mechanism. Cool inspired air can cause congestion and increased resistance.

(h) *Emotional and psychological response:* This causes autonomic imbalance and alteration in the nasal resistance by regulating the erectile tissue.

Protection of the Lower Respiratory Tract

(a) *Filtration:* Vibrissae in the nasal vestibule prevent the large particles in the inspired air from passing through the nasal cavity.

(b) *Air-conditioning of the inspired air:* The temperature and humidity of the inspired air is regulated by the nasal mucosa. The blood flow of the nasal cavity is from the posterior to anterior direction as shown in Fig. 22.4, which is opposite to the flow of inspired air. This mechanism is applied in refrigeration industry and is called as counter-current mechanism. This allows the inspired air to be humidified as it comes in contact with the mucous blanket, which also traps the dust particles. The humidification of the inspired air occurs from the evaporation of mucous blanket. The counter-current effect also allows heating of the inspired air that gets pretreated in the nasal chamber. This air-conditioning function is controlled by the autonomic nervous system.

(c) *Mucociliary function:* Respiratory mucosa is coated by a thin layer of mucous secretions called mucous blanket, which

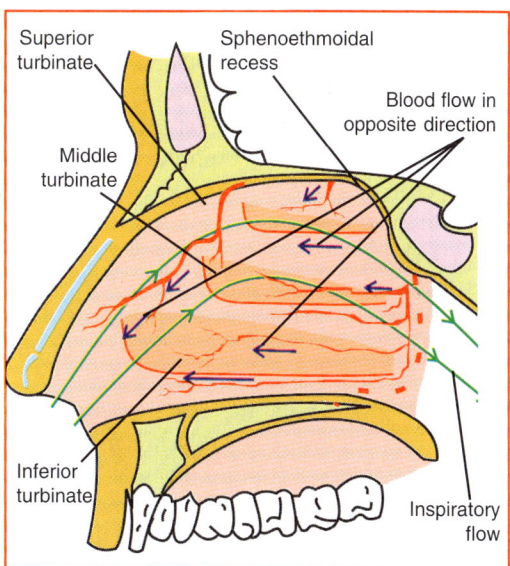

Fig. 22.4: The counter-current mechanism of the air-conditioning function of the nose. Blue arrows show the direction of the blood supply and green arrows show the direction of the inspiratory airflow

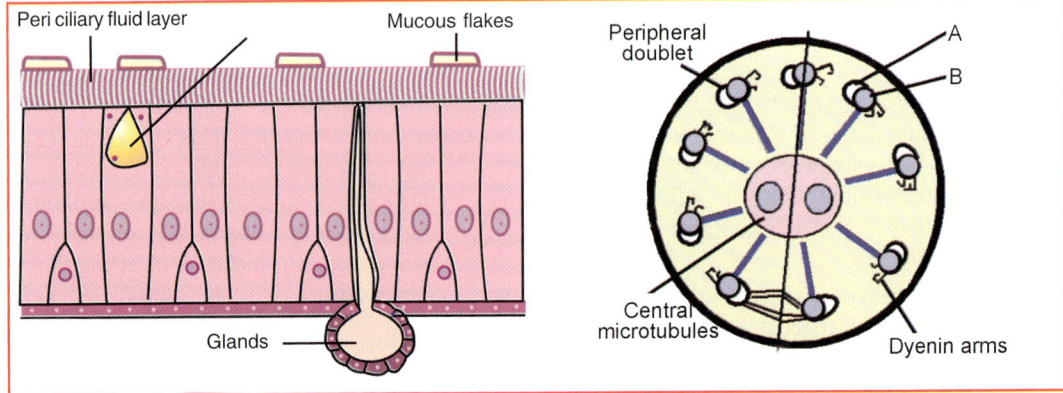

Figs 22.5a and b: (a) Mucous blanket (b) Microstructure of the cilia (cross section)

helps in cleaning the fine particulate matters that are trapped in it during the inspiratory phase. It consists of superficial thick mucous layer (gel) and deep thin periciliary layer (sol) (Fig. 22.5).

The mucous secreting glands and goblet cells of the nasal and sinus mucosa secrete the mucous. The mucous is rich in lysozymes, an important enzyme that initiates bacterial destruction. In addition, it contains secretory IgA, which neutralizes allergens and bacterial toxins. The cilia of the respiratory epithelium beats in a specific manner and direction. It propel the mucous blanket towards the pharynx, where it is swallowed (Fig. 22.6). The cilia are composed of multi-structural axonema which is made up of nine doublets of peripheral microtubules and two single central microtubules (9 + 2 pattern). Among the paired microtubules one (A) contains two dyenin arms (outer and inner) extending towards the other microtubule (B). These dyenin arms contain ATPase responsible for the ciliary movement (Fig. 22.5b).

(d) *Nasal reflex function and protection:* Clinical observation suggests the existence of poorly characterized reflex pathway between upper and lower respiratory pathway. Sneezing is also a protective function in response to irritants and harmful stimuli.

Vocal Resonance

The nasal cavities and the sinuses add nasal tone to the articulated voice by acting as resonators.

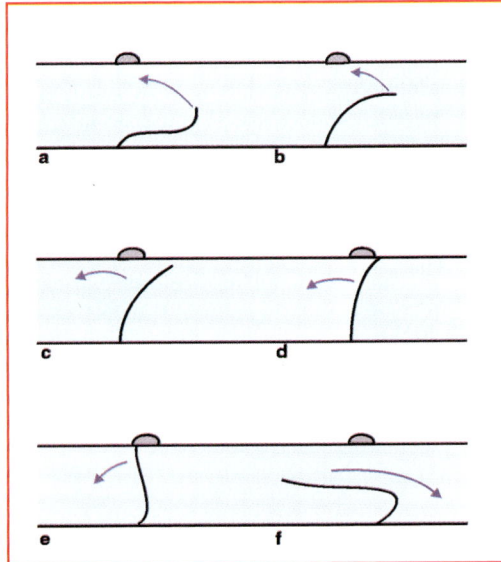

Fig. 22.6: (a) Initiation of beat of cilia. (b, c, d, e) Propelling of cilia making the mucous blanket to move. (f) Recovery stage

Nasal speech (rhinolalia), results due to nasal or nasopharyngeal obstruction (rhinolalia clausa) or due to abnormal communication between the oral and nasal cavities as in cleft palate and palatal paralysis (rhinolalia aperta).

Olfaction

It is defined as a mechanism by which the smell is perceived. The olfactory area of the nasal cavity as described earlier is responsible for this function of the nasal cavity. The main functions of olfaction are

1. Regulation of the food intake and perception of flavour and palatability.
2. Regulation of reproductive behavior (more developed in lower animals)
3. *Protective function*: Detection of the noxious and toxic substances.

Mechanism of Olfaction

Olfactory receptors situated in the upper part of the nasal cavity above the level of the superior turbinate senses the odorant particles in the inspired air. Each olfactory receptor neuron has 8 to 20 cilia that are whip-like extensions of 30 to 200 microns in length. The olfactory cilia are the sites where molecular reception with the odorant occurs and sensory transduction (i.e., transmission) starts. The amount of inspired air reaching this area depends on the nasal anatomy and pathological abnormalities. Sniffing increases the availability of inspired air into the olfactory area. The regulation of the olfactory system is mainly achieved by the olfactory mechanism, which consists of the olfactory epithelium and its central connections and to some extent by the non-olfactory receptors of the V, VII, IX and X cranial nerves. The Vth cranial nerve perceives odor upto 30%.

Olfactory Pathway (Fig. 22.7a and b)

Mechanism of odor perception: Many theories exist to explain the mechanism of odor perception. Among them the lock and key concept of chemical recognition is widely held. According to this concept, odor perception depends on the interaction of the odorant molecules with highly specialized and highly specific olfactory receptor sites in the olfactory cell membrane. The electrical impulse thus generated is transmitted to the higher centers. The odor particles have to cross the mucus to reach the receptor cells, which necessitates it to be water soluble to some extent, but lipid solubility will enhance interaction with the plasma membrane. Because of the pigments like carotenoids which are found in the bowman's glands, a role similar to that of retina has been proposed.

Outlet for Lacrimation Secretion

The nasolacrimal duct drains into the inferior meatus. Blockage of this duct can lead to epiphora.

Function of the Paranasal Sinuses

(a) Warming and moistening of the inspired air occurs in the nasal cavity
(b) Resonance to laryngeal voice

Complex interaction between smell, taste, feeding behavior and reproduction

Olfactory epithelium
↓
Glomerular olfactory bulb
↓
Olfactory tract
↓
Olfactory trigone
↓   ↘
Medial striae   Lateral striae
↓
Hypothalamus ↙
↓
Central connections amygdala and hippocampus

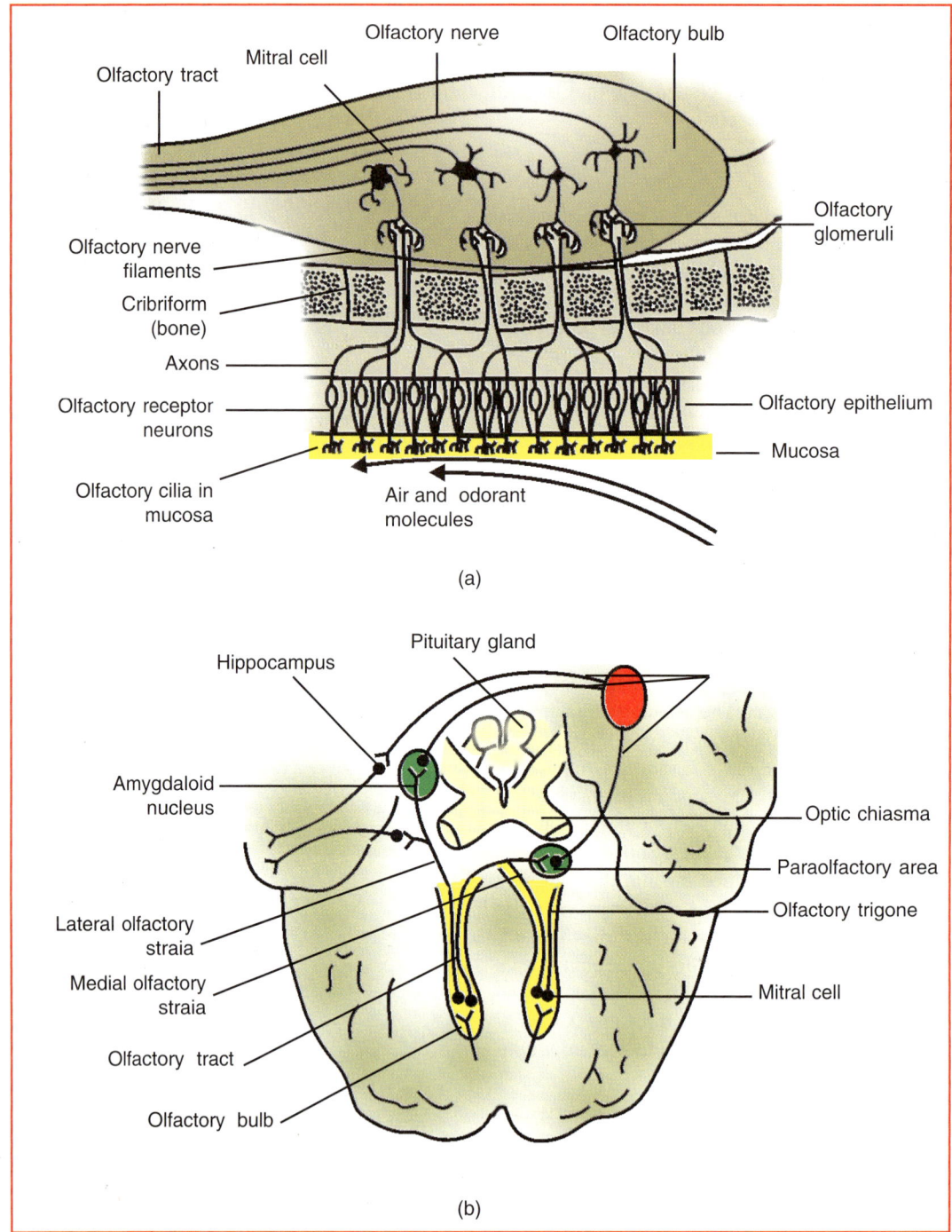

Fig. 22.7: (a) Olfactory pathway (b) Olfactory pathway and connections

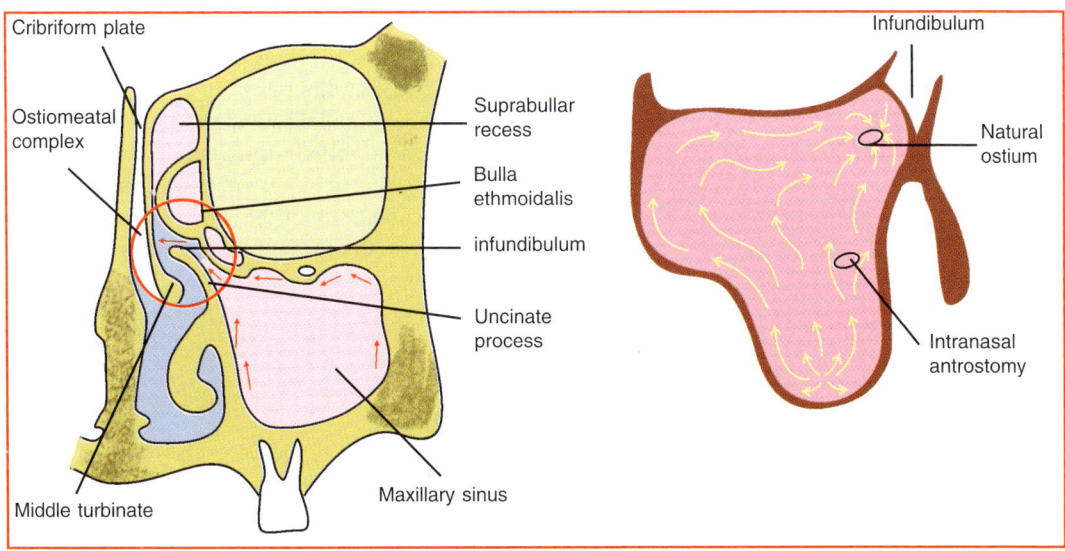

Figs 22.8a and b: (a) Osteomeatal complex and mucociliary pathway towards the ostium (b) Mucociliary clearance of the maxillary sinus towards the natural ostium bypassing the artificially created inferior meatal antrostomy

(c) Temperature buffer
(d) Reducing the weight of the facial bones
(e) Mucociliary clearance.

Mucociliary Clearance

The sinuses act as a constant source of sterile mucous blanket, which is essential to replace the contaminated secretions in the nasal cavity. This is probably the most important function of the paranasal sinuses. Development in nasal endoscopy has revealed more information about the sinus mucociliary clearance activity and in the pathogenesis of sinusitis. Anatomical abnormalities in the nasal cavity especially in the middle meatus can obstruct the outlet of the paranasal sinuses causing persistant inflammatory disease in the sinuses (Figs 22.8a and b).

The secretions from the maxillary sinus start in a star like shape from the floor of the sinus along its wall to reach the inner maxillary ostium at the uppermost and posterior corner of the sinus in the lateral nasal wall. From here it is actively transported through the ethmoid infundibulum over the rear margin of the uncinate process onto the medial surface of the inferior turbinate and then towards the nasopharynx. The secretions never drain through the accessory ostium, rather they move away along its margin and finally proceeds through the natural ostium.

Messerklinger demonstrated the inward transport of the mucous blanket in the frontal sinus along the interfrontal septum, the roof, walls of the frontal sinus laterally, returning to the floor of the sinus and leaving the inner ostium laterally (Fig. 22.9).

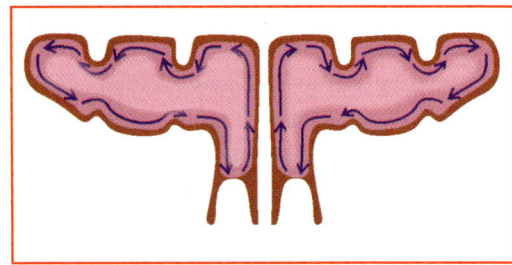

Fig. 22.9: Mucociliary clearance of frontal sinus

Not all the secretions leave the sinus at once. In the frontal recess some of the secretions get back into the frontal sinus and is called as retrograde flow. The secretions from the frontal sinus, enters the ethmoidal infundibulum and finally joins the secretions from the maxillary sinus.

The secretions from the sinuses form two streams of flow. The one from the middle meatus flows along the lateral wall towards the nasopharynx, below the eustachian tube and is called **infratubal stream** (Fig. 22.10) (Blue arrow). The secretions from the superior meatus and sphenoethmoidal recess, goes above the tubal orifice and is called **supratubal stream** (Fig. 22.10) (Green arrow). In acute and chronic infective conditions of the sinuses the secretions may overflow the eustachian tube orifice as shown in the figure 22.10 (Red arrow).

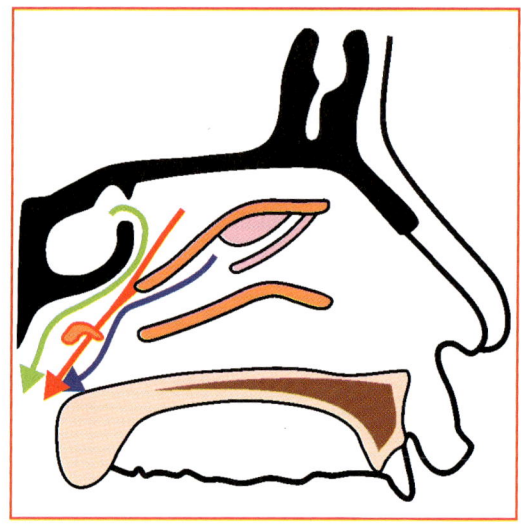

Fig. 22.10: Mucociliary drainage pathways in the nasal cavity from various sinuses

POINTS TO REMEMBER

1. An adult inspires upto 10,000 liters of air daily.
2. The inferior and middle turbinate and the corresponding part of the nasal septum contain errectile tissue, that functions as internal nasal valve.
3. The paranasal sinuses are ventilated only in the expiratory phase.
4. Changes in the nasal mucosa are primarily the result of a vascular response and erectile tissue controlled by autonomic nervous system.
5. Respiratory mucosa is coated by a thin layer of mucous blanket, that helps in cleaning the fine particulate matter including bacteria that are trapped in it during the inspiratory phase.

23

History Taking and Clinical Examination of Nose and PNS*

History Taking

It is very important to take a detail history of the patient before examining in the following order.

Chief Complaint

The common presenting symptoms include:
- Nasal obstruction
- Nasal discharge
- Sneezing
- Epistaxis
- Post-nasal drip (hawking)
- Headache and facial pain
- Swelling and deformity
- Disturbance of smell
- Snoring
- Change in voice- Hyponasal/ hypernasal
- Tinnitus
- Dryness of nose and throat
- Sensation of foreign body in the nose

History of present illness

The flowing questions are asked and the findings are noted.
- What is the reason for consulting the specialist?
- When did the problem start? Acute or insidious?
- How did the problem start and what is the duration?
- Whether it is bilateral or unilateral?
- Whether it is progressive or status quo?
- Is the symptom intermittent (episodic) or continuous?
- If intermittent, what is its frequency and what is the duration of each frequency?
- What are the aggravating and relieving factors of the symptoms?
- Is there any other associated symptom?
- What is the treatment received, if any, and what is its outcome?

Past History

Were there any similar episodes in the past? If so, provide details.

Any other illnesses, the patient is suffering from which may or may not be directly related to the patient's present illness. Example: Diabetes, hypertension, bronchial asthma, history of allergies, etc.

Family History
- Is there any similar illness in the family?

---

*Note: *For detailed and elaborate description, please refer to the same author's book on 'Clinical and Operative methods in ENT and Head & Neck Surgery'.*

Treatment History

What is the treatment received for present or any other illnesses in the past and what were their outcomes?

Menstrual History

When did the female patient attain menarche and if menstruating, whether the cycles are regular and what is the quantity of flow and its duration?

Personal History

Socioeconomic status, habits, addictions, marital status, etc.

General Examination

As described under the section, 'Otology'.

EXAMINATION OF THE NOSE AND PARANASAL SINUSES

Examination of the External Nose

Inspection

External nose: Should be examined to look for any external deformity and skin changes. Common deformities are saddle, hump, deviation and crooked nose.

Nasal vestibule: Best examined by lifting the tip of the nose, digitally using the thumb. Look for furuncle, erythema and fissuring of the skin of the vestibule, caudal dislocation, etc. (Fig. 23.1).

Palpation

1. ***Superficial palpation:*** It is done with thumb and the index finger being applied one on each side of the nose. The bony and soft parts are examined carefully to look for the following:
   (a) Mobility
   (b) Thickness
   (c) Fluctuation
   (d) Temperature
   (e) Pain and tenderness

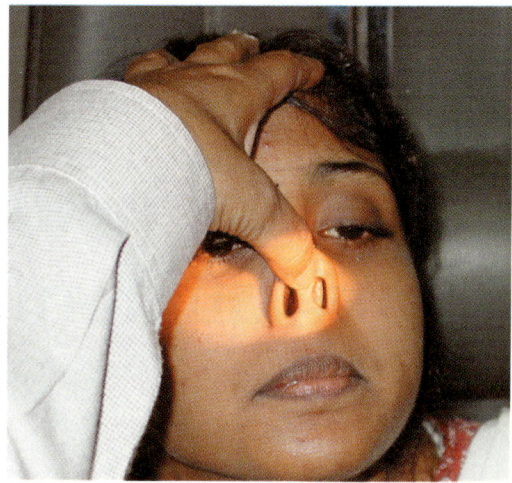

Fig. 23.1: Examination of the nasal vestibule. Caudal dislocation of the septum can be seen

Careful examination is done to check for the following:
- Any change in shape
- Intactness of bony framework
- Any lesion

2. ***Deep palpation:*** Strong pressure is applied with the thumb and the index finger to examine the bony framework of the nose. Crepitus may be present and tenderness may be elicited in fracture of the nasal bone following trauma.

Examination of Nasal Cavity

Cold Spatula Test (Fig. 23.2)

A cold spatula or tongue depressor is kept in front of the anterior nares and the fogging that occurs during expiration is compared with each nostril to detect nasal obstruction.

Anterior Rhinoscopy (Fig. 23.3)

This is done by using a Pilcher's/Vienna (Fig. 23.4) or Thudichum (Fig. 23.5) nasal speculum. The structures that can be seen are nasal septum, anterior part of inferior turbinate, inferior meatus, middle turbinate and middle meatus, floor of the nasal cavity (23.6). Superior meatus, posterior end of septum, posterior end of middle and inferior turbinate cannot be examined by anterior rhinoscopy.

Posterior Rhinoscopy (Fig. 23.7)

This is done by using a posterior rhinoscopy mirror. Structures that can be seen are choana, posterior end of the septum, posterior end of middle and inferior turbinates and the eustachian tube orifices, fossa of Rosenmiiller (Figs 23.8a and b).

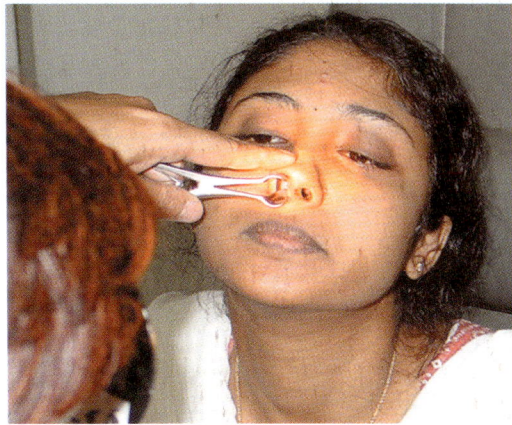

Fig. 23.4: Anterior rhinoscopy with Pilcher's/Vienna nasal speculum

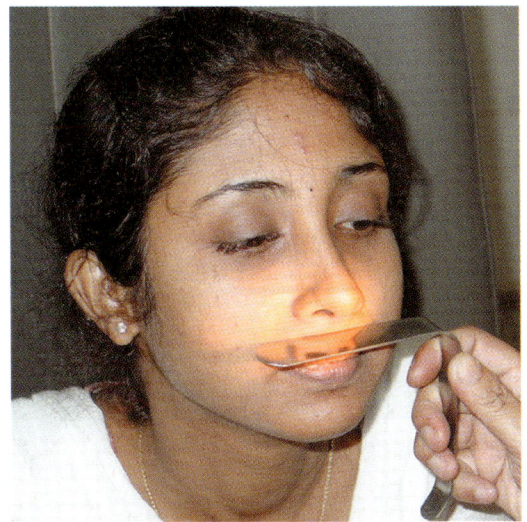

Fig. 23.2: Cold spatula test

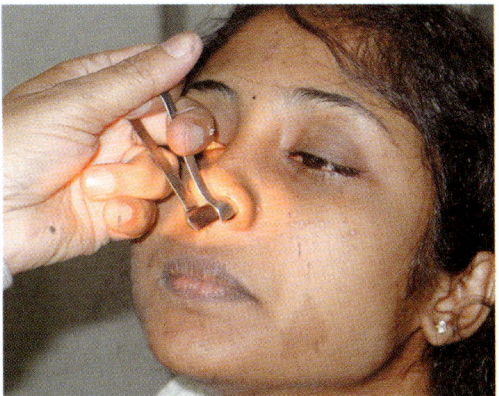

Fig. 23.5: Anterior rhinoscopy with Thudichum nasal speculum

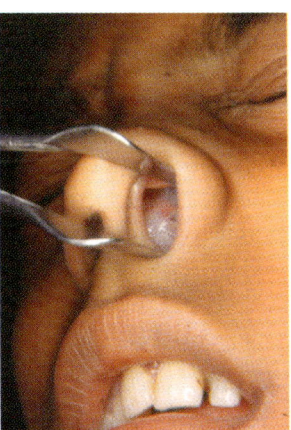

Fig. 23.3: Anterior rhinoscopy showing nasal polyp

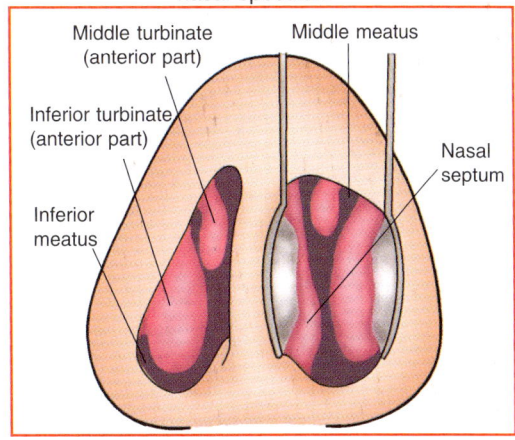

Fig. 23.6: Structure seen on anterior rhinoscopy

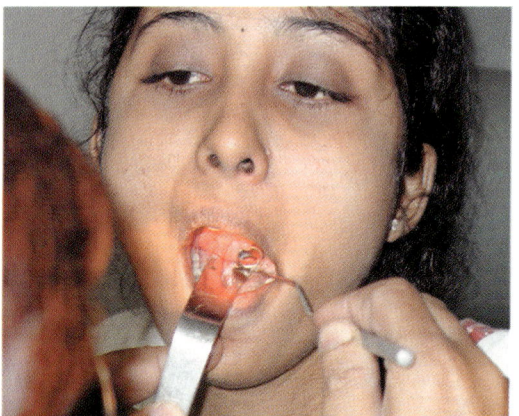

Fig. 23.7: Posterior rhinoscopy

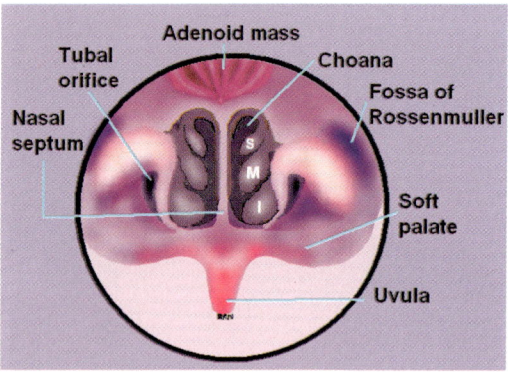

Fig. 23.8a: Telescopic view showing the structures in the postnasal space

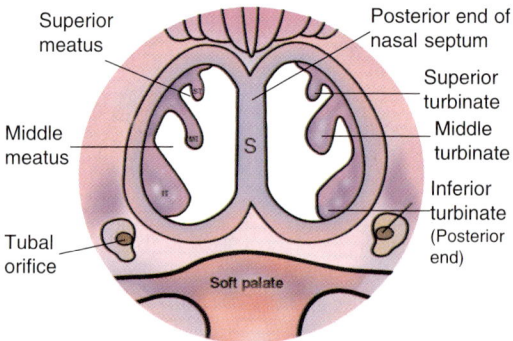

Fig. 23.7b: Diagrammatic view of posterior rhinoscopy examination

Probing

This is a very important nasal examination to confirm and rule out any nasal mass. Using a blunt probe, the nasal mass is probed and the following features are elicited (Fig. 23.9).

1. What is the consistency of the nasal mass?
2. Is the mass mobile?
3. Is the mass sensitiv to touch?
4. Whether it bleeds on touching?
5. Where is the origin of the mass? The probe is passed all around the mass and the possible site of attachment is assessed.

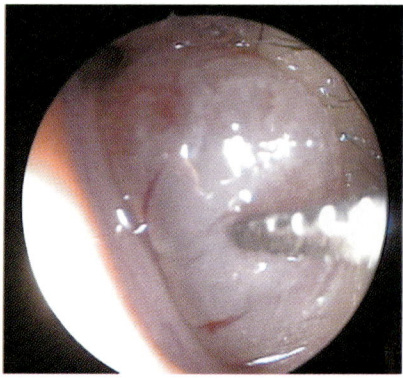

Fig. 23.9: Probing of nasal mass

Examination of the Paranasal Sinuses

Inspection

Look for any swelling/skin changes over the paranasal sinuses. Intercanthal widening may be seen in ethmoidal lesions like ethmoidal polyposis. Also examine the orbit for any lid edema, conjunctival congestion, limitation on extraocular movements, proptosis, visual acuity, etc. Anterior and posterior rhinoscopic examination will reveal discharge from different meatus depending on the sinus involved.

Palpation

Eliciting the Sinus Tenderness

1 Maxillary sinus tenderness is elicited over the canine fossa avoiding the infraorbital nerve (Fig. 23.10).

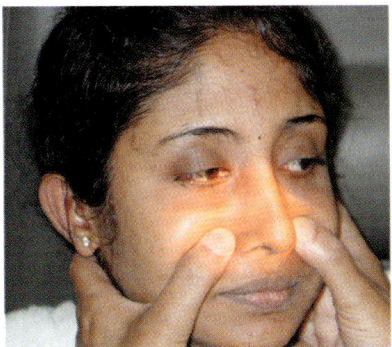

Fig. 23.10: Eliciting the maxillary sinus

- Frontal sinus tenderness is elicited over the floor of the frontal sinus above the medial canthus (Fig. 23.11).
- Ethmoid sinus tenderness is elicited on the medial wall of the orbit just posterior to the root of the nose (Fig. 23.12).

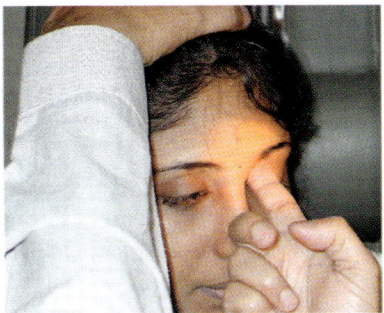

Fig. 23.11: Eliciting the frontal sinus tenderness

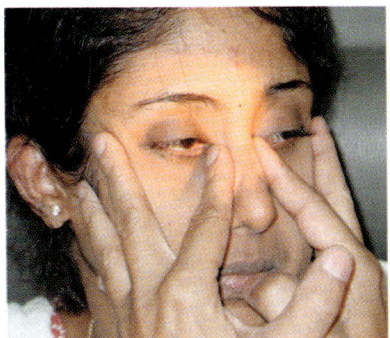

Fig. 23.12: Eliciting the tenderness of ethmoidal sinuses

Transillumination Test

This is rarely done nowadays. In a dark room, bright light is applied on the hard palate in the midline, closing the lips. The 'crescentic' glow is observed bilaterally in the region of the eyelids and over the maxillary sinuses in normal individuals. However, if the maxillary sinus has pus, mucosal thickening or mass, it does not transmit the light resulting in absence or poor glow. Frontal sinuses also may be tested separately by applying the light at the floor of the frontal sinus and the light glow is observed over the anterior wall of the frontal sinus. This is compared with that of the opposite side.

Postural Test

Even this is rarely done nowadays. The middle meatus is observed for appearance of the discharge in various head positions.

Special Examination

1. ***Diagnostic nasal endoscopy (DNE)***
   This is a very useful tool as it allows inspection of various intranasal structures in its every nook and corner with good illumination and various angled nasal endoscopy. Special emphasis is given to evaluation of the middle meatus, superior meatus and the nasopharynx. Even subtle disease in the 'ostiomeatal complex' may be picked up, which may otherwise not be possible by a routine anterior rhinoscopy. Site of bleeding in case of epistaxis can be easily identified and cauterized. Nasal mass deep in the nasal cavity or the nasopharynx can be better evaluated and biopsised (Fig. 23.13).

2. ***Nasopharyngeal examination under anesthesia***
   This is necessary if nasal endoscopy is not available. Under general anesthesia, the patient is positioned as for a tonsillectomy. Boyle-Davis mouth gag is placed and rubber catheters are passed on in each nasal cavity. The catheters are brought out through the mouth and the soft palate is retracted. Using

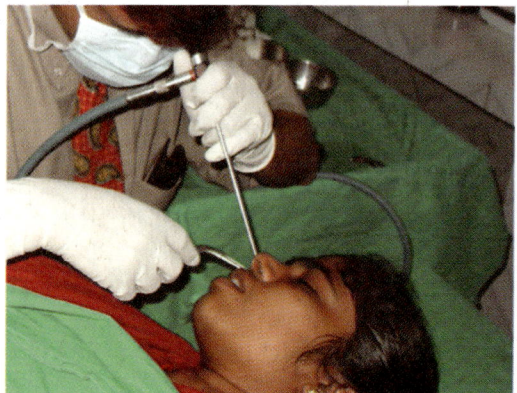

Fig. 23.13: Diagnostic nasal endoscopy under progress

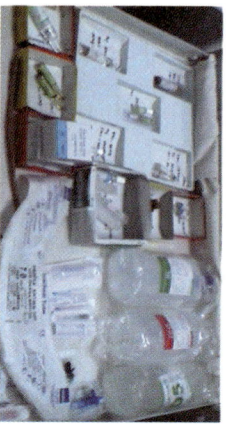

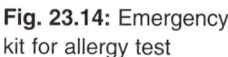

Fig. 23.14: Emergency kit for allergy test

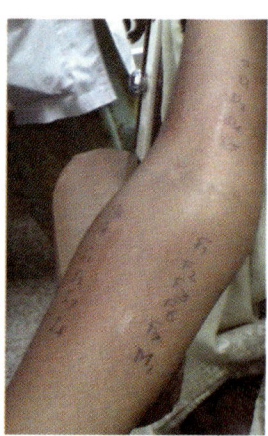

Fig. 23.15: Prick test

angled mirrors, the nasopharynx may be examined.

3. *Tests for the sense of smell*
   Odorous substances like lemon, peppermint, clove, coffee or tea powder may be used to test the sense of smell of the two nasal cavities separately. Quantitative analysis has been described by Elsberg and Duoek. Ethereal substances like spirit and irritant substances are best avoided in the test of olfaction. Ammonia stimulates the fifth cranial nerve and may be used if psychogenic cause is suspected. More sophisticated tests of the sense of smell like UPSIT (University of Pennsylvania Smell Identification test) may be performed but is cumbersome and not practical.

4. *Allergic tests*
   (i) **In vivo tests:** These are done on the patient's body.

   (a) **Skin tests**
   - *Subcuticular tests* (Prick or the scratch tests): This is the most popular, accurate, practical, quick, easy and safe test of nasal allergy. Risk of anaphylaxis is much less compared to the intradermal test as the allergens are inoculated superficially in the sub-cuticular layer of the skin.

Emergency kit should be available while doing the test. (Figs 23.14 and 23.15).

- *Intradermal tests: Refer Chapter 34.*

   (b) **Nasal challenge tests**

   (ii) **Invitro tests:** These are done in the laboratory using the patient's blood sample.

   a. **RAST** (Radio allegrosorbent test)
   b. **PRIST** (Paper radioimmunosorbent test)
   c. **RIST** (Radio immuno sorbent test)

5. *Rhinomanometry*: This is done by calculating the nasal resistance to the airflow by two measurements, i.e. nasal airflow and transnasal pressure. The technique of rhinomanometry includes the following:

   a. **Active rhinomanometry:** This involves generation of nasal airflow and nasal pressure with normal breathing.
   b. **Passive rhinomanometry:** This involves generation of nasal airflow and pressure from an external source, *e.g.*: Fan or pump.

6. *Radiology of the Nose and PNS* (Table 23.1)

   (a) **Plain radiography:** Various views for evaluation of the paranasal sinuses have been described. They are:
   (i) *Water's view (Occipeto-mental):* Ideal for the frontal and maxillary sinuses and is the commonest view taken (Fig. 23.16).

Table 23.1: Investigation in rhinology

- Radiological examination
- X-ray lateral view nose and nasopharynx
- Nasal and sinus endoscopy

• Plain	• Angiography
• Contrast	• Rhinomanometry
• X-ray PNS	• Olfactometry
• CT Scan	• Allergic testing

(ii) *Caldwell view (Occipeto-frontal):* Ideal for the frontal sinus, nasal cavity and the orbit.

(iii) *Lateral view:* Suitable for the ethmoids and the sphenoid sinuses, adenoids (Fig. 23.17).

(iv) *Base skull view (Submento-vertical view):* Suitable for the sphenoid sinus and the ethmoids.

Pathological changes to be looked for are:

- Haziness/cloudiness/opacity of the sinuses
- Fluid level
- Mucosal thickening
- Polyp/ cyst/ mass in the sinus
- Expansion of the sinus

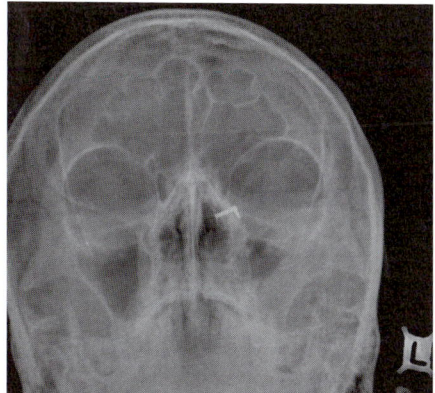

Fig. 23.16: X-ray PNS showing left maxillary sinusitis

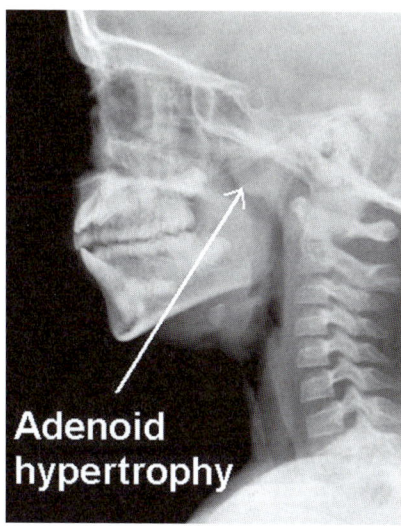

Adenoid hypertrophy

Fig. 23.17: X-ray showing lateral view of the skull. Soft tissue shadow occupying roof of the nasopharynx can be seen (Adenoid)

- Erosion of the bony walls
- Fracture
- Loss of scalloping of the frontal sinuses
- Abnormalities in the nasal cavities like DNS, spur, turbinate hypertrophy, etc. However, these findings are difficult to be evaluated by plain radiographs and needs CT/MR imaging for better evaluation.

(b) **Radiology of the nasopharynx:** Lateral view of the head and neck may be done if adenoid hypertrophy is suspected (Fig. 23.17).

(c) **CT imaging** (Fig. 23.18): Coronal sections of the PNS with special reference to the ostio-meatal complex give the best information an endoscopic surgeon requires like:
- Extent of disease in the various sinuses
- OMC status
- Status of the vital relations of the spheno-ethmoids like the cribriform plate, fovea ethmoidalis, lamina papyracea, optic nerve and the carotid arteries.

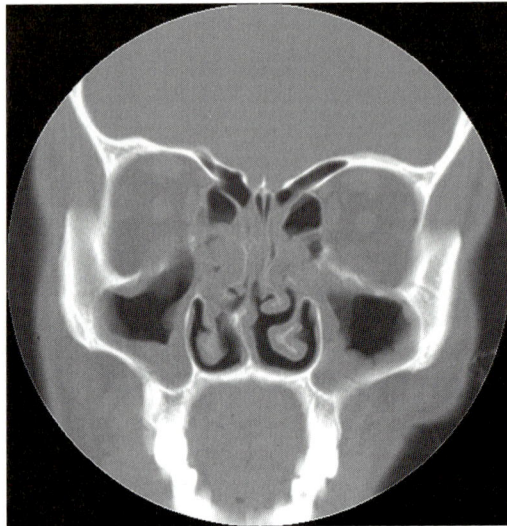

Fig. 23.18: Coronal CT (OMC) of paranasal
sinuses showing PAN sinusitis

POINTS TO REMEMBER

1. Saddle, hump, deviation and crooked nose deformity are the most common types of external nasal deformity.
2. Nasal vestibule should be examined for furunculosis and vestibulitis before using the nasal speculum.
3. Superior meatus and turbinate cannot be examined by anterior rhinoscopy.
4. Probing should be avoided if vascular mass like angiofibroma is suspected.

Congenital Anomalies of Nose and PNS

24

Anomalies of the nose and PNS are rare and it occurs due to failure of fusion of various processes and /or failure of recanalization of the primitive membrane. Knowledge of the embryology of the nose and PNS is necessary to understand and treat these conditions. A brief description of the embryology of nose is given in Chapter 21.

Congenital Malformations

The common congenital anomalies of the nose are as follows (Table 24.1).

- Congenital occlusion of the anterior nares
- Choanal atresia
- Bifid nose
- Nasal meningoencephalocele
- Glioma
- Dermoid
- Fistula/Sinuses

They are caused by either genetic or teratogenic factors in the second month of fetal life. Congenital cysts occur mainly in the midline and a fistula is often present.

Table 24.1: Anomalies of the nose and PNS

Failure of Fusion of Processes	Anomalies
Maxillary/Pre-maxillary	Cleft Lip
Maxillary and lateral nasal process	Facial cleft
Palatine process and nasal septum	Bifid uvula. Submucous cleft Cleft palate. Complete medial cleft leads to cranio-facial abnormality
Failure to develop nasal placode	Complete absence of nose – rare
	Unilateral absence is associated with proboscis lateralis.
Epithelial entrapment in the line of fusion between	Cyst
• Maxillary and medial nasal process	Nasolabial cyst
• Primitive palate and palatine process	Globulo-maxillary cyst

Congenital Occlusion of the Anterior Nares

Etiology

Failure of canalization of the epithelial plug (web) between the median and lateral nasal processes lead to congenital occlusion of the anterior nares.

Types

This can be of two types, i.e.; partial or complete and can be further divided into unilateral and bilateral.

Treatment

Excision of the web or stenosis is done by using the diathermy or laser. A stent can be used to prevent closure and facilitate epithelialization.

Choanal Atresia

Etiology

It occurs mainly due to failure of the bucco-nasal membrane to rupture at the 7th–8th week of gestation.

Types

It can be divided into three types, i.e.

1. Bony
2. Membranous
3. Partly bony and membranous

Degree

Depending on severity and extent of the stenosis this can be divided into;

1. **Incomplete:** Here the postnasal aperture is partially open. The involvement can be:
   - Unilateral
   - Bilateral
2. **Complete:** Here the postnasal aperture is completely occluded. The occlusion can be:
   - Unilateral (Compatible with life) (Fig. 24.1)
   - Bilateral (Dangerous, incompatible with life.)

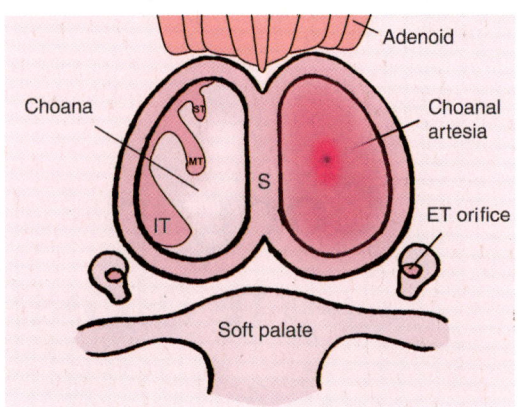

Fig. 24.1: Unilateral choanal atresia with a dimple in the center

Pathology

The partition occluding the choana is attached to basisphenoid, median pterygoid plate, vomer and hard palate which is usually bony, membranous or both.

Clinical features

The severity of clinical features depends on the degree of involvement, i.e. incomplete or complete and whether one or both sides of the postnasal apertures are involved. Normally unilateral choanal atresia does not present any symptoms unless associated with upper respiratory tract infection and the patients are reported late or accidentally found while routine examination is done.

CHARGE Syndrome is a multi-featured disorder characterized by a unique combination of diverse abnormalities. This syndrome was first described in 1979 but the acronym 'CHARGE' was first used in 1981. The acronym 'CHARGE' is used to describe a heterogeneous group of children who exhibit at least four of the features as described below.

C Coloboma are ocular deformities involving an absence of part of the eye like Iris, retina, etc. and their function. Visual impairment may or may not be present. Anophthalmos or microphthalmia may also be present.

H Heart defects include tetralogy of Fallot, patent ductus arteriosus, etc. Choanal Atresia a narrowing or a blockage of the passages between the nasal cavity and the nasopharynx is one of the major criteria for diagnosis. The blockage may be unilateral or bilateral, membranous or bony.

A Atresia of choana is a narrowing or a blockage of the passages between the nasal cavity and the nasopharynx is one of the major criteria for diagnosis of CHARGE syndrome. The blockage may be unilateral or bilateral, membranous or bony.

R Retarded growth may manifest as the child matures.

G Genital anomalies in various forms.

E Ear anomalies can affect the external ear (loop or cup shaped, large, small or absent), middle ear (ossicular malformations, chronic serous otitis, stapedius tendon anomalies), and/or the internal ear (especially high frequency sensori-neural hearing loss). Mixed hearing loss (i.e. conductive loss with sensori-neural loss) is the most common form of hearing loss in CHARGE Association. Malformation or absence of the semicircular canals is fairly common.

Other anomalies that may be associated include

1. ENT abnormalities
   - Abnormal tongue size
   - Cleft lip and/or palate
   - Facial palsy
   - Malformations of the larynx
   - Atresia of the esophagus
   - Tracheoesophageal fistula
2. Renal abnormalities
3. Skeletal abnormalities

Unilateral Choanal Atresia

Patient usually becomes symptomatic when there is complete atresia of one side of the postnasal aperture. The common presenting symptoms are:

(a) Unilateral nasal obstruction

(b) Unilateral persistent glue like nasal discharge

(c) Sometimes symptoms can be presented at a later age

(d) Mouth breathing if the other nasal cavity is blocked due to associated DNS or other nasal pathology.

(e) *Failure to thrive*: If the infant has unilateral involvement associated with nasal pathology on the other side, it can lead to airway obstruction as infants and newborn are obligatory nasal breathers. In such cases emergency airway management is required.

Bilateral Choanal Atresia

Asphyxia: This can be cyclical or suckling.

In **cyclical type**, the child usually cries. This helps in facilitation of breathing. Later when the child becomes exhausted and goes to sleep, it develops features of respiratory distress and cyanosis and again with crying, the symptoms are relieved.

In **suckling type**, the child mainly develops symptoms of asphyxia, including breathlessness and cyanosis during feeding when the child tries to suckle. Otherwise the child will be relatively free from symptoms.

Diagnostic tests

(a) *Probing with the catheter*: It cannot be passed through the nose into the pharynx.

(b) Cold spatula test is more reliable in adults, which shows absence of fogging on the affected side.

(c) Posterior rhinoscopy may be useful in adults where it will show complete occlusion of the choana with a thin plate of membrane or bone with a dimple in its center.

(d) *Air blow test*: Air is blown into the nostrils to check the patency.

(e) Radio-opaque dye is instilled into the nostrils (contrast radiography) and an X-ray is taken to detect choanal atresia.

(f) CT imaging axial cuts shows the type and thickness of atresia (Figs 24.2a and b).

(g) Methylene Blue dye or Indian ink may be used to check the patency of the choana

(h) Diagnostic nasal endoscopy is the most useful method to detect choanal atresia on an outpatient basis. However in infants, it may be difficult to perform under local anesthesia.

Treatment

(a) Transpalatal excision of the atresia and stenting

(b) Transnasal endoscopic excision and stenting. Nasal endoscopic drilling and excision requires partial excision of the posterior end of inferior turbinate and middle turbinate for better visualization followed by elevation of the mucosa of the posterior most part of the septum and floor of the nasal cavity, to identify the bony plate occluding the posterior choanae. Bony plate is removed by drill and fibrous plate can be excised either by KTP 532 laser or by diathermy.

(c) Tracheostomy is required if immediate surgical treatment is not planned for in case of bilateral atresia. Alternatively an oral airway or endotracheal intubation may be done till definite surgery is performed.

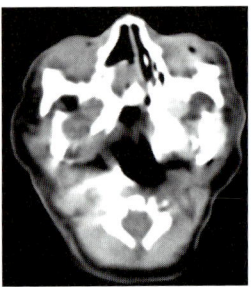
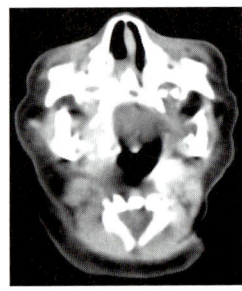

Figs 24.2a and b: CT image of choanal atresia

Bifid Nose

Etiology

It occurs due to the failure of fusion of the fronto-nasal process.

Clinical Features

- Hypertelorism
- Cephalic anomaly
- Mental deficiency

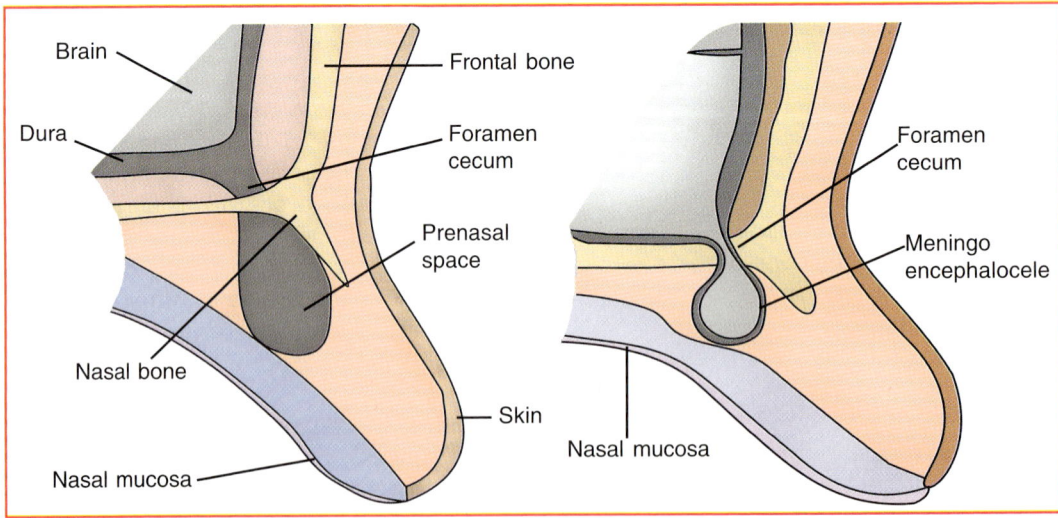

Figs 24.3a and b: Meningo-encephalocele due to persistent foramen cecum

Treatment

Surgical repair with cranio-facial reconstruction.

Nasal Meningocoele/Meningo Encephalocoele

It occurs at the base of the cranium due to local herniation of the glial tissue and meninges. The herniation occurs during the process of development before the foramen cecum is closed and a small extension of the dural tissue may extend to the prenasal space through the foramen cecum. When the foramen cecum fails to close, the herniation persists leading to meningocoele or meningo-encephalocoele. It frequently present as a cystic, polypoidal nasal mass (Figs 24.3a and b).

Types of Meningocoele/ Meningo-encephalocoele

(a) Frontoethmoidal
(b) Ethmoidal
(c) Sphenoidal
(d) Nasal

Clinical Features

It commonly presents with nasal obstruction.

Anterior Rhinoscopic Examination

A soft, cystic bluish, compressible and translucent mass is noted where Frustenberg test is positive [Swelling increases in size in response to coughing].

Investigations

CT scan/ MRI of the skull- coronal and axial sections with contrast and nasal endoscopy. Biopsy should never be attempted. Isolated solitary polypoidal mass arising from the roof should raise the index of suspicion of a meningocoele/ meningoencephalocoele.

Treatment

Transnasal endoscopic excision of the mass is the treatment of choice with less morbidity. Closure of defect is done after removal of the brain tissue if it is not reducible. Bone/ cartilage graft is used along with temporalis fascia and fat to seal the defect.

External approach is adopted for fronto-ethmoidal meningocoele.

Craniotomy is indicated in cases with extensive cranial defect.

Glioma (Fig. 24.4)

It is a congenital malformation associated with isolated heterotopic brain tissue which presents as a nasal mass. It occurs as a result of herniation of brain tissue into the nasal cavity through cranial defect (foramen cecum) during the intrauterine life. Its communication gets detached due to fusion of cranial bones in late intrauterine life. It is attached to the skull by a fibrous stalk near the foramen cecum.

Clinical Features

Usually it manifests in children with nasal obstruction and a bluish nasal mass which is non compressible. Frustenberg's test is negative.

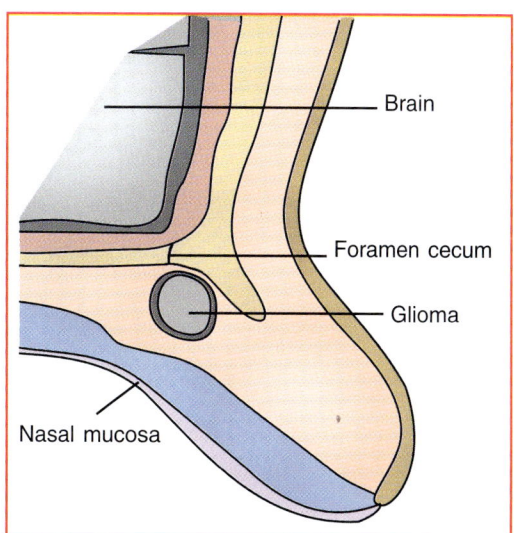

Fig. 24.4: Trapped glial tissue due to closure of foramen cecum after herniation causing glioma

Investigations

As in meningocoele

Treatment

Intranasal mass is excised by endoscopic approach. External approach is adopted if the mass is extra nasal.

Dermoid (Figs 24.5a and b)

This is an ectodermal cyst containing epithelial lining and dermal structure.

Clinical Features (Fig. 24.6)

It is commonly seen over the dorsum of the nose as a fluctuating cystic swelling but can also present as a nasal mass causing nasal obstruction.

The mass is always compressible and non expansible which always present in the midline.

Frustenberg test is always negative.

Treatment

Complete excision of the cyst.

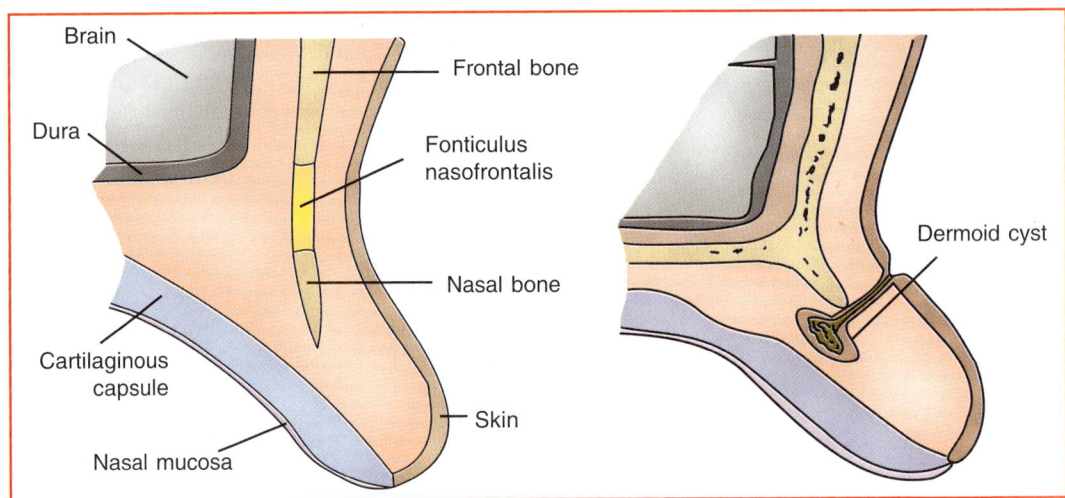

Figs 24.5a and b: Development of a dermoid

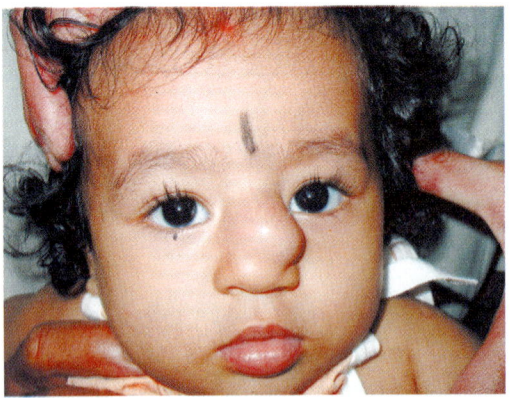

Fig. 24.6: Dermoid cyst of the nose

Congenital Cyst/Fistula (Fig. 24.7)

It is due to failure of separation of ectoderm from dura during the replacement of fonticulus nasofrontalis by bone, leading to entrapment of skin in the pre nasal space. This results in dermoid cyst that may be seen beneath the nasal bone and often connected to a fistula or sinus that opens on the skin surface in the midline. If infected it can be associated with discharge.

Clinical Features (Figs 24.8 and 24.9)

Patient usually presents with a discharging sinus or a fistula which can be confirmed by probing.

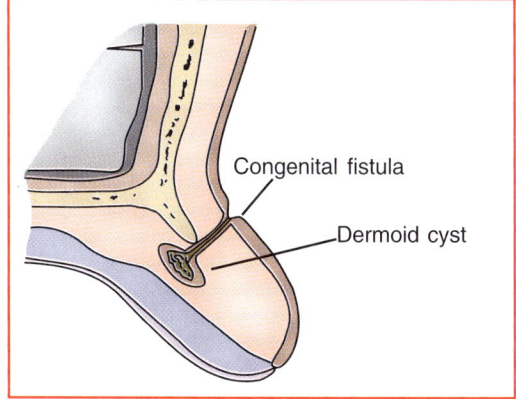

Fig. 24.7: Congenital fistula is often connected to the underlying dermoid cyst beneath the nasal bones

Investigation

- CT Scan is helpful to find out associated dermoid cyst.
- Fistulogram helps to determine the tract.

Treatment

Complete excision of the tract.

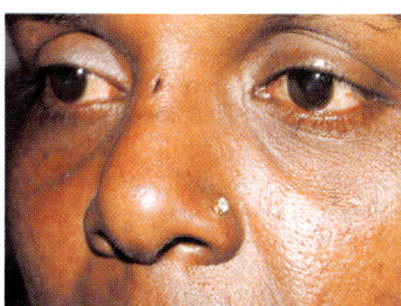
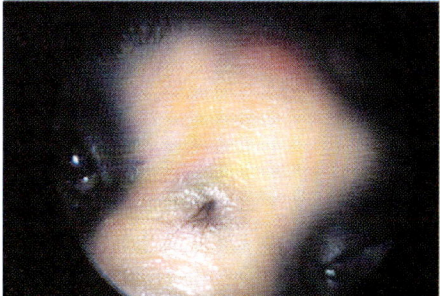

Figs 24.8 and 24.9: Congenital sinus opening on to the skin surface over the root of the nose. Close-up view shows the tuft of hairs emerging from the sinus opening

POINTS TO REMEMBER

1. Bilateral choanal atresia is often fatal as infants are obligatory nasal breathers. Placement of oropharyngeal airway immediately after birth and emergency excision of atretic segment should be carried out.
2. Diagnosis of choanal artesia may be easily made by passing a rubber catheter into the nose and by looking for it in the throat.
3. Meningocele/meningo-encephalocele occurs due to persistence of prenasal space and foramen cecum.
4. Unilateral nasal polyp in a child < 3 years should not be biopsied until meningocele is ruled out.

25

Diseases of the External Nose

Introduction

The diseases of external nose may involve the skin, cartilage or bony framework of the nose which could be:

- Congenital
- Developmental
- Inflammatory
- Traumatic and
- Neoplastic

Congenital anomalies have been described in Chapter 24. The traumatic and developmental abnormalities frequently results in external nasal deformity due to post-traumatic mal-union, distorted bony framework, dislocation, faulty development of facial bone or cartilage due to childhood trauma, etc. The inflammatory conditions usually involve the soft tissue and the skin but rarely can cause destruction of the cartilage or bone of the external nasal framework leading to deformity. Neoplastic lesions also may cause external nasal deformity due to expansion as in benign lesions and destruction and infiltration as in malignant lesions. The most frequent presentation is deformity of external nose for which the patient is often concerned.

Post-trauma/Developmental Defect involving the External Nose

The external nasal deformities may produce the following problems which may indicate a **rhinoplasty** (Reconstruction of the external nose):

- **Cosmetic:** The most common cause is post-traumatic nasal defect which usually occurs due to inadequate treatment of skeletal framework injury. This is often preventable. Grossly deviated nasal septum may lead to external nasal deformity. 'Where the septum goes, there goes the external nose'.
- **Functional:** External nasal deformity can give rise to nasal obstruction due to associated nasal septal deformity or due to reduction in the **Cottle's angle**. Sometimes collapse of the nasal valve at the 'limen nasi' may give rise to nasal obstruction.

The common types of deformity affecting the external nose are the following:

- Midline deformity
  - Hump
  - Saddle nose
  - Tip deformities
- Lateral nasal deformity
  - Crooked nose
  - Deviated nose
  - Alar depression

Hump

This is due to an excess of bony or cartilaginous skeleton and does not produce any functional disturbance. The hump is removed by 'reduction rhinoplasty' where in the excess cartilage or bone is resected by using osteotome or knife and is followed by median and lateral osteotomy to narrow the bridge. If the hump is small it can be rasped. Sometimes a psudohump is formed due to subluxated septal cartilage from the maxillary crest or excessive resection of inferior strip from the maxillary crest causing loss of tip support and collumellar retraction leading to acute nasolabial angle and reduction in nasal height. To reduce pseudohump correction and repositioning of subluxated septal cartilage along with collumellar support is required. In addition, a tip rotation is helpful (Figs 25.1a and b).

Saddle Nose

This is often caused by trauma which may be due to road traffic accident, sports injury, accidental or iatrogenic as in SMR operation and other nasal surgeries. It can also occur due to certain infections like syphilis, tuberculosis and leprosy. It is corrected by an internal or external 'augmentation rhinoplasty' where the defect is augmented by cartilage/ bone/ synthetic materials like silastic. A columellar strut may be required if there is columellar retraction due to loss of caudal end of the septal cartilage (Figs 25.2a and b).

Tip Deformities

These are more difficult to treat surgically. The surgeon should have adequate expertise in rhinoplasty before venturing into tip surgeries. The common types of tip deformities are:
- Bulbous tip
- Narrow or the 'pinched' tip
- Bifid tip
- Under projection
- Over projection
- Rotated tip

The tip correction can be done by internal or external rhinoplasty approach. Bulbous tip is corrected by division of the lateral crurae of the lower lateral cartilages in two strips i.e. medial and lateral. The medial strip is rotated and sutured in the midline to the septum. Interdomal suturing may be required. Reduction of alar dome is done in over projection of tip. Multiple incisions may be required at strategic sites to open up the tip in

case of pinched nose. Bifid nose requires suturing of the two medial crura of the lower lateral cartilages at the dome. Further tip projection can be done using a tip graft (cartilage). Tip rotation is done by an open approach or tip delivery technique.

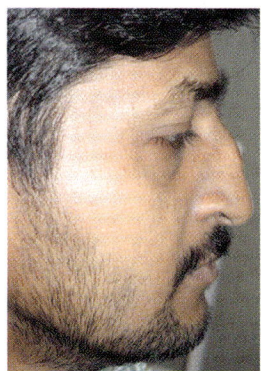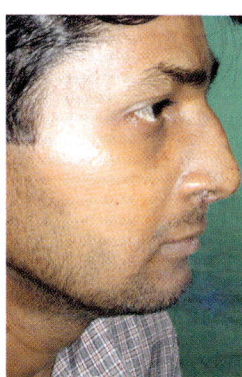

Figs 25.1a and b: (a) Hump before correction, (b) Hump after correction

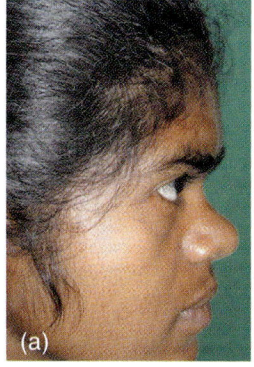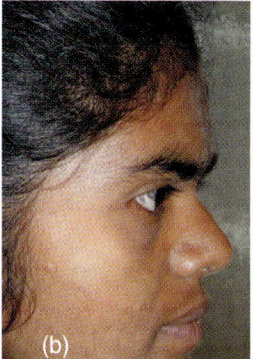

Figs 25.2a and b: (a) Saddle nose before correction, (b) Saddle nose after correction

Crooked Nose

The nasal dorsum is crooked and could be C shaped, S-shaped or undefined. It usually involves both cartilaginous and bony framework. It is corrected by combination of lateral and medial osteotomy and release of the septal cartilage from the upper lateral cartilages by intercartilaginous incision. This can be done by either external or internal rhinoplasty approach (Figs 25.3a and b).

Deviated Nose

The nasal dorsum is deviated away from the midline. It may be cartilaginous or bony-cartilaginous. Simple cartilaginous deviation may be corrected by a proper septoplasty and release of septal cartilage from the lateral nasal cartilage. In case of deviated Bony-cartilaginous framework, in addition to release of upper lateral cartilage, lateral and median/ angular osteotomies are necessary. To work on the dorsum, one has to make inter-cartilaginous incision for exposure in internal rhinoplasty approach.

Details of septorhinoplasty procedure are described under the chapter *Common surgeries of the Nose and PNS* under the heading: septorhinoplasty.

Rhinophyma (Figs 25.4 a and b)

Synonym

Elephantiasis of nose, cystadenofibroma of nose.

Definition

A condition associated with benign nodular enlargement of the tip of the nose due to hypertrophy of the sebaceous gland of the skin as a complication of Acne rosacea leading to potato nose deformity.

This is also called as **elephantiasis** of the nose.

Pathology

- Last stage of acne rosacea.
- Slow growing over a period of 10 to 15 years.
- Nodular enlargement of the skin with dilated blood vessels and tissues.

Histology

1. Greatly increased number and size of sebaceous glands.
2. Fissures containing epithelial debris and sebaceous gland.

Clinical Features

Swelling in the lower half of the nose, especially the nasal tip and the nostril.

Treatment

Decortication of the thickened skin is done by removal of pathologic tissue by taking care not to expose cartilage or bone then regrowth of the skin occurs by remaining skin follicles. If cartilage is exposed, then a skin graft should be placed. Recently dermabrasion has been tried for better contouring of nose. Radio-frequency knife with loop shaving technique has been used recently for the surgery of rhinophyma.

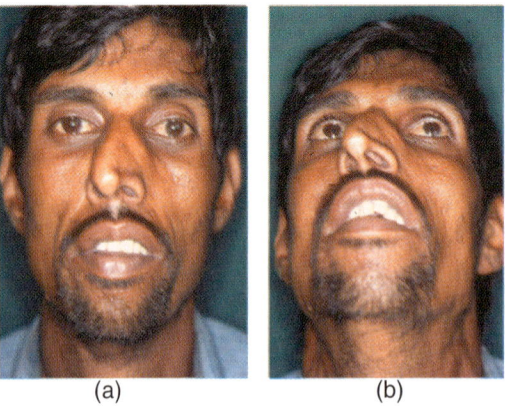

(a)   (b)

Figs 25.3a and b: (a) Frontal view of crooked nose, (b) Basal view of crooked view

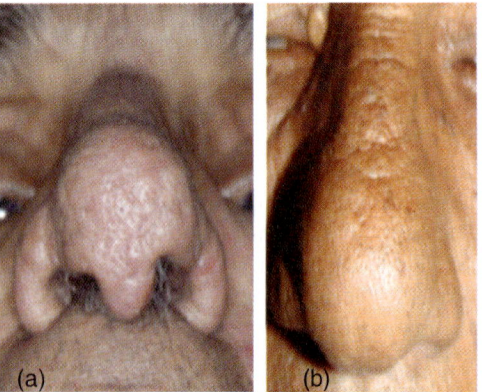

(a)   (b)

Figs 25.4a and b: Rhinophyma of the nose

INFLAMMATORY CONDITIONS OF THE EXTERNAL NOSE

Vestibulitis

A dermatitis in nasal vestibule, frequently results from persistent nasal discharge.

Types

Can be acute and chronic.

Etiology

- Persistent infected discharge from the nose leading to irritation and maceration of the skin of the vestibule.
- Nose picking or rubbing with the finger
- Frequent cleaning of the nasal discharge with handkerchief.
- Traumatic ulceration of the projected skin over a caudally dislocated septum.

Clinical Features

Symptoms

- Itching and irritation of the nose (more common in acute form).
- Pain in the nose

Signs

- Induration over the skin of the vestibule is the cardinal feature.
- Excoriation and painful fissures over the affectd area can be seen commonly in acute form but sometimes can persist with the chronic form.

Treatment

- Nasal discharge should be removed with suction and underlying cause like rhinitis and sinusitis should be treated.
- Local application of soframycin, mupirocin or chlorhexidine cream.
- Application of petroleum jelly to form a protective barrier.
- In chronic form local steroid preparation can be useful.

Furunculosis

Definition

It is a localized inflammatory condition of the nasal vestibule involving the hair follicle caused by *Staphylococcus aureus*.
Causative agent: *Staphylococcus aureus*.

Predisposing factor

1. Trauma
2. Diabetes
3. Immunodeficiency state
4. Long term steroids
5. Agranulocytosis.

Clinical Features

Patient usually complains of mild pain over the affected area and swelling, which may involve the tip of nose depending on the site of the affected hair follicle.

In severe form, pain can be throbbing in nature if the area is touched. In more advanced form it may rupture (Figs 25.5 a and b).

Signs (Fig. 25.6)

Swelling and redness of the affected area may be seen around the hair follicle in the vestibule of the nose. The affected area is usually tender.

Treatment

Antibiotics like cloxacilline, cefaclor, etc. are commonly prescribed as they are Staphylococcal specific. Seratiopeptidase and acelofenac may be given to reduce inflammation and pain.Once the swelling is localized,it can be incised and drained.

Complications

- Cavernous sinus thrombosis.
- Septal abscess

Cavernous Sinus Thrombophlebitis

It is a rare, dangerous, and is historically difficult condition to diagnose and treat.

Septic emboli may spread to:

1. Lungs

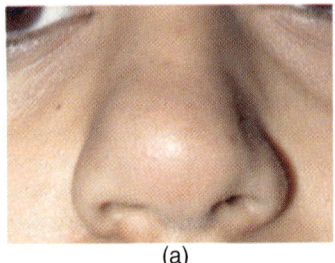 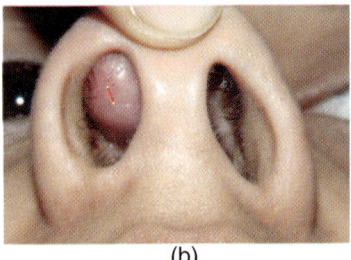 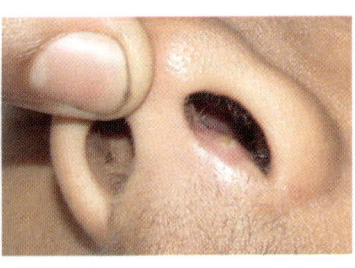

(a) (b)

Figs 25.5a and b: (a) Showing furunculosis of the nasal vestibule associated with swelling of the tip, (b) Same patient showing the furunculosis of the nasal vestibule. The red line shows the site of incision and drainage

Fig. 25.6: Showing furunculosis of the nasal vestibule in the region of columella

2. Kidney
3. Spleen
4. Liver and various other parts of body can occur.

Etiology

Most cases are of septic origin usually following furunculosis of the nose, danger area of the face, acute ethmoiditis, infections in the ear, etc. Aseptic types may follow trauma, local stasis or a failing circulation. Immunocompromised patients are more prone for cavernous sinus thrombosis.

Causative Agent

- Stahylococcus
- Streptococcus

Pathogenesis

Coagulase positive staphylococcus has the toxin coagulase. This toxin has the property to enhance coagulation of the blood and produce marked changes in the intima of veins associated with changes in surrounding tissues. This leads to a septic thrombosis of the cavernous sinus and adds mechanical stasis to the septic factor.

Clinical Features

To begin with, it is often unilateral but later may become bilateral because of the anatomic communications between the two cavernous sinuses by anterior and basilar sinuses, situated on the floor of the sella turcica under the pituitary body.

Symptoms

- High degree pyrexia associated with chills and sweats and occasionally emesis
- Delirium-come often-meningitis supervenes terminally
- Loss of vision
- Pain in region supplied by ophthalmic branch of 5th cranial nerve.
- Rarely trismus.

Signs

Rapid-small and thready pulse

- Engorgement and oedema of face, eyelids, conjuctiva
- Pulsatile proptosis
- Congestion of retinal veins
- Papilloedema.
- 3rd, 4th, 5th, 6th cranial nerve palsy.
- Meningeal signs and altered sensorium
- Signs of raised intra ocular pressure.

Investigations

- CT/MRI with contrast
- Fundoscopy
- Blood culture
- Lumbar puncture and CSF analysis.

Diagnosis

1. Exopthalmus followed by edema and chemosis
2. Presented in the same side of the body as infection near afferent or efferent venous connections with cavernous sinus

3. Involvement of the second eye within forty-eight hours.

If unilateral throughout, an orbital cellulitis should be suspected.

Differential Diagnosis

- Orbital cellulitis—unilateral (hardest to differentiate)
- Cellulitis of cheek and face—accompanies by edema of the eyelids
- Infections of accesory sinuses.
- Exophthalmis goiter (particularly malignant type of exopthalmus)
- Tumors of orbit, optic nerve, lacrimal gland.
- Fractures and trauma to head with sterile thrombi in cavernous sinus.
- Thrombotic process is infected.

Treatment

- Hospitalization and ICU care.
- Intravenous antibiotics like penicillins, the cephalosporins, and metronidazole, etc. can be given.
- Primary infection should be drained (Facial abscess, sphenoid sinusitis).

- Anticoagulant treatment.
- Corticosteroid may help in reducing inflammation.

Erysipelas

An acute spreading cellulitis of the face caused by *Streptococcal dermatitis* of the vestibule.

Clinical Features

- Pyrexia
- Lymphadenopathy
- Red Swollen area of the vestibular skin with sharply defined margin and spreads outwards on to the face and eyelids as the disease advances.
- Nasal mucosa is congested and hemorrhagic and can cause fatal complications like cavernous sinus thrombosis in the presence of diabetes mellitus or other immunocompromised conditions.

Treatment

1. Systemic penicillin
2. Analgesics
3. Anti-inflammatory drugs like seratiopeptidase.

POINTS TO REMEMBER

1. Rhinophyma occurs as a complication of Acne Rosacea that leads to potato nose deformity.
2. Furunculosis of the nose is a localized inflammation involving hair follicle of the nasal vestibule by staphylococcus aureus that can be associated with complication like cavernous sinus thrombophlebitis.
3. Cavernous sign thrombosis has a mortality rate of 30% CT/MRI with contrast is the choice of investigation for diagnosis. Aggressive antibiotic treatment (ceftriaxone with metronidazole) along with anticoagulant and steroid therapy is the mainstay of treatment.

26

Epistaxis

Introduction

Epistaxis is defined as acute hemorrhage from the nostril, nasal cavity, or nasopharynx. It is a very common condition that can present as a life threatening emergency. Epistaxis can be unilateral or bilateral. The site of bleeding varies with a number of factors including age, sex, anatomical and pathological abnormalities, occupation, climate, etc. Both external and internal carotid arteries supply the nose. The dividing line between the area supplied by them is the upper part of the middle turbinate. Above this line the blood supply to both the lateral wall and the septum is mainly from the internal carotid artery whereas, below this line the blood supply is mainly from the external carotid artery. The majority of the blood supply to the nasal cavity is by the sphenopalatine artery and is more commonly involved artery in epistaxis. Hence this is called the *artery of epistaxis*. Younger individuals particularly below the age of 40 years commonly bleed from the anterior aspect of the nose. In contrast, people above this age bleed more commonly from the posterior aspect of the nasal cavity. Epistaxis is rarely seen in infants.

Historical Background

Carl Michel (1871), James Little (1879), and Wilhelm Kiesselbach were the first to identify the nasal septum's anterior plexus as a source of nasal bleeding.

Pilz was the first to surgically treat epistaxis with ligation of the common carotid artery (1869).

Seiffert ligated the internal maxillary artery via the maxillary sinus in 1928. Henry Goodyear performed the first anterior ethmoid artery ligation in the treatment of epistaxis.

Vascular Anatomy of the Nasal Cavity

A rich vascular supply underlies this thin mucosal covering. Nasal erectile tissue results in a large number of venous sinuses, AV anastomoses, and venules, as discussed under 'Anatomy of the nose and PNS'. Multiple arterial vessels fed by the high-pressure carotid system course through the nose. The respiratory mucosa with it's underlying vascular supply serve to regulate heat exchange and humidification during respiration (Fig. 26.1).

The nasal cavity is basically supplied from two main sources (Fig. 26.2).

I. Branches of external carotid artery

(a) Sphenopalatine artery
(b) Greater palatine artery
(c) Superior labial branch of the facial artery.

II. Branches of internal carotid artery

(a) Anterior ethmoidal artery
(b) Posterior ethmoidal artery.

272

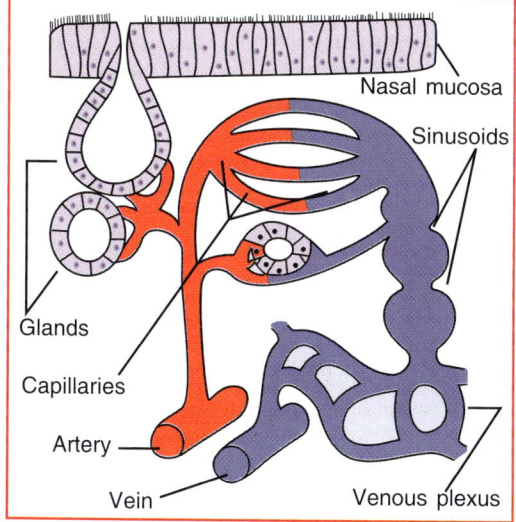

Fig. 26.1: Showing the subepithelial venous plexus (erectile tissue)

These arteries intercommunicate in a rich plexus. There are two areas that are often implicated in nose bleeds - Kiesselbach's plexus (giving rise to anterior bleeds), and Woodruff's plexus (giving rise to posterior bleeds).

The **Kiesselbach's plexus** is situated in the 'Little's area' in the anteroinferior part of the nasal septum (Fig. 26.3a). This plexus is contributed by four arteries of the nasal septum namely,

1. Sphenopalatine artery
2. Greater palatine artery
3. Superior labial branch of the facial artery
4. Anterior ethmoidal artery (Fig. 26.3b).

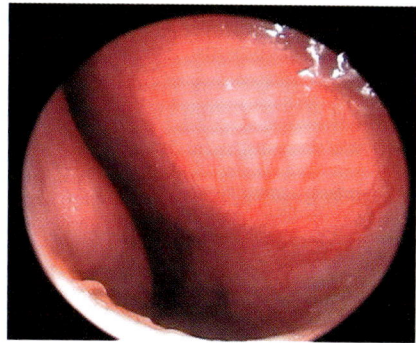

Fig. 26.3a: Endoscopic picture showing the Little's area

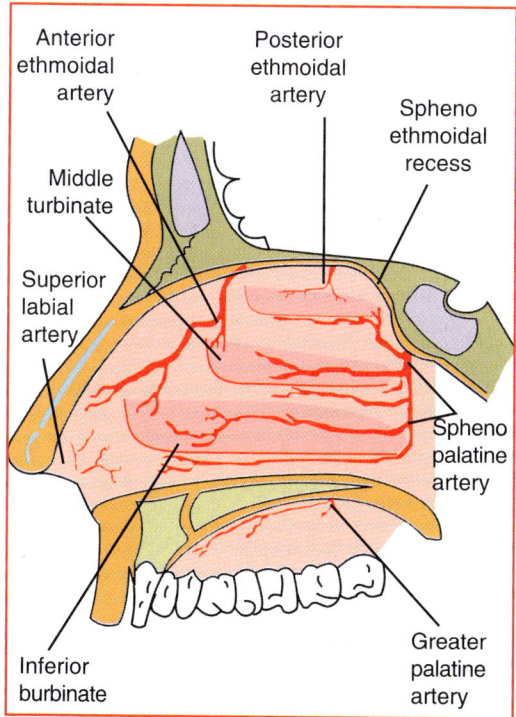

Fig. 26.2: Arterial supply of the lateral wall of nose

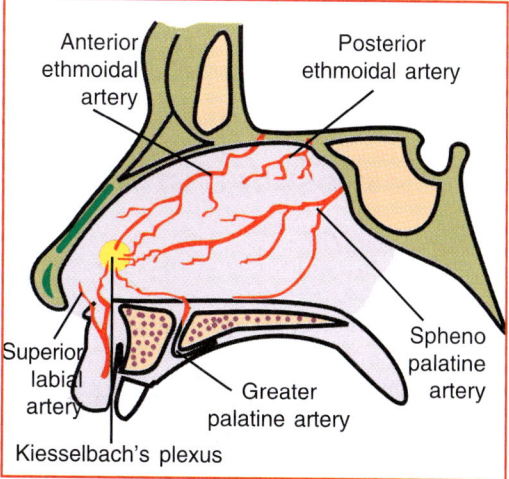

Fig. 26.3b: Arterial supply of the nasal septum

This plexus is the commonest site of bleeding (90% of cases).

The plexus decribed by Woodruff's states the following sites: The posterior 1 cm of nasal floor, inferior meatus, inferior turbinate posterior end, middle meatus, the vertical strip of mucosa anterior to the Eustachian tubecushion, the mucusa lateal and superior to the posterior choana, covering adjacent sphenodi rostrum. Although earlier thought to be an arterial plexus, recent studies suggest it to be a venous plexus with thin walled sinusoids (Fig. 26.4).

The maxillary sinus ostium serves as the dividing line between "anterior" and "posterior" epistaxis. Anterior bleeding is usually easier to access and is, therefore, less dangerous. Posterior epistaxis is more difficult to treat as visualization is more difficult and blood is often swallowed, making it more difficult to gauge the amount of blood loss.

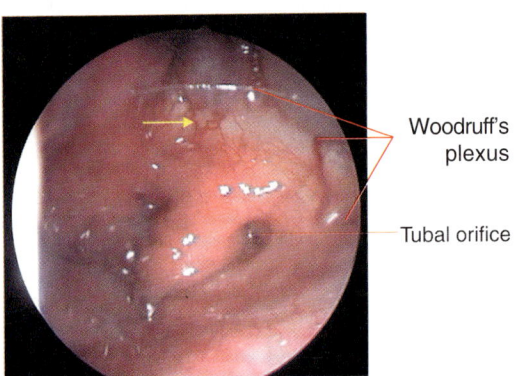

Fig. 26.4: Endoscopic picture showing Woodruff's plexus

ETIOLOGY OF EPISTAXIS

A. Local Causes

1. Congenital
   Hereditary telengectasia (Osler-Weber-Rendu syndrome)
2. Trauma
   - Microtrauma by Nose picking (common in children)
   - Facial and skull base fractures
   - Foreign body in the nose including myiasis
   - Iatrogenic trauma
   - Barotrauma
3. Inflammatory
   - Infective rhinitis
4. Specific
   - Acute infection like diphtheria
   - Chronic granulomatous conditions
     - Tuberculosis
     - Leprosy
     - Syphilis
     - Rhinosporidiosis
     - Rhinoscleroma
     - Wegener's granulomatosis
5. Non-specific
   - Viral- Common cold, influenza, etc.
   - Bacterial- Secondary bacterial rhinitis sinusitis
   - Fungal rhinosinusitis
   - Atrophic rhinitis
6. Neoplastic
   - Benign
     - Juvenile angiofibroma, angioma of the septum, capillary and cavernous hemangioma, inverted papilloma, etc.
   - Malignant
     - Squamous cell carcinoma, olfactory neuroblastoma, nasopharyngeal carcinoma, etc.
7. Miscellaneous causes
   - *Deviated nasal septum and spur*: It causes eddy air currents and dryness of the nasal mucosa and crusting
   - Localized dryness and crusting in rhinitis sicca
   - Spontaneous rupture of tortuous arteriosclerotic vessels
   - Rhinolith
8. Physiological causes
   - High altitude
   - Extreme cold or hot climate

B. Systemic causes

1. Hypertension—Commonest cause of epistaxis in elderly.
2. Cardiac—CCF, mitral stenosis
3. Pulmonary—COPD
4. Cirrhosis—Vit K deficiency

5. Renal—Nephritis
6. Hormonal—Vicarious menstruation, endometriosis, granuloma gravidarum
7. Coagulopathies
   - Clotting disorders like Christmas disease, VonWillibrand's disease, hemophilia, etc.
   - Bleeding disorders like thrombocytopenic purpura
   - Agranulocytosis
   - Leukemia
   - Vitamin K deficiency
   - Exanthematous fevers like measles, mumps, typhoid, etc.

C. Idiopathic

No obvious cause detected clinically and after investigations.

EVALUATION OF EPISTAXIS

In acute active epistaxis, priority is given to control the bleeding before doing the investigations to find out the cause. Hypovolemia and blood loss should be promptly dealt with. Vital signs should be regularly monitored and concentration is given on the following:
- Volume status
- Blood pressure
- Adequacy of airway
- Oral and nasal examination.

FIRST AID

- ABC of emergency management is followed: Airway, Breathing and Circulation
- Make patient sit up; pinch the nose for 5–10 minutes, open mouth and breath
- Ice pack on the nose
- Sedation/sublingual antihypertensives in case of hypertensive epistaxis
- In profuse bleeding aspiration is prevented by (#facial bones) lateral position/intubation with inflated cuff.
- Xylocaine with adrenaline pack is controversial
- Injection or topical use of hemocoagulase (Botropase®)

Detailed medical and treatment history is taken as the patient is being managed and the bleeding is controlled.

Anterior Rhinoscopy

This is the mainstay of evaluation. With good light source using a head mirror or head light, the nasal cavity is inspected using a nasal speculum. Special attention should be paid to the plexus areas as these are areas that often bleed. In case of active bleeding, a suction cannula may be used to determine the site of bleeding. Sometimes a cotton applicator may be used to find the bleeding point. Local anesthetic and vasoconstrictor may be required for better visualization and manipulation. If the bleeding point is identified, cauterization ($AgNO_3$) of the bleeder or anterior nasal packing may control bleeding. Posterior nasal packing may be required if the bleeding is from the posterior part as in hypertensives. Alternatively a Foley's catheter or nasal balloon may be used as a tamponade to control the bleeding.

Posterior Rhinoscopy

Posterior rhinoscopy is often difficult, but is helpful in recurrent mild epistaxis or blood stained nasal discharge following neoplasia, rhinosporidiosis in the nasopharynx or fungal sinusitis.

Nasal Endoscopy

Nasal Endoscopy is a very useful tool in identifying and treating the bleeding point, especially so in difficult cases where the bleeder is too posterior or superior (Fig. 26.5).

Radiological Evaluation

1. X-ray PNS helps in ruling out infective, traumatic and neoplastic conditions.
2. CT scan is more useful in such cases.
3. Digital subtraction angiography is more useful in identification of the bleeding vessels in profuse and recurrent epistaxis. Embolization of the bleeder may be done selectively

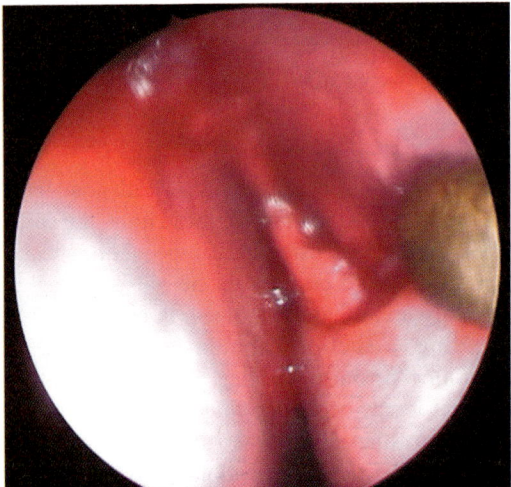

Fig. 26.5: Endoscopic picture showing injury to the lateral nasal wall and the bleeding points

Hematological Investigations

Complete blood picture including:
- Clotting and bleeding profiles
- Blood grouping and cross matching
- Blood counts including total platelet count

MANAGEMENT OF EPISTAXIS

Common local causes to be looked for in children include Little's area bleed, bleeding from retrocolumellar vein, foreign body, etc. In adults the common causes include hypertension and other systemic illnesses. Once the site of bleeding has been located, following steps can control the bleeding.

Compression of the nostrils for 5–10 minutes. Pinching of the nostrils applies pressure over the lateral wall against the nasal septum, thus tamponades the bleeding site. Patient may be put in the sitting position with the head bending forwards with mouth open (Trotter's method). He breathes quietly through the mouth and spits out the blood that collects in the pharynx. This will usually stop the active bleeding arising from the septum. Sometimes after this step, application of cotton wool soaked with vasoconstrictor can be helpful. Placement of ice-cubes over the bridge of the nose may hasten vasoconstriction. If this fails to control the bleeding, the next step should be anterior nasal packing.

If the bleeding stops or reduces, the bleeding point may be cauterized using chemical or electrocautery. Chemical cautery may be done either with 20% silver nitrate, 3% trichloroacetic acid may be more effective because of its more caustic nature.

Anterior Nasal Packing

Technique (Fig. 26.6)

This is usually done by using roller gauze, one meter long, soaked in liquid paraffin, Vaseline or Bismuth iodoform paraffin paste (BIPP). Under vision, using a long bladed nasal speculum and Tilley's nasal dressing forceps, the nasal cavity is packed with multiple loops placed in horizontal layers from below upwards (step-ladder fashion) as shown in the figure. The pack may be kept for 2–3 days. BIPP pack can be kept for a longer period. Alternatively, hemostatic agent like Gelatin sponge (Gelfoam), Merocel$^{(R)}$ or

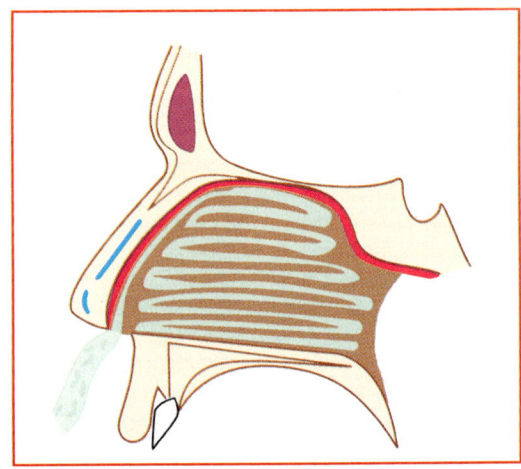

Fig. 26.6: Placement of anterior nasal packing in layers

Surgicel$^{(R)}$ may be used. Gelfoam provides both tamponade to the site of bleeding and also promotes clot formation with early sealing of blood vessels. It need not be removed as it gets absorbed. Prophylactic antibiotics should be used if pack is in a place for more than 24 hours.

A balloon tamponade may be used as an alternative to anterior nasal packing. This is less traumatic and is best suited in epistaxis due to bleeding or clotting disorders. Morbidity is less as it has a breathing tube. Posterior nasal balloon may be inflated if bleeding is from a posterior aspect of the nasal cavity and nasopharynx (Fig. 26.7).

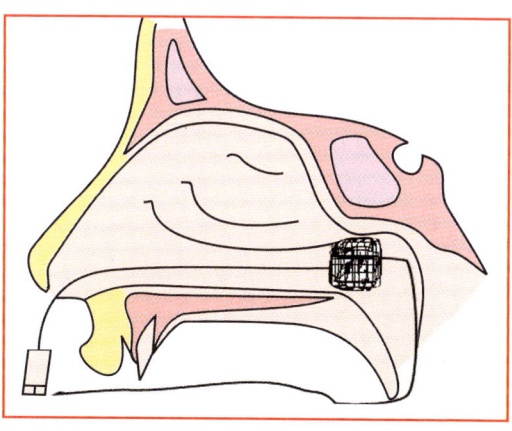

Fig. 26.8a: Postnasal pack with gauze piece

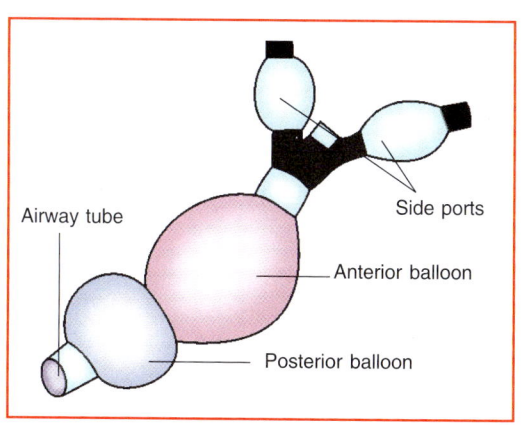

Fig. 26.7: Nasal balloon

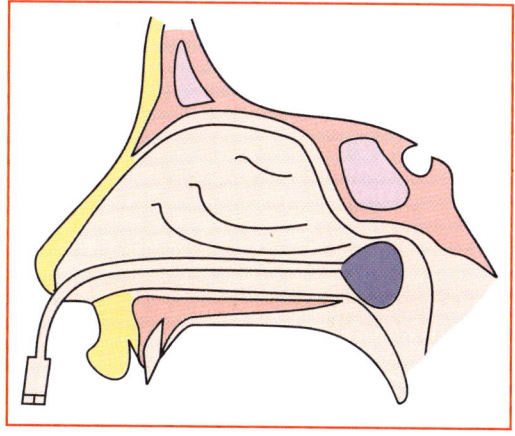

Fig. 26.8b: Postnasal pack with Foley's catheter with balloon inflated

Posterior Nasal Packing

Technique (Fig. 26.8)

This is required in rare instances and can be life saving. This is usually indicated in posterior bleeding. Hypertensive epistaxis, bleeding following angiofibroma excision, etc. are the common indications. A small gauze piece is rolled into a thumb-sized pack and three threads are tied to it, two at its ends and one in the center. The pack is soaked in liquid paraffin or BIPP. Two rubber catheters are passed through the nose and brought through the oral cavity. Each one is tied to the corresponding thread of the pack. The catheters are pulled through the nose and this brings the pack into the nasopharynx. It is kept in place at the posterior end of the septum. The threads are tied against the columella after guarding it with a piece of rubber. The thread tied at the center of the pack comes out through the mouth, which is strapped at the cheek. This thread aids in removal of the pack, which is usually done after 24 to 36 hours.

Alternatively, a postnasal balloon or Foley's catheter may be used as a tamponade in the postnasal space or the nasopharynx.

Surgical Intervention

This is necessary if the epistaxis is refractory to the conservative measures. Following surgical methods may be tried.

1. Nasal endoscopy assisted bipolar cauterization under general anesthesia may be done to coagulate the bleeder (Fig. 26.9).
2. Ligation of the artery may be required only in refractory cases where bleeding fails to stop after packing/ tamponade (anterior and postnasal)
   (a) External carotid artery is ligated distal to the lingual branch after exploring the neck.
   (b) Transantral clipping or ligation of the internal maxillary artery may be done by a sublabial-pterygomaxillary fossa approach.

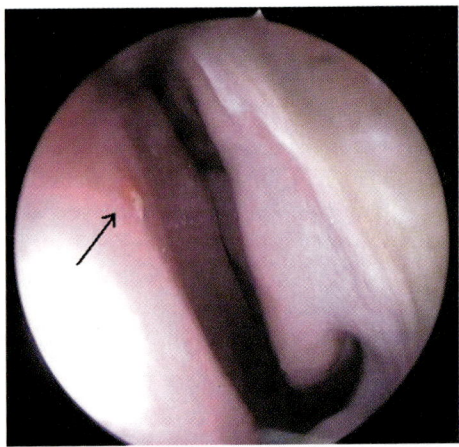

Fig. 26.9: Black arrow showing bleeding point in the Little's area on nasal endoscopy

(c) Bleeding from the upper part of the nose, above the level of the middle turbinate, requires ligation or clipping of the anterior ethmoidal artery by external incision near the inner canthus.

POINTS TO REMEMBER

1. The artery of epistaxis is sphenopalatine artery which is the terminal branch of the external carotid artery.
2. Incidence of epistaxis has a bimodal distribution.
3. Commonest in childhood and old age.
4. Causes are different in the two age groups.
5. Epistaxis may be classified as either anterior or posterior.
6. 80% of cases are anterior and arise on lower part of nasal septum (Little's area).
7. **P**rofuse **P**aroxysms **P**ainless un**P**rovoked epistaxis in adolescent males could be due to juvenile nasopharyngeal angiofibroma.
8. Hypertension is the commonest cause of profuse epistaxis in adults.

Diseases of the Nasal Septum

27

DEVIATED NASAL SEPTUM (DNS)

Definition

Deviation of cartilage and/or bony framework of the nasal septum from the midline associated with nasal symptoms.

Etiology

(a) Trauma
  (i) Birth trauma especially during the face presentation. Kent et al. found DNS even in children born of cesarian section. Thus birth molding/ pressure or trauma during birth is not the only cause for DNS. He also found 4% incidence of septal deviation in neonates, which probably could also be due to genetic cause.
  (ii) Trauma to the nose after birth, which may be due to blow, sports injuries, repeated falling on the face during childhood, etc. This may lead to dislocation of the quadrilateral cartilage from the maxillary crest and subsequent mal-development.
(b) Developmental error
(c) Role of a high arched palate is doubtful. It may be associated with a high arched palate due to the deviation that causes nasal obstruction and subsequent pulling of the palate superiorly. Obstructive adenoid hypertrophy is also associated with high arched palate, probably due to the same mechanism.
(d) *Racial factor:* It is more common in Caucasians than in Negroes.
(e) *Heredity:* It could be genetically predisposed as often several members of the family are found to suffer from a deviated nasal septum.
(f) Other factors like age and sex may have a role to play because of the nature of day-to-day activities.

Site of DNS

- Cartilaginous/bony/both
- Anterior/posterior
- High/low

Types of DNS (Figs 27.1a to f)

(a) **C-shaped deviation:** Both the cartilaginous and the bony septum is deviated to one side.
(b) **S-shaped deviation:** The cartilaginous part is deviated to one side, where as the bony part gets deviated to the opposite side.
(c) **Caudal dislocation:** The caudal end of the septum is projected over the columella on one side because of the subluxation of septal cartilage over the anterior nasal spine and maxillary crest.
(d) **Spur:** It is angulation at the bony cartilaginous junction.

(e) **Thick septum:** Commonly occurs due to overlapping of bone and the cartilage.

(f) **Crooked septum:** Unexplained gross septal deformity following trauma.

Effect of DNS

(a) Compensatory hypertrophy of the turbinates of the opposite side—C-shaped deviation associated with hypertrophy of both inferior and middle turbinates. While a S-shaped deviation is associated with inferior turbinate hypertrophy on one side and middle turbinate hypertrophy on the other side.

(b) *External deformity*—Deviation involving junction of the septal cartilage to upper lateral cartilages can lead to external deviation. Caudal dislocation with subluxation of the septal cartilage over the maxillary crest leads to loss of support to the columella as well as the tip of the nose leading to tip deformity and columellar retraction.

(c) Impairment of drainage to sinuses due to blockage of the ostiomeatal complex.

(d) Secondary atrophic Rhinitis on the roomier side of the nasal cavity due to inadequate humidification.

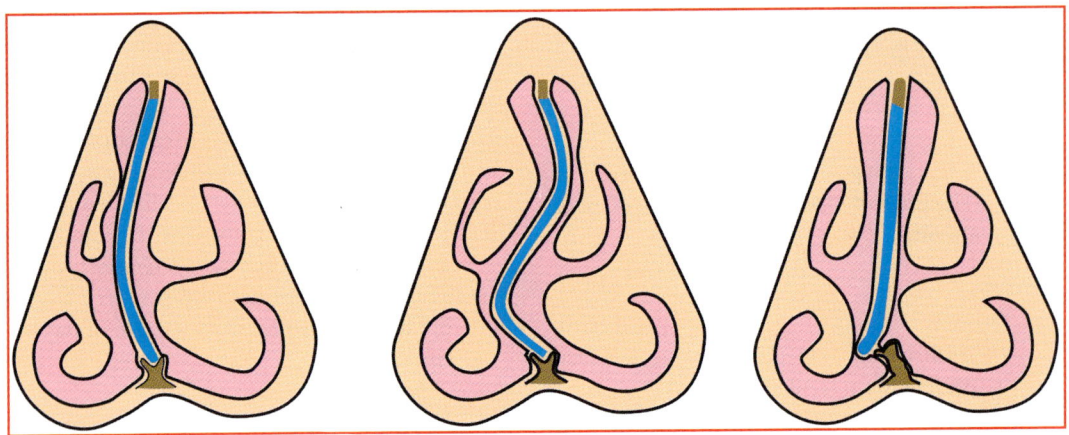

Fig. 27.1a: C-shaped deviation   **Fig. 27.1b:** S-shaped deviation   **Fig. 27.1c:** Subluxation of septal cartilage

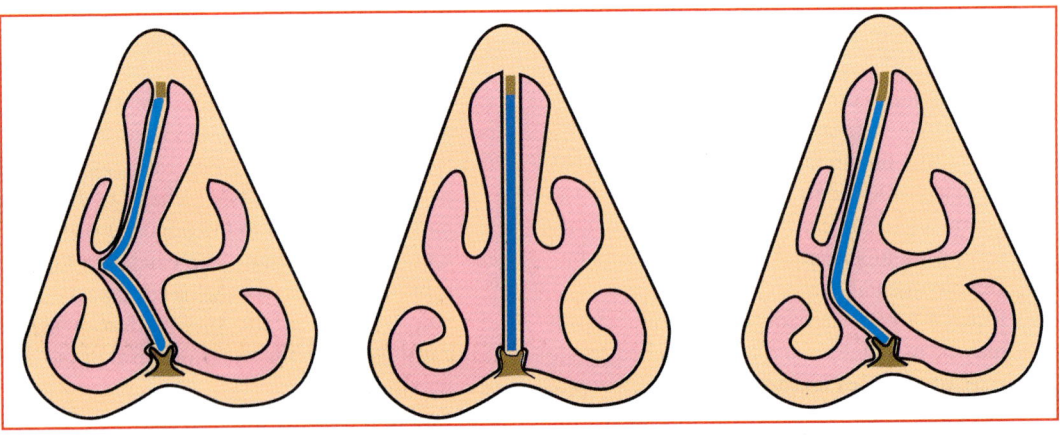

Fig. 27.1d: Septal spur   **Fig. 27.1e:** Normal septum   **Fig. 27.1f:** Anterior deviation

Clinical Features

Symptoms

1. **Nasal obstruction:** May be unilateral in C-shaped deviation or bilateral in S-shaped deviation. Associated rhinitis/ sinusitis can cause increase in nasal obstruction. Bernoulli's phenomena can also play a role in increasing the nasal obstruction.

2. **Headache:** Usually occurs due to associated sinusitis. It can also be due to 'anterior ethmoidal nerve syndrome' wherein contact areas in the nose give rise to referred pain over the vertex.

3. **External deformity:** Septal deviation affecting the dorsal part of the cartilaginous septum, subluxation and caudal dislocation of the cartilage with loss of support to the tip and columella may be associated with external deformity.

4. **Hyposmia/anosmia:** This is seen usually in association with bilateral nasal obstruction. Anosmia due to DNS alone is very rare.

5. **Epistaxis:** It is usually due to spur or crusting of nasal mucosa.

Signs

1. Elevate the tip of the nose to look for caudal dislocation and the vestibule of the nose.

2. Anterior rhinoscopy is done to determine the site and type of deviation as described above, presence of compensatory hypertrophy, status of nasal mucosa, discharge from the meatus, crusting, etc.

3. Local application of decongestant like cocaine/xylocaine with adrenaline helps in better assessment of the deeper areas in the nasal cavity. Middle turbinate and middle meatus area should be inspected for concha bullosa, contact areas, discharge and polyps.

4. Cottle's test– Pulling the cheek outwards at the nasofacial crease improves the nasal patency at the valve area.

Investigations

1. **X-ray PNS (Water's view and Caldwell view):** To look for haziness of the various sinuses. The alignment of the septum and the size of the turbinates may also be assessed.

2. **CT scan of the paranasal sinuses** including the OMC (Ostio-meatal complex) is superior to plain radiographs of the PNS. All the sinuses including their pathology can be evaluated. Contact areas, the status of ostiomeatal complex and the presence of concha bullosa can be identified better.

3. **Diagnostic nasal endoscopy (DNE):** Helps in precise identification of the pathologic site, anatomical variation and abnormalities of the septum and the lateral wall, especially the ostio-meatal complex.

4. **Bleeding and clotting profile:** BT, CT, PT and APTT.

Treatment

Medical treatment for associated rhinitis/ sinusitis

Surgical treatment

- Surgery for the deviated nasal septum
  - Septoplasty
  - Submucosal resection
  - Endoscopic septoplasty
- Surgery for the external nasal deformity with deviated nasal septum (Septorhinoplasty)

This term is used when the septoplasty forms an integral part of rhinoplasty procedure. They can be of two types based on the approach preferred.

1. Internal
2. External.

History of Septal Surgery

Decades have passed since septoplasty was first introduced for the management of nasal airway. Numerous medical descriptions are available regarding the pathology and treatment of deviated nasal septum (Freer, 1902; Metzenbaum, 1929; Galloway, 1946; Cottle et al 1958; Maran 1974).

The submucous resection was popularized and refined by Killian (1904) and Freer (1902). The increased incidence of complications following such radical surgeries led to more and more conservative septal surgery. Metzenbaum in 1929 described the swing door technique for caudal dislocation and subluxation. Galloway (1946) removed the entire septal cartilage and replaced it as a separate auto-graft. Cottle (1958) described pre-maxilla-maxilla approach for the correction by making inferior and superior tunnel on concave side and inferior tunnel on convex side to facilitate necessary resection of cartilage and bone to correct the septal deformity. Maran (1974) has described septoplasty, but used a more radical technique in the terms of removal of bony septum. However, none of these descriptions have highlighted a complete surgical management of this condition to improve the nasal airway. Each surgical procedure has its limitations and cannot deal with all the variants of the deformities of the nasal septum. It is essential to know the biomechanical behavior of the cartilaginous septum (Murakami et al 1982). Kennedy et al (1998) and Nayak et al (1998,2000) described the technique of endoscopic septoturbinoplasty.

An ideal surgical correction of the nasal septum should satisfy the following criteria (Nayak et al, 1998):

- Should relieve the nasal obstruction.
- Should be conservative.
- Should not produce iatrogenic deformity.
- Should not compromise the ostiomeatal complex.
- Should relieve all the contact areas
- Must have the scope for a revision surgery, if required later.

Indications for Septal Surgery

1. Persistent nasal obstruction caused by deviated nasal septum.
2. Deviation as a cause for sinusitis
3. If the deviation is the cause of epistaxis.
4. Access for surgery particularly for functional endoscopic sinus surgery, polypectomy, etc.

5. As an approach for hypophysectomy by doing submucosal resection.
6. For harvesting septal cartilage or bone as graft material.

OPERATIVE TECHNIQUE

Submucosal Resection (SMR)

Surface anesthesia

- By 4% Xylocaine nasal packing.
- Infiltration by 2% Xylocaine and 1 in 100,000 adrenaline on either side of the septum from anterior to posterior or posterior to anterior direction.

Incision

Killian's incision is used which is given at about 1.25 cm behind the columella at the mucocutaneous junction at the convex side of the deflection.

Flap Elevation

The mucoperichondrial flap is elevated with the help of Freer's perichondrial elevator from the septal cartilage and continued posteriorly to elevate the mucoperiosteum from the bony septum (Fig. 27.2).

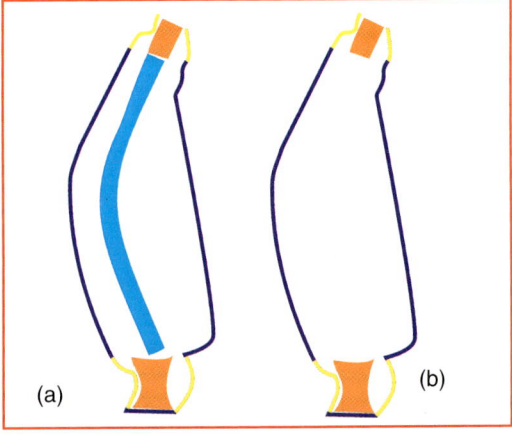

Fig. 27.2: (a) Elevation of the mucoperichondrial—mucoperiosteal flaps on the sides, (b) Resection of the deviated bone and cartilage

Resection of cartilage: The cartilage is incised keeping about 1 cm of the caudal end of the septum to support the columella and a dorsal strip of cartilage to support the dorsum.

Resection of bone: Posterior bony septum is removed by using a bone cutting/Luc's forceps. Maxillary crest is removed by V-shaped nasal gouge (Fig. 27.3).

Nasal packing: Both the septal flaps are apposed and anterior nasal packing/splinting is done in both the sides of nasal septum after the incision site is sutured. The splints may be sutured in place by through and through sutures (Fig. 27.4).

Septoplasty

It is a tissue-sparing procedure where septal deviation is corrected by minimal resection of cartilage and bone, strategic criss-cross incision and repositioning.

Steps of surgery (Fig. 27.5)

Surface anesthesia: By 4% Xylocaine nasal packing.

Infiltration by 2% Xylocaine and 1 in 100,000 adrenaline on either side of the septum from

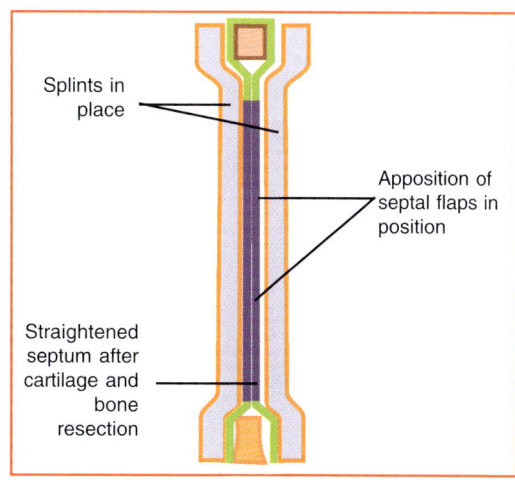

Fig. 27.4: Nasal splints in place after SMR operation

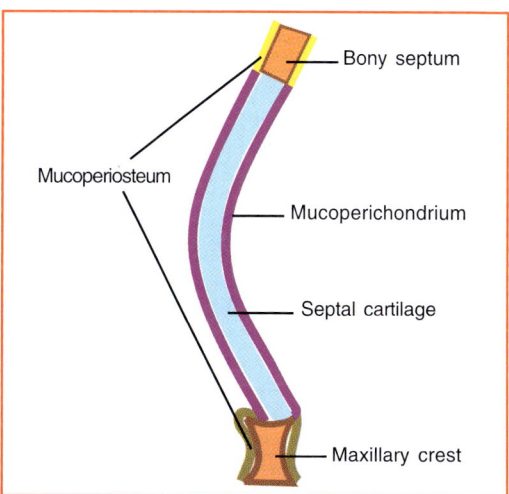

Fig. 27.5: C-shaped DNS before surgery

anterior to posterior or posterior to anterior direction.

Freer's hemitransfixation incision is given at the caudal end of the septum, usually on the concave side of the cartilage (Fig. 27.6).

Flap elevation: The mucoperichondrial elevation is done on the side of incision and three tunnels are created.

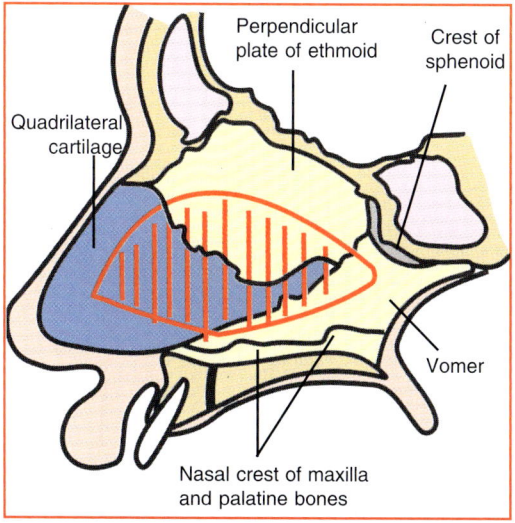

Fig. 27.3: The area of cartilage and bony resection (red shaded area) in SMR, preserving the dorsal and caudal strut of cartilage of about one cm thickness

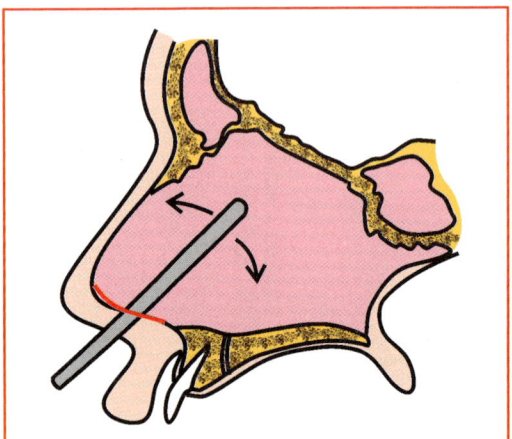

Fig. 27.6: The Freer's incision (red line) made at the mucocutaneous junction and the elevation of the mucoperichondrial–periosteal flap using Freer's elevator

Anterior tunnel: Exposure of the quadrangular septal cartilage is done on the concave side (Fig. 27.7).

Inferior tunnel: Periosteum is elevated and the anterior nasal spine and maxillary crest on both the sides are exposed (Fig. 27.8a and b).

Posterior tunnel: With sharp dissection the bony septum comprising of the perpendicular plate of

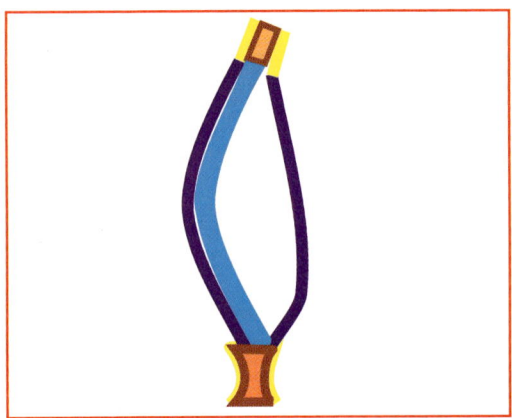

Fig. 27.7: Creation of the anterior tunnel by elevating the mucoperichondrial flap

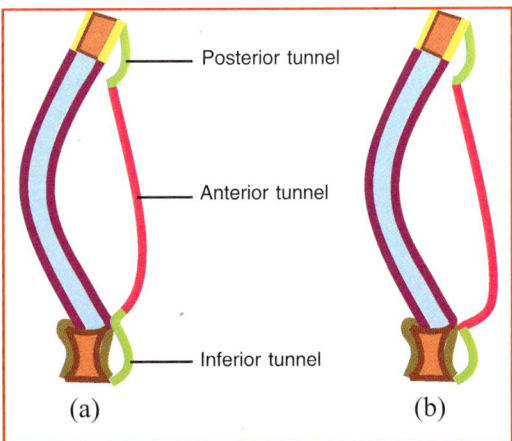

Figs 27.8a and b: (a) Anterior, posterior and inferior tunnels being raised. (b) The tunnels are being combined into a single tunnel

ethmoid and vomer is exposed. A small incision is given at the bony cartilaginous junction to elevate the mucoperiosteum of the opposite side (Fig. 27.9).

Disarticulation of bony cartilaginous junction: The cartilage is freed from the bony attachments.

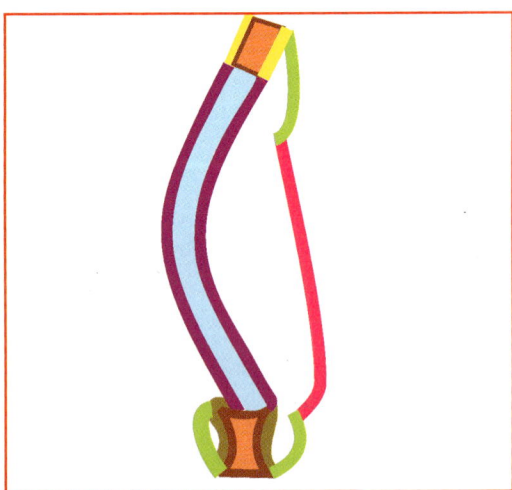

Fig. 27.9: Elevation of the inferior tunnel on the opposite side after disarticulation of the cartilage from the maxillary crest

Cartilage and bony resection: Inferior strip of excess cartilage is resected. The part of the perpendicular plate and the vomerine angulation is removed using bone cutting forceps (Fig. 27.10a and b, Fig. 27.11a and b).

Bone realignment: Fracture realignment of the rest of the bony framework is done.

Cartilage alignment: On the concave side, multiple full thickness criss-cross incisions (Cross cuts) are given in various planes to straighten the cartilage.

Columellar tunneling is done if caudal dislocation is present. Excess caudal end is trimmed and is inserted into the tunnel, which is fixed by figure of 8 sutures through the anterior nasal spine.

Incision is sutured and anterior nasal packing or splitting is done as described in SMR procedure (Fig. 27.11).

Endoscopic Septoplasty and Turbinoplasty

The traditional surgeries of the nasal septum improve the nasal airway but do not fulfill the criteria for an ideal surgical correction (page 306) in most instances. The reasons outlined for this are poor visualization, relative inaccessibility, poor illumination, difficulty in evaluation of the exact pathology, need for nasal packing, unnecessary manipulation, resection and over exposure of the septal framework, reducing the scope for a revision surgery (Nayak et al, 2002). The nasal endoscope allows precise preoperative identification of the septal pathology and its associated lateral nasal wall abnormalities and helps

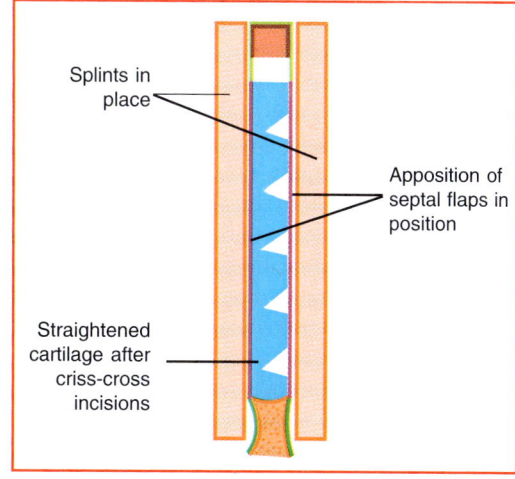

Splints in place

Apposition of septal flaps in position

Straightened cartilage after criss-cross incisions

Fig. 27.11: Splinting after septoplasty

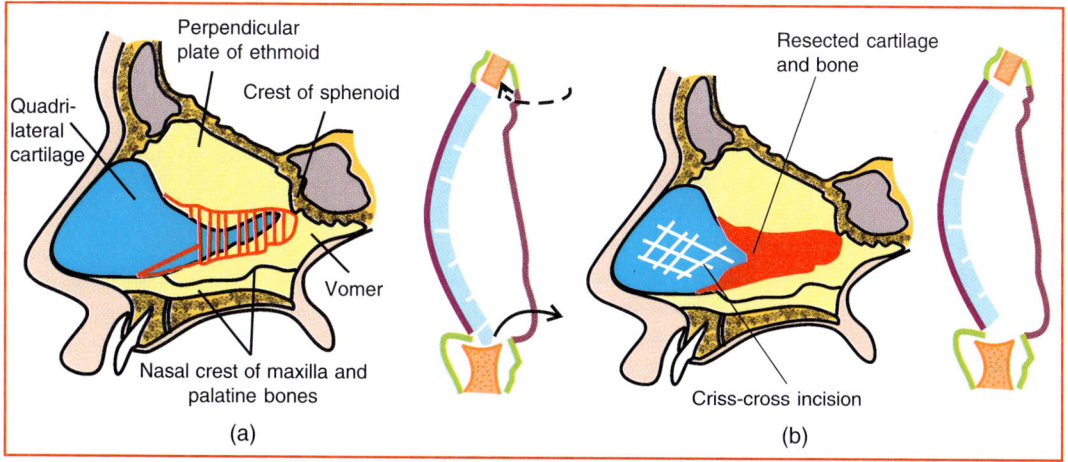

Perpendicular plate of ethmoid

Crest of sphenoid

Quadri-lateral cartilage

Vomer

Nasal crest of maxilla and palatine bones

(a)

Resected cartilage and bone

Criss-cross incision

(b)

Fig. 27.10: (a) Resection of inferior strip of cartilage (arrow) and disarticulation of bony cartilaginous junction (interrupted arrow). Criss-cross incisions are made on the cartilage, (b) After resection of inferior strip of cartilage

in better planning of endoscope-aided septal surgery (Nayak et al, 1998). This technique is ultra conservative and fulfills the above-mentioned criteria of an ideal septal surgery.

Steps of Endoscopic Septoplasty

- Surface anesthesia—Same as for septoplasty.
- Endoscopic infiltration of the nasal septum with 1% Xylocaine with 1 in 200,000 adrenaline on the convex side of the cartilaginous septum along the crest and bony septum on both sides including the spur whenever present.
- Incomplete incision at the caudal end of the septum in its lower half in most cases except when there was a caudal dislocation or anterior buckling (hemi-transfixation).
- Incision is made on the convex side in cases with anterior deviation and on the concave side for subluxation, spur or posterior deviation to expose the abnormality at the bony cartilaginous junction. In cases of an isolated spur, incision is made parallel in the floor on the spur itself (Fig. 27.12 a)
- Elevation of the initial mucoperichondrial flap using Cottle's elevator and Pilchards nasal speculum. Further elevation is done using 0° Hopkins rod nasal endoscope (4 mm) held in left hand, keeping the tip of the endoscope between the mucoperichondrial flap and the septal cartilage. The right hand is used for instrumentation. Flap elevation in the correct cleavage plane is required to minimize bleeding. The exposure is limited to the 'target area'. The traditional anterior and inferior tunnels, described by Cottle et al (1958) are not followed in the endoscopic method.
- Excess of cartilage at the maxillary crest, which usually overlaps the crest/ vomer is precisely shaved endoscopically (Figs 27.12 b, c and d).
- In case of posterior deviation or a deviation at the ethmochondral junction, the bony septum is fractured to realign in the midline or a minimum resection of the caudal end of the ethmoidal plate is performed. Dislocation of the ethmochondral junction should be avoided; especially in a child and a deviated septum here is precisely shaved using the Bard-Parker Knife.
- A C-shaped cartilaginous deviation is dealt with by precise multiple wedge resections aided by the endoscope, placing them on strategic sites and planes. Criss-cross incisions are made on the cartilage on the concave side.
- A spur without any other deviation of the septum is resected after incision and exposure made directly over the spur.

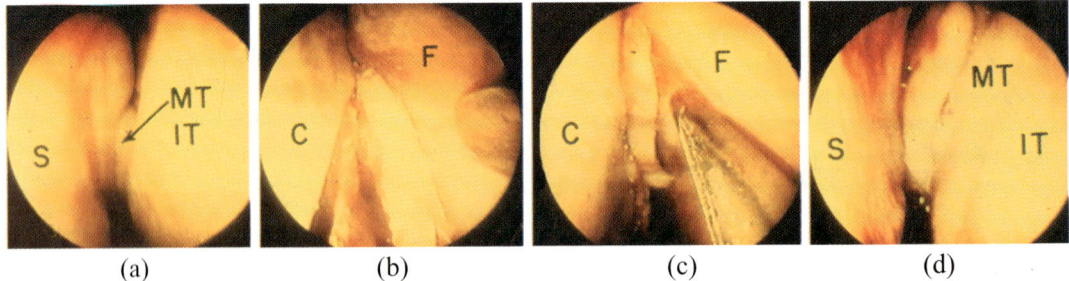

(a)   (b)   (c)   (d)

Figs 27.12a to d: (a) Posterior DNS with subluxation (Left) of cartilage, (b) Precise resection of overlaping inferior strip of cartilage (c) Shaving of the cartilage and wedge resection at the bony cartilaginous junction, (d) After correction

    Septum (S); Middle turbinate (MT); Inferior turbinate (IT); Muco-perichondrial/periosteal flap (F)

- Turbinoplasty may be done to reduce the size of the inferior or middle turbinate using bipolar cautery, laser or a microdebrider wherein the precise posterolateral resection is done for hypertrophied turbinates or a concha bullosa. (Nayak D. R. et al 2001& 2002). Alternatively a submucosal resection of the inferior concha may be performed.
- Splinting of the nasal septum is done using wax plates or silastic sheets. This acts like a splint, tamponade and prevents synechia formation. It can be kept in-situ for 5-7 days in children. Alternatively anterior nasal packing may be done. Limited septal surgeries like spur reduction does not require splinting or packing.

Complications of Septal Surgery

(a) Septal perforation
(b) Septal hematoma
(c) Septal abscess
(d) Saddle nose deformity
(e) Columellar retraction
(f) Flapping of septum
(g) Epistaxis
(h) Synechia

Nasal Synechia

They commonly occur due to adhesions between septum and the lateral wall and/or between middle turbinate and the lateral wall following nasal surgery and nasal packing. They can be prevented by doing proper postoperative cleaning and proper lubrication of nasal pack before insertion. Use of septal splints following surgery helps in prevention in formation of synechia.

Clinical Features (Fig. 27.13)

Nasal obstruction is the most common presenting feature. Synechia between middle turbinate and lateral wall can cause impairment of drainage of the sinuses leading to sinusitis and headache.

Treatment

They can be excised and released using diathermy/bipolar cautery/laser. A spacer like dental wax

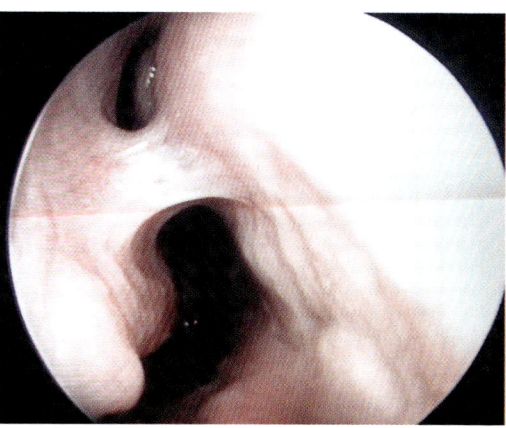

Fig. 27.13: Showing synechia between the septum and the inferior turbinate

plate, silastic sheets, etc. is kept between the two epithelial surfaces to prevent further adhesions for about one week.

Septal Hematoma

Causes

- Traumatic
  - Blunt injuries- Boxers, sports, RTA
  - Iatrogenic- SMR, septoplasty
- Non-traumatic
  - Bleeding/clotting disorders

Clinical Features (Fig. 27.14)

1. Bilateral constant usually acute nasal obstruction following trauma
2. Mouth breathing
3. Pain
4. Septum thickened and bulging to both sides completely obstructing the nasal cavity.

Investigations

1. Bleeding, clotting and prothrombin time
2. ESR
3. Complete blood picture
4. X-ray PNS

Management

1. Wide bore needle aspiration

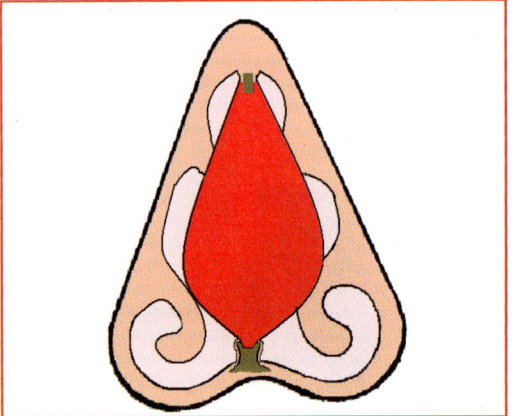

Fig. 27.14: 'Septal hematoma' as a result of collection of blood within the nasal septal flaps following SMR surgery

2. Incision and drainage
3. Anterior nasal packing or quilting sutures to prevent re-accumulation
4. Antibiotics, analgesics, etc.

Complications
Septal abscess and its consequences

Septal Abscess

Definition
It is defined as collection of pus within the septum.
   Table 27.1 lists the differences between Septoplasty and SMR.

Causes
- Traumatic
  - Usually follows septal hematoma
- Non-traumatic
- Furuncle of the nasal vestibule
- Immunocompromised states.

Clinical Features

Symptoms
- Nasal obstruction, which is usually bilateral
- Pain in the nose
- Fever with chills and rigors
which commonly occurs as a result of infection of a septal hematoma.

Signs
- Tenderness +
- Pus pointing +/–
- Rupture with purulent discharge +/–
- External nasal deformity +/–

Management
- Incision and drainage/ wide bore needle aspiration
- Anterior nasal packing
- Antibiotics, analgesics, etc.

Complications
1. Spread of infection
   - Meningitis

Table 27.1: Difference between Septoplasty and SMR	
Septoplasty	**SMR**
• Conservative	• Radical
• Reconstructive/ realignment procedure	• Resective procedure
• May be done for any DNS	• Posterior DNS
• Complications less	• Complications more
• Can be done in children	• Contraindicated in children
• Can be combined with rhinoplasty	• Combination with rhinoplasty is difficult
• Can be revised	• Difficult to revise

- Facial cellulitis/ abscess of the upper lips
- Cavernous sinus thrombophlebitis

2. External nasal deformity
   - Saddle nose/columellar retraction
3. Septal perforation

Septal Perforation

Causes

- Traumatic
  - Mechanical-RTA, assault, sports, etc.
  - Chemical-Chrome perforation (occupational)
  - Thermal/ radiation trauma
  - Finger nail trauma
  - Iatrogenic-SMR
- Septal hematoma/abscess
- Atrophic rhinitis
- Chronic granulomatous conditions
- Nasal myiasis

- Neoplasm of the septum
- Cocaine addicts

Clinical Features

- Epistaxis if due to granulomatous conditions
- Small perforation:
  - Whistling/hissing noise during nasal breathing (Fig. 27.15)
- Big perforation
  - Atrophic changes and consequent crusting, epistaxis, dry feeling in the nose, etc. (Fig. 27.16).

Management

- Asymptomatic – No treatment is necessary
- Small perforation:
  - Obturator/ septal buttons can be used.
  - Surgical closure
- Large perforation:
  - Surgical closure—Nasal/ buccal/ skin flaps

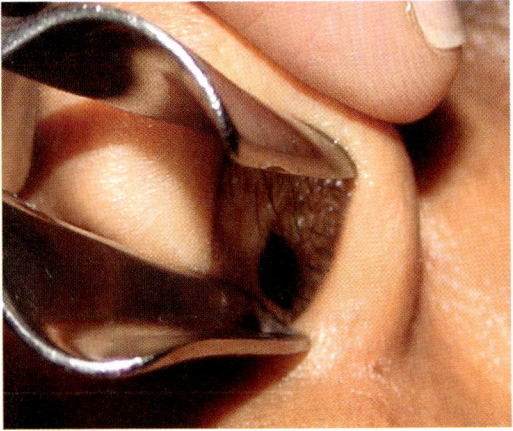

Fig. 27.15: Showing nasal septal perforation on anterior rhinoscopy

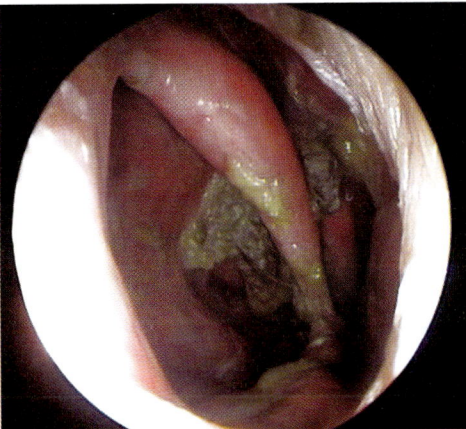

Fig. 27.16: Endoscopic picture showing septal perforation and atrophy of nasal mucosa

28

Acute Inflammatory Conditions of the Nasal Cavity

ACUTE NON-SPECIFIC RHINITIS (COMMON COLD)

This common cold (acute coryze) is a contagious, viral infectious disease of the upper respiratory system, caused primarily by rhinoviruses and coronaviruses.

Etiology

Predisposing Factors

- Climate—Temp/Chills/Humidity
- Environment—Over crowding
- Immune status—Diabetes, HIV
- Nutrition and vitamin deficiency
- Fatigue, fitness and exercise
- Nasal obstruction/Foci of chronic infection
- General diseases.

Causative Agent

Viruses are the primary pathogens. Common viruses involved are the Rhino/Corona, influenza, adeno and echo viruses. Many viruses and different strains of each may affect the nose thus making eradication difficult.

Bacterial infection is often secondary to the viral attack.

Mode of Transmission

- Air borne 'Droplet' infection
- Through contact

Pathology

Vasoconstriction of nasal mucosa occurs initially causing dry feeling followed by reflex vasodilatation which leads to mucosal edema causing nasal obstruction and rhinorrhea.

Clinical Features

Prodromal stage (Ischemic stage)

1. Dryness of nose, fever, body ache, etc.
2. Itching of nose.

Reactive stage (stage of vasodilatation) (Figs 28.1 and 28.2)

1. Increased muco-ciliary action (runny nose)
2. Dry cough due to post nasal drip.
3. Ciliary paralysis with stasis of secretion.
4. Thick viscid mucous blanket.
5. Venous stasis and secondary bacterial invasion

Stage of Resolution

1. Improved ciliary function
2. Mucosal edema subsides
3. Nasal airway patency improves
4. Symptoms subside

Complication

- Pharyngitis
- Sinusitis

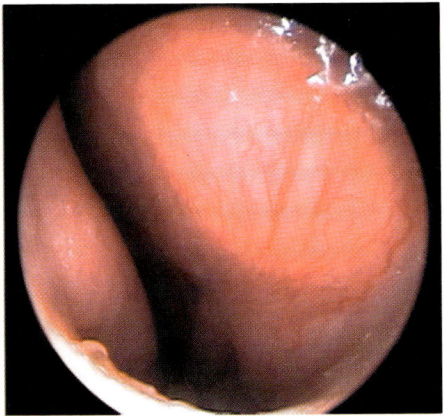

Fig. 28.1: Endoscopic photograph showing grossly congested nasal mucosa in acute rhinitis

- Otitis media
- Tonsillitis
- Lymphadenitits
- Lower respiratory tract infection
- Nephritis
- Otitis media
- GI infection
- Rheumatism.

Differential Diagnosis

- Allergic rhinitis
- Vasomotor rhinitis
- Chronic rhinitis

Treatment

- General—Bedrest in warm well ventilated room.
- Systemic antibiotic
- Decongestants like pseudoephidrine hydrochloride, etc.
- Antipyretics, Analgesics
- Local treatment—Decongestant/Saline nasal drops
- Steam Inhalation.

Indications for Starting Antibiotics

- Mucopurulent discharge
- Stridor in children can occur due to spread

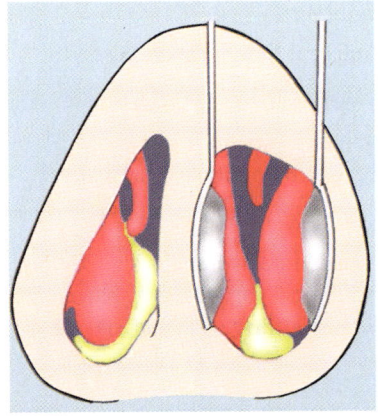

Fig. 28.2: Anterior rhinoscopy showing congested nasal mucosa and mucopurulent exudate in both nasal cavity

of infection to larynx and lower respiratory tract

INFLUENZAL RHINITIS

This is a severe form of viral infection of upper air way associated with severe morbidity and mortality

Etiology

- It is a form of viral infection of the upper respiratory tract
- Causative agent–Influenza–Type A/B/C.

Pathology

- Necrosis of ciliated epithelium
- Secondary bacterial invasion

Symptoms

- It is a more severe form of acute rhinitis than common cold .

General Symptoms
- Fever
- Malaise
- Joint pain

Local Symptoms
- Rhinorrhea.
- Acute respiratory obstruction in children

Investigation
- Antiviral titre in severe case.

Complication
- Acute respiratory disease
- Severe morbidity and mortality.

Treatment
1. Amantidine hydrochloride 200 mg/day.
2. Antibiotics for secondary bacterial infection.

Prevention: Influvac vaccine may be given.

ACUTE SPECIFIC RHINITIS

Diphtheric Rhinitis (Nasal diphtheria)

Causative agent

Corynebacterium diphtherae.

Pathology

A greyish white membrane is formed over inferior turbinates, nasal floor and septum. This membrane is not adherent to the underlying structures and does not bleed easily on removal unlike in faucial diphtheria. These patients are usually carriers.

Symptoms

General
- Fever

- Malaise
- Joint pain.

Local
- Nasal obstruction
- Serofibrinous exudate
- Offensive discharge (occasionally)

Signs
- Nasal discharge is purulent
- Greyish white patch can be seen covering the inferior turbinates. This pseudomembrane can be removed easily unlike faucial diphtheria. The mucous blanket covering the ciliated epithelium prevents its attachment and absorption of toxins. Thus the toxic features are less in nasal diphtheria.

Differential Diagnosis

- Chronic specific rhinitis
- Atrophic rhinitis
- Influenzal rhinitis

Investigations

- Nasal swab for culture and staining.
- X-ray PNS

Treatment

1. Isolation
2. Anti-Diphtheric Serum
3. Inj. Crystalline Penicillin.

POINTS TO REMEMBER

1. Acute nonspecific rhinitis or common cold commonly occurs primarily as a viral infection caused by Rhino virus.
2. Influenzal Rhinitis is caused by Influenza virus type A/B/C. This is frequently associated with morbidity and mortality.
3. Diphtheric rhinitis or nasal diphtheria is caused by Corynebacterium Diphtherae. These patients are usually carriers of diphtheria.

29

Chronic Non-specific Inflammation of the Nose

It is an advanced stage of an unresolved acute rhinitis due to the presence of predisposing factors.

Predisposing Factors

1. Neighbouring infection
2. Vasomotor rhinitis
3. Nasal obstruction
4. Metabolic factors.

Pathology

1. Chronic Hyperemia
2. Engorgement of cavernous spaces
3. Loss of cilia and goblet cells (Reversible)

Symptoms

1. Nasal obstruction
2. Nasal discharge
3. Postnasal drip
4. Headache
5. Anosmia.

Signs

Anterior Rhinoscopy

(a) Secretion in the floor of the nose

(b) Mucous membrane is swollen.
(c) May be pale red or bright red elastic looking (Fig. 29.1)
(d) Septum is congested and velvetty
(e) Middle turbinate is enlarged and shiny.

Posterior rhinoscopy

Pinkish and shiny posterior end of inferior turbinate.

Diagnosis

It is based on history and clinical examination.

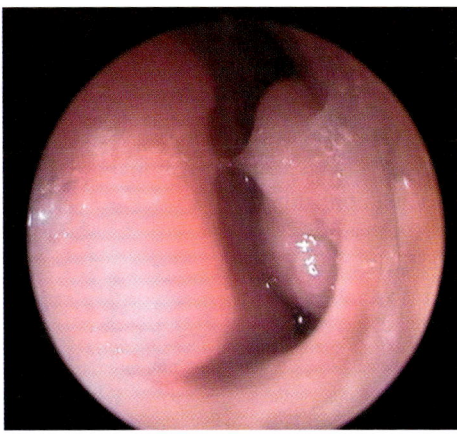

Fig. 29.1: Chronic simple rhinitis with muco-purulent discharge on nasal endoscopic examination

293

Treatment

General

1. Correction of the predisposing factors.
2. Antibiotics may be required during acute exacerbation

Local

1. Saline or alkaline nasal douche
2. Mild vasoconstriction
3. Topical steroid
4. Antibiotics

CHRONIC HYPERTROPHIC RHINITIS

Definition

It is an advanced stage of simple chronic rhinitis with irreversible mucosal and submucosal changes

Etiology

Predisposing factors are same as simple chronic rhinitis.

Pathology

- Permanent hypertrophy changes
- Thick nodular mucosa
- Fibrosis.

Clinical Features

Symptoms

- Excessive nasal secretion
- Nasal obstruction, more at night
- Mouth breathing
- Hyperemia
- Thick voice
- Hawking.

Signs

Anterior rhinoscopy

- Diffuse hypertrophy with papillary surface on anterior end of the inferior turbinate (Figs. 29.2a and b).

- Diffuse/circumscribed hypertrophy of the rest of the inferior turbinate.
- Middle turbinate appears dull red with polypoidal changes.

Posterior rhinoscopy (Fig. 29.3)

- Mulberry enlargement of the posterior end of the inferior turbinate.

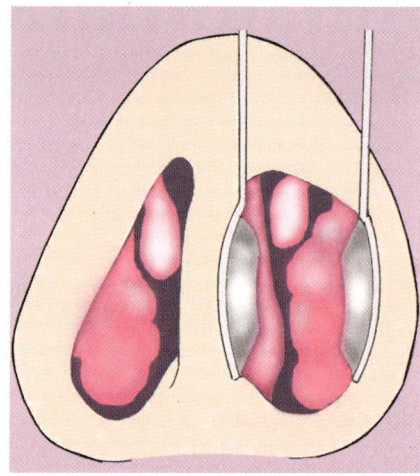

Fig. 29.2a: Anterior rhinoscopy showing papillary hypertrophy of inferior turbinate and pale edematous middle turbinate

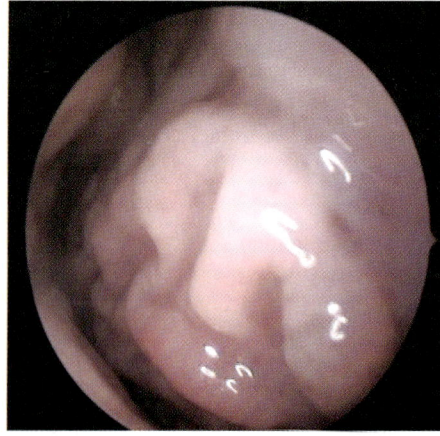

Fig. 29.2b: Endoscopic picture showing diffuse papillary hypertrophy of anterior end of inferior turbinate

Investigation

- Diagnostic nasal endoscopy
- X-ray PNS

Treatment

1. Electrocauterization
2. Submucosal diathermy and coagulation
3. Cryosurgery- Laser
4. Surgical trimming

Complications of Chronic Non-specific Rhinitis

1. Chronic sinusitis
2. Chronic pharyngitis
3. Polyposis

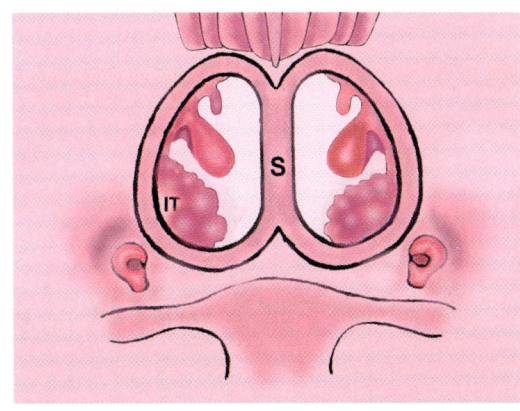

Fig. 29.3: Mulberry hypertrophy of the posterior end of inferior turbinate (IT) seen in case of chronic hypertrophic rhinitis

POINTS TO REMEMBER

1. Both chronic simple rhinitis and hypertrophic rhinitis can cause persistent nasal obstruction.
2. Chronic hypertrophic rhinitis is commonly associated with gross hypertrophy of turbinates.
3. Papillary hypertrophy of anterior end and mulberry hypertrophy of the posterior end of the inferior turbinate is the characteristic appearance.

30

Rhinitis Sicca, Caseosa and Medicamentosa

RHINITIS SICCA

Definition

It is condition of the nose associated with dirty black crust in the anterior aspect of the nasal cavity seen in persons exposed to dry and dusty environment.

Etiology

More common in people exposed to dry and dusty work environment as in farmers, miners, etc.

Precipitating Factors

- Alcohol
- Nutrition
- Dusty and dry environment
- Nasal surgery.

Pathology (Fig. 30.1)

- Squamous metaplasia of ciliated columnar epithelium
- Periglandular fibrosis
- Viscid and stagnant mucous blanket
- Crust formation

Symptoms

- Nasal obstruction

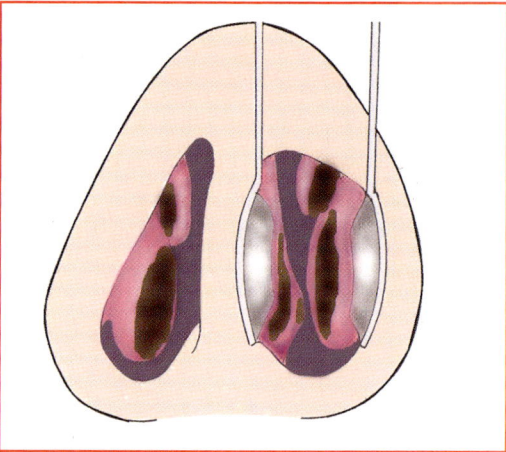

Fig. 30.1: Dirty black crust seen in the anterior part of the septum and inferior turbinate and anterior aspect of middle meatus

- Discharge of dirty black crusts
- Epistaxis

Signs (Fig. 30.2)

- Dry mucosa more in the anterior part of the nasal cavity
- Dirty black crust is seen over the anterior end of inferior turbinates, middle meatus and septum. Unlike atrophic rhinitis there is absence of fetor and atrophy of bone.

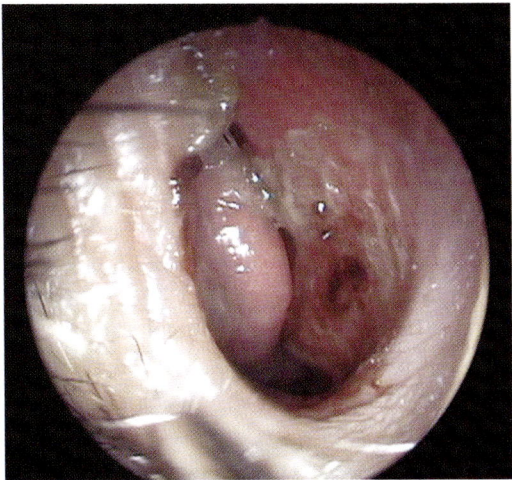

Fig. 30.2: Dirty black and gray crusts seen in the anterior aspect of nasal cavity involving the septum and the turbinates. Removal of crusts frequently causes epistaxis

- Excoriation over septum.
- Perforation of anterior septum

Treatment

- Change of place of work and residence if possible
- Ointment to prevent crusting
- 25% glucose in glycerine nasal drops
- No decongestant nasal drops

RHINITIS CASEOSA (NASAL CHOLESTEATOMA)

Definition

Chronic inflammatory condition of the nose due to the obstruction to nasal passage, and/or all major sinuses due to stenosis, adhesions or synechia, etc. leading to stagnation of the secretion and constant exfoliation of nasal mucosa. The discharge thus accumulated along with collected debris undergoes chemical changes and putrefaction resulting in the formation of caseous material in the nasal cavity.

Etiology

- Nasal stenosis/ obstruction
- More common in the 3rd and 4th decade
- This is commonly associated with suppurative sinusitis
- Foreign body/ rhinolith can cause nasal obstruction leading to stagnation of secretions
- Fungal infection may be associated.

Pathology

- Stagnation of secretion and secondary infection occurs following nasal obstruction.
- Continued excoriation of nasal mucosa cause accumulation of debris, which undergo mechanical and chemical changes.
- Secondary infection due to stagnation and debris collection undergo putrefaction and gets transformed to caseous material.

Symptoms

1. Nasal obstruction
2. Fetid discharge
3. Offensive odor
4. Headache
5. Deformity
6. Anosmia/cacosmia
7. Defective taste/halitosis.

Signs

- Cheesy material may be seen in the nasal cavity or in the meatus.
- Perforation and destruction of nasal septum or lateral nasal wall.
- Ulceration of the mucosa may be seen especially if associated with foreign body or rhinolith.

Investigations (Fig. 30.3)

- Nasal endoscopy and biopsy
- Fungal culture
- X-Ray PNS—Complete opacity of the affected sinus may be seen

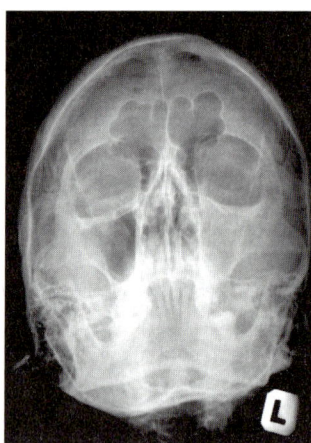

Fig. 30.3: X-ray water view showing left maxillary sinus opacity in a case of rhinitis caseosa

- CT Scan—Unilateral sinus opacity is seen often
- Biopsy and fungal culture should be done to rule out fungal sinusitis

Complication

- Intracranial spread of infection.
- Orbital complications as described under the chapter – Sinusitis

Treatment

Medical
Antibiotics are given to treat secondary infection

Surgical
Endoscopic removal of foreign body/ rhinolith

Relieving Nasal Obstruction
Establishment of drainage by endoscopic sinus surgery / intranasal antrostomy.

Drug Induced Rhinitis

Several medications have been implicated in the development of rhinitis. They include local and systemic drugs.

Examples

Local
- Topical nasal decongestant (Rhinitis medicamentosa)
- Inhaled cocaine

Systemic

Antihypertensives: Angiotensin-converting enzyme inhibitors, reserpine, guanethidine, phentolamine, methyldopa, beta-blockers.

Ergot alkaloids: These produce peripheral vasodilatation and nasal obstruction.

Aspirin: This inhibits the cyclo-oxygenase pathway, which leads to preferential lipoxygenase metabolism and increase leucotrienes and slow reacting substances production. Aspiration intolerance can lead to bronchial asthma and polyposis.

Drugs with anticholinergic activity like

- Neostigmine
- Chlorpromazine
- Gabapentin
- Penicillamine
- Non-steroidal anti-inflammatory drugs
- Exogenous estrogens
- Oral contraceptives.

Rhinitis Medicamentosa

This is due to prolonged use of local nasal decongestants (more than a week).

Pathology

- Initial vasoconstriction and ischemia due to vasoconstrictor effect of the nasal decongestants leading to localized anemia.
- Reflex vasodilatation and rebound congestion occurs due to secondary hyperemia a few hours after.
- This is associated with increased vascularity with sinusoidal engorgement causing nasal obstruction. This further encourages the patient to use more nasal decongestants.

- Long standing use probably reduces the effect of the nasal decongestants (tachyphylaxis) due to desensitization of mucosal vessels with loss of alpha-adrenergic tone. Further irritation of the mucosa and dryness can occur with suppression of nasal cycle for up to 6 months after cessation of treatment.
- Persistent use gives rise to subepithelial interstitial fibrosis.

Clinical Features

- Nasal obstruction (worse at night)
- Headache may be due to obstruction to the sinus ostia which gives rise to either vacuum headache or secondary infection causing sinusitis.

Signs (Fig. 30.4)

- *Anterior rhinoscopy*: Diffuse papillary hypertrophy of the anterior end of inferior turbinates
- *Posterior rhinoscopy*: Mulberry hypertrophy of the posterior end of the inferior turbinate.

Diagnosis

Based on history of prolong use of nasal decongestants and clinical findings.

Treatment

- Discontinue nasal decongestants
- Nasal and systemic steroids
- Turbinate reduction procedures like SMD, turbinoplasty, partial turbinectomy.

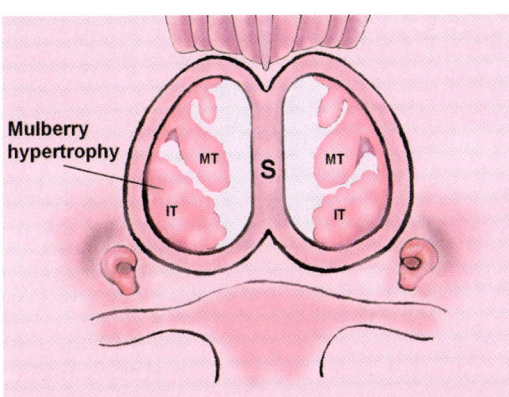

Fig. 30.4: Pale mulberry hypertropy of the posterior end of inferior turbinate in rhinitis medicamantosa

POINTS TO REMEMBER

1. Rhinitis sicca is a condition which occurs in drug and dusty atmosphere characterized by dirty black crust formation in the anterior aspect of nasal cavity.
2. Rhinitis caseosa occurs following obstruction to the nasal passage or draining of sinuses due to adhesions and stenosis, characterized by formation of caseous material in the nasal cavity. Fungal sinusitis should be ruled out in such cases.
3. Rhinitis medicamentosa occurs due to prolonged use of local nasal decongestant.
4. Certain topical and systemic drugs can cause chronic rhinitis, polyposis leading to nasal obstruction.

31

Atrophic Rhinitis

Definition

Atrophic rhinitis (AR) is a debilitating nasal mucosal disease of unknown etiology and is defined as a chronic inflammatory condition of the nose associated with progressive atrophy of the nasal mucosa, characterized by greenish yellow crust formation, roominess of nasal cavity and with characteristic fetor and paradoxical nasal congestion.

History

Dr. Spencer Watson (London) called it Ozoena in 1875.

Dr. Bernhard Fraenkel (1876) described what we now recognize as the triad of atrophic rhinitis, namely fetor, crusting, and atrophy of the nasal structures.

Types

Primary: It is also called idiopathic atrophic rhinitis, as the primary cause is not known. Primary atrophic rhinitis has decreased markedly in incidence in the last century. This probably relates to the increased use of antibiotics for chronic nasal infection.

Secondary: It occurs secondary to some known pathology conditions like tuberculosis, syphilis,

leprosy, etc. Secondary atrophic rhinitis resulting from trauma, surgery, granulomatous diseases, infection, and radiation exposure accounts for the majority of cases encountered by the rhinologist today. Excessive turbinate surgery has been both acquitted and accused in the literature as an etiology for secondary atrophic rhinitis.

Causes of Secondary Atrophic Rhinitis

- DNS (Unilateral)
- Chronic sinusitis
- Chronic granulomatous conditions (described under chronic specific rhinitis)
  1. Tuberculosis.
  2. Leprosy
  3. Syphilis
  4. Rhinoscleroma
  5. Wegener's granulomatosis
- Iatrogenic (Fig. 31.1).

Primary Atrophic Rhinitis

Etiology

- ***Coccobacillus foetidis/Klebsiella ozenae:*** Primary AR is almost always associated with a single organism *K. ozenae*.
- ***Endocrine imbalance:*** Disease has been reported to be aggravated with menstruation or pregnancy.

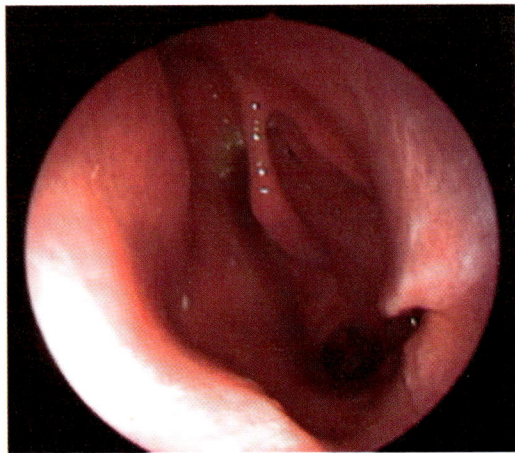

Fig. 31.1: Iatrogenic atrophic rhinitis due to extensive nasal surgery

- More common in females
- *Hereditary and racial influence:* A strong family history, hereditary influence has been reported. Sibert and Barton (1980) found eight of 15 children of an Irish family suffering from primary atrophic rhinitis with an affected father and proposed an autosomal dominant inheritance pattern.
- *Poor nutrition:* Han-Sen found hypo-cholesterolemia to be present in 50 percent of his patients, also found symptomatic improvement in 84 percent treated with Vitamin A. Disease is more common in poor socioeconomic group.
- *Iron deficiency anemia:* Bernat found benefit in 50 percent of patients given iron therapy.
- *Surfactant deficiency:* Significant change in the phospholipid profile in the nasal aspirate has been found which suggests a possible role for surfactant deficiency in the etiopathogenesis of cases of primary atrophic rhinitis (Sayed et al 2000).
- *Autoimmune disease:* The role of cellular immunity has been studied by Fouad et al (1980), in patients with atrophic rhinitis using the in vitro leukocyte migration and the spontaneous rosette tests. Cellular hypersensitivity to crude nasal homogenate was detected in 90 percent of cases associated with a decrease in the absolute number of T-lymphocytes. Altered cellular reactivity or loss of tolerance to nasal tissues may be precipitated primarily by virus infection, malnutrition and/or immuno-deficiency which trigger a destructive autoimmune process with the release of antigen(s) of nasal mucosa into the circulation.

Pathology

- Squamous metaplasia
- Atrophy of the glands
- Atrophy of the nerves
- Dilated capillaries/Endarteritis and periarteritis.

Two types

1. *Type I:* This is associated with Endarteritis and periarteritis
2. *Type II:* This is associated with vasodilatation of capillaries with increased alkaline phosphatase activity that leads to bone resorption and roominess of the nasal cavity and crusting.

Symptoms

- Offensive smell (Ozaena) perceived by others near the patient, than the patient himself/ herself known as merciful anosmia
- Anosmia/Hyposmia due to atrophy of the olfactory receptors.
- Nasal obstruction occurs due to the crusts though the nasal cavities are roomy.
- Discharge of greenish yellow thick crusts
- Epistaxis may be seen due to dislodgement of crusts.

Signs (Fig. 31.2)

- Presence of fetor
- Roomy nasal cavity due to atrophy of the turbinates/bony resorption following type II

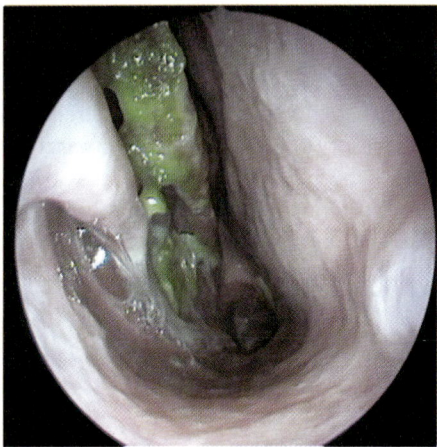

Fig. 31.2: Endoscopic picture showing features of primary atrophic rhinitis

atrophic rhinitis as a result of increased alkaline phosphatase activity.
- Greenish yellow crust formation due to drying of the stagnant secretions due to loss of ciliary motility.
- Dryness and atrophy of nasal mucosa
- Atrophy of all the turbinates and nasal septal mucosa

Investigations

- Complete blood picture, Serum proteins and Iron
- *X-ray PNS/CT Scan:* CT Scan is more informative and may show the following changes;
  – Mucoperiosteal thickening of the paranasal sinuses
  – Loss of definition of the ostiomeatal complex secondary to resorption of the ethmoid bulla and uncinate process.
  – Hypoplasia of the maxillary sinus
  – Enlargement of the nasal cavities with erosion and bowing of the lateral nasal wall.
  – Bony resorption and mucosal atrophy of the middle and inferior turbinates.

- *Nasal swab:* To rule out infective granulomatous conditions caused by acid-fast bacilli.
- *Chest X-ray:* To rule out tuberculosis
- Serological test for syphilis and other granulomatous conditions
- Nasal biopsy.

Treatment

The overall therapy encompasses two main goals: restoration of nasal hydration, and minimization of crusting and debris. To achieve these goals, several broad classes of therapies may be used; i.e. conservative (topical or local, systemic) or surgical.

Conservative

1. 2% Alkaline nasal douche / irrigation. This is prepared by using 2 parts of sodium chloride, one part of sodium bicarbonate and one part of sodium biborate.
2. Periodic nasal cleaning/ crust removal under anterior rhinoscopy/ nasal endoscopy.
3. 25% glucose in glycerin nasal drops
4. Kemicitine anti-ozaena solution
5. Potassium iodide is given orally
6. Submucosal injection of placental extract
7. Estrogen is tried in Type I atrophic rhinitis with limited success
8. Vitamin A, D, E replacement may be helpful.

Surgical

1. Young's operation–The anterior nasal aperture is closed completely surgically (Fig. 31.3).
2. Modified Young's operation–The anterior nasal aperture is closed surgically except a small opening of three mm to facilitate breathing (Fig. 31.4)
3. Lauten-Slauger's operation with bone/ cartilage/teflon implantation has been done in the past to reduce excessive roominess in the nasal cavity with limited success.

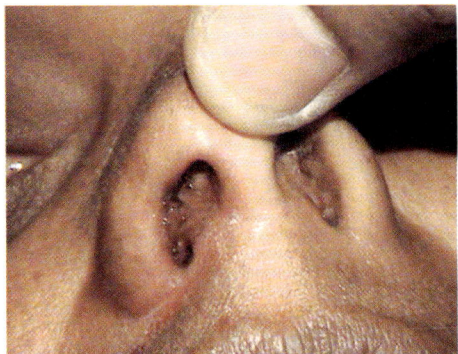

Fig. 31.3: Post Young's operation showing complete closure of anterior nares

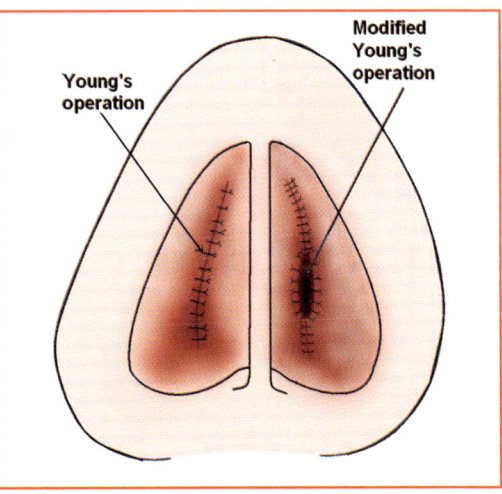

Fig. 31.4: Surgical procedure for atrophic rhinitis

4. Dermofat implantation over the inferior turbinate has been tried to reduce the size of the nasal cavity.
5. Stellate ganglion block may be done to increase nasal secretion.

6. Stenson's duct has been reimplanted into the maxillary sinus in the past with limited success.

POINTS TO REMEMBER

1. Atrophic rhinitis is common is low socioeconmic groups or may occur secondary to granulomatous conditions of nasal cavity.
2. Type I is associated with endarteritis/periarteritis and type II with vasodilation.
3. Granulomatous condition should be ruled out be through clinical evaluation and serological/histopathological tests.
4. Modified Young's operation is the surgical of choice if conservative treatment is not successful.

32

Chronic Specific Rhinitis

Chronic specific rhinitis refers to certain specific granulomatous conditions with classical clinical presentation.

GRANULOMAS OF THE NOSE

Granuloma is a tumor like mass of nodular granulation tissue with actively growing fibroblasts and capillary buds due to chronic inflammatory process associated with vasculitis.

Classification

1. Bacterial
   (a) Tuberculosis, lupus vulgaris, sarcoidosis
   (b) Leprosy
   (c) Rhinoscleroma
2. Spirochetal
   (a) Syphilis
3. Fungal
   (a) Rhinosporidiosis
   (b) Mucormycosis-rhinocerebral/rhino-cerebro-orbital
4. Idiopathic
   (a) Wegener's granulomatosis
   (b) Stewart's granuloma
   (c) Sarcoidosis
5. Miscellaneous:
   (a) Foreign body granuloma
   (b) Eosinophilic granuloma

These granulomatous conditions commonly present in various clinicopathological stages. They include:

1. Catarrhal (prodromal) stage
2. Nodular stage
3. Ulcerative stage
4. Cicatrization stage.

TUBERCULOSIS OF THE NOSE

It is a chronic inflammation of the nasal cavity caused by mycobacterium tuberculosis. During the past 2 decades, tuberculosis-both pulmonary and extrapulmonary has re-emerged as a major health problem worldwide and is attributed to increased incidence of HIV disease.

Etiology

It is a very rare condition, usually occurs secondary to pulmonary tuberculosis. Primary tuberculosis of the nose is rare. The first case of primary tuberculosis of the upper respiratory tract and nose was presented to the Pathological Society of London by Clarke in 1852. In 1997, Butt found only 35 cases of primary nasal tuberculosis in the medical literature.

Pathology

It affects the anterior part of the nasal cavity

consisting of the cartilaginous part. Nasal septum is the most common site.

The stages include

1. **Catarrhal (prodromal) stage:** There is marked inflammation of the mucosa with congestion.
2. **Nodular stage:** The granuloma appears and is seen as a tumor like swelling with central caseation (***tuberculoma***). This usually affects the septum, which is swollen bilaterally.
3. **Ulcerative stage:** The swelling subsequently ruptures with ulceration and may perforate the cartilaginous septum.
4. **Cicatrization stage:** The lesion heals with fibroblastic proliferation with subsequent cicatrization, stenosis and adhesion.

HISTOPATHOLOGY

The lesion is characterized by presence of epitheloid cells, ***Langhan's gaint cells*** and extensive caseation. Acid-fast bacilli are present in the granuloma. Biopsy confirms the diagnosis.

Clinical Features

Symptoms

- Discharge—Serosanguinous nasal discharge. It may be blood stained at the later stages.
- Nasal obstruction due to swelling of the nasal septum and subsequent stenosis. Crusting of the lesion increases the nasal obstruction.
- Pain is seen in the ulcerative stage due to exposed nerve endings.

Signs (Fig. 32.1)

- Bright red nodular thickening of the septum with or without ulcer.
- Perforation may be present in the cartilaginous septum.
- Adhesions and stenosis may be seen due to cicatrization.

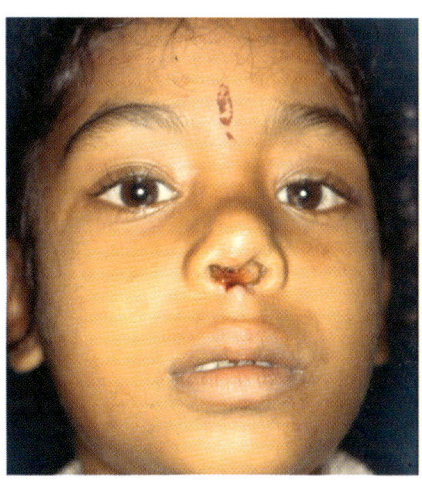

Fig. 32.1: Tubercular lesion of the nose involving the columella and the septum. There is loss of skin and cartilage in the affected part

Investigation

- Biopsy of the nodular or ulcerative mass
- Swab may show the acid-fast bacilli. Culture may be helpful in doubtful cases.
- Other tests may be done to rule out pulmonary focus, like chest X-ray, sputum for AFB, ESR, Montoux test, etc.
- X-ray—PNS may show secondary sinusitis.

Treatment

Antitubercular drugs (Rifampicin, ethambutol/ streptomycin, isoniazid, pyrazinamide) may be given for a minimum period of 6 months and the patient is evaluated at regular intervals.

Surgical reconstruction may be required for vestibular stenosis or other cicatrisation changes, once the patient is disease free.

Lupus of the Nose

It is an indolent and chronic form of tuberculosis infection.

Female: male ratio is 2:1. Commonest site of involvement is mucocutaneous junction.

Pathology (Fig. 32.2)

Granuloma formation is seen in the vestibular region with subsequent fibrosis and cicatrization and stenosis of the nasal cavity. External nose and face may be affected.

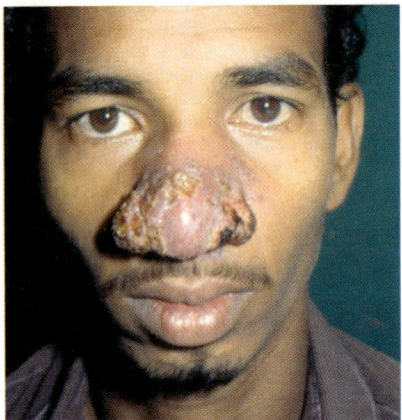

Fig. 32.2: Lupus of the nose

Clinical Features

- Deformity of the nose
- 'Butter fly appearance' of the facial skin

Symptoms

- Foul smelling nasal discharge
- Crusting
- Nasal obstruction
- Epistaxis
- Nasal deformity due to ulceration, fibrosis and distortion of ala nasi, nasal tip and nasal vestibule.

Signs

- Typical lesion is a reddish brown gelatinous nodule
- Cutaneous lesion involving the external nose has a typical *butterfly appearance*.
- Stenosis of the nasal cavity and perforation in the cartilaginous part of the nasal septum
- Crust formation

Diagnosis

1. Diascopy – Blood is squeezed out of the surrounding tissue with a glass slide by applying pressure on the skin thus making a reddish brown nodule more evident by contrast (*apple jelly nodule*).
2. Bacteriological examination of nasal discharge and sputum.
3. Biopsy – Typical tubercle with sparse caseation necrosis
4. Mantoux test is strongly positive
5. Chest X-ray – To rule out pulmonary tuberculosis.

Complication

1. Atrophic rhinitis
2. Chronic dacryocystitis
3. Lupus of the face and nasopharynx

Treatment

Specific Anti-tubercular drugs as a short course may be given for a period of 6 months.

- Calciferol (Vit D2) 1,50,000 U/day for 6-9 months
- Reconstructive surgery of residual nasal deformity may be done after the arrest of the disease.

Leprosy of Nose (Hansen's Disease)

It is a chronic granulomatous infection which attacks the skin, peripheral nerves and mucous membranes (eyes, respiratory tract). It is more common in warm, wet areas like the tropical and subtropical countries. Leprosy is also known as Hansen's disease because the bacillus which causes it was discovered by G.A. Hansen in 1873.

Etiology

Causative agent – *Mycobacterium leprae*. This is common in Asia, Africa and Central/ south America

Mode of Transmission

- Prolonged human to human contact.

- Droplet infection can occur in active stage of the disease (rhinitis).

Pathology

Types: Tuberculoid, lepromatous and borderline (intermediate)

Site of Involvement

Superficial peripheral nerves, skin, mucous membranes of the upper respiratory tract, anterior chamber of the eyes, and testes.

These areas tend to be cooler parts of the body.

Pathophysiology

Reduced cell-mediated immunity enhances spread and multiplication of the lepra bacilli. Associated immunological reactions (ie, lepra reactions) leads to tissue damage including the nerves.

Histopathology

A nodule shows perivascular cellular infiltration of the tissue and contains vacuolated giant cells and bacilli arranged in parallel bundles.

Clinical Features

Catarrhal stage: Usually associated by coryza due to the bacterial infiltration following nose picking into the septum by the finger nail. This is the most infective stage of the disease. Symptoms include sneezing, rhinorrhea and nasal obstruction. The discharge is often profuse serous/ mucoid.

Nodular stage: Nodular thickening of the affected area in the septum occurs usually after an interval of 10 years. Features of *secondary atrophic rhinitis* may be seen in the nasal cavity (Fig. 32.3).

Ulcerative stage: The nodule ulcerates leading to *septal perforation* which progresses further leading to complete destruction of the nose. Palate and the larynx may be involved. Loss of skeletal framework can lead to *saddle nose*

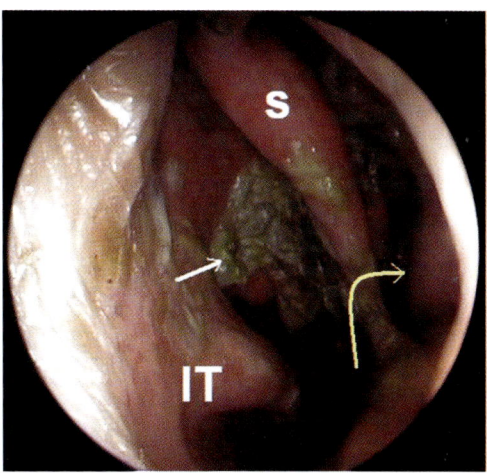

Fig. 32.3: Nasal endoscopic photograph showing secondary atrophic rhinitis (white arrow) and septal perforation (yellow arrow) in a case of leprosy. Septum (S); Inferior turbinate (IT)

deformity. Ulceration usually produces fetid, blood stained nasal discharge and may be associated with crusting. Nasal obstruction may be seen due to the crusts/ granuloma.

Cicatrization stage: Affected area can undergo fibrosis and may lead to stenosis of the vestibule.

Diagnosis

This is based on biopsy, tissue scrapping and smear for acid-fast bacilli and by Lepramin test.

Treatment

Medical: Clofazimine, rifampicin and dapsone for long periods

Surgical: Plastic reconstruction may be done once the patient is disease free.

Rhinoscleroma

Syn: Mikulicz disease

It is a granulomatous condition of the respiratory tract often affecting the external nose and nasal cavity caused by ***Klebsiella rhinoscleromatis***.

Etiology

- Young adults (second/ third decade) are commonly affected.
- Females are more often affected
- Endemic areas—Eastern Europe, South America, Middle East, Africa, some parts of India and Indonesia
- This condition is more common in lower socio-economic status. Probably poor nutrition and hygiene plays a role in its causation.
- Causative agent is *Klebsiella rhinoscleromatis* (**Frisch Bacillus**), a capsulated gram-negative coccobacillus.

Pathogenesis

Exact mode of infection is not known. Air borne infection is suspected. Direct inhalation of the droplets or contaminated material is said to be the mode of transmission. Patients are usually immunologically normal, however cellular immunity may be impaired. Ineffective phagocytosis of the organism by the **Mikulicz cells** has been noted. Mucopolysaccharides of the bacterial capsule probably contribute to inhibition of phagocytosis

Pathology

Gross

Vestibule of the nose is often first affected. It can occur in nose, pharynx, larynx, trachea, etc. Hence this condition is also called scleroma respiratorium.

Lesion has a characteristic woody feeling on palpation.

Histopathology

Bacteria may be seen by special stains like PAS, Giemsa, Gram, and silver stains. The characteristic histologic features are:

1. Accumulation of plasma cells, lymphocytes and eosinophils in submucosa.

2. Engulfment of bacilli by scattered macrophages leads to the formation of large foam cells (Mikulicz cells) that are found containing Frisch bacilli which are found in the prodromal stage of the disease.
3. Presence of Russell bodies–vacuolated cytoplasm with nucleoli.

Microbiology

Klebsiella rhinoscleromatis is a gram-negative, encapsulated, nonmotile, diplobacillus member of the family Enterobacteriaceae. A positive culture in MacConkey agar medium is diagnostic of rhinoscleroma but the cultures are positive in only 50 percent of the cases.

Clinical Features

It depends on the stages, which are as follows.

1. **Prodromal/catarrhal stage:** It is associated with infiltration and congestion of nasal mucosa. It mainly presents as purulent rhinorrhea that can be mistaken for common cold.
2. **Atrophic stage:** It follows the catarrhal stage. Nasal block is the main presenting feature. It is frequently associated with crusting and atrophic changes. Epistaxis may be present.
3. **Nodular stage/Granulomatous stage:** Multiple rubbery nodules non-ulcerative are formed which appears pale and rubbery. These nodules coalesce together to form pale and hard granuloma. Severe cases may lead to broadening of the nose due to thickening of the skin with characteristic **'Hebra nose'**. Laryngeal involvement may cause dyspnea/stridor (Fig. 32.4).
4. **Stage of cicatrization:** Fibrosis of the involved area may lead to vestibular stenosis, nasopharyngeal stricture, stenosis of pharynx, larynx, etc. The fibrotic deformity of the extenal nose is called the 'Tapir nose'.

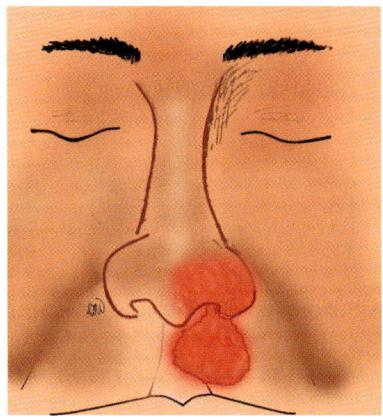

Fig. 32.4: Nodular lesion involving the vestibule and extending to the external nose and adjacent upper lip- 'Hebra nose'

Complications of the Disease

Disease can extend to the sinuses, lacrimal sac, nasopharynx, trachea and main bronchi of the respiratory tract. Spread to the lymph node may be present and can cause blockade of the lymphatic system. Bone may be extensively involved. Malignant changes can occur rarely.

Diagnosis

1. Classical clinical presentation should raise the suspicion
2. Histopathology confirms the diagnosis.

Treatment

Prolonged antibiotic course with tetracycline/ streptomycin/ Amoxicillin may be given for 6 to 8 weeks. Tetracycline is the drug of choice. Ciprofloxacin and rifampicin has also been found to be effective. Steroids help in reducing acute inflammatory reaction. Stenosis may be released by laser after the medical treatment.

Some with variable success have tried radiotherapy for this condition.

Nasal reconstruction may be done after achieving complete resolution of the disease.

Syphilis of Nose

This is a spirochetal infection caused by *Treponema pallidum*. The commonest form of syphilis manifestation in the nose is tertiary syphilis associated with 'Gumma'.

Stages of Syphilis

- Primary
- Secondary
- Tertiary

Primary

It presents as a hard, non-painful, ulcerated papule called the 'chancre'. This is often solitary swelling or an ulcer with indurated edges. This is associated with an enlarged rubbery node 3 to 4 wks after contact. The lesion disappears spontaneously.

Secondary

This occurs 6 to 10 weeks after inoculation. This is the most infective form of syphilis and one has to be very careful during examination of ENT.

Symptoms

Features of simple catarrhal rhinitis associated with rhinorrhea and crusting. Non-pruritic maculopapular eruptions in the skin and mucosa.

Signs

The presenting feature is mucocutaneous patch. The patch may be seen in the nose, oral cavity and the pharynx. Anterior rhinoscopy shows features of rhinitis.

Crusting and fissuring of nasal vestibule is often seen.

Tertiary

Pathology

The presenting lesion is known as *'Gumma'*. It affects the bony part of the nose. Commonest site is the septum. It can lead to septal and palatal perforation and collapse of the nasal bridge due to destruction. Commonli involves the mucous membrane, periosteum and bone.

Histologically it is characterized by edema, infilteration of the stroma with lymphocytes, plasma cells, and endothelial cells. Perivascular cuffing may be present with endarteritis, which leads to necrosis and ulceration.

Symptoms

- Pain and headache which become worst at night
- Offensive nasal discharge
- Bleeding and crusting

Signs

- Swelling of the bony part of the septum, perforation may be seen
- Gumma appears as ulcers with *'wash-leather'* floor.
- Presence of scarring and crust formation in the posterior part of the nasal cavity with features of *secondary atrophic rhinitis*.
- Saddle nose deformity may be present.

Congenital Syphilis

Infant snuffles

At birth – the child presents as simple catarrhal rhinitis

Secondary fissuring and excoriation of the nasal vestibule.

Delayed:

- At puberty – Gumma formation
- Saddle nose deformity
- Other stigmata of syphilis

Treatment

Adults

- Injection procaine, penicillin 1gm I.M. for 10–15 days
- Benzathine penicillin 1.8 gm I.M. 1–3 injections at weekly intervals
- Doxycycline 100mg orally t.d.s for 21 days
- Amoxycillin 3.0gm twice daily for 14 days (with 1gm probenecid orally daily)

Congenital Syphilis

- Benzyl penicillin 50 mg/kg I.M.I. or I.V.I. in 2 divided doses for 10 days
- Procaine penicillin 50 mg/kg I.M.I. for 10 days

RHINOSPORIDIOSIS

Definition

Rhinosporidiosis is a chronic granulomatous infection of the mucous membranes caused by *Rhinosporidium seeberi* and it manifests as vascular friable polyps that arise from the nasal mucosa or mucosal surfaces including nasopharynx, larynx, pharynx, trachea, conjunctiva, etc and rarely the skin.

Malignant rhinosporidiosis is described as disseminated form of the disease with systemic involvement.

History

First described by Guillermo Seeber in 1900 in a patient in Argentina. It is endemic in India, Srilanka, Africa and South America

Ashworth described the life cycle of the organism in 1923.

Etiology (Fig. 32.5)

This is caused by *Rhinosporidium seeberi*, which was thought to be a fungus. Molecular biological

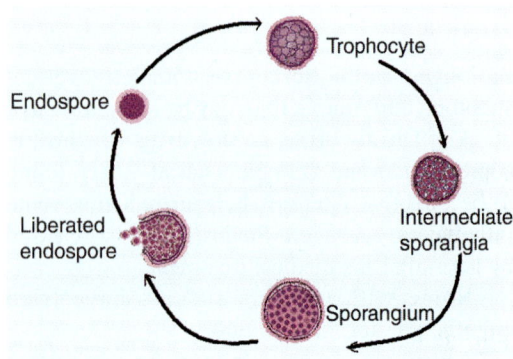

Fig. 32.5: Life cycle of *Rhinosporidium seeberi*

techniques have more recently demonstrated that this organism is an aquatic protistan parasite. It is currently included in a new class, the Mesomycetozoea, along with organisms that cause similar infections in amphibians and fish.

More common in young males (15–40 years of age)

Mode of Transmission

- Water borne: This is the Commonest route of transmission. It is common in farmers and country dwellers and was thought to be due to bathing in infected ponds used to bathe animals like cattle, horse, etc. The spores get deposited in the traumatized part of the nasal cavity/ other areas and continues its life cycle and produces sporangia.
- Air borne: Rare.

Pathology (Fig. 32.6)

Bleeding polyps with

1. Vascular fibromatous structure consisting of sporangia in various stages from trophocytes to mature sporangia
2. Mature sporangium is about 100-300 microns in size and contains numerous spores of 1.5 to 3 microns in size

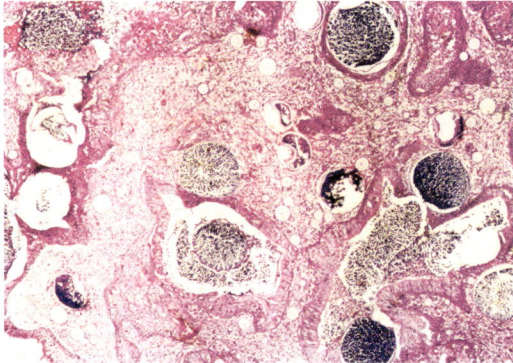

Fig. 32.6: Histopathology of rhinosporidiosis showing sporangia in different stages of development

3. Sporangium has a thick chitinous wall with an apical pore.

Symptoms

1. Epistaxis
2. Nasal obstruction
3. Postnasal drip
4. Hyposmia

Signs (Figs 32.7 and 32.8)

Present as a leaf like, pinkish granular mass with strawberry appearance and its surface is studded with whitish spots. The mass is friable pedunculated and bleeds on touch.

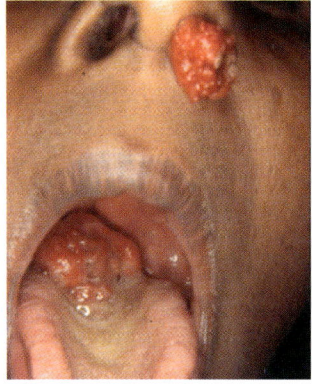

Fig. 32.7: Nasal and pharyngeal rhinosporidiosis

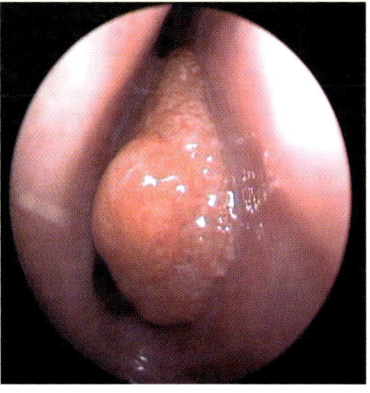

Fig. 32.8: Endoscopic picture showing rhinosporidial mass in the nasal cavity

Diagnosis is based on clinical features and it can be confirmed by biopsy and histopathological examination.

Investigation

Nasal endoscopy is help in locating the site of attachment.

Treatment

Recurrence is common. Complete excision of the mass with cauterization of the base offers the best satsfactory mode of treatment. Results of laser excision are promising.

Midline Non-healing Granuloma

Two main types are seen

- Wegener's granulomatosis
- Stewart's (idiopathic midline destructive diseases) granuloma

Wegener's Granulomatosis

It is an autoimmune condition with systemic manifestation involving the nasal cavity and the respiratory tract. The condition is associated with a generalized vasculitis and a focal form of glomerular nephritis.

Clinical features depend on the staging and site of involvement. The nasal cavity is often the first site to be involved.

The various stages are

- **Stage I:** Ulceration and crusting of the nose gradually involving the upper respiratory tract
- **Stage II:** Involvement of the lower respiratory tract with more systemic symptoms eg: hemoptysis and cavity formation on chest X-ray
- **Stage III:** Multiple organ failure

Manifestations in the Nose and Paranasal Sinuses

1. Associated epistaxis, nasal obstruction, excessive crusting with blood stained discharge, septal destruction and nasal collapse
2. There is no other condition which can give larger crusts than Wegener's granulomatosis.
3. There is no gross destruction of the mid-facial skin as seen in Stewart's granuloma (nasal T-cell lymphoma) and basal cell carcinoma.

Pulmonary Manifestations

- Cough, hemoptysis, pleuritic pain, cavities in the lungs (on chest X-ray), etc.

Renal Manifestations

- Urine microscopic picture shows casts and red cells. Patients often have impaired renal function.

Otological Manifestations

- Otitis media—with Conductive and/or sensorineural deafness.

Oral Manifestations

- Hyperplastic granular lesions of gingival

Laryngotracheal Manifestations

- Laryngotracheal stenosis and obstruction.

Other Manifestations

- Skin ulceration, conjunctivitis, polyarthritis, polymyalgia, etc.

Investigation

1. ESR
2. Urine microscopy – For casts and red cells
3. Chest X-ray – Cavity formation
4. ANCA test (Anti–Neutrophil Cytoplasmic Antibody test)–Negative does not rule out Wegener's granulomatosis
   It is 90 percent sensitive in type 3 (systemic vasculitis)
   65 percent sensitive in type 1 and 2

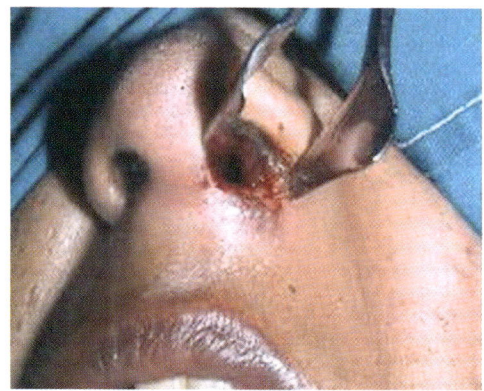

Fig. 32.9: Wegener's granuloma presenting as a non healing ulcer involving the nasal vestibule and floor of the nasal cavity

30 percent sensitive in complete remission Positive denotes microscopic polyanginitis
5. Biopsy – Should be deep and from the margin of the ulcer of the nasal cavity involving both healthy and involved tissue.
   Features seen are: Vasculitis, which is mandatory for diagnosis, fibrinoid vascular necrosis, evidence of granuloma
6. If biopsy comes as negative then drill biopsy can be done and if necessary a kidney biopsy can also be taken.

Differential Diagnosis

- Nasal drug abuse like cocain snif, people who use snuff
- Sinonasal lymphoma.

Treatment

- Prednisolone – 60 to 80mg/day for 3 mth
- Cyclophosphamide – 2mg/kg body weight
- Zathioprine – 200mg/day
- Cotriamoxazole DS—Once daily for indefinite period.

Stewart's granuloma (Lethal midline granul ma)

It is also known as midfacial lymphoma. It is a rare T-cell lymphoma that gradually ulcerates the cartilage and bone of the nose and mid-face.

Synonyms

Non-healing midline granuloma, lethal midline granuloma, Stewart's granuloma, midline granuloma syndrome (Pleomorphic), midline malignant reticulosis

Depending on the mode of presentation it can be divided into three types

1. Generalized lymphoma of the sinonasal tract
2. Malignant lymphoma of the Waldeyer's ring.
3. Peripheral sinonasal T-cell lymphoma-responsible for the slow-growing progressive destruction of the nose and paranasal sinuses.

On Examination

Complete destruction of the mid-facial region can be noted.

Investigation

- Biopsy most often reports as inconclusive because of massive necrosis of the tissue.
- Deep and repeat biopsy may often be necessary to get a proper diagnosis.
- Nasal T-cell lymphomas should be considered as a distinct clinicopathological entity, strongly associated with EBV, and with cytotoxic features in most cases. No prognostic parameters were detected to predict dissemination and response to therapy.

Treatment

Treatment of choice is with radiotherapy and surgical excision of necrotic tissue.

Difference between Wegener's and Sinonasal lymphoma is given in Table 32.1.

Table 32.1: Differences between Wegener's granulomatosis and sinonasal lymphoma

Wegener's granulomatosis	Sinonasal lymphoma
• Diffuse ulceration	• Focal ulceration
• Pulmonary and renal involvement is common	• Rare
• Histopathological examination—Vasculitis	• Pleomorphic lymphoid infiltration and angio-invasive features

POINTS TO REMEMBER

1. Tuberculosis of the nose commonly affects the cartilaginous part of the nasal septum.
2. Lupus of the nose commonly affects the nasal vestibule. It is an indolent and chronic form of tuberculosis.
3. Leprosy of the nose commonly affects the cartilaginous part of the nasal septum and anterior nasal spine.
4. Rhinoscleroma commonly affects the vestibule of the nose and the lesion has a characteristic woody feeling.
5. Rhinosporidiosis is a chronic granulomatous infection caused by Rhinosporidium seeberi/ Rhinosporidium kineli. The organism is now included under the class Mesomycetozea.
6. Wegener's granulomatosis is an autoimmune condition associated with systemic manifestation. The condition is associated with generalized vasculitis.
7. Stewart's granuloma is a rare form of nasal T-cell lymphoma.

Vasomotor Rhinitis

33

Definition

It is a chronic condition of the nasal cavity associated with nasal blockage and rhinorrhea as a result of an imbalance in the autonomic system with parasympathetic over activity (Fig. 33.1).

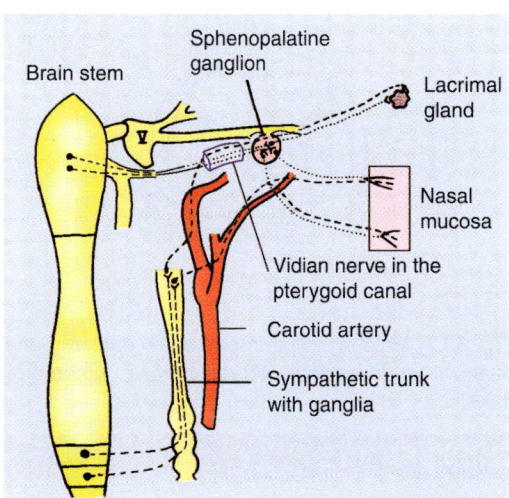

Fig. 33.1: Autonomic supply to the nasal cavity

Etiology

Predisposing Factors

1. **Age:** Common in younger age group.
2. **Sex:** Women with vasomotor rhinitis have

been shown to have higher rates of anxiety and depression when compared to healthy women without rhinitis.

3. Heredity
4. Infection
5. Constitutional make-up
6. Psychological
7. Endocrine
8. Sensitive loci in the nasal mucosa
9. Septal deflection
10. Drugs, etc.

Precipitating Factors

1. Atmospheric change
2. Fumes, inhaled irritants and strong odors
3. Alcohol
4. Reflex
5. Stress

Pathology

- Nasal mucous membrane is normal unlike allergic rhinitis, where it is swollen.
- Turbinates may be hypertrophied due to sinusoidal engorgement in the erectile tissue.

Clinical Features

- Sneezing is most frequently associated with exciting factors like exposure to cold, emotional disturbances, etc.

- Rhinorrhea is the most predominant symptom
- Alternating nasal obstruction
- Patients with profuse rhinorrhea and those with predominant nasal congestion are known by using the terms runners and blockers, respectively.
- Postnasal drip

Signs (Figs 33.2 and 33.3)

- Nasal mucosa appears to be normal and shining.
- It can be sometimes congested.
- The turbinates are usually hypertrophied
- Posterior end of inferior turbinate may be grossly hypertrophic to give a 'Mulberry appearance'.

Differential Diagnosis

- Allergic rhinitis
- Infective rhinitis

Treatment

Medical

- Avoidance of the precipitating factors.
- Antihistamines
- Decongestants are less satisfactory and prolonged use can cause rhinitis medicamentosa.
- Ipratropium bromide nasal spray helps to control rhinorrhea.
- It is used to reduce the excessive nasal secretions and can be used for prolonged period but can cause excessive dryness of the nasal mucosa and epistaxis.

Surgical

1. Reduction in the size of the turbinates may be done by submucosal diathermy, cryotherapy, bipolar cauterization, laser turbinoplasty, partial turbinectomy, etc.
2. Vidian neurectomy is done in refractory cases, which can be approached through the maxillary antrum.

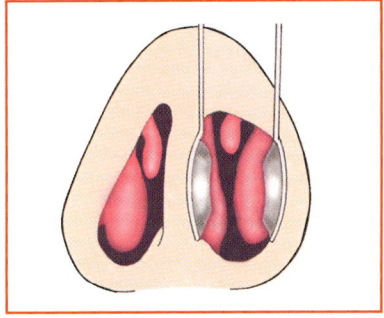

Fig. 33.2: Hypertrophic turbinates with normal mucosa in vasomotor rhinitis

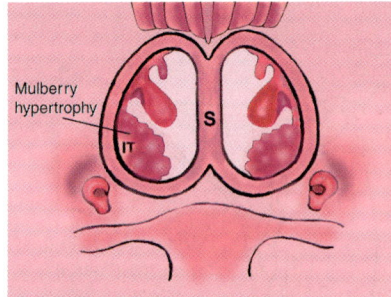

Fig. 33.3: Mulberry hypertrophy of the posterior end of the inferior turbinate (IT) in chronic vasomotor rhinitis

POINTS TO REMEMBER

1. Vasomotor rhinitis is due to overactivity of the parasympathetic system.
2. Alternating nasal obstruction, early morning rhinorrhea are its characteristic symptoms.
3. Precipitating factors include climate changes, exercise and emotional factors and endocrine changes.
4. Nasal mucosa appears normal but may be sometimes congested. Mulberry Hypertrophy of the turbinate are seen in long standing cases.
5. Vidian neurectomy is the surgical treatment of choice. Turbinate reducing procedures are also helpful.

Allergic Rhinitis

34

Definition

It is an acute IgE mediated, type-1 hypersensitivity reaction of nasal mucosa in response to antigenic substance [allergen] associated with episodic attacks of sneezing, watery rhinorrhea and watering of the eyes. Patient may also present with tightness of chest due to subclinical bronchospasm.

Types

1. Seasonal
2. Perennial
3. Mixed

Etiology

Allergic rhinitis is the commonest chronic disease. Its causation is multifactorial. Manifestation is multifocal. The symptom of patient and the type of allergy depends on a number of factors.

Precipitating Factors

(a) *Aerobiological flora:* This is determined by the allergens present in that environment of which inhalant allergen is more common.
(b) *Nasal physiology:* Altered nasal cycle.

Predisposing Factors

(a) *Age:* Patient with any age are susceptible for allergy. However, young patients are more affected. About 70 percent of the cases present with symptoms of nasal allergy before 30 years of age (Yadav et al).
(b) *Sex:* Males are more commonly affected with male to female ratio of about 3:2. Some report equal predilection.
(c) *Industrialization and urbanization:* Incidence of allergic rhinitis is ever increasing because of industrialization and urbanization responsible for environment pollution. Reported incidence of allergic rhinitis is 1.4 to 39.7 percent of population in the western countries. In UK there is four-fold increase in incidence of allergic rhinitis in last thirty years.
(d) *Genetic predisposition* plays a significant role in allergic manifestation. Chances of getting allergic rhinitis are more if one or more parents are suffering from allergy.
(e) *Focal sensitivity* of nasal mucosa can trigger the allergic reaction.
(f) *IgA deficiency* state makes the patient more prone for allergy.
(g) *Psychological factors*
(h) *Living conditions:* Residential and workplace conditions play a significant role in the etiology. Crowding, dusty environ-ment, air-conditioned rooms may predispose. Dust may accumulate in the carpets, curtains, bed sheets, bookshelves, store shelves, etc. and its exposure may precipitate the allergic response in genetically predisposed individuals. Allergy may be an

occupational hazard wherein the individual is exposed to allergen in his workplace. Example: Librarian, storekeeper, factory worker, etc.

(i) ***Environmental factors:*** Depends on the aerobiological flora of the particular environment. Climatic conditions including season, altitude can affect the manifestation of the symptoms. Based on this the allergic manifestations may be classified into

(a) Seasonal and

(b) Perennial allergic rhinitis.

In seasonal allergic rhinitis, the symptoms are more in a particular season. Example: Pollens in spring, fungus in rainy season, etc. In perennial the symptoms are present throughout the year. Common examples: House dust mite, pets, etc. (Fig. 34.1)

Common Allergens

I. Inhalant – Commonest cause.

(a) Pollen and dust including house dust mite – 75 percent

(c) Fungus

(d) Animal dander

(e) Miscellaneous

II. Food allergy:

Egg, sea food, etc.

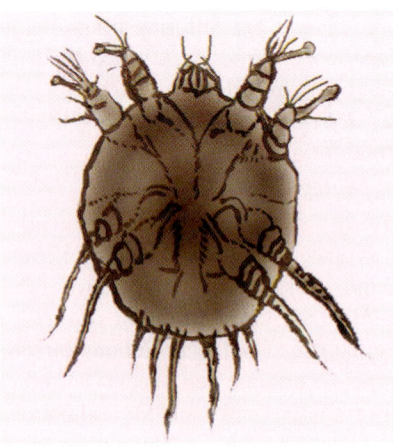

Fig. 34.1: House dust mite

Pathophysiology

Primary Response

This is also called 'Priming'. After initial exposure to the allergen (antigen), in genetically predisposed individual, specific antibody is produced which gets fixed to the mast cells and basophils. This sensitizes the nasal mucosa to this allergen. Allergic challenge occurs in less than 24 hrs and the reversal starts 48 hrs after. It is mainly mediated by histamine.

Local Phenomenon

It occurs in response to the chemical mediators leading to mucosal edema associated with sneezing

Key to abbreviation

PCI–Prostaglandin E

SRS–A–Slow reacting substance of anaphylaxis.

ECF–Eosinophils chemo tactic factor

NCF–Neutroplulic chemo tactic factor. and rhinorrhea.

Non-specific Response

It occurs due to non-specific stimuli like pollutants, salicylates, cold weather, air-conditioning, etc. This can initiate a response similar to priming and can precipitate symptoms.

Mechanism of allergic rhinitis is given in (Fig. 34.2).

Clinical Features

Symptoms

The symptoms may be seasonal or perennial. All symptoms are simply a manifestation of the body's defense mechanism to the allergen.

Classical: Mainly seen in seasonal allergic rhinitis. This includes paroxysmal bouts of sneezing, watery rhinorrhea and nasal obstruction with itching of the nose on exposure to known or unknown allergen. This may be associated by non-nasal manifestations like watering and itching of the eyes, itching of the palate and skin and in some

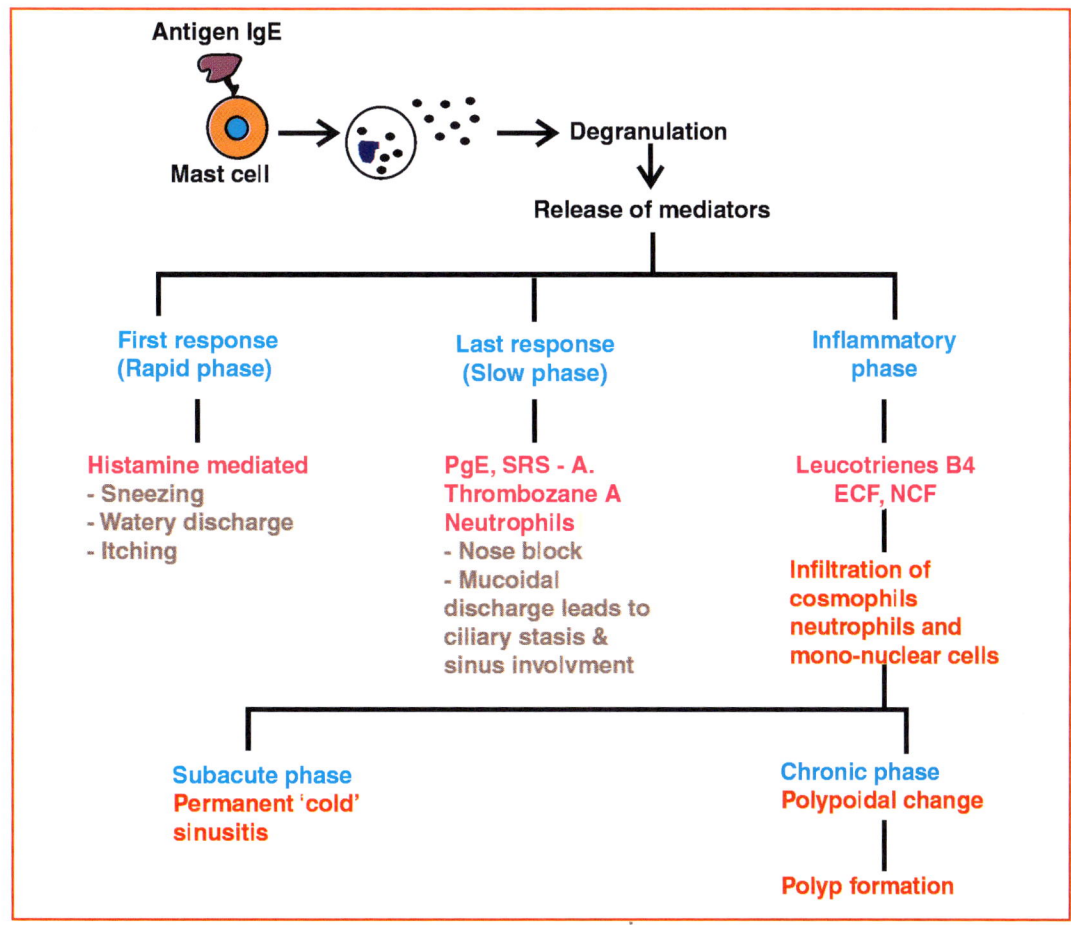

Fig. 34.2: Mechanism of allergic rhinitis. Prostaglandin E (PGI); Slow reacting substance of anaphylaxis (SRS-A); Eosinophilic chemotactic factor (ECF); Neutrophilic chemotactic factor (NCF)

it may be associated with bronchospasm, which may be subclinical. Patient may complain of hyposmia or anosmia depending on the severity of the disease.

In perennial allergy the symptoms are usually less severe and may present as recurrent 'cold' or nasal stuffiness with sneezing and watery rhinorrhea.

Signs
- Pale bluish edematous nasal mucosa (Fig. 34.3)

- Bulky edematous turbinates with bluish/ purplish tinge of the mucosa.
- Mucosa coated with clear/ mucoid secretions
- In advanced cases the mucosa of the middle turbinate may be polypoidal and frank polyposis may be seen in the middle meatus (Fig. 34.4).
- Septum may be thickened due to mucosal swelling.

Classical signs associated with allergic rhinitis
- Overriding maxillary incisors
- High arched palate

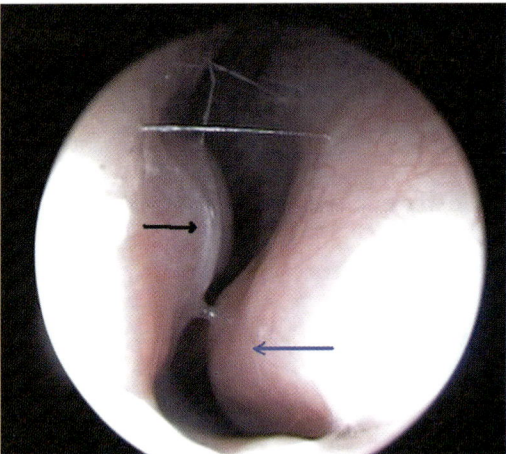

Fig. 34.3: Endoscopic picture showing the pale edematous turbinates with septal spur coated with clear mucoid secretions

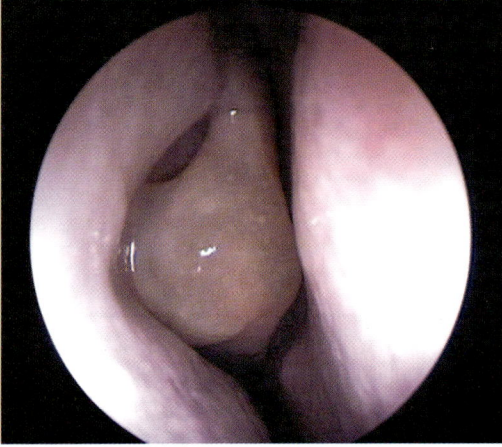

Fig. 34.4: Middle turbinate showing polypoidal changes

- Allergic shiners (Fig. 34.5)
- Allergic salute—Child frequently rubs the nose with his palm because of itching sensation.
- Transverse crease above the tip of nose and lower eyelids (Fig. 34.6)
- Conjunctival congestion
- Periorbital swelling

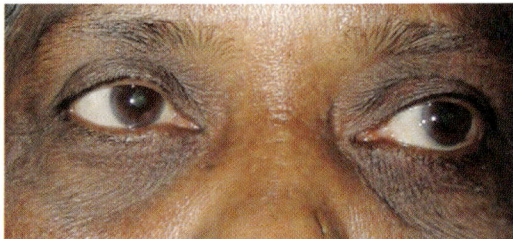

Fig. 34.5: Showing allergic shiners (dark circles around the eyes)

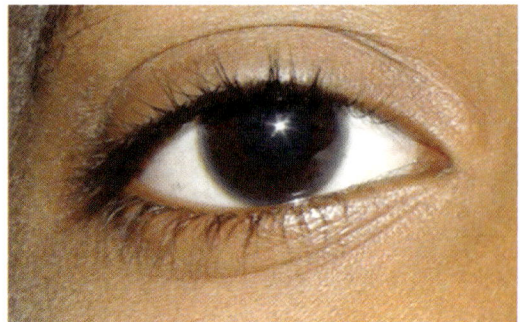

Fig. 34.6: Transverse crease below the lower eyelid (Dennies line)

Investigations

To Confirm Allergy

Non specific

- Nasal smear for eosinophils
- Total WBC count and differential count
- Absolute eosinophil count
- Histamine test

Specific (Qualitative and quantitative tests)

In vivo tests

- *Skin Tests*
  1. **Subcuticular test** (Prick/ scratch test): This is the most popular, practical and safe test. It may be used as a screening test. Prick test is more preferred. This test is more readily reproducible, has lower incidence of false positive results, is more accurate and has less risk of anaphylaxis. In this test, a drop of test extract solution

(allergen with histamine and saline as control) is placed on the unprepared skin of the medial aspect of forearm. Using a lancet at about 45 degrees to the skin, through the drop the epidermis is pricked with a lifting motion. Care is taken not to penetrate the dermis. The area is examined after 10 minutes for histamine control and after 20 minutes for the allergen. Wheal response around the prick is measured and compared with standardized scales. In India, Shivapuri criteria are used to quantify the severity of the wheal response. Prick test is contraindicated in cases with dermographism, patients with antihis-taminic, anti-inflammatory or decon-gestant treatment (Refer chapter 23 on clinical examination of nose and PNS).

2. *Intradermal skin test:* This has higher chances of anaphylaxis and has to be done only with resuscitation drugs and equipment ready.

3. *Skin end-point titration tests:* This is a quantitative intradermal skin test for specific allergen. This test is done using a dilute and known concentration of an allergen, which is injected intradermally, and the response is noted. The dose is increased gradually

- *Nasal Challenge (Nasal Provocation) Test:* Not a very popular test due to potential risks of anaphylaxis and has limited clinical applications. The test dose is delivered in a nebulizer using a specific allergen.

- *Nasal Cytology:*
It can be done using a dry wipe technique without surface anesthesia. The specimen is applied to the slide with a firm rolling action. The smear is fixed immediately with 95 percent alcohol and is stained with Wright-Giemsa stain. Following cell types are noted.

(i) Eosinophils
(ii) Mast cells/basophils/both
(iii) Epithelial cells
(iv) Lymphocytes
(v) Neutrophils
(vi) Goblet cells

In allergy, patients have increased eosinophils of more than 10 percent

In vitro Tests

1. *Radio-allergo-sorbant test (RAST):* This is very useful test especially in case with dermographism. This is less sensitive than skin prick test but is more expensive.

2. *Fluoro-allergo-sorbant test (FAST)*

3. *Paper immuno-allegro-sorbant test (PRIST)*

Other Tests

These are done to rule out associated sinus pathology and polyposis.

(a) X-ray PNS
(b) CT OMC
(c) Diagnostic nasal endoscopy.

Treatment

Medical

1. **Avoidance of Allergen**
This is ideal but is not always possible. Some of the known allergens can be avoided, like-paper dust, house dust, animal dander, etc., by avoiding pets, washing curtains regularly, keeping less articles in the living room, changing bed-sheets and pillow covers frequently, use of ironed bed sheets, pillow covers before use, use of mask/ nasal filters while cleaning the house, prefer vacuum cleaning or wet mopping to dry mopping, avoidance of carpets, etc., will control most of the aero-allergens effectively. Seasonal and environmental allergen can be avoided to certain extent by knowing and avoiding the aero-biological flora of that particular environment. Allergic skin tests may be useful in identifying the allergens.

2. Pharmacotherapy

(a) **Anti-histaminic:** This is the mainstay of treatment for allergic rhinitis, when avoidance of allergens is not possible. It is most preferred during the acute attack. These are basically H-1 receptor antagonists and block the effect of histamine on the receptors. Various anti-histamines are available and the recent ones like fexofenadine, loratidine, rupatidine levocetrizine, etc., have faster onset of action, longer duration and with less side-effects like sedation and cardiovascular changes and anti-cholinergic effects. Antihistamines like azelastine can be used as a nasal spray with no long term side effects.

(b) **Steroids:** They act by inhibiting the inflammatory reaction. Systemic steroids can be given in short course in seasonal or perennial allergic rhinitis. Steroid nasal sprays like beclomethasone, budesonide, fluticasone, mometasone, etc., are particularly useful as they have lesser side-effects and may be used for longer period. Reduction in middle meatal edema may facilitate drainage of the sinus secretions. Long term use may cause crusting and fungal colonization.

(c) **Sodium chromoglycate:** This stabilizes the mast cells and prevents its degranulation. It is available as nasal drops or nasal spray and is used for prophylaxis and therefore should be used regularly and before the attack.

(d) **Decongestants:** This is useful to reduce nasal obstruction and mucosal edema and rhinorrhea. Oral preparations are available with anti-histamines. Long term use of topical decongestants is best avoided as they can cause 'rhinitis medicamentosa' and should not be given for more than 4 to 5 days. Oral preparations include pseudoephidrine hydrochloride, phenylephrine hydro-chloride, etc. Topical decongestants include oxymetazoline, Xylometazoline, ephidrine in saline, etc.

(e) **Saline irrigation of the nasal cavities:** This helps in removing secretions and prevent secondary infection.

3. Immunotherapy

The role of immunotherapy is limited especially in case of multiple allergens. However, people with allergy to limited number of allergens may find it useful. It is effective only in about 40 percent of cases. It is administered by giving sub-cutaneous inactions in diluted form at weekly intervals. The dose is gradually increased till the optimal level is achieved. RAST/ skin end point titration based immunotherapy is more effective since the quantitative analysis can be done and the patient can receive higher dose without the fear of anaphylaxis. Hence they get an early response. Immunotherapy helps in reducing the specific serum IgE level and a decrease in basophil sensitivity and increase in IgG blocking antibody level which helps in preventing the allergen from reaching the mast cells and thus preventing their degranulation.

Surgical

Role of surgery is limited to reduction of the size of the turbinates, correction of septal deviation and limited endoscopic sinus surgery if sinuses are involved. The inferior and the middle turbinates are trimmed by infero-lateral partial resection using micro-debrider or turbinectomy scissors. Septal deviation should ideally be dealt with limited ultraconservative endoscopic approach. Limited sinus surgery with preservation of uncinate process may reduce postoperative postnasal discharge, which is often seen following traditional Functional endoscopic sinus surgery (FESS) for allergy associated chronic sinusitis (Nayak et al, 2001). Anti allergy treatment should continue even after surgical intervention.

POINTS TO REMEMBER

1. Allergic rhinitis is an IgE mediated type I hypersensitivity reaction of the nasal mucosa and antigenic substance (allergen).
2. Genetic predisposition play a significant role in allergic manifestation.
3. Pollen and house dusts are the common inhalant allergent (75%).
4. Prick test is the most popular, practical and safe test for nasal allergy screening.
5. Sodium chromoglycate prevents mast cell degranulation.

35

Sinusitis

DEFINITION

Sinusitis refers to inflammation of the mucosa of one or more paranasal sinuses where the mucociliary clearance function is affected as a result of anatomical or pathological abnormalities leading to blockage of the sinus ostium. Depending on the site of involvement, it can be described as:

- Frontal sinusitis
- Maxillary sinusitis
- Ethmoidal sinusitis
- Sphenoidal sinusitis
- Pansinusitis—All sinuses are involved which could be unilateral or bilateral.

In the past, sinusitis was addressed individually with respect to site. The etiopathogenesis, clinical features, investigations and treatment were individualistic. More emphasis was given to maxillary sinus as the most common site of infection. With clear understanding of ostiomeatal complex anatomy and its role in the pathogenesis of chronic sinusitis and with the availability of nasal endoscope and CT imaging for study of sinus pathology, the concept of sinus pathology and its treatment has changed rapidly. The intimate relationship of the sinus system to the nasal cavity and also that of upper and lower respiratory tracts, the role of ostiomeatal complex and middle meatus in the etiopathology of chronic infection of the major sinuses has been better understood and changed the treatment policy. Conventional procedures like intranasal antrostomy, Caldwell-Luc operation, etc. have become almost obsolete and are reserved only for irreversible disease. Present treatment is directed at the disease causation than the result. The ostiomeatal disease is endoscopically dealt with and the physiological sinusotomies are created. Example: middle meatal antrostomy for treatment of maxillary sinusitis, frontal recess clearance for frontal sinusitis, etc.

For this reason the etiopathogenesis and the management has been discussed in common. The clinical features of individual sinuses and their specific treatment have been discussed separately.

ETIOLOGY OF SINUSITIS (IN GENERAL)

Predisposing Factors

1. Mechanical obstruction
2. Focal infection
3. Decreased mucociliary function
4. Allergy
5. Immunodeficiency state
6. Autoimmune and hormonal imbalance
7. Granulomatous conditions
8. Iatrogenic.
9. Idiopathic.

I. Mechanical Obstruction

Anatomical and pathological obstruction in the region of the ostiomeatal complex leads to impaired mucociliary clearance, inadequate drainage of sinuses, stagnation of secretions and persistent secondary infection. Ethmoid is the key area in disease causation, which acts as a reservoir of infection, besides its pathological changes can lead to mechanical obstruction.

II. Focal Infection

1. Rhinogenic: Nasal infection is the most common cause for sinusitis. The causative agents can be viral, bacterial or fungal.
2. Adenotonsillitis.
3. Dental: Extraction, infection of roots (especially P2 and M1, 2).
4. Trauma: Injury/ Surgical/ Barotrauma/ Hemoantrum leading to bacterial infection.

III. Mucociliary Clearance Abnormality

- Primary ciliary dyskinesia: Kartageners, 1933 (Sinusitis + Azoospermia + Bronchiectasis).
- Disturbance of ciliary beating and immobility:
  - Young syndrome
  - Cilia abnormality
- Abnormal thick mucosa
- Secondary to viral URTI (upper respiratory tract infection)

IV. Allergy

Allergic rhinitis can cause mucosal edema and hyperplasia associated with blockage of ostium and stagnation of secretion, which further leads to secondary bacterial infection.

V. Immunodeficiency

Body defense mechanism is suppressed in:

1. AIDS
2. Polyhypogammaglobulinemia (Mackey et al, 1983)
3. Patients on immunosuppressive drugs
   - Anti-malignant CT
   - Long-term steroids.

VI. Autonomic Imbalance

Seen in conditions like:

- Emotional disturbances
- Stress (Lee 1981)
- Thermal changes, change in humidity
- Drug induced rhinitis

VII. Hormones

The hormonal changes in certain conditions can cause vasomotor imbalance, which can be responsible for sinusitis like:

- Pregnancy, puberty, menstruation
- Sexual excitement (Honeymoon rhinitis)
- Oral contraceptives. (Toppozadactel 1984)
- Myxoedema—Old mans drop.

VIII. Granulomatous Conditions

The nasal manifestations of various granulomatous conditions can usually present with rhinitis and secondary sinusitis as follows:

- Wegeners granulomatosis
- Sarcoidosis
- Amyloidosis
- Tuberculosis, leprosy, syphilis
- Rhinoscleroma
- Churg Strauss syndrome.

IX. Iatrogenic

- Rhinitis medicamentosa
- Aspirin intolerance
- Drugs–Guanethedine
- Neostigmine
- Isoprenaline
- Ergots

X. Idiopathic

Pathogenesis of Sinusitis

It can be described in three stages

I. Acute stage: This stage usually starts with an acute upper respiratory infection which is followed by secondary bacterial infection. The inflammatory process and pathological changes associated with sinusitis are:

- Leukocytic infiltration
- Release of chemical mediators
- Edema and vasodilatation of the submucosa
- Blockage of ostium.

II. Subacute stage: It occurs between 3 weeks to 3 months period if the acute sinusitis is not resolved completely or inadequately treated. It is associated with thick sinus secretion leading to postnasal discharge and nasal obstruction.

Pathological Changes

1. Infiltration of lymphocytes and proliferation of fibroblast.
2. Proliferation of immature cells.
3. Replacement of ciliated columnar epithelium with non-ciliated epithelium (reversible).

III. Chronic stage: Refers to persistent subacute infection in the sinuses for more than 3 months and usually involves the ostiomeatal complex.

Pathogenesis

1. Persistent venous and lymphatic obstruction.
2. Thick hyperplastic proliferation of mucosa with polypoidal changes.
3. Frank polyp formation in the middle meatus/ethmoids which blocks the ostium of major sinuses.
4. Pathological obstruction in middle meatus. and stagnation of sinus secretions setting a vicious cycle of infection within the ostiomeatal complex.

Pathology

- Epithelial hyperplasia
- Squamous metaplasia
- Increased number of goblet cells
- Edema and infiltration of inflammatory cells
- Ciliary damage
- Subepithelial interstitial fibroblastic prolifertation with lymphatic obstruction and frank polyposis.

CLINICAL FEATURES OF ACUTE SINUSITIS

Depends on the sinus involved.

Acute Frontal Sinusitis

Frequently acute infection of anterior ethmoidal cells causes obstruction of the frontal recess due to mucosal edema, which further leads to frontal sinusitis. Isolated frontal sinusitis is uncommon and most often the patients present with acute fronto-ethmoiditis.

Etiology

Infection is often rhinogenic in origin. Secondary bacterial infection usually follows a viral infection. For more details, refer to the general description of etiology and pathogenesis.

Symptoms

- Headache—Usually severe and periodic in nature and is confined to the frontal region. It starts in the morning and subsides in the afternoon and hence is called as 'office headache'. Bending, straining or coughing can precipitate this headache. In severe cases patients may complain of throbbing or pulsatile headache, which may be unbearable. It can be unilateral or bilateral. Usually it affects the medial canthus region and the root of the nose.
- Swelling of the upper eyelid may involve the forehead and orbit in severe cases. In children, acute ethmoiditis is more common and can present with orbital swelling.
- Nasal discharge is absent initially. It may later present as purulent and may be bloodstained on forceful blowing of the nose.
- Nasal obstruction may be present which may be unilateral or bilateral.
- Pyrexia may be present in severe cases.
- Anosmia or hyposmia is usually present due to mucosal edema and/or secretional obstruction.
- Altered taste sensation.
- Symptoms of otitis media or effusion may be present such as blocking sensation and deafness.

Signs

- Swollen nasal mucosa.
- Presence of pus high in the middle meatus

- Tenderness over the frontal bone, especially on the roof of the orbit and at a point medial to the supraorbital notch. Percussion on the anterior wall of the sinus can be painful.
- Edema of the upper eyelid.

Differential Diagnosis

1. Early herpes zoster infection involving the supraorbital nerve.
2. Erysipelas.
3. Insect bite.
4. Acute ethmoiditis.

Investigations

- **Diagnostic nasal endoscopy:** Shows discharge from the upper part of the middle meatus, edema of the uncinate process, attachment of the middle turbinate and bulla ethmoidalis at frontal recess.
- **CT scan of the Ostiomeatal complex:** This is the radiological investigation of choice. It may show fluid level, mucosal edema and involvement of the anterior ethmoids (Figs 35.1a and b).
- **X-ray PNS:** May show loss of bony definition in the superior frontal sinus margin in association with frontal sinus opacity.

Treatment

Medical: Main stay of treatment is medical.

- Broad spectrum antibiotic like amoxycillin with clavulanate is preferred. Metronidazole may be given if anaerobic infection is suspected.
- Observation for complications.
- Systemic decongestants like pseudo-ephedrine hydrochloride in combination of mucolytic like bromohexine promotes drainage.
- Local decongestants like oxymetazoline or xylometazoline should be instilled in head down forward position.
- Analgesics like aceclofenac can be given as anti-inflammatory and analgesic.

Surgical

This is limited for severe form of sinusitis with threatened complications or unbearable pain.

Frontal sinus trephination is indicated if the pain is severe and persistent in spite of antibiotic treatment. Endoscopic sinus surgery limited to frontal sinus may be done as an alternative procedure.

Endoscopic frontal recess clearance.

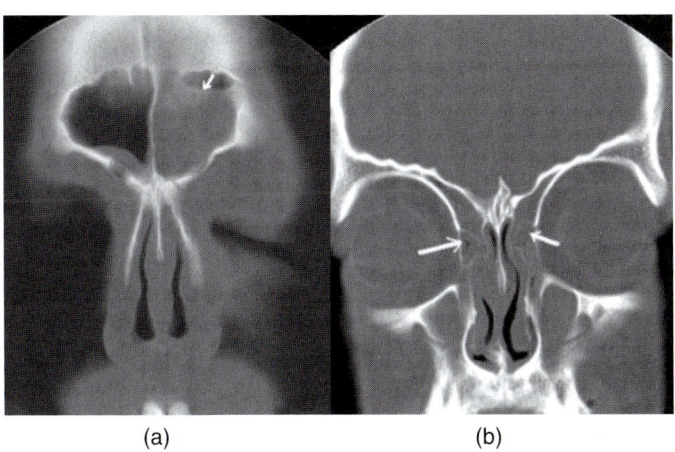

(a)   (b)

Figs 35.1a and b: (a) CT Showing acute frontal sinusitis with fluid level (Left), (b) Showing extensive disease in the frontal recess, ethmoid and maxillary sinus (acute pansinusitis)

Acute Maxillary Sinusitis

It is the most common form of sinusitis to present as a single entity. The infection is rhinogenic in origin in 90 percent of cases.

Etiology

The main etiological factors are as follows:

1. **Nasal infection:** Infection follows mostly after an attack of upper respiratory tract infection of viral etiology with secondary bacterial invasion.
2. **Dental infection**
   • Following dental extraction.
   • Following apical abscess.
   • An acute dental sac infection in infancy.

Clinical Features (Fig. 35.2)

• Pain over the check following upper respiratory infection, which may radiate to the teeth or the frontal region. Pain is aggravated on straining or bending forwards.
• Nasal discharge—This may be initially

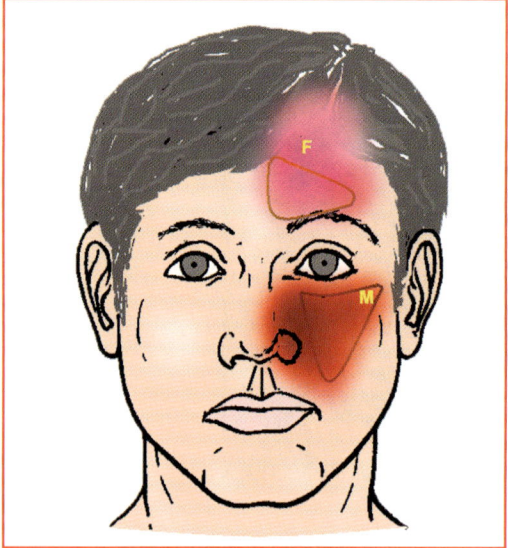

Fig. 35.2: Showing area of distribution of pain in frontal and maxillary sinusitis

absent. It later becomes purulent and blood-stained on forceful blowing of the nose.
• Nasal blockage.
• Sense of smell may be reduced or the patient may experience foul smell in the nose.
• Swelling over the cheek may be evident in children.
• Pyrexia may be present occasionally.

Signs

• Tenderness over the canine fossa.
• Edema of the cheek may be seen in children
• On anterior rhinoscopic examination, the nasal mucosa may be found to be swollen especially in the region of the middle meatus with associated mucopurulent discharge.
• Associated dental infection has to be ruled out, in such case there may be foul smelling and discharge in the nose due to anaerobic infection.
• Factors like deviated nasal septum, parado-xically curved middle turbinate, etc. contri-buting to the infection should be looked for.

Investigations

• Diagnostic nasal endoscopy.
• X-ray of PNS where the maxillary sinus may be found to be hazy. Rarely fluid level may be seen.
• Diagnostic proof puncture is less often being done presently, as better diagnostic tools are available (Fig. 35.3).
• CT imaging may show fluid level/comlete opacity and very useful in complicated cases, where the extent of disease can be evaluated and if fungal sinusitis is suspected (Fig. 35.4).

Treatment

• Medical treatment remains the mainstay of treatment. Infection of dental origin should be treated by antibiotic coverage for anaerobic infection.

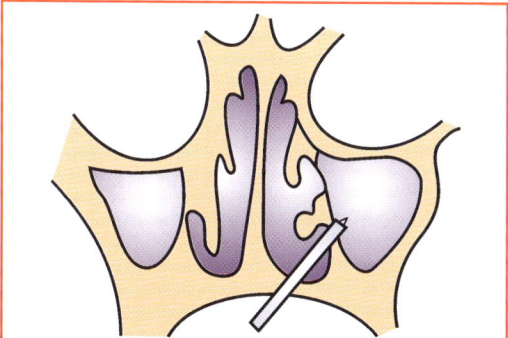

Fig. 35.3: Diagnostic proof puncture

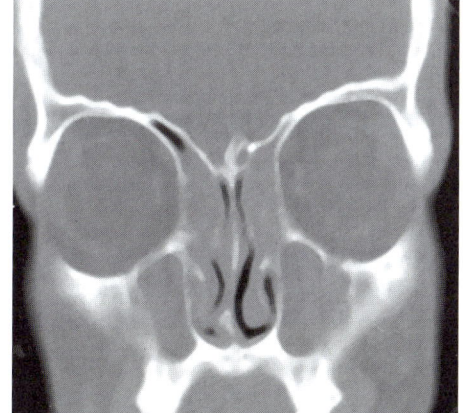

Fig. 35.4: Disease in the ethmoid and maxillary sinus

- Surgical intervention is done if the infection fails to resolve with the medical treatment. Middle meatal maxillary sinusostomy can be performed endoscopically to facilitate drainage through the natural ostium. Alternatively the maxillary sinus may be irrigated with isotonic saline by an antral puncture (Figs 35.5a and b).
- Infected tooth, if any, should be extracted/ treated.

Acute Ethmoiditis

It is the most common sinus involved in children. In adults, isolated acute ethmoiditis presenting as a separate clinical entity is rare.

Etiology

Same as the etiology described under sinusitis in general.

Clinical Features

Symptoms (Fig. 35.6)

- Pain between the eyes associated with frontal headache. Discharge may be present from the nose which is usually purulent.
- There may be postnasal drip which may be associated with nocturnal cough in children.

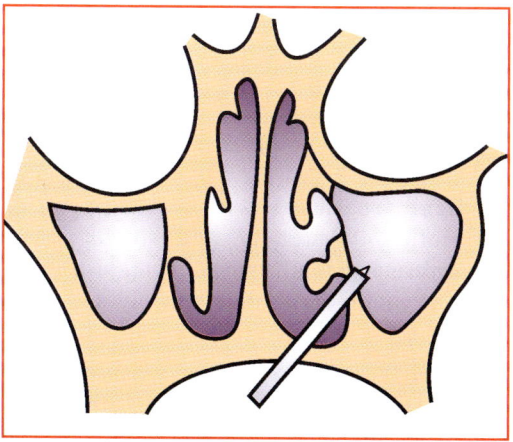

Fig. 35.5a: Antral puncture

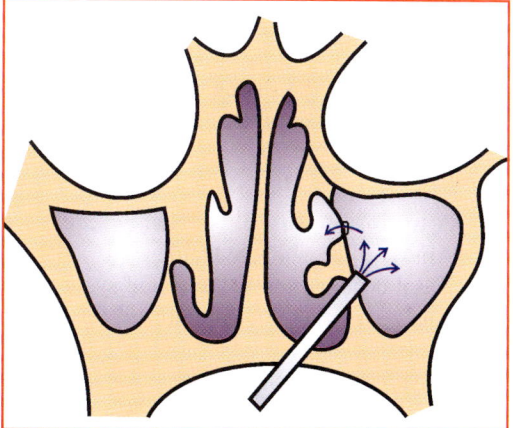

Fig. 35.5b: Irrigation of the antrum after removal of trocal, while keeping cannula in-situ

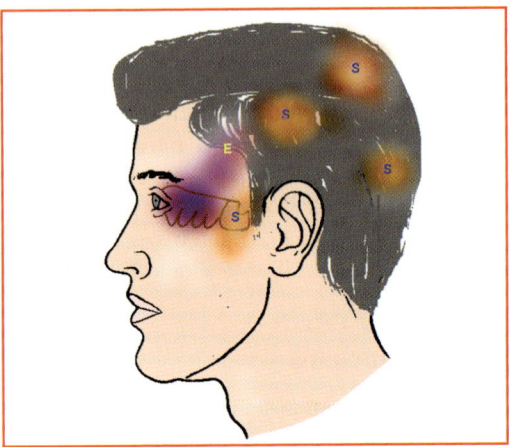

Fig. 35.6: Distribution of pain in ethmoidal sinusitis (E) and in sphenoidal sinusitis (S)

- Constitutional symptoms like fever and bodyache may be present particularly in children.

Signs

- Tenderness in the intercanthal region.
- Anterior rhinoscopy may reveal discharge from the middle meatus.
- Posterior rhinoscopy—Discharge from the middle meatus and superior meatus can be seen.

Investigations

- CT Scan of the ostiomeatal complex will show the extent of the disease.

Treatment

- Antibiotics for 3 weeks. Preferably Amoxycillin with clavulanic acid.
- Nasal decongestants: Local and systemic.
- Analgesics and anti-inflammatory agents.

Acute Spheniodal Sinusitis

Etiology

Isolated sphenoidal sinusitis is rare. It presents usually as part of 'pansinusitis', and sometimes can be associated due to infection involving the posterior ethmoids.

Pathology

As described earlier, it follows acute ethmoiditis. Occasionally fractures of the skull base involving the sphenoethmoids can give rise to secondary sinusitis.

Symptoms

Headache may be vertical, frontal, occipital or central. Occasionally the pain may radiate to the temporal region.

Postnasal drip and hawking may be present.

Signs

Posterior rhinoscopy: Presence of discharge from the superior meatus can be seen in posterior ethmoidal sinusitis and discharge above the superior turbinate, from the sphenoethmoidal recess in case of sphenoidal sinusitis. This is also seen flowing down the roof and posterior wall of the nasopharynx (Supratubal stream of discharge).

Investigation

CT scan imaging or Water's view with mouth open (Pierre's view) will show fluid level or mucosal edema of the sphenoid sinuses. Nasal endoscopy helps better visualization of the disease and discharge in the superior meatus/ sphenoethmoidal recess (Fig. 35.7).

Treatment

Medical treatment with broad-spectrum antibiotics, systemic and local nasal decongestants, anti-inflammatory, anti-histamines, nasal irrigation with saline, mucolytics, steam inhalation, etc. may be tried.

Surgical treatment: This is indicated if the disease is refractory to medical treatment. Endoscopically the anterior wall of the sphenoid sinus is perforated (endoscopic sphenoidotomy) to drain the sinus.

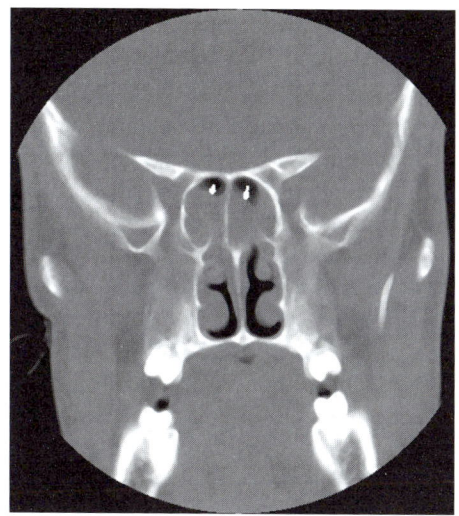

Fig. 35.7: CT coronal cut showing air fluid level in both sphenoidal sinuses suggestive of acute sphenoidal sinusitis

CHRONIC SINUSITIS

Chronic Maxillary Sinusitis

Etiology and pathogenesis: Same as described above under sinusitis.

In children, adenoid hypertrophy is a common associated factor.

Pathology

- Chronic inflammatory cellular infiltration around the vessels.
- Increased number of seromucinous glands and goblet cells.
- Fibrosis of lamina propria.
- Small multiple abscesses in the thickened mucosa.

Symptoms

- Headache is less severe than acute sinusitis and more evidenced towards afternoon.
- Nasal obstruction is usually persistent and more at night.
- Loss of taste and cacosmia.

- Reduced sense of smell.
- Nasal discharge is more viscid and mucoidal.
- Hawking sensation due to postnasal drip.

Signs

- Tenderness on percussion can be elicited over the canine fossa.
- Anterior rhinoscopy–Presence of discharge is seen in the middle meatus which is usually mucoid or mucopurlent.
- Posterior rhinoscopy–Discharge is seen in the middle meatus.

Investigation

- X-ray PNS will show haziness of the affected maxillary sinus with evidence of thickened mucosa (Figs 35.8 and 35.9).
- CT scan of PNS with particular reference to ostiomeatal complex will show opacity of the affected maxillary sinus and also detect associated anatomical and pathological abnormality.
- Diagnostic nasal endoscopy will confirm discharge from the middle meatus and may detect any abnormality like accessory ostium, polyp, etc.
- Antroscopy—Allows direct visualization of the maxillary sinus mucosa. Biopsy and culture can be taken in suspected cases of fungal sinusitis.

Treatment

Medical: Acute exacerbations are treated like acute sinusitis. Steroid nasal spray may be helpful in certain cases.

Antral lavage: This is done by performing an antral puncture in the inferior meatus with the help of Tilly-Litchwitch trocar and cannula. The cannula is left in situ for irrigation while the trocar is being removed. This helps in removing the purulent discharge from the sinuses and maintaining patency of the sinus ostium temporarily.

Intranasal antrostomy: This is done by making a window in the inferior meatus to facilitate

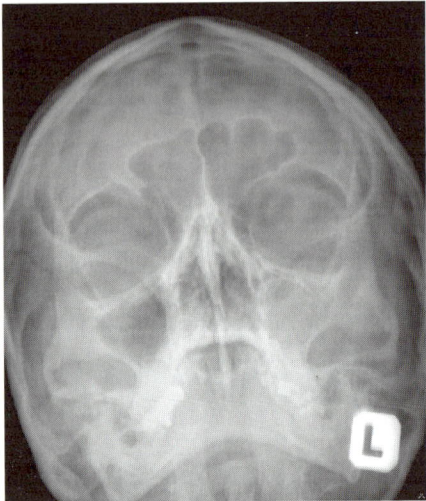

Fig. 35.8: X-ray PNS (Water's view) showing right maxillary mucosal thickening and left maxillary opacity

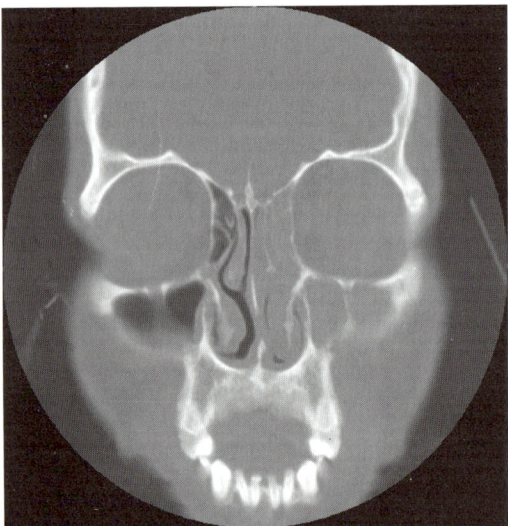

Fig. 35.9: CT of ostiomeatal complex showing left maxillo ethmoidal sinusitis

drainage through gravity and aeration of the sinus. Since the sinuses drain through the natural ostium a middle meatal antrostomy is preferred and a traditional intranasal antrostomy is seldom being done these days.

Endoscopic middle meatal antrostomy: This is the treatment of choice for management of chronic maxillary sinusitis. The steps of surgery include:

1. *Infundibulotomy:* The uncinate process is removed to open the ethmoidal infundibulum.
2. Clearance of anterior ethmoidal disease by exenteration of anterior and middle ethmoidal cells after removal of bulla ethmoidalis to relieve permanent focus of infection.
3. *Middle meatal antrostomy:* The natural ostium of the maxillary sinus is enlarged by using a back biting forceps. The accessory ostium if any is joined with the natural ostium.

Since the endoscopic sinus surgery removes the cause of the disease process as well as treats the sinusitis by facilitating natural drainage of the sinus through its ostium, and as it normalizes the mucosal changes by providing adequate ventilation it is called as 'functional endoscopic sinus surgery. Caldwell-Luc operation is rarely done these days.

Chronic Frontal Sinusitis

Etiology and pathogenesis same as described above under sinusitis. In elderly children, persistent adenoid hypertrophy may predispose to this condition. Isolated frontal sinusitis is rare and is usually associated with chronic ethmoiditis.

Symptoms

Headache: This is usually less severe than acute frontal sinusitis but may be quite irritating for the patient. The headache is of 'dull aching' type or feeling of heaviness of the head. It is more in the morning and reduces by afternoon (office headache).

Anosmia or hyposmia: May be associated with due to mucosal edema in the region of the middle turbinate. Cachosmia may be present due to purulent discharge following anaerobic infection.

Postnasal drip and hawking sensation: This is commonly seen and can lead to pharyngitis or laryngitis.

Nasal obstruction: May be occasionally present if associated with deviated nasal septum.

Signs

Frontal tenderness may be present during acute exacerbations.

Anterior rhinoscopy may reveal discharge in the middle meatus.

Investigations

- X-ray PNS: The views taken usually are the Caldwell view (occipito-frontal) or 'Water's view' (Occipito-mental view). Haziness or opacity, mucosal thickening can be seen.
- CT imaging of the PNS (coronal sections) in the region of the ostiomeatal complex is radiological investigation to find out the anatomical and pathological changes in the ostiomeatal complex. Affected sinus may show opacity or fluid level.
- Diagnostic nasal endoscopy shows discharge and mucosal edema in the upper part of middle meatus in the region of the frontal recess.

Treatment

Functional endoscopic sinus surgery is the treatment of choice, which includes frontal recess clearance. Surgeries done in the past to treat the frontal disease include external fronto-ethmoidectomy (Lynch-Howarth operation), Patersons operation, osteoplastic flap operation with or without obliteration of the frontal sinus, etc. These are seldom done now-a-days.

Medical treatment can only give temporary relief as discussed in acute sinusitis.

Chronic Ethmoiditis

The ethmoidal labyrinth consists of small tiny air cell system. These tiny cells often get infected in relation to anatomical and pathological abnormalities. Inadequately treated acute infection and in the presence of these abnormalities, the infection tends to persist within the anterior ethmoidal cells. This tiny air cell system is prone to harbor chronic inflammatory focus within its mucosa and cause persistent or recurrent infection in the major sinuses. Thus the anterior ethmoidal air cell system within the middle meatus is considered to be the 'key' area for causation of chronic sinus disease. The anterior ethmoid contains tiny micro channels through which the major sinuses like the maxillary and frontal drain. The disease associated within the middle meatus especially involving the anterior ethmoidal cells is called ostiomeatal complex disease, which blocks the drainage of the major sinuses.

Clinical Features

Because of the anatomical site and the nature of infection that it is associated with, frequently involves multiple sinuses. Hence a combination of symptoms may be present. Isolated chronic ethmoiditis is uncommon.

Symptoms

Headache: This is usually a dull and persistent and is more of a pressure symptom than true headache. The site of the pain is between the eyes. As it is often associated with other sinus involvement, the site of headache may be varied.

Nasal obstruction: Persistent disease with polypoidal changes can cause nasal obstruction.

Hawking and postnasal discharge is frequent. It may be associated with sore throat, ear block, etc.

Signs

Tenderness may be elicited in the region of the intercanthal area during acute exacerbation. Frequently tenderness of other sinuses may be elicited.

Anterior rhinoscopy may reveal discharge and mucosal changes in the middle meatus.

Posterior rhinoscopy may reveal discharge in the middle and/ or superior meatus depending on the group of the ethmoids involved.

Investigation

CT scan of the ostiomeatal complex and diagnostic nasal endoscopy are the two investigations, which can pick up ethmoidal disease. Plain radiographs are not of much use. Hence this condition is often under-diagnosed.

Diagnosis

Based on the nasal endoscopy and the CT scan findings, the disease is diagnosed and is called 'ostiomeatal complex disease'. The term chronic sinusitis refers to the disease of the ethmoid where the major sinuses are often involved secondarily.

Treatment

Presently functional endoscopic sinus surgery (FESS) is the treatment of choice. Other surgeries performed in the past are obsolete now. They include intranasal, external or transantral ethmoidectomies. Newer developments have made this surgical procedure more safe and effective, especially after the development of image-guided technology. Micro-debrider and laser may be used as tools for precise and conservative surgery. The principle of FESS is to eradicate the disease from the anterior ethmoid and facilitate drainage of the major sinuses through the natural ostia. The mucociliary drainage of the sinuses is preserved.

Basic steps of FESS include the following. The surgery is tailor-made depending on the sinuses involved.

1. Infundibulotomy (uncinectomy)
2. Anterior ethmoidectomy
3. Middle meatal antrostomy
4. Frontal recess clearance
5. Posterior ethmoidectomy, sphenoidotomy and trimming of the middle turbinate may be done, if indicated.

Chronic Sphenoidal Sinusitis

Etiology

Isolated sphenoidal sinusitis is rare. It presents usually as part of 'pansinusitis', and sometimes can be associated due to infection involving the posterior ethmoids. In isolated sphenoidal sinusitis, a fungal cause should be suspected.

Pathology

As described earlier, under the 'pathology in general'. It is associated with chronic ethmoiditis. Occasionally fractures of the skull base involving the sphenoethmoids can give rise to secondary sinusitis.

Symptoms

Headache is usually vague and may be vertical, frontal, occipital or central. Occasionally the pain may radiate to the temporal region. Postnasal drip and hawking may give rise to vague throat and ear symptoms. Cacosmia and halitosis may be present.

Signs

Posterior rhinoscopy: Presence of supratubal stream of discharge.

Investigation

CT scan imaging or Water's view with mouth open (Pierre's view) will show fluid level or mucosal edema of the sphenoid sinuses. Nasal endoscopy helps better visualization of the disease and discharge in the superior meatus/ sphenoethmoidal recess.

Differential Diagnosis

- Sphenoidal mucocoele
- Pituitary adenoma.

Treatment

Medical treatment is usually ineffective. Broad-spectrum antibiotics, systemic and local nasal decongestants, anti-inflammatory, antihistamines, nasal irrigation with saline, mucolytics, steam inhalation, etc. may be tried.

Surgical treatment

FESS including the posterior ethmoidectomy and the sphenoidotomy.

Endoscopic sphenoidotomy in isolated sphenoidal disease.

COMPLICATIONS OF SUPPURATIVE SINUSITIS

Types

- Extracranial
- Intracranial.

Pathogenesis

Spread of infection may occur through the following routes.

1. Direct spread through the wall of the sinus— This occurs through preformed pathway or due to disease process like Osteitis or osteomyelitis (in acute sinusitis) and osteoporosis following polyposis.
2. Venous spread—This occurs through subepithelial venous plexus.
   - Septic venous thrombosis (osteomyelitis)
   - Thrombosis of veins within sinus mucosa
   - Septicemia and pyemia.
3. Lymphatic spread.
   - Perivascular lymphatics spreads the infection to the subperiosteal plane.
4. Spread through perineural spaces of olfactory nerve.

Extracranial Complications

1. Mucocele especially of frontal sinus
2. Cellulitis of the face
3. Abscess over the face
   - Bridge of nose, over the cheek, above/ below medial canthus.
4. Orbital complications (Fig. 35.10)
   - Subperiosteal abscess of orbital cavity.

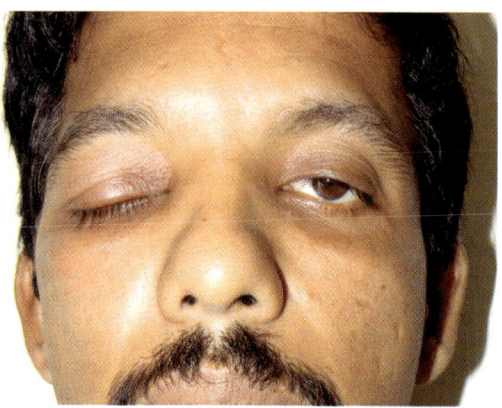

Fig. 35.10: Preseptal orbital cellulitis due to acute sinusitis in the stage of recovery

- Orbital cellulitis
  - Intraorbital abscess
  - Cellulitis of eyelids.
5. Osteomyelitis.
6. Sinus disease may act as septic focus for the flowing conditions:
   - ASOM
   - CSOM
   - SOM
   - Pharyngitis
   - Tonsillitis
   - Laryngitis
   - Bronchitis
   - Bronchiectasis

Intracranial

1. Meningitis
2. Encephalitis
3. Abscess
   - Subdural
   - Extradural
4. Cavernous sinus thrombosis (sphenoidal sinusitis).

Investigations

1. X-ray PNS
2. Nasal endoscopy

3. CT Scan of OMC
4. Diagnostic proof puncture.

Mucocele/Pyocele: This is a cystic swelling of the sinus lined by mucosa and occurs as a result of permanent/chronic obstruction of the sinus ostium or the duct of the mucous gland. This leads to collection of secretions of the gland/sinuses resulting in retention cyst. It is more commonly seen in ethmoid and frontal sinus. Secretions are usually sterile and if its gets infected it forms a pyocele.

Frontal sinus mucocele: This commonly occurs as a result of obstruction to the frontal ostium due to chronic disease of the frontal recess or due to postsurgical/traumatic fibrosis causing blockage. In most of the cases it involves the superior medial wall of the orbit. Due to expansion this wall becomes thinner and leads to displacement of the orbit. If it expands posteriorly it can displace the dura. Rarely does it involve the anterior wall causing swelling in the forehead.

Clinical Features

Symptoms

- Supraorbital swelling usually above and lateral to the medial canthus.
- Diplopia may be present due to proptosis.
- Headache is usually confined to the frontal region and is mild and dull.

Signs

- Proptosis (forward, downward and lateral displacement of the eyeball).
- Swelling is usually cystic and non-tender and egg-shell crackling may be elicited.

Investigations

- X-ray PNS–Show cloudiness of the affected frontal sinus with loss of scalloping.
- CT scan of the ostiometal complex and PNS shows the same features and shows the extact extension of the cystic swelling in relation to the orbit, intracranium and the ethmoids.

- Diagnostic nasal endoscopy—There may be a swelling at the region of the attachment of the middle turbinate.

Treatment

Presently endoscopic sinus surgery with frontal recess clearance and uncapping of the mucocele is the treatment of choice. Alternatively and external frontoethmo-diectomy (Lynch-Howarth operation) or osteoplastic flap operation by bi-coronal incision may be done to excise/marsupialize the cyst and a passage is created into the middle meatus. Stent may be placed in the region of frontonasal duct to maintain the patency till the epithelialization is complete. In case of a pyocele a course of antibiotics should be given prior to the surgical intervention.

Mucocele of the ethmoids: This causes expansion the cyst towards the least resistance, i.e. lamina papyraeica. This leads to displacement of the orbital contents, outwards and laterally. Clinical features include proptosis, diplopia and rarely decreased vision if posterior ethmoids are involved. Investigations nasal endoscopy reveals a bulge in the middle meatus. Detailed extension can be confirmed by a CT scan Treatment is endoscopic sinus surgery/external fronto-ethmoidectomy.

Mucocele of the maxillary sinus usually presents as a retention cyst commonly in the floor of the sinus one expansion and erosion are rare. This may be marsupialized by endoscopic sinus surgery if symptomatic.

Sphenoethmoidal mucocoele is very rare and it usually extends to retrobulbar area causing exophthalmos by occupying the space or by interfering with the venous drainage of the orbit. Visual disturbances may be encountered due to pressure on the optic nerve. It may be associated with superior orbital syndrome with involvement of the fifth cranial nerve. The patients may complain of the headache in the region of the occipital region/vertex. CT scan helps in confirming the diagnosis. It may be treated by endoscopic sphenoidotomy or by external sphenoethmoidectomy.

2. Cellulitis of the Face

Orbitial cellulites may extend to the face in acute ethmoiditis especially in children. It can lead to abscess of the face involving the bridge of nose, over the cheek and above/below medical canthus.

3. Orbital Complications

The common orbital complication include the following and can be dangerous if adequate parenteral antibiotics and timely surgical intervention is not made.

- *Orbital cellulitis and subperiosteal abscess of orbital cavity:* This is the most common orbital complication and it occurs as a result of extension of infection from any of the paranasal sinuses as described under pathogenesis. Patients present with proptosis, lid edema, pain, chemosis of the conjunctiva and progressive limitation of the eye movements. Constitutional symptoms like fever and headache may be present. This is common in acute ethmoiditis especially in children. If not treated early with proper abtibiotics, it can lead to a subperiosteal abscess and if infection spreads to orbital contents it leads to intraorbital abscess. Fluctuation may be present in such cases. Marked proptosis and opthalmoplegia may be present along with features of orbital cellulitis. Orbital CT imaging is the most important investigation and should be done as an emergency to confirm the diagnosis. If the abscess is confirmed, and exploratory operation should be done.
- Cellulitis of eyelids is common in acute ethmoiditis and rarely in acute frontal sinusitis.

4. Osteomyelitis

This is an infection of the bone where the bone marrow is involved. It should be differentiated from ostitis which usually involves the compact bones. Ostiomyelitis usually involves the frontal and the maxillary sinus.

Etiology

The causative agents are *staphylococcus aureus,* B-hemolytic streptococci, pneumococci and the anaerobic species. Suppurative sinusitis and trauma are the commonest cause for the osteomyelitis. This is more common in females than in males.

Pathology

Infection may get transmitted directly or by hematogenous spread through thrombophlebitis (frontal sinus).

Clinical Features

Frontal osteomyelitis is more often seen in adults as the frontal sinus is not well developed in infants and children. In acute fulminating type, fever, headache. Edema of upper eyelids on the affected site, and later a soft doughy swelling appears in the frontal region (Pott's-puffy tumor) or pericranial abscess. If the treatment is delayed, it may spread to intracranial structures and can spread rapidly leading to death due to severe toxemia and meningitis.

A chronic localized form without breach of the internal table can be associated with a low grade fever, malaise and localized tenderness may be elicited. Later sequestrum may be formed. Doughy swelling may be present. Purulent discharge from the bone may be present if it ruptures through the skin. Fungal sinusitis should be ruled out. CT imaging is helpful and can ruleout other intracranial complications. Treatment is by exploration of the frontal sinus by external frontoethmoidectomy approach with a bicoronal incision (Osteo-plastic flap).

Osteomyelitis of the maxilla: This is common in children. It is usually secondary to dental infection and in infants sometimes secondary to buccal infection Acute maxillary sinusitis is the primary cause of osteomyelitis in infants.

Pathology

Infection can spread in three ways:

(a) Through the fascial surface with swelling of the soft parts of the check leading to abscess formation.

(b) Through the palatine and alveolar process leading to a fistulous tract to the oral cavity.

(c) Through the zygomatic process leading to necrosis and extended infection into the pterygopalatine fossa causing absecess.

Treatment

Parenteral antibiotics and sequestrectomy.

5. **Sinus disease may act as septic focus for the flowing conditions:**
   - ASOM
   - CSOM
   - SOM
   - Pharyngitis
   - Tonsillitis
   - Laryngitis
   - Bronchitis
   - Bronchiectasis

Intracranial Complications

1. Meningitis
2. Encephalitis
3. Abscess—Intracranial / subdural / extradural.

   These are similar to that in otology
4. Cavernous sinus thrombosis (sphenoids) as described under diseases of external nose.

FUNGAL SINUSITIS

Definition

It is a distinct clinical entity characterized by inflammation of the sinus mucosa due to a fungal infection, and may be seen in immunocompetent or immunocompromised hosts.

Etiology

Causative Agents

1. Aspergillus
2. Mucormycosis
3. Paecilomyces
4. Candida
5. Penicillium species, etc.

Aspergillosis is the most common associated fungus causing sinusitis.

Causative Factors

- Immunocompromised patients and in diabetics, patients with chronic renal failure, HIV infection, prolonged systemic steroids, chemotherapy, etc.
- Prolonged use of steroid nasal spray.
- Occupational—In farmers, garbage cleaners, etc. may be prone to develop opportunistic fungal infection.

Pathology

There are four types of fungal sinusitis:

1. Mycetoma Fungal Sinusitis produces clumps of spores, a "fungal ball," within a sinus cavity, most frequently the maxillary sinuses. The patients are usually an immuno-competent host and the disease is often non-invasive.

2. Allergic Fungal Sinusitis (AFS) is an allergic reaction to environmental fungi that is finely dispersed into the air. This is often seen in immunocompetent patients and present with history suggestive of allergic rhinitis. Anti-inflammatory medical therapy and immunotherapy are typically prescribed to prevent AFS recurrence.

3. Chronic Indolent Sinusitis is an invasive form of fungal sinusitis in immunocompetent hosts. This is common in lower socio-economic group of patients. Microscopically, chronic indolent sinusitis is characterized by a granulomatous inflammatory infiltrate (nodular shaped inflammatory lesions). A decreased immune system can increase the risk for this invasive disease.

4. Fulminant Sinusitis is usually seen in the immunocompromised patients. The disease leads to progressive destruction of the sinuses and can give rise to intra or extracranial complications.

Symptoms

Depends on the type of fungal sinusitis, immune status of the patient and age. The disease often progresses from months to years and presents symptoms that include chronic headache and progressive facial swelling that can cause visual impairment.

- Thick purulent nasal discharge, which may be blood stained occasionally.
- Nasal obstruction
- Epistaxis
- Swelling of the cheek or orbit
- Proptosis, diplopia, visual impairment may be present
- Headache is severe if intracranial extension is present.
- Halitosis and cacosmia may be present
- Features of allergic rhinitis in AFS.

Signs

- Swelling of the cheek or orbit or proptosis
- Thick purulent nasal discharge may be seen in the middle meatus on anterior rhinoscopy.

- Polyposis may be seen which is often unilateral.
- Mass in the middle meatus associated with purulent discharge should raise the suspicion of fungal sinusitis.

Investigations

1. Diagnostic nasal endoscopy.
2. Nasal swab for fungal culture.
3. CT imaging of the paranasal sinuses and intracranium or X-ray of the paranasal sinuses. This often shows areas of hyperattenuation due to calcareous deposits (Fig. 35.11).
4. MRI Scan is also useful in detecting invasive fungal sinusitis (Figs 35.12a and b).
5. Biopsy, if nasal mass is present. Histopathological examination with special stains will help in ruling out fungal granuloma/invasive fungal sinusitis.

Treatment

Medical

Anti-fungal treatment—Depends on the fungus isolated and the pathological type.

Oral anti-fungal drugs available are:

Fluconazole—Effective against candida.

Itraconazole—Effective against aspergillus, palcilomyces

Intravenous anti-fungal drug– Amphotericin B– Effective against mucormycosis, aspergillosis, etc.

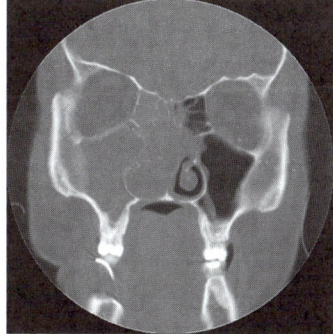

Fig. 35.11: CT of ostiomeatal complex showing fungal sinusitis involving right maxillary and ethmoid sinuses.

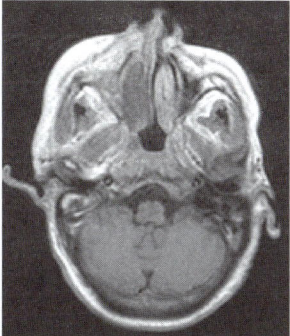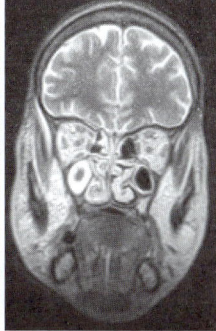

Figs 35.12a and b: (a) Axial, (b) Coronal, MRI showing features of fungal sinusitis in right side involving maxillary and ethmoid sinuses

In allergic fungal sinusitis, medical treatment as for allergic rhinitis may be tried. The mainstay of treatment is to facilitate drainage, which may be achieved surgically. Functional endoscopic sinus surgery is the treatment of choice today. Role of anti-fungal treatment is limited in such cases.

Surgical

Objective of surgical treatment is debridement and establishment of drainage (Fig. 35.13).

The recommended therapies for both chronic indolent and fulminant sinusitis are aggressive surgical removal of the fungal material and intravenous anti-fungal therapy.

Complications

- Orbital cellulitis (Fig. 35.14)
- Orbital abscess
- Intracranial invasion causing meningitis and brain abscess
- Cavernous sinus invasion commonly occurs from sphenoid sinus causing thrombosis.

Sinusitis in Children

Although sinusitis is commonly thought as disease that affect adults, both chronic and acute sinusitis also affect a large population of children each year.

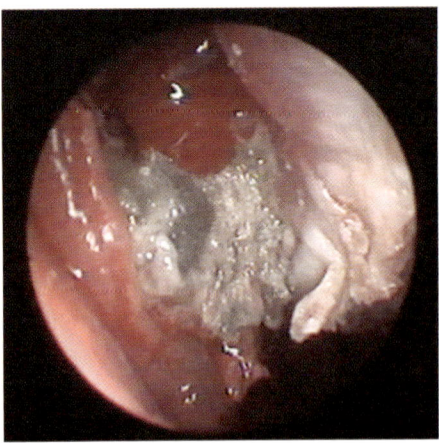

Fig. 35.13: Endoscopic intraoperative picture showing cheesy material in the middle meatus in fungal sinusitis

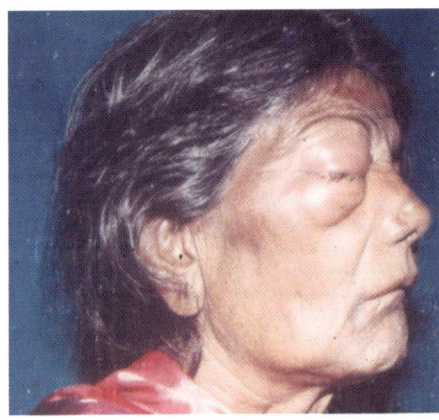

Fig. 35.14: Oribital cellulitis secondary to fungal sinusitis (aspergilosis–invasive)

The structure of a child's sinuses differs from that of an adult's. A child's sinus cavities are smaller and are still developing during childhood. The sinuses are incompletely developed at birth, and become fully developed by puberty.

Symptoms

In young children: Halitosis, rhinorrhea, cough are common.

In older children: Purulent rhinorrhea, nasal obstruction, periorbital pain.

The common presenting symptoms are as follows:

- Runny nose or "cold" lasting more than 10 to 14 days should be suspected for sinusitis.
- Child may have low-grade fever.
- Weakness and tiredness are common, and child may be irritable.
- Cough may be more severe at night due to post-nasal drip.
- Headache is seen usually in children age six or older.

Signs

- Purulent postnasal drip.
- Thick greenish yellow nasal discharge on anterior rhinoscopy.
- Eyes may be swollen.
- Child may have features of adenoid facies.

Investigations

- Diagnostic nasal endoscopy.
- CT-scan/ X-ray PNS.
- X-ray soft tissue neck lateral view to rule out enlarged adenoids.

Treatment

Medical: Acute sinusitis should be treated with broad-spectrum antibiotics for a period of 2 to 3 weeks. Nasal decongestants–both systemic and local are helpful in drainage. Steam inhalation/saline irrigation are helpful to clear the secretions.

Surgical: It is indicated in chronic sinusitis or when adenoid hypertrophy is present. In acute sinusitis surgical intervention is indicated if there is orbital or intra-cranial complications.

Recent Advantages

Sinus balloon catheter system: Ballon sinuplasty uses a catheter based system and is a minimal invasive endoscopic technique to dilate. Balloon sinuplasty technology was intended by Josh Makower in 2005, a former chronic sinusitis sufferer.

Balloon sinuplasty technique: Using a sinus guide catheter and a flexible sinus guidewire the targeted sinus is entered (Fig. 35.15). After confirming with C-Arm/Relieva LUMA system, the sinus balloon catheter is advanced over the sinus guidewire. The ballon is placed at the site of obstruction/stenosed ostium and is dilated (Figs 35.16 and 35.17).

Advantages:
- Safe and effective
- Minimal invasive
- Minimised bleeding
- Early recovery
- Revision possible
- Short hospital stay/Office based procedure

Disadvantages:
- Disposable catheter and balloon.
- Expensive
- Long term results yet to be assertained.

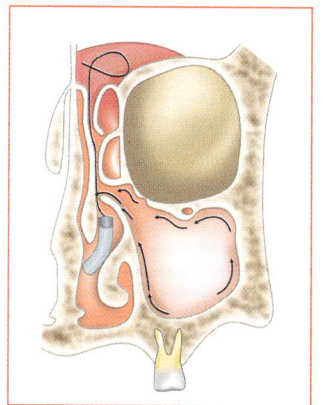

Fig. 35.15: Guide wire being passed along with ballon catheter inside the frontal sinus

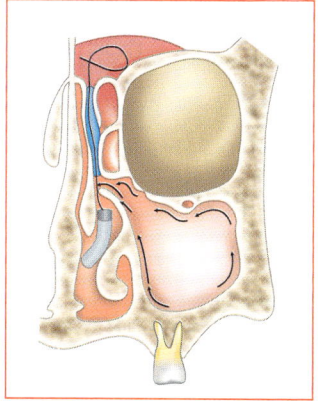

Fig. 35.16: Balloon is inflated at the level of frontal sinus ostium

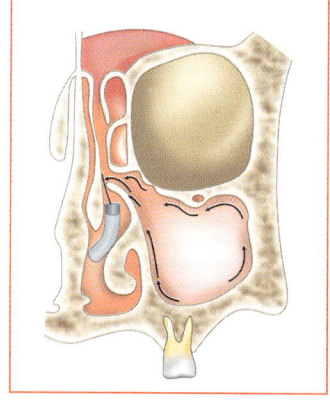

Fig. 35.17: Balloon catheter has been withdrawn alongwith guide wire after dilating the frontal ostium and recess

POINTS TO REMEMBER

1. Anatomical and pathological obstruction in the region of ostiomeatal complex leads to impaired mucocilliary clearance stagnation of secretions and persistent infection in the dependent sinuses.
2. Ethmoid is the key area in the disease causation and acts as a reservoir of infection.
3. Office headache is characteristically seen in frontal sinusitis.

36

Nasal Polyposis

Introduction

Polyposis means 'many feet'. Nasal polyp is an inflammatory condition of unknown etiology, consists of edematous mucosa involving usually the ethmoid sinus and rarely the maxillary sinus. It presents as soft, jelly-like over growth of the lining of the sinus wall. The ethmoidal polyps appear like grapes on the end of a stalk.

Definition

Nasal polyp is an inflammatory condition of unknown etiology and occurs as an apparent new growth. It is defined as a prolapsed, edematous, pediculated nasal mucosa, which may arise from the sinuses or the nasal cavity.

Clinical Types

The polyp can be divided into following types:

Common
1. Ethmoidal
2. Antrochoanal

Rare
1. Sphenochoanal
2. True choanal

Ethmoidal Polyp

They arise from the multiple air cells of the ethmoidal labyrinth. They present as multiple grape-like masses, which can be best seen on anterior rhinoscopic examination.

Etiology

Exact etiology of nasal polyp is not known and precise mechanism of polyp formation is incompletely understood. Causation of nasal polyp appears to be multi-factorial.

Incidence

The overall prevalence rate of nasal polyposis ranges from 1 to 4 percent, 7 percent have associated asthma, 2 percent of chronic rhinitis patients have nasal polyp. 10 percent of children with cystic fibrosis may have nasal polyp. Ethnoidal polyp is commonly seen in middle aged men. Recently number of publications associate polyp as due to allergic fungal sinusitis. Lot of other conditions including malignant lesion are often diagnosed as nasal polyps clinically but histologically are found to be inverted papilloma, angiofibroma, olfactory neuroblastoma, angioma of the septum, meningocoele, etc.

Etiological factors postulated are:

1. *Heredity:* Hereditary factors may play an important role in the development of nasal polyposis in diseases like cystic fibrosis and ciliary dyskinesia.
2. *Bernoulli's phenomenon:* Bernoulli's principle says that increased air velocity produces decreased lateral pressure. More the velocity more is the drop in lateral pressure. When air passes through narrow passages, its velocity increases. Polypi are more seen in the stenotic areas of nasal cavity like the middle meatus (Fig. 36.1).
3. *Allergy:* Approximately 30% of patients with nasal polyps test positive for environmental allergies.
4. *Infection*
5. *Vasomotor response*
6. *Polysacharide metabolism disorder*
7. *Endocrine*
8. *Polypeptide theory:* Polypeptides like p-factors are released in the contact areas of the nasal cavity. They produce increase in vascular permeability and polyp formation.
9. Increased incidence in children with cystic fibrosis and persons with known aspirin hypersensitivity.
10. Allergic fungal sinusitis is found to be associated with recurrent ethmoidal polyposis, which was poorly diagnosed in the past.

Aspirin hypersensitivity, nasal polypi and bronchial asthma is known as Samter's triad

Pathogenesis

There is no single etiological factor that is responsible for the development of nasal polyposis. In 1990, Tos reported 10 pathogenic theories of nasal polyp formation:

- Adenoma and fibroma theories
- Necrosing ethmoiditis theory
- Glandular cyst theory
- Mucosal exudate theory
- Cystic dilatation of the excretory duct and vessel obstruction theory
- Blockade theory
- Periphlebitis and perilymphangitis theory
- Glandular hyperplasia theory
- Gland new formation theory
- Ion transport theory

Inflammation still remains to be the central major factor for all nasal polyps. Activation of epithelial cells, mast cells, and macrophages by various factors (bacteria, virus, allergens, altered amino acid metabolism, altered aerodynamics) results in the release of inflammatory mediators.

High tissue TGF- [beta] 1 quantity in healthy nasal mucosa without its active form on the cell surface and its low quantity in polyps may reflect its essential role in the inhibitory mechanisms of nasal polyposis. Interleukin-5 plays a key role in the eosinophil recruitment and activation, and both atopic and non-atopic pathways might activate this process. The main sources of IL-5 and TGF-[beta]1 are the eosinophils and macrophages. Immediate hypersensitivity besides other mechanisms might be related to atopic polyps, but the involvement of other, local allergic mechanisms in IgE production of nonatopic polyp tissue cannot be excluded. Hirschberg A (2003).

Pathology

The nasal polyp may be multiple or solitary. The nasal polyps are found to commonly arise from

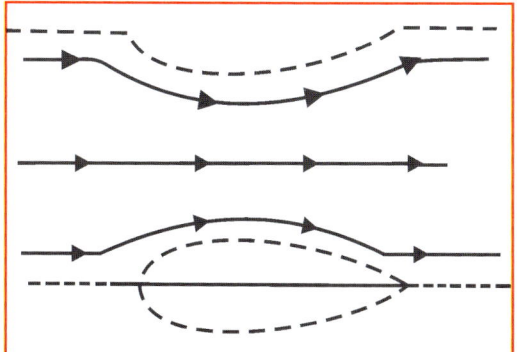

Fig. 36.1: Bernoulli's phenomenon: Negative pressure produced at the stenotic site facilitates accummulation of edematous fluid in the submucosa

the mucosa of the ostia, clefts, and recesses in the ostiomeatal complex where the initial stage of sinonasal polyposis seems to take place (Larsen and Tos, 2004).

The pathological changes that occurs are:

- Round cell infiltration of submucosa
- Edema of the lamina propria
- Bulging of the mucosa
- Prolapse of the mucosa, giving rise to polyp formation
- Increase in intraepithelial glandular structures
- *Polyp can be of two types:*
  - Edematous type with little glandular structure
  - Glandular and cystic type
- Long standing polyposis leads to cystic degeneration with fibrosis giving the polyp a fibrous appearance histologically with less glandular tissue (Fig. 36.2).

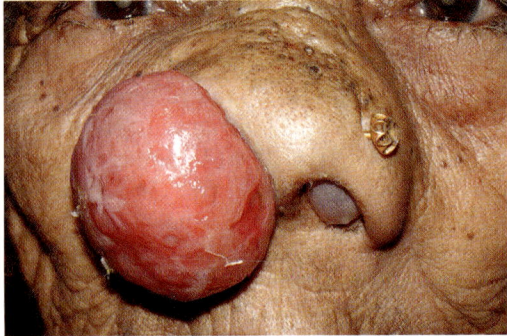

Fig. 36.2 Right infected ethmoidal polyp presenting as a reddish nasal mass (right nostril) with increase vascularity and protruding polyp (left nostril)

Histopathological Features

- Polyp is lined by respiratory epithelium with less ciliary activity.
- In long standing cases the mucosa may undergo squamous metaplasia.
- Edematous stroma with few goblet cells and submucous glands.

Histologically there are 2 types:

1. *Neutrophil type:* Seen with purulent secretions and in association with Kartagener's syndrome/ cystic fibrosis.
2. *Eosinophil type:* Predominant cell is eosinophil. Associated with serous secretions in asthma, allergy and aspirin intolerance.

Clinical Features

Symptoms

- Nasal obstruction: Often bilateral, which may be partial or complete. May be associated with mouth breathing.
- Hyposmia or anosmia depending on the severity.
- Nasal discharge usually mucoid in nature and may become purulent if associated with secondary infection involving the sinuses.
- Hawking sensation due postnasal discharge
- Altered or reduced sensation of taste.
- Symptoms of nasal allergy like sneezing, itchy nose, watery rhinrrhea may be present.
- Broadening of the nose in long standing cases
- Headache due to secondary sinusitis
- May be associated with itchy throat, hoarseness, cough, wheezing, etc. due to associated allergic pharyngitis/ laryngitis and/or bronchial asthma.
- Hyponasal voice (rhinolalia clausa)
- Snoring and sleep apnea may present

Signs

External Examination

- Widening of the intercanthal distance with 'frog face' deformity in extensive ethmoidal polyposis.
- Signs of nasal allergy as described under 'allergic rhinitis' may be present.
- Cold spatula test reveals reduced or absence of fogging.

Anterior Rhinoscopic Examination

- Multiple pale grayish or bluish white, 'grape-like' masses arising from the middle meatus
- Infected polyposis may have a vascular pinkish appearance due to increased vascularity
- On probing the masses are insensitive to touch, soft, mobile and pedunculated. The probe can be passed all around the mass. They are non-friable mass and do not bleed on touch.
- Polyp tend to present more anteriorly (Figs 36.3a and b).

Differential Diagnosis

Congenital conditions like meningocoele, meningo-encephalocoele, glioma, etc.

Mucosal polyp like antrochoanal polyp, sphenochoanal polyp, polypoidal middle or inferior turbinate, etc.

Granulomatous polyp: Examples—Rhinosporidiosis, rhinoscleroma, tuberculosis, etc.

Neoplastic polyp: Examples—Inverted papilloma, angiofibroma, plasmacytoma, olfactory neuroblastoma, and other malignancies.

Investigations

Diagnostic nasal endoscopy: The polyp can be traced up to its stalk in the middle or superior meatus. Associated anomalies in the ostiomeatal complex can be diagnosed which helps in treatment planning (Fig. 36.4).

Radiological: X-ray PNS, CT imaging of the ostio-meatal complex (coronal sections): Exact extent of the disease in the sinuses and the ostiomeatal complex can be assessed. Relation of the various vital landmarks of the sphenoethmoids can be better seen which helps in preventing certain operative complications.

Allergy tests including prick test/ intradermal skin test/ RAST.

Nasal swab for fungal culture: Increased incidence of fungal infection is found especially in recurrent ethmoidal polyposis. Systemic antifungal treatment has shown to reduce the recurrence rates following surgery.

Biopsy if neoplasm or granulomatous condition is suspected.

Routine investigations like complete blood picture, absolute eosinophil count, etc.

Treatment

Endoscopic sinus surgery is the treatment of choice. However, the causative factor like allergy

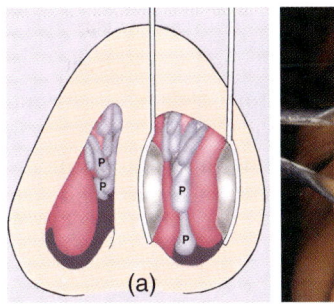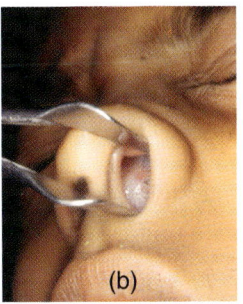

Figs 36.3a and b: Anterior rhinoscopy showing bilateral ethmoidal polyposis (P) presenting as multiple grape like mass

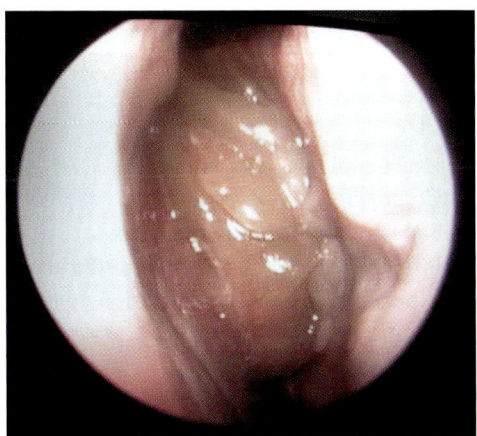

Fig. 36.4: Diagnostic nasal endoscopy with 30° Hopkin's rod endoscope showing multiple ethmoidal polyposis

should be treated adequately by medical measures or desensitization to prevent recurrence. Medical treatment following surgery with steroid nasal spray helps in preventing recurrence. Antifungal treatment should be given if allergic/ invasive fungal sinusitis is suspected or proved. Conventional treatment, which were popular in the past including intranasal polypectomy by snare, intranasal ethmoidectomy, external ethmoidectomy, transantral ethmoidectomy etc., have become obsolete after the evolution of functional endoscopic sinus surgery. Image guided endoscopic sinus surgery, better tools like micro-debrider and laser have made this surgery more conservative, safe and effective.

ANTROCHOANAL POLYP

Synonym: Killian's polyp

Definition

It is defined as a polyp originating in the maxillary sinus, protruding in the middle meatus through the ethmoidal infundibulum or an accessory ostium and further extending posteriorly through the choana into the nasopharynx/ oropharynx.

Thus antrochoanal polyp has three parts which include : (a) Antral part (b) Nasal part (c) Choanal part.

Etiology

- Exact etiology is not known.
- Commonly seen in children.
- Seen both in males and females.
- Probably caused by infection of the sinus.
- Proetz attributed the causation to faulty development of the maxillary ostium. Accesory ostium is frequently associated in such cases.
- Bernoulli's phenomenon may play a role.
- Often unilateral but can be bilateral occasionally.
- Symptoms of allergy are usually not elicited.

Pathogenesis

Possible reasons for posterior extension of the antrochoanal polyp are:

1. Ostium of the maxillary sinus is situated more posteriorly, more so the accessory ostium.
2. Sloping of the inferior turbinate is postero-inferiorly, on which the polyp slides, aided by gravity.
3. Anteroinferior part of the middle turbinate is more bulbous and is often associated with a concha bullosa. This part of the middle turbinate is anterior to the maxillary ostium. It probably prevents anterior extension of the polyp.
4. The mucocilliary transport is from anterior to posterior due to effective beating of the cilia from anterior to posterior.
5. Posterior choana is larger in comparison to the anterior nasal aperture.
6. The inspiratory current is more forceful than the expiratory current.
7. Suction effect during swallowing probably pulls the polyp posteriorly.

Pathology

It is usually dumb-bell shape and emerges usually through the accessory ostium or rarely through the natural ostium. The polyp is constricted at the ostium giving it a dumb-bell shape. In the antrum, it arises usually from the floor or the lateral wall.

Microscopic Pathology

Epithelium is respiratory type with normal basement membranes. No eosinophils are seen in the interstitium. Rest of the features in the interstitium is similar to the other polyposis.

Clinical Features

Symptoms

1. Unilateral nasal obstruction is the most common symptom. The obstruction is usually during the expiration due to ball-

valve effect (valvular obstruction). Obstruction may become bilateral if it blocks both the choana in the nasopharynx. Bilateral antrochoanal polyp may be suspected in such cases.
2. Nasal discharge and postnasal drip may be present.
3. Headache or heaviness in the head may be associated in the affected site.
4. Anosmia or hyposmia is not common.
5. Symptoms of allergy are not common.

Signs

1. Polyp may be missed on anterior rhinoscopy as the bulk of the mass lies in the posterior part of the nasal cavity and in the nasopharynx. Early antrochoanal polyp may present as solitary unilateral nasal mass in the middle meatus. Probe cannot be passed around the mass as it arises in the lateral wall (Fig. 36.5).
2. Posterior rhinoscopy will reveal a large polyp, which is pale white and translucent in the choana of the affected side. Sometimes it comes out into the oropharynx, pushing the soft palate downwards. Here it can be diagnosed without the need for posterior rhinoscopy. Postnasal drip may be seen which is usually mucoid in nature (Fig. 36.6).

Investigations

1. *X-ray PNS:* Unilateral opacity of the maxillary sinus and obliteration of the nasal airway may be seen. In early cases antral polyp may be seen with the convexity of the mass directed upwards or medially.
2. *X-ray of the neck lateral view* showing the nasopharynx (soft tissue exposure) may show the radioluscent mass with an air column above it- known as *Crescent sign*.
3. *CT scan* of the ostiomeatal complex (coronal sections are preferred): Mass can be occupying the maxillary sinus and extending into the nasopharynx, can be studied through different cuts. The attachment site in the antrum may be identified.
4. *Diagnostic nasal endoscopy:* The stalk of the polyp may be traced into the accessory ostium in the middle meatus. The posterior extension to the nasopharynx may be better appreciated by passing through the opposite side.

Differential Diagnosis

- Juvenile nasopharyngeal angiofibroma
- Meningocoele
- Hamartoma
- Hypertrophied posterior end of the turbinate

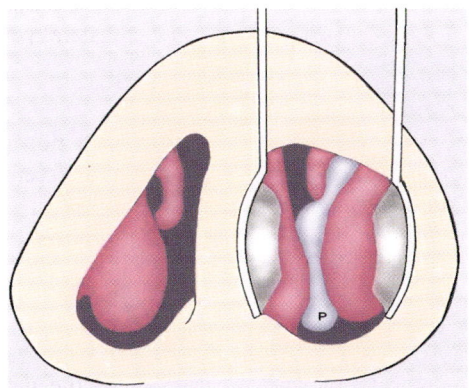

Fig. 36.5: Anterior rhinoscopy showing nasal part of antrochonal polyp (P)

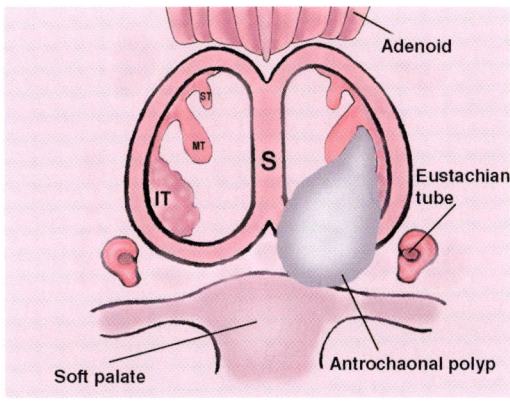

Fig. 36.6: The choanal part of the antrochoanal polyp (P) on posterior rhinoscopy

- Sphenochoanal polyp
- Nasopharyngeal rhinosporidiosis
- Thronwaldt's cyst
- Rathke's pouch tumors like cranio-pharyngioma.

Treatment

Complete surgical removal of the polyp transnasally or transorally is the commonly employed treatment and incomplete resection is associated with a relatively high recurrence rate.

Endoscopic polypectomy with a middle meatal antrostomy by joining the accessory and natural ostia together is the present treatment of choice. The entire polyp from the antrum can be removed under direct vision using giraffe's or angled forceps. Microdebrider also may be used to remove the antral part completely.

Caldwell-Luc operation, which was done frequently in the past, was associated with more morbidity. It is indicated only in recurrent polyp if endoscopy is not available. It is contraindicated before the second molar tooth erupts, i.e. 18 years of age.

POINTS TO REMEMBER

1. Common types of nasal polyps include ethmoidal and antrochoanal.
2. Antrochoanal polyp is commonly seen in children.
3. Ethmoidal polyp is common in middle aged men.
4. Histologically ethmoidal polyps are of two types, i.e. neutrophil type and eosinophil type.
5. Exact etiology of antrochoanal polyp is not known.
6. Frog face deformity of nose is associated with ethmoidal polyp.

37

Foreign Body and Myiasis

FOREIGN BODY IN THE NOSE (FB)

Foreign bodies in the nose are not uncommon and are more common in children than in adults.

Etiology

They can enter the nose through both routes, i.e. anterior and posterior routes.

Accidental: It is the commonest etiological factor and is seen mostly in children. Usually small foreign bodies are pushed through the anterior nares into the nose.

Food particle can enter the nose through the posterior choana while coughing at the time of eating or during an attack of vomiting. Swabs or cotton wool may be left behind while cleaning.

Penetrating: Through penetrating injuries foreign bodies can enter the nose.

Infection: Conditions like suppurative sinusitis and atrophic rhinitis can attract flies to deposit eggs, which usually hatch within 24 hours to produce maggots.

Malignancy of nose/ PNS and post-radiation osteo-radionecrosis may cause foul smelling nasal discharge, which may cause maggots.

Pathology

Foreign bodies in the nose can be of two types:
Animate: Maggots, Leach, etc.

Inanimate: Pebbles, beads, buttons, rubber, paper, chalk piece, etc.

An inflammatory reaction may be seen in association with nasal discharge. The site of impaction is usually in the lower part of the nose. Long standing foreign bodies can be associated with atrophic changes and sometimes calcium and magnesium salts may be deposited over it, leading to formation of a rhinolith.

Clinical Features

Symptoms

- Unilateral nasal discharge which is usually blood stained, purulent and foul smelling.
- Bleeding from the nose.
- Pain may be present initially after introduction.
- Sneezing may be present due to irritation.

Signs

Foreign body (FB) may be seen on the floor of the nasal cavity and may be obscured by inflammatory exudates, mucosal edema or granuloma.

Investigation

X-ray PNS and lateral view of the head: Radio-opaque FB may be seen.

Diagnostic nasal endoscopy: Helps to inspect the nasal cavity thoroughly and to locate a clinically non visible nasal FB (Figs 37.1 and 37.2).

Treatment

Removal of the foreign body is done by using a foreign body hook for inanimate foreign bodies which can be seen under anterior rhinoscopy (Fig. 37.3)

Larger impacted foreign bodies require removal under general anesthesia. Nasal endoscopy can be very useful for removal under better visualization.

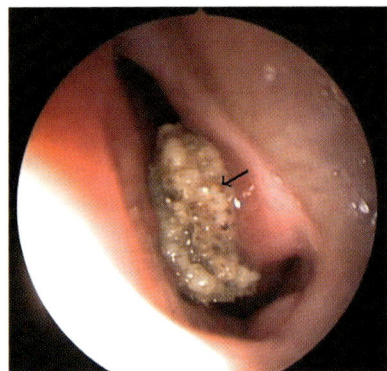

Fig. 37.1: Endoscopic view of foreign body (rubber) in the nasal cavity (←)

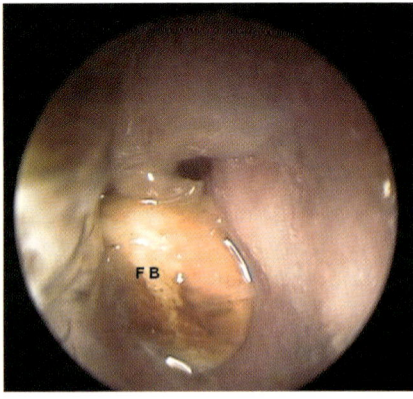

Fig. 37.2: Endoscopic view of vegetable foreign body (FB) in the right nostril

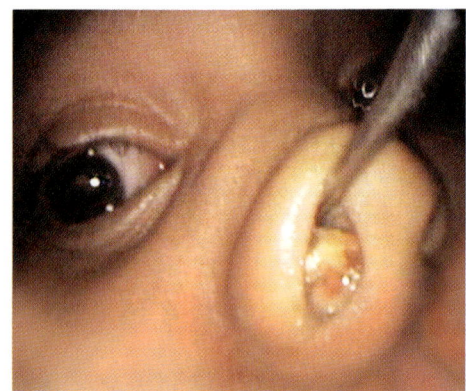

Fig. 37.3: Showing removal of foreign body by using a foreign body hook

NASAL MYIASIS (MAGGOTS IN THE NOSE)

Definition

Myiasis is well recognized as an infestation in humans and vertebrate animals with dipterous larvae, which, at least for a certain period of time, feed on the host's dead or living tissue, liquid body substances, or ingested food. These diptera are medically classified into three groups according to the site of the lesions:

- *Specific:* Whose larva stage can occur only in the living tissue of animal or human host.
- *Semi-specific:* Larvae of these flies parasitize wounds and other damaged tissues, and some species further invade living tissues adjacent to the wound.
- *Accidental myiasis:* Occurs when egg-stage flies are ingested on contaminated food or come in contact with the genitourinary tract.

Nosocomial myiasis, although rare, is sometimes reported in debilitated patients with diabetes and immunocompromised states.

Etiology

Nasal myiasis is rare in the world, but India being a tropical country this disease is not uncommon and extremely demoralizing for the patients. The common etiological factors are:

1. Poor hygiene
2. Atrophic rhinitis
3. Suppurative sinusitis
4. Comatosed patients
5. Uncontrolled diabetes mellitus and other immunocompromised states.
6. Malignancy of the maxilla
7. Osteoradionecrosis following radiotherapy
8. Granulomatous conditions like leprosy, syphilis, Wegener's granulomatosis, etc.

Pathogenesis (Figs 37.4 and 37.5a to d)

Foul smelling discharge in the nose attracts flies; especially genus *Chrysomyia bezziana*, which lay eggs in the nasal cavity in the affected area. The eggs hatch into larvae within 24 hours. These larvae are called maggots, which penetrate into the surrounding tissues. The maggots secrete proteolytic enzymes that are capable of causing extensive tissue destruction. The maggots may find their way into the soft tissues of the face, orbit, oral cavity, paranasal sinus, intracranium, etc.

Pathology

This is an inflammatory response to maggots. Analysis of tissues exhibiting infestation reveals a high concentration of lymphocytes, giant cells, neutrophils, eosinophils, and plasma cells. Secondary infection by bacteria is uncommon, because "bacteriostatic activity in the gut of the larva seems to prevent undesirable overgrowth of pyogenic bacteria" (MacNamara and Durham).

Clinical Features

Symptoms

1. Tickling sensation in the nose caused due to the movement of the maggots. It produces intense irritation and sneezing.
2. Nasal obstruction occurs due to inflamed mucosa with gross swelling of the soft tissues.
3. Epistaxis/bloodstained discharge may be present following invasion and destruction of the surrounding soft tissues.

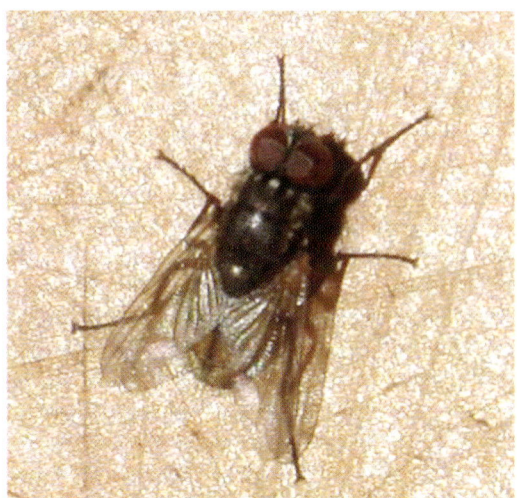

Fig. 37.4: Adult house fly

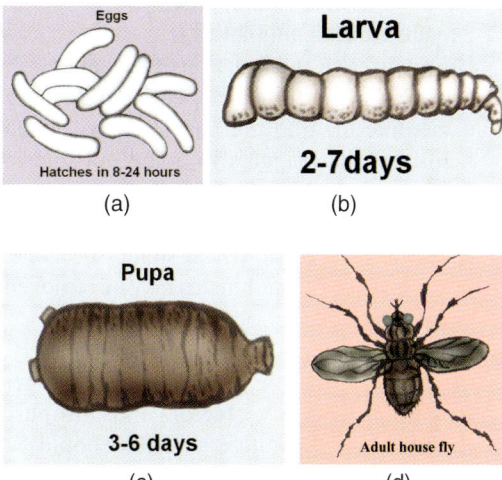

Figs 37.5a to d: Stages of development of house fly

4. Diffuse swelling around the nose and eyes associated with epiphora.
5. Pain over the root of the nose, vertex and occiput.
6. Offensive nasal discharge.
7. Patient may complain of seeing wormlike 'maggots'.

8. Psychological impact—Due to associated social stigmata in certain community, cases of suicide have been reported

Signs

1. Congested and edematous nasal mucosa with swelling of the surrounding subcutaneous tissue in the external nose.
2. Necrotic material with embedded maggots can be seen.
3. Ulceration of the mucosa may be seen.
4. Can be associated with septal perforation and perforation of the palate due to excessive tissue necrosis and destruction caused by the maggots.
5. Associated sepsis and infection can cause meningitis.

Treatment

- Injection tetanus toxoid
- Broad-spectrum antibiotics.
- Hospitalization and isolation of the patient.
- Insertion of cotton pledgets soaked with turpentine oil into the nasal cavity, which facilitates the maggots to come out due to suffocation, and thus can be easily removed. These maggots are then burnt.
- Removal of necrotic tissue should be done. Intranasal necrotic turbinates may be removed endoscopically.
- After the maggots are removed completely, the patient's hygiene is improved by proper irrigation. Causative factors like atrophic rhinitis and suppurative sinusitis should be treated adequately.
- Patient should be counseled carefully due to the stigmata attached to the condition.

RHINOLITH

Definition

Rhinoliths are calcarious concretions that are formed by deposition of calcium and magnesium salts on an untreated foreign body or inspissated mucous in the nasal cavity.

Etiology

Chronic foreign body in the nose or thick mucous can act as a nidus over which deposition of calcium and magnesium salts occur over a long period. It occupies the space available inside nasal cavity and acquires variable size and shape.

Clinical Features

- Unilateral nasal obstruction
- Headache due to neuralgia
- Fetid blood stained rhinorrhea
- Epistaxis
- Anterior rhinoscopy shows brown-black mass in nasal cavity with griffy feeling on probing.

Investigations

- X-ray PNS—Shows radio-opaque shadow in the nasal cavity.
- Diagnostic nasal endoscopy confirms the location and extent of the rhinolith.

Treatment

Endoscopic removal, in toto or piecemeal, anteriorly or posteriorly under local or general anesthesia.

Complication

Oroantral fistula.

POINTS TO REMEMBER

1. Foreign body of the nose are more common in children and are mostly accidental in nature.
2. Myiasis is the infestation of human and vertebrate animals with dipterous larvae (House fly) especially genus *Chrysomyia bezziana*.
3. Rhinolith is calculus of nasal cavity due to deposition of salt over chronic foreign body or inspissated mucous.

38

Maxillofacial Trauma

With increase in number of road traffic accidents, injury to the face and facial skeleton has become more common. The injuries could be of the soft tissue, bone or both. The type and extent of injuries and their depth should be noted. The nature of the objects that could have caused should be documented. *These cases are often medico-legal in nature and hence require proper documentation and reporting after careful evaluation.*

SOFT TISSUE INJURY

Abrasion

This refers to superficial loss of epithelium. The areas should be cleansed with antiseptic solution like povidone iodine or savlon and any foreign body, dust particles should be removed. The wound can be left dry or may be covered with gauze impregnated with petroleum jelly for protection during epithelialization (Fig. 38.1a).

Laceration

Laceration is an injury involving penetration of the skin, in which the wound is deeper than the superficial skin level. The defect usually has irregular edges and is often contaminated by dirt. Areas of skin may be avulsed from the edges or

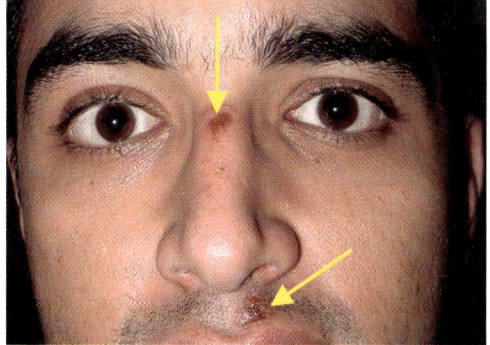

Fig. 38.1a: Superficial abrasions in the dorsum of the nose upper lip and nasal filtrum

can be associated with tissue loss. Exact nature of tissue loss especially of deeper structures like cartilage, muscle, etc. should be carefully noted.

Deep laceration of the skin may involve even the oral/nasal mucosa (Fig. 38.1b). Devitalized tissue should be removed and irregular skin margins should be trimmed after thorough saline and antiseptic irrigation. Wound should be closed in layers. Proper suturing of skin defect helps in minimizing the facial scar. Larger skin defect may require closure with local flap (like naso-labial flap) or a split skin graft.

Incised wound: Primary suturing is done after proper decontamination as described above.

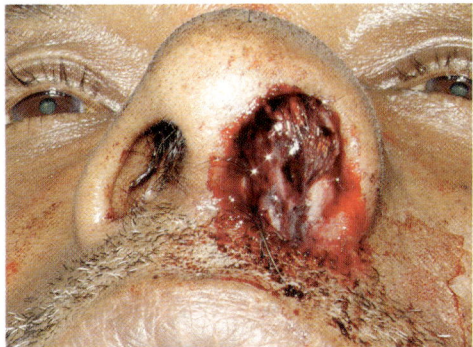

Fig. 38.1b: Laceration involving skin of the nasal vestibule and mucosa of the inferior turbinate and nasal septum

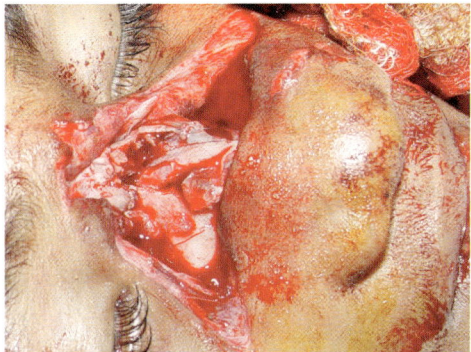

Fig. 38.1c: Avulsion of the nose from the root with the associated injuries to bone and cartilages of the external nose

Avulsion of Nose

Avulsion of the nose is not uncommon and the nose may be avulsed from below upwards, above downwards or from lateral to medial. This may be associated with cartilage and bone injury including the nasal septum (Fig. 38.1c). Treatment is same as for a laceration. Wound should be closed in layers after removal of devitalized tissue. Mucosal closure, closure of the nostrils with proper apposition of the skin is essential to prevent subsequent nasal stenosis. Stenting/splinting or nasal packing may prevent stenosis.

Hematoma

This refers to accumulation of blood within the soft tissue of the face or the nasal septum. If not treated, it may get infected and form an abscess. This can be evacuated by an incision and drainage or by aspiration. Medicated wick may be inserted after incision and drainage if re-accumulation is anticipated. Septal hematoma may require splinting/nasal packing after evacuation to prevent re-accumulation.

Orbital Injury

Injury to the orbit is often associated due to its proximity to the nose and paranasal sinuses (Fig. 38.1d). One should look for the following injuries:

1. Rupture of the globe.
2. Ocular muscle entrapment.
3. Abrasion or laceration of the eyelids, cornea, sclera, and conjunctiva.
4. Sub-conjunctival hemorrhage.
5. Conjunctival edema.
6. Foreign bodies in the eye.
7. Impaired visual acuity.

   CT imaging of the orbit is essential to assess the extent of the lesion and type of surgical intervention required like endoscopic orbital/optic nerve decompression.

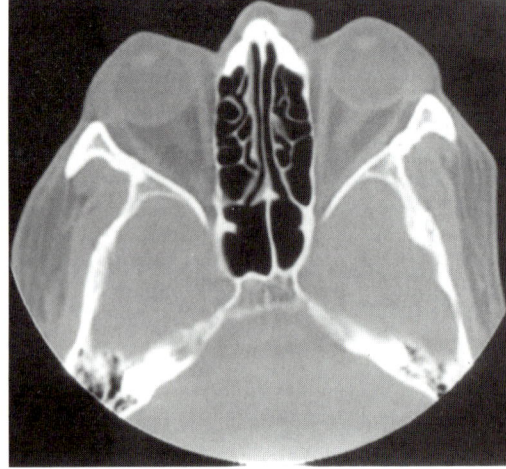

Fig. 38.1d: Axial CT showing the right and left orbits in relation to ethmoids

Facial Nerve Injury

This requires neural repair under an operating microscope using 9–0 monofilament suture like prolene after proper trimming and approximation. Nerve loss may require cable grafting using great auricular or sural nerve.

Parotid Gland/ Duct Injury

This is common in injury between the tragus of the ear and the mid cheek. Milking the parotid gland and observing the flow of saliva from the Stensen duct may help assess patency of the parotid duct. The wound is explored to identify the duct and its cut edges. The duct is repaired by microsurgical technique and stenting.

Vascular Injury

Vessels commonly involved are the facial and internal maxillary artery. Refractory bleeding may require exploration and ligation. Facial artery may be ligated in the neck and the internal maxillary artery can be clipped by a trans-antral approach.

Bony Injuries

For descriptive purposes, the facial skeleton can be divided into 3 parts:

  I. Upper third formed by the frontal bone.

  II. Middle third by the maxilla, malar-zygomatic complex and naso-ethmoidal complex.

  III. Lower third by the mandible.

  Fracture of the middle and lower third of the face can be associated with compromised airway. Injury to the facial bone is often associated with head and spine injuries, which requires a neurosurgical and orthopedic evaluation. Le Fort fractures of the maxilla are usually associated with airway obstruction.

Evaluation of Facial Fractures

1. The first objective should be to establish the airway by an endotracheal intubation/tracheostomy.

2. Hemorrhage should be controlled and hypovolemia corrected.
3. Head and spinal injuries should be ruled out.
4. Neurological evaluation should be done and appropriately managed.
5. Injuries to the other parts of the body should be looked for and be evaluated by respective specialty constituting a 'multidisciplinary trauma team'.
6. The wound areas should be thoroughly cleaned with antiseptic like povidone iodine. Blood clots and foreign body to be removed. Antibiotics and tetanus toxoid should be given.
7. Injuries should be noted and documented carefully as this case may be of medico-legal interest.
8. Examination of facial skeleton should include:
   a. Evaluation and bidigital examination of the mandible to detect fractures and malocclusion.
   b. Evaluation of the maxilla to look for its stability.
   c. Evaluation and palpation of the malar-zygomatic and the naso-ethmoidal complex to rule out fracture.
   d. Orbital margins should be palpated and orbital soft tissue injuries including visual acuity should be assessed.

Fracture of the Middle of the Face

Fracture involving the part of the face between supra orbital ridge and upper teeth. This may be characterized by:

1. Mobility or displacement of the palate.
2. Mobility of the nose in association with the palate.
3. Epistaxis.
4. Mobility of displacement of the entire third of the face.

Le Fort's Fractures

Le Fort's classification of maxillary fractures is satisfactory for both diagnosis and therapeutic purposes.

Le Fort-I (Guerin's fracture): This is a low transverse fracture of the maxilla involving the palate only and is characterized by mobility or displacement of the maxillary dental arch and palate, dental malocclusion is usually present. The fracture line involves lower part of the maxilla, which runs along the lower edge of the pyriform aperture extending further to the alveolar process of maxilla and finally to the lower part of the pterygoid process of the sphenoid bone (Fig. 38.2).

Le Fort-II: (Pyramidal fracture): This is the commonest type of Le Fort fractures. It involves fracture en block of the palate and middle third of the face, including the nose. The fracture line starts at the mid part of the nasal bone extending to the lacrimal bone and orbital floor and the infraorbital margin. It runs onto the zygomatico-maxillary suture line and extends further laterally to the mid-portion of the pterygoid process.

This commonly occurs following road-traffic accidents and is often a complex fracture, as a result of more severe trauma (Fig. 38.3).

Le Fort-III (Craniofacial dysjunction): This is a type of fracture where the bony facial framework gets completely separated from its cranial attachment (Craniofacial dysjunction) and is usually a result of severe frontal violence and is often fatal. The fracture line starts from the root of the nose and extends along the nasofrontal, maxillofrontal, zygomaticofrontal and ethmoido-frontal suture lines. It then extends to the upper part of the pterygoid process of the sphenoid bone. The entire zygomatico-maxillary complex may be mobile and displaced (Fig. 38.4).

Symptoms

- Facial swelling
- Facial deformity
- Malocclusion
- Epistaxis
- Elongated face (in type 2 and 3)
- Nose block
- CSF rhinorrhea may be present in type 3 fractures.

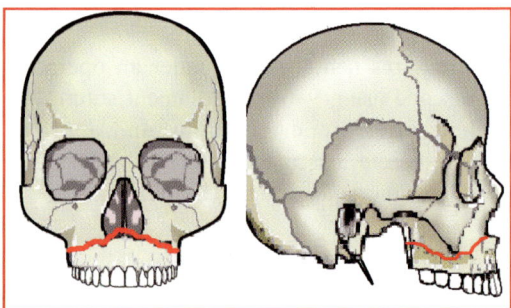

Fig. 38.2: Le Fort-I fracture shown in red line

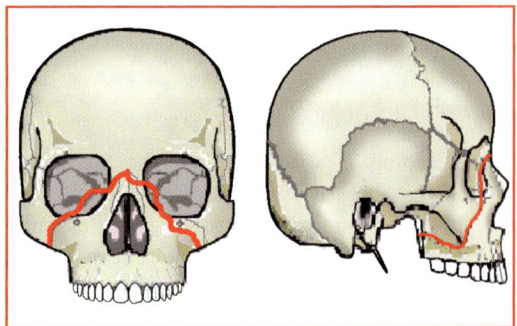

Fig. 38.3: Le Fort-II fracture shown in red line

- Diplopia and other orbital symptoms may be present in type 2 and 3 fractures.
- Infra-orbital paresthesia especially in type 2 fractures.

Signs

- Orbital ecchymosis, proptosis, limitation of extra-ocular movements may be present in type 2 and 3
- Malocclusion
- Periorbital edema
- Dish-face deformity in type 2 and 3
- Step deformity
  - At the orbital rim and nasal bones in type 2
  - At the nasal bones in type 3
  - Pyriform aperture and palatal region in type 1

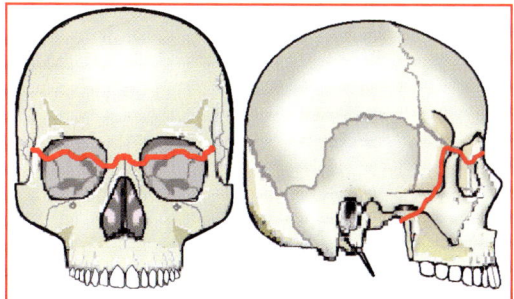

Fig. 38.4: Le Fort-III fracture shown in red line

- Crepitus on palpating/moving the fractured segments.
- Trismus may be present and is more common in type 2 and 3 due to spasm of pterygoid muscles.

Investigations

- X-ray skull lateral views and X-ray PNS-occipitomental and occipitofrontal views. Submentovertical (base skull) view is valuable but should be taken only after ruling out fracture of the cervical spine.
- X-ray nasal bones.
- CT scan with 3 D reconstruction.
- Nasal endoscopy is useful in the evaluation of CSF rhinorrhea.

Treatment

Open reduction with internal fixation of fracture segments by mini-plates or intermaxillary fixation. Dental cap splints or Box frame with pin fixation may be employed. Soft tissue lacerations should be carefully repaired to avoid scarring. Epistaxis and CSF rhinorrhea should be managed as described under corresponding chapters.

Fracture of Nasal Bone

This is the commonest fracture of the facial skeleton due to its prominent position in the face. This may be due to a simple blow to the front or side of the nose, sports injury or road traffic accidents. Occasionally it could be an occupational injury. It is often associated with septal fracture and displacement/septal hematoma. Nasal bone fracture may be associated with other fractures of the mid-face including cribriform plate, ethmoids and frontal bone.

Types (Fig. 38.5)

Depending on the amount of force

1. Un-displaced fracture (greenstick): Fracture line seen without displacement of the fracture segments.
2. Displaced fracture

Depending on the direction of the force applied to the nose

1. Depressed fracture or 'open book' fracture occurs due to frontal force and causes flattening of the nasal dorsum. Saddle nose deformity may be associated with.

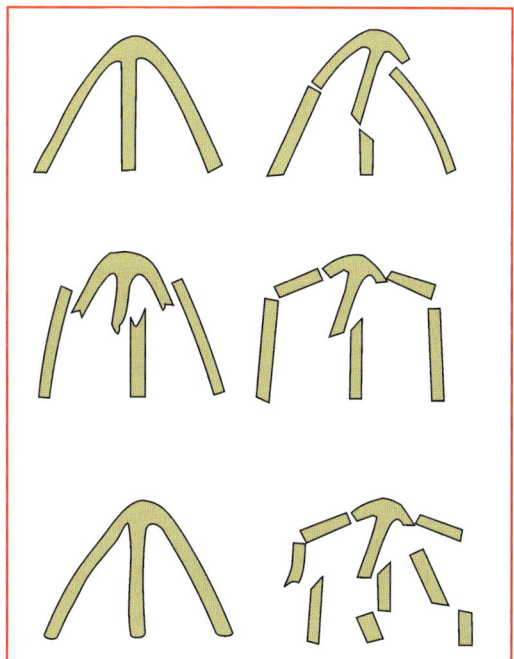

Fig. 38.5: Common types of nasal bone fractures

2. Angulated fracture occurs due to lateral force and causes 'Crooked nose'.

Depending on the soft tissue injury involved overlying the nasal bones it may be classified into:
1. Open fracture
2. Closed fracture

Symptoms

Depends on recent or late injury:
- Epistaxis
- Pain and swelling
- Black eye
- Deformity
- Nose block.

Signs (Fig. 38.6)
- Swelling over the external nose
- Nasal deformity like flattening of the nose (depressed fracture), crookedness of the bridge (displaced fracture).
- Crepitus and tenderness may be felt.
- Periorbital and subconjunctival ecchymosis can be noted.

Investigation: X-ray of nose - AP, Lateral (Fig. 38.7).

Treatment

- It depends on the duration of the injury.

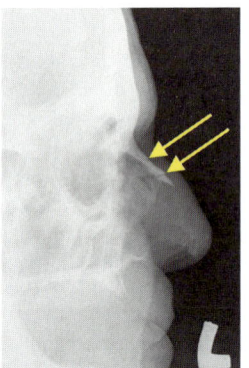
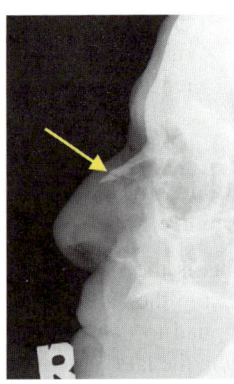

Fig. 38.7: X-ray of the nasal bones showing fracture lines (yellow arrows)

- If the patient presents immediately before the swelling over the nose appears, surgical intervention with reduction of the fracture can be done immediately using a Asche's or Spencer Wells forceps after disimpaction of the fractured bone followed by realignment by using digital pressure. Walsham's forceps may be required for disimpaction (Figs 38.8a and b).
- If swelling has already appeared over the external nose, the fracture reduction should be delayed until the swelling subsides. After about 7–14 days fracture can be reduced as described earlier. Procedure can be done under local or general anaesthesia.

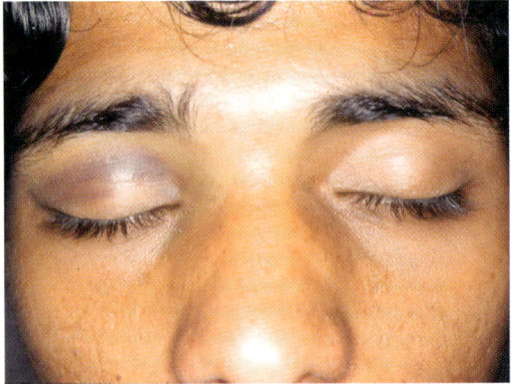

Fig. 38.6 Showing periorbital ecchymosis and swelling of the external nose

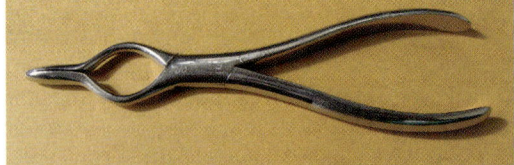

Fig. 38.8a: Walsham's forceps

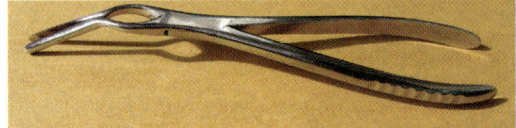

Fig. 38.8b: Asche's septal forceps

- For delayed, neglected, mal-united fracture rhinoplasty is required (discussed under chapter Common Surgeries of the Nose and PNS).

Lateral

Malar-Maxillary Complex Fracture (Tripod fracture) (Fig. 38.9)

This is the second most common facial fracture next to the nasal bones. This occurs due to force applied to the malar bone or the zygomatic arch from the lateral aspect leading to displacement of fracture segments consisting of the malar bone backwards and downwards into the antrum. There are three sites of fracture namely zygomatico-maxillary, fronto-zygomatic and the zygomatic arch. Hence it is called tripod fracture.

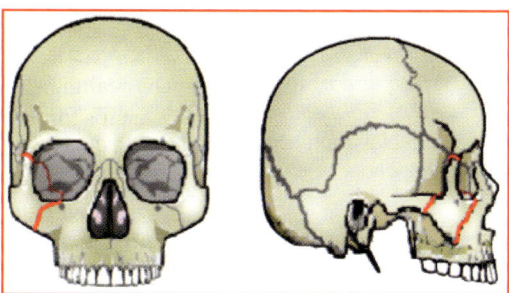

Fig. 38.9: Malar zygomatic fracture shown in red line

Clinical Features

- Flattening of malar eminence is noticed immediately after the fracture. This may get masked later as the facial swelling develops.
- Peri-orbital ecchymosis is often present.
- Diplopia is present in some cases.
- Step-deformity of the infra-orbital rim may be palpated.
- Paresthesia of the cheek may be present due to infra-orbital nerve entrapment.
- Epistaxis
- Trismus may be seen due to entrapment of temporalis muscle or due to associated fracture of coronoid process of the mandible.

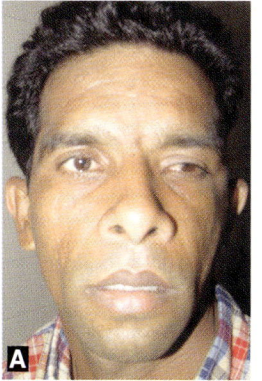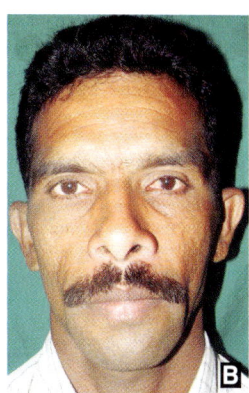

Fig. 38.10 a and b: (a) Flattening of the mallar eminance in the left eye associated with narrow palpebral fissure, (b) Post-operative picture of the same patient following fracture reduction

- Oblique/narrow palpebral fissure if lateral canthal ligmant is pulled infero-laterally as shown in the Figs 38.10a and b.

Investigations

- X-ray PNS- Water's and Caldwel view- show the fracture segments and hemoantrum
- Hirtz view or the base skull view is suitable to show the zygomatic arch.
- CT scan is most preferred investigation which shows the fracture segments better especially with respect to the posterior wall of maxilla (Figs 38.11a and b).

Treatment

Open reduction and internal fixation by wiring or plating under general anesthesia. Sublabial approach may be employed (Figs 38.12a and b). Incision on the temporal region behind the hairline may be useful in reduction of zygomatic arch fractures.

Blow-out Fracture of the Orbital Floor (Fig. 38.13)

This occurs due to blunt injury to the orbit. The sudden pressure raise in the orbit causes fracture

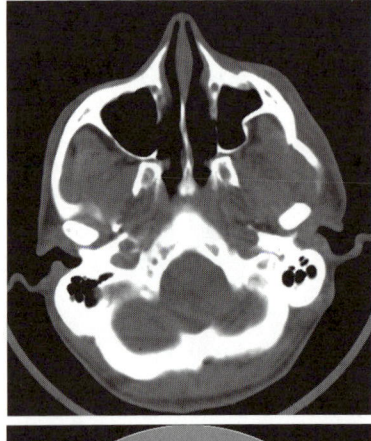

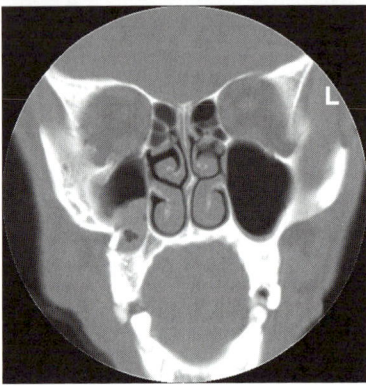

Figs 38.11a and b: Axial and coronal scans showing malar-maxillary fracture of the left side (arrow)

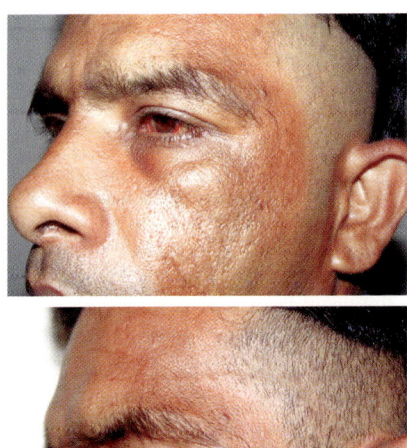

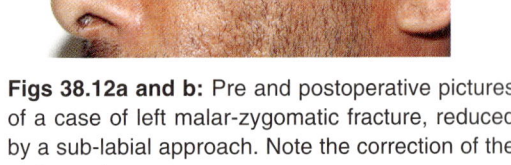

Figs 38.12a and b: Pre and postoperative pictures of a case of left malar-zygomatic fracture, reduced by a sub-labial approach. Note the correction of the malar eminence

of the weak orbital floor and consequent herniation of the orbital contents into the maxilla. It may be associated with entrapment neuropathy (infra-orbital nerve) or entrapment myopathy (inferior rectus/inferior oblique muscles). Muscle entrapment causes inability of the eye to move downwards and outwards and diplopia.

Clinical Features

1. Enophthalmous (eyeball is pushed inwards) due to herniation of orbital contents.
2. Infra-orbital paresthesia.
3. Vertical diplopia may be present.
4. Forced reduction test is done by passively moving the globe in all directions after instillation of topical anesthesia to the

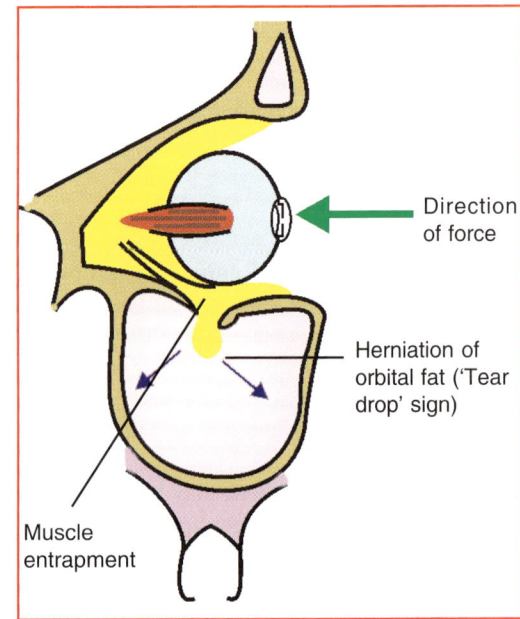

Fig. 38.13: The mechanism of blow-out fracture

cornea. In case of muscle entrapment, globe cannot be passively moved.

Investigation

X-ray PNS/coronal CT scan shows the classical 'tear drop' sign due to herniation of orbital fat.

Treatment

Open exploration and release of the orbital nerve/muscles. Repair of the floor may be done using cartilage/nasal septal bone grafts.

CSF RHINORRHEA

Definition

It refers to leak of cerebrospinal fluid (CSF) from its intracranial location through the nose. Incidence of CSF rhinorrhea in rhinological practice is becoming more because of better diagnostic tools like diagnostic nasal endoscopy and CT scan. At present, its treatment has become more rhinological than neurosurgical.

CSF rhinorrhea may be classified as traumatic and non-traumatic cause. It has been reported that between 2 and 9% of the cases of nasal trauma are complicated by CSF rhinorrhea, and in those involving the paranasal sinuses, the incidence rises to 25%. Trauma to the floor of the anterior cranial fossa must have disruption of the arachnoid, a tear in dura and fracture of bone (as well as tear through the periosteum and mucosa) to result in a fistula. The bone of the anterior skull is thin with densely adherent dura and hence fractures here often result in dural tears. The T-shaped mass of the crista galli and the cribriform plate is strong and moves as a single unit. Thus, a fracture in the medial fovea ethmoidalis is most common. Atraumatic fistulae occur commonly in the cribriform area through the olfactory tracts.

Middle cranial fossa fractures are less common injuries that can cause leakage into the nose via the sphenoid sinus or eustachian tube. CSF leak may also occur from the posterior fossa in fracture of the clivus allowing CSF into the sphenoid sinus, and fracture of the petrous temporal bone allowing fluid to enter the mastoid air cell system and hence the eustachian tube (in the presence of intact TM).

Post traumatic CSF is immediate in majority of the cases. When delayed it appears within 3 months in 95% of cases. The pathophysiology of this is not clearly understood and it is said that edema and inflammation can temporarily obstruct the flow of CSF. As this resolves in the first week after injury 70% of fistulae have already manifested. In delayed fistulae, disrupted blood supply causes resorption of bones and tissue which weakens the pia and arachnoid seal leading to elevation in ICP with delayed fistula formation and ending up with leak. 16% of CSF leak is due to surgeries in nose, paranasal sinuses and skull base.

Etiological Factors

The etiological factors of CSF rhinorrhea have been best described by Ommaya (1976). The classification is described as follows:

1. **Traumatic**
   - Accidental: Acute or delayed onset
   - Iatrogenic: Acute or delayed onset
2. **Non-traumatic**
   High pressure
   - Tumors
     Direct: Due to invasion by the tumor
     Indirect: Due to increase in intracranial pressure
   - Hydrocephalus
   Normal pressure
   - Congenital
   - Focal atrophy: Olfactory or sellar
   - Osteomyelitic erosion
   - Idiopathic

Location of CSF Rhinorrhea

Leakage is seen mostly in the floor of the anterior cranial fossa at the levels of cribriform plate which may be either anterior or posteriorly placed.

Anteriorly placed leaks are in the frontoethmoidal junction or cribriform plate and posteriorly placed leaks in the sphenoethmoidal junction and sphenoid sinus.

Clinical Features

1. Recurrent watery clear non-sticky discharge from the nose, often unilateral (Refer Table 38.1).
2. Hyposmia and anosmia in 80% of cases.
3. Headache in 20% of cases.
4. Recurrent meningitis may be associated with CSF rhinorrhea.

Investigations

- Diagnostic nasal endoscopy is useful to locate site of leak, i.e. middle meatus, superior meatus, sphenoethmoidal recess.
- Wet handkerchief test.
- Positional change or jugular compression can increase the flow.

- Reservoir sign—after being supine for some time, the patient is brought to upright position with the neck flexed. A sudden rush of fluid occurs.
- Halo sign (Target sign or double ring sign) - when the CSF rhinorrhea is blood stained and dries out with a central blood stain surrounded by a clear ring.
- Estimation of glucose content in the nasal discharge. Increase of 30 mg per ml is significant.
- Immunoelectrophoretic identification of $\beta2$ transferrin is most widely used test.
- Glucose oxidase impregnated strips—not reliable as false positive test may be given lacrimal and nasal mucous secretions.
- Metrizamide computer tomographic cisternography (MCTC).
- Injection of color dye in subarachnoid space like methyl blue, indigocarmine, toludine blue.
- Radioactive isotope injection

Table 38.1: Differences between allergic rhinorrhea and CSF rhinorrhea

	Allergic rhinorrhea	CSF rhinorrhea
Clinical features	Features of allergies like sneezing, nasal block and itching are present	These associated features are absent
Etiology	Allergen	Traumatic (Accidental or Iatrogenic) Spontaneous
Discharge	Mucous-like or clear, which is not increased by raising intra-abdominal pressure and intracranial pressure but discharge can be sniffed back	Thin and watery which increases on bending forwards and cannot be sniffed back
Taste	Salty	Sweet
Handkerchief test	Discharge is dried up and cloth becomes stiff	No such effect
Halo sign	Absent	Present in traumatic cases
Lab	Sugar content less than 10 mg/dl $\beta2$ transferrin absent	More than 30 mg/dl $\beta2$ transferrin present
CT scan	Normal skull base	Shows bony dehiscence in anterior skull base

- Contrast CT/MRI. CT scan with contrast (Omnipaque) intrathecally by lumbar puncture. The scan is taken usually 3 hours after this injection contrast and reveals the leak better (Fig. 38.14).
- Intrathecal fluroscein injection is useful in locating the site of leak.

HRCT—Coronal/Sagittal/Axial

Treatment

Depends on the cause.

In traumatic CSF rhinorrhea the following measures are taken:
1. Prophylactic antibiotic.
2. Bed rest in head up position.
3. Avoid coughing, sneezing and nose blowing.
4. Mild laxative to prevent constipation.
5. Repeated or continuous lumbar puncture.
6. Traumatic cases heals with medical management (diuretics, manitol, etc.)

Surgical Treatment
1. Extracranial.
2. Intracranial.

Extracranial Surgical Repair

The middle turbinate is resected inferolaterally (a concha bullosa is excised on its lateral aspect) for better visualization of middle meatus. An infundibulotomy is performed by resecting the uncinate process. Bulla is identified and opened in the same way as done in endoscopic sinus surgery. The anterior ethmoidal cells are exenterated completely to expose the dome of the ethmoid. The anterior ethmoidal artery is identified. If the posterior ethmoid and the sphenoid are sites of leakage, they should be opened further, keeping the ethmoid as the landmark. The anesthesiologist is asked to hyperventilate the patient and raise the CSF pressure which facilitates in identifying the CSF leak. The dura is exposed further at the site of the leak. A piece of temporalis fascia harvested from the postauricular region is placed over the defect which is anchored between the dura and bone. The graft is further covered with subcutaneous fat, which is well supported further with surgicel and gel foam. The middle meatus is then packed with BIPP pack. This can be removed on 10th postoperative day. The cavity should be re-inspected after 1 month. CSF pressure should be controlled during post-operative period till the healing is complete.

Use of nasal endoscope has taught us how to be delicate, precise, conservative and at the same time result oriented while dealing with the micronasal pathology.

Today's fiberoptic Hopkin's rod endoscope is a highly sophisticated one and use of its various accessories like endovision camera have vastly widened the scope of the indications of endoscopic sinus surgery. Repair of CSF rhinorrhea, removal of meningocoele, anterior cranio-facial resection, excision of acoustic tumor through posterior fossa keyhole approach etc. becomes possible without doing craniotomy in most of the cases.

Endoscopic Technique

This is done by endoscopic approach via transnasal route. The mortality and morbidity in this approach is absolutely minimal in comparison to intracranial

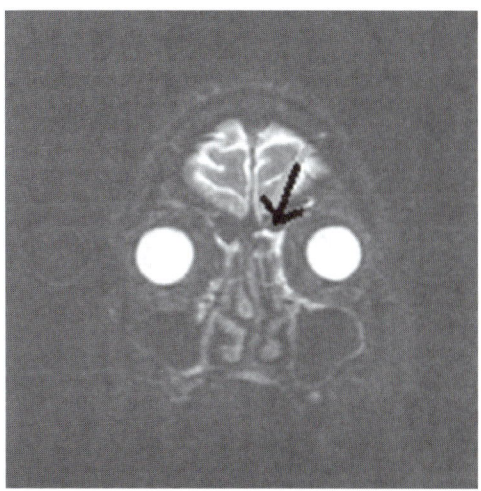

Fig. 38.14: MRI scan showing the site of CSF leak (←)

approach. It gives high success rate of closure. This approach can be done in very elderly patient also without having any fear of developing cerebral anoxia. That is why this approach is gaining more and more popularity among surgeons and also with patients (Figs 38.15a to c)

CSF rhinorrhea can be adequately managed by transnasal endoscopic approach. However, infrastructure like good radiologist with CT and MRI scan facilities and adequate surgical expertise is required.

Neuro Surgical Approach

This is done by an intracranial approach through bicoronal craniotomy. It is done through bicoronal craniotomy or mini craniotomy approach. Repairing of the defect is done transcranially by using bone and fascia lata graft.

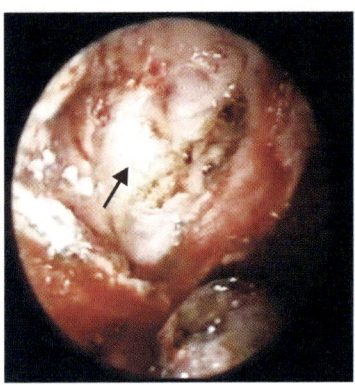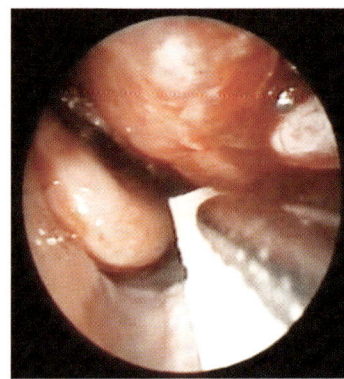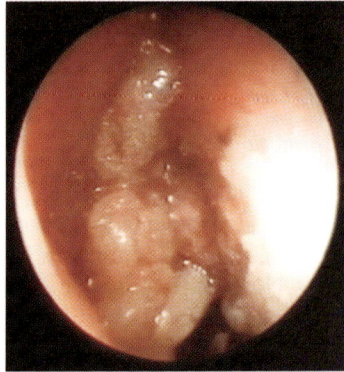

Figs 38.15a to c: Endoscopic technique of repair of CSF rhinorrhea, (a) Site of leak is identified, (b) A piece of cartilage (autograft) is used to seal the leak, (c) Ethmoid cavity is packed with fascia temporalis

POINTS TO REMEMBER

1. Nasal bone is the most common facial bone to be fractured, followed by zygoma.
2. Pyramidal fracture (Type II) is the most common type of Le-Fort fracture.
3. 'Tear drop' sign is characteristic radiological feature of blow-out fracture of orbit.
4. Majority of traumatic CSF rhinorrhea heal with conservative management. Presently endoscopic endonasal repair and CSF rhinorrhea has replaced the morbid neurological approach.

Benign Tumors and Tumor Like Conditions of the Nasal Cavity and PNS

39

Classification

Epithelial

- Odontogenic
  - Dental cyst
  - Dentigerous cyst
- Non-odontogenic
  - Squamous papilloma
  - Inverted papilloma
  - Salivary adenoma
  - Nasopalatine and nasolabial cyst
  - Dermoid cyst

Non-epithelial

- Odontogenic
  - Dentinoma
  - Cementinoma
- Non-odontogenic
  - Fibro-osseous dysplasia
  - Myxoma
  - Lipoma
  - Chondroma
  - Osteoma
  - Hemangioma

COMMON CYSTS OF THE NOSE AND PARANASAL SINUS

1. ODONTOGENIC CYSTS

They are derived from odontogenic epithelium (ameloblasts, cementoblasts, odontoblasts) around impacted or unerupted teeth, or from epithelial rests or remnants of dental lamina.

(a) Dental Cyst (Radicular Cyst)

This occurs around the root of erupted tooth and is due to infection of the periapical epithelium leading to cystic changes.

Etiology

- *Incidence:* Most common cyst of the jaw (60% of all dental cysts)
- Infection around the root is the primary cause
- It is intimately associated with root of the tooth and hence it is called *radicular cyst*.
- It can present as a lateral periodontal cystwhen inflammation occurs in the gingival pocket.

Pathology

- Infection initiates cystic degeneration
- Secretes a variety of interleukins, which cause bone resorption and facilitates further expansion of the cyst.
- After reaching sufficient size, it can predispose to pathological fractures.

Histopathology

- Squamous lining with 6 to 20 cells thick and cyst contains cholesterol crystals.

Clinical Features (Fig. 39.1)

- Swelling around an erupted tooth preceded with pain.

365

- Egg-shell crackling may be elicited when the bone is thin.

Investigation

Radiological: Occlusal view/ orthopantomogram shows round or ovoid cyst associated with tooth root.

Treatment

Enucleation of cyst with extraction or apicectomy of the infected tooth.

Prognosis: Has a tendency to recur

(b) Dentigerous Cyst (Follicular Cyst)

Definition

Cyst developing around an unerupted permanent tooth in young adults

Incidence

- 13% of all dental cysts
- *Peak incidence:* 10-35 years of age
- 1% with complete dental radiographs

Pathology (Fig. 39.2)

- Fluid accumulates between ameloblasts (epithelium that produces the crown) and unerupted tooth.

- Usually involves permanent third molars and maxillary cuspids
- Slow growing cyst causing bone expansion and thinning and teeth displacement.
- Recurrence suggests incomplete excision.

Histopathology

- Lined by thin flat cuboidal epithelial lining
- Cyst contains cholesterol crystals

Clinical features: Painless, slowly progressive facial swelling in the region of upper jaw.

Investigation: X-ray occlusal view/ orthopantomogram: unilocular cyst associated with crown of unerupted tooth

Treatment: Enucleation with tooth of origin.

2. NON-ODONTOGENIC CYSTS

Non-odontogenic cysts associated with faulty fusion of embryological elements that form the maxilla:

Medial Group

- Median alveolar cyst
- Median palatal cyst
- Nasopalatine cyst.

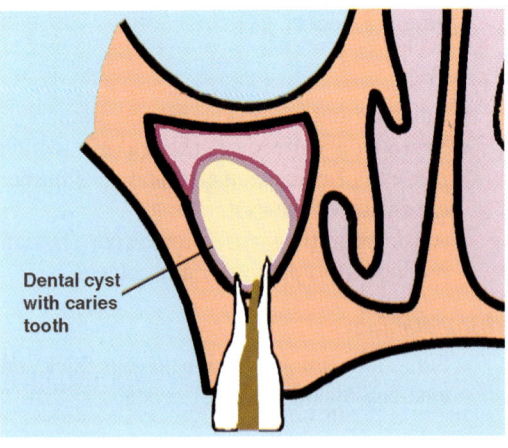

Fig. 39.1: Dental cyst (radicular cyst) arising from erupted caries tooth

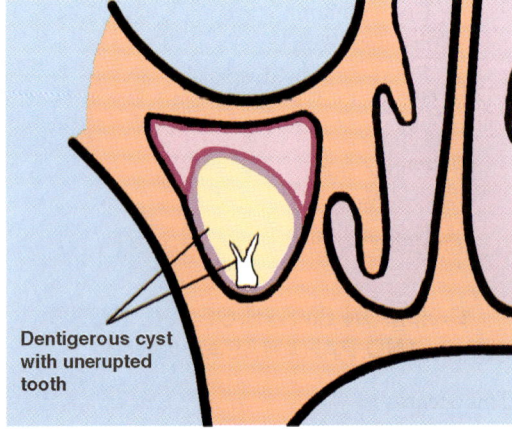

Fig. 39.2: Dentigerous cyst arising from unerupted tooth

Lateral Group

- Lateral alveolar cyst
- Nasoalveolar cyst (nasolabial cyst)

(a) Nasopalatine Cyst

- Due to enclavement of vestigial oronasal cysts

Incidence:

- Usually ages 30 to 60 years
- More common in males with ratio 3:1

Pathology: May develop entirely within bone, within incisive papilla of anterior palatal gingiva or within bone and soft tissue.

Histopathology: Lined by stratified squamous or respiratory epithelium and may contain prominent neurovascular bundle within connective tissue wall.

Radiology: More than 7 mm round or heart shaped cyst between upper and central incisors

Treatment: Enucleation

(b) Nasoalveolar Cyst (Nasolabial cyst)

- Formed due to defective fusion of maxillary and globular processes, may develop from caudal end of nasolacrimal rod or duct
- Arises in soft tissue of upper lip or lateral aspect of nose, may be bilateral
- More common in blacks and women
- Often becomes infected, obliterates nasolabial fold

Microscopic feature: Llined by stratified squamous or respiratory epithelium

Treatment: Enucleation

COMMON BENIGN TUMORS OF NOSE AND PNS

Squamous Papilloma (Fig. 39.3)

This occurs mainly in the skin of the nasal vestibule and septum. They are usually solitary pedunculated or sessile warty lesions. If large enough, it can cause nasal obstruction. This may be excised

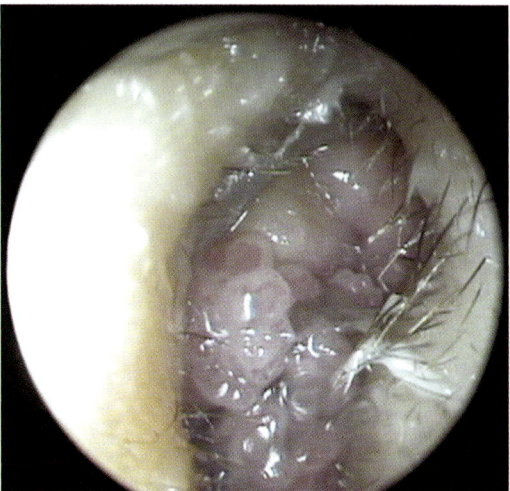

Fig. 39.3: Endoscopic view of nasal papilloma

surgically under endoscopic supervision using diathermy or laser.

Inverted Papilloma

Synonyms

Ringert's tumor, transitional cell papilloma, fungiform papilloma, cylindrical cell papilloma, Schneiderian cell papilloma, epithelial papilloma.

Inverted papillomas are benign tumors of nose and PNS that often arise from the lateral wall of the nasal cavity especially in the region of middle meatus. Less common sites are the vestibule, the septum, the floor of the nasopharynx, sphenoid and frontal sinus, and the lacrimal sac.

Etiology

It is a rare tumor occurring in approximately 0.5 percent of the nasal tumors, thus representing approximately 4 percent of all nasal polyps

Exact etiology is not known. Viruses have been implicated due to the well described finding in recurrent respiratory papillomatosis. A recent study has shown the presence of the human papilloma virus in specimens of inverted papilloma hybridized in situ with RNA probes to

HPV 6, 11,16, and 18. No definite correlation has been found with subtype and dysplasia.

Pathology

Gross

Inverted papilloma grossly looks like a polyp, but is usually firmer with significant bulk and has more of a granular mulberry type appearance. They are a variety of colors from red to pale pink. They are usually more vascular than the average polyp.

Histopathology

Microscopically the lesion has a thickened epithelial covering with extensive invasion of the hyperplastic epithelium into the underlying stroma. Hence it is called inverted papilloma. The behavior of the invasion into the underlying stroma has been theorized to be due to an origin from the **Schneiderian membrane**. The tumor appears to invaginate or infold into the surrounding underlying bone yet does not invade in the absence of malignancy.

Extension to all of the sinuses as well as the cranial base is possible. While inverted papillomas are considered benign tumors, approximately 10% undergo malignant change into squamous cell carcinoma. Hence a complete surgical resection is mandatory.

Clinical Features

Symptoms

The main symptoms include the following:
1. Nasal obstruction
2. Facial swelling
3. Hyponasal speech
4. Epistaxis or blood stained nasal discharge
5. Pressure and pain
6. Rhinorrhea
7. Orbital symptoms like proptosis, diplopia and epiphora
8. Hyposmia/anosmia

Signs

They usually present as a polyp and are mistakenly treated as a polyp. They are reddish or pinkish, solitary, sometimes granular, friable mass arising in the region of the middle meatus in the lateral wall of the nose. It may bleed on touch. Extension to the surrounding sinuses and the orbit can lead to facial swelling and proptosis. If there is evidence of bone erosion, malignancy should be suspected.

Diagnosis

This is usually based on clinical presentation and histopathological examination. Serial section studies should be done as there is possibility of malignancy in certain areas.

Differential Diagnosis

Antrochoanal polyp, allergic fungal sinusitis, squamous cell carcinoma, adenocarcinoma, esthesioblastoma, inverted papilloma and other rare tumors.

Investigations

1. *Radiological:* X-ray PNS may show involvement of sinuses with associated bone erosion. CT scan imaging (both coronal and axial) helps in depicting accurate extensions of the tumor and in proper treatment planning.
2. Diagnostic nasal endoscopy and biopsy.

Treatment

Usually a medial maxillectomy (Figs 39.4a and b Figs 39.5a and b) including the medial aspect of maxilla and the ethmoids, is done with lateral rhinotomy with or without Lynch extension or by a mid-facial degloving approach. Small lesions may be excised endoscopically using laser. If histopathology shows associated malignancy, it should be treated as carcinoma of maxilla as described under the malignant tumors.

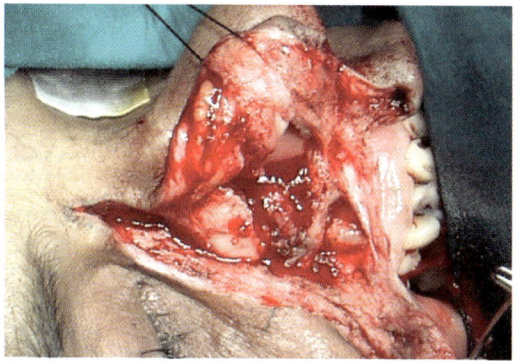

Fig. 39.4a: Exposure of the tumor mass after lateral rhinotomy

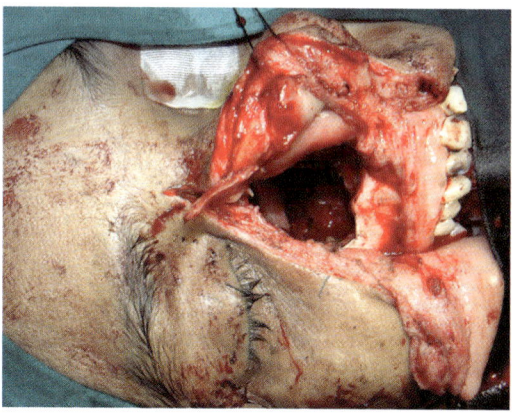

Fig. 39.4b: Defect after medial maxillectomy and tumor removal

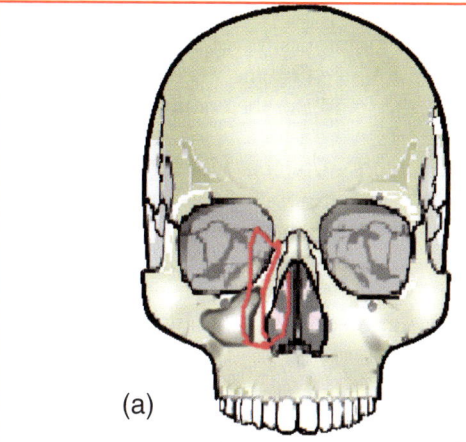

(a)

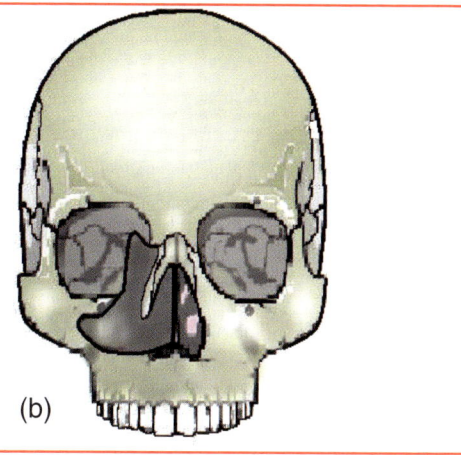

(b)

Fig. 39.5a: Osteotomy mark (red line) for medial maxillectomy approach

Fig. 39.5b: Defect after the medial maxillectomy and ethmoidectomy

Juvenile Nasopharyngeal Angiofibroma (JNA)

They are uncommon, benign, slow growing tumors. JNAs most commonly arise from the sphenopalatine foramen or the posterolateral wall of the roof of the nose. These tumors are difficult to manage because they are typically locally destructive causing invasion into the nasal cavity, maxillary sinuses, the orbit and even the intracranium.

Nasal obstruction, epistaxis (nosebleed), rhinorrhea (nasal drainage), facial swelling, displacement of orbital contents, and headache are the most common presenting symptoms. The etiology of JNAs is not known but they are found almost exclusively in males with the highest prevalence in teenagers and young adults.

Treatment

Treatment of JNAs is primarily surgical, but in some situations radiation therapy may be used.

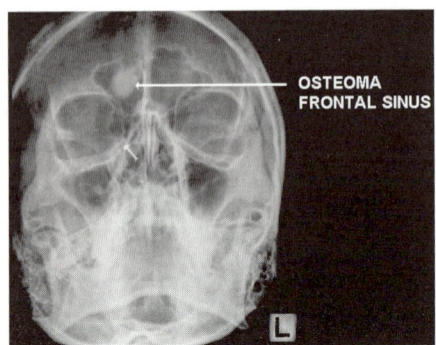

Fig. 39.6: Radiography shadow in right frontal sinus suggesting an osteoma

For more details refer to Chapter 54 under section pharynx.

Osteoma (Fig. 39.6)

This is a benign osteogenic tumor which is slow growing and contains mature bone. In order of frequency, osteoma is more common in frontal sinus than in the ethmoid and rarely in the maxillary sinus. Sphenoidal osteoma is extremely rare.

Most often they are found incidentally on radiological examination. When it enlarges to obstruct the ostium of the affected sinus causing secondary sinusitis, patients call for medical attention. Sometimes the patient may come with mucocele of the affected sinus with external swelling. It is more common in 15 to 40 years of age. It is often pedunculated. Ethmoidal osteoma can present with proptosis as they invade the orbit. It can also involve the sphenoid sinus and the optic nerve.

Gardner's syndrome is an autosomal dominant condition in which 50 percent of the offspring are affected by osteoma. Classical symptom complex is a hard and soft tissue tumor associated with polyposis of the bowel and osteoma of skull and facial bone as a constant feature. Treatment is excision by osteoplastic flap approach or through Lynch-Howarth external frontoethmoidectomy approach.

Ossifying Fibroma

Synonym: Fibrous osteomas, osteofibromas.

Definition

Ossifying fibromas are encapsulated, slow-growing benign fibro-osseus neoplasms, composed of fibrous tissue mixed with varying amounts of mature bone.

Etiology

They tend to affect women more than men and can occur over a wide age range, but are frequently seen in the third and fourth decades of life.

Pathology

The most common sites of occurrence are the mandible followed by the maxilla. Lesions that occur in the sinuses or the cranial base tend to be more aggressive.

These types of tumors typically do not cause symptoms and are often diagnosed incidentally by radiographic examination.

A variant of ossifying fibroma is juvenile active ossifying fibroma. These tumors may behave aggressively with local destructive capabilities.

Clinical Features

1. Facial swelling
2. Deformity
3. Proptosis
4. Malocclusion

Treatment

Surgical excision is the treatment of choice.

Prognosis is excellent after complete excision. Treatment of juvenile active ossifying fibroma variant needs a complete surgical excision with a more radical approach.

Fibrous Dysplasia

This is a skeletal developmental abnormality wherein the medullary bone is replaced by fibro-osseous tissue. There are four types: Monoostotic, polyostotic, craniofacial form and cherubism.

Etiology

- Unknown
- **Age:** Usually presents in age of 3 to 15 years. Most of the cases present before 20 years of age. Some may present even in later age group.
- **Sex:** More common in females. Some reports show equal sex predilection.
- **Race:** No specific racial predilection exists

Pathology

Three histological types

1. **Active form:** Rich in cellular connective tissue with numerous mitotic figure. Seen in younger patients. Involved bone does not contain any lacunae or osteoblasts.
2. **Quiescent form:** Associated with more mature connective tissue, fewer mitosis and bone component is prominent.
3. **Inactive form:** Degeneration of connective tissue and matrix associated with lamellar bone and osteoblastic rimming.

Clinical Features

Painless swelling of the bone. Maxilla is more commonly associated than mandible. Common site in maxilla is canine fossa area or zygomatic area. Alveolus is frequently involved.

Swelling can produce cosmetic or functional disability (Fig. 39.7).

Functional Disability

- **Orbital:** Proptosis, diplopia, impaired vision if optic nerve is compressed, epiphora, etc.
- **Oral:** Dysarthria, difficulty in chewing, malocclusion
- Polyostotic form with cutaneous pigmentation and endocrine abnormality is called 'Albright's syndrome'.

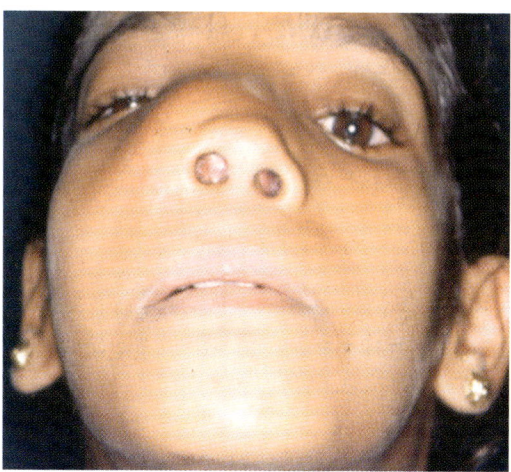

Fig. 39.7: Swelling on the right side of the face due to fibrous dysplasia

- Familial variant involving the cranio-facial region is called 'Cherubism'.

Investigation

X-ray of PNS/CT imaging shows classical 'ground glass' appearance of the tumor. CT may show obliteration of the sinuses with obliteration of infraorbital margin.

Treatment

Surgery is the treatment of choice and is only indicated in symptomatic patients. The surgery should be as conservative as possible and is confined to cosmetic or function trimming/ paring. Irradiation is dangerous as it can promote malignant transformation.

Hemangioma

Hemangioma and angioma are common in the nasal septum. It can also arise from the turbinates, nasopharynx and rarely in the external nose. Most common presenting feature are nasal obstruction and epistaxis. Delayed treatment can cause broadening of the nose and deformity. Nasal tip is the common site in the external nose. Excision

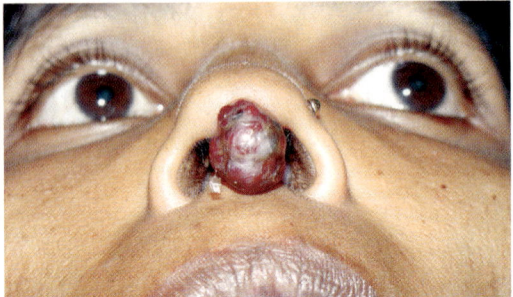

Fig. 39.8a: Hemangioma involving the columella and nasal tip

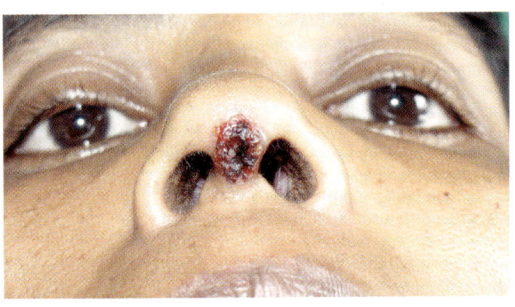

Fig. 39.8b: Post laser excision of hemangioma. Healing is by epithelialization with minimal scarring

using laser is the best treatment. Injection of sclerosing agents may be tried (Figs 39.8a and b)

Bleeding Polypus

Bleeding polypus of the nasal septum is a benign pedunculated bleeding mass arising from the nasal septum. Most common type is angioma and it commonly arises from the Little's area of the nasal septum (Fig. 39.9) and occurs at the age of 20 to 50 years predominantly in females.Laser excision of the polypus is the treatment of choice.

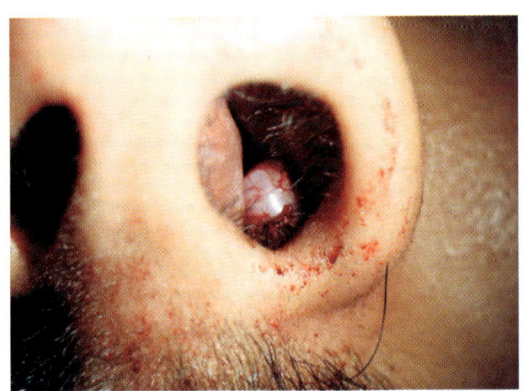

Fig. 39.9: Bleeding polypus of the nasal septum

POINTS TO REMEMBER

1. Dental cyst ocurs around root of erupted tooth and dentigerous cyst develops around unerupted permanent tooth .
2. Inverted papilloma may undergo malignant transformation in about 10 percent of cases.
3. Medial maxilectomy is treatment of choice for inverted papilloma
4. Fibrous dysplasia of the facial bone is common in young females and the surgical treatment of choice is cosmetic functional sharing or parring of the tumor.

Malignant Tumors of Nose and Paranasal Sinuses

40

Cancer of nasal cavity and paranasal sinuses are uncommon. Cancer of the skin of the nose is probably the commonest of the facial cancer. Cancer in the maxillary and ethmoid sinus is more common than cancer in the sphenoid and frontal sinus.

MALIGNANT TUMORS OF NASAL CAVITY AND PNS

Etiology

Incidence: It comprises of 0.5 percent of all malignancy and 3 percent of all head and neck tumors.

Predisposing Factors

1. Infection
- Chronic sinusitis
- Protracted polyposis

2. Occupation
- People working in wood industries are prone to develop adenocarcinoma of ethmoid.
- People working in nickel and chrome industries have an increased risk of developing paranasal sinus cancer.
- People working in leather industries also can develop cancer of the ethmoid.

3. Habits: Snuff use is an well recognized etiological factor.

4. Iatrogenic: Post-irradiation

5. Inverted papilloma may undergo malignant transformation.

Pathology

Around 80 percent of tumors affecting nose and paranasal sinuses are of squamous cell carcinoma. These tumors are graded from well differentiated to undifferentiated. About 60 percent of them are of antral, 30 percent in the nasal cavity and 10 percent seen in the ethmoid sinus. The incidence of cervical lymph node involvement is about 15 percent. It is primarily a male disease and present mainly in sixth decade of life, it has no close relationship with known carcinogens that have been described. Spreads outside the sinus wall are common.

Squamous Cell Carcinoma

Squamous carcinoma is the commonest tumor to affect the maxillary and ethmoid sinus. They are commonly associated with bone erosion of lateral nasal wall, the palate and the alveolus. It can also involve some important area like pterygoid plate, the orbit, the posterior ethmoids and the cribriform plate in the advanced stage with relatively poor prognosis. Lymphatic spread from maxillary sinus are commonly to submandibular area through retropharyngeal lymph nodes and those from ethmoids to jugulodiagstric and subdigastric group.

Adenocarcinoma

It is second commonest tumor after squamous cell carcinoma to affect the maxillary and ethmoid sinuses. They are more common in ethmoid sinus and has been thought to be due to known carcinogen like wood dust, nickel, etc. It presents in the same way like squamous cell carcinoma.

Rare malignant tumors of nose and paranasal sinus

- *Transitional cell carcinoma:* It is a non keratinizing type of squamous cell carcinoma and has a close relationship with inverted papilloma. Rarely it can arise directly from benign inverted papilloma.
- *Anaplastic carcinoma:* It is a rare tumor and has similar histological picture with that of lymphomas, olfactory neuroblastoma, rhabdomyosarcoma.
- *Malignant melanoma*: Comprise of 1 percent of nasal and paranasal cancers and commonly arise from septum or the lateral nasal wall. Often present as polypoidal swelling that may be grey, blue or black.
- *Olfactory neuroblastoma:* Also known as esthesioneuroblastoma or neuroendocrine tumors that resembles like an anaplastic carcinoma. It arises in the upper part of nasal cavity from the stem cells of neural crest origin that subsequently differentiate into olfactory sensory cells. It is the slow growing tumor which may become large and destructive. Commonly presents as a nasal mass which is reddish in color, friable, and bleeds on touch. It is considered to be a neuroendocrinal tumor, should be evaluated for vanillylmandelic acid (VMA) which can be associated with hypertension.
- *Adenocystic carcinoma*: It arises from minor salivary gland within the nasal cavity and maxillary antrum. Histologically three distinct type are seen, i.e. Tubular, Cribriform and Solid. Tubular form is least aggressive. These tumor in nose and PNS have worst prognosis than any other area of head and neck, and have the characteristic feature of perineural invasion. Vascular invasion is also common.

- *Metastatic carcinoma*
- *Malignant osseous tumor*: It is rare tumor in nose and PNS. Osteogenic sarcoma is most common bony tumor which frequently affects maxilla. Rare tumor involving sphenoid bone has been reported in literature (Hazarika & Nayak et al).
- Malignant connective tissue tumor
- *Chondrosarcoma:* Its prognosis is bad if present in posterior part of nose and PNS and often associated with skull base erosion and destruction
- **Rhabdomyosarcoma:** This is common in children and its prognosis is improved due to advancement in chemotherapy
- *Hemangiopericytoma:* This is vascular tumor and arises from pericyte of capillary. It grows locally due to limited infiltration
- *Lymphoma:* It usually affects males in 5th and 6th decade. Commonest types is histiocytic lymphoma. Nasal T cell lymphoma has a very bad prognosis and commonly associated with necrotizing midfacial lesion. They should be differentiated from Wegeners granulomatosis.
- *Malignant oncocytoma:* They are rare tumors of the minor salivary gland which may involve the nasal cavity.

Classification of Squamous Cell Carcinoma

It is very difficult to classify malignant tumors of the nose and PNS satisfactorily. It is important to know where the tumor starts, where it goes and what it has invaded. Problem also exists in relation to converting a dimensional picture in to a dimensional verbal plan. **Ohngren** classified the maxillo-ethmoidal complex carcinoma by drawing an imaginary plane extending between the medial canthus of the eye to the angle of the mandible. Growth present above the line was described as suprastructure and below the line as infrastructure is now no more followed.

In 1969, Lederman classified the tumor using 2 horizontal lines; one passing through the floor of the orbit and the other one passing through the floor of the antrum. These divide the upper jaw into upper suprastructure, middle mesostructure and lower infrastructure. His classification is as follows.

T1 : Tumor limited to one sinus or a tissue of origin, e.g. turbinate, septum or nasal vestibule.

T2 : Tumor limited to horizontal spread to the same region or to adjacent vertically related regions.

T3a : Tumor involving three regions, with or without orbital involvement

T3b : Tumor extension beyond the upper jaw. e.g. nasopharynx, cranial cavity, skin, buccal cavity or pterygopalatine fossa.

Carcinoma Nasal Cavity and Ethmoidal sinus (UICC and AJC Joint Committee 2004)

Tx : Primary tumor cannot be assessed

T0 : No evidence of primary tumor

Tis : Carcinoma in situ

T1 : Tumor restricted to any one subsite of nasal cavity or ethmoid sinus, with or without bony invasion

T2 : Tumor invading two subsites in a single region or extending to involve an adjacent region within the nasoethmoidal complex, with or without bony invasion

T3 : Tumor extends to invade the medial wall or the floor of the orbit, maxillary sinus, palate or cribriform plate

T4a : Tumor involving / invades any of the following: anterior orbital contents, skin of nose or cheek, minimal extension to anterior cranial fossa or pterygoid plates

T4b : Tumor invades any of the following: orbital apex, dura, brain, middle cranial fossa, cranial nerves other than V2, nasopharynx or clivus.

Carcinoma Maxillary Sinus (UICC and AJC Joint Committee 2004)

Tx : Primary tumor cannot be assessed

T0 : No evidence of primary tumor

Tis : Carcinoma in situ

T1 : Tumor limited to maxillary sinus mucosa with no erosion or destruction of bone

T2 : Tumor causing bone erosion or destruction including extension to the hard palate and/or the *middle nasal meatus*, except extension to the posterior wall of maxillary sinus and pterygoid plates

T3 : Tumor invades any of the following: bone of the posterior wall of maxillary sinus, subcutaneous tissues, medial wall or the floor of the orbit, pterygoid fossa and/or ethmoid sinuses

T4a : Tumor involving anterior orbital contents, skin of cheek, pterygoid plates, infratemporal fossa, cribriform plate, sphenoid or frontal

T4b : Tumor invades any of the following: orbital apex, dura, brain, middle cranial fossa and/or cranial nerves other than V2, nasopharynx or clivus.

Tumor Extensions

1. Local spread

Tumor usually extends through the thin wall of the sinuses and also through preformed routes due to passing of nerves and vessels and congenital/ acquired dehiscence.

Malignancy of the maxillary sinus: It commonly involves the ethmoids, lamina papyracea, orbit, lateral wall of the nose, anterolateral wall of the maxillary sinus into the skin and the floor to the alveolus. The posterior wall and pterygo-palatine fossa involvement is not uncommon and has poor

(Figs 40.4 and 40.5) prognosis. Infratemporal fossa extension is rare and tumor has multiple route of exit.

Malignancy of the ethmoid sinus: Tumor can extend to the maxillary sinus and into the nose. It can extend to the frontal sinus antero-superiorly. Superiorly it can extend to the cribriform plate and the anterior cranial fossa. It may involve the optic nerve posteriorly, which is closely related to the posterior ethmoid and sphenoid sinuses.

The periosteum of the orbit resists the tumor spread initially and hence most of the time the eye can be saved during surgical resection.

2. **Lymphatic spread:** Paranasal sinus tumors usually spread into the retropharyngeal nodes and from there into the subdigastric nodes of the deep jugular chain. Skin involvement gives rise to submandibular node, which is commonly seen in maxillary cancer.

3. **Distant metastasis:** This is extremely rare and is commonly associated with sarcomas.

Clinical Features

Symptoms depend on the wall of the sinus involved and the extent. Symptoms may be classified into:

- *Facial:* Swelling of the cheek, pain, paresthesia, nasal deformity (Fig. 40.1).
- *Orbital:* Swelling of the lids, proptosis, diplopia, loss of vision, etc.
- *Nasal:* Unilateral nasal obstruction, blood stained nasal discharge, epistaxis, hyposmia, etc.
- *Neurological:* Multiple cranial nerve involvement
- *Oral:* Loosening of the tooth, ill-fitting denture, palatal swelling, trismus due to pterygoid muscle involvement (Fig 40.2).
- *Otological:* Blocked ear due to eustachian tube dysfunction, referred otalgia, etc.
- *Cervical:* Swelling in the neck due to lymphatic metastasis and is usually associated with olfactory neuroblastoma, rhabdomyosarcoma, melanoma and carcinoma if it involves the skin or alveolus.

Clinical Signs

Patient should undergo complete ENT, head and neck examination including the orbit and the nervous system.

- *Anterolateral wall:* Skin involvement and infraorbital nerve paresthesia should be looked for. Extent of the facial swelling should be noted with respect to the orbital rim, gingivo-buccal sulcus for fullness or any fistulous tract.

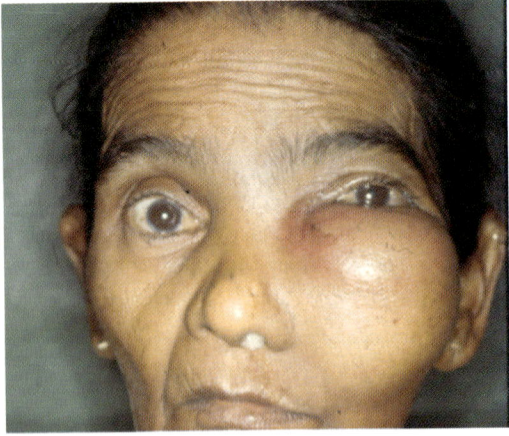

Fig. 40.1: Swelling of the left cheek due to cancer of the maxillary antrum

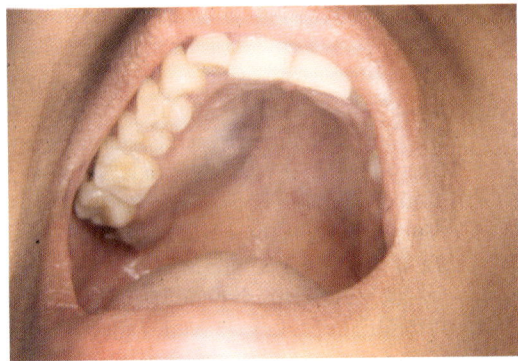

Fig. 40.2: Showing the palatal swelling secondary to maxillary malignancy

- **Inferior wall:** Palatal swelling, gingivo-buccal sulcus for loosening or absence of tooth, bulge, ulcer, growth, oroantral fistula, etc. Trismus may be present due to involvement of pterygoid muscles.
- **Posterior wall:** Extension occurs to the infratemporal fossa and then to the cheek which can be confirmed by digital palpation.
- **Superior wall (orbit):** Orbital rim and floor should be palpated for any periosteal thickening, fullness or bone destruction. Restriction of extraocular movement, visual acuity and visual field should be assessed. Presence of proptosis should be looked for and its type should be noted. The proptosis will be directed upward and laterally in cases of maxillary sinus malignancy and downward and laterally in ethmoidal sinus malignancy.
- **Nasal cavity:** Anterior and posterior rhinoscopy may show tumor extension as bulge or a fleshy mass in the nasal cavity. The mass is usually reddish, friable and bleeds on touch especially in case of olfactory neuroblastoma, which arises from the roof of the nasal cavity.

Neck: Should be palpated for any cervical lymph node metastasis.

Investigations

Nasal Endoscopy: To examine the middle meatus, posterior extent in nasal cavity and nasopharynx. Biopsy may be taken from the mass/ bulge. Maxillary mass biopsy may be done through the inferior meatus.

Radiological

1. Radiograph of PNS shows sinus opacity with or without bone erosion.
2. CT imaging done in both axial and coronal planes gives valuable information with respect to the tumor spread.
3. MR imaging shows better soft tissue delineation and thus the extension of the tumor to the pterygopalatine, infratemporal and orbit can be assessed.

Biopsy: Should be taken through inferior meatus. If frank growth is seen in **FNAC.**

Treatment

- Depends on the tumor extent and the type of malignancy.

Modalities available are

1. Surgery
2. Radiotherapy
3. Chemotherapy

Treatment is usually combined modality which is often surgery followed by radiotherapy.

Surgery: Tumor confined to infrastructure can be treated by partial maxillectomy. Often a total maxillectomy (Fig. 40.3) is required which may be combined with orbital exenteration if the orbital contents like fat is involved.

If tumor extends to the ethmoid or in case of primary tumor of ethmoid or maxilloethmoidal complex, a ***craniofacial resection*** (Anterio skull base approach) is done for complete enblock resection. It is the surgery of choice for olfactory neuroblastoma (Figs 40.6 to 40.9).

Tumor extension to infratemporal fossa is dealt with extended Weber-Fergusson incision (Figs 40.4 and 40.5) followed by condylectomy and resection of the tumor including the pterygoid plate and the muscles **(Barbosa technique).**

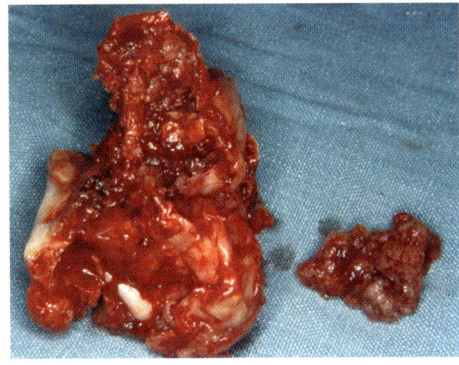

Fig. 40.3: Maxillectomy specimen after removal of the tumor

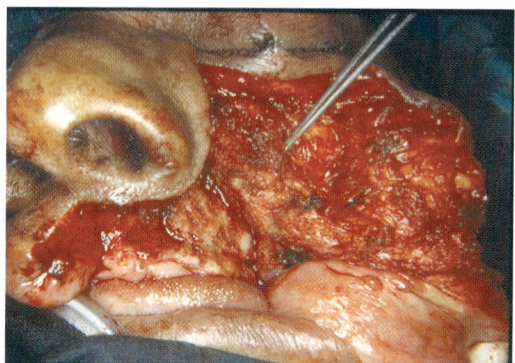

Fig. 40.4: Elevation of skin flap after Weber Fergusson incision

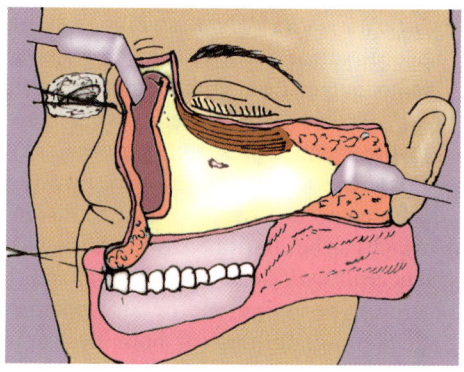

Fig. 40.5: Bony exposure of the anterior and lateral wall of the maxlla after Weber Furgusson incision

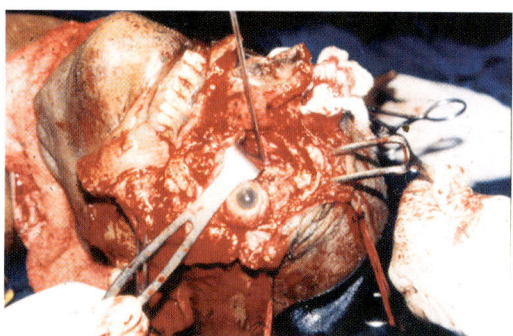

Fig. 40.6: Intraoperative photograph showing exposure for medial maxillectomy with ethmoidectomy and orbital exenteration with faciocranial resection (exposure after extended lateral rhinotomy with Lynch extension) for maxillo-ethmoidal complex malignancy

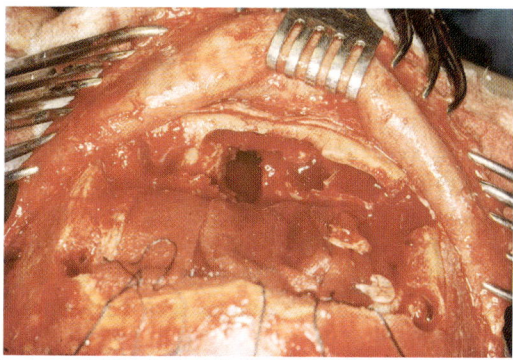

Fig. 40.7: Resected area after craneotomy (which include cristagalli, cribriform plate and ethmoidal roof) for craniofacial resection

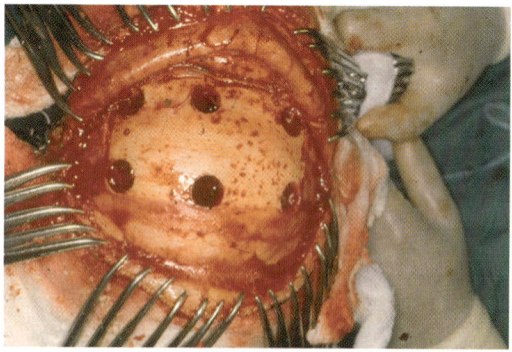

Fig. 40.8: Frontal craniotomy in progress for anterior CFR

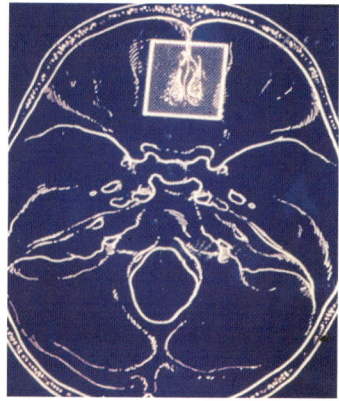

Fig. 40.9: Area of intracranial resection in anterior CFR

Neck dissection is done if neck nodes are involved. Nasopharyngeal involvement may need an anterolateral skull base approach.

Various surgical approaches to the tumors of nose and paranasal sinuses are discussed in the chapter 'Surgery of the Nose and Paranasal Sinus'.

Radiotherapy: Telecobalt or linear accelerator 6500 rads in divided fraction over 5 weeks. Brachytherapy may be of use if surgical treatment is not possible.

Chemotherapy: Cisplatinum and 5-flurouracil may be used in advanced cases concurrent with radiotherapy. Intra-arterial chemotherapy has been tried with mixed success.

MALIGNANT TUMORS INVOLVING THE SKIN OF THE EXTERNAL NOSE

These are the most common malignant tumors of the face. It should be treated like any other skin cancer of the face. The most common types include:

1. Basal cell carcinoma
2. Squamous cell carcinoma.

Basal Cell Carcinoma
(Figs 40.10a and b)

External nose is a very common site for basal cell carcinoma and is thirty times more common than squamous cell carcinoma. Its clinical presentation may vary. It may be a small nodular or ulcerative growth with rolled border. Treatment is aggressive local excision as recurrences are common. Skin tumors of the nose should not be treated by dermatologists by cautery and curettage, this apparently leads to resolution in short term but recurrences are very common and when it does occur, it is difficult to differentiate the tumor extent.

Squamous Cell Carcinoma of The External Nose (Figs 40.11a and b)

Skin tumors affecting the tip of the nose can penetrate quite deep before affecting the bone and the cartilage whereas those affecting the dorsum may quickly involve the upper lateral cartilage or the periosteum of the caudal ends of the nasal bone. The tumor may spread to the peri-facial, submandibular and jugulodigastric nodes. Radiotherapy is very effective in treating such tumors unless there is no nodal metastasis. If there is advanced tumor involvement of bone and cartilage, it requires surgical excision followed by radiotherapy. Reconstruction of the defect can be done by midline forehead flap/ naso-labial flap or by prosthesis. Tip of the nose is a very difficult area to reconstruct and it often involves the vestibular skin and vice versa.

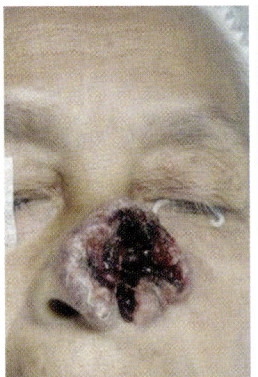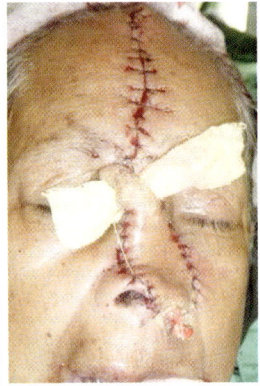

Figs 40.11a and b: (a) Squamous cell carcinoma of the external nose with complete destruction of the left side of the external nose (b) Postoperative appearance after resection and reconstruction using forehead flap

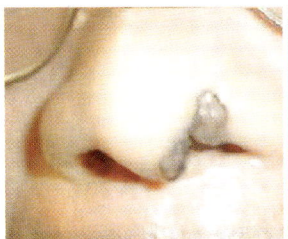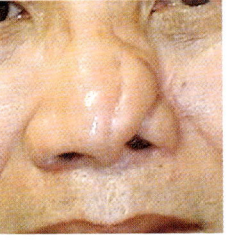

Figs 40.10a and b: (a) Basal cell carcinoma of the nose involving nasal tip, vestibule and ala (b) Postoperative appearance after resection and reconstruction using naso-labial flap

POINTS TO REMEMBER

1. Inverted papilloma may undergo malignant transformation.
2. 80 % of malignant tumors of nose are squamous cell carcinoma
3. Cranio-facial resection is the treatment of choice for maxillo-ethmoidal complex malignancy.
4. Olfactory neuroblastoma is a neuroendocrine type of malignant tumors.

41

Disorders of Olfaction

Applied Anatomy and Physiology

Detailed anatomy, physiology and clinical evaluation of olfaction have been described in the respective chapters.

Olfactory epithelium is derived from olfactory placode at around first month of fetal life. The lamia propria contains the branched tubuloalveolar glands of Bowman which produces a thin fluid covering the olfactory surface. This fluid contains odorant binding proteins. To sense the smell a substance has to be soluble in both water and lipids. The olfactory mucus unlike respiratory epithelium is not propelled by underlying cilia but possibly pulled by traction of nearby respiratory cilia. The olfactory neuroepithelium is located above the level of superior turbinate and corresponding part of the nasal septum and is about 100 to 400 mm² on either side.

The olfactory mucosa is constantly being renewed in a cycle of 30 to 40 days. This is the only neuroepithelium which is exposed directly to the external environment. The olfactory mucosa contains flask shaped microvilli cells. There are no cilia or basal bodies. At the lower end of the cell a long slender cytoplasmic process extends towards the basement membrane which resembles an axon. Similar cells are seen in vomeronasal organ of animals. This vomeronasal organ is vestigial in humans and is present in the anteroinferior part of the nasal septum. It serves as a neuroendocrine organ and its role in humans

is uncertain. In animals it serves as a receptor to pheromones (Fig. 41.1).

Causes of Olfactory Disorders

- *Obstructive nasal and sinus disease (NSD):* This is the most common cause of olfactory dysfunction. Space between the nasal septum and the middle turbinate below and anterior to the cribriform plate is the critical nasal area required for optimal olfaction. Obstruction in this area due to mucosal edema, polyps, or scarring can decrease olfactory ability even when the rest of the nasal cavity is normal. Common causes include allergic rhinitis, nasal polyp, deviated nasal septum, intranasal tumors, etc.
- *Post upper respiratory tract infection:* Viral, HIV infection, acute rhinitis, acute ethmoiditis, atrophic rhinitis, etc.
- *Head injury and trauma:* Shearing of the olfactory nerves at the cribriform plate can cause anosmia and CSF leak may be present. Total anosmia is 5 times more likely with occipital blow than frontal blow.
- *Aging:* The impaired sense of smell due to aging associated with degeneration from 2nd to 3rd decade onwards is termed as presbyosmia.
- *Physiological:* Alteration in female olfaction is seen in different phases of menstrual cycle and also pregnancy. Hunger, nausea and

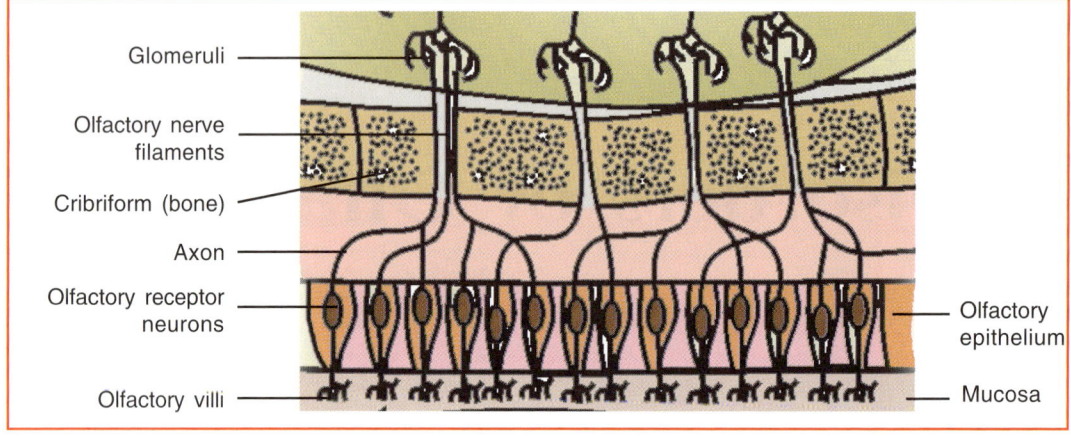

Fig. 41.1: Olfactory mucosa and olfactory neurons

obesity increase the olfactory acuity whereas satiety diminishes it. Increase in humidity and temperature also increases the acuity.

- **Toxins:** Carbon dioxide, sulphur dioxide, trichloroethylene, nicotine, etc. can cause olfactory dysfunction.
- **Congenital anosmia:** This is due to certain craniofacial developmental abnormalities like cleft lip/ palate, choanal atresia, etc.
- **Medications:** Antiamebics, anti-histamines like chlorpheneramine maleate, antibiotics like ampicillin, ethambutol, streptomycin, etc., and antithyroid drugs like thiouracils, antiepileptics like phenytoin, anti-cancer drugs like methotrexate, etc.
- **Tumors:** Olfactory neuroblastoma, meningioma, pituitary tumors can cause olfactory dysfunction. Olfactory hallucinations may be seen in temporal lobe tumors.
- **Psychiatric:** Schizophrenia, hysteria, malingering are the common causes.
- **Neurological:** Multiple sclerosis, Parkinsonism, strokes, epilepsy, etc.
- **Iatrogenic:** Surgery in the form of craniofacial resection, repair of CSF rhinorrhea, rhinop- lasty, radiotherapy to head and neck, after total laryngectomy, etc.
- **Endocrine:** Diabetes is the commonest endocrine cause to decrease olfactory acuity.

Other conditions include Turner's syndrome and Kallmann's syndrome, Addisons disease, Cushing's syndrome, hypothyroidism, etc.

- **Nutrition:** Vitamin A, B12, zinc deficiency.
- **Miscellaneous:** Cirrhosis and chronic renal failure is also associated with olfactory dysfunction.

Types of Olfactory Disorders

- *Anosmia:* Complete loss of smell
- *Hyposmia:* Partial loss of sense of smell
- *Parosmia:* Altered (perverted) or abnormal or qualitative changes in the olfactory response.
- *Cacosmia:* Subjective sensation of an unpleasant odor.
- *Phantosmia:* Continuously perceives unpleasant odor.

Parosmia and phantosmia often accompany brain or psychiatric disease and is common in women.

Evaluation and Diagnosis

History

- Determining the olfactory ability prior to the loss
- Careful history of the chemosensory complaint

- Taste versus smell
- Decreased sensitivity versus distorted perception
- Prior treatment for nasal or sinus disease
- Nasal symptoms including allergy
- Events that might have taken place before the loss like
  - Head trauma
  - Upper respiratory tract infection
  - Toxins
  - Others
  - Medical disease if any
  - Aging
  - Any psychological problem
- Left versus right nostril
- Inhalation versus exhalation

Physical examination includes anterior and posterior rhinoscopy, corda tympani involvement. Oral cavity if any disease is present, neurological examination.

Investigations

1. Diagnostic nasal endoscopy
2. CT/ MRI imaging of the nasal cavity and the sinus (coronal cuts)
3. Olfactory tests
   (a) *Threshold tests:* The measurement of the threshold attempts to quantify the most dilute concentration of a particular odorant that the individual can detect.
   (b) *Identification tests*
   - Scratch and sniff test for olfaction – Booklets containing 40 microencapsulated odorants are very popular method of smell identification. The patient is given a choice of 4 answers and therefore a chance performance would be 25 percent correct. Thus anyone scoring less than this should be considered malingering (UPSIT- University of Pennsylvania Smell Identification test).
   - **Odorant confusion matrix:** 10 single chemical odorant representing common household items and one blank are presented to the subject in random order.

The subject has a list of 10 odorants and must choose one of the words for each presentation. The same sequence is then presented 9 more times in the same order so that the group of odorant is administered 10 times. The result can be represented on a matrix. The total and individual correct scores can be calculated from the diagonal as well as trends showing improvement or decrement (fatigue/ adaptation) during the test.

- **T and T olfactometer:** This is another standard test used in all parts of the world especially in Japan. It is a rack containing 8 concentrations of 5 different odors. From this both detection and recognition thresholds can be determined which can be charted on a graph similar to an audiogram.
   (c) *Electro-olfactogram:* This is objective test which measures the electric potential across the olfactory epithelium by placing electrodes over it. When a odorant stimulates the receptor cells a slow negative sweeping voltage is seen.
   (d) *Brain electric activity monitoring (BEAM):* This technique can display color topographic maps of the cortical activity while events such as sniffing re occurring. Thus it can display an individual response to a particular odorant.
4. Biopsy from olfactory and taste epithelium.

Management

- Treatment of obstructive causes responds well following medical/surgical management depending on the cause.
- Topical steroid is helpful.
- For patients placed in the other diagnostic category does not respond well. No proven therapy is available in such cases.
- Vitamin A is found to be effective in certain cases especially in nutritional deficiency.
- Zinc and other nutrients like gincoba biloba, vitamin B12, zinc copper, etc., may be given if nutritional deficiency is detected.

- Aminophylline is useful for anosmic and hyposmic patients, but corroborative evidence for this is not available.
- Phantosmia may be treated with cocaine hydrochloride or by olfactory bulbectomy via craniotomy approach but surgery removes the olfactory ability permanently.

These patients especially with anosmia should be reassured.
- Precautions are necessary in these patients to avoid 'spoilt food' consumption or smoke detection which helps them in cases of fire.
- Understanding of the disease by the relatives and friends is essential.

POINTS TO REMEMBER

1. Olfactory surface is covered by a thin fluid secreted by glands of Bowman.
2. Olfactory mucosa is constantly renewed in a cycle of 30 to 40 days.
3. Vomero-nasal organ is vestigial in humans and is present in the anterior inferior part of the nasal septum.
4. Presbyosmia refers to impaired sense of smell due to aging.
5. Obstructive nasal and sinus disease is the most common cause of olfactory dysfunction.

Sleep Apnea Syndrome

42

The sleep apnea syndrome was described by Guilleminault, Eldride and Dement in 1973.

Definition

It is defined as an intermittent cessation of airflow at both nose and mouth during sleep. Normal healthy individual can have apneic episodes of less than 10 seconds several times an hour without significant clinical disturbances. In sleep apnea syndrome, apneic episodes may last for 20 to 30 seconds to as high as 2 to 3 minutes. Significant disturbances are noted about 15 times or more per hour.

These disturbances of respiration is associated with

- Reduction of breathing (hypopnea)
- Cessation of breathing (apnea)

Sleep apnea can be classified as:

1. Obstructive
2. Central
3. Mixed

- The term *obstructive sleep apnea* is used when the symptom of sleep apnea is produced by obstruction to the upper airway. If the cause of sleep apnea is in the brain it is called *central sleep apnea*. One of the classical features of the sleep apnea is the vigorous effort made by the patient to overcome the obstruction during cessation of airflow. Often noise is generated from the upper airway due to partial upper airway obstruction and the term *snoring* is used.

- *Apnea:* Cessation of airflow at the nostrils and mouth for 10 seconds
- *Apnea index:* Number of apneas per hour of sleep.
- *Hypopnea:* 50 percent reduction in thoraco abdominal movement lasting for 10 seconds.

Obstructive Sleep Apnea

Etiology

Incidence is more in male. Elderly are more commonly affected than young. It is more common in obese individuals.

The obstruction can be at three levels including

1. Nasal cavity and nasopharynx
2. Oral cavity and oropharynx
3. Larynx and hypopharynx

Causes in the nasal cavity and nasopharynx

- DNS
- Ethmoidal polyposis
- Antrochoanal polyp
- Nasal packing
- Rhinitis
- Nasopharyngeal tumors
- Enlarged adenoids

Causes in oral cavity and oropharynx

- Enlarged palatine tonsils
- Enlarged lingual tonsil
- Large tongue
- Micrognathia or retrognathia

Causes in larynx and hypopharynx

- Tumors
- Congenital anomalies e.g. laryngomalacia
- Laryngeal edema

Systemic causes

- Myxoedema (causing large tongue)
- COPD

Pathophysiology of Sleep Apnea

In normal individuals the muscles of the oropharynx and hypopharynx maintains the airway by the tonic activity of dilators which includes genioglossus, geniohyoid, palatoglossus and medial pterygoid. This increase in tonicity is maintained by behavioral response when the individual is awake. When the individual goes to sleep, the behavioral response is decreased causing relaxation of these muscles with resultant hypotonicity which results in narrowing of the airway.

In case of obstruction of the airway at various levels due to structural abnormality, the hypotonicity during sleep (REM) further reduces the airway causing the obstruction which is also associated with a number of factors including venturi effect leading to rapid flow of inspiratory air through the narrow passage. This is superadded with Bernoulli effect caused by the flow of air within the narrow airway leading to fall in pressure around the wall of hypopharynx. The hypotonicity of the musculature of the pharynx during REM sleep facilitates collapse of the lumen of the pharynx leading to further obstruction of the airway. This obstruction leads to negative intrathoracic pressure causing increased cardiac output. Increased cardiac output is associated with decreased oxygenation causing stimulation of respiratory center and cerebral cortex causing the

patient's arousal which facilitates better ventilation and the patient goes to sleep again.

Persistent obstruction to the airway causes increased load on the heart due to increased cardiac output to maintain saturation. This results in left ventricular hypertrophy. Persistent decrease in oxygenation leads to polycythemia, pulmonary hypertension and COPD leading to cor pulmonale and sudden death.

Clinical Features

Symptoms

1. Snoring and obstructive episodes
2. Excessive day time sleepiness
3. Morning headaches
4. Intellectual deterioration and personality changes
5. Abnormal body movements
6. Nocturnal enuresis and impotence
7. Obesity

Signs

1. Snoring
2. Features of airway obstruction in children due to adenoids, kissing, tonsils, etc.
3. Obese patients with short neck, bulky tongue, micrognathia with hypoplasia of mandible, craniofacial abnormalities, excessively bulky soft palate with redundant mucosa, large tongue (Fig. 42.1).
4. Other obstructive causes due to space occupying lesions.

Investigations

1. Complete blood picture
2. Thyroid function profile
3. Chest X-Ray
4. ***Polysomnography:*** This is the gold standard investigation in diagnosis of OSA. Though not completely standardized a polysomnogram (PSG) will have measurements including an electroencephalogram (EEG), electrooculogram, submental and tibial electromyogram (EMG), nasal or oral

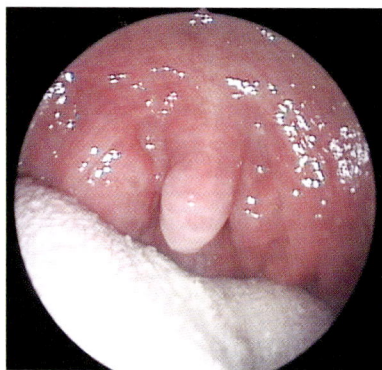

Fig. 42.1: Endoscopic picture showing the classical snorer's throat with redundant mucosa of the uvula, soft palate and the tonsillar pillars

airflow, respiratory movement or effort, oximetry, electrocardiogram (ECG), and sleeping position. Some may also include measurements of penile tumescence and multilevel esophageal manometry.

5. **Diagnostic nasal endoscopy** to rule out nasal pathology

6. **Muller's maneuver:** With flexible naso-pharyngoscope visualizing the nasopharynx, the patient is asked to breath with nose and mouth closed to see the actual site of collapse in the nasopharynx/oropharynx/hypo pharynx.

7. **Cephalometry:** Various dimensions and angles are measured using the lateral view radiography.

8. **Multiple sleep latency test** (MSLT)

Management

1. **Physical:**
   - Reduction of weight
   - Avoidance of alcohol and sedatives
   - Physiotherapy

2. **Medical**
   - Nasal continuous positive airway pressure (C-PAP)
   - Control of alcohol ingestion
   - Medroxyprogesterone or Protriptyline
   - Tongue retaining devices

3. **Surgical**
   - Correction of obstructive causes like DNS, polyps adenoid and tonsil hypertrophy, etc.
   - Uvulo-palato-pharyngo-plasty (UPPP) (Fig. 42.2)
   - KTP-532 laser assisted uvulo-palatoplasty (LAUP) (Fig. 42.3)
   - Hyoid advancement
   - Mandibular osteotomy and advancement
   - Genioglossal advancement and hyoid myotomy and suspension
   - Maxillary/mandibular osteotomy and advancement
   - Laser assisted wedge excision of tongue base
   - Radiofrequency ablation
   - Tracheostomy

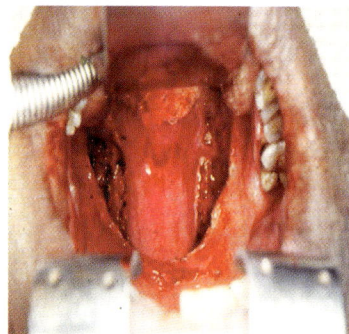

Fig. 42.2: Intraoperative picture following UPPP

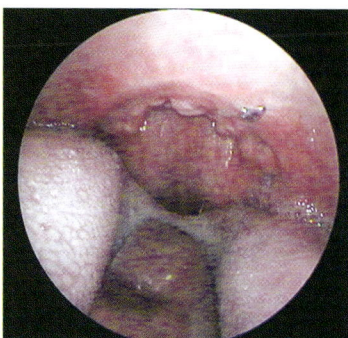

Fig. 42.3: Postoperative endoscopic picture following LAUP

POINTS TO REMEMBER

1. Sleep apnea refers to an intermittent cessation of airflow at both mouth and nose during sleep.
2. Obstructive sleep apnea is used when symptom of sleep apnea is produced by obstruction to the upper airway.
3. Sleep apnea is common in obese patient.
4. Polysomnograph is the gold standard investigation in diagnosis of obstructive sleep apnea.
5. Surgical treatment modality depends on the site and type of obstruction. LAUP is the most commonly performed surgery for snoring and sleep apnea.

43

Headache and Facial Pain

Headache and facial neuralgias are common but quite disturbing for which the patients move from specialty to specialty for the proper treatment. This may vary from ENT, psychiatry, neurology, internal medicine, ophthalmology, etc. Proper and careful history and thorough clinical examination and certain diagnostic tools often help in correct diagnosis.

DEFINITION

Headache

Headache is defined as a pain or discomfort between the orbit and the occipital region arising from extracranial and/or intracranial pain sensitive structures.

Facial Neuralgia

Neuralgias are extremely painful conditions distributed along the course of the cutaneous supply, commonly seen to arise via the trigeminal nerve (trigeminal neuralgia), glossopharyngeal nerve (glossopharyngeal neuralgia), cervical plexus (cervical neuralgia), etc.

Origin of Headache and Facial Pain

It can be either intracranial or extracranial.

Intracranial pain sensitive structures:

- Venous sinuses
- Cortical veins
- Basilar arteries and its branches
- Dura

These pain sensitive structures are present in the anterior, middle and posterior cranial fossa. The anterior and the middle fossa are innervated by first and second branch of the fifth cranial nerve. The pain from this region is referred to the forehead (anterior cranial fossa) and the temporal region (middle cranial fossa).

Extracranial pain sensitive structures

- *Mucous membrane*
  - Nose and the paranasal sinuses
  - Middle ear cleft
- *Skin of the external auditory canal*
- Extracranial muscles
- Scalp vessels
- Orbital contents
- Teeth and gums

The onset of headache may be divided into

- Sudden onset
- Insidious onset

The patient may describe the headache to be sharp, dull, throbbing type of headache which could be unilateral or bilateral; the attack may be acute, chronic or recurrent. Diurnal variation is often seen in headache of the paranasal sinus origin like acute frontal sinusitis. Precipitating factors like coughing, posture, etc. are suggestive of sinus headache. History of associated features like nausea, vomiting, visual disturbances, its relation to the medication, loss of consciousness, etc., should be noted. The examination should include complete general examination, local examination including ear, nose, oral cavity, throat and neck. Ophthalmologic assessment should include the assessment of visual acuity, intraocular pressure and visual fields. Complete neurological examination is mandatory.

Etiology

The common causes of headache include:

Naso-sinus causes
- Sinusitis
- Contact neuralgia (Sluder's neuralgia)
- Vacuum headache
- Sinonasal tumors
- Trauma

Ear Causes
- Complications of otitis media
- Malignant otitis externa
- Malignancy of the ear
- Herpes zoster oticus

Ophthalmic
- Refractive error
- Eye strain
- Glaucoma
- Retrobulbar neuritis
- Dacryocystitis
- Orbital tumors

Vascular
- Migraine
  - Common migraine
  - Classical migraine
  - Cluster headaches
- Temporal arteritis

Neuralgias
- Trigeminal neuralgia
- Para-trigeminal neuralgia
- Glossopharyngeal neuralgia
- Pterygopalatine neuralgia
- Cervical neuralgia
- Dental neuralgia
- Sluder's syndrome

Dental
- Malocclusion
- Temporomandibular joint dysfunction
- Caries teeth
- Apical abscess

Tension Headache
- Muscle contraction headache
- Head injury
- Psychological

Intracranial
- Tumors
- Meningitis/ encephalitis
- Brain abscess
- Space occupying lesions
- Benign intracranial hypertension
- Hemorrhage
- Hydrocephalus

Systemic Causes
- Hypertension
- Endocrine
- Renal
- Hypoglycemia
- Hypercalcemia
- Hypoxic state
- Post-convulsion
- Hangover reaction (post-alcohol withdrawal)

Drugs
- Vasodilators
- Oral contraceptives
- Caffeine
- Monosodium glutamate
- Tyramine

Migraine

This is the most common cause of headache. Headache is of throbbing type along the arteries which could be unilateral or bilateral. Headache comes in paroxysms and the frequency and duration of each attack is variable. Aura is usually present in classical migraine. Patient may have nausea and vomiting. Intolerance to light (photophobia) and sound (phonophobia). Precipitating factors include physical and mental stress and certain diet like chocolate, cheese, etc. Relieving factors are rest, sleep and staying in silent and dark room. This is twice more common in females than males. It is suspected to be of neurovascular in origin and is thought to be a disorder of sensory dismodulation that involves the trigeminovascular system and CNS modulation of pain producing structures of the cranium. It is said to be due to defect in the neurotransmitters like serotonin. Analgesics and antiemetics (metaclopromide with paracetamol/aceclofenac) are given in acute attacks. If not responding, vasoconstrictors like ergot alkaloids are given with caution. Sumatryptan has been used more successfully. Prophylaxis of migraine may be achieved by topiramate, flunarizine, propranol, etc.

Cluster Headache

This is also called Horton's cephalgia or histamine cephalgia. It is less common than migraine. Pain is more severe than migraine and there is no aura. The attack comes in clusters of 1 to 7 each day for a period of week or more and then there is symptom-free interval for weeks or months. Males are commonly affected than females. The headache is characterized by severe unilateral pain around the eye associated by conjunctival injection, rhinorrhea and a transient Horner's syndrome occasionally.

Mechanism

Serum histamine level is raised during the attack and hence it is called histamine cephalgia.

Treatment

Ergotamine and Methisergide may be useful. Some improve with inhalation of 100 percent oxygen. Sumatryptan may be helpful. Prednisolone 30 mg. daily for 10 days may be tried in refractory cases.

Tension Headache

This is a common form of headache and is experienced by most people at some stage of life.

The headache is characterized by diffuse dull aching band like headache worse on touching the scalp aggravated by noise associated with tension but not with other physical symptoms. The condition may last from few hours to few days, it is worse towards the end of the day. It may persist for long periods. The headache is due to persistent contraction of scalp and posterior neck muscles like clinching of teeth, particular posture for long periods, etc. Headache is bilateral and frequently localizes to the occipital nuchal area. Non-steroidal anti-inflammatory medications, short course of diazepam, reassurance are helpful. Antidepressants are rarely necessary.

Temporal Arteritis

This is common in elderly. It is associated with severe throbbing type of headache that involves overlying vessel and usually involves the superficial temporal artery. It can involve any intra or extracranial or multiple arteries. The patient may complain of pain while chewing or talking due to ischemia of the masseter muscle following jaw claudication. There may be associated blindness and diplopia. Other symptom may be weight loss, lassitude and polymyalgia rheumatica (generalized muscle aches).

Mechanism

Large and medium sizes vessels undergo giant cell infiltration and fragmentation of lamina and narrowing of the lumen. Occlusion of the important arteries can occur and can cause blindness if it involves ophthalmic artery.

Investigation

ESR is raised; C-reactive and protein hepatic alkaline phosphatase may be elevated. Biopsy is diagnostic.

Treatment

Prednisolone should be started to prevent eye complication at the dose of 60 mg. daily and is gradually reduced to 5 mg. daily.

Post-traumatic Headache

This follows head injury and is more similar to the migraine or tension type of headache. The patient may complain of light headedness, irritability and difficulty in concentration. Underlying neurological defects should be looked for and appropriate treatment should be given.

Ramsay Hunt Neuralgia

This is rare and occurs due to involvement of the geniculate ganglion by the Herpes zoster virus. This is described under the section otology.

Temporomandibular Joint Dysfunction

The patient may have malocclusion, improper positioning of the mandibular condyle within the glenoid fossa. It occurs due to contraction of the masticatory muscles. Bruxism may play part. Unequal bite may cause spasm. Treatment is NSAIDs, massage; joint rest, muscle relaxant exercise, condylectomy for joint ankylosis, etc.

Para-trigeminal Neuralgia (Raeder's syndrome)

The neuralgia is characterized by retro-ocular pain and may be associated with dilated pupil. It may occur due to encroachment into the para-trigeminal region by vessel. Treatment is neuroendoscopic surgical decompression.

Trigeminal Neuralgia

Synonym: Tic Douloureux, suicide disease

Definition

The disorder is characterized by episodes of intense, stabbing, electric shock-like pain in the areas of the face where the branches of the trigeminal nerve are distributed – lips, eyes, nose, scalp, forehead, upper jaw, and lower jaw (Figs 43.1a and b).

A less common form of the disorder called "Atypical Trigeminal Neuralgia" may cause less intense, constant, dull burning or aching pain,

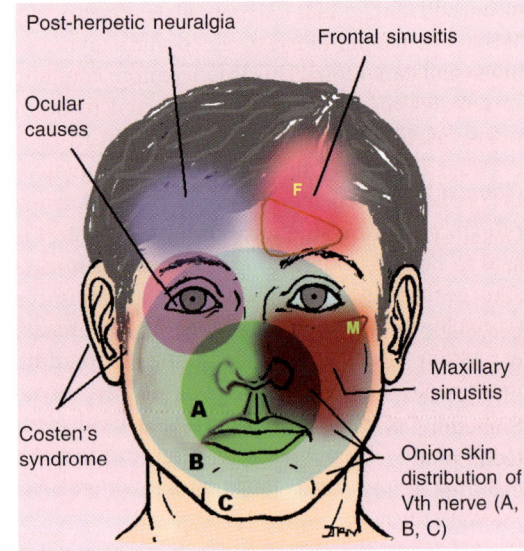

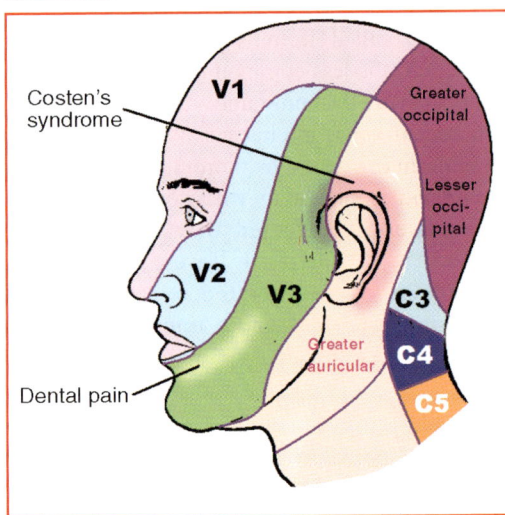

Figs 43.1a and b: Distribution of pain sensation and headache in various conditions

sometimes with occasional electric shock-like stabs. Both forms of the disorder most often affect one side of the face, but some patients experience pain at different times on both sides.

Etiology

The exact cause is not known. Idiopathic neuralgia may be due to abnormal loop of vessels over the nerve intracranially and micro-vascular decompression has shown to relieve the pain. Aneurysms, tumors, chronic meningeal inflammation, or other lesions may irritate trigeminal nerve roots and cause secondary neuralgia.

Clinical Features

Onset of symptoms occurs most often after the age 50 years, but cases are known in children and even infants. Pain is along the distribution of the nerve and is sharp shooting type as described in the definition. Usually it is triggered by the effect of trigger factors on trigger zones in the face. Something as simple and routine as brushing the teeth, putting on makeup or even a slight breeze can trigger an attack, resulting in sheer agony for the individual. It is universally considered to be the most painful affliction known to medical practice.

Treatment

Trigeminal neuralgia is usually treated by anticonvulsant drugs, such as Tegretol or Neurontin. Some antidepressant drugs may have pain relieving effects. If medication is ineffective or if it produces undesirable side effects, neurosurgical procedures to relieve pressure on the nerve or to reduce nerve sensitivity may be useful.

Some patients report having reduced or relieved pain by means of alternative medical therapies such as acupuncture, self-hypnosis, meditation etc. Trigeminal blocks or radiofrequency thermocoagulation of the nerve has been shown to be useful.

Glossopharyngeal Neuralgia

Except for the location this is similar to trigeminal neuralgia. The pain may get radiated to vagus nerve causing vagopharyngeal neuralgia. The triggering zone is often in the tonsillar area and extends to the ipsilateral area. The pain may also be felt in the back of the tongue or the posterior pharyngeal wall. The pain is precipitated by swallowing, eating or irritation of the tonsillar region. Xylocaine test may be helpful in reducing the pain. Stylalgia is glossopharyngeal neuralgia due to elongated styloid process and is described under pharynx. Treatment is similar to that of trigeminal neuralgia. Intracranial section of the IX nerve may be necessary. Carbamazepine alone or in combination with phenytoin is tried.

POINTS TO REMEMBER

1. Headache is a pain or discomfort between the orbit and the occipital region arising from extracranial and/or intracranial pain sensitive structures.
2. Neuralgias are extremely painful conditions distributed along the course of the cutaneous supply.
3. The commonly seen neuralgias are trigeminal and glossopharyngeal.
4. Migraine is the most common cause of headache
5. Aura is usually present in classical migraine
6. Migraine is more common in females where as cluster headache (Histamine headache) is more common in males.
7. The trigeminal neuralgia can be due to an abnormal loop of vessels over the trigeminal nerve intracranially. Microvascular decompression in such cases are effective.

Orbit in ENT Diseases

The orbit is closely related to the paranasal sinuses. The ethmoid sinus is separated from the orbit by a papery thin plate of bone called lamina papyracea. The lateral wall of the sphenoid sinus is closely related to the orbital apex and the optic nerve. Frontal sinus is related to the roof of the orbit and if over-pneumatized, the frontal sinus may even form the entire roof of the orbit. The roof of the maxillary sinus forms the floor of the orbit. Any inflammatory, traumatic or neoplastic lesion of the paranasal sinuses may complicate the orbit and similarly an orbital lesion may present in or could be surgically accessed through the sinuses.

ORBITAL ANATOMY

- Orbit is a quadrilateral pyramid with its base facing forwards, laterally and slightly inferiorly.
- Average volume of orbit – 30 ml, of which 70 percent is occupied by retrobulbar structures.

Orbit is made up of 7 Bones

1. Sphenoid
2. Lacrimal
3. Palatal
4. Maxillary
5. Ethmoid
6. Frontal
7. Zygomatic

Orbit has 7 Important Contents

1. Globe (7 ml)
2. Extraocular muscles (EOM)
3. Optic nerve
4. Cranial nerves – III, IV, V and VI
5. Blood vessels
6. Lacrimal gland and sac
7. Orbital fat.

The Orbit Consists of 4 Walls

- Medial
- Lateral
- Superior (Roof)
- Inferior (Floor)

Medial Wall

- It is composed of
  – Frontal process of maxilla
  – Lacrimal bone
  – Lamina papyracea of ethmoid
  – Body of sphenoid
- At the frontoethmoid suture, where the medial wall meets the roof, foramina for anterior and posterior ethmoidal vessels and nerves are located.
- Ethmoid foramina are also indicators of level of cribriform plate
- Rule of 24-12-6 (Rontal et al)
  – Distance from anterior lacrimal crest to anterior ethmoid foramen 24 mm

– Distance from anterior to posterior ethmoid foramen – 12 mm
– Distance from posterior ethmoid foramen to optic canal – 6 mm
- Lacrimal fossa for lacrimal sac lies between anterior and posterior lacrimal crests
- As the medial wall is thin in parts and could be dehiscent, there is risk for orbital cellulitis, from spread of paranasal sinus infection or mucocele.

Lateral Wall

- It is composed of
  – Greater wing of sphenoid
  – Orbital surface of zygoma
  – Zygomatic process of frontal bone
- Posterior boundaries of lateral wall could be taken as the superior and inferior orbital fissures
- Superior orbital fissure is about 28 mm from the frontozygomatic suture at the orbital rim
- Optic nerve lies 8 mm behind the medial edge of the superior orbital fissure (SOF)
- SOF extends posteriorly to the cavernous sinus
- Lateral wall is encountered in
  – Orbital decompression
  – Lateral craniotomy
  – Infratemporal fossa surgery
  – Lateral orbitotomy
  – Exploration of fractures

Superior Wall (roof)

- It is triangular in shape
- It is composed of:
  – Orbital plate of frontal bone
  – Lessor wing of sphenoid
- In the superomedial area of roof, 5 mm posterior to the orbital rim is the trochlea – a connective tissue sling anchoring the tendinous part of the superior oblique muscle to the orbit. Avoid injury to trochlea during surgery to prevent vertical diplopia.
- Supraorbital notch/foramen in the superior orbital margin transmiting supraorbital vessels and nerves.

- Superior walls is encountered in
  – Frontal sinus trephination
  – External frontoethmoidectomy
  – Orbital decompression
  – Orbital fracture repair
  – Orbital clearance/exenteration

Inferior Wall (floor)

- It is composed of:
  – Orbital plate of maxilla
  – Zygomatic orbital plate (anterolaterally)
- The infraorbital canal which transmits infraorbital nerve and artery is the thinnest and hence weakest part of the floor. It leads to the infraorbital foramen.
- Anteromedially just behind the orbital rim is a shallow depression for the origin of the inferior oblique muscle. Disruption of I.O. causes vertical diplopia.
- Floor is separated from lateral wall by inferior orbital fissure. It transmits – infraorbital nerve and artery, inferior ophthalmic vein and anterior/posterior superior alveolar nerves.
- It is encountered in
  – Orbital decompression
  – Repair of orbital floor fractures
  – Maxillectomy

Periorbita

- It is the periosteum lining the bony orbital walls
- It is continuous with the dura mater at the optic foramen and superior orbital fissure
- Inferiorly and medially it splits to line the fossa and to invest the lacrimal sac
- Superiorly it forms the pulley of the superior oblique tendon
- Septa pass from the periorbita to divide the orbital fat into lobules.

Orbital Septum /Palpebral Fascia

- It is a fibrous sheet that stretches across the entrance of the orbit and is continuous with the periorbita at the rim (Fig. 44.1).

- It is related to the posterior aspect of orbicularis oculi muscle.
- In the upper lid, it unites with the levator aponeurosis and in the lower lid it fuses with the tarsus and sheath of the inferior rectus.

Bulbar Fascia/Tenon's Capsule

- Fibrous sheath surrounding the globe, except the cornea.

Muscular Fascia

- Made up by the fusion of the fibrous sheaths of the EOM.
- Surgical space between the periosteum and the muscular fascia—peripheral space.
- Surgical space deep to the muscular fascia, within the muscle cone – central space.

Orbital Vessels

- Main blood supply to orbit—ophthalmic artery branch of internal carotid artery. It enters through optic foramen.
- Anterior/posterior ethmoid arteries are branches from the ophthalmic artery.
- Parts of inferior orbit are supplied by the infraorbital artery, branch of interior maxillary artery.
- The superior ophthalmic vein and superior branch of inferior ophthalmic vein drain into cavernous sinus through superior orbital fissure
- Inferior branch of inferior ophthalmic vein communicates with pterygoid plexus by passing through inferior orbital fissure.

Lacrimal System

A. Secretory System

- Basic secretors
  1. Goblet cells in conjunctiva
  2. Accessory lacrimal glands of subconjunctiva of upper lid
  3. Tarsal Meibomian glands
- *Reflex secretors* – Lacrimal gland – in the lacrimal fossa in the lateral orbit superiorly and anteriorly.

B. Excretory System

- In each lid there is an opening located medially – Punctum
- Punctum leads to canaliculus
- Canaliculus has
  - Vertical component - 2 mm in length
  - Horizontal component - 8 mm in length
- They join together to form common canali that empties into lacrimal sac.
- Lacrimal sac is situated in lacrimal fossa situated in anterior part of medial orbital wall
- Lacrimal sac empties into nasolacrimal duct
- Canaliculi and sac are lined with stratified squamous epithelium.

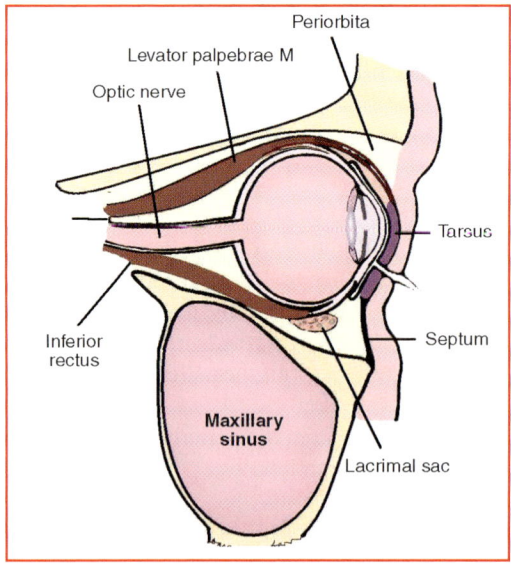

Fig. 44.1: Intraorbital structures and relation to maxillary sinus

EVALUATION OF THE ORBITAL LESIONS

History

- Fever
- Pain

- Diplopia, visual loss
- Allergies, sinus infections, epistaxis, nasal discharge /obstruction, tearing
- History regarding thyroid disorders, granulomatous diseases and neoplasms
- History regarding blunt/penetrating head trauma.

External Examination

- Lid retraction, lid lag, injection of blood vessels over EOM – endocrine (graves) cause.
- Pulsations of globe – AV malformation / carotid cavernous fistula
- Palpation of thrill, auscultation of bruit, or discoloration of lids (bluish hue) – vascular lesion.
- Warmth, erythema, fluctuance of lids – inflammatory lesion
- Direction of displacement of proptosis eye
  - Down and laterally – acute inflammation / chronic mucopyocele of frontal / ethmoid sinuses
  - Upwards – Tumors or maxilla
  - Medially – Lacrimal gland tumor/mass in the temporal fossa
  - Axial – Tumors within the muscle cone, e.g., optic nerve glioma, graves disease.

Ophthalmologic Examination

- Intraocular pressure measurement (tono-metry)
- Hertel exophthalmometer – Distance of corneal apex to lateral orbital wall at the lateral canthus
- Decreased visual acuity – Intraorbital lesion close to optic nerve / retina
- Visual field defects – Optic chiasmal lesion
- Ocular motility limitation – Involvement of III, IV or VI cranial nerves in their pathway, mechanical impingement of EOM/globe by orbital mass or intrinsic involvement of muscles as in endocrine exophthalmos
- Papilledema/optic atrophy (fundoscopy) – Tumor pressure / infiltration of optic nerve

Otolaryngologic Examination

- Inflamed mucosa, purulence or polyps in nose and nasopharynx (NP) – Sinusitis, mucopyocele.
- Black necrotic eschar along the turbinates – mucormycosis
- Thyroid enlargement – Graves ophthal-mopathy
- ET dysfunction with serious middle ear effusion—mass lesion/inflammation in nasopharynx / ethmoid sinuses.

Lab Investigation

- C.B.P. – Increased WBC count, increased ESR – Inflammation
- Hypercalcemia – Neoplastic process, sarcoidosis
- T3, T4, TSH, TRH (thyrootropin releasing hormone).

Radiologic Studies

- Ground glass appearance of maxillary bone – Fibrous dysplasia
- Dehiscence of orbital floor/lamina papyracea – Mucocele of frontoethmoid region
- Bone displacement without destruction– Benign tumor – Hemangioma, dermoid
- Focal calcification within orbit– Retinoblastoma.

Arteriography

- To detect the feeding vessel to a tumor, e.g. JNA (Juvenile NP angiofibroma)
- Rapid filling of superior ophthalmic vein – carotid cavernous sinus fistula.

CT Scan

- It uses the differential X-ray absorption of orbital muscles and neurovascular tissues – 35 hounsfield units, and the surrounding fat – 100 hounsfield units.
- With thin slice CT imaging (1.5 mm cuts) and computer software programs, 3-D reconstruction is possible.

- Coronal images useful in diseases of paranasal sinuses.
- Enlarged EOM's with involvement of tendinous insertion—Inflammatory pseudotumors.
- Enlarged EOM's without involvement of tendinous insertion—Grave's ophthalmopathy. C.T./MRI evaluation useful in evaluation post trauma visual loss and optic nerve injury (Figs 44.2a and b).

Ultrasound

- Based on reflection of high frequency sound energy projected through soft tissues of orbit.
- 'A' mode—"ONE" dimension (Ultra sonography).
- 'B' mode - "TWO" dimension (Ultrasonography)

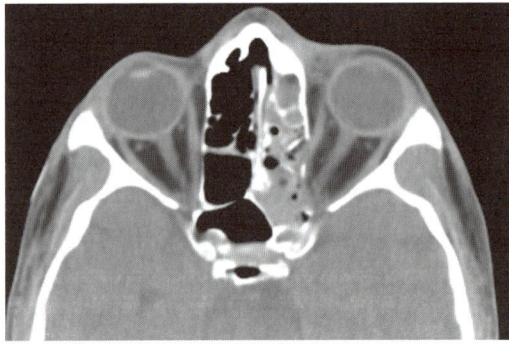

Fig. 44.2a: CT scan of the orbit in a case of orbital trauma

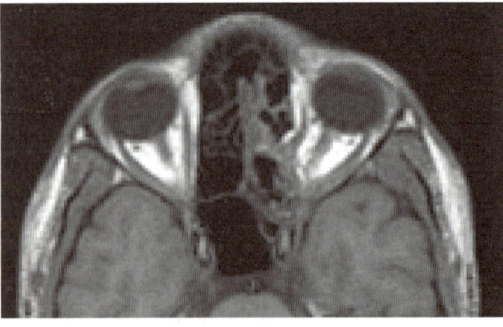

Fig. 44.2b: MRI scan of the same patient after endoscopic decompression

- Four patterns of mass lesion are identified:
  1. Cystic – Dermoid's
  2. Solid – Glioma
  3. Angiomatous – Hemangioma
  4. Infiltrative – Lymphoma.

MRI Scan

- Takes advantage of differences in magnetic properties of various tissues and pathophysiologic processes
- Useful to distinguish between paranasal sinus tumor and mucosal thickening/fluid retention which the tumor may cause.

PROPTOSIS

Definition

Proptosis refers to forward displacement of the globe due to any disease process within /adjacent to the orbit as a consequence of the rigid confines of the orbital wall.

Exophthalmos is any abnormal protrusion of the eye. It is more specific to the organ involved. The two words can be used interchangeably.

Pseudoproptosis refers to simulation of abnormal protrusion of the eye or a true abnormal protrusion that does not originate from a mass, an inflammation or a vascular disorder.

The average volume of an adult orbit is 30 ml. An increase of orbital volume of any 4 ml will produce 6 mm of proptosis.

Clinically significant proptosis is any forward displacement of one globe 2 mm greater than the other as measured by Krahn/Hertel exophthalmometer.

Causes of Unilateral Proptosis

1. Neoplastic
- Cavernous hemangioma
- Rhabdomyosarcoma
- Optic glioma
- Meningioma

- Carcinoma – Secondary from adjacent nose, sinus/brain
- Carcinoma – Metastatic
- Neurofibroma, melanoma, teratoma, lymphangioma
- Lymphoma, leukemia
- Lacrimal gland tumor
- Fibro-osseous lesions, e.g. fibrous dysplasia, ossifying fibroma, osteoma.

2. *Vascular*
   - Anteriovenous malformation
   - Aneurysm
   - Orbital varix
   - Carotid – Cavernous sinus fistula

3. *Traumatic*
   - Penetrating injury
   - Foreign body
   - Subdural hematoma

4. *Metabolic/Inflammatory*
   - Grave's ophthalmopathy
   - Orbital cellulites/abscess
   - Paranasal sinusitis/mucocele
   - Orbital pseudotumors
   - Other granulomatous disorders

5. *Congenital Development Cysts*
   - Dermoid, teratoma and
   - Microphthalmos with cyst

Vasclar Exophthalmos

- Venous (Varix)
- Arterial – Dural sinus fistula (low flow shunt)
- Carotid cavernous fistula (high flow shunt)

Venous Varix
- Positional proptosis or proptosis induced by valsalva maneuver
- Observation is the most prudent therapy

Arterial – Dural Sinus Fistula
- Insidious onset of proptosis
- Headache, tinnitus
- Fistula often closes spontaneously
- Selective carotid angiogram—Both diagnostic and therapeutic

- Embolization with small detachable balloons therapeutic

Carotid Cavernous Fistula
- Spontaneously, following trauma
- Bruits, proptosis, chemosis, ophthalmoplegia
- Arteriolized conjunctival vessels that approach the limbus in a corkscrew fashion characteristic
- Shunt closure with either detachable balloon/ carotid artery ligation.

Inflammatory – Infectious Exophthalmos

- Pseudotumor – is an idiopathic inflammatory process that mimics an orbital tumor
- Explosive onset – Proptosis, chemosis, pain, edema, decreased visual acuity
- *CT scan – 4 forms*
  1. Infiltrative
  2. Tumefactive
  3. Muscle enlargement and enhancement
  4. Uveoscleral thickening and enhancement
- *Myositis*
  - May involve one or more EOM.
  - Involved muscle is enlarged with inclusion of tendinous insertion.
- *Acute Dacryoadenitis*
  - Upper outer lid tender on palpation
  - S-shaped lid
  - CT – enhancing mass in lacrimal fossa
- *Perioptic Neuritis*
  - Simulates optic neuritis
  - Pain with retropulsion of globe
  - CT – Optic nerve enlarged
- *Orbital Cellulitis*
  - Commonly occurs as a complication of sinusitis

Neoplastic Exophthalmos

- *Tumors within muscle cone:* Axial proptosis, extraconal tumors – proptosis in direction opposite to that of lesion.
- *Important feature:* Lack of pain, except adenoid cystic carcinoma of lacrimal gland because of perineural invasion.

Capillary Hemangioma

- They grow until 2 to 3 years of age and then spontaneously involute
- Benign, invasive, unencapsulated, strawberry red appearance
- Deeper lesions – Proptosis
- Conservative management
- Diffuse lesions–Systemic/intralesional steroids

Rhabdomyosarcoma

- Most common childhood primary malignancy of childhood
- Involves superior orbit causing proptosis with downward displacement
- *Types*: Embryonal –80%, alveolar, botryoid, pleomorphic
- *Treatment*: High dose local radiation followed by chemotherapy (VAC), vincristine, adriamycin and cyclophosphamide.

Glioma

- Juvenile pilocytic astrocytoma of orbital optic nerve
- Loss of vision, papilledema/optic atrophy, strabismus, proptosis–Axial and downwards
- 25 to 50 percent have systemic neurofibromatosis
- *CT scan*–Fusiform enlargement of optic nerve and concentric enlargement of optic canal
- *Treatment* is controversial

  Conservative? Total excision?
- *Metastasis* 6th to 7th decade
- *Primary* schirrous adenocarcinoma, oat cell carcinoma, renal cell carcinoma, prostate carcinoma.

SURGICAL APPROACH TO ORBITAL TUMORS

1. Lateral Orbitotomy (Maroon and Kennerdell)

Uses

- Lesions in lacrimal fossa, lesions temporal to optic nerve both intraconal and extraconal and above/below the optic nerve can be approached
- No danger to any important orbital structure.
- No functional/cosmetic defect is present

Steps

- *Incision*–LAZY-S/HOCKEYSTICK shaped along the lateral orbital rim
- Temporalis fascia is cut posteriorly. Temporalis muscles is detached.
- Periosteum of lateral orbital rim is cut and reflected off.
- With a malleable retractor protecting the periorbita, the lateral orbital rim is divided above the frontozygomatic and body of zygoma. The bone flap is out fractured.
- Additional lateral wall upto anterior wall of middle cranial fossa can be removed with rongeurs

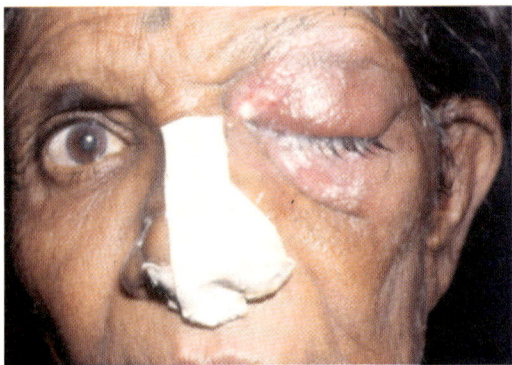

Fig. 44.3: Left sided orbital cellulitis with abscess following fungal sinusitis (aspergillosis) treated by endoscopic sinus surgery and endonasal drainage and decompression

- Lateral rectus is used for identification
- Periorbita is incised over the tumor and tumor can be removed by blunt dissection or cryoprobe.
- Before skin closure, bone flap is reinserted and periosteum closed over it
- Skin closed in 2 layers

2. Medial Orbitotomy

- Used for lesions that are medial to the plane of the optic nerve
- *Two Types*
  - Anteromedial (conjunctival) with disinsertion of medial rectus muscle (intraconal lesion)
  - Lynch/lateral rhinotomy type approach (extraconal lesion)

SINUS DISEASES THAT CAN PRODUCE PROPTOSIS

Inflammatory Causes

1. *Bacterial Infection*
   - 75 percent of bacterial infections in the orbit are caused by paranasal sinusitis
   - Spread by two routes
   - Venous through valveless veins (periphlebitis/thrombophlebitis)
   - Direct spread through paper plate of ethmoid
   - *Organism – Streptococcus pneumoniae, H.influenzae*, Beta hemolytic Streptococci, *Staphylococcus aureus*
   - *Sites* – Ethmoid sinus (in children)
     - All sinuses (in adults)
   - Classification (Chandler and Associates)
     - Preseptal cellulitis
     - True orbital cellulitis
     - Subperiosteal abscess
     - Orbital abscess
     - Cavernous sinus thrombosis

Treatment

- High dose, broad spectrum, IV antibiotics until signs of inflammation have resolved followed by oral antibiotics for 2 more weeks
- Nasal decongestants
- Surgical decompression and drainage which is described later

2. **Mucormycosis**
   - Organism – Fungus – Rhinocerebral phycomycosis
   - Rhizopus/absidia/mucor organisms
   - Patient profile
     - Poorly controlled diabetes
     - Immunodeficiency syndromes
     - Malnutrition
     - Chronic renal failure
     - Cirrhosis
     - Long term antibiotic/steroid therapy
   - *Pathology*: Fungi are part of normal respiratory flora in sinuses and orbit. They invade arterioles producing thrombosis and ischemic infarctions
   - *On examination*: Black, crusted and necrotic areas over turbinates and nasal septum are seen
   - Frontal sinus is usually spared and ethmoid sinuses are commonly involved

Treatment

- Correction of hyperglycemia and keto-acidosis
- IV amphotericin B
- Wide surgical debridement.

3. **Aspergillosis**

   - *Organism* – Fungus found in soil and decaying fruits/plants – aspergillus
   - *Site* – Antrum and ethmoids
   - *Predisposing factor* – Polyp disease with recurrent sinusitis in tropical setting
   - In the orbit fibrosis causes rigid proptosis and optic nerve damage

Treatment

- Wide surgical excision with exteriorization

4. **Wegener's disease**
   Wegener's disease is described under chronic specific rhinitis.

Benign tumors and tumor like growths of sinuses affecting the orbit

- Mucocele
- Inverting papilloma
- Osteoma
- Fibrous dysplasia
- Juvenile nasopharyngeal angiofibroma
- Ameloblastoma

Malignant Sinus Tumors that may involve the Orbit

- Sites of origin
  - Maxillary sinus   –   55%
  - Nasal cavity   –   35%
  - Ethmoid sinus   –   09%
- Most sinus tumors with orbital signs and symptoms are advanced tumors with bad prognosis. This has been discussed under neoplastic conditions of the Nose and PNS.

THYROID AND THE ORBIT

Graves Ophthalmopathy

- *Definition* A condition of altered thyroid metabolism that causes protein depositions within the EOM's, increasing their bulk by as much as tenfold along with an increase in orbital fat. It is a bilateral disease.

- There is abnormal autoimmune response with abnormal antibody receptor site complexes in the tissues. T-lymphocyte is the main culprit.
- *Clinical Features*
  - Lid retraction
  - Lid lag
  - Lid edema
  - Temporal flare of upper lid
  - Injection and chemosis of conjunctiva
  - Myopathy
  - Proptosis and diplopia, exophthalmos
  - Optic neuropathy
- Enlarged EOM is the main cause of proptosis in order of involvement – IR, MR, SR and LR
- *CT Finding*
  - Enlarged EOM's - "Fusiform" with sparing of tendinous insertions.
  - Bulging orbital septum due to protruding fat
  - Dilated superior ophthalmic vein.

Differential Diagnosis

- Pseudotumor cerebri
- Lymphoma of orbit
- Metastatic tumor
- Vascular anomaly
- Neurofibroma

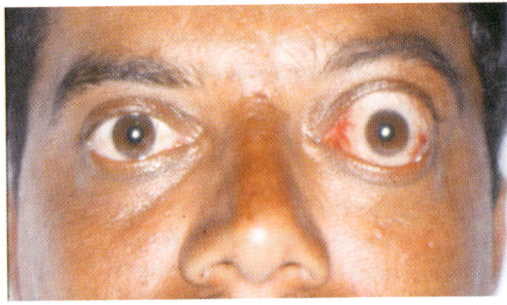

Fig. 44.4: Proptosis of the left eye ball due to malignant tumor of the maxilloethmoidal complex

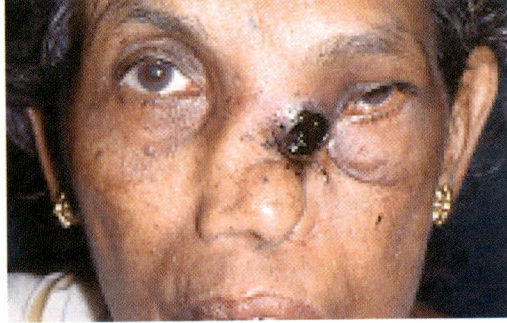

Fig. 44.5: Proptosis of the left eye ball due to malignant melanoma of the maxilloe- thmoidal complex

- Retinoblastoma
- Congenital shallowness of orbit.

Treatment Decisions (Table 44.1)

Orbital Decompression

- **Concept:** There is too much tissue in a bony space and either tissue should be removed or space enlarged. Removal of tissue not practical, so space must be enlarged.
- **Indications**
  - Decreased visual acuity
  - Visual field defects
  - Abnormal visual evoked potentials
  - Disc edema
- **Approaches**
  - Superior – Naffziger
  - Inferior – Hisch and Urbanek (1930)
  - Medial – Sewell
  - Lateral – Kronlein
  - Combined medial and inferior—Walsh and Ogura

– Endoscopic intranasal orbital decompression is most popular today.

Walsh-Ogura Antral – Ethmoidal Decompression

Advantages

- Largest space for decompression
- Utilizes gravitational force for D.C.
- Extracranial approach
- No facial incisions
- Surgical anatomy and operative technique is easily mastered by otolaryngologist
- Immediate reduction of proptosis
- Dramatic vision improvement within 24 hours post-op.

Steps

- Patient position – Semi-sitting position with knees slightly flexed—15 degree reverse Trendelenburg position.

Table 44.1: Treatment decisions	
Therapy	*Indication*
Non-surgical treatment	
High dose steroids	Rapid visual deterioration
Immunosuppressive agents	
(Cyclophosphamide, Cyclosporine)	Experimental
Radiation therapy (200 cGy)	Slowly progressive visual loss
Surgical treatment	
Medial decompression	Mild exophthalmos (2–3 mm)
Lateral decompression	-Do-
Inferior decompression	Mild to moderate
Superior decompression	Congenital orbitopathy
Two wall decompression	Moderate exophthalmos (3–5 mm)
Three wall decompression	Severe exophthalmos (5–7 mm)
Endoscopic medial decompression	By experienced endoscopist
Eyelid retraction surgery	Widened palpebral fissure and exposure
Strabismus surgery	Diplopia

- Sublabial/Cadwell – Luc incision is made and a large antrostomy (in max antrum)
- Bone is removed from the area superomedial to infraorbital nerve.
- Microscope introduced and transantral ethmoidectomy done
  - *Site of entry:* At junction of medial posterior and superior walls of maxillary sinus
  - *Angle of entry:* 45 degree upward, directed to the medial canthus of opposite eye
  - Ethmoid cells are removed upto the cribriform plate and back to the sphenoid sinus with preservation of lamina papyracea and attachment of middle turbinate.
- Floor of orbit is fractured away with curette/chisel. Care should be taken to avoid injury to periorbita. Lamina papyracea is fractured medially and removed.
- Longitudinal incisions are made in the periorbita. Succeeding cuts are made more laterally. 4 to 6 incisions suffice. The orbital fat will herniate through them.
- Nasal antrostomy is performed
- Incisions are closed.

Complications of Orbital Decompression

- Corneal abrasion
- Optic nerve compromise
- Retrobulbar hematoma
- Nasolacrimal duct obstruction
- CSF rhinorrhea
- Oroantral fistula
- Diplopia
- Ectropion

- Infraorbital nerve injury
- Retinal vascular occlusion
- Blindness
- Infection
- Retrobulbar hematoma
- Retinal vascular occlusion (sight threatening emergencies)
- Corneal ulcer

OTHER SURGICAL INTERVENTIONS OF THE ORBIT BY ENT — HEAD and NECK SURGEONS

1. Endoscopic dacryocystorhinostomy (Endonasal endoscopic DCR)
2. Endoscopic orbital decompression
3. Endoscopic optic nerve decompression
4. Transnasal endoscopic orbital biopsy
5. Orbital exenteration for sinonasal malignancy involving the orbit (Fig. 44.6)

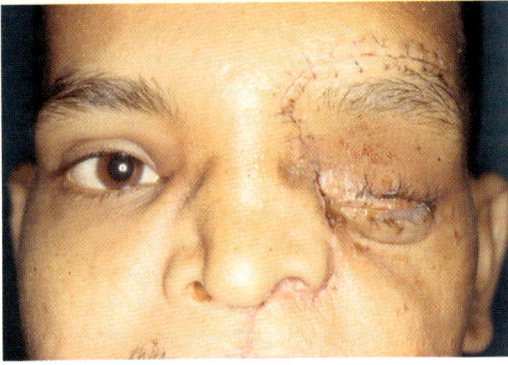

Fig. 44.6: Orbital exenteration after faciocranial resection for maxilloethmoidal malignancy

POINTS TO REMEMBER

1. All paranasal sinuses are related to the orbit.
2. Orbit is made up of 7 bones and has seven important contents.
3. Proptosis refers to forward displacement of globe due to any disease process within or adjacent to the orbit.

45

Common Surgical Procedures of the Nose and Paranasal Sinuses

The common surgeries of the nose and paranasal sinuses include the following:

Nasal Septum

- Septoplasty
- Submucosal resection (SMR)
- Septorhinoplasty.

Inferior Turbinate

- Submucosal diathermy
- Partial turbinectomy
- Laser turbinoplasty
- Microdebrider/radiofrequency assisted turbinoplasty
- Out-fracture of the turbinate
- Bipolar cautery of the turbinate
- Cryosurgery

Middle Turbinate

- Concha bullosa partial resection
- Bipolar cautery

Maxillary Sinus

- Antral puncture
- Intranasal antrostomy (INA)
- Endoscopic sinus surgery – Middle meatal antrostomy (MMA)
- Caldwell-Luc operation

Ethmoid Sinus

- Intranasal ethmoidectomy (Mosher's)
- External ethmoidectomy (Howarth's operation)
- Transantral ethmoidectomy
- Endoscopic sinus surgery – Ethmoidectomy.

Frontal Sinus

- External frontoethmoidectomy (Lynch-Howarth's operation)
- Endoscopic sinus surgery—Frontal sinusostomy
- Osteoplastic flap method
- Frontal sinus obliteration procedure

Sphenoid Sinus

- External sphenoethmoidectomy
- Endoscopic sinus surgery: Sphenoethmoidectomy/ sphenoidotomy

Surgeries for nose and paranasal sinus neoplasm

- Lateral rhinotomy (medial maxillectomy)
- Total maxillectomy
- Partial maxillectomy
- Craniofacial resection

Intranasal Antrostomy

After the inferior meatus is anesthetized with

surface anesthesia (4 percent xylocaine with 1 in 200,000 adrenaline), inferior turbinate is elevated superiorly using Freer's elevator and a cottonoid strips soaked in 4 percent xylocaine with 1 in 200,000 adrenaline is placed in the inferior meatus to facilitate decongestion. Using a Tilley's Antral Harpoon (Fig. 45.1) nasoantral wall is opened. Alternatively Myle's nasal antral perforator can be used to perforate the nasoantral wall in the inferior meatus. The opening can be enlarged further by using the reverse cutting edge of the Myle's perforator. To create a large nasoantral window Ostrum's backwards cutting forceps or Stamburger's antrum punch can be used.

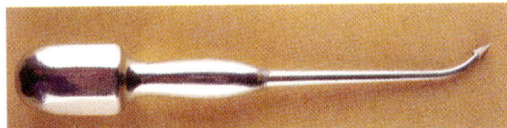

Fig. 45.1: Tilley's antral harpoon

Indications

1. Chronic suppurative sinusitis associated to Kartagener's syndrome/immotile cilia syndrome, etc.
2. In chronic sinusitis, though it is now largely replaced by FESS (Functional endoscopic sinus surgery) which is the treatment of choice.
3. To take biopsy through antral window in suspected cases of malignancy through antral window.
4. Sometimes a small opening is made to facilitate passing of instrument for the removal of antral polyp/stalk of the antral polyp attached to the floor/cyst/pyocele under endoscopic guidance when it is not accessible in addition to middle meatal antrostomy.
5. Prior to radiotherapy in cases of malignancy of maxilla and maxilloethmoid complex where surgery is deferred.

Caldwell-Luc Operation

- (Synonym: Radical antrostomy, canine fossa antrostomy)

Definition

It is defined as a sublabial approach to the maxillary sinus through the canine fossa wherein the maxillary mucosa is radically excised and drainage is established by creating an intranasal antrostomy.

Technique (Fig 45.2)

- This procedure can be done under local anesthesia (2% xylocaine with 1 in 200,000 dilution adrenaline) by infiltrating above the buccogingival sulcus in the region of the canine fossa. Also, a strip of cottonoid soaked with 4 percent xylocaine with adrenaline is kept below the inferior turbinate.
- General anesthesia is given in non-compliant patients.
- *Incision:* A bone deep horizontal incision is made in the gingivobuccal sulcus well above the roots of the teeth between canine and second molar.
- Periosteal flap is elevated till the infra orbital foramen exposing the canine fossa. Care is taken not to injure the infraorbital nerve during elevation and retraction. The flap is retracted superolaterally to prevent injury to the nerve.
- The canine fossa is opened using a burr or a gouge. After making the initial opening further enlargement is done using Kerrison's bone cutting forceps.

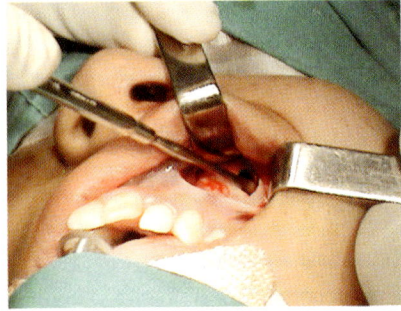

Fig. 45.2: Caldwell-Luc operation in progress (Sublabial radical antrostomy)

- The mucosa of the antrum is inspected and cyst/ polyp or benign tumors are removed by elevating the affected mucosa using a suitable elevator. Alternatively a micro-debrider can also be used for the removal of a polyp or a cyst. Benign tumors are better removed by blunt dissection as adequate tissue is available for histopathological examination. Normal mucosa should be spared in such cases.
- Irreversible diseased mucosa of the antrum can be removed completely.
- Intranasal (inferior meatal) antrostomy is done as described earlier.
- A pack is placed in the antrum with its one end brought out through the intranasal antrostomy into the nasal cavity.
- The mucoperiosteal flap is sutured in 2 layers with 4-0 vicryl.
- The pack is removed intranasally after 48 hours.

Indications

- Chronic maxillary sinusitis with irreversible mucosal changes which is refractory to other modalities of treatment.
- Recurrent antro-choanal polyp if the patient is more than 18 years old (after eruption of the second molar tooth).
- Removal of benign tumors/ dentigerous cyst.
- As an approach for Vidian neurectomy
- As an approach for maxillary artery ligation.
- Invasive fungal sinusitis of the maxillary sinus
- Hemoantrum
- Blow-out fracture of the orbit

Complications:
(Mnemonic SHOOT pain)

- Swelling of the cheek
- Hemorrhage
- Oroantral fistula
- Osteomyelitis of the maxilla
- Tooth root damage
- Infraorbital paresthesia

Submucous Resection and Septoplasty

They are the most common surgical procedures of the nose where deviated septal framework is corrected by either radical resection of the septal cartilage and the bones (submucosal resection) or by minimal resection of the cartilage and selective removal of the deviated bone and realignment of the septal framework to correct the septal abnormality (septoplasty). It has been discussed in detail in the chapter deviated nasal septum.

Septorhinoplasty: (Greek; Rhinos, "Nose" + Plastikos, "to shape")

- This surgery is used to improve the function (reconstructive surgery) or appearance (cosmetic surgery) of a person's nose. According to Indian literature the origin of rhinoplasty goes to Sushruta.
- However in the present era first intranasal rhinoplasty was performed by John Orland Roe in 1887
- When a rhinoplasty is performed for deviation of the external nose, most of which are post- traumatic, it is very essential to correct the septal deviation to get the desired results. In case of cosmetic rhinoplasty it should be avoided.
- Depending on the type of approach it can be divided into:
  - External approach
  - Internal approach
- Though the approaches are different the basic principle of surgical technique and correction are same. When an "external" incision, meaning an incision on the outside skin, is used, the operation is called an "open or external" rhinoplasty. A "closed or internal" rhinoplasty is when no incision on the outside skin is made.
- External approach provides the surgeon with the best chance for symmetric reconstruction
- Each patient has a different configuration of nose and requires individual planning for surgical reconstruction which may vary from patient to patient. This includes the amount

of tissue to be excised/augmented, area of anatomical correction , thickness of skin associated ,nasal pathology (trauma).

- *The principle of septorhinoplasty includes the following steps:*
- Septoplasty
- Tip correction which may include remodeling , projection or rotation (discussed in Chapter Diseases of external nose)
- Removal of the hump (discussed in Chapter Disease of external nose)
- Narrowing of the nose with osteotomies
- Final correction of the deformities

Steps of Septorhinoplasty

- *External Approach* (Figs 45.3 and 45.4)
- *Incision:* A transcollumellar incision in a form of inverted V to minimize the resultant scar which usually is invisible post operatively after healing. The incision is then extended posteriorly along the margin of the lower lateral cartilage. (As shown in the Figs 45.4b)
- A skin flap is elevated with the help of sharp scissors to expose the nasal tip and lower lateral cartilage
- For correction of the septal deformity, fibrous tissue between the two lower lateral cartilages are separated to expose the caudal end of the septum .The perichondrial incision is given at the caudal end to elevate the

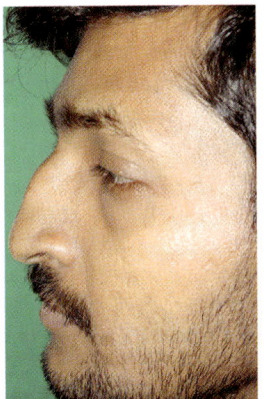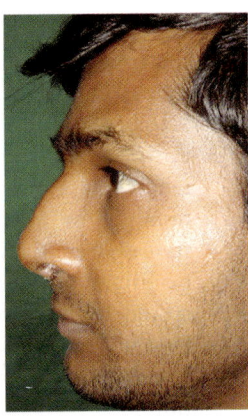

Figs 45.3a and b: Pre and immediate postoperative pictures (lateral views) following external rhinoplasty for deformity following previous septal surgery

mucoperichondrial flap. The rest of the surgical technique is as described in the chapter 'deviated nasal septum' under SMR and septoplasty.

- To correct the deviated nose, elevation of the septal flaps is done on both the sides and the septal cartilage is separated from the lower and upper lateral cartilages. If necessary, to correct the dorsal deformity incision and excision of a portion of upper lateral cartilages may be necessary. Hump can be directly visualized and should be corrected before doing other procedures including septal surgery.

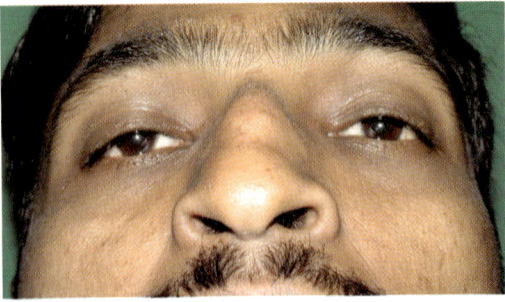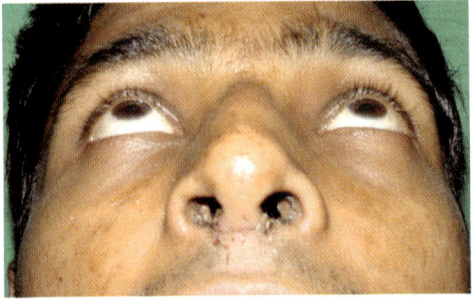

Figs 45.4a and b: Pre and postoperative pictures (basal views) following external rhinoplasty for the same patient. The correction was done by major septal repair and by cartilage graft for tip and columellar support in addition to tip surgery for projection and rotation. Rib cartilage graft was used for reconstruction

- Osteotomies are very important to correct the bony deviation. A median oblique osteotomy followed by a lateral osteotomy is done till the level of the frontomaxillary suture line at the root of the nose. Both the lateral osteotomies are joined together in the midline. Thus the cartilage and bony framework can be mobilized easily and can be brought to the midline to correct the deformity.

- Sometimes a hump is in fact a pseudohump which is due to depressed tip as a result of previous septal surgery due to excessive resection of the inferior strip of cartilage or gross subluxation or fractured nasal septal cartilage. In such cases tip correction is necessary as described under diseases of external nose.

- The hump removal is done by reduction rhinoplasty already described under hump chapter 'Diseases of external nose'.

- When the surgery is complete, a splint is applied to help the nose maintain its new shape. Nasal packs or soft plastic splints also may be placed in nostrils to stabilize the septum.

Internal Approach

- *Incision:* This approach includes complete hemi-transfixation incision, elevation of mucoperichondrial flap of septum is done on the concave side.

- *Intercartilaginous/Transcartilaginous incision:* Transcartilaginous incision is preferred when tip refinement, volume reduction and tip projection is necessary. The approach is simple and easy to perform and technique is called 'tip non-delivery' approach. In 'tip delivery' technique the intercartilaginous incision is given and dissection is carried out between the upper lateral cartilage and lateral process of the lower lateral cartilage to separate nasal cartilage from the overlying skin. Overlying soft tissue and the periosteum over the bony

framework is done by using the periosteal elevator after the periosteum is incised over the nasal bone.

- The hemitransfixation incision is then joined with the intercartilaginous incision and septum is separated from upper lateral cartilage by sharp dissection. When there is external deformity involving the cartilaginous framework it is ideal to separate both the lateral cartilage from the septum. The septum is corrected before proceeding to correct the external deformity. Septal correction is very important part in scoliotic/ deviated/ crooked nose.

- The cartilaginous deviation is corrected first before proceeding to bony deformity. Strategic wedge resection/incision may be required to correct the upper lateral cartilage.

- Cartilaginous hump is corrected before the bony portion of the hump, by reduction of cartilaginous portion by knife, caudally from the nasal bone to the caudal end of the septum. To reduce the height of upper lateral cartilage straight iris scissor is used.

- Correction of bony hump is done then by using 4 mm osteotome. Small bony humps can be reduced by using a rasp after elevation of the periostium from the nasal bone (Figs 45.5a and b).

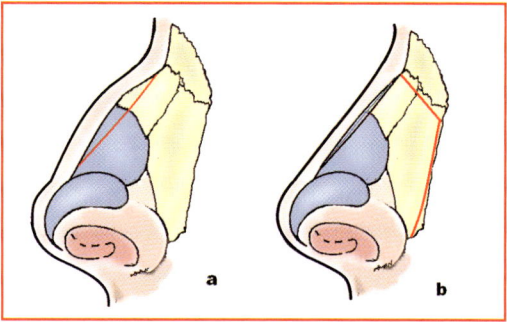

Figs 45.5a and b: (a) Shaded line showing the area of bony and cartilaginous hump to be resected (b) Results to be obtained after resection of hump (red line indicates the line of osteotomy to be performed after hump reduction)

- Correction of bony framework and narrowing is done by osteotomies after the hump excision to appose the flat dorsum thus created. The median osteotomy should be short and should be directed laterally along the line of intended fracture. Curved low lateral osteotomy is done to prevent trauma to surrounding structure. Lateral osteotomies are carried out through pyriform aperture. A small incision is given in pyriform aperture and the small periosteal tunnel is created, a guarded osteotomy is preferred to do the lateral osteotomy. The lateral osteotomy should be as near as to medial canthus and care should be taken not to injure the lacrimal sac and osteotomy should be kept lateral to that. Alternatively to facilitate the low lateral osteotomy medial oblique osteotomies angled laterally, approximately 15 to 20 degree from vertical midline is preferred. This technique results in less trauma, prevents asymmetries and less manual pressure is necessary unlike a low curved lateral osteotomies alone. Multiple / triple osteotomies are required for post-traumatic scoliotic or crooked nose to facilitate proper bony realignment. The realigned bony fragments usually stay attached to each other without getting displaced by fibrosis.
- After the osteotomies are over, the nasal framework should be realigned, septal splinting is given followed by external nasal splint to support and keep nasal framework in place and protect external nose.

Augmentation Rhinoplasty

- To correct the saddle nose deformity it is very important to asses the defect in order to select the proper graft material. The basic principles that should be kept in mind are
  1. The nose is hazardous recipient area.
  2. There is no single best graft material.
  3. Synthetic material tend to extrude and the need to have a good thick layer of soft tissues that should separate them from internal or external surface

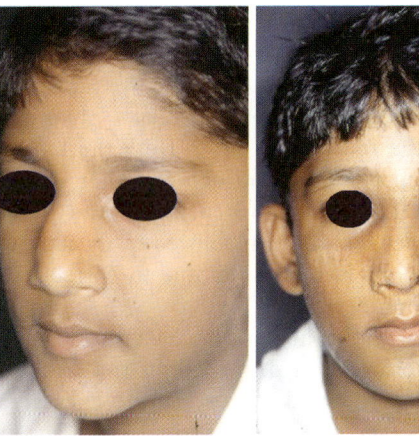

Figs 45.6a and b: (a) Deviated (scoliotic) nose, (b) Showing postoperative photograph after correction

4. All natural materials like cartilage and bone get adsorbed to some degree, particularly the cartilage gets absorbed in contact with the blood. The graft and its bed are always subjected to frequent trauma. Commonly used graft materials for augmentation are:

- **Bone:** commonly iliac crest bone graft and tibial bone grafts are taken. Tibia is excellent for saddle deformity of dorsum and it gives a natural contour.
- **Cartilage:** Can be taken from the septum and conchal cartilage of the ear. The septal cartilage is good for the correction of the dorsum and also is ideal material for collumellar strut and important to give tip projection. But the problem encountered with septal cartilage is that, it is some time not adequate enough particularly if the septal surgery is done before. Most of the septal deformities that come following post SMR/ Septal surgeries or post traumatic where the septal cartilage may have necrosed due to associated hematoma at the time of trauma. Rib cartilage can also be used for the reconstruction of the cartilaginous part and for augmentation.
- **Synthetics:** May get extruded. Commonly used material are sialastics teflon, etc.

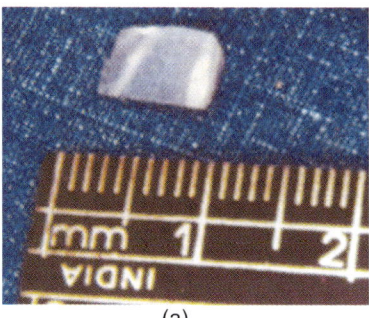

(a)

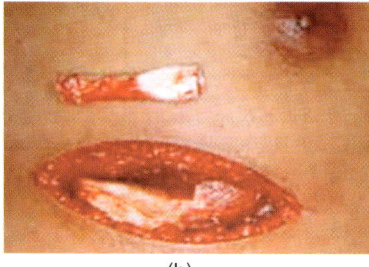

(b)

Figs 45.7a and b: Silastic block can be fashioned and used for implantation to reconstruct the nasal defect

(Figs 45.7a and b) telfon, etc. Preformed nasal graft nasal materials are available. They should not have any sharp edge. They are easy to place and can be rejected easily unless thickness of nose is evaluated properly

Indications of Augmentation Rhinoplasty

The common indications are:
- Saddle nose deformity due to bony saddle, cartilaginous saddle, bony and cartilaginous saddle
- Retracted columella
- Systemic disease like tuberculosis, leprosy, syphilis after treatment of the under lying disease

Steps

External rhinoplasty approach is preferred over internal rhinoplasty to prepare the graft bed. The over lying skin and columella is lifted up adjacent to the caudal end of the septal cartilage, after a routine external rhinoplasty approach with the help of a dorsal retractor. Alternatively intercartilaginous incision is given as described in the internal rhinoplasty approach and the overlying skin, soft tissue is retracted from the dorsum with the help of a dorsal retractor. The soft tissue over the nasal bones are dissected and separated with the help of a sharp elevator. Bony surface is made raw occasionally medial and lateral osteotomies may be necessary for reshaping. After the nasal bed is prepared the suitable graft material is harvested or a preformed synthetic graft material can be used instead in case of non-availability of natural graft. The graft should be prepared according to the length and height required. It should be shaped in such a way that it comes down to the septal angle and no further. The graft is gently inserted into the target area and the incision sites are closed by catgut (3'0) for transcartilaginous/ intercartilagin- ous incision. 6'0 prolene is used for external rhinoplasty incision (Figs 45.8, 45.9a and b).

Functional Endoscopic Sinus Surgery (FESS)

Better understanding of the pathophysiology of chronic sinusitis and the role of ethmoid and the ostiomeatal complex in the disease causation and with the availability of better diagnostic procedures like CT scan and diagnostic nasal endoscopy, it has now been possible for us to treat sinusitis more effectively and conservatively. Functional endoscopic sinus surgery deals with the ostiomeatal complex obstruction and helps in restoring the mucociliary drainage of the paranasal sinuses. All the sinuses can be dealt with by this approach and being ultraconservative the morbidity of this procedure is very minimal with minimal hospitalization.

The salient steps of FESS are:
- Uncinectomy (infundibulotomy)
- Middle meatal antrostomy
- Frontal recess clearance
- Anterior ethmoidectomy
- Posterior ethmoidectomy and sphenoido-tomy are done only if it is indicated.

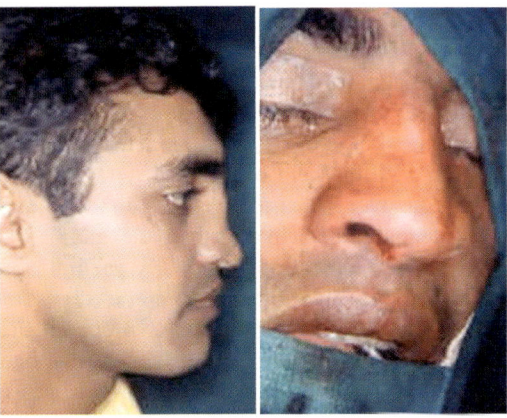

Figs 45.8 a and b: Pre and postoperative photographs following augmentation rhinoplasty. Rib cartilage graft is used for reconstruction

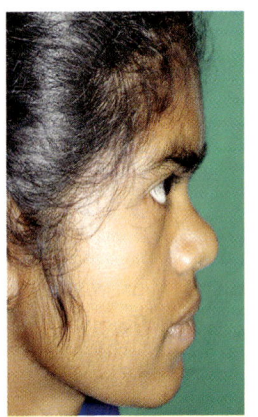 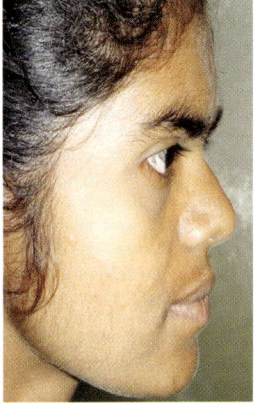

Figs 45.9a and b: Pre and postoperative photographs following augmentation rhinoplasty

Technique

1. Anesthesia: This can be done either under local anesthesia or general anesthesia, but local anesthesia is preferred. The nose is initially packed with cottonoid strips soaked in 4 percent lignocaine with adrenaline (1:50,000 dilution) for 5 to 10 minutes. Later 2 percent lignocaine with adrenaline (1:100,000 dilution) is injected under endoscopic vision into the uncinate process, bulla ethmoidalis, middle turbinate as shown in the Fig. 45.10 (black dots).

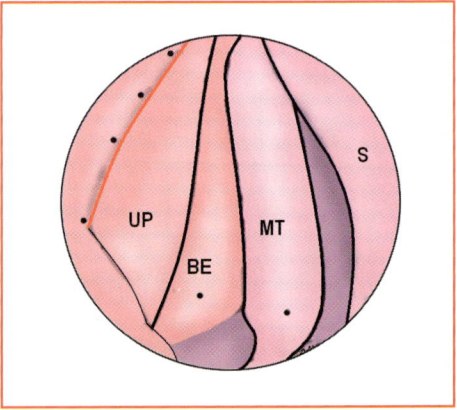

Fig. 45.10: Sites of injection of the local anesthetic for FESS (black dots). UP: uncinate process, BE: bulla ethmoidalis, MT: middle turbinate and S: septum

2. Uncinectomy (infundibulotomy): Incision is given circumferentially over the mucosa immediately anterior to the uncinate process using a sickle knife and the incision follows the course of the uncinate process. The knife is directed inferiorly and parallel to the lateral nasal wall to prevent injury to the lamina papyracia while separating the uncinate process (Fig.45.21).

The uncinate process is subluxated medially using a straight perichondrial elevator from its superior to inferior attachments (Fig 45.11). Then the subluxed uncinate process is removed using straight Blakesly forceps (Fig. 45.12). This opens the infundibulum and exposes the bulla ethmoidalis.

3. Anterior Ethmoidectomy: The natural ostium of the maxillary sinus is identified. Often the inferior part of the uncinate process prevents the visualization of the natural ostium and its careful removal will help to visualize the natural ostium. The bulla ethmoidalis is opened antero-infero-medially (Fig. 45.13) by gently pushing the straight Blakesly Weil forceps or a suction tip. After identifying the lumen entire bulla can be

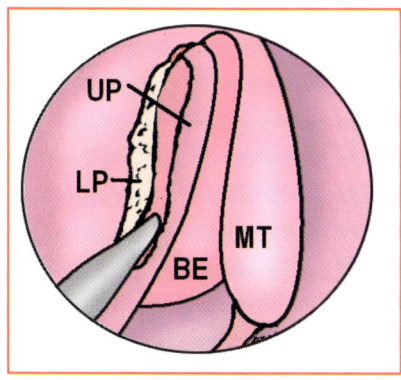

Fig. 45.11: Incision and subluxation of the uncinate process

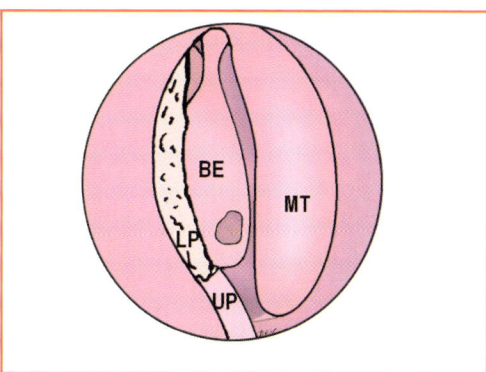

Fig. 45.13: Opening of the bulla ethmoidalis. UP: Residual uncinate process inferiorly, BE: bulla ethmoidalis, LP: lamina papyracea and MT: middle turbinate

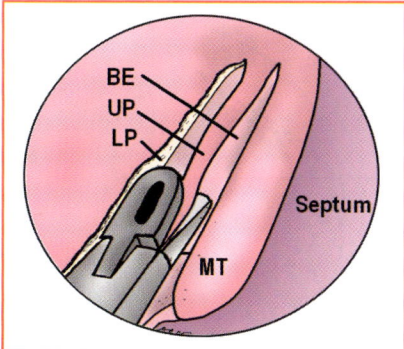

Fig. 45.12: Removal of the subluxated uncinate forceps using a straight Blakesly forceps. UP: Uncinate process, BE: bulla ethmoidalis, LP: lamina papyracea and MT: middle turbinate

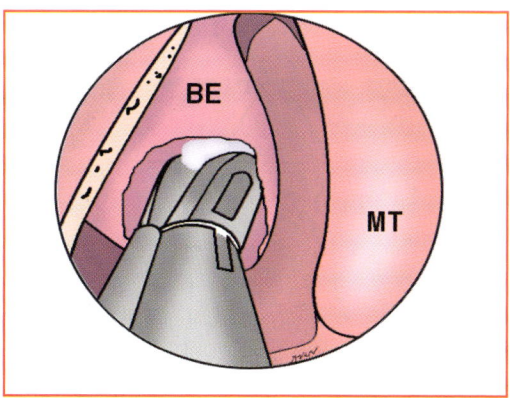

Fig. 45.14: Opening of the bulla ethmoidalis. BE: bulla ethmoidalis and MT: middle turbinate

resected step by step (Fig. 45.14). This is followed by removal of anterior and superior cells to bulla and sinus lateralis. The anterior ethmoidal artery is a useful landmark to identify the roof of the ethmoid, i.e. the anterior skull base as shown in the figure. The ground lamella (posterior wall of the bulla separating the anterior and the posterior ethmoids) is not opened routinely, unless indicated (Figs 45.15, 45.16, 45.23).

4. ***Middle meatal antrostomy:*** The maxillary sinus ostium is not enlarged routinely if the ostium is well patent. If accessory ostium of the maxillary sinus is present, the natural and accessory ostia are connected. If the ostium is stenosed, it can be enlarged towards the anterior fontanelle using a back-biting forceps as shown in the Figs 45.19, 45.21, 45.24.

5. ***Exploration of the frontal recess:*** This can be done after removal of the anterior ethmoidal cells including the bulla and after identification of the ethmoidal roof. Angled Blakesly forceps is used with 30 degree or

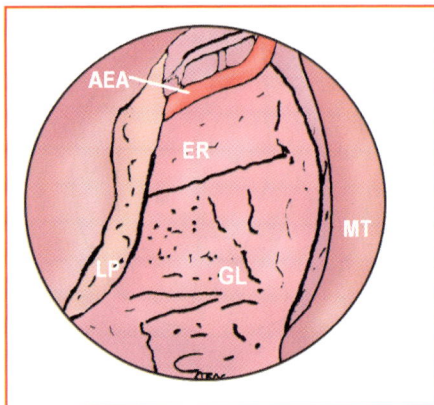

Fig. 45.15: FESS cavity after complete anterior ethmoidectomy exposing the ground lamella (GL). LP: lamina papyrecea and MT: middle turbinate, GL: Ground lamella, ER: ethmoidal roof, AEA: anterior ethmoidal artery

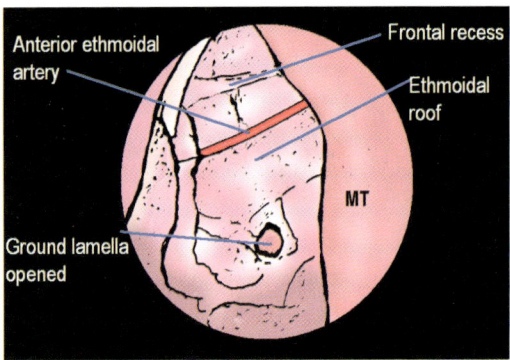

Fig. 45.16: Opening of the ground lamella

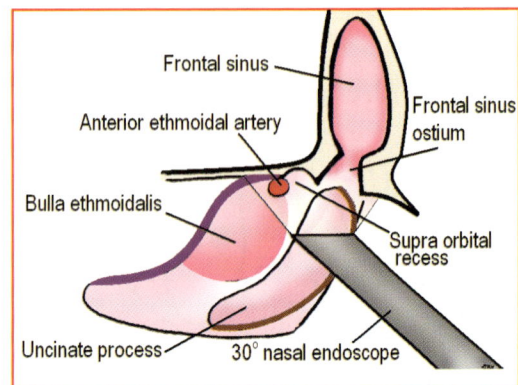

Fig. 45.17: Visualization of the frontal recess area using a 30 degree nasal endoscope

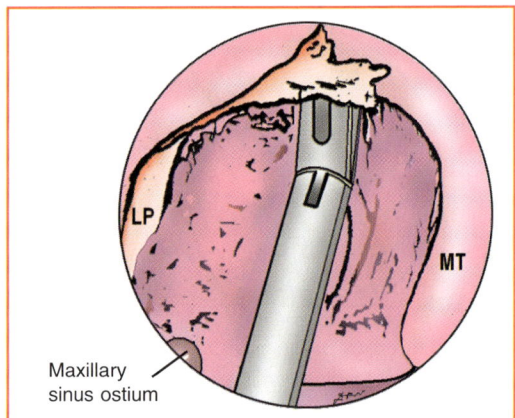

Fig. 45.18: Clearance of the frontal recess using upturned Blakesly forceps. LP: lamina papyrecea and MT: middle turbinate

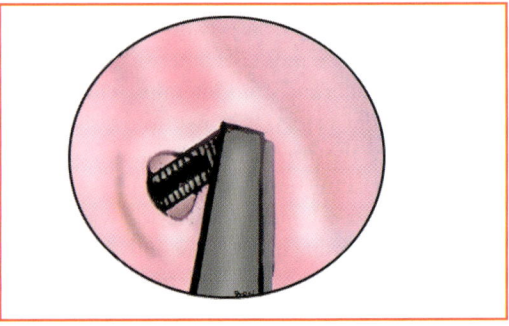

Fig. 45.19: Widening of the natural maxillary ostium using a backward cutting forceps

45 degree endoscopes to explore and clear the disease (Figs 45.17 and 45.18).

There may be varied anatomical variation including the non-development of the frontal sinus. The frontal sinus can be opened after removal of the cranial part of the uncinate process. The anterior ethmoidal artery is the most important landmark to the frontal recess which is situated anterior to the supraorbital recess (Figs 45.17 and 45.24).

6. ***Posterior ethmoidectomy and sphenoido-tomy:*** To enter the posterior ethmoid the

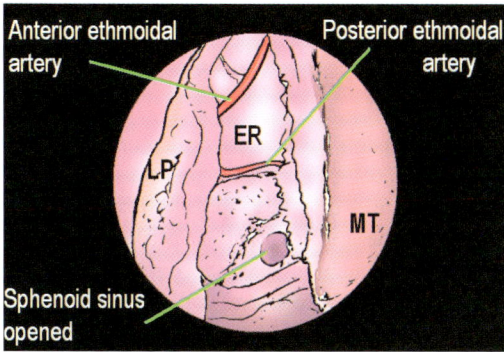

Fig. 45.20: Opening the sphenoid sinus inferomedially. LP: lamina papyrecea, MT: middle turbinate, ER: ethmoidal roof

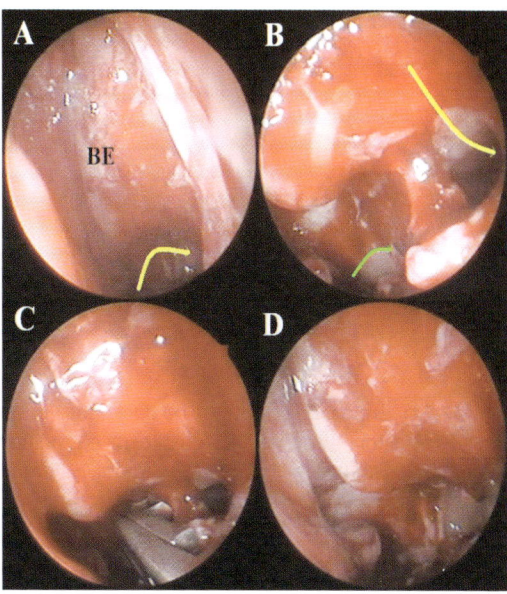

Fig. 45.22a to d: Intraoperative endoscopic picture showing middle meatal antrostomy being performed. (a) Bulla ethmoidalis (BE) and the natural maxillary ostium (yellow arrow) seen after uncinectomy, (b) Natural maxillary ostium (yellow arrow) and the accessory maxillary ostium (green arrow), (c) The two ostia are being connected by backward cutting forceps and (d) after middle meatal antrostomy

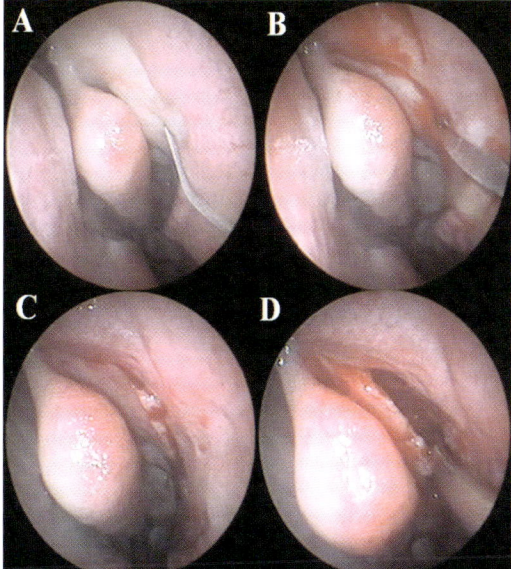

Figs 45.21a to d: Intraoperative endoscopic picture showing infundibulotomy in progress. (a) Injection of the local anesthetic into the uncinate process, (b) and (c) Incision of the uncinate process, (d) Subluxation of the uncinate process

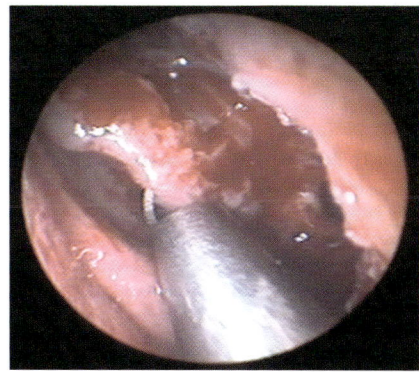

Fig. 45.23: Intraoperative endoscopic picture showing bulla ethmoidalis being opened using a microdebrider

ground lamella is opened inferomedially (Fig. 45.16). A small portion of the ground lamella is removed and the posterior ethmoidal cells are exenterated if they are diseased. After exenteration of the posterior ethmoids the bulge of the sphenoid sinus is visible is then opened inferomedially under

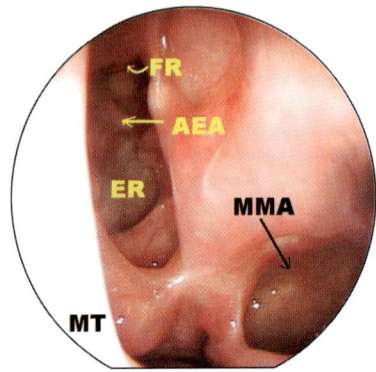

Fig. 45.24: Endoscopic view of healed post-FESS cavity. FR: Frontal recess, AEA: anterior ethmoidal artery, ER: Ethmoidal roof, MMA: Middle meatal antrostomy and MT: middle turbinate

direct vision. A measuring rod may be passed to confirm the anterior and posterior wall of the sphenoid. The interior of the sphenoid sinus will show the bulge of the optic and the carotid artery in its inferolateral aspect (Fig. 45.20).

Lateral Rhinotomy

The traditional lateral rhinotomy incision was popularized by Moure in 1902 and was first described by Michaux in 1848. It has proved to be a versatile approach for the mid-facial skeleton. Suitability of this technique is to approach the wide variety of pathologic conditions that occur in the mid-facial structures. It provides excellent exposure of the interior of the nose, the paranasal sinuses, and the nasopharynx with minimal postoperative deformity.

Incision

The classical lateral rhinotomy incision Fig. 45.25 (a) starts midway between the bridge of the nose and the medial canthus at the level of the upper border of the pupil. It then continues downwards in the nasomaxillary groove and curves medially below the lower ala towards the midline upto the base of columella as shown in the Fig. 45.25.

This can be used for medial/ partial maxillectomy. This is often used as the facial component for craniofacial resections (CFR).

The incision can be extended superiorly as a Lynch extension Fig. 45.25(c) and/or extending downwards following along the ala nasi at the collumella and dividing upper lip by splitting incision in the midline Fig. 45.25(b), to raise the flap laterally that gives excellent exposure to hard, soft palate and antero lateral wall of maxilla. The Lynch extension gives excellent exposure for the medial wall of the orbit.

The surgery is proceeded by deepening the incision upto the bone and elevating the soft tissue from the anterolateral wall of maxillary antrum. Diathermy can be used to cut the soft tissues after initial clean incision. Periosteum is then elevated followed by the clipping or ligation of the anterior ethmoidal vessels.

For lateral rhinotomy alone the nasal bone and part of the frontal process of maxilla can be chiseled and raised as a flap as is done in lateral osteotomy to retract the bone flap for good exposure as in the Figures 45.26 a and b.

Indications for Lateral Rhinotomy

- Benign tumors like inverted papilloma
- Angiofibroma confined to nasal cavity
- Medial maxillectomy as an approach
- Facial component for craniofacial approach
- Repair of septal perforation

Median Maxillectomy
(Figs 45.25 to 45.30)

This is a surgical procedure where the medial part of the maxilla is removed en bloc along with the lateral wall of the nose including the ethmoids, medial orbital rim and the lamina papyracea.

After the exposure of the anterolateral wall of the maxilla, medial orbital wall and the nasal bones by a Fergusson incision (a+b) in the Fig. 45.25. Incision (c) may be given if floor of the frontal sinus has to be opened) (Fig. 45.27).

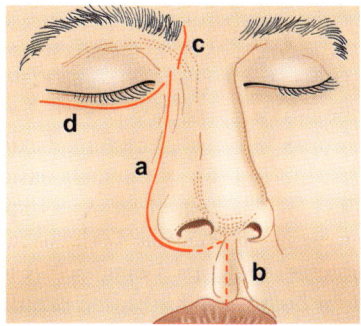

Fig. 45.25: Various incisions for maxillectomy. (a) Moore's lateral rhinotomy, (b) Lip splitting incision (Fergusson), (c) Lynch extension, (d) Weber Fergusson (connection of a, b and d)

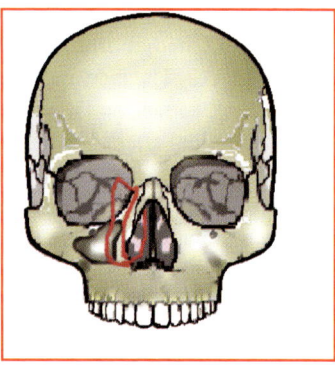

Fig. 45.28: Bony cuts for medial maxillect omy (red line)

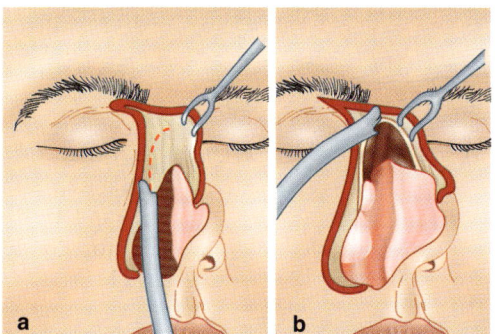

Figs 45.26a and b: (a) Exposure of nasal cavity and bony frame work. Dotted line denotes the area of bony cut to be made with osteotome. (b) Exposure of the bony cut is being made following lateral rhinotomy incision

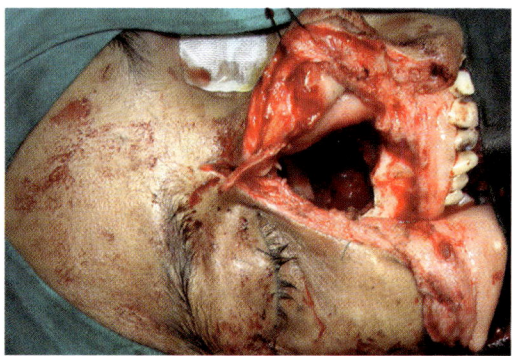

Fig. 45.29: Bony defect after resection of inverted papilloma by medial maxillectomy approach

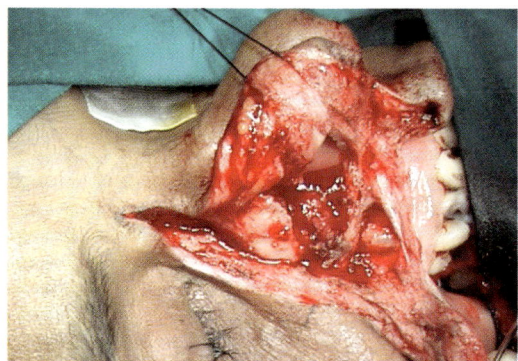

Fig. 45.27: Exposure of the tumor and bony surface of the lateral rhinotomy

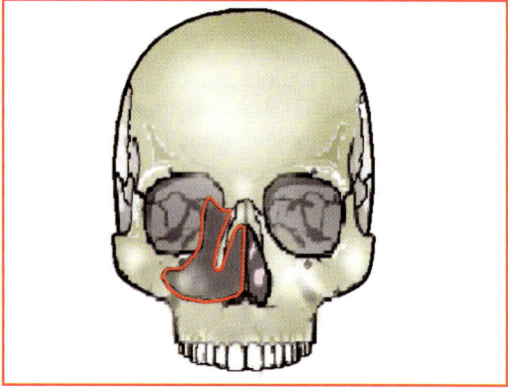

Fig. 45.30: Bony defect following medial maxillectomy. Maxilloethmoidal cavity is communicated with nasal cavity (red line)

The orbital periosteum should be carefully separated from the medial orbital wall including the lamina papyracea. The lacrimal bone is drilled exposing the sac. The lacrimal duct is transected. The anterior ethmoidal artery and the angular vein may be ligated if necessary. Bleeding can be controlled by bipolar cautery. With a fissure bur a cut is made in the anterior wall of the antrum below the orbital floor medial to the infraorbital foramen.

A 7 mm osteotome may be used after that to cut upto the frontonasal suture line which marks the cribriform plate. The next cut should be given on the frontoethmoidal suture line away from the posterior ethmoidal artery, to prevent damage to the optic nerve. The dissection is continued downwards to completely excise the lateral wall of the nose by giving a cut in the lateral wall of inferior meatus along the floor of the nasal cavity (Figs 45.28 and 45.29).

The lateral wall of the nose can be better removed with the Mayo's scissors that allows enbloc resection of the specimen. Sphenoid and remnant of the posterior ethmoids should be inspected for any residual tumor and should be completely excised (Figs 45.29 and 45.30).

Indications for Medial Maxillectomy

- Inverted papilloma
- Columnar cell papilloma
- Angiofibroma with extension to maxillary sinus
- Other benign tumors
- Extensive fungal sinusitis of the maxilloethmoidal complex with orbital complications.
- Early malignancy confined to lateral wall of the nose especially adenocarcinoma.

TOTAL MAXILLECTOMY
(Figs 45.32 To 45.37)

Incision

Weber-Fergusson's incision as shown in the Fig. 45.31. The mucosal incision is given after the splitting of the upper lip and is continued sub-labially till the tuberosity of the maxilla This provides a wide exposure to the affected maxilla, orbit and the incision can be extended laterally to expose the infratemporal fossa.

Alterative incision is midfacial degloving approach which consists of a sublabial incision along with complete transfixation incision of the nasal septum and the incision is extended laterally like an internal rhinoplasty approach. The entire midface on both the sides can be exposed. The limitations are poor exposure to the frontal sinus, orbit and beyond zygomatic arch and infratemporal fossa.

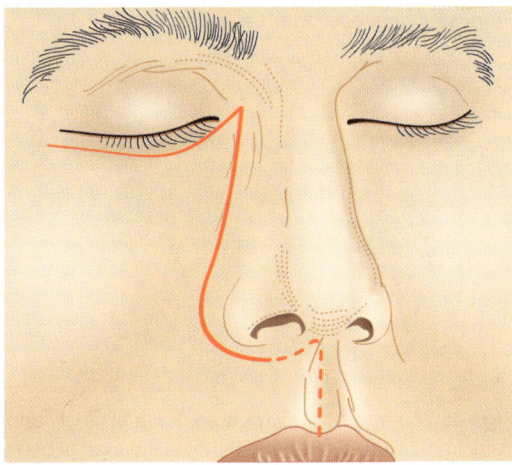

Fig. 45.31: Weber-Fergusson's incision for total maxillectomy (red line)

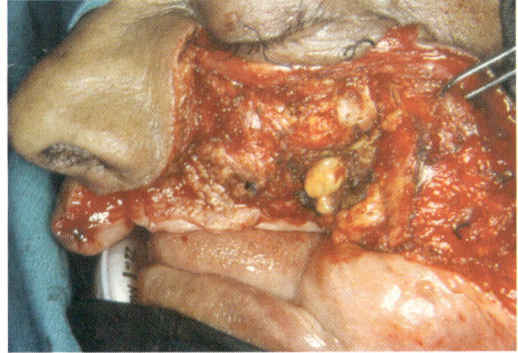

Fig. 45.32: Exposure after elevation of the plap following Weber-Fergusson's incision

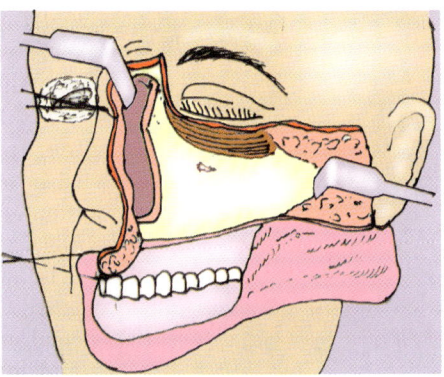

Fig. 45.33: Exposure after elevation of the flap following Weber-Fergusson's incision (diagrammatic)

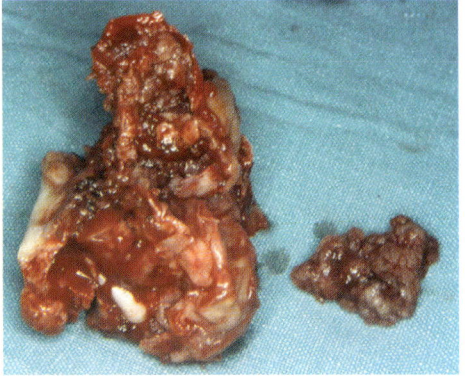

Fig. 45.36: Maxillectomy specimen

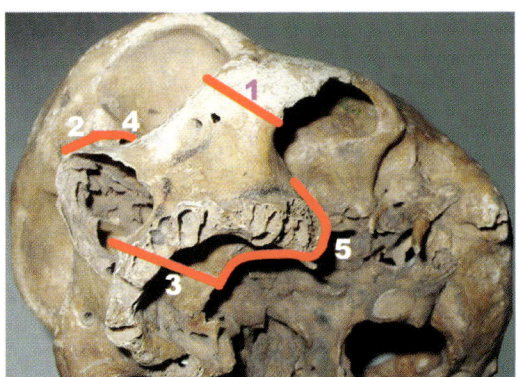

Fig. 45.34: Various bony cuts being made for total maxillectomy as shown in the red line as labelled

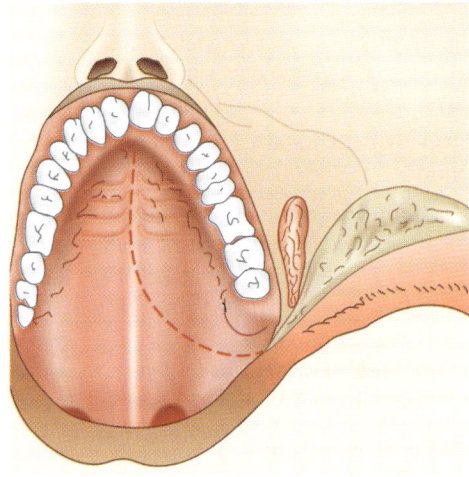

Fig. 45.37: Palatal osteotomy

After the exposure of the maxilla and the floor of the orbit by elevating the periosteum on affected side, the bony suture lines are marked to make the following bony cuts:

1. *Zygoma from the infraorbital fissure using a giggle's saw or osteotome.*
2. *Nasofrontal process of the maxilla using an osteotome.*
3. *Midline of the palate after removing the first incisor.*

This can be done by making a cut at the midpoint between the hard and the soft palate and by passing a right angles artery forceps to bring out an end of the giggle saw to facilitate the cut along

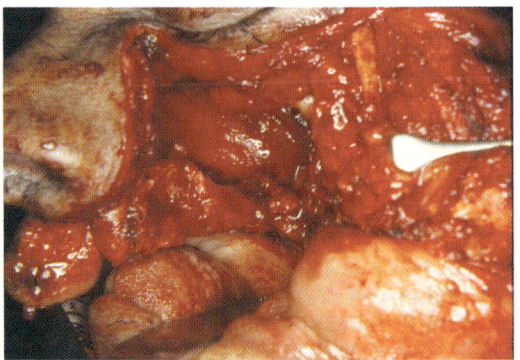

Fig. 45.35: Showing post- resection deformity and resected specimen

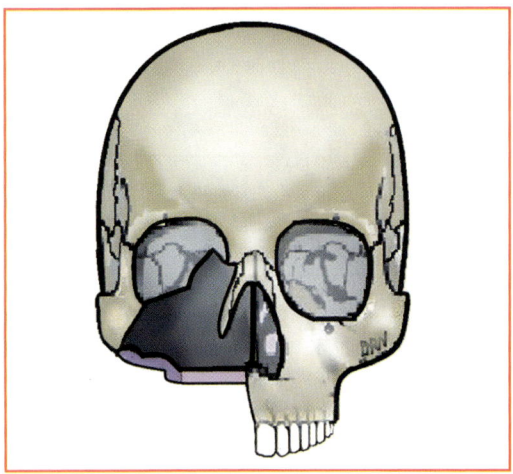

Fig. 45.38: Defect following total maxillectomy on the right side

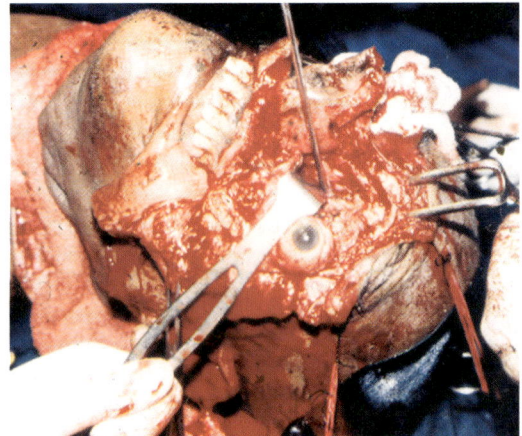

Fig. 45.39: Facio-cranial approach (inferior approach for CFR)

the floor of the nasal cavity lateral to the nasal septum.

4. *Along the plane of anterior and posterior ethmoidal artery* and carried out posteriorly till the sphenoid. This cut is made at the level of the cribriform plate to include the ethmoid in the resection.

5. *Pterygomaxillary cut* to detach the maxilla from the pterygoid plates. Soft palate can be separated from the hard palate using diathermy upto the maxillary tuberosity. This facilitates better exposure of the attachment of the pterygoid plates to the maxilla.

Orbital exenteration may be required if tumor involves the orbital periosteum and the periorbital fat.

Indications for Total Maxillectomy

1. T2 or T3 tumors of the maxilla without ethmoidal involvement.
2. Radioresidual tumors of the maxilla.

Craniofacial Resection

This surgery is done along with a total maxillectomy/medial maxillectomy to include the cribriform plate of the ethmoid and the ethmoidal

complex by doing a craniotomy or through inferior approach (Fig. 45.39).

The craniotomy may be performed by a bi-coronal incision or by a midline incision extended upwards from that of lateral rhinotomy (Fig. 45.40).

The facial incision is same as that for lateral rhinotomy with Lynch extension for ethmoidal tumors without lateral extension to the maxillary sinus. A Weber-Fergusson incision is given for tumor involving the maxilloethmoidal complex with significant involvement of the maxillary sinus (T3 and T4 lesions). Bony cuts are done for medial maxillectomy/total maxillectomy as described earlier depending on the tumor extent. At his stage a craniotomy is performed as follows.

After the bicoronal incision, the galleal flap is created to reconstruct the cranial defect. The craniotomy is done by doing multiple burr holes. A shield or square shaped frontal bone is removed to expose the cranium. Care is taken not to injure the dura and the saggital sinus. The dura is lifted up from the anterior cranial floor including the cribriform plate upto the level of the optic foramen. It can be carried out with careful bipolar cautery and continuous suction irrigation to

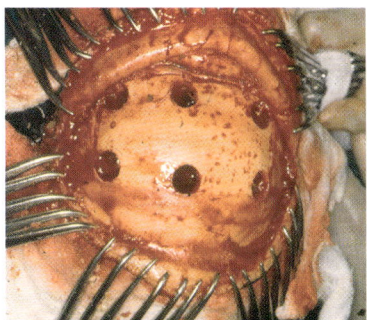

Fig. 45.40: Frontal craniotomy being performed by doing multiple burr holes after bicoronal flap has been elevated anteriorly

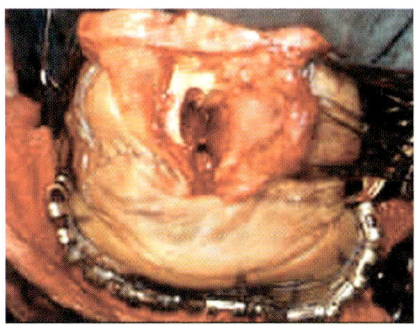

Fig. 45.42: Cranial defect after removal of the specimen following anterior craniofacial resection

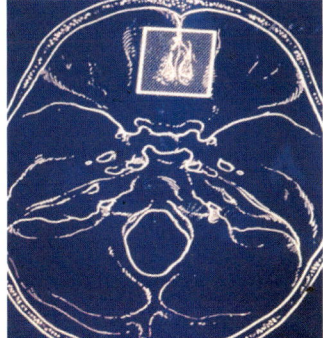

Fig. 45.41: Area of resection of cranial bone including cribriform plate of ethmoid as shown in dotted area

prevent thermal damage. The frontal lobe is then retracted gently and the bony cuts are made through the fovea on each side and then through the posterior border of the cribriform plate. Thus a rectangular window is made as shown in the Fig. 45.42. Then the tumor mass is resected enblock consisting of the cranial bone including the cribriform plate the attached superior, middle and inferior turbinates along with medial maxilla (medial maxillectomy)/total maxillectomy. The dural defect is closed by duroplasty using fascia lata. The wound is closed in layers.

Pharynx and Esophagus

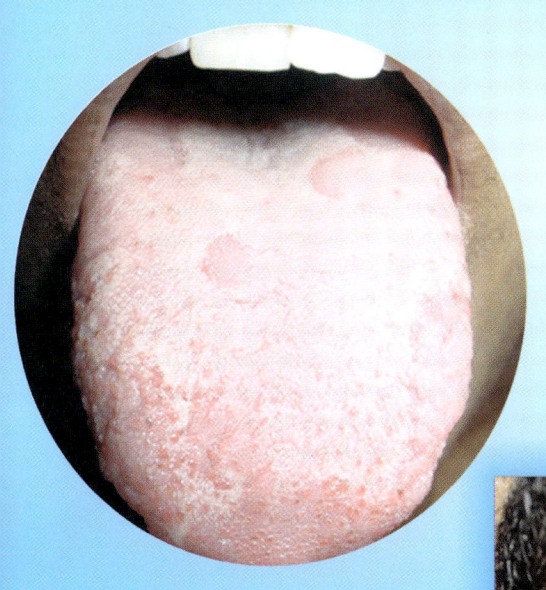

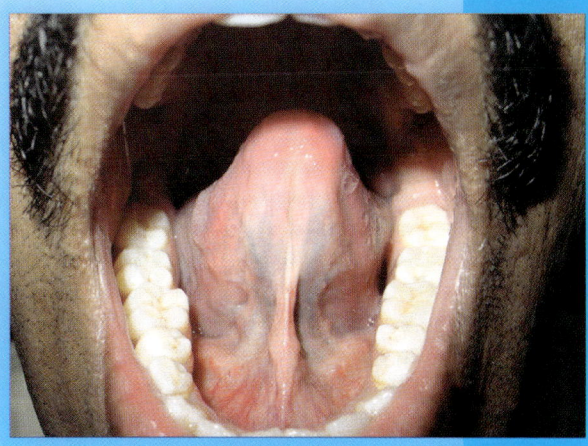

46

Anatomy of Oral Cavity and Pharynx

EMBRYOLOGY

The most typical feature of the head and neck is that it is formed by the branchial or pharyngeal arches. These appear in the 4th and 5th weeks of development of the embryo.

The branchial apparatus consists of bars of mesenchymal tissue lined by ectoderm outside and endoderm inside. The arches are separated by deep clefts known as branchial or pharyngeal clefts on its outer aspect. Along with these, pharyngeal pouches also develop in the most cranial part of foregut. Thus branchial apparatus has clefts in between the arches externally and pouches internally. The pharyngeal arches also contribute in the formation of the face (Fig. 46.1).

Pharyngeal Arches and their Derivatives

First Arch (Mandibular Arch)

Bone

- Incus
- Malleus
- Premaxilla, maxilla
- Part of temporal bone
- Sphenomandibular ligament

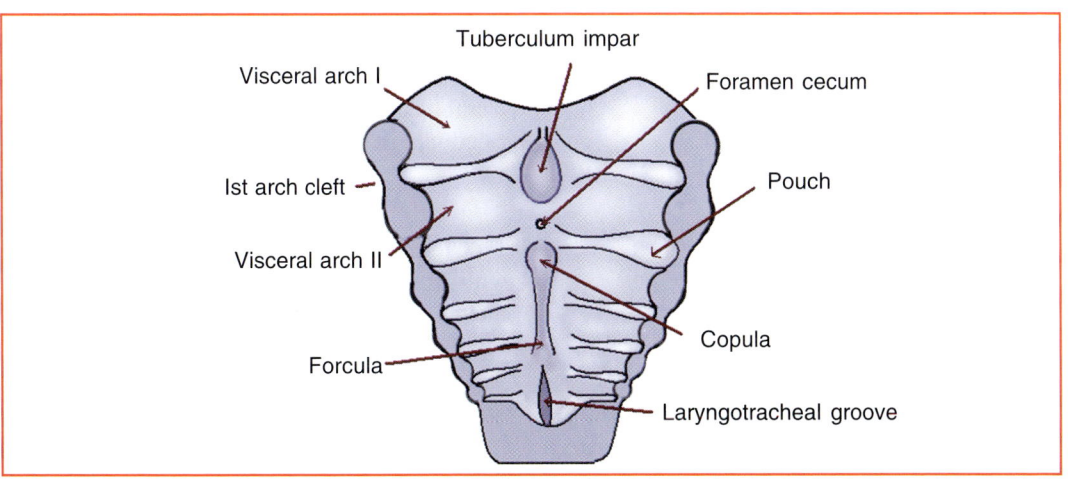

Fig. 46.1: Branchial apparatus with its various arches, clefts and pouches

Muscles

- Muscles of mastication—Masseter, temporalis, medial and lateral pterygoids
- Anterior belly of digastric
- Myelohyoid
- Tensor tympani
- Tensor palatini

Nerve

- Mandibular branch of trigeminal nerve

Second Arch
(Hyoid Arch- Reichert's Cartilage)

Bone

- Stapes
- Styloid process of temporal bone
- Stylohyoid ligament
- Hyoid bone – lesser horn and upper part of body of hyoid

Muscles

- Stapedius
- Posterior belly of digastric
- Stylohyoid
- Auricular muscles
- Muscles of facial expression

Nerve

- Facial nerve

Third Arch

Bone

- Hyoid bone (Greater horn and lower part of hyoid body)

Muscle

- Stylopharyngeus

Nerve

- Glossopharyngeal nerve

Fourth and Sixth Arches

Fuse to form the cartilages of the larynx i.e., thyroid, cricoid, arytenoid, cuneiform and corniculate.

Fourth Arch

Muscles

- Cricothyroid
- Levator palatine
- Constrictors of the pharynx

Nerve

- Superior laryngeal branch to pharyngeal plexus (vagus nerve)

Sixth Arch

- Muscles – Intrinsic muscles of larynx
- Nerve – Recurrent laryngeal branch of vagus nerve.

Pharyngeal Pouches

Five pairs – Each with a ventral and dorsal section

1st Pouch – Develops into external auditory meatus, middle ear cavity, eustachian tube.

2nd Pouch – Develops into:

(a) Partly Eustachian tube
(b) Palatine tonsils
(c) Nasopharyngeal tonsil
(d) Lingual tonsil

3rd Pouch

(a) Thymus gland
(b) Inferior parathyroid gland

4th Pouch: Superior parathyroid gland

5th Pouch: Ultimobranchial body (gives rise to parafollicular 'C' cells of parathyroid which secrete calcitonin in the adult).

Pharyngeal Clefts

1st Cleft: External auditory meatus. It also, along with 1st pharyngeal pouch forms the tympanic membrane.

2nd, 3rd, 4th Clefts: Form a temporary cavity called the cervical sinus. This sinus usually disappears completely. If 2nd arch fails to fuse then this sinus is seen persisting as branchial fistula.

Development of Oral Cavity

The mouth or the oral cavity is derived partly from the stomodeum and partly from the foregut. Hence its epithelial lining is partly ectodermal and partly endodermal. The primitive pharynx is derived from the cranial part of the foregut. Both oral cavity and primitive pharynx are separated by a membrane called buccopharyngeal membrane which disappears later.

A series of mesodermal thickening bronchial arches also appears in the wall of the cranial most part of the foregut (Fig. 46.1). The first arch and the second arch mainly contributes to the structures of the mouth and oral cavity.

In the region of the floor of the mouth the mandibular process takes part in the formation of the lower lip, lower jaw and tongue.

The tongue develops in relation to the pharyngeal arches in the floor of the developing mouth. The medial most part of the mandibular arches proliferates to form two lingual swellings.

The lingual swellings are partially separated from each other by another swelling that appears in the midline known as ***tuberculum impar.*** Immediately behind the tuberculum impar, the epithelium proliferates to form the ***thyroglossal duct*** from which the thyroid gland develops. The site of this downgrowth is called ***foramen cecum***.

Another midline swelling is seen in relation to the medial end of second, third and fourth arches. This is called ***hypobranchial eminence***. The anterior two thirds of the tongue is formed by the fusion of tuberculum impar and the two lingual swellings. The posterior one third of the tongue is formed from the cranial part of the hypobranchial eminence. This explains the dual nerve supply of the tongue.

Development of Pharynx

After the establishment of the branchial apparatus and its various derivatives, the primitive pharynx is converted into the definitive pharynx. At the cephalic end, the ventral wall of the pharynx communicates with the stomodeum after the rupture of the buccopharyngeal membrane.

The pharynx then divides into the nasal and the oral cavity by the development of the permanent palate. At the caudal end, the ventral wall of the definitive pharynx communicates with the laryngeotracheal tube through furculla. Thus the pharynx is now subdivided into three parts – nasal, oral and laryngeal.

ANATOMY OF THE ORAL CAVITY

The cavity of the mouth is divided into vestibule and oral cavity proper (Fig. 46.2). The vestibule or labial cavity lies between the lips, cheeks, gums and the teeth. The upper and lower lip together forms the anterior most part of the vestibule. The skin and mucous membrane becomes continuous with each other at the free margin of the lip. The muscular layer constitutes to the chief bulk of the lip and mainly formed by the orbicularis oris. In each lip there is an arterial arc formed by the labial branch of the facial artery. The lymph vessels of the lower lip join the submental and submandibular lymph node. Upper lip drains into the submandibular and superficial parotid group of lymph nodes.

The oral cavity (buccal cavity) proper is bounded by the dental arches consisting of teeth,

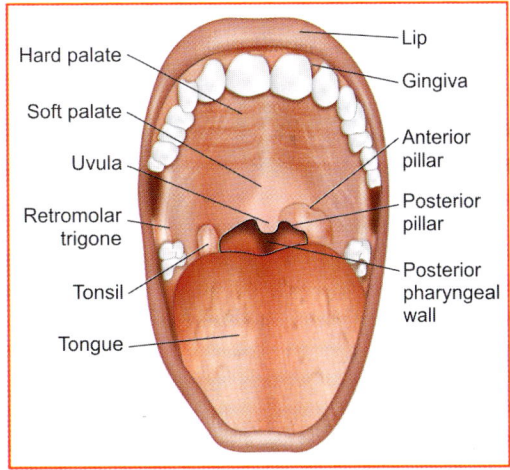

Fig. 46.2: Showing different parts of the oral cavity

gums and alveolar process. The oral cavity communicates posteriorly to the oropharynx through the oropharyngeal isthmus at the level of palatoglossal arch. The roof of the buccal cavity is formed by hard palate and anterior part of the soft palate.

The floor is formed by the dorsal surface of the anterior two thirds of the tongue and by the mucous membrane which connects the tongue with the inner surface of the mandible. It is into the mouth proper that the submandibular duct and the sublingual duct open. The important structures found in the floor of the mouth are the sublingual fold and the frenulum linguae. At the sides of the frenulum, the opening of the submandibular duct on the summit of the sublingual papilla is seen (Fig. 46.3).

Blood Supply

Mouth is supplied by the branches from the facial artery, inferior alveolar artery, maxillary artery, infraorbital and posterosuperior alveolar arteries.

Lymphatic Supply

- Buccal aspect of both upper and lower gum along with deeper tissues of the cheek drain into the submandibular node.
- The inner aspects of the gum of the upper

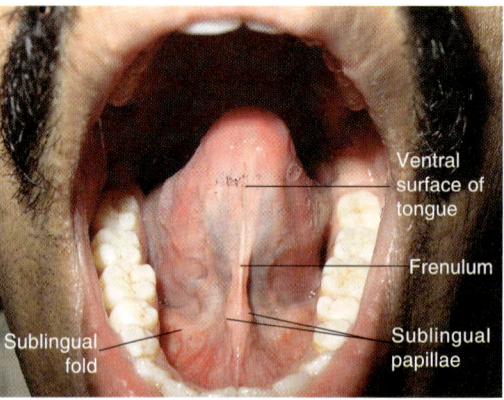

Ventral surface of tongue

Frenulum

Sublingual fold

Sublingual papillae

Fig. 46.3: Showing different parts of the floor of the oral cavity

jaw along with the hard and soft palate drain into the upper deep cervical nodes. Some vessels may drain into the retropharyngeal nodes.
- Gums of the lower incisor drain into the submandibular lymph nodes.

Nerve Supply

- From the maxillary and mandibular nerve.

Palate

The palate forms the roof of the mouth. The anterior 2/3rd is rigid known as the hard palate formed by the palatine process of the maxillary bone. The posterior 1/3rd constitute the soft palate which is movable fibromuscular partition attached to the posterior margin of the hard palate and the side wall of the pharynx.

The soft palate consists of a dense fibrous framework called the palatine aponeurosis formed by the expanded tendon of the tensor palati muscle. To this aponeurosis, other palatine muscles are attached. Inferior surface and posterior margin, a variable part of the superior surface are covered with stratified squamous epithelium. Rest of the superior surface is covered by pseudostratified ciliated columnar epithelium.

Laterally, the soft palate blends with the pharyngeal wall, passing downward from the palate are the palatoglossal fold formed by the palatoglossus muscle, posterior one is the palatopharyngeal fold formed by the palatopharyngeal muscle. The soft palate is attached to the skull base by the tensor palati and the levator palatini muscle. Posteriorly, the soft palate has a free margin. At the midline the posterior margin goes backwards and downwards as a rounded projection called uvula formed by musculus uvulae. The soft palate helps in swallowing, breathing and phonation by regulating the nasopharyngeal and oropharyngeal isthmus.

Palate receives blood supply from the branches of ascending palatine of the facial, lesser palatine from the maxillary, and a palatine branch from the ascending pharyngeal artery.

Venous drainage runs mainly into the tonsillar and the pterygoid plexus and from there to the anterior facial vein and then to the deep facial vein.

Nerve Supply

All the muscles of the palate are supplied by the cranial part of the accessory of the pharyngeal plexus where as, tensor palatini is from the mandibular nerve. Sensory supply is derived from the lesser palatine branches of the sphenopalatine ganglion and from the branches of the glossopharyngeal nerve.

Soft palate is a movable muscular fold, suspended from the posterior border of hard palate. It separates the nasopharynx from the oral cavity and oropharynx.

It has two surfaces and two borders namely.

- **Anterior surface** which is concave marked by median raphe. Main bulk is due to mucous glands.
- **Posterior surface** convex, is continuous superiorly with the floor of the nasal cavity.
- **Superior border** attached to the posterior border of hard palate.
- **Inferior border** free and bounds the pharyngeal isthmus.

From the middle hangs the uvula. On each side palatoglossus and palatopharyngeal arches and its muscles are present.

Muscles of Soft Palate

- Tensor palati
- Levator palati
- Palatoglossus
- Palatopharyngeus

Blood Supply

- Greater palatine branch of maxillary artery
- Ascending palatine branch of facial artery
- Palatine branch of ascending pharyngeal arteries

Venous Drainage

- Veins pass into the pterygoid and tonsillar plexus of veins

Lymphatic Drainage

- Drains into the upper deep cervical and retropharyngeal lymph nodes

Nerve Supply

- *Motor:* All muscles are supplied by pharyngeal plexus except tensor palati which is supplied by the mandibular nerve.
- *Sensory:* Middle and posterior palatine nerves
- *Secretomotor:* Derived from superior salivary nucleus through the greater petrosal nerve.

Gums and Teeth

Gums are composed of dense fibrous tissue covered with smooth and vascular mucous membrane. They are attached to the alveolar margin of the jaw and closely embraced by the neck of the teeth. In the adult there are 16 teeth in each jaw. From the median plane backward on each side there are 2 incisors, 1 canine, 2 premolars and 3 molars. The teeth are normally arranged in each jaw to form an arched curve without projection inwards or outwards of individual teeth. Arc formed by the upper teeth is elliptical where as arc in the lower is parabolic.

Nerve supply of the upper teeth is by the alveolar branch of the maxillary nerve and that of the lower jaw is by inferior alveolar branch of the mandibular nerve.

Tongue

Tongue is a muscular organ situated in the floor of the mouth and in the anterior wall of the pharynx. Its main functions are mastication, deglutition, speech, touch and taste. It has a free portion called mobile part and main mass or body with a free rounded body as far back as last molar teeth. It is attached by muscle to the hyoid bone below, mandible in front, styloid process posterolaterally, palate above and also mucous membrane attachment to the floor of the mouth, lateral wall of the pharynx and epiglottis.

The dorsum of the tongue is subdivided by a V – shaped groove, i.e. sulcus terminalis into the anterior palatine part (anterior two third) and posterior pharyngeal part (posterior one third/ **base of tongue**). Foramen cecum lies in the apex of sulcus terminalis, where as circum-vallate papillae are found anterior to it.

Anterior portion of the tongue is developed from the 1st pharyngeal arch and is supplied by the lingual nerve and the chorda tympani nerve. Pharyngeal portion is derived from the 2nd and 3rd pharyngeal arch and is supplied by the glossopharyngeal and branch from superior laryngeal nerve.

Structure of the Tongue

The tongue consists of:

  (a) Mucous membrane
  (b) Mucous glands
  (c) Lymphoid tissue
  (d) Fat
  (e) Striated muscle fibers
  (f) Fibrous tissue

A median connective tissue septum divides tongue into right and left half. Mucous membrane is covered by stratified squamous epithelium. In the healthy individuals, the oral part of mucous membrane is pink and studded with numerous small projections known as papillae. The posterior part is smoother and shows nodular elevations due to underlying lymphoid nodules and mucous glands. The posterior part is also covered by thin whitish fur. From base of the tongue, the mucous membrane passes backwards to the epiglottis forming glossoepiglottic fold and also passes laterally to form pharyngoepiglottic fold. Between these two folds there is a depression called the vallecula.

Papillae

They are projections consisting of connective tissue pore covered with stratified squamous epithelium. There are three types of papillae:

  • Circumvallate papillae
  • Fungiform papillae
  • Filiform papillae

    – Circumvallate papillae are arranged in a row parallel to and in front of sulcus terminalis. These papillae are surrounded by a circular groove.

    – Fungiform papillae are more globular in shape. They are numerous near the tip and the margin of the tongue. These papillae have rich blood supply and look bright red because of the vascularity.

    – Filliform papillae are prevalent on the dorsum of the tongue arranged in rows parallel to the sulcus terminalis.

Taste Buds

Associated with the papillae are the microscopic taste buds, each of which is somewhat flask shaped with a wide base and a short narrow neck opening at the taste pore. Each bud has two kinds of cells: supporting and neuroepithelial taste cells.

Lingual Tonsils

Numerous lymphoid tissue or lingual tonsils are found in the posterior part of the tongue along with various serous and mucous glands.

Muscles

Muscles of the tongue are paired and grouped into extrinsic and intrinsic. Main extrinsic muscles on each side are: genioglossus, hyoglossus, and styloglossus.

Intrinsic muscles are arranged in four groups:

  • Superior longitudinal
  • Inferior longitudinal
  • Transverse
  • Vertical

Arteries and Veins

Major blood supply to the tongue is derived from the lingual artery. This artery runs forward immediately above the hyoid bone passing deep to the hyoglossus and continued to the tip as profunda artery. Veins from the tongue drain into the internal jugular vein.

Lymphatic Drainage

The tongue is drained by lymph vessels which may be divided into 4 groups:

- Apical vessel
- Marginal vessel
- Central vessel
- Basal vessel
- *Apical vessels:* Lymphatic vessels from the tip of the tongue drain into submental and supraomohyoid glands.
- *Marginal vessels:* They drain from the side of the tongue to submandibular and then to deep cervical group of lymph nodes. Many of these vessels pass down to the outer surface of the hyoglossus muscle. There may be lymph nodes lying on the hyoglossus known as lingual glands.
- *Central vessels:* These are vessels draining the tongue on either side of the median raphe and then drain to both sides of the deep cervical glands.
  - *Basal vessels:* These vessels drain from the posterior part of the tongue and pass freely from one side of the tongue to the other before draining into deep cervical group of lymph nodes.

Nerve Supply

- *Motor: All the muscles of the tongue except palatoglossus are supplied by hypoglossal nerve.*
- *General sensation:* Lingual nerve
- The taste sensation is carried by Chorda tympani from the anterior 2/3rd and by the glossopharyngeal nerve from the posterior 1/3rd.

ANATOMY OF PHARYNX

Pharynx is a wide fibromuscular membranous tube and is about 12 cm in length extending from the base of the skull to the lower border of the cricoid cartilage. It is the upper part of the respiratory and digestive tract and is a crossroad of the air and the food passages (Fig. 46.4). Each major crossroad may be closed by muscular sphincter.

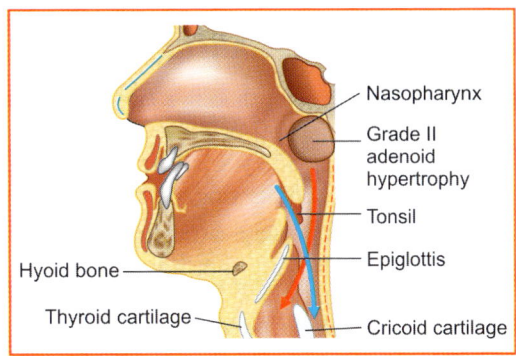

Fig. 46.4: Pharyngeal crossway of the air and food passage (red and blue arrow)

Routes of Communication

1. Nasal cavity through the posterior nasal aperture (choana)
2. Mouth through the oropharyngeal isthmus
3. Middle ear through the Eustachian tube
4. Larynx and tracheobranchial tree through the Glottis
5. Esophagus through the upper esophageal sphincter (Cricopharynx)

Boundaries of The Pharynx

Superiorly: Base of skull including posterior part of body of sphenoid and basilar part of occipital bone.

Inferiorly: Level of 6th cervical vertebrae or lower border of cricoid cartilage where it is continuous with the esophagus.

Posteriorly: Pharynx glides freely on the prevertebral fascia, which separates it from the cervical spine.

Anteriorly: Communicates with nasal cavity, oral cavity and larynx.

Divisions of Pharynx (Fig. 46.5)

Depending on its site, the pharynx can be divided into the following.

1. Nasopharynx (Postnasal space)
2. Oropharynx
3. Laryngopharynx (Hypopharynx).

NASOPHARYNX

This is situated behind the nose and above the lower border of the soft palate and Passavant's ridge. It is respiratory in function and is characterized by the following.

- It is lined by pseudostratified columnar ciliated epithelium (respiratory epithelium)
- The walls are rigid and non–collapsible
- It opens anteriorly into the nasal fossae bounded above by the base of skull (anteroinferior surface of the body of sphenoid bone and basilar part of the occipital bone).
- Below it is limited by the soft palate.
- Inferiorly it communicates with the oropharynx at the nasopharyngeal isthmus (Figs 46.4 and 46.5) which is bounded by:
  - The lower border of soft palate
  - The posterior wall of pharynx (Passavant's muscle).

Lateral Wall Presents

- Pharyngeal opening of the auditory (Eustachian) tube
- Tubal elevation (Torus tubaris) bounds the tubal opening
- Salpingopharyngeal fold of the mucous membrane running downwards from the posterior margin of tubal elevation
- Another fold passes from the anterior edge of the tubal opening onto upper surface of soft palate cased by levator palati muscle
- Behind the tubal elevation lies the pharyngeal recess (Fossa of Rosenmüller)

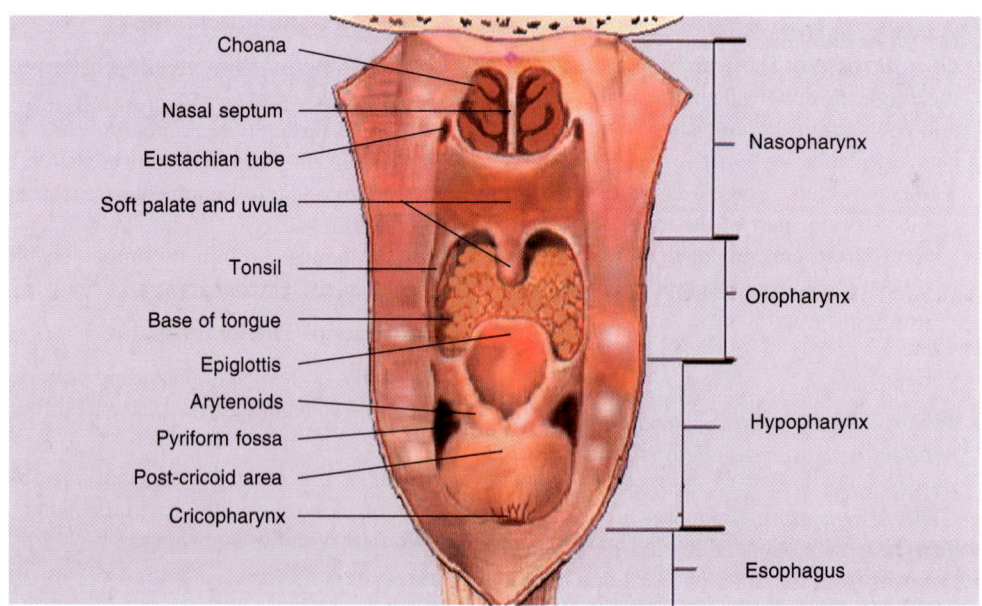

Choana
Nasal septum
Eustachian tube
Soft palate and uvula
Tonsil
Base of tongue
Epiglottis
Arytenoids
Pyriform fossa
Post-cricoid area
Cricopharynx

Nasopharynx
Oropharynx
Hypopharynx
Esophagus

Fig. 46.5: Showing the extent of the pharynx and its divisions

Roof and Posterior wall

Forms a continuous slope opposite the posterior part of body of sphenoid, basiocciput and anterior arch of atlas. Under the mucous membrane, opposite to basiocciput, there is a collection of lymphoid tissue called the nasopharyngeal tonsil or the adenoids. When pathologically enlarged it can cause nasal and tubal obstruction.

Nasopharyngeal isthmus leads the nasopharynx into oropharynx. It is closed during swallowing by using soft palate and contraction of the palatopharyngeal sphincter.

Fossa of Rosenmuller (Pharyngeal recess)

This is the commonest site of origin for nasopharyngeal cancer. This is a deep recess in the region of the base-skull and is not entirely visible even on a nasopharyngoscopy (Fig. 46.6).

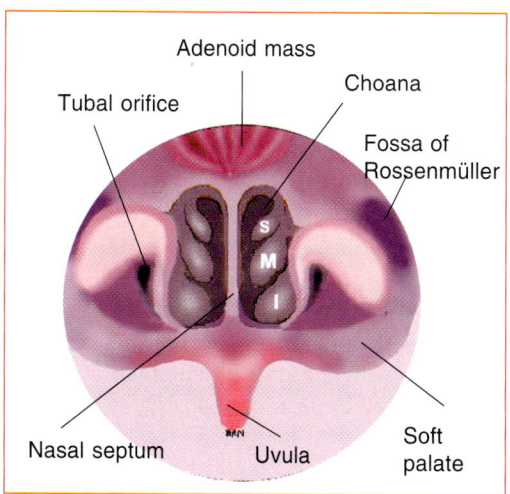

Fig. 46.6: Posterior rhinoscopic view showing the structures of the nasopharynx

Boundaries

Anteriorly: Eustachian tube and levator palati muscle

Posteriorly: Posterior pharyngeal wall mucosa overlying the pharyngobasilar fascia and retropharyngeal space containing lymph nodes of Rouvier.

Medially: Nasopharyngeal cavity

Superiorly: Base of the skull till the foramen lacerum and floor of the carotid canal

Postero-lateral (apex): Carotid canal opening and petrous bone apex posteriorly (foramen ovale and spinosum laterally)

Laterally : Tensor palatini muscle and mandibular nerve in the prestyloid compartment of parapharyngeal space.

Oropharynx (Figs 46.5 and 46.7)

This is the middle part of the pharynx. It extends from the lower edge of the soft palate to the tip of the epiglottis or to the laryngeal inlet.

Boundaries

Superior Wall

- Formed by inferior surface of soft palate and uvula
- It communicates with the nasopharynx through the nasopharyngeal isthmus

Anteriorly the superior wall is continuous with the oral cavity through the oropharyngeal isthmus. It is demarcated from oral cavity by uvula, anterior pillar and circumvalate papillae on each side.

Posterior wall: This is related to:

- The body of axis (2nd cervical vertebra)
- Upper part of 3rd cervical vertebra.

Lateral wall presents palatine tonsil in the tonsillar fossa, which lies between the palatoglossal and the palatopharyngeal muscles forming the anterior and the posterior pillars respectively. The supratonsillar fossa is triangular area of the mucous membrane that lies above the tonsil in the region of the angle between the anterior and posterior pillars. The tonsil in this area is separated from the superior constrictor muscle by loose areolar tissue and the area is less vascular. Hence this area is used as a cleavage plane for tonsillectomy.

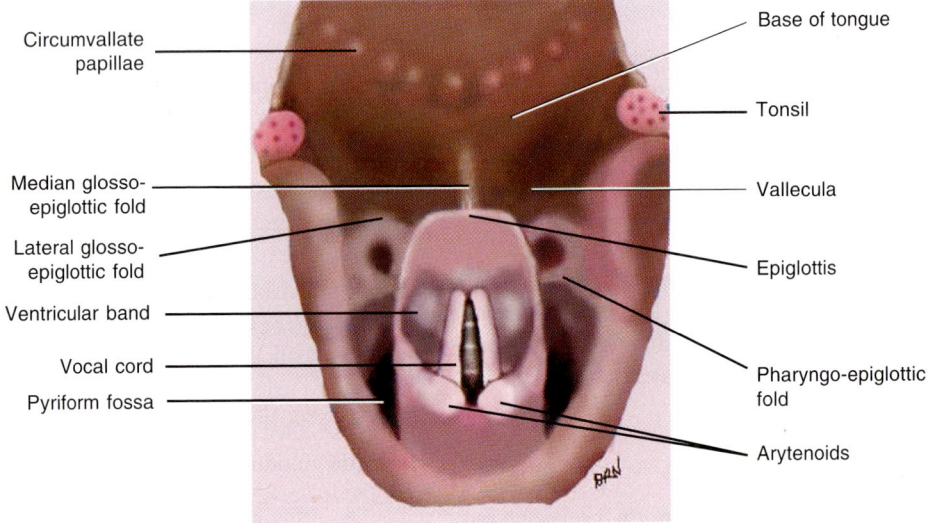

Fig. 46.7: Showing parts of the larynx, oropharynx and laryngopharynx

Inferiorly is the glossoepiglottic area, which is formed by the posterior 1/3rd of tongue (base of the tongue) till the circumvallate papillae. At the lower part of this wall, the paired valleculae are present.

The valleculae are separated from each other in the midline by the median glossoepiglottic fold passing from base of the tongue to anterior or lingual surfaces of epiglottis.

Laterally, each vallecula is bounded by the lateral glossoepiglottic fold, which lies in relation to the tonsillolingual sulcus.

The wall of the oropharynx is formed mainly by the superior constrictor, the palatoglossus and the palatopharyngeus muscles. The tonsillopharyngeus muscle refers to fibers of the lateral part of the palatopharyngeus, which is attached to the capsule of the tonsil at the junction of the upper and the lower lobes.

The oropharynx is lined by non-keratinizing stratified sqamous epithelium.

Hypopharynx

- It lies behind the larynx and partly to each side where it forms the pyriform fossa.

- It is continuous above with the oropharynx and below with the esophagus at the lower border of the cricoid cartilage through the cricopharyngeal sphincter.
- It extends from the upper border of epiglottis to the lower border of cricoid cartilage.

Posterior wall: 3rd, 4th, 5th and 6th cervical vertebrae

Anterior wall: Lies in the larynx with its oblique inlet. The inlet is bounded anteriorly and superiorly by the upper part of epiglottis. Posteriorly, by the elevations of arytenoid cartilage and laterally by the aryepiglottic fold.

It is divided into three anatomic sites:

- The pyriform sinus (fossa)
- The postcricoid area
- Posterior pharyngeal wall

Pyriform sinus (fossa): Extends from the pharyngoepiglottic fold to the upper end of esophagus. It is bounded laterally by the mucosa covering the thyrohyoid membrane and thyroid cartilage and medially by the surface of aryepiglottic fold and mucosa of arytenoid and cricoid cartilages.

Postcricoid area: Extends from the level of the arytenoid cartilages and the connecting folds to the inferior border of the cricoid cartilage.

Posterior pharyngeal wall*:* Extends from the level of the floor of the vallecula to the inferior level of the cricoarytenoid joints.

Deep to the mucous membrane of the lateral wall of the pyriform fossa lies the internal branch of superior laryngeal nerve (accessible for local anesthesia).

STRUCTURE OF PHARYNX

Pharyngeal wall consists of layers – from inwards to outwards:

- Mucous membrane
- Pharyngobasilar fascia
- Muscle layer
- Buccopharyngeal fascia

1. MUCOUS MEMBRANE

This is continuous with mucous membrane of the:

- Eustachian tubes
- Nasal fossae
- Mouth
- Larynx
- Esophagus

Nasopharynx is lined by pseudostratified columnar ciliated epithelium upto the level of the lower border of soft palate.
Oropharynx and hypopharynx are lined by non-keratinizing stratified squamous epithelium.

Between nasopharynx and oropharynx, it is lined by stratified columnar and transitional epithelium.

Subepithelial lymphoid tissue of pharynx is scattered collections of lymphoid tissue (Waldeyer's ring) and is widely distributed beneath the pharyngeal mucosa and are called tonsils. They have efferent lymph vessels but no afferent vessels.

Waldeyer's ring – Consists of (Fig. 46.8)

1. ***Palatine tonsil***: situated between the anterior and posterior pillars of fauces on each side of the oropharynx.

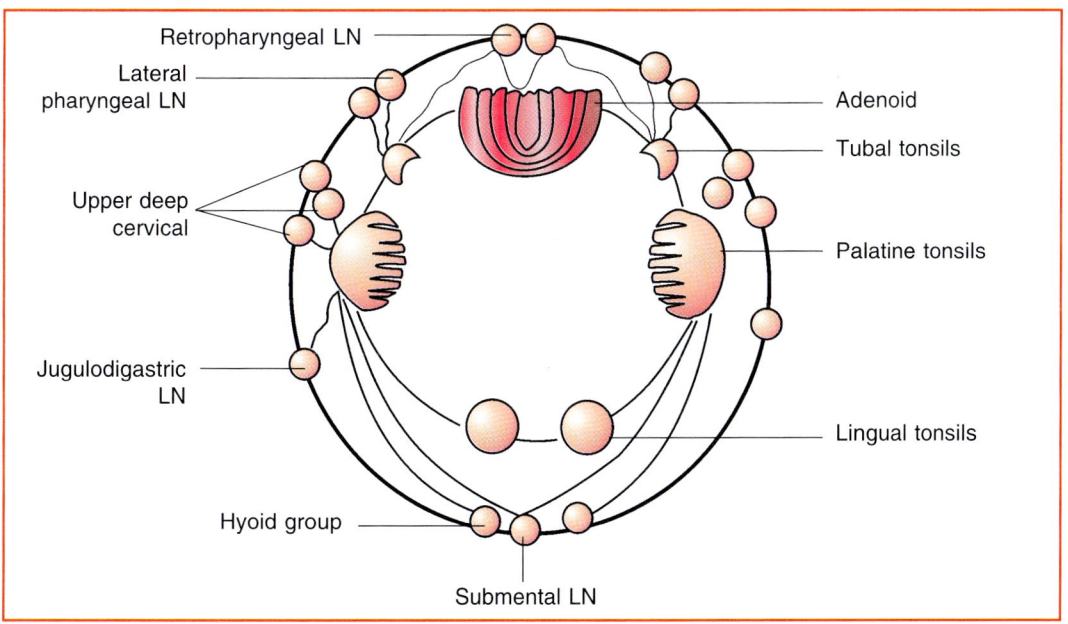

Fig. 46.8: Showing the Waldeyer's ring and its constituents

2. *Nasopharyngeal tonsil (Adenoid):* lies at the junction of roof and upper part of the posterior wall of the nasopharynx in the midline.
3. *Lingual tonsils*: clothes upper surface of the base of tongue (posterior 1/3rd of tongue), one on either sides. They are continuous with the lower ends of palatine tonsils.
4. *Tubal tonsils*: Lie in the fossa of Rosenmüller, behind the pharyngeal opening of eustachian tube.
5. *Lateral pharyngeal bands*: Descend from tubal tonsil, behind the posterior facial pillars.
6. *Discrete nodules*: Occur in the subepithelial layer of posterior pharyngeal wall.

Functions of Waldeyer's Ring

1. Formation of lymphocytes
2. Body immunity and antibody formation especially in early years of life.
3. Protection to the lower respiratory tract by guarding the entry to air passage.
4. Formation of plasma cells
5. Continuous monitoring of different varieties of infective bacteria in incoming air and food and warns the body accordingly.

2. PHARYNGOBASILAR FASCIA

It is a fibrous sheet which lies between the mucous membrane and the pharyngeal muscle layers. It is thick above and attached superiorly to basilar region of occipital bone. Posteriorly, it is strengthened by a strong band (median raphe) which gives attachment to the constrictors.

3. MUSCULAR LAYER

It is arranged into inner longitudinal layer and outer circular layer (Fig. 46.9).

1. *Inner longitudinal muscle layer are:*
   - Stylopharyngeus
   - Palatopharyngeus
   - Salpingopharyngeus
2. *Outer circular layer muscles are:*
   - Superior constrictor

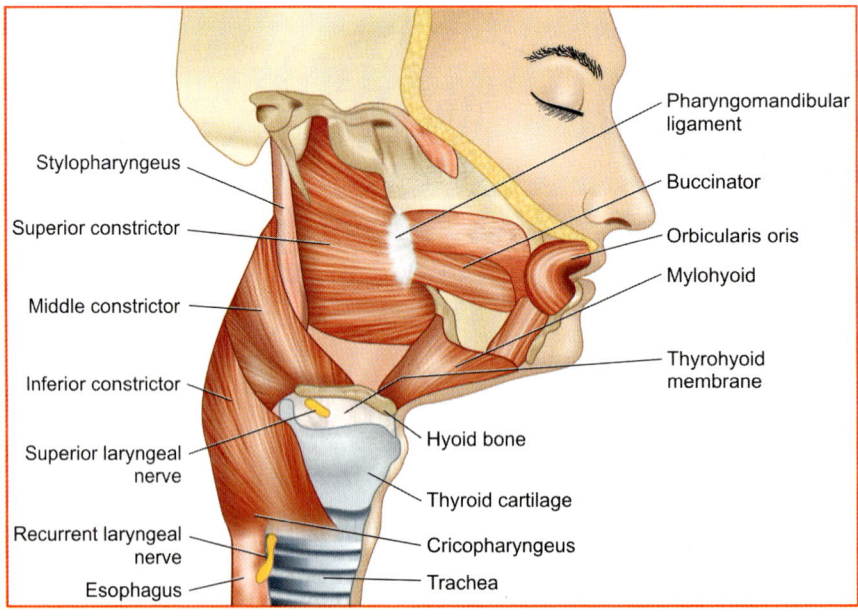

Fig. 46.9: Showing various muscles of the pharynx

- Middle constrictor
- Inferior constrictor

Each constrictor muscle's lower end is surrounded by upper fibers of the one below. All the constrictor muscles are inserted into the median raphe.

During deglutition, the constrictor muscle contracts in a co-ordinated way to propel the bolus through the oropharynx into the esophagus. The longitudinal muscles elevate the larynx and shorten the pharynx during this movement.

Killian's dehiscence: A potential gap between the thyropharyngeus and cricopharyngeus. A pharyngeal pouch may be caused at this dehiscence.

4. BUCCOPHARYNGEAL FASCIA

It covers the outer surface of the constrictor and extends forwards over the pterygomandibular ligament on the buccinator muscle.

Posteriorly, it is loosely attached to the prevertebral fascia

Laterally, it is attached to the styloid process, its muscles and to the carotid sheath.

Superiorly, above the upper border of the superior constrictor it is firmly united with the pharyngobasilar fascia. Here the fascia forms a single layer.

Structures Entering / Leaving the Pharynx

Above the Superior Constrictor

- Cartilaginous part of the eustachian tube
- Tensor palati, levator palati muscles
- Palatine branches of ascending pharyngeal artery

Between Middle and Superior Constrictor Muscles

- Stylopharyngeus muscle
- Glossopharyngeal nerve

Between Middle and Inferior Constrictor Muscles

- Internal laryngeal nerve

- Superior laryngeal vessels pierce the thyrohyoid membrane and come to lie submucosally on the lateral wall of pyriform fossa.

Below the Inferior Constrictor

- Recurrent laryngeal nerve
- Inferior laryngeal artery passes between cricopharyngeal part of inferior constrictor and esophagus behind the articulation of the inferior horn of the thyroid cartilage with the cricoid cartilage.

Blood Supply of Pharynx

Arteries supplying pharynx are all branches of external carotid artery:

- Ascending pharyngeal artery
- Ascending palatine and tonsillar branch of facial artery.
- Branches of internal maxillary artery chiefly the ascending palatine
- Dorsalis linguae branch of lingual artery.

Veins form a plexus which communicates above the pterygoid plexus and drains into the common facial vein to the internal jugular vein.

Nerve Supply of Pharynx

The pharynx is supplied by the pharyngeal plexus of nerves, which is situated in the buccopharyngeal fascia surrounding the pharynx.

The Plexus is Formed by:

- Pharyngeal branch of vagus
- Pharyngeal branch of glossopharyngeal
- Pharyngeal branches of superior cervical sympathetic ganglion.

Vagal fibers are chiefly motor. Glossopharyngeal fibers are mainly sensory and sympathetic is vasomotor.

Motor Fibers

These are derived from the cranial accessory nerve through the branches of vagus. They supply all the muscles of the pharynx except stylopharyngeus, which is supplied by the 9th cranial nerve.

These plexus also supply all the muscles of soft palate except tensor palati which is supply by the mandibular nerve.

Sensory Fibers

Sensory fibers for pharynx are derived from the:

1. Branches of glossopharyngeal nerve
2. Branches of vagus nerve

Nasopharynx is supplied by the pharyngeal branches of maxillary nerve through pterygo-palatine ganglion and the soft palate and the tonsil by the lesser palatine and the 9th nerve.

Taste Sensations

From the vallecula and epiglottic area pass through internal laryngeal branch of vagus and from the posterior one third of the tongue it passes along the glossopharyngeal nerve. The *parasympathetic secretomotor* fibers to the pharynx are derived from greater petrosal nerve through the lesser palatine branches of pterygopalatine ganglion.

Lymphatic Drainage of Pharynx

The vessels pass to the deep cervical nodes either directly or indirectly (Fig. 46.8).

Retropharyngeal Nodes

These are situated between the buccopharyngeal and prevertebral fascia. Efferent vessels pass to the upper deep cervical nodes.

Tonsillar Nodes

This is the jugulodigastric node. It is one of the deep cervical nodes and is situated along the internal jugular vein, where it is crossed by the posterior belly of digastric muscle.

Nasopharyngeal tonsil: Drain into the upper deep cervical group mostly retropharyngeal nodes.

Palatine tonsil: Drain into upper deep cervical group– jugulodigastric nodes.

Epiglottis – Drain into infrahyoid lymph nodes.

Rest of pharynx – Drain into deep cervical nodes, either directly or indirectly into retropharyngeal and paratracheal nodes.

Deep Neck Spaces

There are two important potential spaces in relation to the posterior and lateral aspects of pharynx. They are:

- Retropharyngeal space
- Parapharyngeal space

For more details please refer to the Chapter 'Deep Neck Space Infections'.

RETROPHARYNGEAL SPACE

This is a potential space behind the pharynx and is also known as *space of Gillete*.

Boundaries (Fig. 46.10)

Anteriorly – Buccopharyngeal fascia covering the constrictor muscles

Posteriorly – Alar fascia and prevertebral fascia (covers cervical vertebrae and muscle)

Superiorly – Base of skull

Laterally on each side by the carotid sheath and the parapharyngeal space. Carotid sheath encloses:

- Internal jugular vein
- Vagus nerve
- Ansa cervicalis

Inferiorly – Passes into the superior mediastinum (known as *Lincoln's highway*)

Contents

The space is filled with loose areolar tissue and 2 groups of retropharyngeal group of lymph nodes, the nodes of Rouveior and Krause.

The prevertebral fascia covers the prevertebral muscles (longus capitis and longus cervicis)

Suppuration in the retropharyngeal lymph node with the formation of pus may push the

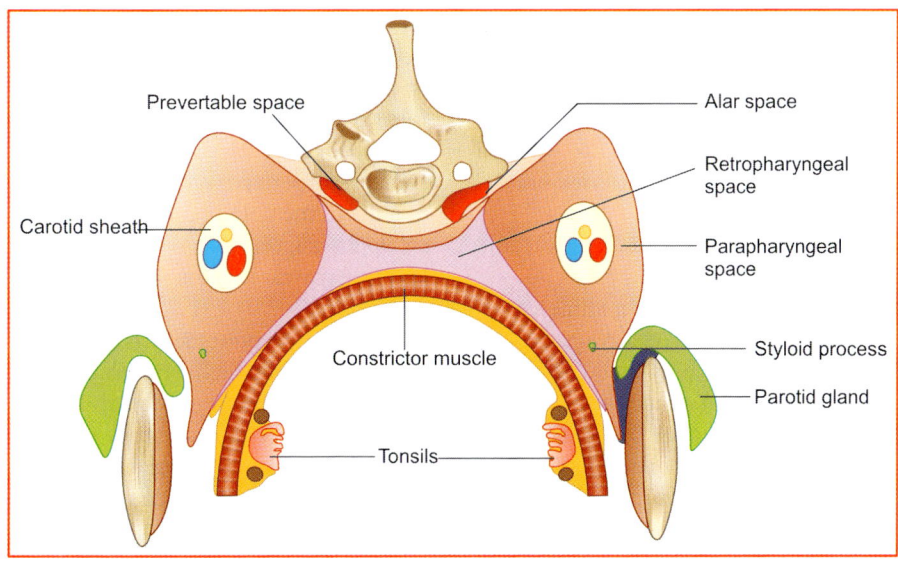

Fig. 46.10: Showing the retropharyngeal and the parapharyngeal spaces

posterior pharyngeal wall forward and present as retropha- ryngeal abscess. It is common in infants where in infection can spread downwards to the superior mediastinum. Infection with suppuration behind the prevertebral fascia presents as a median swelling in the posterior pharyngeal wall and it commonly occurs following tuberculosis of the cervical spine.

PARAPHARYNGEAL SPACE

It is triangular in cross-section. It lies lateral to the pharynx on each side. It extends above from the base of the skull to the level of hyoid bone below.

Boundaries (Fig. 46.10)

Anteromedial wall: Formed by the buccopharyn-geal fascia.

Posteromedial wall: Consists of the transverse process of cervical vertebrae, covered by the prevertebral muscles and fascia.

Lateral Wall

1. *Upper part*

- The ascending ramus of the mandible in front
- The parotid gland and the pterygoid muscles behind.

2. *Lower part*
   - Sternocleidomastoid muscle
   - The strap muscles of the neck
   - The intervening deep fascia.

Contents

1. Great vessels of the neck like internal carotid artery and internal jugular vein.
2. Ascending palatine and ascending pharyngeal artery
3. Deep cervical lymph nodes
4. The last four cranial nerves
5. The cervical sympathetic trunk
6. Styloid process and styloid group of muscles.

The styloid process divides the para-pharyngeal space into two compartments namely, the pre-styloid and the poststyloid.

Applied Anatomy

1. **Spread of infection**: This usually enters the space from infection of the tonsils or teeth

(particularly the third lower molar). It may spread:

- From base of skull to mediastinum within the space
- Into the skull, along side the internal carotid artery, IJV or posterior cranial nerves
- Down to paraesophageal region and superior mediastinum.

It does not spread across the midline, as the median raphe of the buccopharyngeal fascia is firmly united to the prevertebral fascia.

2. **The parapharyngeal space tumors** in the prestyloid compartment are commonly salivary gland in origin, whereas those in the post-styloid compartment are commonly neurogenic in origin.

PALATINE TONSIL

Embryology

The tonsil pillars are formed from 2nd and 3rd branchial arches, through dorsal extension of mesenchyme into the forming soft palate. The tonsillar crypts develop by 3 to 6 months as solid ingrowths from surface epithelium (the crypts forms, branches, rebranches and even regress after birth). Lymphocytes appear near epithelium during 3rd month, but organizes to nodular form after 6 months. By 5th month, tonsillar capsule is formed from mesenchyme.

Lingual tonsil represents the lymphoid infiltration into base of tongue concomittant with the development of palatine tonsil.

During 4 to 6 months of intrauterine life, development of lymphatic tissue also forms within the posterior wall of nasopharynx to become nasopharyngeal tonsil (adenoid).

Anatomy

Tonsil is an almond shaped mass of specialized subepithelial lymphoid tissue situated in the tonsillar fossa bounded by palatoglossal and palatopharyngeal folds. The upper pole is almost free. The lower pole is embedded besides the base of tongue. In late fetal life, a fold of mucous membrane extends posteriorly from the palatoglossal fold to cover anteroinferior part of tonsil. In childhood, this fold is invaded by lymphoid tissue and is incorporated into tonsil. A semilunar fold of mucous membrane extends from upper part of palatopharyngeal arch towards upper part of tonsil and separates it from base of uvula (plica semilunaris).

In the lower pole, the lymphoid tissue is continuous with subepithelial lymphoid tissue on base of tongue called as lingual tonsil. Tonsillolin-gual sulcus separates tonsil from base of tongue. Tonsils are larger in childhood, when it is more active, and gradually become smaller during puberty.

Structure of Tonsil

The tonsil consists of lymphoid follicles supported in a fine connective tissue framework. The lymphocytes are less densely packed in the center -'the germinal center'. Multiplication of lymphocytes occur in this area.

On the medial surface of tonsil, there are 15 to 20 openings irregularly placed over surface. These are tonsillar crypts. These may penetrate nearly whole thickness of tonsil. These crypts contain desquamated epithelial cell debris. Usually, these debris are automatically cleared off. Sometimes it becomes yellow and hardened. Both medial surface and crypts are lined by stratified squamous non-keratinized epithelium.

In the upper part of tonsil, there is a deep intratonsillar crypt extending laterally and inferiorly towards the lower pole of tonsil, within its capsule. It may represent the persistent ventral portion of 2nd pharyngeal pouch. Some believe it to be 'supratonsillar fossa', which is the area of mucous membrane above the tonsil between palatopharyngeal and palatoglossal folds. Tonsillolith can occur in this region.

The lateral surface is lined by a capsule. The deep part of the tonsil is separated from the wall of oropharynx by loose areolar tissue. This provides the easy dissection of tonsil from tonsillar fossa. Suppuration of this peritonsillar space can cause 'peritonsillar abscess'.

Relationships of Tonsil

Medial surface is free and faces towards the oropharynx covered by mucosa

Anterior: Palatoglossal fold with palatoglossal muscle.

Posterior: Palatopharyngeus muscle in palatopharyngeal fold.

Some fibers of palatopharyngeus muscle (tonsillopharyngeus) are seen attached to the tonsillar capsule.

Inferiorly: The capsule is firmly connected to the side of the tongue and superiorly it extends to the edge of soft palate.

Laterally: Bed is formed by pharyngobasilar fascia. Deep to it on the upper part, there is superior constrictor muscle and below it styloglossus muscle passing forward into the tongue.

Lateral to superior constrictor is buccopharyngeal fascia. The glossopharyngeal nerve and the stylohyoid ligament pass obliquely downwards and forwards beneath the lower edge of superior constrictor in the lower part of tonsillar fossa.

Palatine vein and external palatine or paratonsillar vein descends from soft palate across lateral aspect of capsule and pierce the pharyngeal wall to open into the pharyngeal plexus.

The tonsillar artery pierces superior constrictor muscle and reaches the tonsil accompanied by two tonsillar veins. A fibrous band is noted at this point, between tonsillar capsule and tonsillar bed on dissection.

More distant lateral relations of lower part of the tonsil are posterior belly of digastric muscle and submandibular salivary gland with facial artery arching over them. Further laterally medial pterygoid and angle of mandible is related to the tonsil.

Clinical Importance

A penetrating oropharyngeal injury directed posterolaterally travels the tonsillar bed and the superior constrictor muscle enters the 'parapharyngeal space'. In this region, the structures that can be injured are internal jugular vein, internal carotid artery, nerves associated with carotid sheath at this point (X, XI, XII) and sympathetic trunk.

If penetration is more lateral, parotid gland, posterior facial vein, external carotid artery and one of the trunks of the facial nerve are involved.

BLOOD SUPPLY OF THE TONSILS
(Fig. 46.11)

Arterial Supply

- Main artery supplying the tonsil is ***Tonsillar artery*** – Branch of facial artery.
- Tonsils receive arterial supply from the following:
  1. **Facial artery** (tonsillar and the ascending palatine branches)
  2. **Ascending pharyngeal artery**
  3. **Internal maxillary artery** (descending palatine branch)
  4. **Lingual artery** (dorsalis linguae branch)

(Remember the Mnemonic: **FAIL**)

Venous Drainage

- Paratonsillar vein

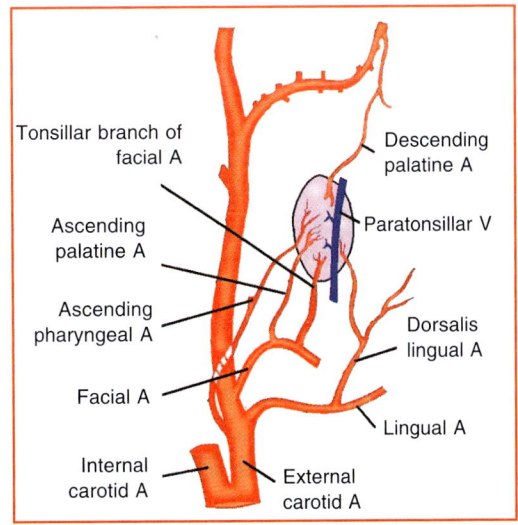

Fig. 46.11: Showing the blood supply of the tonsil

- Pharyngeal plexus
- Facial vein

These communicate with pterygoid plexus and eventually into common facial and internal jugular veins.

Lymphatic Drainage

Tonsillar fossa drain into upper deep cervical nodes. Anterior pillar drain into upper deep nodes along with internal jugular vein and into submaxillary gland and rarely into posterior triangle nodes (jugulodigastric).

Posterior pillar area drain into upper deep cervical nodes, posterior triangle nodes and nodes around the spinal accessory. Tonsil has no afferent lymphatic vessels.

Innervations

Sensory supply is mainly from tonsillar branch of glossopharyngeal nerve. The upper part of the tonsil near soft palate supplied by lesser palatine branches of maxillary division of trigeminal nerve, received by way of pterygopalatine ganglion.

Sympathetic fibers from superior cervical ganglion.

Applied Anatomy

Referred pain in the ear following tonsillectomy is due to common nerve supply. The sensory branches of glossopharyngeal nerve have its cell bodies located in the inferior ganglion of IX cranial nerve. Also located here are the cell bodies of tympanic nerve (Jacobson's nerve) which provides general sensation to medial surface of tympanic membrane and middle ear mucosa. Both oropharyngeal and tympanic nerves project proximally via trigeminal tract to the ventral posteromedial nucleus of thalamus. These common central projections account for the simultaneous perception of pain in ear and oropharynx.

ADENOIDS (PHARYNGEAL TONSIL)

This is submucosal lymphoid tissue in the nasopharynx. It arises from the junction of roof and posterior wall of nasopharynx and is composed of vertical ridges of lymphoid tissue separated by deep clefts. It has no crypts. It has no capsule and is covered by ciliated pseudo-stratified columnar epithelium (respiratory). Adenoids are present at birth and continue throughout the childhood. The atrophy of adenoids usually occurs at puberty.

Adenoids occasionally extend laterally to lie in close relation to the opening of the eustachian tube (tubal tonsil). Rarely it extends into the pharynx and project below the soft palate.

Blood Supply of the Adenoids

Ascending palatine branch of a facial artery

- Ascending pharyngeal branch
- Pharyngeal branch of maxillary artery

Tubal Tonsils (Gerlach's Tonsil): This is the extension of pharyngeal tonsil into lateral pharyngeal wall.

LINGUAL TONSILS

Lingual tonsils are raised papilliform masses on the posterior 1/3rd of tongue between vallate papilla in front and epiglottis behind. Each mass has a single opening on the mucosal surface, that form tubular gland or crypt. Lined by squamous epithelial cell crypts contain cellular debris and bacteria.

Applied Importance: Hypertrophy may occur after tonsillectomy or in women after menopause. If swelling is large it will cause a feeling of lump in the throat. Inflammation or abscess can even occur.

Blood supply to other tonsils is not significant, since it is from regional small arteries. Venous drainage occurs through pharyngeal plexus into internal jugular vein.

PHYSIOLOGY OF WALDEYER'S RING

The tonsils are sites of lymphocytes formation. So it is immunologically important. But the role of tonsils and adenoids in the process of immunology is controversial. In certain immune deficient states, e.g. *agammaglobulinemia* tonsils are poorly developed, when compared with normal individuals. On the other hand, patient having repeated infection and tonsillar hypertrophy does not prove alteration in IgG. So also, no significant alteration of susceptibility of infection following tonsillectomy is noted.

Recent study shows that it is involved in IgA production, which provides local immunity. Other works prove that both tonsils and adenoids may produce IgE (mediating reaginic hypersensitivity reaction).

Mechanism of Production of Immunoglobulins by Tonsils and Adenoids

The lymphocytes of tonsils receive messages from antigen processing cells. It induces the production of IgM, the pentamer of IgM5 is first produced. Consequently, IgG and IgA are produced by γ and α cells respectively. There is no active transport of immunoglobulin in tonsils. Some immunoglobulin may leak into the lumen of pharynx, and the extra cellular leakage is favored by inflammation. Some cells produce immunoglobulin, while some divide and form memory clones. Some enter the circulation to populate other glandular areas like adenoids. The migrating cells recognize paragland- ular lymphoid tissue by antigen expressed on the wall of post-capillary venule. In adenoids, penta-metric IgM5 and dimeric IgA2

are elaborated, which has chains so it is actively secreted through epithelial cells into the pharynx, which gives local immunity. The secretion of IgE is passive leakage only. During infection, the leakage is more.

Adenoid hyperplasia is a common cause of nasal obstruction in children. As a part of Waldeyer's ring, adenoids occupy a key position in the development of immune process. Adenoids are small at birth, and increase in size by 1 to 3 years of age and when active immunity gets established, it may regress by puberty.

In the nasopharynx, they are in constant contact with inspired air, and are continually bathed by nasal mucous secreted from posterior chonae by naso-cilliary mechanism. They are thus continually exposed to inhaled antigens. They react by forming their own complement of antibodies to these antigens.

It has been postulated that they modify the micro-organisms encountered and release them or their toxin into reticuloendothelial system of the body to produce active immunity. This activity causes increase in size of adenoids during infections.

Children may inhale from 10,000 to 15,000 liters of air/day. Much of this air is polluted with CO, Ozone, SO_2, Ketones, ammonia, cigarette smoke, etc. These cause increased mucous secretion. The increased nasal airway resistance leads to increased pulmonary resistance and alveolar hypoventilation which is mediated by naso-pulmonary reflexes which may result in hypoxia.

POINTS TO REMEMBER

1. Pharynx is a fibromuscular organ, that extends from the base of the skull to the lower border of cricoid cartilage.
2. Fossa of Rosenmüller is the commonest site for nasopharyngeal cancer.
3. Waldeyer's ring is a scallered collection of subepithelial lymphoid tissue arround the aerodigestive tract.
4. Tonsils have efferent lymph vessels but no afferent
5. Killian's dehiscence is a potential gap between thyropharyngeus and cricopharyngeus.
6. Tonsilar branch of facial artery is the main artery supply to the tonsil.

47

Physiology of Pharynx

Pharynx is a crossroad of the air and the food passages and serves the following functions:

Functions of Pharynx

- Deglutition
- Protection from aspiration
- Part of respiratory and food passage
- Speech: Pharynx adds resonance to the voice
- Waldeyar's ring is involved in immunity and is described in the previous chapter.
- Taste sensation in oropharynx from the posterior one third of the tongue
- *Mucociliary clearance*: The mucus from the respiratory passage is swallowed
- Eustachian tube ventilates and drains the middle ear cleft into the pharynx

PHYSIOLOGY OF DEGLUTITION

Deglutition refers to the process of propulsion of bolus of food from oral cavity to the stomach. It is controlled by neuromuscular activity which could be voluntary or involuntary.

3 Phases of deglutition are:

1. **Oral phase:** Voluntary
2. **Pharyngeal phase:** Both (mostly involuntary)
3. **Esophageal phase:** Involuntary

Oral Phase

Movement patterns depend on consistency of material swallowed.

- **Solids:** Chewed, mixed with saliva, made into appropriate size bolus
- **Liquids:** Poured or sucked into and is maintained as bolus
- Lip is closed using the orbicularis oris muscle (supplied by facial nerve)
- Rotatory and lateral jaw and tongue movement helps in grinding and mixing the bolus with saliva
- Bolus is held between tongue and anterior hard palate
- Anterior to posterior tongue movement (1 sec).

Pharyngeal Phase (1 sec)

As the bolus slips into the oropharynx, there is closure of nasopharyngeal isthmus (soft palate raised)

With the action of the pharyngeal constrictors the bolus is pushed through the pharynx to the cricopharyngeal sphincter at the top of the esophagus.

This is associated with tilting, elevation and closure of the larynx at all three sphincters (epiglottis/aryepiglottic folds, false vocal folds, and true vocal folds) to prevent food from entering the airway.

Simultaneously there is relaxation of the cricopharyngeal sphincter to allow material to pass from pharynx into the esophagus.

Gravity also plays a part while in prone position or when lying on one side.

Esophageal Phase (8–20 sec)

Primary Peristalsis

Sequential contraction of the circular muscle of the esophageal body, which results in a contractile wave that migrates toward the stomach can be documented by esophageal manometry (Fig. 47.1). As the bolus reaches the lower end of esophagus there is relaxation and opening of the lower esophageal sphincter. The entire process of this phase is under involuntary control mediated through the Vagus nerve.

Secondary peristalsis

A peristaltic sequence that occurs in response to distention of the esophagus (not associated with cricopharyngeal sphincter (VES) relaxation or deglutition)

Neural Regulation of Swallowing

Pharyngeal: Stimulation of receptors (7th, 9th, and 10 cranial nerves). Efferent (motor) function (9th, 10th cranial nerves). Cricopharyngeal sphincter opening is reflexive

Esophageal
- Primary peristalsis
  - Proximal– striated– contracts first
  - Distal– smooth– contracts later
- Secondary peristalsis
  - Intrinsic plexus: Auerbach's myentric plexus.

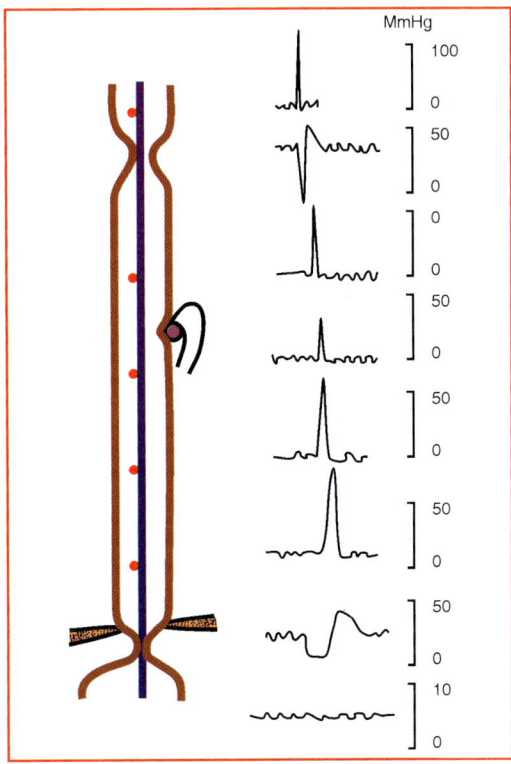

Fig. 47.1: Showing pressure changes in the esophagus during swallow

Cranial Nerves and their Role in Deglutition

CN V and XII: Chewing and tongue movements

CN VII: Sensation of oral cavity through nervus intermedius and taste to anterior two-third of tongue and motor supply to orbicularis oris.

CN IX: Taste to posterior tongue, sensory and motor functions of the pharynx

CN X: Taste to oropharynx, and sensation and motor function to larynx and laryngopharynx and airway protection.

POINTS TO REMEMBER

1. The three phases of deglutition are oral phase (voluntary), pharyngeal phase (both but mostly involuntary) and esophageal phase (involuntary).
2. Multiple cranial nerves are involved in deglutition.

48

Clinical Evaluation of Oral Cavity and Pharynx

A thorough history taking is very much essential prior to clinical examination of the oral cavity and the pharynx. Collection of information of basic data like, name, sex, address, occupation, etc are essential to identify the concerned patient and also the specific presentation of certain diseases may be related to the above. Nasopharyngeal angio-fibroma occurs in adolescent males, Plummer-Vinson syndrome and postcricoid malignancy are more common in females. Extranasal scleroma and rhinosporidiosis occurs more commonly in certain geographical situations and certain diseases like allergic pharyngitis and other inflammatory conditions may be related to the occupation and the environmental conditions of the patient.

The chief complaints should be presented in the chronological order as per the presentation. In the history of presenting illness, each symptom should be described in relation to its onset, duration, progression, aggravating and relieving factors and the details of the treatment received for the same symptom. Past history of similar complaints or diseases like diabetes, hypertension, tuberculosis, syphilis, Hansen's disease, trauma, etc should be noted. Family history of major illnesses or similar illness should be noted. In children, history of immunization should be elicited. Personal history of habits like tobacco/betel nut chewing, smoking, alcohol, extramarital sexual exposure and other important personal history like diet, bowel and bladder habits, etc should be noted.

Common Oral and Pharyngeal Symptoms

1. *Pain in the oral cavity:* Often seen in acute inflammatory and traumatic conditions and advanced cancer of the oral cavity especially of the tongue. Dental pain may present sometimes as referred otalgia and one should look for dental caries and eruption of wisdom tooth.

2. *Swelling/ulcerations in oral cavity:* Swelling may be related to certain benign lesions like ranula, mixed salivary tumors of the palate, lingual thyroid, papilloma, hemangioma, etc. Malignant tumors are often associated with ulceration. Traumatic ulcer may be due to sharp tooth. Malignant ulcers are initially painless but later become painful, whereas traumatic ulcers and apthous ulcers are painful from the beginning.

3. *Trismus:* This is commonly associated with submucous fibrosis (betal nut/ ghutka chewer), tetanus, inflammatory conditions like peritonsillitis and peritonsillar abscess, para-pharyngeal abscess, advanced cancer of the oral cavity and pharynx, fracture of the mandible, etc.

4. *Bleeding gums:* Often related to scurvy and hematological and liver diseases.

5. *Disturbances of salivation:* Xerostomia can be associated with mouth breathing, Sjogren's syndrome, post-radiotherapy for head and neck cancer, etc. Increased salivation is often seen in oral ulcers and poor orodental hygiene.

6. *Halitosis:* Can be associated with periodontitis, dental sepsis, tonsillitis, etc.

7. *Disturbances of taste:* Can be associated to injury to corda tympani nerve during ear surgery, tobacco chewing, involvement of glossopharyngeal nerve, tumors in oral cavity, Bell's palsy, vitamin deficiency, etc.

8. *Difficulty in speech* is often due to ankyloglossia and tongue tie. Sometimes muffled voice is associated with mass in the base tongue.

9. *Mouth breathing:* It may be associated with pathology in the nose and nasopharynx like adenoids and nasopharyngeal tumors.

10. *Snoring and sleep apnea:* It can be associated with bulky tongue, short chin, adenoids and tonsillar hypertrophy.

11. *Sore throat:* Commonly seen in pharyngitis and tonsillitis.

12. *Dysphagia:* Pharyngeal and esophageal pathology like achylasia cardia, cricopharyngeal web, stricture esophagus, neoplasms of esophagus, etc should be suspected.

13. *Odynophagia:* is commonly associated with acute inflammatory conditions like peritonsillitis, acute tonsillitis, acute retropharyngeal abscess, etc and cancer of the base tongue.

14. *Foreign body/sticky sensation:* is often seen in case of ingested foreign body or pharyngitis.

15. *Lump in throat:* pharyngeal tumors may obstruct the food passage.

16. *Cough:* May be due to postnasal drip, reflux pharyngitis and laryngeal pathology.

17. *Aspiration:* It is often due to neurological conditions including vagal paralysis or obstruction to cricopharynx/upper esophagus.

18. *Choking spells:* Often due to reflux laryngitis or due to aspiration.

EXAMINATION OF ORAL CAVITY AND PHARYNX

This should be done in a systematic manner and includes:

- Lips
- Angle of mouth
- Mouth opening
- Buccal mucosa
- Gums and teeth
- Buccogingival and gingivolabial sulcus
- Tongue
- Floor of the mouth
- Hard and soft palate
- Anterior and posterior tonsillar pillar and uvula
- Tonsillar fossa
- Posterior pharyngeal wall

Nasopharynx and laryngopharynx should be examined with postnasal and laryngeal mirrors respectively (Figs 48.1 and 48.2). For more details on postnasal examination and indirect laryngoscopy please refer to the respective chapters under *Nose and Larynx.*

During clinical examination of the oral cavity and pharynx the following mucosal changes should be noted:

- Asymmetry/swelling
- Growth
- Ulceration
- Discoloration
- Restriction of movement
- Tenderness.

Inspection

Lips: Look for fissures, congenital deformities, discoloration as seen in jaundice and cyanosis, any

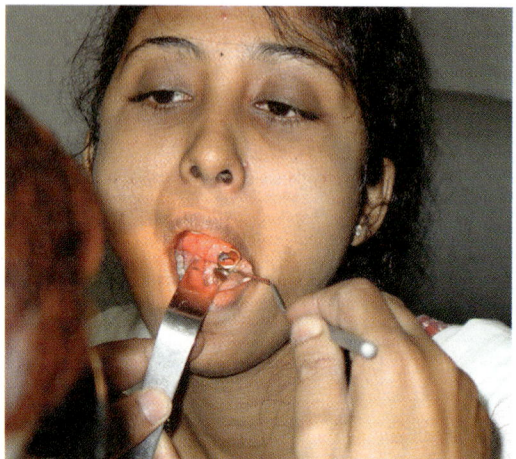

Fig. 48.1: Postnasal examination in progress

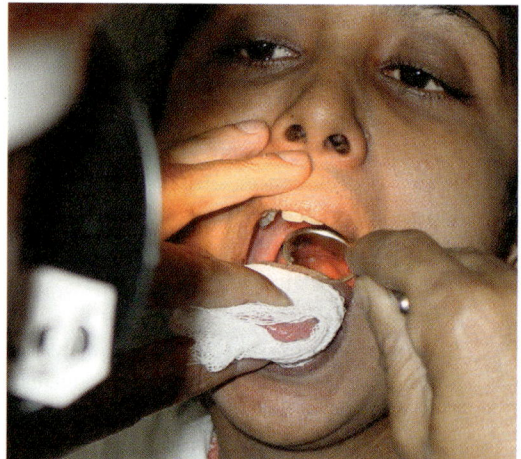

Fig. 48.2: Indirect laryngoscopy in progress

hypertrophy if associated with clefts. Tumor like swelling may be seen in hemangioma. Ulceration should be suspected for malignancy.

Angle of mouth: Look for ulcerations as seen in angular stomatitis and malignancy.

Mouth opening is restricted in trismus or painful conditions of the oral cavity.

Buccal mucosa: Abnormalities in the opening of the Stenson's duct should be noted and redness of the opening is seen in parotitis. Look for leukoplakia, submucous fibrosis or mucosal changes (Figs 48.3 and 48.4).

Buccogingival and gingivolabial sulcus should be carefully opened using a tongue depressor and look for mucosal changes. Malignancy here is often overlooked during quick oral cavity examination.

Gums and teeth: Look for hemorrhage, fistula, dental status, pyeriodontitis, malocclusion, loose teeth, ill-fitting denture, widening of the alveolar margins, etc.

Tongue is examined by asking the patient to open the mouth keeping the tongue in its position for any mucosal changes like staining, discoloration, ulcers, swelling, etc. Movements of the tongue and fasciculation's of the tongue are looked for.

Palate: Look for mucosal changes and perforation, bullae, clefts, ulcerations; swelling, neoplasm, torus palatinous, etc. are looked for.

Floor of the mouth: Look for tongue tie, swellings like dermoid cyst, ranula, etc. Cystic dilatation of the Wharton's duct due to sialolithiasis or sialectasis, etc. (Figs 48.4a and b).

Retromolar trigone: Look for inflammation, submucous fibrosis, ulcerations, growth, etc. (Fig. 48.3b).

Oropharynx: This is examined by asking the patient to open the mouth widely and relax the tongue. Tongue depressor is used to depress the anterior two thirds of the tongue. Palatal movements are observed as the patient phonates 'aah' (Fig. 45.5).

Tonsillar fossa with its pillars are observed on both sides and looked for any swelling or hypertrophy of the tonsils, any pus pockets or membrane over the crypts, any asymmetry between the two tonsils, mucosal changes like ulceration, growth, etc. Pillars are looked for congestion, ulceration, etc.

Soft palatal and uvular redness and edema is seen in peritonsillitis/ abscess.

Posterior pharyngeal wall: Look for granular pharyngitis, bulge as in retropharyngeal abscess, postnasal drip, ulcerations, growth, etc.

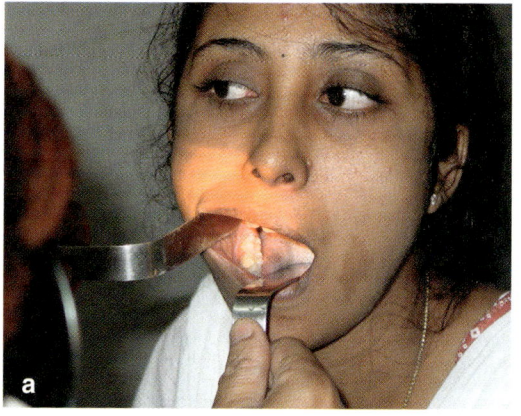
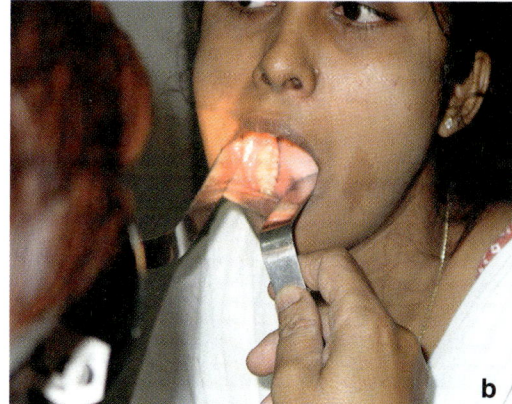

Figs 48.3a and b: Examination of the oral cavity using two tongue depressors

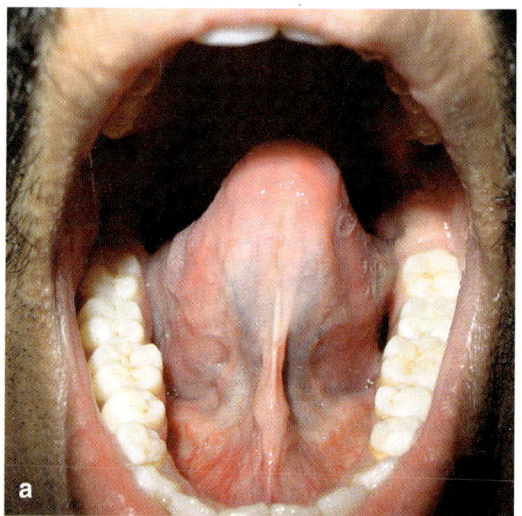

Fig. 48.4a: Normal floor of the mouth

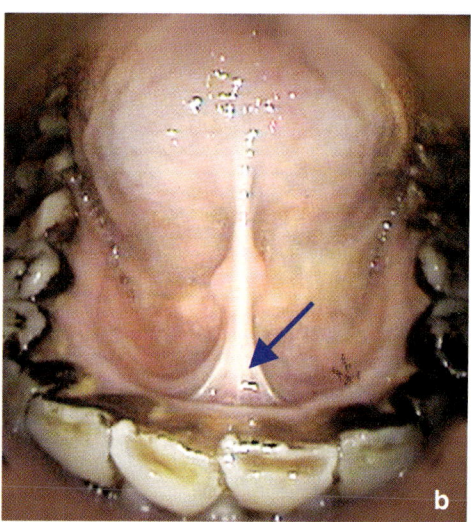

Fig. 48.4b: A tongue tie (blue arrow)

Base of the tongue, vallecula, pharyngo-epiglottic fold can be examined by indirect laryngoscopy (Fig. 48.2).

Palpation

Inspection findings are confirmed by palpation using tip of index finger with gloves (Fig. 48.6).

Patient is explained about the procedure and is done usually if a pathological lesion is suspected. It is very important to palpate specific sites like base of tongue, vallecula, tonsillolingual sulcus, retromolar trigone and floor of the mouth.

Look for

- Induration
- Tenderness
- Calculus
- Consistency and mobility of the mass
- Periosteal thickening if growth is close to mandible/ maxilla in which case the bucco-gingival sulcus may become shallow.

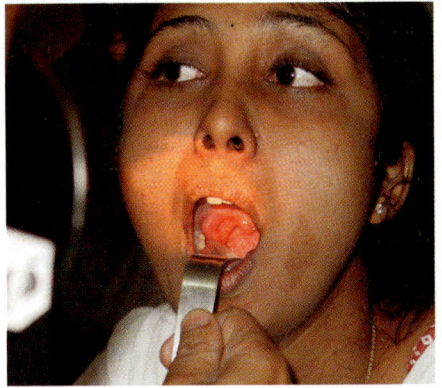

Fig. 48.5: Examination of the oropharynx by depressing the anterior two thirds of the tongue

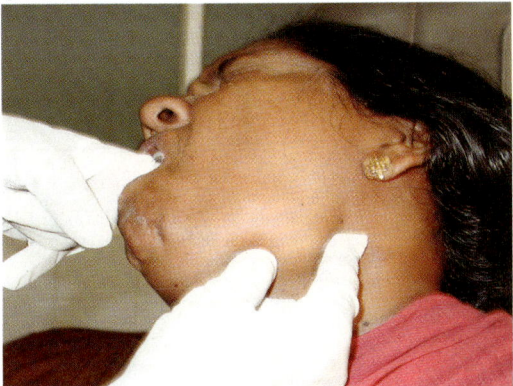

Fig. 48.6: Palpation of the oral cavity and oropharynx

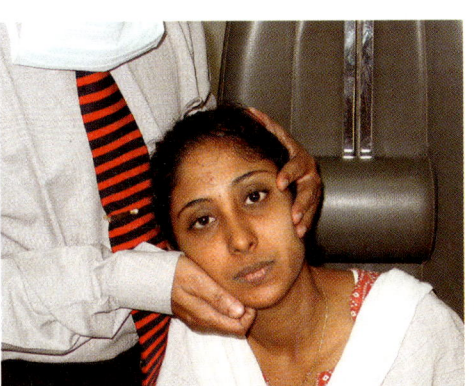

Fig. 48.7: Examination of the submandibular region

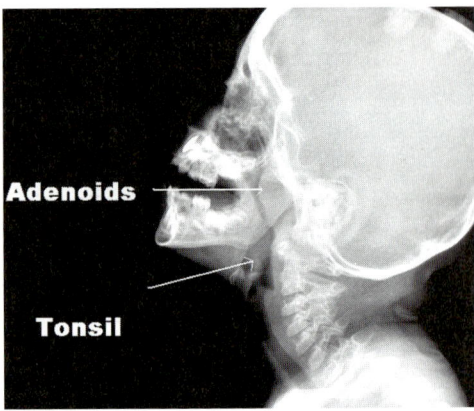

Fig. 48.8: X-ray lateral view of the head and neck showing adenoid hypertropy occluding the nasopharyngeal airway

- Malignancy in the tonsillolingual sulcus (coffin corner) may be overlooked and missed if palpation is not done.

Neck has to be palpated for any inflammatory condition as in tonsillitis where jugulodigastic nodes are enlarged or malignant conditions for metastatic diseases in the neck (Fig. 48.7).

Investigations for Oral and Oropharyngeal Conditions

Specific

1. Throat swab for culture and sensitivity test

2. Radiological investigation (X-ray soft tissue neck AP and lateral view) (Fig. 48.8)
3. X-ray base of the skull
4. CT-scan imaging or MRI
5. Barium swallow
6. Coagulation profile
7. Endoscopy
   - Nasopharyngoscopy
   - Laryngoscopy
   - Rigid telescopy of the larynx and laryngopharynx and base of the tongue
   - Hypopharyngoscopy.

Non-specific

1. Complete blood picture
2. Urine routine for protein, sugar microscopic, etc.

3. RBS—Random blood sugar
4. ECG
5. LFT—Liver Function test, etc.
6. Serological tests for syphilis and Mantoux.

POINTS TO REMEMBER

1. Malignancy of oral cavity and pharynx is common in India and detail personal history of tobacco chewing, smoking, alcohol and nutritional status are important.
2. Digital palpation of oral cavity and oropharynx is mandatory during the course of clinical examination.
3. Systematic neck examination is necessary in cancer of oral cavity and pharynx.

49

Common Benign Lesions of the Oral Cavity

Classification of Benign Lesions

1. Developmental conditions

- Median rhomboid glossitis
- Dermoid cyst
- Torus
- Hereditary hemorrhagic telengectasia

2. Non-inflammatory conditions

- Coated tongue
- Fissured tongue
- Geographic tongue
- Fordyce spots

3. Inflammatory and ulcerative conditions

- Reactive
  - Linea alba
  - Granuloma fissuratum
  - Reparative granuloma
  - Leucoplakia
  - Mucositis
    - Radiation
    - Drug-induced
- Infective
  - Acute herpetic gingivitis
  - Herpetic stomatitis
  - Apthous stomatitis
  - Candidiasis

4. Traumatic conditions

- Cheek bite
- Sharp tooth and traumatic ulcer of tongue

5. Benign tumors and tumor-like lesions

- Papilloma
- Fibroma
- Pleomorphic adenoma
- Hemangioma
- Neurofibromatosis
- Lymphangioma
- Mucocele/ retension cyst of the oral mucosa
- Ranula
- Salivary calculus

Coated Tongue

This is also called hairy tongue and is seen on the dorsal surface as a darkly stained shag carpet as a result of hyperkeratosis and elongated filiform papillae.

Etiology

- Prolonged antibiotic therapy
- Reduced normal bacterial flora of the oral cavity
- Secondary pigment producing bacteria

Pathology

Hyperkeratosis and hypertrophy of the filiform papillae associated with discoloration of the mucosa.

Clinical Features

Dark stained coating of the tongue

Investigation

Biopsy will confirm the condition

Treatment

- Good oral hygiene
- Withdrawal of the antibiotic treatment if not absolutely necessary
- Brushing of the tongue with a tooth brush.

Fissured Tongue

Synonym: Scrotal tongue

This is a common non-pathologic abnormality associated with fissures of variable size and depth on the dorsal surface of the tongue with no discoloration of the tongue.

No treatment is required unless inflamed.

Cleaning the oral cavity with 3 percent hydrogen peroxide solution may be helpful.

Fordyce's Spots

They are functioning sebaceous glands that are found frequently on the buccal surface of the oral cavity in older patients.

Clinical Features

- It appears as a cluster of small white raised lesions
- Usually the patient is asymptomatic
- No treatment is indicated and the patient is reassured regarding the nature of the lesion.

Geographic Tongue

Synonym: Benign migratory glossitis

This presents as a map-like well defined margin on the dorsal surface of the tongue.

Etiology

- Exact cause is not known
- Stress may be one of the factor.
- Common in females than males.
- Menstrual cycle may exacerbate the condition

Clinical Features

- Burning and itchy sensation on the surface of the tongue.

- The lesions are non-indurated patchy spots which are devoid of filiform papillae (Fig. 49.1).

Treatment

- Benzydamine (tantum) may be used as a gargle/ mouth wash in concentrated form which reduces pain and itching.
- Chlorhexidine gargling may be tried
- The condition is self limiting.

Torus Palatinus

This is a bony midline exostosis of the hard palate. Sometimes torus mandibularis also may be seen on the lingual surface of the inferior alveolus.

Etiopathology

- Common around puberty
- It occurs as a failure of the palatal and the mandibular bone to stop developing after fusion.

Clinical Features

It appears as a hard firm swelling of the palate or the lingual surface of the mandible and is prone for trauma. It is associated with secondary inflammation. They may create problem in wearing dental prosthesis.

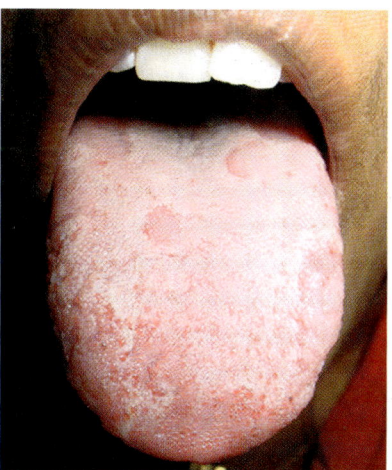

Fig. 49.1: Showing geographic tongue

Treatment

Excision may be required if it interferes with use of dental prosthesis.

Epulis (Reparative Granuloma)

This is a benign, localized swelling of the gingiva. There are many types of epulis. Fibrous and giant cell epulis are the common types.

- **Fibrous Epulis**
  - This usually presents as a slowly growing, smooth, soft or firm reddish lump that generally emerges between two teeth. It may bleed on touch.
  - It usually develops in response to trauma and infection.
  - It is a fibrous tissue tumor that arises from the periodontal membrane
  - This lesion is treated by excision and curettage of the lesion.
- **Giant Cell Epulis**
  - This presents as a gingival lump emerging between two teeth, however unlike the fibrous type, it grows more quickly as an irregular red fleshy mass which may invade local bone. The mass may ulcerate or bleed (Fig 49.2).

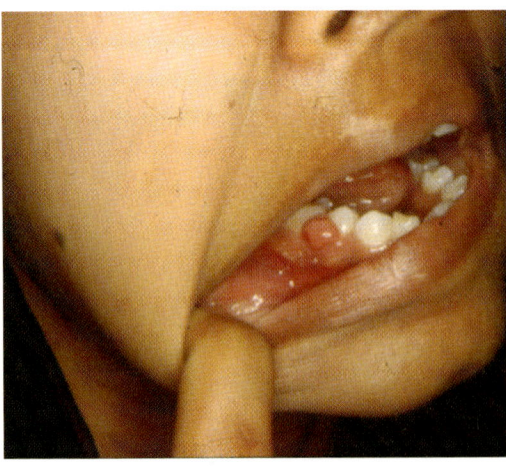

Fig. 49.2: Showing gaint cell epulis

- Histopathologically it consists of giant cells in a vascular stroma and shows features of osteoclastoma.
- Treatment is extraction of associated teeth and excision and curettage of local bone.
- **Pregnancy granuloma**
  - This often occurs during the 2nd month of gestation. Hormonal influence may be the causative factor.
  - Pain, bleeding mass in the gingiva is the common presenting features.
  - It can be observed as it resolves spontaneously after delivery.
  - If bothersome, it may be excised.

Herpes Stomatitis

Recurrent herpes stomatitis is a distinct Herpes simplex infection from that of primary herpetic gingivitis.

Causative Agent

Type I Herpes simplex virus

The lesion is commonly found in the mucocutaneous junction. The lesions of the herpes simplex, herpes zoster and varicella zoster has an identical appearance. A change in specific neutralizing antibody titre occurs in primary lesions and not in recurrent lesions. After primary infection the virus is not generally eliminated but lies in a sensory ganglion. Periodically external stimulus like fever, stress, sunlight, trauma, etc. may reactivate the virus that is conducted by peripheral nerves fibers and manifests in the skin or mucous membrane of the oral cavity.

Clinical Features

Symptoms: They commonly present as a cold sore or blister at the mucocutaneous junction of the lip. The lesions are generally painful. The disease is self limiting unless the patient is immunocompro- mised.

Signs: The site of the lesion is associated with formation of the papule that forms vesicles. Later these vesicles may become purulent. It ruptures spontaneously between 7 to 10 days (Fig 49.3).

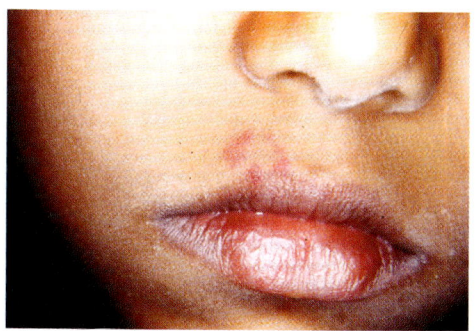

Fig. 49.3: Herpes labialis

Treatment

Supportive care is given that include topical anesthetics and mouth washes. Vitamins and good nutrition should be given. Steroids should be avoided as it can aggravate the disease.

Leucoplakia

This is a sharply outlined milky white patch in the mucosa which does not peel and is without induration and pain. For more details please refer to the chapter 'Neoplasms of the oral cavity and pharynx'.

Oral Candidiasis (Moniliasis)

Candida albicans is a yeast like fungus and is a normal commensal of the oral cavity and can be pathogenic under certain circumstances.

Predisposing conditions are

- Prolonged use of antibiotics and corticosteroids
- Diabetes mellitus
- Radiotherapy and chemotherapy
- Debilitated states

Symptoms: The lesions are painful and interfere with swallowing and chewing.

Signs: They appear as soft white plaques attached to the mucosa. It has to be distinguished from leucoplakia. There is often associated inflammation in the surrounding area.

Direct examination with KOH demonstrates the branching hyphae, characteristic of this fungus. Grams staining may confirm.

Treatment

Nystatin oral solution may be given as gargle or cotrimazole oral paint may be applied.

Recurrent Aphthous Stomatitis

This is a benign painful condition of the oral cavity often referred to as canker sore.

Etiology

Exact etiology is not known.

Possible causative factors are

- Hypersensitivity to a transitional L-form of an alpha-hemolytic streptococcus
- An autoimmune response to a oral sub epithelium
- Herpes simplex infection
- Food allergy
- Emotional stress.

Clinical Features

- Painful ulcers often multiple affecting the oral or pharyngeal mucosa. Initially they are in the form of small vesicles which quickly becomes an ulcer.
- Increased salivation
- Painful mastication, swallowing or articulation.
- Minor aphthae are usually 2 to 5 mm in size with slough-covered floor and erythematous margins.
- Major aphthae can be large and often more than 10 cms in size.

Treatment

- Analgesic gel/ lozenges/ mouth washes may be given.
- 2 percent lignocaine gel may be applied 4th hourly.
- Levamisole has been tried with an intent to restore the cell mediated immunity

- Steroid lozenges or paste to facilitate early resolution may be tried.
- Oral hygiene should be maintained.
- Avoid spicy and hot food
- Vitamin supplementation
- The condition is usually self limiting and resolves within 4 to 5 days. In case of delayed resolution or major aphthae short course of oral steroids may be given.

Retention Cyst/ Mucocoele

This is a common lesion of the oral cavity and often affects the lower lips or the buccal mucosa. The lesions appear as small cystic swellings (Fig 49.4). It can lead to mucous retention cyst or rupture of mucous gland or duct leading to extravasation of the fluid into the tissue. Cysts are pale and bluish in color and are usually

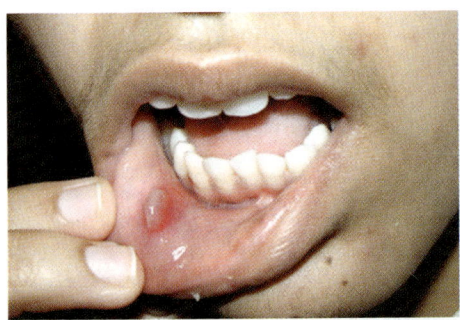

Fig. 49.4: Mucus retention cyst of the lip

painless. It often ruptures and gets self marsupialized. Large cysts need surgical excision.

Ranula and Salivary Calculi

These are described under respective chapters later.

POINTS TO REMEMBER

1. Scrotal tongue refers to fissured tongue, which is a benign condition and require no treatment unless inflamed.
2. Fordyc's spots are functioning sebacious gland found frequently on the buccal surface of the oral cavity.
3. Epulis is a benign localized swelling of the gingiva.
4. Prolong use of antibiotics and corticosteroids can cause oral candidiasis.

50

Inflammatory Conditions of the Pharynx

PHARYNGITIS

Definition

Pharyngitis is a mucosal and submucosal inflammation of the pharynx that can include the oropharynx, nasopharynx, hypopharynx, adenoids, and tonsils.

Infection may or may not be a component of the disease. Because of high concentrations of lymphoid tissue, these sites are prone to reactive changes, especially in response to pathogenic viral or bacterial organisms.

NASOPHARYNGITIS

It is of two types:

1. Acute—Viral or bacterial
2. Chronic
   (i) Non-specific
   (ii) Specific
   (iii) Atrophic.

I. Chronic Non-specific Nasopharyngitis

- Secondary to rhinitis or sinusitis
- Secondary to excessive exposure to dust

Clinical Features

- Postnasal and palatal irritation
- Mucopurulent sticky postnasal discharge
- Occasional blood stained discharge may be present
- On postnasal examination, congestion of the mucosa and sticky mucopurulent discharge in the postnasal space can be seen

Differential Diagnosis

- Allergic rhinitis with pharyngitis
- Chronic maxillary sinusitis
- Psychoneurosis

Treatment of the underlying cause

II. Chronic Specific Nasopharyngitis

- **Syphilitic lesions** hardly ever seen in the nasopharynx
- **Tuberculous deposits** may occur in miliary spread and also secondary to pulmonary tuberculosis due to deposition of the infected sputum.
- **Scleroma**
  - Spreads into the nasopharynx from the nasal cavities
  - Rare disease but common in certain geographical locations like North Africa, Eastern Europe and Central America.
  - *Sites of predilection* posterior end of septum, eustachian cushions
  - *Gothic palate* dense scar tissue formation after initial catarrhal and granulomatous stage which affects the soft palate

retracting it upwards. The nasopharynx becomes almost closed off with scar tissue.
– Treatment is with systemic tetracyclines or streptomycin

III. Chronic Atrophic Nasopharyngitis

• Occurs as an extension of atrophic rhinitis
• Postnasal mirror examination shows dry crusts adhering to dry looking mucous membrane.

OROPHARYNGITIS

It is of two types:

1. *Acute*
   • Acute non-specific oropharyngitis
   • Acute specific oropharyngitis
2. *Chronic*
   • Chronic non-specific oropharyngitis
   • Chronic specific oropharyngitis

Acute Oropharyngitis

This is usually due to viral infection which is followed by secondary bacterial infection. The inflammation involves the pharynx including the mucosa covering the tonsils. This often results from generalized upper respiratory tract infection.

Etiology

1 ***Causative agents***
   – **Viruses:** Adeno, rhino, respiratory syncytial virus and rarely influenza and parainfluenza virus. Can be part of exanthematous fevers like varicella and measles.
   – **Bacterial:** *Streptococcus hemolytics*, non-hemolytic streptococcus, pneumococcus, *hemophilus influenzae*.
• ***Etiological factors***
   – Climatic conditions like cold and damp weather, sudden change of temperature can affect low immune individuals.
   – Local trauma and corrosive injury.
   – Environmental pollution like exposure to smoke, dust, chemicals, etc.

Clinical Features

This can occur in mild or severe forms:

1. *Mild form*
   • Sore throat is common
   • Low grade fever
   • Enlargement of regional cervical lymph nodes which may be tender.
2. *Severe form*
   • Associated with high grade fever (usually 100–105°F)
   • Rigor may preceed the attack
   • Uvula and soft palate are usually edematous
   • Mucopurulent exudate is usually seen and it can be associated with a non-adherent membrane mimicking diphtheria and may involve whole of the pharynx and the oral cavity.
   • Circumoral pallor and flushed face are common.
   • Patient may develop scarlet fever if associated with streptococcal infection.

Complications

• Otitis media
• Laryngitis
• Bronchitis
• Edema of the glottis especially in children
• Acute supraglottic laryngitis (if *H. influenzae* infection is present)
• Ludwig's angina if infection spreads to submandibular space
• Septicemia, pericarditis, meningitis and nephritis are rare in the antibiotic era.

Differential Diagnosis

• Acute tonsillitis
• Diphtheria
• Vincent's angina
• Leukemic angina
• Monocytic angina (infectious mono-nucleosis)
• Exanthematous conditions
• Blood dyscrasias

Investigations

- Complete blood picture including total and differential count and peripheral smear for hemopoietic disorders.
- Throat swab should be taken to rule out diphtheria and to isolate the causative agent in case of secondary bacterial infection.

Treatment

- Systemic broad spectrum antibiotics in more severe cases
- Anti-inflammatory antipyretics like paracetamol, aceclofenac, ibuprofen, etc.
- Antiseptic gargles may be helpful
- Throat lozenges may be given for soothing effect
- Treatment of complications, if present (discussed under respective chapters)

ACUTE SPECIFIC PHARYNGITIS

DIPHTHERITIC PHARYNGITIS

Synonym: Faucial diphtheria

Definition

A severe contagious and life threatening infection of the pharynx and the faucial area including the tonsils caused by *Corynebacterium diphtheriae.*

Incidence

Rare nowadays due to effective immunization program.

Etiology

- *Causative agent:* The causative agent is *Corynebacterium diphtherae.* This produces endotoxins that is absorbed from the membrane into the blood stream and is responsible for its severity of symptoms and complications-neurological and cardiac.
- *Mode of transmission:* Close contact with patient's discharges and by droplet infection like coughing and sneezing.

- Incubation period: 2 to 4 days
- *Types:* It can be in three forms depending on the strain. Gravis, intermedius and Mitis
- Staining is by Albert's stain which shows the characteristic *'Chinese letter pattern'* of the bacilli.

Pathology

There is formation of greyish white membrane over the tonsils, pillars and the posterior pharyngeal wall. Membrane is more adherent to the underlying structures and bleeds easily on removal.

Symptoms

- *General*
  - Fever of 101°F with pulse raised out of proportion
  - Features of toxemia is marked
  - Malaise
  - Joint pain
- *Local*
  - Sore throat
  - Odynophagia
  - Stridor if it spreads to the larynx

Signs

- Greyish white patch can be seen covering the tonsils and adjacent structures. This pseudo-membrane cannot be removed easily unlike nasal diphtheria (Fig. 50.1).
- False membrane may be absent in atypical cases which may simulate streptococcal infection.
- Toxic features are severe compared to nasal diphtheria
- Palatal paralysis, peripheral nerve paralysis and myocarditis are seen in some cases due to toxins and usually is seen after 2 to 3 weeks after infection.
- Cervical lymph nodes are markedly enlarged giving Bull neck appearance

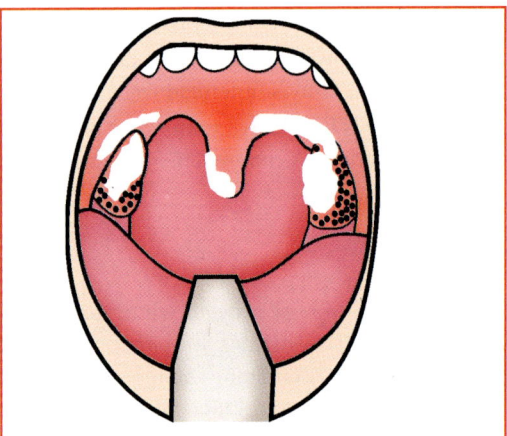

Fig. 50.1: Greyish white patch over the tonsils and uvula

Differential Diagnosis

- All forms of membranous pharyngitis as discussed under membrane over the tonsils

Investigations

- Complete blood picture
- ESR
- Throat swab is very important. Culture and staining is done to confirm the diagnosis. *Culture media:* Loffler's serum slope or blood agar.

Treatment

- Hospitalization and isolation
- Anti – Diphtheric Serum of about 40,000 to 100,000 units should be started immediately when the infection is suspected.
- Inj. Crystalline Penicillin is the drug of choice to control primary and secondary infection.
- Intubation/ tracheostomy may be needed if associated with airway obstruction or paralysis of the chest muscles.

Prevention

Routine vaccination of both children and adults is essential to prevent the re-emergence

VINCENT'S ANGINA

Synonym: Trench mouth

Definition

It is an acute ulcerative lesion of the pharynx that involves one or both tonsil and usually extends to fauces, soft palate and gums.

Etiology

- *Causative agent:* Two organisms namely *Fusiform bacillus* and *Spirocheta denticola*
- *Epidemiology:* Was common in troops during world war-I due to overcrowding in trenches (trench mouth)
  Other predisposing factors
  - Caries teeth
  - Pyorrhea
  - Poor diet

Clinical Features

- Sudden onset
- Sore throat
- Pain is usually severe
- Fetor oris
- High grade fever
- Cervical adenitis
- Associated area is covered with greyish membranous slough, which on separation is associated with considerable loss of tissue. Base of the ulcer usually bleeds and the slough reforms after removal (Fig. 50.2).
- Though the acute symptoms subside in 4 to 7 days, the ulcers may persist for few weeks.

Investigations

- Swab for staining and culture
- Gentian violet-stained smear of the pharyngeal exudate demonstrates the presence of Fusobacterium and spirochetes

Treatment

- Systemic antibiotics including Metro-nidazole, Penicillin or Clindamycin and

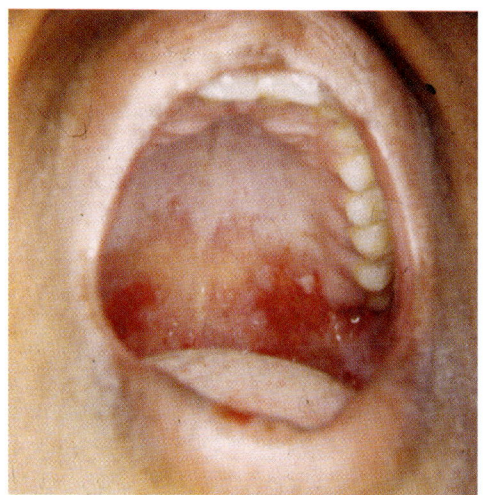

Fig. 50.2: Vincent's Angina

surgical debridement are the recommended treatment.
- Antiseptic mouth wash
- Antiseptic paint over fauces and gums

A. CHRONIC NON-SPECIFIC OROPHARYNGITIS

Chronic pharyngitis may be due to a primary infection in the pharyngeal tissues but more commonly the pharynx becomes infected as a result of disease in other parts of the upper respiratory tract or other systems.

- The usual age group to be affected is 15 years onwards
- Both the sexes are equally affected

Predisposing Factors

1. *Endogenous*
- *Nose and paranasal sinuses:* Allergic rhinitis and chronic sinusitis.
- *Oral cavity and oropharynx:* Chronic tonsillitis, dental sepsis, post-tonsillectomy complication, dyspeptics complaining of pharyngeal symptoms like gastritis, water brash or eructation after aerophagy

- *Respiratory tract:* Chronic bronchitis and bronchiectasis
- Gastroesophagial reflux disease (GERD)

2. *Exogenous*
- Tobacco
- *Atmospheric pollutants*—smoke, industrial waste products (irritant fumes)
- Alcohol
- Habitual use of condiments and highly spiced foods

3. *Functional*
- Emotional factors are sometimes responsible
- Pharyngeal neurosis leading to excessive hawking
- Faulty or excessive use of voice

4. *Miscellaneous*
(a) ***Mouth breathing:*** When the air is breathed in through the mouth, it is not subjected to humidification, warming and cleansing which normally takes place during its passage over the nasal mucosa. Thereby, the pharyngeal mucosa becomes dry, and is subjected to an abnormal degree of infection. Causes are as follows:
(*i*) *Nasopharyngeal*
- In young patients due to adenoid hypertrophy
- In older patients, tumors of nasopharynx or antrochonal or ethmoidal polyp.
(*ii*) *Nasal*
- Nasal obstruction maybe due to maldevelopment, congenital atresia of the posterior chonae, or due to structural defects like deflection of the nasal septum or large turbinates
- Inflammatory conditions such as acute or chronic rhinitis causing thickening of the nasal mucosa, as also in allergic states.
- Nasal polyp
- Rarely tumors causing complete obstruction
- Narrowing of nasal airway due to scarring after acute infections, syphilis, lupus or leprosy

(*iii*) *Dental:* Protruding teeth prevents lips from coming into apposition thus preventing the normal development of the alveolus and palate with aggravation of the dental condition

(*iv*) *Habitual*
- In those whose organic nasal obstruction has been relieved
- Treatment is breathing exercises

(*b*) ***General condition of the patient*** like diabetes and immunocompromised states

Clinical Types

1. ***Simple:*** In which there is dusky red congestion of the mucosa or a pale mauvish edema due to engorgement of vessels which may be seen coursing over the posterior pharyngeal wall. There are thickened anterior pillars of the fauces. The uvula may appear enlarged or elongated. There is increased secretion of mucous, and the walls of the pharynx maybe covered with frothy fluid (Chronic hyperemic pharyngitis).

2. ***Hypertrophic:*** Small nodules of hypertrophied lymphoid tissue are scattered over the pharyngeal wall, giving a granular appearance which may coalesce to form large masses (Figs 50.3 and 50.4). The lateral pharyngeal bands may be very prominent (Granular pharyngitis).

3. ***Follicular:*** Usually accompanied by similar infections in the tonsils when present. Small yellowish cysts are seen, commonly in the valleculae, which often escape notice.

Symptoms

- Dry cough and retching
- Irritation due to foreign body sensation in throat
- Dryness and discomfort on waking up oftendue to mouth breathing
- Pain in throat
- Early voice fatigue
- Snoring.

Treatment

- Rest
- Avoid coughing and hawking
- Stop smoking, alcohol and spices
- Voice rest
- Warm saline gargles and steam inhalation
- Cryosurgery may be useful if done on the hypertrophied lymphoid tissue
- Oral cavity care

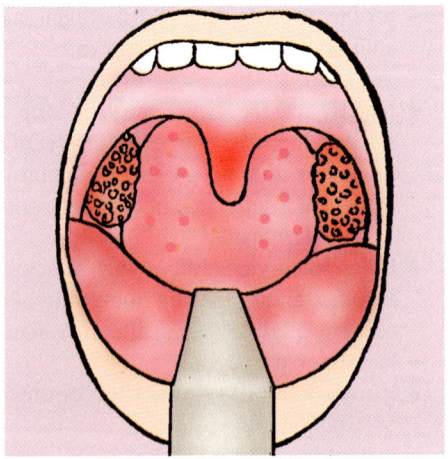

Fig. 50.3: Prominent lymphoid follicles in the posterior pharyngeal wall

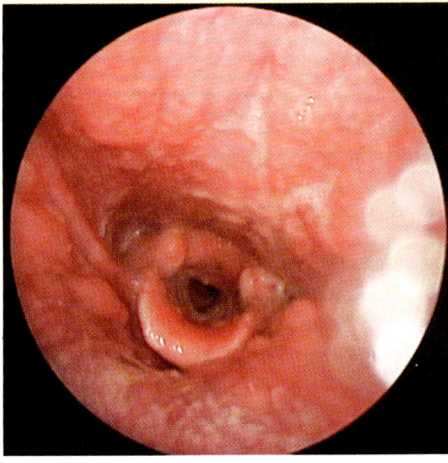

Fig. 50.4: Endoscopic picture of a patient with severe granular pharyngitis

- Regulated diet and eating habits
- Treat the underlying factors like GERD, naso sinus sepsis, dental sepsis, bronchiectasis, etc.

CHRONIC ATROPHIC PHARYNGITIS

Etiology

- It is associated with atrophic rhinitis
- It is regarded as direct extension of disease from the nose. It can spread to laryngopharynx and may involve larynx and trachea.
- In its mild form it is known as pharyngitis sicca. It may follow granular pharyngitis or conditions that lead to mouth breathing.
- It is sometimes associated with diabetes mellitus or gout.

Symptoms

- Irritation of throat
- Dryness of throat (relief on taking sips of water).
- Constant coughing and hawking due to the presence of crusts.
- Talking aggravates the condition

Signs

- Dry parchment like appearance of pharynx due to atrophy of pharyngeal mucosa and mucous glands.
- Glazed surface which becomes wrinkled when the muscle contracts
- Fetor oris due to secondary infection of the crusts formed.
- Pharyngeal lumen appears large due to thinning of walls and cervical spine outline may be clearly seen.

Treatment

- Saline gargles
- Removal of crusts with the help of oily applicator or hydrogen peroxide.
- Alkaline lotions should be sprayed on pharynx three times a day.

- 10 per cent glucose in glycerin improves the condition of nose.
- Potassium iodide administration in 325 mg. dose to promote secretion of mucous for short periods.
- Treatment of atrophic rhinitis by Young's or Modified Young's surgery.
- Other treatment as in chronic pharyngitis.

Chronic Specific Oropharyngitis

Chronic specific pharyngitis is usually due to granulomatous conditions of the pharynx that may be infectious, non-infectious or due to systemic diseases and in neoplasms.

A granuloma is a chronic inflammatory process characterized by the presence of modified macrophages (or epithelioid histiocytes) usually surrounded by other inflammatory cells and fibroblasts. Coalescence of these epithelioid histiocytes result in the formation of giant cells.

Infectious Causes

- *Bacterial:*
  - Tuberculosis
  - Leprosy
  - Syphilis
- *Parasitic:*
  - *Leishmania brasiliensis*
  - *Toxoplasma gondii*
- *Miscellaneous:*
  - Sarcoidosis

Non-infectious Causes

- Foreign bodies
- Tonsillolith

Systemic Causes

- Wegener's granulomatosis
- Crohn's disease

Neoplasms

- Hodgkin's lymphoma
- Non-Hodgkin's lymphoma
- Malignant lymphomas
- Metastatic tumors

TUBERCULAR PHARYNGITIS

- Infection caused by *Mycobacterium tuberculosis*
- Involvement of pharynx is rare
- It often occurs due to expectoration of infected sputum from a pulmonary focus.
- It occurs secondary to disease in the lungs, larynx, nose or mouth.
- Seen often in young males
- It occurs in three forms:
  – Widespread acute miliary tuberculosis
  – Chronic forms with infiltration, ulceration or tuberculoma
  – Extremely chronic form of lupus vulgaris.

(a) Acute Miliary Form

- Systemic spread of tubercle bacilli by blood stream.
- Eruption of tubercles on the fauces, soft palate, base of tongue or buccal mucosa. These tubercles coalesce and break down to form superficial grey ulcers with crenate margins with surrounding inflammatory reaction
- Symptoms of acute pain, dysphagia, tendency to bleed and excessive salivation, a muffled voice from swollen palate, continued fever, sepsis, hemorrhage, exhaustion. The general condition of the patient deteriorates rapidly.

(b) Chronic Tuberculous Ulceration

- Always associated with advanced pulmonary tuberculosis
- Sputum laden with tubercle bacilli
- Initial pale grey or red soft infiltrations form in one or more areas about the fauces or posterior pharyngeal wall, with slight surrounding inflammation. Slow or more rapid ulceration occurs with the formation of superficial ulcers covered with grey granulations and pus with 'mouse-nibbled' margins and undermined soft bleeding edges.
- In the nasopharynx, a tuberculoma may form which is a soft red tumor which bleeds on probing and which later rapidly ulcerates.
- It shows a tendency for recurrent infection
- Symptoms of severe pain, dysphagia, otalgia and change in voice (nasal voice) may be seen.

Diagnosis

- Pus from ulcers showing tubercle bacilli.
- Biopsy shows tuberculous nature of lesions
- Sputum AFB and Culture and Sensitivity-positive
- X-ray Chest to confirm tuberculosis
- Mantoux test

Treatment

- Mouth washes
- Analgesics
- Anti-tubercular treatment

(c) Lupus Vulgaris

- It is uncommon and is a cutaneous manifestation of tuberculosis
- Associated with lupus of face or nose and it is secondary to latter
- Occasionally lupus of larynx is also seen
- Disease runs a chronic course
- Most common in young women
- Most common site is anterior end of nasal septum.

Symptoms

- Voice change due to fixation of palate
- Difficulty in swallowing
- In early stages, burning sensation and slight degree of sore throat.
- In advanced stages, regurgitation of fluids through nose.

Pathology

- In the pharynx, the soft palate and the fauces may be affected, but rarely with tonsils.
- There is associated disease in the nose, larynx and infrequently in the chest.
- There is considerable surrounding reaction because of marked infiltration of lymphoid cells.

- Eruption of apple-jelly nodules that soon become grey and appear more solid, microscopically they resemble tubercles.
- In rare cases, hard palate is affected; bone may be exposed but is not involved in the disease process.
- Scarring is present in the palate
- Uvula may reduce in size or may vanish
- There will be no cervical adenitis

Differential Diagnosis

- Tertiary syphilitic ulceration
- Leprosy
- Lymphoma
- Scleroma

Investigation

- Biopsy

Treatment

- *Local:* UV rays application as from a cold generator
- Oral hygiene
- *General*: Good hygiene, proper diet, rest
- *Systemic*: Antitubercular treatment for 18–24 months
- Regular follow–up is necessary to detect relapses.

Tuberculosis of Tonsils and Adenoids

- Mode of infection is unknown, it could be due to bovine type of tubercule bacillius which has gained entrance in milk
- Typical tubercles in the depths of lymphoid follicles
- Exclusively in children and young adults
- Tuberculous cervical glands are characteristic

Symptoms

- None
- There may or may not be usual hyperplasia of lymphatic structures

Management

- Should be suspected when tuberculous cervical glands are present.

- Microscopic examination of excised tonsil and adenoids are confirmatory.
- Anti–tubercular treatment is required in addition to removal of tonsils and other suspected lymphoid tissue. This should be the rule when tuberculous cervical lymph nodes are present.

Atypical Mycobacterial Pharyngitis

- It has become prevalent in the last decade.
- It is less virulent than *M.tuberculosis* or *M.bovis*
- It infects persons with altered host defenses, especially patients with AIDS in whom atypical mycobacteria disease (especially *M.aviumintracellular*) involves lower respiratory tract and gastrointestinal tract.
- In children, cervical lymph node enlargement is seen and its usual cause is *M. scrofulaceum.*

SYPHILIS OF THE PHARYNX

Syphilitic lesions of the pharynx occur at any stage of the disease but in the secondary stage, the spirochates are widely distributed throughout the body and thus the manifestations of it are seen.

(a) Primary Syphilis: Chancre of Pharynx

- Most common site for extragenital chancre is the lip and mouth.
- Chancre may be situated on the tonsil, or cheek and may be mistaken for carcinoma or Vincent's infection.
- It is unilateral in nature.
- It runs an indolent course and persists for weeks.

Symptoms

- Hard infiltration of the upper pole of the tonsil and pillars, with some difficulty in swallowing. Erosion and slight soreness and redness of surrounding mucosa.
- The lesion presents the typical feature of primary chancre with the 'cartilagenous' base and ulceration with dirty slough but may remain small due to the relative absence of secondary infection.

- Characteristic rubbery feel of enlarged regional lymph nodes usually on the same side.

Diagnosis

Wasserman test is not usually positive till the secondary stage. Examination under dark ground illumination of smear taken from lesion reveals *Treponema pallidum* which has to be differentiated from spirochaetes that normally inhabit the mouth (Vincent's organisms).

Differential Diagnosis of Chancre

- Quinsy
- Tuberculosis
- Lymphoma
- Sarcoma
- Agranulocytosis
- Vincent's angina
- Diphtheria

(b) Secondary Syphilis

- Usually arises in 6 to 8 weeks
- Spirochaetes are widely distributed throughout the body
- Most infective state of disease
- Multiple mucous patches are found on the lips, inside the cheeks, edges of the tongue, the tonsillar pillars and the fauces, pharyngeal wall and base of tongue. They appear as slightly raised round or oval bluish or pearly lesion on a slightly congested mucosa. They disappear or reappear in crops.
- Symmetrically placed snail track ulcers with dirty grey color.
- Rare condyloma, a warty grey thickened patch occurring in protected areas such as the inside of the cheek or nasopharynx.
- Cervical glands are enlarged and there may be skin eruptions.
- Rash distribution all over the body and when forehead is involved it is called corona veneris.
- Associated anemia and alopecia may be present.

Symptoms

- No local symptoms
- Low grade sore throat due to erythema without fever lasting for weeks.
- Pain when mucous patches ulcerates on taking hot or spicy foods or by smoking.

Differential Diagnosis of Secondary Syphilis

- Aphthae
- Herpes
- Pemphigus
- Lichen ruber planus
- Mercurial stomatitis

Diagnosis

- Dark field smear will demonstrate *Spirochaeta pallida*
- Positive Wasserman test
- Other serological tests will be positive.

(c) Tertiary Stage – Gumma of Pharynx

- Occurs as a localized mass where there is more diffuse infiltration.
- Manifestation occurs with secondary stage or may occur many years later.
- Sites of lesion are: Soft and hard palate, posterior surface of the velum, the posterior surface of the nasopharynx, the region below the auditory tube, mouth and rarely tonsil or tongue.
- Lesions tend to be multiple or maybe in successive crops which may form years apart.

Symptoms

- Painless mass for months causing mechanical interference with swallowing or speech.

Pathology

Chronic infection of tissues with endarteritis of arterioles leading to necrosis in the area of their distribution.

Secondary infection leads to:

- Formation of punched out ulcer with a wash leather slough at the base.
- Bone is commonly involved.

- Thus, there maybe perforation of the hard palate.
- Soft tissues are also affected; there maybe ulceration of tonsil and pharynx which is often seen.
- Since nerve endings are destroyed early there is little pain and ulceration of palate and fauces.
- Regional lymph nodes become affected; cervical and epitrochlear adenitis is present.

Differential Diagnosis

- Large pharyngeal tuberculous ulcer maybe present which maybe painless.
- May resemble peritonsillar abscess or subacute type of fusospirochaetal infection.
- It could be malignancy for which a biopsy is required.
- Perforation of palate due to trauma or lupus vulgaris
- Scleroma
- Wegener's granulomatosis
- Actinomycosis

Diagnosis

- From the history of the disease.
- Positive Wasserman's test or other specific test in blood or spinal fluid.

(d) Congenital Syphilis

- Pharynx may be involved in gummatous infiltration owing to infection acquired in utero. Lesions resemble those seen in tertiary syphilis but progress more slowly with considerable scarring in consequence. There maybe perforation of palate.
- Permanent teeth may be affected, especially upper incisors and produce a deformity— Hutchinson's teeth wherein the cutting edges are eroded and tend to become semilunar; while the whole tooth is malformed and becomes like a peg.

Treatment

- Local—Gargle with hydrogen peroxide or alkaline solutions

- Systemic penicillin is administered.
- Treatment as described under *Syphilis of the Nose.*

Scleroma of Pharynx

- It is a rare chronic inflammatory disease occurring in parts of Eastern Europe, North Africa, Central America.
- Causative organism has been described by Frisch is the *Klebsiella scleromatosis.*
- Disease usually begins in the nose, spreading from there to nasopharynx, pharynx and larynx.
- Histological appearance is characterized by Mikulicz cells, Russell bodies and Gram negative bacteria.

Clinical Features

- Painless, hard almost cartilaginous induration replaces the pharyngeal wall.
- Usually spreads down from nasopharynx that may become closed off by the bulky tissue and by cicatrization.
- No ulceration is seen.

Differential Diagnosis

- Lupus
- Syphilis
- Leprosy
- Tuberculosis
- Lymphoma
- Malignant disease

Treatment

- *Systemic antibiotics:* Tetracyclines and Streptomycin and are often used together with systemic steroids.
- *Surgery:* Obstructive tissue may be removed surgically from the nasopharynx ideally using laser.

Leprosy of Pharynx

- It is a chronic inflammatory disease that is caused by *Mycobacterium leprae.*
- Site of predilection is the nose, eventually the disease may involve the skin and peripheral nerves as well as mucous membranes.
- Tuberculoid leprosy is a low grade lesion affecting an area of skin and its nerve supply

while lepromatous leprosy is a more florid form of the disease with massive infection of the dermis of the skin. It can affect the nasal cavities, nasopharynx and also the testis and lymphoreticular system.

Clinical Features

- Leprous nodules become ulcerated and then healing occurs, leaving pale stellate scars on the pharynx and palate.
- Uvula becomes granular and ulcerated and may be destroyed.
- Perforation of the palate may occur.
- The leprous lesion is painless.

Diagnosis

- It can be made on clinical grounds by physical examination.
- In early stages, the copious mucoid nasal discharge contains huge numbers of *M.leprae*
- Demonstration of bacilli in lesions.
- Histological examination of thickened skin or nervous tissue in tuberculoid type.
- Lepromin skin test is positive in tuberculoid type of leprosy and is negative in lepromatous type of leprosy

Treatment

- Long-term chemotherapy with rifampicin, clofazime and dapsone.

Toxoplasmosis

- Common disease of birds and mammals caused by protozoan *Toxoplasma gondii.*
- Infection is transmitted to humans by the ingestion of cysts in uncooked meat or food contaminated with animal feces.
- In immunocompetent humans, acquired toxoplasmosis may give rise to no symptoms but in immunocompromised patients it may eventually result in multisystem failure and death.
- Disease is usually self-limiting.

Clinical Features

- Sore throat

- Fever with malaise lasting for several weeks
- Cervical lymphadenopathy
- Multisystem involvement such as lungs, myocardium, pericardium, liver, brain and skeletal muscles.

Diagnosis

- *Serological tests:* Indirect dye or fluorescent antibody test
- Biopsy of lymph nodes
- Histological study showing follicular hyperplasia and typical epitheloid cells.

Treatment

- Usually not necessary
- In those with severe systemic manifestation or in immunodeficient patients, a combination of pyrimethamine and sulfadiazine is indicated.

FUNGAL INFECTIONS

Candidiasis

- *Candida albicans* is a part of the flora of oral cavity or oropharynx in 30 to 40 percent of normal individuals.
- Any local change like lichen planus, leucoplakia or systemic change in the host will result in symptoms due to the pathogenic organisms.
- Therefore, it is known as the disease of the diseased.
- Systemic antibiotic administration may change the oral flora sufficiently to disturb the local balance and allow overgrowth of candida.
- Various other factors such as radiotherapy to the oral cavity and pharynx and the chronic ill-health of the patient is often complicated by candida.
- Thus, diabetes mellitus, acquired immunodeficiency syndrome (AIDS), lymphoma and treatment with immuno- suppressive agents predispose to candidiasis.

Clinical Features

- Usually asymptomatic

- Severe pain with dysphagia is sometimes the presenting feature.
- On examination, white patches are seen in the oral cavity and the pharynx, which when removed leaves an erythematous ulcer.

Treatment

Local

- Antifungal agents such as Nystatin 100,000 units 6th hourly.
- Cotrimazole (candid) oral paint is often beneficial
- Miconazole cream may be applied locally every 6th hourly

Systemic

- Ketoconazole or fluconazole 100 mg. twice daily is more effective.
- Amphotericin B 100,000 units 6th hourly is given only in severe cases in immuno-compromised patients.

Actinomycosis

- Rarely occurs in the pharynx.
- As elsewhere, deep ulcers and sinuses occur containing sulphur granules.
- Laboratory investigation of this material will be diagnostic.
- Treatment is long course of large doses of penicillin, continuing treatment for at least 2 months after clinical cure.

Blastomycosis

- Very rare but serious fungal infection which may involve the pharynx
- Formation of shallow granulating ulcers.
- Treatment is with amphotericin suspension 1 ml. 4 times daily held in contact with the lesions.
- Systemic treatment may be required if other areas are involved.

Sarcoidosis (Boeck's disease)

- This is a rare chronic granulomatous condition which occassionally involves the palate.
- It is a multisystem disorder of unknown etiology
- It commonly presents with hilar lymphadenopathy, pulmonary and cutaneous involvement.
- Extranodal head and neck involvement by sarcoidosis includes the ear and temporal bones, sinonasal region, salivary glands, pharynx, tonsils and larynx.
- Pharyngeal or tonsillar involvement may initially present as an inflammatory process and tonsillar hyperplasia may be observed.

Symptoms

- Chronic cough
- Dysphagia

Clinical Features

- Painless nodules appear which are white, brown or bluish with an injected areola.

Histopathological Findings

- Multiple non-caseating granulomas consisting of nodules of epitheloid histiocytes surrounded by mixed inflammatory infiltrate.
- Langhan's giant cells maybe present with a variety of cytoplasmic inclusions including star-shaped or calcific laminated bodies called asteroids and Schaumann bodies, respectively.
- Though these pathological features are characteristic they are not specific for sarcoidosis.

Diagnosis

- Biopsy
- Kviem's test maybe positive

Treatment

- Corticosteroid therapy: In such patients the prognosis is good with as many as 70 percent improving or remaining stable after therapy.
- Vitamin D

Tonsillolith (Calculus of tonsil)

- These are calculi created by deposition of lime salts (i.e. calcium and magnesium carbonates and phosphates) in any of the lingual, palatine and pharyngeal tonsillar crypts to form a hard mass.
- These formations are associated with crypts harboring *Leptothrix buccalis.*

Symptoms

- Halitosis
- Sore throat
- Discomfort
- Fever

Clinical Features

- Affected tonsillar tissue is frequently enlarged with stone producing chronic inflammation and discharge.

Treatment

- Removal of tonsillar tissue
- Reccurent stones in the tonsil is treated by tonsillectomy.

Wegener's Granulomatosis

- This is a rare disorder, considered to be an autoimmune disease, is characterized by acute necrotizing lesions on the respiratory tract, focal necrotizing vasculitis, and renal disease in the form of focal glomerulitis or diffuse glomerulonephritis.
- The disease begins in the upper airway, especially the sinuses in the pharynx, larynx or trachea.
- Affects adults, rarely seen in children.
- Peak incidence is seen in the 4th and 5th decades of life.
- The most frequent clinical presentation of Wegener's granulomatosis is in the nasal cavity and paranasal sinuses and less commonly in the pharynx.
- Other sites involved are the eye, orbit, palate and middle ear.

Histopathological Examination

- Poorly formed granulomas consisting of scattered multinucleated giant cells in and around areas of 'ischemic' necrosis.
- Vasculitis of small and medium sized arteries, lymphocytes and histiocytes.
- Non-specific inflammatory changes associated with neurons are often the most prominent features.

Symptoms

- Granulomatous involvement of oropharynx or larynx may result in hoarseness, sore throat or inspiratory stridor from upper airway obstruction.
- Patient often presents with persistent nasal discharge that is blood-stained.

    A modified or limited form of presentation of Wegener's granulomatosis primarily involving the nose, running a relatively benign history has been reported by Friedmann (1995) wherein patient complains of nasal obstruction, crusting and epistaxis and an initial diagnosis is of atrophic rhinitis. At such a point, nasal secretions will often grow *Staphylococcus aureus* and nasal biopsy is necessitated. Patient maybe going into crucial renal failure and renal biopsy is essential for early diagnosis and treatment.

Diagnosis

- Nasal biopsy
- Renal biopsy
- Autoantibody estimation by antineutrophil cytoplasmic antigens (ANCA) to differentiate between polyarteritis nodosa where their antigenic target is perinuclear and in Wegener's antigenic target is cytoplasmic. The specificity of this test is 85 to 98 percent. The titer of c-ANCA correlates well with activity of the disease and allows monitoring of therapy.
  - c-ANCA +ve – Diagnostic (True for acute phase of disease)
  - c-ANCA -ve—does not exclude the disease.

Treatment

- High steroid doses (40–60 mg. prednisolone /day)
- Cyclophosphomide used in doses of 2mg/kg/day.
- Azathioprine (3mg/kg/day)
- Regular irrigation and use of glucose in glycerine nose drops to reduce crusting.
- Surgery for sinus drainage maybe required.
- Correction of common saddle nose deformity is best left until control of disease is well established.

Differential Diagnosis

- Angiocentric malignant lymphoma has similar clinical and morphological presentation.

Crohn's Disease

- It is a granulomatous inflammatory process of unknown etiology
- Primarily affecting the small and large intestines.
- Pharyngeal involvement by Crohn's disease maybe be seen in 9 percent of the patients during course of disease which usually follows intestinal manifestations
- Infrequently, pharyngeal Crohn's disease precedes that of intestinal manifestation and is rarely the sole manifestation of the disease.

Treatment

- Cytotoxic drugs may be used
- Surgery is not curative.

51

Inflammation of the Lymphoid Follicles of the Waldeyer's Ring

Chronic Adenoiditis

Synonym: Adenoid hypertrophy, adenoids

Definition

Chronic inflammation/enlargement of the adenoids causing obstruction to the nasopharyngeal airway (Fig. 51.1) and consequent recurrent nasosinus infections, otitis media or maldevelopment of the face (adenoid facies).

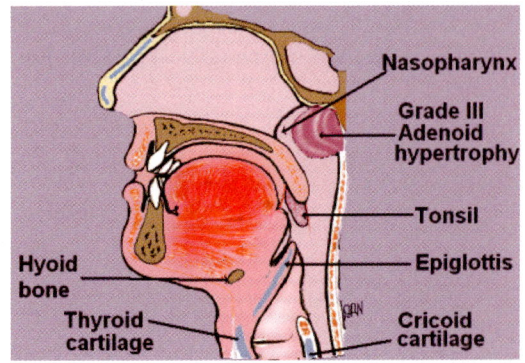

Fig. 51.1: Adenoid hypertrophy

History

In the late 1800s, Willhelm Meyer of Copenhagen, Denmark, proposed that adenoid vegetations were responsible for nasal symptoms and impaired hearing.

Etiology

- Common in children (Immunologically active age)
- Physiological hypertrophy—Peak 2–4 years
- Recurrent upper respiratory tract infections/allergy
- Low socioeconomic status
- Environmental factors—crowding, environmental pollution, etc.
- *H. Influenzae* infection has been commonly implicated in adenoid and tonsillar

hyperplasia. By about 6 months of age, various organisms including lactobacilli, anaerobic streptococci, actinomycosis, Fusobacterium species, and Nocardia species are present. Normal flora include alpha-hemolytic streptococci, enterococci, Corynebacterium species, coagulase-negative staphylococci, *Neisseria species*, *Haemophilus species*, *Micrococcus species*, and *Stomatococcus species*. The adenoids can become infected and harbor pathogenic bacteria, which may lead to the development of disease of the ears, nose, and sinuses. Recent studies show that the most commonly cultured bacteria in adenoiditis are *Haemophilus influenzae*, group A beta-hemolytic Streptococcus, *Staphylococcus aureus, Moraxella catarrhalis*, and *Streptococcus pneumoniae*, usually in that order.

- Tuberculosis can rarely affect the adenoids
- Adenoid hypertrophy in adults though not uncommon, should raise the suspicion of lymphoma.

Pathology and Immunology

Apart from physiological hypertrophy, the size of the adenoid has been found to be directly proportional to aerobic bacterial load and the number of B and T cells.

The distribution of dendritic cells, antigen presenting cells, is altered during disease, with fewer dendritic cells in the surface epithelium and more in the crypts and extrafollicular areas.

Clinical Features

Symptoms

- ***Nasal symptoms:*** (Due to obstruction/ recurrent nasosinus infection)
  - Nasal obstruction which may be associated with mouth breathing and snoring is the most common symptom.
  - Anterior nasal discharge which may be mucoid or mucopurulent
  - Postnasal discharge is also common
  - Obstructive sleep apnea may be seen in severe cases
  - Hyponasal speech (Rhinolalia clausa)
  - Epistaxis is rare and present due to acute exacerbations

Aural symptoms: (Due to ET dysfunction/ AOM/ SOM/ CSOM)

- Recurrent otalgia, deafness, ear discharge, etc.

Throat symptoms: (Due to recurrent pharyngitis/ tonsillitis/ mouth breathing)

- Recurrent sore throat, dysphagia, change in voice, poor eaters, malnutrition

- ***General Symptoms:***
  - Mental dullness
  - Nocturnal eneurisis
  - Night terrors

Signs

Nasal

- Discharge is usually seen in the floor of the nasal cavity and in middle meatus if associated with sinusitis
- Cold-spatula test shows decreased fogging on both the sides.
- Mucosal congestion and edema may be noted.
- Postnasal mirror examination in elderly children may reveal enlarged adenoid (Fig. 51.2).

Aural

- Retracted or bulging drum depending on the severity
- Fluid level may be present
- Tuning fork tests reveal conductive deafness
- Features of acute otitis media or chronic otitis media are not uncommon.

Throat

- Mucosal congestion of the pharynx
- Granular posterior pharyngeal wall
- Postnasal drip may be noted.

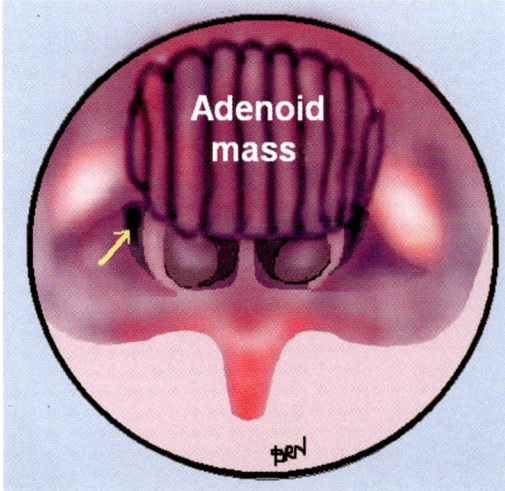

Fig. 51.2: Adenoid hypertrophy partially occluding the left eustachian tube orifice. Yellow arrow showing right eustachian tube orifice

Neck

- Cervical lymphadenopathy is commonly present involving upper deep cervical and posterior triangle nodes.

Facial Features (Adenoid Facies)

Chronic adenoid hypertrophy leads to long standing nasal obstruction which can cause following facial characteristics and abnormalities.

- Pinched nose
- Mouth breathing
- Dribbling of saliva
- Flat nasal arch
- Malar hypoplasia
- Elongated face
- Dull 'idiotic' appearance
- Loss of nasolabial fold
- Short protruding upper lip
- Crowding of teeth especially of the upper jaw
- High arched palate
- Deafness—Inattentive child

General Features

- Growth retardation
- Recurrent LRTI

- Frequent diarrhea
- Low nutritional status
- Pigeon shaped chest
- Protuberent abdomen
- Enuresis +/–

Investigations

- *Diagnostic nasal endoscopy:* This is a very useful tool in visualizing the degree of hypertrophy and the compromise in the nasopharyngeal airway especially in relation to the choana and the eustachian tube orifice (Figs 51.3a and b).
- *X-ray nasopharynx* (Lateral view of the head and neck—Soft tissue exposure) (Fig. 51.4).
- Sleep studies if sleep apnea is suspected

Treatment

Mild/ infrequent symptoms– Medical management

- Control of recurrent respiratory/aural infections
- Antihistamines and decongestants
- Steroid nasal spray like Mometasone may betried
- Improve nutritional status
- Breathing exercises

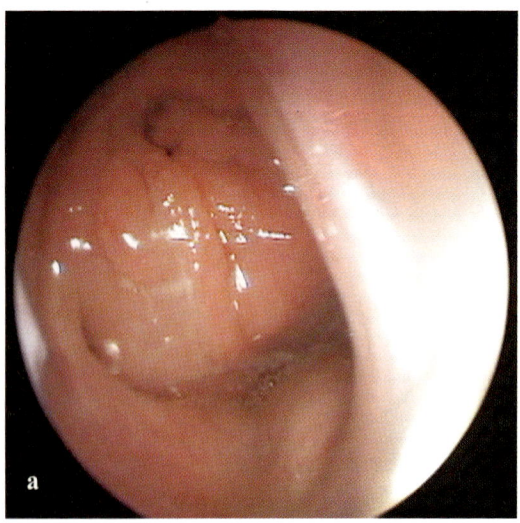 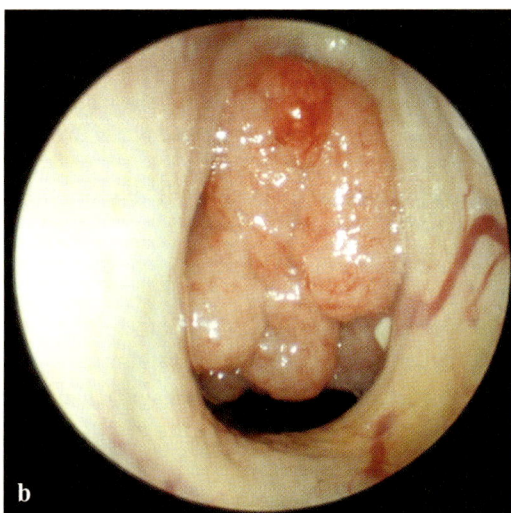

Figs 51.3a and b: Endoscopic view of small and large adenoid mass respectively

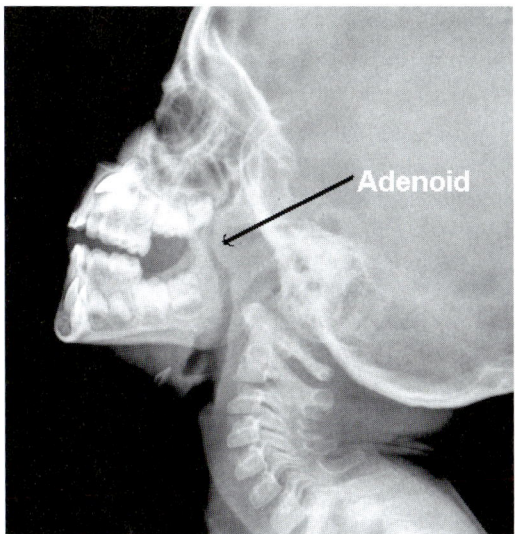

Fig. 51.4: X-ray lateral view of the neck showing adenoid hypertrophy occluding the nasopharyngeal airway

Moderate-severe/Persistent Symptoms

- Adenoidectomy
- Myringotomy and grommet insertion may be required if associated with otitis media with effusion.

Adenoidectomy

Indications

- Adenoid facies
- Adenoids causing nasal obstruction and mouth breathing
- *Septic focus*: Otitis media, chronic rhinosinusitis
- Snoring
- Sleep apnea syndrome

Contraindications

- Age < 3 years
- Bleeding disorders
- Acute infection
- Cervical spine pathology like unstable spine, mucopolysaccharidosis, etc.
- Epidemic of poliomyelitis

Technique

Types:

- *Conventional:* Curettage
- *Endoscopic:* Transnasal or transoral.

Steps of Adenoidectomy Curettage

- Orotracheal intubation.
- *Position*: Supine with extention of neck and atlantoaxial joint
- Place the Boyle-Davis mouth gag in position and the bipod stand is not used
- Palpate the nasopharynx to confirm the size of adenoid with respect to the choana and the septum.
- St. Clair Thomson's adenoid curette with/without cage (Fig. 51.5) is used.
- Insert the curette behind the soft palate till the posterior end of septum is felt (Fig. 51.6).
- Neck is flexed to avoid cervical lordosis thus preventing injury to the anterior spinal ligament during curettage.
- Push curette backwards to trap adenoids inside the curette
- Curette with sweeping motion—Downwards and forwards
- Curettage is repeated till choanae one patient on palpation.

Complications

- *Hemorrhage:* Primary and reactionary. Secondary hemorrhage is very rare.

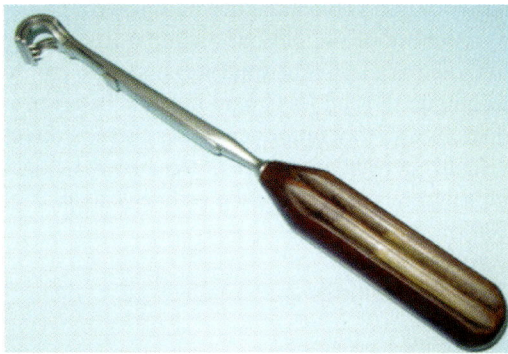

Fig. 51.5: St. Clair Thomson's adenoid curette with cage

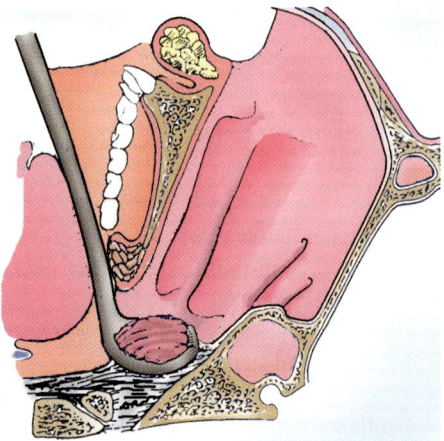

Fig. 51.6: Adenoid curettage in progress

- Aspiration
- *ET orifice injury*: Otitis media with effusion, suppurative otitis media
- Injury to soft palate, posterior pharyngeal wall, etc. may occur.
- Injury to anterior longitudinal ligament causing subluxation of the atlanto-occipital joint which may lead to quadriplegia.

Endoscopic Adenoidectomy

This is the recent development in the surgical management of adenoid hypertrophy. It was first described by Nayak et al in 1998 for a case of Scheie syndrome (MPS I S) which is associated with instability of the atlanto-axial joint and a traditional adenoidectomy is contraindicated as it needs proper positioning of the patient. Comparative study between the conventional versus endoscopic technique showed less blood loss and better post operative airway improvement as there is direct visualization and clearance of the airway without injuring the eustachian tube orifice (Nayak et al 2005).

Acute Tonsillitis

Definition

Acute inflammatory condition of the faucial tonsils often caused by *Streptococcus Hemolyticus,*

hemophilus influenzae or specific infections like diphtheria.

Types

- *Acute tonsillitis (Non-specific)*
- *Acute specific tonsillitis* (this has been discussed under specific pharyngitis) like:
  - *Diphtheretic tonsillitis*
  - *Infectious mononucleosis*
  - *Vincent's angina.*

Acute Tonsillitis (Non-specific)

Definition

Acute inflammatory condition of the fancial tonsil which may involve the mucosa, crypts, follicles and/ or tonsillar parenchyma.

Etiology

- *Causative Agents*
  - *Viral:* Initially starts with viral infection which is followed by secondary bacterial infection. Viruses commonly isolated include influenza, para-influenza, adenovirus and rhinovirus.
  - *Bacterial: Streptococcus hemolyticus, Hemophilus influenzae*, pneumococcus, *M. catarrahalis*, etc.

Pathology and pathogenesis: Usually it starts in childhood when there is a low immune status developed due to reduction in maternal immunity which initially protects the child during infancy and an inadequately developed child's own immunity which makes the child more prone for infection, especially viral. In fact the recurrent childhood infection involving the waldeyer's ring helps in future production of antibodies as the first line defense mechanism. Depending on the progress of the disease, this can be classified further into the following types (Fig. 51.7).

1. **Catarrhal tonsillitis:** It occurs due to viral infection of the upper respiratory tract, involving the mucosa of the tonsil.
2. **Cryptic tonsillitis:** Following viral infection, secondary bacterial infection supervenes and gets entrapped within the crypts leading to a

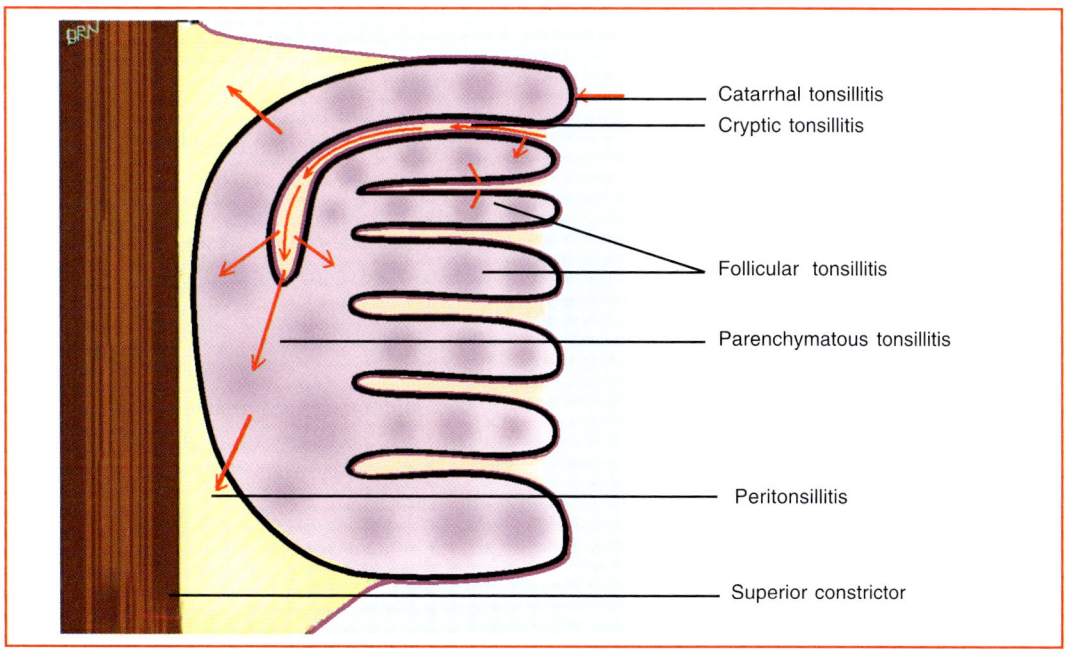

Fig. 51.7: Pathogenesis of various types of tonsillitis (Red arrows show the routes of spread of infection in various types of tonsillitis)

localized form of infection. The mucosa within the crypts gets swollen and is associated with inflammatory excudate which occupies the crypts.

3. **Acute follicular tonsillitis:** In severe form of infection of the tonsils caused by virulent organisms' like *streptococcus hemolyticus*, *Hemophilus influenzae*, etc. it causes spread of inflammation from tonsillar crypts to the surrounding tonsillar follicles. The follicles become inflamed and swollen. This inflammation is more commonly seen in adults. The surface of the tonsils appears irregular with crypts filled with yellowish white exudates which may coalesce to form a coating which gives an appearance of a false membrane (acute membranous tonsillitis).

4. **Acute parenchymal tonsillitis:** In children, the tonsillar parenchyma is loosely arranged with inadequate septae. Following the viral infection the immune status becomes significantly low. This allows the secondary bacterial infection to invade the crypts and that rapidly spreads into the tonsillar parenchyma. The tonsils appear swollen and uniformly enlarged.

Clinically mainly acute follicular and parenchymatous types of tonsillitis are encountered because of their characteristic clinical feature. The catarrhal and cryptic tonsillitis are often overlooked with upper respiratoy infection. Localized cryptic tonsillitis does not produce any significant symptom and rather helps in production of antibodies.

Recurrent acute infection of the tonsil can lead to spread of infection from the tonsil to the peritonsillar space causing peritonsillitis/peritonsillar abscess.

Clinical Features

Symptoms

- Fever which is always high grade
- Generalized malaise and bodyache

- Odynophagia (pain during swallowing)
- Dry cough
- Sore throat

Signs

- Congested and edematous tonsils
- Tonsils may be diffusely swollen in parenchymatous tonsillitis.
- Crypts can be seen filled with pus with swollen follicles in follicular tonsillitis (Fig. 51.8).
- When the pus from the crypts coalesce it gives a membranous appearance and is often termed as membranous tonsillitis (Fig. 51.9).
- Examination of the neck can reveal enlarged and tender jugulodigastric lymph nodes. There may be signs of generalized upper respiratory tract infection including adenoiditis in children.

Investigations

- Throat swab for culture and sensitivity
- Peripheral smear—To rule out hemopoeitic disorders like leukemia, agranulocytosis, etc.

- Paul-Bunnel test may be required if a membrane is seen to rule out infectious mononucleosis.
- X-ray of the paranasal sinuses (Water's view) to rule out nasosinus septic focus.
- X-ray soft tissue of nasopharynx to rule out adenoid hypertrophy.
- CT imaging of the sinuses and neck if sinus focus or complications of acute tonsillitis are suspected.

Treatment

If the symptoms are severe and if a membrane is present, it is necessary to hospitalize the patient for proper diagnosis and to prevent the complications.

Medical

- Penicillin is the drug of choice usually, especially for streptococcus. B-lactamase producing hemolytic streptococci should be treated with amoxicillin+clavulanic acid combination. Erythromycin should be preferred in patients sensitive to penicillin

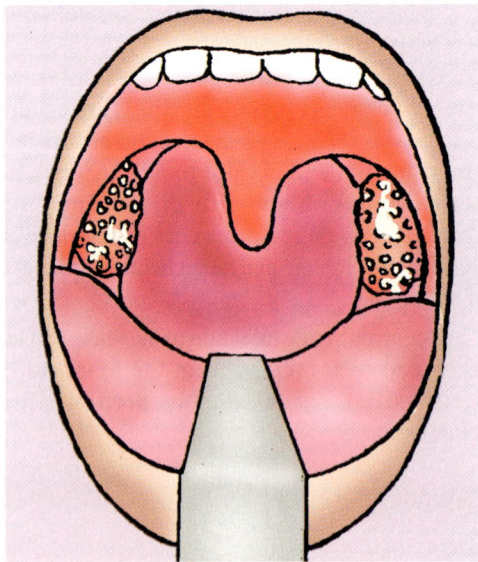

Fig. 51.8: Multiple follicles on the medial surface of both the tonsils and signs of acute inflammation

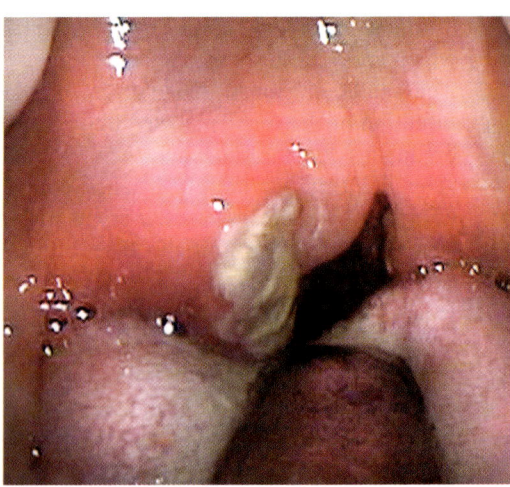

Fig. 51.9: Acute staphylococcal pseudo-membranous tonsillitis with unilateral hypertrophy of the right tonsil. This condition has to be differentiated from other causes of white patch on the tonsil (Table 51.2)

Table 51.1: Causes of white patch on the tonsil

Viral

- Infectious mononucleosis
- Herpes simplex
- HIV (secondary manifestation)

Bacterial

- Acute non-specific
  - Follicular tonsillitis
  - Staphylococcal pseudomembranous tonsillitis
- Acute specific
  - Faucial diphtheria
  - Vincent's angina
- Chronic non-specific
  - Keratosis of the tonsil
- Chronic specific
  - Tubercular tonsillitis
  - Secondary syphilis as mucous patch/ snail track ulcers

Fungal

- Candidiasis

Autoimmune

- Lichen planus
- Wegener's granulomatosis

Trauma

- Post–tonsillectomy
- Surgical trauma causing slough
- Foreign body
- Corrosive poisoning
- Thermal injury
- Post-radiation

Pre-malignant lesions

- Leukoplakia
- Submucous fibrosis

Tumor or tumor-like conditions

- Tonsillar cyst
- Tonsillolith
- Papilloma
- Fibroma of the tonsil
- Malignancy of the tonsillar fossa

Systemic

- Leukemia
- Agranulocytosis
- Aplastic anemia
- Blood dyscrasias

group of antibiotics. Injectable penicillin's like crystalline penicillin and co-amoxyclav, should be given in severe cases. Most of the patients respond to the antibiotics. Full course of the antibiotics should be given to prevent developing antibiotic resistance.

- Antiseptic gargles and throat lozenges may be given. Mandl's throat paint may alleviate pain.
- Paracetamol/ nimesulide for fever (nimesulide should be avoided in children). Anti-inflammatory for pain and inflammation.

Differential Diagnosis (Table 51.2)

- Scarlet fever
- Diphtheria
- Vincent's angina
- Agranulocytosis
- Infectious mononucleosis and
- Other causes of membrane over the tonsil

Complications: Have been discussed under chronic tonsillitis.

Chronic Tonsillitis

Definition

It is the chronic inflammation of the palatine (faucial) tonsils which occurs as a result of repeated attacks of acute tonsillitis or due to inadequately resolved acute tonsillitis.

Etiopathogenesis

- The most frequent etiological agent is β-hemolytic streptococcus
- It follows as a complication of acute tonsillitis. Pathologically microabscesses walled off by fibrous tissue have been seen in lymphoid follicles of tonsils.
- It may be a subclinical infection of tonsils without an acute attack.

- Mostly affects children and young adults.
- Predisposing factor maybe chronic infection in sinuses or teeth.

Clinicopathological Types

(a) *Chronic follicular tonsillitis:* Tonsillar crypts are full of infected cheesy material that shows on the surface as yellowish spots. This is more common in adults and results from repeated attacks of acute tonsillitis.

(b) *Chronic parenchymatous tonsillitis:* Following repeated attacks of acute tonsillitis the lymphoid follicles of tonsillar parenchyma undergo hyperplasia leading to uniform enlargement of the tonsil. The tonsils may be grossly enlarged causing obstruction to food and air passages. These patients may also have adenoid hypertrophy causing snoring and sleep apnea and later cor pulmonale. Tonsils are enlarged and may interfere with speech, deglutition or respiration.

(c) *Chronic fibrotic tonsillitis:* Here the tonsils are small due to atrophy, but the remnants may get infected leading to recurrent attacks.

Clinical Features

Symptoms

- Sore throat (recurrent attacks)—Three to four times a year
- Cough
- Hawking if there is associated adenoid hypertrophy or chronic sinusitis.
- Halitosis
- Bad taste in the mouth due to pus in crypts
- Thick speech
- Difficulty in swallowing
- Sleep apneic episodes
- Acute exacerbations produce symptoms similar to acute tonsillitis.

Four Cardinal Signs

1. Persistent congestion of the anterior pillars
2. Positive tonsillar squeeze (Ervin-Moore sign). A tongue depressor is placed on the anterior pillar and pressed against the tonsil

to squeeze. If purulent yellowish cheesy discharge escapes out from the crypts, the test is positive.

3. The jugulodigastric lymph node on either sides are usually enlarged but non-tender.

4. In chronic parenchymatous type of tonsillitis (Fig. 51.10), the tonsils are enlarged and may be graded into 4 types depending on this size.
   - **Grade I:** Tonsils are congested but are located within the tonsillar fossa.
   - **Grade II:** Tonsils hypertrophies till the brim of the tonsillar fossa.
   - **Grade III:** Tonsillar hypertrophy extends beyond the pillars but does not touch each other.
   - **Grade IV:** The tonsils are in contact with each other (Kissing tonsils) causing respiratory and deglutition problems.

Complications of Tonsillitis

- Peritonsillar abscess
- Parapharyngeal abscess
- Intratonsillar abscess
- Tonsillolith
- Tonsillar cyst
- Focus of infection in renal failure, acute glomerulonephritis, eye and skin disorders.

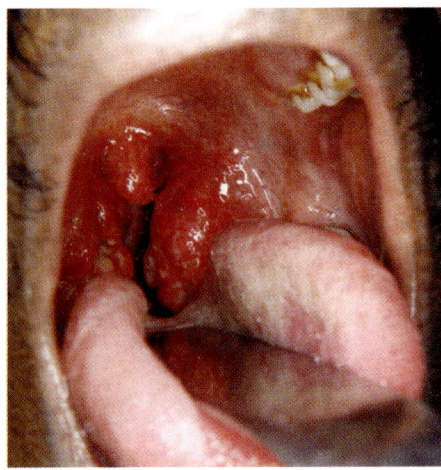

Fig. 51.10: Enlarged tonsils in chronic parenchymatous tonsillitis

Investigations

1. Complete blood picture including hemo-globin, total/differential count, ESR, platelet count and peripheral smear
2. *Bleeding:* Straight clotting and prothrombin and activated prothrombin time
3. Blood grouping
4. ASO titer
5. Throat swab for culture and sensitivity in acute exacerbations.
6. Evaluation of renal and cardiac functions if rheumatic disease is suspected
7. X-ray chest PA view
8. ECG may be required in elderly patients
9. X-ray lateral view neck/diagnostic nasal endoscopy to rule out co-existent adenoid hypertrophy

Treatment

- *Conservative*—General health, diet and treatment of co-existing infection of tooth, nose and sinuses. Treatment of acute exacerbations as in acute tonsillitis.
- *Surgical*—Tonsillectomy.

Tonsillectomy

Types

- Dissection method
- Cryosurgery
- Monopolar cautery assisted tonsillectomy
- Bipolar cautery assisted tonsillectomy with or without aid of microscope
- Laser assisted tonsillectomy
- Coblation tonsillectomy (Radiofrequency ablation)
- Harmonic scalpel assisted tonsillectomy
- Microdebrider assisted tonsillectomy
- Guillotine tonsillectomy

Indications

Absolute Indications

- Respiratory obstruction
- Peritonsillar abscess (4–6 weeks)
- Sleep apnea syndrome

Relative Indications

- Chronic tonsillitis
  - Not responding to medical treatment
  - More than 4 to 6 acute tonsillitis per year
  - Associated with cervical lymphadenopathy
  - Acting as septic focus for rheumatic heart disease, glomerulonephritis, arthritis, etc (β-hemolytic streptococcus)
  - Failure to thrive due to excessively enlarged tonsil
- Primary tuberculosis of the tonsil
- Carrier of diphtheria
- Tumors of tonsils
  - Benign—Papilloma
  - Malignant—Small tumors confined to tonsils
  - Suspected lymphoma in unilateral tonsillar enlargement
- Tonsillar cyst, tonsillolith, embedded FB in the tonsils, etc.
- Surgical approach
  - Elongated styloid process
  - Resection of ossified stylohyoid ligament
  - Glossopharyngeal neurectomy
  - As part of Uvulo-palato-pharyngo-plasty (UPPP).

Contraindications (ABCDEF)

- **A**ctive infection/**A**cute exacerbation, **A**neurysm of internal carotid artery, **A**ge below three years, **A**ctive menstruation.
- **B**leeding and clotting disorders
- **C**ervical spine pathology
- **D**iphtheritic tonsillitis. **D**rugs: Patients under aspirin, oral contraceptives, etc.
- **E**ndemic of polio
- **F**ailure to control systemic diseases like hypertension, diabetes, bronchial asthma, LRTI, etc.

Technique

- General anesthesia is preferred, though few centers perform tonsillectomy under local anesthesia in compliant patients

- Nasotracheal/orotracheal intubation with tube fixed in the midline.
- *Rose position:* Supine with extension of the neck and extension of the head at atlanto-occipital joint
- Boyle-Davis mouth gag is placed after choosing the correct size tongue blade so as to retract the base of the tongue and expose both the tonsillar fossae. Specialized tongue blade with groove for the endotracheal tube (Doughty's tongue blade) may be used in case of orotracheal intubation which avoids compression of the endotracheal tube (Fig. 51.12).
- Draffin's bipod stand is used to stabilize the Boyle-Davis mouth gag in position (Fig. 51.11).
- Superior pole of the tonsil is held using Dennis-Browne tonsil holding forceps or Luc's forceps and the tonsil is gently pulled medially to facilitate retraction of the tonsil from the anterior pillar and in showing a thin white line between the pillar and the tonsil (loose areolar tissue plane).
- Incision is given along that line using a 11 number blade and the incision is converted into a U shaped passing through the upper pole and the pillars (Fig. 51.12).
- Using a Mollison's tonsillar dissector with anterior pillar retractor, the tonsillar capsule is exposed and the tonsil is dissected along the loose areolar cleavage plane till the inferior pole of the tonsil is reached as shown in the Fig. 51.13.
- Tonsillar scissors may be required to divide tough fibrous band attached to the tonsillar capsule from the fossa. Fibrous band is divided close to the tonsillar capsule (Figs. 51.14 and 51.15).
- Eve's tonsillar snare is applied with its loop around the inferior pole and the tonsillar attachment is divided as shown in the Fig. 51.16.
- Hemostasis is achieved either by bipolar cautery or by catching the bleeder using a

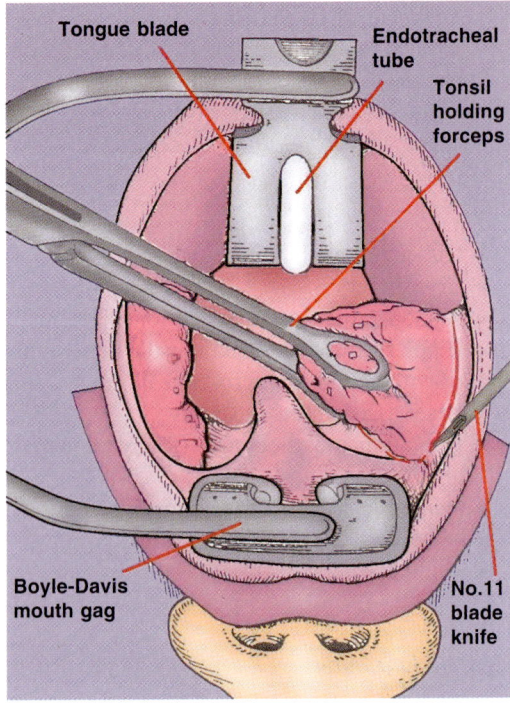

Fig. 51.12: Incision being given along the anterior pillar using No.11 blade knife

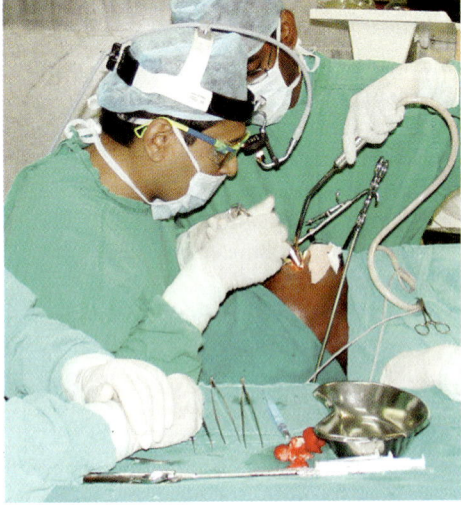

Fig. 51.11: Tonsillectomy being performed

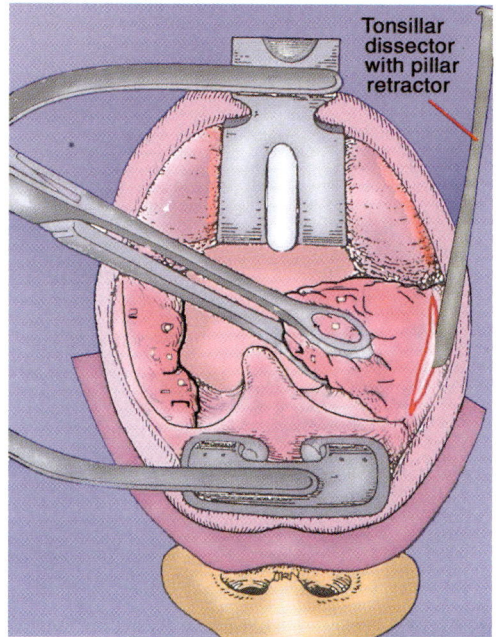

Fig. 51.13: Tonsil being dissected from the tonsillar bed using Mollison's tonsillar dissector

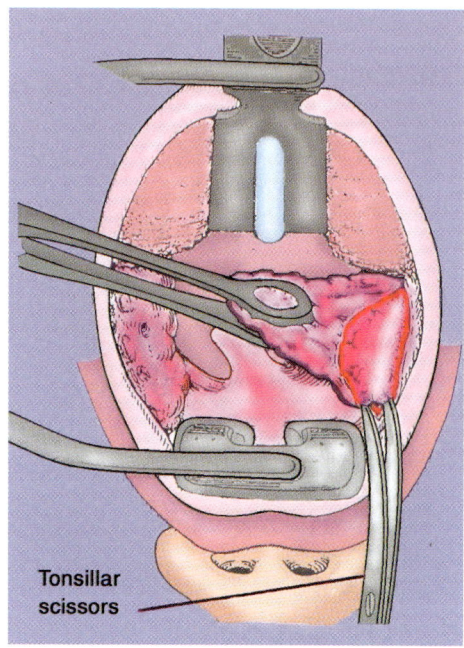

Fig. 51.14: Tonsil being dissected from the tonsillar bed using tonsillar scissors

straight tonsillar hemostat and then replaced by Negus curved tonsillar artery forceps which helps in ligation of the bleeder. The silk knot can be carried to the site using a Negus ligature carrier as shown in the Fig. 51.17.

Postoperative Care

- Lateral position: In the postoperative period the patient is placed in the lateral position to avoid any aspiration.
- Vital signs are monitored frequently. Look for tachycardia, weak and rapid pulse and increased respiratory rate, blood pressure, fever, etc.
- Look for frequent swallow reflex which if present may suggest bleeding in the tonsillar fossa.
- Oral or parenteral antibiotics and analgesics are given.
- Cold feeds after 4 hours which helps in vasoconstriction.

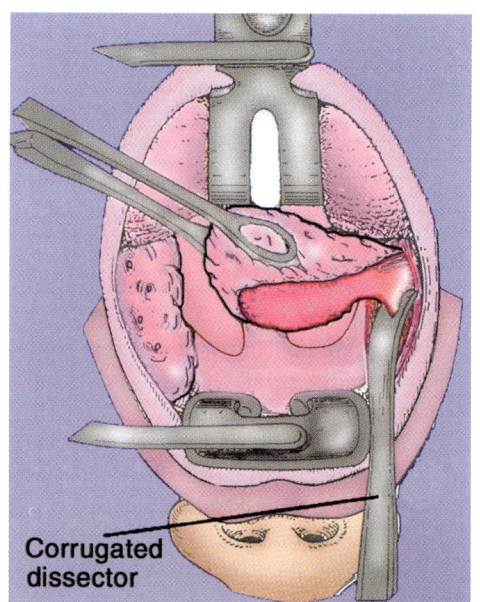

Fig. 51.15: Tonsillar dissection being continued till the inferior pole of the tonsil

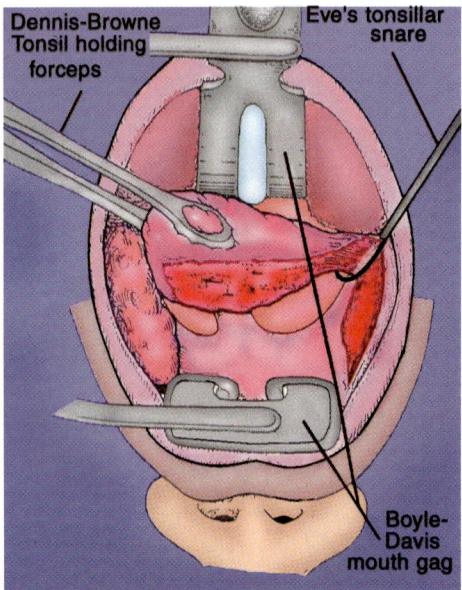

Fig. 51.16: Application of the loop of Eve's tonsillar snare at the inferior pole of the tonsil

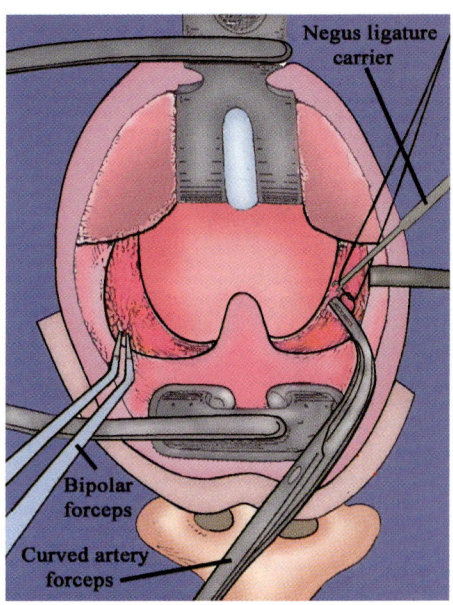

Fig. 51.17: Ligation of a bleeder during tonsillectomy using angled forceps and ligature carrier

- Saline or dilute hydrogen peroxide gargles may be advised to keep the operated site clean.
- Maintain good hydration

Complications

Immediate

- Primary and reactionary hemorrhage
- Aspiration of blood/saliva
- Injury to structures—Teeth, lips, gums, palate, etc.
- Injury to posterior pillars may cause change in speech and nasopharyngeal reflux
- Pain throat with or without referred otalgia
- Dehydration
- Fever is not common and is usually related to local infection
- Postoperative airway obstruction may occur because of uvular edema, hematoma, aspirated material
- Pulmonary edema
- Secondary hemorrhage occurs usually on 5th– 7th day.

Delayed

- Lingual tonsillitis (compensatory hypertrophy) (Fig. 51.18).
- Nasopharyngeal stenosis
- Velopharyngeal insufficiency
- Residual tonsillitis

Tonsillectomy Hemorrhage

Hemorrhage may be classified into primary, reactionary and secondary.

Prim\ary Haemorrhage

- This occurs during surgery often from the paratonsillar veins.
- This is often due to
  - Poor selection of the case: (patient with acute attack of tonsillitis or pharyngitis, bleeding disorders, hypertension or if the patient is on NSAIDS including aspirin, anticoagulant therapy and oral contraceptives, etc).
  - Improper technique (dissection not in the proper cleavage plane, injury to the

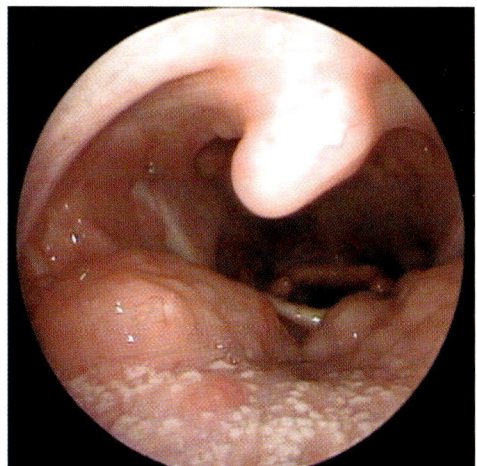

Fig. 51.18: Lingual tonsillitis following tonsillectomy

superior constrictor muscles and para-tonsilaar veins, presence of tonsillar remnants and mucosal tags)

- To stop primary hemorrhage the fossa is packed with wet gauze and wait for 5 minutes till the bleeding and clotting time is over. This will stop the bleeding in most of the cases.
- If bleeding persists, ligate/ cauterize the bleeding vessel

Reactionary Hemorrhage

This occurs in the postoperative within 24 hours. Usually it occurs within 6 to 8 hours after the surgery.

This can be due to the following:

- Failure to ligate all vessels
- Slippage of sutures
- Hypotensive anesthesia—BP returns to normal postoperatively
- Increased arterial or venous pressure during recovery
- Clot in the fossa—Prevents contraction and retraction of the vessels and can precipitate bleeding
- Injured muscle may cause diffuse ooze after recovery from anesthesia.
- Mismatched blood transfusion

Management: Remove the clot and apply pressure with a small pack held in an artery forceps. Usually the bleeding stops. Hydrogen peroxide gargle is helpful in removing the clot postoperatively and is also a mild cauterizing agent. Vital signs should be maintained. Treat hypovolumia and blood loss. If bleeding persists, shift patient to operation theater and ligate/ cauterize the bleeding vessels.

Secondary Hemorrhage

- This is due to sepsis of the tonsillar fossa and usually occurs on 5th to 7th postoperative day. Premature separation of the slough may precipitate this bleeding.
- Management—Start parenteral broad spectrum antibiotics including tinidazole or metronidazole.
- Cold liquid diet
- General management is as for reactionary hemorrhage.
- In case of persistent bleeding, shift patient to operation theater and inter-pillar suturing may be required in extreme cases.

Peritonsillitis and Peritonsillar Abscess (Quincy)

Definition

Peritonsillitis is defined as an acute inflammatory process associated with cellulitis involving the loose areolar tissue in the peritonsillar space which lies between superior constrictor muscle and the tonsillar capsule. The resultant spread of infection involving looser areolar tissue causing collection of pus within the space is called quincy or peritonsillar abscess.

Etiology

1. Recurrent attacks of acute tonsillitis
2. Penetrating trauma or foreign body
3. Common in adults in the 2nd and 3rd decade and is rare in infants and young children.
4. Dental infection like periodontitis
5. Tonsillolith or cyst
6. Infectious mononucleosis

7. Leukemia and other causes of immuno-compromised state.
8. Inflammation of accessory salivary tissue called Weber gland that is situated just above the superior pole in the soft palate, has been recently implicated for.

Pathogenesis

Recurrent attacks of acute tonsillitis may cause crypta magna to be obstructed leading to intratonsillar abscess and subsequent spread of infection to the peritonsillar space. Though this has been well accepted in the past, recent studies shows that the supratonsillar space of the soft palate, immediately above the superior pole of the tonsil and the surrounding muscles, especially the internal pterygoids can be site of initial infection. Group A beta-hemolytic streptococcus is frequently isolated.

Clinical Features

Symptoms

General: Fever, chills and rigor, malaise, bodyache and toxic features are often present.

Local

1. Acute severe unilateral odynophagia
2. Refered otalgia
3. Neck pain
4. Trismus due to pterygoid muscle spasm
5. Muffled speech (hot-potato speech)
6. Dribbling of saliva

Signs

- Anterior pillar cannot be distinguished easily from the rest of the tonsils due to odema and swelling of the overlying mucosa
- Tonsil is pushed medially and downward due to involvement of supratonsillar space.
- Involved tonsil is often congested and follicles/ membrane may be present at the crypts
- Uvula is congested, edematous and deviated to the opposite side
- Mucosa is edematous (Fig. 51.19).

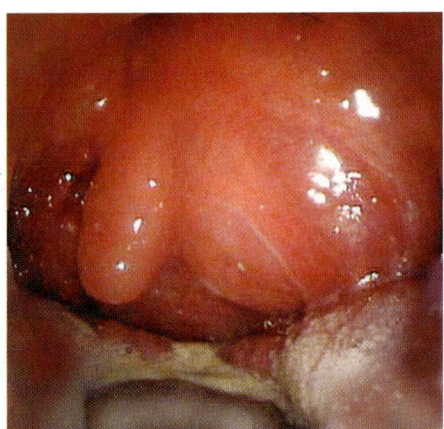

Fig. 51.19: Showing classical clinical presentation of peritonsillar abscess

- Trismus causes difficulty in further examination.
- Tender, enlarged, discrete cervical lymphadenitis may be seen.
- If untreated, the abscess may rupture causing puruilent fetid discharge.

Differential Diagnosis (Table 51.2)

- Peritonsillar cellulitis (Peritonsillitis)
- Parapharyngeal abscess
- Parapharyngeal neoplasm
- Severe tonsillitis

Investigations

- Throat swab for culture and sensitivity
- Complete blood picture
- Rule out diabetes mellitus
- CT imaging if there is suspicion of a parapharyngeal abscess

Treatment

- IV antibiotics and analgesics
- *If dysphagia is severe*: Hospitalization and IV fluids
- Wide bore needle aspiration
- *Incision and drainage:* This is done using a quinsy knife or an ordinary Bard-Parker knife with only about a centimeter of the tip of the knife exposed and the rest covered by

Table 51.2: Causes of unilateral tonsillar enlargement

Inflammatory	Tumor and tumor-like conditions
• *Acute:*	• Papilloma
– Peritonsillitis	• Fibroma
– Peritonsillar abscess (Quincy)	• Tonsillolith
– Intratonsillar abscess	• Tonsillar cyst
– Parapharyngeal abscess	• Parapharyngeal tumors
• *Chronic:*	• Aneurysm of the internal carotid artery
• Tuberculosis of the tonsil and	• Non-Hodgkin's lymphoma
• Other granulomatous conditions	• Kaposi's sarcoma
Trauma	• Squamous cell carcinoma
• Surgical trauma	
• Hematoma	
• Foreign body in the tonsil	

a plaster to prevent deep penetration of the knife. A stab incision is given at one of the following points:

1. Imaginary horizontal line drawn at the base of the uvula which intersects at a vertical line drawn along the anterior pillar. Incision is given at the point of intersection of these two lines.
2. At the point of maximum bulge in the supra-tonsillar area (Fig. 51.20).

• *Hot (abscess) tonsillectomy:* Some people advocate tonsillectomy during the active abscess stage. Others defer it for the fear of excessive bleeding and dissemination of infection and conventionally it is preferred to perform interval tonsillectomy after 6 weeks.

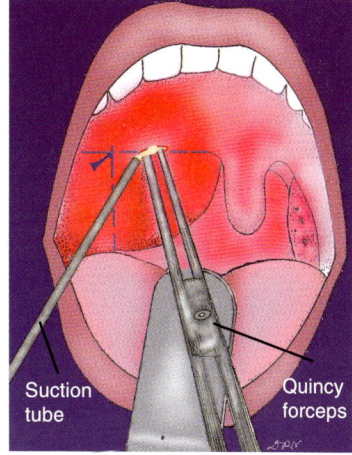

Fig. 51.20: Site of incision for drainage of peritonsillar abscess

POINTS TO REMEMBER

1. Adenoid hypertrophy can cause symptoms in the nose, throat and ear besides general symptoms.
2. Removal of adenoid can cause damage to the Eustachian tube.
3. A white Patch over the tonsil can have various underlying pathology and should be investigated.
4. Abscess of the peritonsilar space is known as quinsy.

52

Deep Neck Space Infections and Pharyngeal Abscess

"Pus in the neck calls for surgeon's best judgment, his best skill and often for all his courage"— Mosher.

Deep neck space infections pose various challenges to the treating surgeon. These infections may rapidly spread in hours and can cause fatal respiratory obstruction. Securing the airway by endotracheal intubation or tracheostomy may be often difficult. Various spaces may intercommunicate facilitating the spread of the infection. The abscess lies deep in the neck and in close proximity to the neurovas cular structures, mediastinum and the base skull. Knowledge of this vital anatomy is a must before venturing into its surgical treatment.

ANATOMICAL CONSIDERATIONS

Fascia of Head and Neck

Neck has 2 portions

1. Larger– Cervical spine and musculature
2. Smaller – Visceral segment. All serious infections occur here.

Cervical fascia is divided into:

1. Superficial cervical fascia
2. Deep cervical fascia

Superficial Cervical Fascia (Tela Subcutanea)

This is a continuous sheet extending from head and neck into thorax, shoulders and axilla. It contains voluntary muscles platysma in the neck and the muscles of facial expression in the face. This contains a potential fascial space (space I) within the fatty tissue superficial to platysma and also between platysma and deep fascia. Infections in these spaces are rare, but involve entire length of neck. They are treated successfully with local incision and drainage and parenteral or oral antibiotics.

Deep Cervical Fascia

This is made up of 3 layers namely: superficial, middle and deep.

Superficial Investing Layer

This is also known as external layer, enveloping layer, anterior layer or 'Mother' of cervical fasciae.

Superiorly it is attached to the nuchal ridge, mandible, zygoma, mastoid, and hyoid bones. Inferiorly, it is bounded by the clavicles, sternum, scapula and acromion. Anteriorly it spreads to face. It invests sternocleidomastoid, trapezius and masseter muscles and envelops parotid and submaxillary glands. About 1 to 3 cm superior to the sternum the fascia divides into two layers forming a space "Suprasternal space of Burns" which contains loose areolar tissue, lymph nodes and sternal heads of sternocleidomastoid muscle.

The investing layer forms the floor of the submental region and the stylomandibular ligament. This fascia creates 4 spaces:

1. Submental space in the midline
2. Submandibular space laterally
3. Parotid space
4. Masticator space

Middle Visceral Layer

This has two divisions.

1. **Muscular division:** This surrounds the strap muscles.
2. **Visceral division:** This encloses all viscera of neck like the thyroid, trachea esophagus and the pharyngeal constrictors.

It is attached anterosuperiorly to hyoid bone and the thyroid cartilage, posteriorly to the skull base and inferiorly to the sternum, clavicle and the scapula. It is continuous with fibrous pericardium, covering of thoracic trachea and the esophagus. Portion of this fascia lying posterior to pharynx and buccinator from skull base to cricoid cartilage is called 'Buccopharyngeal fascia'. The portion lying anterior to thyroid is called Prethyroid fascia and the portion lying anterior to trachea is known as 'Pretracheal fascia'.

Deep Layer

This has two layers, pre-vertebral and the alar layers.

Alar layer: This is superficial portion and lies between middle layer and the prevertebral division. It extends from transverse process of one side to the other and from base skull to T2, where it fuses with the visceral layer. It forms posterior boundary of retropharyngeal space and anterior wall of danger space.

Prevertebral layer: This lies anterior to vertebral bodies and spreads laterally from transverse processes. It is attached to spinous processes posteriorly and extends from base skull to coccyx. It forms anterior wall of vertebral space and posterior wall of danger space.

Retropharyngeal space (space III) lies between visceral layer and alar division. This was called Lincoln's highway by Mosher as it is a pathway for spread of infection into mediastinum.

Danger space lies between alar and prevertebral fasciae.

Vertebral space is present between prevertebral fascia and vertebral bodies.

Carotid Sheath: This is condensation of all 3 layers and extends from skull base to clavicle. It contains the carotid artery, internal jugular vein, vagus nerve, cervical sympathetic chain in separate sheaths. Below clavicle it fuses with covering of great vessels at root of neck and fibrous pericardium.

Etiopathology of Deep Neck Space Infections

1. Patients at risk for deep neck space infections:
   - Immunocompromised—HIV, chemotherapy, etc.
   - Diabetes
   - Intravenous drug abusers
   - Infants
2. Precipitating causes:
   - In the pre-antibiotic era, tonsillitis and pharyngitis accounted for 70 percent of cases and often affected the lateral pharyngeal space (parapharyngeal space).
   - Odontogenic causes: This is presently the most common cause.
   - Salivary gland infections
   - URTI
   - Trauma
   - Foreign body
   - Instrumentation
   - Spread of infection from other areas
   - Previously undiagnosed congenital deformities
   - Pott's disease
   - Retropharyngeal lymphadenitis
   - Peritonsillar cellulites/abscess
   - Intravenous or subcutaneous drug abuse
   - Unknown causes – 20 percent cases.

Microbiology

Mixed flora of aerobes and anaerobes are often encountered (Table 52.1).

β-hemolytic Streptococci and staphylococci and other aerobes are the most common organisms encountered especially in IV drug abusers. Common anaerobes include *B. melaninogenicus,* Peptostreptococcus, *Eikenella corrodens* and Fusobacterium.

General symptoms and signs (Table 52.2).

SPECIFIC SPACES

Neck spaces are divided into

Table 52.1: Microbiology of deep neck space infections

Aerobes		Anaerobes	
Streptococci		Acteroides	23
- α not group D	23	Melaninogenicus	13
- group D	02	Oralis	03
- β group A	11	Others	09
- not A/B/D	07	Peptostreptococcus	15
- γ not group D	03	Peptococcus	06
- microaerophilic	04	Eubacterium	06
		Fusobacterium	06
		Eikenella corrodens	05
		Unidentified Gram +ve cocci	05
		Unidentified Gram -ve bacilli	09
Staphylococcus	11		
Aureus	04		
Epidermidis	07		
Diptheroids	03		
Neisseria	03		
K. pneumoniae	02		
H. influenzae	01		
Pseudomonas	01		

Table 52.2: General symptoms and signs

Symptoms		Signs	
Pain	76%	Swelling	90%
Fever	94%	Dental abnormality	29%
Swelling	62%	Fluctuance	27%
Dysphagia /Odynophagia	42%	**Oropharyngeal**	
Trismus	14%	Abnormality	22%
Respiratory difficulty	14%	Trismus	18%
Dental	8%	Laryngeal abnormality	18%

I. Spaces of Face

A. Maxillary space
   - Buccal
   - Canine
B. Mental space

II. Spaces of Neck (Fig. 52.1)

A. Spaces involving entire length of neck
   1. Superficial space – Space 1
   2. Deep spaces
      Retropharyngeal – Space 3 Posterior visceral space
      - Danger space 4
      - Prevertebral space – Space 5
      - Visceral vascular space (within carotid sheath)
B. Suprahyoid Spaces
   1. Mandibular space
      - Submandibular space
      - Submental space
      - Sublingual space
      - Space of body of mandible

   2. Masticator space
   3. Lateral pharyngeal space
   4. Peritonsillar space
   5. Parotid space
C. Infrahyoid space
      Pretracheal space

I. SUPERFICIAL SPACE INFECTION

This was originally described by Meleny and is often caused by mixed organisms including streptococci and staphylococci. This is also known as 'Streptococcal gangrene' or 'Necrotising Fascitis'.

Clinical Features

- Systemic disease like diabetes or immuno-compromised states may be present.
- Preceding history of trauma is often elicited.
- Eyelids, neck, scalp are the most common sites

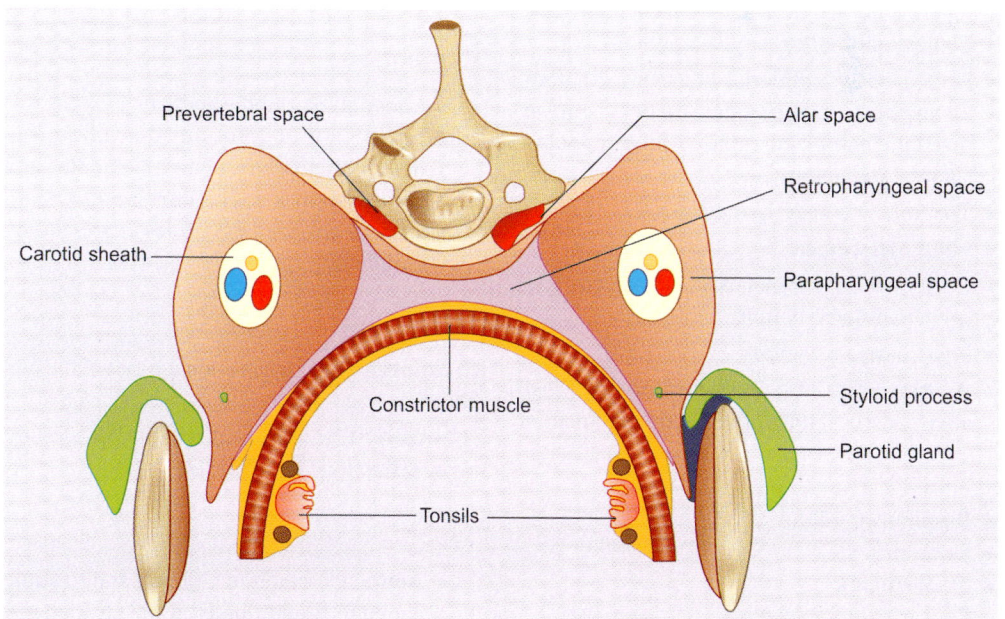

Fig. 52.1: The retropharyngeal and parapharyngeal spaces

- Initially erythema, swelling, warmth and disproportionate tenderness
- Thrombosis of skin vessels leads to skin discoloration
- Cutaneous nerve involvement may give rise to hypoaesthesia/ anesthesia which is suggestive of underlying necrosis
- Frank gangrene.
- Systemically prostration +
- Tachycardia disproportionate to temperature rise
- Hypocalcemia
- Hepatocellular dysfunction

Diagnosis

- Necrosis of subcutaneous tissue and superficial fascia
- CT – For diagnosis of soft tissue gas
- Gram's stain of culture from wound
- Blood culture

Management

- Early diagnosis
- Careful aggressive debridement. May need repeated explorations and frequent dressings. Topical antibiotics may be applied.
- High dose IV antibiotics like penicillin upto 20 million units per day or pencillinase resistant penicillin (methicillin)/cephalosporins are advocated.
- Treatment of underlying cause
- Fluid replacement
- Correction of (a) metabolic (b) electrolyte (c) hematologic deficits
- Hyperbaric O_2 therapy
- Airway control by Tracheostomy—almost always done at time of initial debridement.

Complications

- Respiratory failure
- Delirium
- Mediastinitis
- Pericardial tamponade
- DIC

- Neuropathy
- Sepsis + multiorgan failure + hemodynamic collapse.

II. DEEP NECK INFECTIONS

A. RETROPHARYNGEAL SPACE INFECTION (Fig. 52.1)

Retropharyngeal space is also known as 'Posterior visceral space', 'Retroesophageal space', 'Retrovisceral space', 'space of Gillette' or the 'Lincoln's highway'.

Boundaries

- *Anterior*: Buccopharyngeal fascia
- *Posterior*: Alar fascia
- *Lateral:* Carotid sheath/ parapharyngeal space
- *Medial:* Midline septum divides it into 2 spaces
- *Superior:* Base skull
- *Inferior:* Extends to superior mediastinum where the alar fascia fuses with the visceral fascia (buccopharyngeal fascia).

Contents

- Loose areolar tissue and fat
- Lymph nodes draining adjacent muscles, nose, nasopharynx, pharynx, middle ear and paranasal sinuses. These are more commonly seen in children (as nodes regress during childhood).

Causes

In children: Infection in drainage area of the lymph nodes.

In adults: FB, vertebral fracture, esophageal instrumentation, TB spine, etc.

Types

- **Acute:** Common in children and in adults it is due to foreign body at the cricopharynx/ upper esophagus.

- **Chronic:** This is due to tuberculosis of the cervical vertebrae.

Acute Retropharyngeal Abscess

- Common in children (often <4years) following adenoiditis/ tonsillitis or in adults following foreign body impaction in the cricopharynx or upper esophagus.
- Abscess can spread directly into mediastinum (anterior, posterior) and danger space via alar fascia.
- Hence it is the most dangerous of all neck space infections.
- Especially seen in children of parents with TB, syphilis children with rickets or following URTI.

Symptoms

- Rapidly increasing sore throat
- Acute odynophagia– Children refuse to take feeds
- Fever
- Hot potato voice
- Deep pain
- Lymphadenopathy may cause neck swelling
- Slight neck rigidity – Neck tilts to involved side, finally hyperextended with inability to flex neck.
- Laryngeal edema – Noisy breathing and respiratory difficulty
- No trismus unless secondary to odontogenic infection

Signs

1 *Systemic*– Fever, toxic look of the child
- *Local*
  - Paramedian bulge in the posterior pharyngeal wall
  - Grossly inflamed mucosa
  - Dribbling and pooling of saliva
  - Trismus is often absent
  - Larynx and trachea may be pushed forwards
  - Stridor +/–

Differential Diagnosis

- Croup
- Acute epiglottitis
- Peritonsillar abscess
- Eosinophilic granuloma of cervical spine.

Investigations

1. Lateral neck radiographs
2. CT scan imaging or MRI
   Normal width of radiological prevertebral soft tissue shadow at C2 is 3.5 mm (Widened if >7 mm at C2 and if >14 mm in child and if >22 mm in an adult at C6). Radiological features of acute retropharyngeal abscess include (Fig. 52.2).
   (a) Prevertebral widening: Prevertebral soft tissue shadow is more than 50% of width of vertebral body.
   (b) Displacement of the larynx and the trachea forwards
   (c) Straightening of the cervical spine due to prevertebral muscle spasm.
   (d) Air shadow in the prevertebral space with or without fluid level.

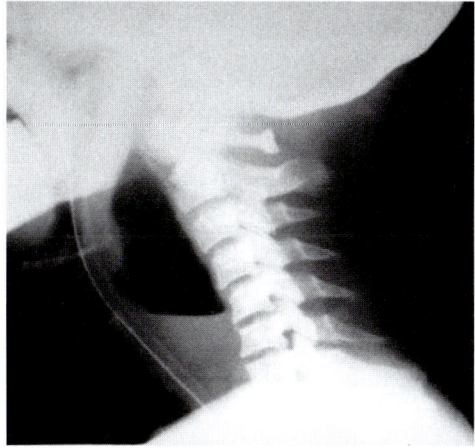

Fig. 52.2: X-ray lateral view showing prevertebral space shadow widening with air fluid level suggestive of acute retropharyngeal abscess. Also note straightening of cervical spine, which is a characteristic feature

Treatment

- Hospitalization
- IV fluids and antibiotics
- If stridor is present, the airway should be secured by tracheostomy or endotracheal intubation (if an experienced anesthetist is available). Intubation is often difficult due to displaced and inflamed larynx, posterior pharyngeal wall bulge and non-compliant child. During intubation there is a risk of rupture of the abscess and aspiration of the pus into the respiratory tract.
- Incision and drainage of the abscess is done by a transoral route. Patient is positioned supine with head low or in Rose position (neck – extreme extension with vertex head dependant). A small vertical incision is made over the most prominent bulge in the posterior pharyngeal wall.

Complications

- Meningitis
- Hemorrhage
- Laryngeal spasm
- Bronchial erosion
- Septicemia
- Metastatic abscess
- Jugular vein thrombosis
- Rupture with aspiratin pneumonia
- Pericardial tamponade
- Mediastinitis
- Acute hemiplegia of childhood
- Spread into other spaces like lateral pharyngeal space, parotid space, masticator space, submandibular space, superior mediastinum and posterior mediastinum.

Chronic Retropharyngeal Abscess

This is due to tuberculosis of the cervical spine. This may initially involve the prevertebral space alone and later to the danger space and the retropharyngeal spaces.

Clinical Features

Symptoms

- The throat symptoms are not severe compared to acute retropharyngeal abscess.
- Insidious onset
- Systemic features of TB +/– (chronic cough, evening rise in temperature, night sweats, loss of appetite and loss of weight)
- Painless lump in the throat
- Dysphagia
- Cervical pain may radiate to the upper limbs with or without sensory/ motor neurological deficits.

Signs

- Median bulge on the posterior pharyngeal wall
- No signs of acute inflammation
- Signs of cervical spine or lymph node tuberculosis and neurological radiculo-pathies may be present

Investigations

Plain radiograph, CT or MRI scan of the cervical spine show caries of the spine with collapse of the body of vertebrae. Prevertebral widening may also be seen (Fig. 52.3).

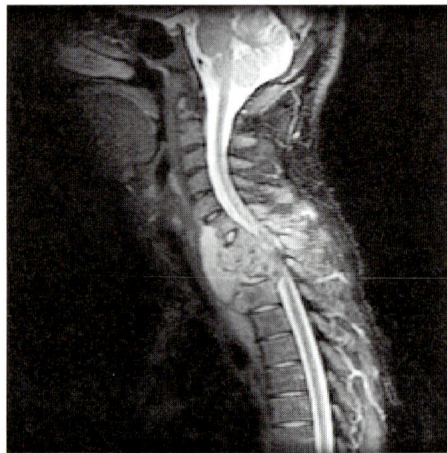

Fig. 52.3: MRI showing destruction of cervical vertebrae with widening of prevertebral space due to tuberculosis of cervical spine

FNAC or cytology of the drained fluid may show acid fast bacillus and the cultures may be positive for tuberculosis.

Treatment

(i) *Anti-tubercular treatment*

(ii) *Incision and drainage* is done by a trans-cervical approach. Oblique cervical incision and exposing the retropharyngeal spaces is done. Sequestrectomy may be performed by orthopedic surgeons or the neurosurgeons, once the acute stage tides over.

Complications

Pus from various spaces can extend caudally

1. *Danger Space (Alar Space)*

   This lies between alar layer and prevertebral layers of deep layer of deep cervical fascia, laterally limited by attachment to transverse process and extends from skull base to posterior mediastinum till the diaphragm. Thus pus may track down the posterior mediastinum and to the thorax.

2. *Prevertebral Space*

   This space is located between the cervical vertebrae and the prevertebral layer and is laterally limited by fascial attachment to transverse process. It extends from the skull base to the coccyx below. Thus the pus can track down till the coccyx without involving the posterior mediastinum.

B. VISCERAL VASCULAR SPACE INFECTIONS

- From base of skull above, through pharyngo-maxillary space, along prevertebral fascia below hyoid and into chest below clavicle.
- Carotid artery, internal jugular vein, Vagus have separate sheaths. Sympathetic chain in a fascial reflection from deep surface – Posterior wall. Infections of neck may involve these.
- Infections are initially localized but spreads fast as there is scanty areolar connective tissue.

- Most common space causing carotid sheath involvement is lateral pharyngeal space.

Clinical Features

1. Persistent tenderness and induration deep to sternocleidomastoid and torticollis.
2. Features of septicemia–Spiking fevers, chills, sweats and shock.
3. Fundoscopy–Disk edema, dilated veins, retinal thrombosis.
4. Edematous pitting on deep pressure suggests internal jugular vein (IJV) involvement.
5. Repeated hemorrhage–Small volume into ear and pharynx suggest erosion of internal carotid artery (ICA).

Mortality rate is about 85%. Hence urgent surgical exploration is indicated.

Investigations

- Ultrasound
- CT with contrast
- MRI helps in assessment of extent of abscess spread and the status of the great vessels.
- Blood cultures during spikes of fever

Treatment

1. Stabilizing patient
2. Treatment of complications
3. Drainage of abscess—Only by external approach (Peroral drainage may result in hemorrhage that may be uncontrollable).
4. Selected cases—Anticoagulants
5. Ligation of IJV—If thrombus is present.

Complications

1. IJV thrombosis – Septicemia
2. Erosion of ICA.

C. PARAPHARYNGEAL SPACE INFECTIONS (Figs 52.1) (ABSCESS)

Synonyms

- Pharyngomaxillary space
- Lateral pharyngeal space

Anatomy

This potential space lies just lateral to the pharynx (Fig. 52.1). It communicates with all other major fascial spaces. In the pre-antibiotic era, this was the most common space involved. This space has a shape of an inverted pyramid with its base formed by the base of skull and apex at the level of hyoid bone. Carotid sheath traverses this from its base to the apex.

Boundaries

- *Anterior:* Interpterygoid fascia and the pterygomandibular raphe
- *Posterior:* Prevertebral division of the deep layer and by the posterior aspect of the carotid sheath.
  - *Medial:* Middle layer of deep cervical fascia around the pharyngeal constrictor and the fascia of the tensor and levator muscles of the velum palatini and the styloglossus.
  - *Lateral:* Superficial layer of the deep cervical fascia that overlies the mandible, medial pterygoids and parotid.

Compartments

Parapharyngeal space is divided by styloid process into:
- Anterior (or) Pre-styloid compartment
- Posterior (or) Post-styloid compartment.

Contents

- *Pre-styloid compartment:* Fat, loose areolar tissue, lymph nodes, internal maxillary artery.
- *Post-styloid compartment:* Carotid artery, IJV, cervical sympathetic chain, cervical nerves IX, X, XI and XII.

Clinical Features

- History of odontogenic disease/tonsillitis/sialadenitis/ lymph node suppuration

- Firm induration, erythema seen lateral and anterior to sternocleidomastoid muscle.
- Difficulty in flexing and turning neck
- Trismus – Secondary to pterygoid involvement, dysphagia, dyspnea
- Bulging of lateral pharyngeal mucosa / tonsil / soft palate

Differential Diagnosis

- Peritonsillar abscess
- Cervical adenitis
- Masticator space infection
- Submandibular space infection

Investigations

- CT for location and extent of abscess and to identify complications (Fig. 52.4)
- Needle aspiration for Gram's stain
- Chest X-ray and CT scan to ascertain mediastinal spread
- Dental evaluation to rule out odontogenic source.

Treatment

- IV antibiotics
- Airway protection
- Early surgical drainage transcervical by incision at level of hyoid across sternocleidomastoid muscle and blunt dissection above hyoid.

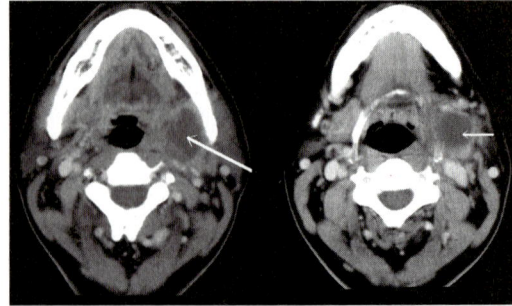

Fig. 52.4: CT imaging showing evidence of right parapharyngeal abscess (white arrow)

Complications

- Most common vascular complication is IJV thrombosis
  - Shaking chills, spiking fever, prostration.
  - Tenderness at angle of mandible and along sternocleidomastoid muscle.
  - Associated with bacteremia, pulmonary emboli, suppurative subclavian phlebitis, lateral sinus thrombosis, brain abscess, metastatic abscesses.

This is treated by prolonged IV antibiotics, surgical drainage of main abscess, ligation of involved segment of vein.

2. *Carotid artery rupture:*
   - By false aneurysm formation
   - Herald bleeds occur before major bleed
   - ICA more commonly involved.
3. Laryngeal edema
4. Mediastinitis

D. MANDIBULAR SPACE INFECTIONS

Spaces about mandible are

- Submandibular space
- Space of body of mandible

Infection here is often caused by odontogenic infection or direct trauma.

Other factors include mandibular fractures, lacerations of floor of mouth, migrating foreign bodies, mandibular tumors, floor of mouth tumors, sialadenitis, lymphadenitis, etc.

Submandibular Space

- This space lies between mucosa of the floor of the oral cavity above and skin, platysma, superficial layer of deep fascia below
- This space is further divided into two inter - communicating spaces namely:
  - Submaxillary or submental space below the mylohyoid muscle
  - Sublingual space above the mylohoid muscle
  - Posteriorly they communicate with each other round the mylohyoid muscle.

SUBMANDIBULAR SPACE INFECTION (LUDWIG'S ANGINA)

Definition

Ludwig's angina is a condition characterized by rapidly spreading infection of the sublingual space initially and later the submaxillary space and is often dentogenic in origin (Fig. 52.5).

Unlike other neck space infection where the abscess formation is the rule, here in Ludwig's angina, it has characteristic cellulitis without lymphatic involvement causing massive swelling of the tongue and floor of the mouth. Unless early surgical intervention is done the disease can be fatal due to respiratory obstruction.

Etiology

- More common in the age 20 to 50 years
- Dental caries especially that of the lower 2nd and 3rd molars are the main source of the infection. Infection from the apex of the tooth can directly involve the submaxillary space.
- Infection following trauma of the tongue, floor of the mouth
- Lingual tonsillitis
- Infection following dental extraction
- Post-radiotherapy osteo-radio-necrosis of the mandible.

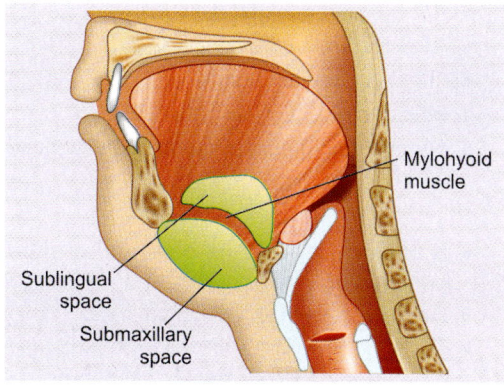

Fig. 52.5: Site of involvement in case of Ludwig's angina

Clinical Features

- Most commonly from second or third lower molar infections. History of recent tooth extraction or trauma may be given by the patient.
- Patient looks toxic, with high fever and malaise
- Disease is rapidly progressive and presents with painful neck swelling in the region below the mandible.
- Dysphagia, difficulty in opening the mouth, dysarthria and dyspnea

Signs

- Signs of sepsis—Fever, rapid pulse and toxic appearance
- Rapidly increasing cellulitis with induration, erythema below the mandible obliterating mandibular line
- Trismus
- Absence of lymphadenitis
- Baruny edema of the floor of the mouth and tongue pushing the tongue posteriorly
- Laryngeal edema forces patient to sit up and lean forwards
- Drooling of saliva
- Dyspnea and stridor

Differential Diagnosis

- Submental space infection
- Acute submandibular sialadenitis
- Acute cervical lymphadenitis
- Infected plunging ranula
- Infection of a necrotic tumor mass
- Tumors/granulomas of submandibular gland.

Diagnosis

- It is based mainly on classical clinical presentation
- Dental X-rays to assess dental status
- CT scan to know the extent of disease, extension to other neck spaces and the patency of the airway.

Treatment

- Intravenous antibiotics, fluids and analgesics
- Serratiopeptidase can be given along with anti-inflammatory analgesics.
- Tracheostomy if stridor is present or in case of threatened airway obstruction.
- Surgical drainage is done via horizontal incision 2 finger breadth below the mandiblar margin from one angle of the mandible to the other over the area of induration. Pus is often not seen as seen in other abscess rather edematous fluid collection may be drained. The incision provides decompression as this allows fluid from edematous tissue to drain. Drainage tube or antibiotic soaked ribbon gauge is placed and the incision is not closed. Daily dressing is done and the wound is allowed to heal by secondary intention (Fig. 52.6).
- Treatment of underlying cause like dental sepsis, diabetes, if any.

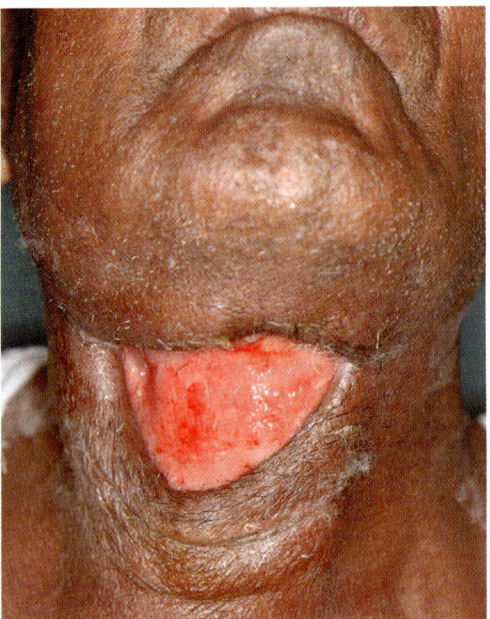

Fig 52.6: The site of incision in Ludwig's angina after drainage with unsutured wound

Complications

- Airway obstruction requiring tracheostomy which may be difficult
- Aspiration pneumonia
- Lung abscess formation
  Fluid and electrolyte imbalance
- Tongue necrosis
- Spread to other spaces like parapharyngeal space, retropharyngeal space, mediastinitis, etc.

Submental Space

- Infection of the inframylohyoid space of the submandibular space which is laterally bound by anterior bellies of digastric muscles.

Clinical Features

- Odontogenic sources (anterior teeth)
- Erythema, induration of skin in submental region, causing board like stiffness similar to Ludwig's angina but no swelling of the floor of the mouth unlike Ludwig's angina.
- Pain, odynophagia, airway compromise
- Minimal respiratory distress and moderate dysphagia may be noted.

Investigation

- CT scan

Treatment

- Intavenous antibiotics, fluids and anti-inflammatory.
- Horizontal incision is given at the site of maximum bulge after the infection localises.

E. MASTICATOR SPACE INFECTIONS

Masticator space is formed as the deep cervical fascia covers the massetter muscle laterally and the pterygoid muscle medially.

Contents

- Masseter
- Ramus and part of body of mandible
- Medial and lateral pterygoids
- Tendon of insertion of temporalis

Causes

- Infected tooth– root of 2nd and 3rd molar
- Infection following local anesthesia if asepsis is not maintained for inferior alveolar nerve block.

Pathology

Masticator space is subdivided into 3 spaces.

Temporal Space

- This lies posterior and superior to masseteric and pterygomandibular spaces. It is divided into superficial and deep spaces by temporalis.
- Both spaces open into masseteric and pterygomandibular spaces.
- Deep space contains interior maxillary A, mandibular nerves and vessels.
- Temporal space infection leads to trismus and induration over temporal area posterior to orbital rim.

Masseteric Space

- Lies on the lateral aspect of mandible and masseter.
- Source of infection is from III molar tooth or from buccal space.
- Patients have induration of posteroinferior portion of face and mild trismus.

Pterygomandibular Space

- Lies between medial aspect mandible and medial pterygoid
- Source of infection third molar tooth or spread from sublingual/submandibular space
- Marked trismus without any induration.

Clinical Features

- Dysphagia, odynophagia, marked trismus
- Posterior sublingual tissue induration
- Swelling over ramus of mandible

- If one space is involved rest of 3 spaces also may get involved eventually.

Treatment

- IV antibiotics
- Incision and drainage – Incision externally below and behind angle of mandible deepened to bone.
- If abscess points lingually – Vertical intraoral incision along anterior border of ramus of mandible.
- If temporal space is also to be drained, incision is given behind brow through skin and temporal fascia.

F. PAROTID SPACE INFECTIONS

This space lies in between the enveloping layers of deep cervical fascia covering the parotid gland.

Contents

- Parotid gland
- VII nerve
- Lymph nodes
- External carotid artery
- Posterior facial vein
- Medical dehiscence adjacent to pharyngomaxillary space

   Stylomandibular ligament separates parotid from submaxillary space.

Clinical Features

- This is often seen in postsurgical patients (surgical mumps), debilitated, dehydrated patients.
- Drugs decreasing salivary flow. e.g: Antihistamines, diuretics, barbiturates, tricyclic antidepressants, etc.
- Severe otitis externa spreading through fissures of Santorini.
- Marked swelling of jaw.
- No trismus/pharyngeal swelling seen.
- Mimics lateral pharyngeal space infection.
- Pain and induration over parotid gland, characteristic pitting edema over gland

- High temperature
- No fluctuation.

Diagnosis

- Aspiration with 18 bore needle can be diagnostic
- Ultrasound or CT/MRI can differentiate between parotitis and abscess.

Treatment

1. Drainage over prominence of parotid swelling parallel to branches of VII nerve if the abscess is small.
2. If abscess is large a modified Blair incision is given to drain the abscess

Complications

- Involves lateral pharyngeal space through superomedial dehiscence
- Later it may involve other deep neck spaces and finally may even involve the mediastinum.

G. PERITONSILLAR SPACE INFECTIONS

- This space lies between the fibrous capsule of palatine tonsil medially and the superior constrictor muscle forming the tonsillar bed laterally. It contains loose connective tissue.
- This is discussed in detail under the Chapter 51.

H. PRETRACHEAL SPACE INFECTION

- Also known as 'Anterior visceral space'
- Extends from thyroid cartilage above to anterior portion of superior mediastinum at about upper border of arch of aorta
- Anterior boundary: Strap muscles
- Posterior boundary: Retropharyngeal portion of visceral compartment
- Continuous with posterior visceral space.

Etiology

Source of infection could be:

- Tonsils

- Trauma to hypopharynx or esophagus
- Laryngeal trauma
- Thyroid gland infections

Clinical Features

- Hoarseness and muffled voice
- Dyspnea and asphyxia
- Dysphagia
- Tenderness over larynx
- Pitting edema +
- Subcutaneous crepitus indicating perforation of hollow viscous
- On indirect laryngeal examination unilateral swelling first involving hypopharynx pyriform sinus is seen.

Investigations

- X-ray lateral neck may show thickened retropharyngeal tissue and gas in soft tissue.

- Gastrograffin defects to show site of perforation of esophagus.

- Endoscopy to diagnose FB/laryngeal fracture.

Management

- IV antibiotics
- Securing airway
- Surgery: Incision and drainage.

Complications

- Laryngeal edema
- Airway obstruction
- Pulmonary infection and edema
- Mediastinitis
- Empyema.

POINTS TO REMEMBER

1. Deep neck spaces may intercommunicate and facilitate spread of infection.
2. Retropharyngeal space lies between visceral layer and alar division is called as 'Lincoln's high way, as the infection here can spread to mediastinum.
3. Parapharyngeal space is divided into pre-styloid and post-styloid compartment.
4. Submandibular space is divided into sublingual and submaxillary space by mylohyoid muscle.

53

Neoplasm of the Oral Cavity and Oropharynx

Neoplasm of the oral cavity and the pharynx can be diagnosed early as the patients often present with definite symptoms like oral lesions, dysphagia and foreign body feeling in the throat. Meticulous history and clinical examination using proper instrumentation often helps us in identifying the lesions at an early stage.

Certain areas where early lesions may be missed include tonsillolingual sulcus, base of the tongue, valleculae and the post-cricoid area. Premalignant conditions/lesions should be looked for especially in high risk individuals like chronic smokers, tobacco/betel nut chewers, etc.

With early identification and proper treatment the cure rates and preservation of function for oral and pharyngeal malignancies are quite good and late presentation, diagnosis and management is often associated with high morbidity and mortality due to very poor disease control rates.

Clinical outcome is determined primarily by histology, extent of disease, and treatment modality.

PREMALIGNANT LESIONS AND CONDITIONS

Lesions

- Leukoplakia
- Erythoplakia
- Submucous fibrosis
- Lichen planus.

Conditions

- Plummer–Vinson syndrome
- Syphilis

LEUKOPLAKIA (Fig. 53.1)

Leukoplakia refers to white patch in the mucosa that does not rub off and cannot be clinically identified as another entity. Most cases of leukoplakia are a hyperkeratotic response to an irritant and are asymptomatic, but about 20 percent of leukoplakic lesions show evidence of dysplasia or carcinoma at first clinical recognition. However, some anatomic sites (floor of mouth and ventral tongue) have rates of dysplasia or carcinoma as high as 45 percent. Erythroleukoplakia refers to

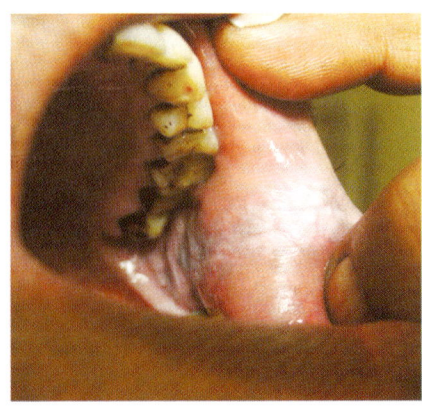

Fig. 53.1: Leukoplakia of the buccal mucosa

leukoplakia with reddish areas and has a higher malignant transformation rate (25%) as compared with a 6.5 percent rate for lesions that are homogeneous.

Types of Leukoplakia

The following three types are seen clinically.

- Amorphous
- Speckled
- Candidial

A greater risk of malignant change has been associated with the following factors:

1. Erythroplakia within a leukoplakia
2. A proliferative verrucous appearance
3. Location at a high-risk anatomic site such as the tongue or floor of mouth,
4. The presence of multiple lesions.
5. Hairy leukoplakia, which is commonly associated with HIV infection can go on to develop lymphoma when associated with HIV.

Approximately 75 percent of carcinoma in situ cases evolve into full-blown carcinoma.

Erythroplakia

Erythroplakia is a red lesion that cannot be classified as another entity. Far less common than leukoplakia, erythroplakia has a much greater probability (91%) of showing signs of dysplasia or malignancy at the time of diagnosis. Such lesions have a flat, macular, velvety appearance and may be speckled with white spots representing foci of keratosis.

Oral Submucous Fibrosis (OSF)
(Fig. 53.2)

This is a well recognized pre-malignant condition seen commonly in India and is due to fabricated betel nut (ghutka) chewing. Betel quid or pan is a preparation of betel leaf (Piper betel), areca nut (the fruit of the areca palm tree, often termed betel nut), tobacco, lime, and catechu. In patients with OSF, betel nut was chewed alone more frequently than it was chewed in combination with pan. Sub-epithelial inflammatory response to the irritants

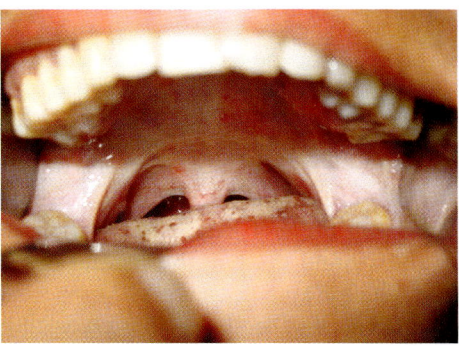

Fig. 53.2: Submucous fibrosis involving the retromolar trigone anterior tonsilar pillars and soft palate on both sides

is presumed to be the cause of OSF. Arecoline, an active alkaloid found in betel nuts, is said to stimulate fibroblasts to increase production of collagen by 150 percent. Role of other factors like genetic predisposition, nutritional deficiencies and autoimmune response is also being considered as probable etiological factors. OSF is found to continue even after cessation of areca nut chewing.

Clinical Features

The lesion appear as white fibrotic bands extending from the retromolar trigone to the soft palate, buccal mucosa, tongue and pharynx and is often associated with trismus, ankyloglossia and restriction of soft palate movements and dysphagia. The patients initially often complain of difficulty in chewing and oral pain/ burning sensation in the oral cavity especially on consuming spicy food. Some experience increased salivation, change in taste sensation, nasal intonation and dry feeling in the mouth and throat. Rarely eustachian tube dysfunction may cause symptoms of otitis media.

Clinical Staging of OSF (Pindborg, 1989)

Stage 1

Stomatitis includes erythematous mucosa, vesicles, mucosal ulcers, melanotic mucosal pigmentation, and mucosal petechia.

Stage 2

Fibrosis occurs in ruptured vesicles and ulcers when they heal, which is the hallmark of this stage.

- **Early lesions** demonstrate blanching of the oral mucosa.
- **Older lesions** include vertical and circular palpable fibrous bands in the buccal mucosa and around the mouth opening or lips, resulting in a mottled marble-like appearance of the mucosa because of the vertical, thick, fibrous bands running in a blanching mucosa. Specific findings include the following:
  - Reduction of the mouth opening (trismus)
  - Stiff and small tongue
  - Blanched and leathery floor of the mouth
  - Fibrotic and depigmented gingiva
  - Rubbery soft palate with decreased mobility
  - Blanched and atrophic tonsils
  - Shrunken budlike uvula
  - Sinking of the cheeks, not commensurate with age or nutritional status

Stage 3

Sequelae of OSF are as follows:

- Leukoplakia is found in more than 25 percent of individuals with OSF.
- Speech and hearing deficits may occur because of involvement of the tongue and the eustachian tubes.

Investigations

Diagnosis is often based on classical clinical presentation. However investigations may be done to assess the nutritional status and to rule-out malignant transformation. Toludine blue staining of the suspicious area help in selecting more representative site for biopsy.

Treatment

Medical

- *Injection hyalase* with hydrocortisone may be given intra-lesionally at multiple sites and may be repeated at weekly intervals.

- *Antioxidants* may be of help in preventing dysplastic changes.
- *Nutritional supplementation* like multi-vitamins may be tried.

Surgical

- Fibrotic bands may be divided using KTP-532 or CO_2 laser at multiple sites.
- Excision of the fibrotic area and skin grafts or local flaps may be tried in multiple sittings.

Lichen Planus

The premalignant or malignant potential of lichen planus is in dispute. Some believe that the occasional epithelial dysplasia or carcinoma found in patients with this relatively common lesion may be either coincidental or evidence that the initial diagnosis of lichen planus was erroneous. However it is prudent practice to biopsy the lesion at the initial visit to confirm the diagnosis and to monitor it thereafter for clinical changes suggesting a premalignant or malignant change. The lesions appear as white lace like patterns often in the buccal mucosa.

Other Premalignant Lesions

Premalignant changes arising in other oral lesions are uncommon. White lesions such as linea alba, leukoderma, and frictional keratosis are common in the oral cavity but have no definite propensity for malignant transformation.

Diagnosis

Verifying the premalignant status of an oral lesion requires a biopsy. Supravital staining like use of toludine blue helps in taking the biopsy from a more representative area. The suspicious area is stained with toludine blue for 20 seconds and then the area is washed with saline. Punch or excision biopsy of the stained area is done.

Treatment

If the histopathological examination proves carcinoma-in-situ, entire area of involvement is excised ideally by using CO_2 or KTP-532 laser.

Chemoprevention

In case of epithelial dysplasia, beta-carotene and the retinoids may be used as antioxidant supplements for chemoprevention of oral cancer. Several clinical trials have found that treating oral leukoplakia solely with beta-carotene supplements is associated with clinical improvement; rates have ranged from 15 to 70 percent.

Estimated relative risk of developing oral cancer from various oral pre-cancers is given in Table 53.1.

MALIGNANCY OF THE ORAL CAVITY

Oral cancer accounts for about 3 to 4 percent of all cancers. Of all oral cancers, 96 percent are carcinomas and 4 percent are sarcomas. The most common type of oral cancer is squamous-cell carcinoma, constituting about 90 percent of oral malignancies. Chewing or smoking tobacco is the main cause of oral cancer, a condition which claims the lives of 10,000 people each year, more than cervical cancer. Because of late presentation, it has one of the worst survival rates of all cancers, less than 50 percent of patients survive more than 5 years after diagnosis. Yet, if it is detected and treated early, survival of oral cancer is better than those of most cancers. Thus, clinicians should look for any mucosal lesions by meticulous inspection and palpation for the early detection of cancerous changes in the mouth.

Anatomical Considerations

Various sites of oral cavity include the following. Lips, buccal mucosa, gingiva alveolus, buccogin gival sulcus and gingivolabial sulcus, hard and the soft palate, floor of the mouth, anterior two thirds of the tongue and the retromolar trigone. All these areas should be examined using a tongue depressor or a spatula. The tongue and the floor of the mouth are rich in lymphatics. The drain to both the sides and muscular action of the tongue may facilitate lymphatic spread. Vestibule of the oral cavity refers

Table 53.1: Estimated relative risk of developing oral cancer from various oral pre-cancers

Disease Name	Malignant Transformation Potential
Proliferative verrucous leukoplakia (PVC)	******
Nicotine palatinus in reverse smokers #	******
Erythroplakia	*****
Oral submucous fibrosis	*****
Erythroleukoplakia	****
Granular (verruciform, rough) leukoplakia	****
Laryngeal keratosis (leukoplakia)	***
Actinic cheilosis	***
Smooth, thick leukoplakia	**
Lichen planus (erosive forms)	**
Smooth, red tongue of Plummer-Vinson disease	**
Smokeless tobacco keratosis	*
Smooth, thin leukoplakia	+/−

 # reverse smoking: Smoking with the lit end of the cigarette in one's mouth

(**Reference:** Modified from: Bouquot JE. The pathology and progression of oral premalignancy. Proceedings, Epithelial Dysplasia Symposium, 5th International Congress on Oral Cancer, Royal College of Physicians, London, United Kingdom; September, 1997).

to the space between buccal mucosa-lips and gingival-teeth. Due to close proximity, retromolar trigone malignancies tend to involve the mandible and the pterygoid muscles early to produce trismus. The oropharynx is separated from the oral cavity by a line joining uvula, anterior pillars and the circum-vallate papillae.

Types of Malignancy

- Squamous cell carcinoma: >90 percent
- Verrucose carcinoma (Ackerman's tumor)
  - A less virulent form of squamous cell carcinoma thought to be caused by human papilloma virus.
- Salivary tumors– Adenocarcinoma, adenoid cystic carcinoma, mucoepidermoid carcinoma, etc.
- Sarcoma– Rare
- Lymphoma– More common in oropharynx

Squamous cell carcinoma: Commonest type of oral malignancy.

Etiology

1. **Tobacco:** At least 75 percent of oral cancer patients use tobacco in any form like smoking and tobacco chewing. Reverse smoking is common in certain areas of India and can cause palatal cancers.
2. **Alcohol:** Those who smoke and consume alcohol have 15 times higher risk of developing oral cancers compared to general population. Tobacco and alcohol act synergistically.
3. **Age:** More common above 40 years of age
4. **Sex:** Male: Female:: 6:1. Probably related to the lifestyle and habits.
5. **Race:** Black: white:: 2:1. (5-year survival is 33%:55%)
6. Genetic predisposition is not clear.
7. Prolonged exposure to sunlight and the use of sunscreens for protection are implicated as causative factors for cancer of the lips.
8. The human papilloma virus, particularly HPV16 and 18 have been implicated in some oral cancers.

9. *Nutritional deficiencies*: Diet low in fruits and vegetables have been blamed by some studies to predispose to oral cancer. Conversely diet rich in these could be preven- tive due to the presence of antioxidants.
10. Premalignant lesions like leukoplakia/ erythroplakia/submucous fibrosis. Six 'S' described to cause these are:
    - Smoking
    - Spices
    - Sepsis
    - Spirit
    - Sharp tooth
    - Syphilis

Pathological Types

Gross

- *Proliferative (Exophytic):* Cauliflower-like growth, irregular, friable and bleeds on touch.
- *Ulcerative (Endophytic):* Ulcer with everted and irregular edges bleeds on touch.
- Ulceroproliferative
- *Infilterative:* Lesion spreads deep and may appear as bulge/ edematous mucosa. Palpation reveals induration.

Microscopy

Squamous cell carcinomas are characterized by epithelial pearls and clusters of neoplastic squamous cells. They are differentiated into various

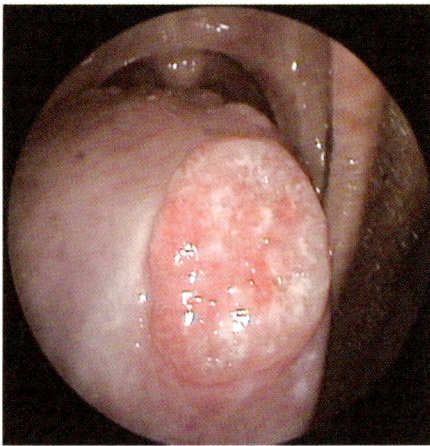

Fig. 53.3: Squamous cell carcinoma involving the left dorsum of the tongue extending to the lateral border

types depending on the number of cells that resemble the squamous cells.

- Verrucous carcinoma (Most well differentiated squamous cell carcinoma)
- Well differentiated squamous cell carcinoma: >75% differentiation
- Moerately differentiated squamous cell carcinoma: 50 to 75% differentiation
- Poorly differentiated squamous cell carcinoma: 25 to 50% differentiation
- Anaplastic carcinoma: <25% differentiation

Sites of Oral Malignancy

- Lips
- Buccal mucosa
- Lower alveolar ridge
- Upper alveolar ridge
- Retromolar trigone
- Hard palate
- Soft palate
- Floor of the mouth
- Anterior two thirds of the tongue—Lateral border/tip/dorsum/under surface (non-villious surface)

The most common site is the posterior ventrolateral border of the tongue followed by the floor of the mouth. Together with the retromolar region, these areas form a horseshoe-shaped zone of increased cancer susceptibility and this is the location of about 75 to 85 percent of all intraoral cancers.

Clinical Features

Symptoms

- In initial stages it may be asymptomatic or patient may experience burning/ discomfort or numb feeling over the site of lesion.
- Loose tooth or ill-fitting dentures
- Increased salivation
- Difficulty in mastication, (a tongue, retromolar trigone)
- Difficulty in articulation (in Ca tongue)
- Dysphagia/ odynophagia (Tonsilar toss Ca tongue)

- Abnormal taste may be present
- May notice a growing lesion in the oral cavity like fullness of the alveolus, ulcer or growth in the oral cavity.
- Pain radiating the ear (referred otalgia mediated through the trigeminal nerve) - Indicates advanced stage
- Facial asymmetry or cheek swelling which may ulcerate and fungate.
- Pain over the mandible.

Signs

- Characteristic growth may be seen which may be ulcerative/ proliferative/ulcero-proliferative or infilterative as described earlier.
- Note the inspectory and palpatory extent of the lesion.
- Evidence of leukoplakia/ erythroplakia or submucous fibrosis may be present.
- Mandibular involvement—Early sign would be periosteal thickening. Later stages may show widening of the alveolus or the tooth socket, tenderness or pathological fractures.
- Look for involvement tongue—Tongue movement may be restricted or may be fixed (ankyloglossia)
- Orodental status should be assessed.
- Cervical metastasis should be looked for both ipsilateral and contralateral sides.

Staging of Oral Malignancies

Stage I

Lesion is less than 2 centimeters in size (about 1 inch), and has not spread to lymph nodes in the draining areas.

Stage II

Lesion is more than 2 centimeters in size, but less than 4 centimeters (less than 2 inches), and has not spread to lymph nodes in the draining area.

Stage III

One of the following may be true: Lesion is more than 4 centimeters in size. Lesion is of any size but has spread to only one lymph node on the same side of the neck as the primary and is less than 3 centimeters in maximum dimension.

Stage IV

One of the following may be true:

(a) Lesion has spread to tissues around the lip and oral cavity. The lymph nodes in the area may or may not contain cancer.

(b) The cancer is any size and has spread to
  - More than one lymph node on the same side of the neck as the cancer
  - To lymph nodes on opposite or both sides of the neck,
  - To any lymph node that measures more than 6 centimeters (over 2 inches).

(c) The cancer has spread to other parts of the body.

Residual malignancy: Persistent lesion in spite of the treatment or reappearance of the lesion within 4 months in the same area. Persistent mucosal edema for more than 4 months in the site of the lesion treated should raise suspicion of residual malignancy.

Recurrent malignancy: Recurrent disease means that the cancer has come back (recurred) after it has been successfully treated. It may come back in the lip and oral cavity or in another part of the body.

The TNM staging system: T describes the tumor, N describes the lymph nodes, and M describes distant metastasis.

Primary Tumor Status

- TX Primary tumor cannot be assessed
- T0 No evidence of primary tumor
- Tis Carcinoma in situ
- T1 Tumor 2 cm or less in greatest dimension
- T2 Tumor more than 2 cm but not more than 4 cm in greatest dimension
- T3 Tumor more than 4 cm in greatest dimension
- T4 (lip) Tumor invades adjacent structures (e.g., through cortical bone, inferior alveolar nerve, floor of the mouth, skin of face, i.e., chin/ nose.)
- T4a (Oral cavity) Tumor invades adjacent structures (e.g., through cortical bone, into deep [extrinsic] muscle of tongue, maxillary sinus, skin of face)
- T4b (Oral cavity) Tumor invades masticator space, skull base, pterygoid plates and/or encases the internal carotid artery.

Nodal Status

Same as oropharynx which is discussed in page 489.

Distant Metastasis

- MX Presence of distant metastasis cannot be assessed
- M0 No distant metastasis
- M1 Distant metastasis

Differential Diagnosis

- Granulomatous conditions like TB/ Syphilis/ Hansens, etc.
- Eosinophilic granuloma
- Accessory salivary malignancy
- Pyogenic granuloma
- Granular cell myoblastoma.

Investigations

- Biopsy –Punch/excision/incision or wedge biopsy. Biopsy should be taken from the margins of the lesion. Supravital staining is helpful in case of leukoplakia.
- FNAC of the lymph nodes
- X-ray mandible/ orthopantomogram/ CT scan or Technitium bone scan to rule out mandibular involvement.
- Chest X-ray to rule out pulmonary metastasis and assess pulmonary status.

Management

Modalities of treatment include

- Surgery
- Radiotherapy
- Chemotherapy

Surgery

Wide excision with at least 1.5 to 2 cm of normal tissue all around including the depth of the tumor along with *en bloc* resection of the level I, II, III and IV nodal clearance in case of N0 neck (extended supraomohyoid neck dissection). If metastasis is seen (N1/ N2/ N3) a modified or radical neck dissection is required. Marginal mandibulectomy may have to be done if the growth is close to the mandible without periosteal involvement. Segmental or hemimandibulectomy is required for mandibular involvement depending on its extent. In case of the cancer of the anterior two third of the tongue, partial/ hemiglossectomy with or without tip sparing is done. Total glossectomy may be needed if tumor is crossing the midline or adjacent base tongue but functional reconstruction is often difficult and is more morbid. Surgical defect is reconstructed by primary closure or by using local flaps/ myocutaneous flaps/ free flaps (radial forearm with or without bone depending on the mandibular resection). Radial/ fibular bone along with skin and soft tissue free flaps is commonly used for mandibular reconstruction and the surgical defect of the tongue, floor of the mouth, etc. Stress is given on the experience of the surgeons for reconstruction. The possible reconstruction of the defect within the oral cavity is:

1. Mucosal lining
2. Mucosal lining plus bulk
3. Mucosal lining plus bone
4. Mucosal lining plus bulk plus bone

Myocutaneous flap reconstruction for oral cavity defects:

- Pectoralis major myocutaneous flap
- Latissimus dorsi flap
- Sternocleidomastoid myocutaneous flap
- Trapezius myocutaneous flap
- Platysma myocutaneous flap

Free tissue transfer options for intraoral reconstruction:

- Radial free forearm flap
- Lateral arm flap
- Latissimus dorsi free flap
- Rectus abdominus free flap
- Deep circumflex iliac artery free flap
- Scapular free flap
- Fibular free flap

Radiotherapy

Teletherapy (distance beam radiation) alone or in combination with brachytherapy is used. Approximately 6500 rads of radiation is given in about 28 fractions over 5 weeks. *Brachytherapy* (near beam radiation) is given in the form of needles, seeds, wires or catheters containing radioactive substances like Iridium-192, Cesium, Palladium, etc. may be given alone or in combination with teletherapy. Iridium is now more often used as needles in plastic tubing inserted into the tumor. Osteoradionecrosis is a common complication if radiation is given for tumors involving bone. In such cases radiation is preferred after surgical resection.

Chemotherapy has only adjuvant role along with other modalities. Cisplatinum and 5-Fluorouracil and Methotrexate are the common chemotherapeutic drugs used.

In early stages: T1 or T2, surgery or concomitant chemoradiotherapy alone may be employed and surgery if often preferred due to better disease control and less morbidity. Radiotherapy is given if results can be matched with that of surgery. In lip cancer if the commissure is involved, radiotherapy is preferred due to better functional/ cosmetic results. In advanced disease, stage III and IV, combined modality of treatment is often employed. Retromolar trigone cancers are better treated with surgery followed by radiotherapy due to early bone involvement.

Prognosis

57 percent survive 5 years for oral cavity cancer in the US 1992–99 (Cancer Facts and Figures, American Cancer Society, 2004)

Malignancy of the Oropharynx

Oropharyngeal malignancies are frequently associated with lymph node metastasis due to their rich lymphatic drainage. The lymphatics drain to both the sides and hence frequently associated with both occult and obvious metastatic nodes which are often bilateral.

Surgical Anatomy and Pathology

The detailed anatomy has already been described under the chapter 'Anatomy of the pharynx'. The oropharynx extends from the level of hard palate superiorly to the level of the hyoid bone inferiorly. The anterior-most part is the palatoglossal arch but the mucosa over it is continuous with that of the retromolar trigone. The main components are:

- *The anterior wall:* Base tongue (tongue posterior to the foramen cecum), vallecula and the lingual surface of the epiglottis. Tumor of the base of the tongue can involve the genioglossus and the hyoglossus muscles and can extend to the vallecula, epiglottis, larynx and the pre-epiglottic space.
- *The lateral wall:* Formed by the tonsillar fossa bounded by palatoglossal and the palatopharyngeal arches. The parapharyngeal space lies lateral to this wall. Any tumor infiltration here can involve this space and may infilterate all the structures here including the carotid sheath and its neurovascular structures. Roof is formed by the palatoglossus, palatopharyngeus, levator palati and tensor palati.
- *Posterior wall* which extends from the level of the hard palate to the level of the hyoid bone corresponds to second and third cervical vertebra and is bounded by the superior and inferior constrictor muscle. Tumors can extend to the nasopharynx above and to the hypopharynx below.
- Tumors of the tonsil, tonsillar pillar and soft palate, although anatomically located close to one another, behave quite differently from each other. Tumors of the tonsillar pillar tend to be more superficial and tend to spread over a broad region. By comparison, tonsillar fossa cancers often present with advanced, bulky tumors. Tumors of the soft palate often

are less aggressive. Soft palate tumors linger in early stages and remain superficial for longer periods.
- The lymphatics of the oropharynx drain into the jugulodigastric (level-2), jugulo-omohyoid (level-3) and the retropharyngeal group of lymph nodes frequently. Lower deep cervical nodes (level-4) also may be involved in advanced stages.

Etiology (Sqamous Cell carcinoma)

- Same as for oral cancers.
- Men are more affected than females by 5 to 8 times
- More common between 50 to 70 years

Pathological Types of Malignancy

- *Squamous cell carcinoma*: Commonest
- *Lymphoma:* Common in the tonsil
- Accessory salivary gland malignancies seen commonly in the soft palate like adenoid cystic carcinoma and mucoepidermoid carcinomas.

Sites of Oropharyngeal Malignancy

- *Lateral wall:* Commonest oropharyngeal tumor (50%) and it often involves the tonsil.
- Base of the tongue and vallecula is the second commonest site (40%)
- Other sites are rare.

Clinical Features

Symptoms

- Sore throat—Most common feature
- Lump in the throat
- Feeling of ulcer in the throat
- Odynophagia/dysphagia
- Neck selling due to lymph node metastasis
- Trismus
- 'Hot potato speech'
- Increased salivation and dribbling of saliva
- Otalgia mediated through the glossopharyngeal nerve.
- Pain in the neck

Classical presentation is described as 'a patient sitting in the out–patient department with hand over the ear due to pain and dribbling of the saliva, spitting frequently to a hand kerchief". This should raise the suspicion of oropharyngeal malignancy especially that of the base tongue.

Signs

Meticulous examination of the oral cavity and oropharynx should be done with special reference to anterior pillar, tonsillolingual sulcus, tonsillar fossae, base tongue and soft palate. Mirror examination will help in inspecting the hidden areas of the base of the tongue, valleculae and the tonsill- olingual sulcus as well as the nasopharyngeal surface of the soft palate.

Common Types of the Lesions

- Ulceroinfilterative lesions are common in base tongue and the vallculae.
- Endophytic lesions may sometimes be seen submucosally presenting as a simple indurated bulge especially in the base of the tongue with not frank ulcer on the surface.
- Proliferative (exophytic) are common in the posterior pharyngeal wall and sometimes in the tonsillar fossa and the soft palate.
- Assess the size and extent of lesion by both inspection and palpation
- Presence of unilateral smooth tonsillar mass should be suspected for lymphoma
- Tongue movements may be restricted or fixed (ankyloglossia)
- Palpation of the tonsilolingual sulcus, base of the tongue and vallecula are important for eliciting the induration.
- Careful examination for the lymph nodes should be made with special reference to the levels I, II, III, IV and V.

Investigations

- Biopsy –Punch biopsy should be taken from the margins of the lesion. Sometimes the biopsy may have to be done under general anesthesia if there is trismus or severe pain or lesions of the base tongue/ vallecula or the tonsillolingual sulcus. Incisional biopsy is preferred in such cases. If lymphoma is suspected in the tonsillar fossa, tonsillectomy should be done for tissue typing. Obtaining biopsy from base of the tongue can frequently cause problem
- Panendoscopy to rule out second primary
- FNAC of the lymph nodes
- CT/ MRI / PET-CT scan gives more information about the exact extent of the lesion especially with respect to its depth and tumor volume. It also gives more accurate information regarding the neck metastasis. PET-CT scan is very useful for pre and post treatment evaluation and to pick up occult primaries.
- Ultrasound of neck may be done for evaluation of the cervical node metastasis.
- X-ray mandible/ orthopantomogram/ CT scan or Technitium bone scan if mandibular involvement is suspected.
- Chest X-ray to rule out pulmonary metastasis and assess pulmonary status.

TNM Staging System (AJC 2002)

T describes the tumor, N describes the lymph nodes, and M describes distant metastasis.

Primary Tumor Status

- **TX** Primary tumor cannot be assessed
- **T0** No evidence of primary tumor
- **Tis** Carcinoma in situ
- **T1:** Tumor 2 cm or less in greatest dimension
- **T2:** Tumor more than 2 cm but not morethan 4 cm in greatest dimension
- **T3:** Tumor more than 4 cm in greatest dimension
- **T4a:** Tumor invades the larynx, deep/ extrinsic muscle of tongue, medial pterygoid, hard palate, or mandible.
- **T4b:** Tumor invades lateral pterygoid muscle, pterygoid plates, lateral nasopharynx, or skull base or encases carotid artery.

Nodal Status

- **NX** Regional lymph nodes cannot be assessed

- **N0** No regional lymph node metastasis
- **N1** Metastasis in a single ipsilateral lymph node, 3 cm or less in greatest dimension
- **N2** Metastasis in a single ipsilateral lymph node, more than 3 cm but not more than 6 cm in greatest dimension; in multiple ipsilateral lymph nodes, not more than 6 cm in greatest dimension; in bilateral or contralateral lymph nodes, not more than 6 cm in greatest dimension
- **N2a** Metastasis in single ipsilateral lymph node more than 3 cm but not more than 6 cm in greatest dimension
- **N2b** Metastasis in multiple ipsilateral lymph nodes, not more than 6 cm in greatest dimension
- **N2c** Metastasis in bilateral or contralateral lymph nodes, not more than 6 cm in greatest dimension
- **N3** Metastasis in a lymph node more than 6 cm in greatest dimension

Distant Metastasis

- **MX** Presence of distant metastasis cannot be assessed
- **M0** No distant metastasis
- **M1** Distant metastasis.

Treatment

Modalities of treatment include:

- Surgery
- Radiotherapy
- Chemotherapy
- Combined

Treatment Objectives

- **Curative:** Surgery/ Radiotherapy/ Surgery +postop radiation
- **Palliative:** Radiotherapy/ Radiotherapy + Chemotherapy/ Tracheostomy

The oropharyngeal tumors are often advanced with neck metastasis. They often require combined modality of treatment.

Base of Tongue (Figs 53.5 and 53.7)

For early stage tumors of the base of tongue, organ preservation is attempted with concomitant chemo-

radiotherapy. Small lesions may be excised microscopically using KTP-532 or CO_2 laser. Either surgery or radiation may be used as primary therapy with equally good results. Extended supraomohyiod neck dissection including level IV is done in N0 neck. In clinically positive neck nodes modified or radical neck dissection is done. For more advanced (T3 and T4) disease a combined treatment of surgery and radiotherapy is advocated. Alternatively a concomitant chemorad- iation therapy may be more advantageous over mutilating and often futile surgery. Early trials have shown encouraging results.

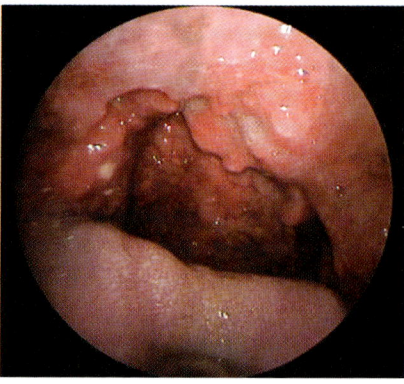

Fig. 53.4: Extensive ulcero-prolierative growth involving the soft palate, tonsil and the posterior pharyngeal wall. The soft palate is destroyed by the tumor

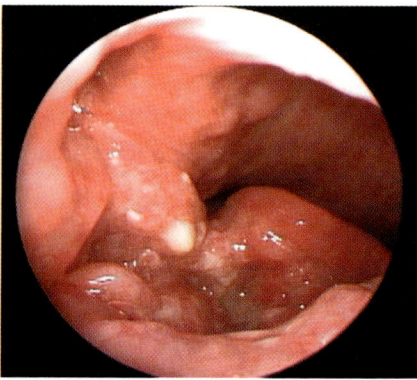

Fig. 53.5: Endoscopic picture showing an ulcero-proliferative growth involving the vallecula, lingual surface of the epiglottis and the base of tongue

Tonsil, Tonsillar Pillar and Soft Palate
(Figs 53.4 and 53.6)

For early lesions either surgery or radiation is advocated. Small tumors are easily amenable to laser excision. Due to the high risk of the disease spreading to nearby lymph nodes, treatment of the neck should be considered in all such patients. Advanced disease usually requires surgical intervention (Commando's operation) followed by postoperative radiation therapy. Mandibular preservation techniques have been advocated of late and it has changed the quality of life in such patients dramatically. However, treatment primarily with radiation followed by surgical treatment of the neck also may be an option.

Commando operation includes a mandibular swing approach (paramedian mandibulotomy) and lip splitting. Incision is extended to the neck either as 'Y', 'T' or inverted hockey stick to carry out simultaneous neck dissection. The surgical specimen includes

- Widely resected primary tumor with 1.5 to 2 cm margins along with the soft tissue with segmental mandibulectomy
- Continuous (en bloc) or discontinuous neck dissection including level I, II, III, IV for N0 neck and radical or modified neck dissection for a positive neck.

Surgical approaches and reconstruction methods are given in the Tables 53.2 and 53.3 (Fig. 53.8).

Posterior Pharyngeal Wall

For early stage disease, either radiation or surgery is contemplated. Surgery for even early stage

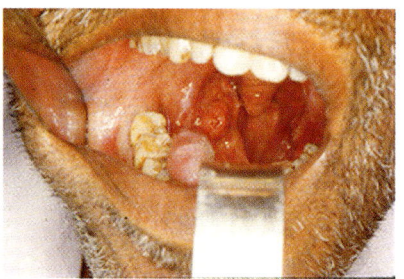

Fig. 53.6: Tonsillar malignancy

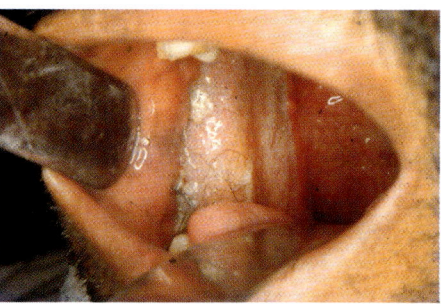

Fig. 53.8: Postoperative photograph of recons-tructed oropharyngeal defect by a pectoralis major myocutaneous flap

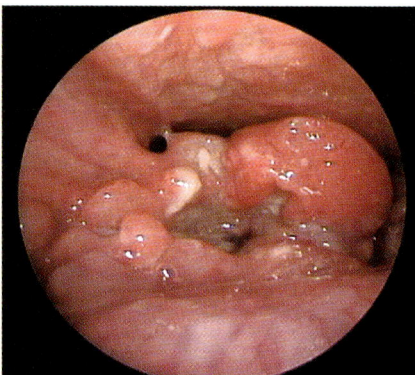

Fig. 53.7: Endoscopic picture showing ulcero-proliferatve growth involving the base of the tongue, vallecula and supraglottis

Table 53.2: Common surgical approaches for oropharyngeal cancer
• Peroral microscopic laser excision for T1 lesions
• Midline or paramedian mandibulotomy approach
• Angled mandibulotomy approach
• Suprahyoid median pharyngotomy approach
• Lateral pharyngotomy approach
• Mandibular sparing procedures.

Table 53.3: Reconstruction procedures following oropharyngeal resection

- Primary closure
- Local flaps using tongue flaps, masseteric muscle cross over flaps, temporoparietal fascial flaps
- Myocutaneous flaps like pectoralis major and latissimus dorsi are useful in reconstruction following Commando operation.
- **Free flaps:** Latissimus dorsi and rectus abd- ominus free flaps, radial forearm free flaps including skin and bone. Free scapular and fibular flaps can also be used for soft tissue and bone reconstruction.

disease typically calls for bilateral (both sides) neck dissections. Small tumors may be resected by a transhyoid or a lateral pharyngotomy approach. In advanced disease multimodality therapy should be considered.

Prognosis

In general oropharyngeal malignancies have a poor prognosis due to late presentation and early lymph node metastasis.

POINTS TO REMEMBER

1. Premalignant conditions of oral cavity and oropharynx are leukoplakia, erythroplakia, submucous fibrosis, lichen planus, plummer–Vinson syndrome, etc.

2. Leukoplakia refers to white patch in the mucosa that does not rub off and cannot be clinically identified as another entity. They should be excised and sent for histopathological examination to rule out malignancy.

3. Alcohol, chewing/smoking tobacco, human papilloma virus infection, etc. can cause cancer of oral cavity and oropharynx.

54

Neoplasms of the Nasopharynx

BENIGN TUMORS OF NASOPHARYNX

Benign tumors of nasopharynx are rare and the commonest form is angiofibroma.

Other Benign Tumors of the Nasopharynx

- Chondroma
- Dermoid
- Teratoma
- Hamartoma
- Epignathi
- Branchial cyst

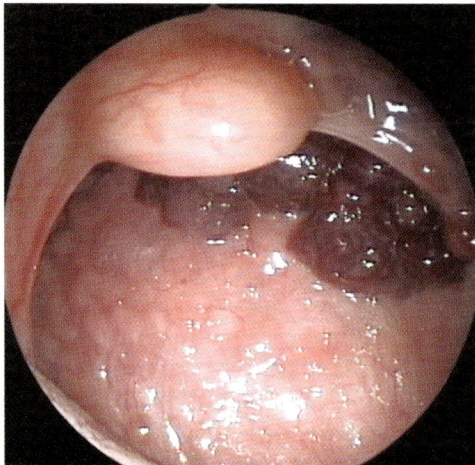

Fig. 54.1: Hemangioma of the nasopharynx

- Rhabdomyoma
- Hemangioma (Fig. 54.1)
- Hemangiopericytoma
- Craniopharyngioma.

JUVENILE NASOPHARYNGEAL ANGIOFIBROMA

Definition

Juvenile nasopharyngeal angiofibroma (JNA) is a histologically benign yet locally aggressive vascular tumor occupying the nasopharynx exclusively seen in adolescent males and is characterized by unprovoked paroxysms of painless profuse epistaxis.

Incidence

It is the commonest benign tumor of the nasopharynx and represents only 0.05% of all head and neck tumors.

Etiology

Exact cause was not known. Though it is common in adolescent males it may also be occasionally seen in adult males. Legouest in 1865 first reported its predilection in males. The term angiofibroma was first introduced by Friedberg in the year 1940.

Popular Theories of Etiopathogenesis

- Abnormal growth of embryonal fibrocartilage between the basiocciput and the basisphenoid
- Hormonal theory: Testosterone acting on a hamartomatous nidus of inferior turbinate tissue mislocated in the nasopharynx similar to the midline erectile tissue like penis. There is evidence of increased androgen receptors of tumors and successful tumor regression after anti-androgen therapy.
- Tumor growth from normal nasopharyngeal fibrovascular stroma.
- Desmoplastic response of the nasopharyngeal periosteum
- Origin from nonchromaffin paraganglionic cells of the terminal branches of the maxillary artery has also been suggested.
- Comparative genomic hybridization analysis of these tumors revealed deletions of chromosome 17, including regions for the tumor suppressor gene p53 as well as the Her-2/neu oncogene.
- Other suggested etiologies include trauma, inflammation, infection, allergy, and heredity.

PATHOGENESIS OF TUMOR SPREAD

The tumor can spread to various anatomical sites in and around the sphenopalatine foramen from where the tumor originates. Since the tumor does not have a definitive capsule it invades locally and behaves like a locally malignant tumor. The tumor extends usually along the path of least resistance and the thin plates of bone can easily be eroded to facilitate the tumor expansion further.

Medial

This is the earliest and the commonest extension where the tumor after originating from the sphenopalatine foramen enters the nasal cavity and the nasopharynx. This is associated with secondary attachments to the roof of the choana, posterior part of middle turbinate, nasal septum and the nasopharynx as the tumor enlarges further.

Lateral Spread

It occurs late and the tumor extends to the pterygopalatine fossa from where it can erode the posterior wall of the maxilla and thus can enter the maxillary sinus. Further lateral extension allows the tumor to involve the infratemporal fossa via the pterygomaxillary fissure and later into the cheek.

Posterior Spread

In the sphenopalatine foramen the tumor destroys the median pterygoid plate which forms the posterior margin of the foramen and then the lateral pterygoid plates and enters via the vidian canal.

Anterior Spread

Through the infraorbital fissure it spreads into the orbit and through the pterygopalatine fossa into the maxillary sinus.

Superior Spread

After entering the nasal cavity at the floor of the sphenoid sinus from the sphenopalatine foramen the tumor extends superiorly into the sphenoid sinus.

Intracranial Spread

It occurs commonly through the sphenoid sinus from where it can extend laterally to involve the cavernous sinus and superiorly to the sella and the middle cranial fossa. The tumor can extend anterolaterally from the sphenoid to the posterior ethmoids, orbital apex and the anterior cranial fossa. From the orbital apex the tumor can directly extend to the middle cranial fossa. The tumor from the pterygopalatine/ infratemporal fossa can erode the greater wing of sphenoid and extend into the middle cranial fossa.

Pathology

Though it was earlier thought to be arising from the roof of the nasopharynx, it is now confirmed to have its origin from a point above the superior margin of the sphenopalatine foramen and the base of medial pterygoid plate. Thus it tends to spread laterally into the pterygopalatine fossa.

- **Gross**
  - Lobulated, firm, non-encapsulated mass
  - Usually pink-grey or purple-red
  - Sessile or pedunculated
  - Secondary attachments usually, complicating resection in continuity.
- **Histopathology:** The characteristic histological features include:
  - It has no capsule.
  - Tumor composed of thin-walled vessels of varying caliber in a mature connective tissue stroma
  - The vessels are primitive embryonic in type and typically have a single endothelial cell lining without a muscularis or elastic layer, which probably explains the tumor's propensity for hemorrhage
  - Discontinuous vascular basal laminae, focal lack of pericytes, and pronounced irregularity of the smooth muscle layers. In thick smooth muscle layers and pads, the orientation of muscle cells is frequently disturbed, and the individual cells differ in size and shape. Occasionally, the muscle layers disperse peripherally into individual cells, creating the impression of vessel-independent smooth muscle cells within the stroma. (Beham et al, 2000).

Clinical Features

Symptoms

- This condition is seen exclusively in adolescent males but may rarely manifest at a later age.
- Average age of onset of symptoms: 14–18 years

- *Nasal and nasopharyngeal manifestations:*
  - Nasal obstruction, nasal discharge (100%). —This is unilateral initially and later may become bilateral due to obstruction to both choanae.
  - Profuse, painless, unprovoked paroxysms of epistaxis (60%)
  - Anosmia/hyposmia
  - Mouth breathing and snoring
  - Rhinolalia clausa
- *Extra-nasopharyngeal manifestations:*
  - **Facial:** Frog-face deformity, cheek swelling and proptosis is seen in advanced stage (Fig. 54.2).
  - **Otological:** Hearing loss, tinnitus, blocked feeling in the ear and recurrent otalgia may be present due to eustachian tubal orifice obstruction in the nasopharynx.
  - **Ophthalmological:** Symptoms include eye pain, lacrimation, proptosis, diplopia and rarely blindness.
  - **Neurological:** Tumor involving the cavernous sinus may cause multiple cranial nerve paralysis like involvement of trigeminal causing neuralgic pain; occulomotor nerve and trochlear nerve involvement may give rise to diplopia and optic nerve involvement in the orbital

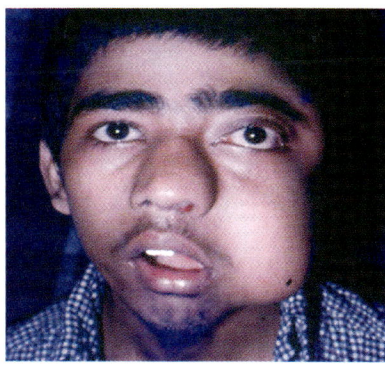

Fig. 54.2: Tumor showing extranasopharyngeal extension to the cheek and infratemporal fossa. Broadening of the nose on left side can also be seen

apex/ optic chiasma can give rise to blindness. Headache, blurring of vision and projectile vomiting suggest raised intracranial pressure.

– **General:** Sexual underdevelopment.

Signs

- Anterior rhinoscopy sometimes show the characteristic globular pinkish mass in the posterior part of the nasal cavity between the middle turbinate and the septum which is often pushed to the opposite side.
- Nasopharyngeal mass, usually pink-to-purple and globular with dilated blood vessels on its surface on postnasal examination (Fig. 54.3).
- *Probe test:* Contraindicated.
- Soft palatal bulge may be seen and is more prominent when the tumor occupies most of the nasopharynx (Fig. 54.4).
- Digitally palpation of the tumor is contraindicated
- Swelling of the cheek over the zygoma may be present
- Otological examination often show evidence of otitis media with effusion
- Proptosis
- Neurological signs as described under symptoms.

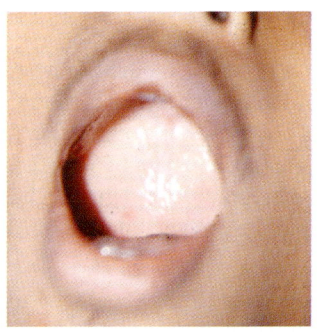

Fig. 54.4: Buldging of soft palate following compression

Investigations

- Diagnosis by clinical suspicion
- Diagnostic nasal endoscopy
- Biopsy contraindicated (Fig. 54.5)
- *Radiology*
  – Plain radiographs
  – CT scan/MRI
  – Vascular 'dumb-bell' shaped mass in nasal cavity/nasopharynx and pterygopalatine fossa with constriction at pterygopalatine foramen
  – Anterior bowing of maxilla and posterior bowing of pterygoids (Holman-Miller sign)
  – *Other extensions:* Intracranial and extracranial.

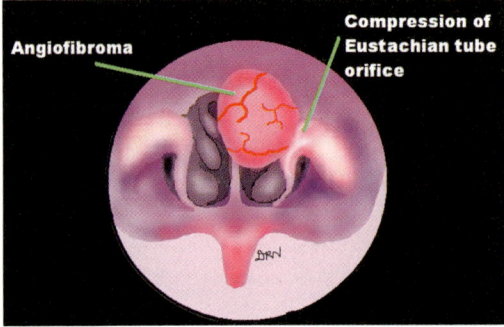

Fig. 54.3: Postnasal examination showing a pinkish globular vascular mass in the nasopharynx (angiofibroma) occupying the left choana, compressing the eustachian tube orifice

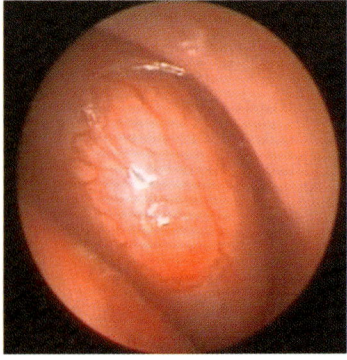

Fig. 54.5: Nasal endoscopic picture showing reddish vascular mass typical of a juvenile nasopharyngeal angiofibroma

- *Digital subtraction angiography*
  - Characteristic tumor blush is often seen.
  - Feeding vessels usually ipsilateral internal maxillary-may be embolised pre-operatively (Fig. 54.6).
  - Materials that can be used for embolization include Gelfoam, spring coils, etc. Non-absorbable polyvinyl alcohol particles are now the preferred materials that are used today.
- Findings suspicious for intracranial extension include blood supply of tumor from internal carotid artery.

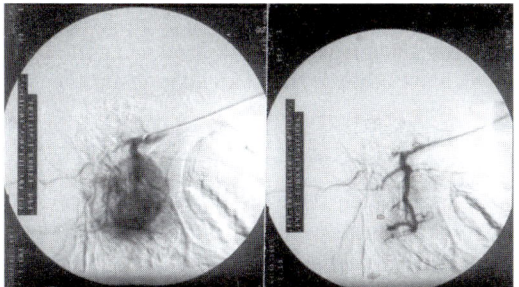

Fig. 54.6: Pre- and postembolization pictures for nasopharyngeal angiofibroma

Staging

- Classification according to Sessions
  - *Stage IA:* Tumor limited to posterior nares and/or nasopharyngeal vault
  - *Stage IB:* Tumor involving posterior nares and/or nasopharyngeal vault with involvement of at least one paranasal sinus
  - *Stage IIA:* Minimal lateral extension into pterygomaxillary fossa
  - *Stage IIB:* Full occupation of pterygomaxillary fossa with or without superior erosion of orbital bones
  - *Stage IIIA:* Erosion of skull base (i.e., middle cranial fossa/pterygoid base); minimal intracranial extension
  - *Stage IIIB:* Extensive intracranial extension with or without extension into cavernous sinus

- Classification according to Fisch
  - *Stage I:* Tumors limited to nasal cavity, nasopharynx with no bony destruction
  - *Stage II:* Tumors invading pterygomaxillary fossa, paranasal sinuses with bony destruction
  - *Stage III*: Tumors invading infra-temporal fossa, orbit and/or parasellar region remaining lateral to cavernous sinus.
  - *Stage IV:* Tumors invading cavernous sinus, optic chiasmal region, and/or pituitary fossa.

Treatment

- *Excision of the tumor:* Treatment of choice
- Adequate blood should be kept ready
- Preoperative embolization or external carotid clamping before excision to reduce bleeding
- Approach depends on the extent
- Complete excision should be done to prevent recurrence.

Surgical Approaches

- *Transpalatal:* Suitable for tumor limited to nasopharynx. This was originally described by Wilson. U-shaped incision is made about 2.5 cm anterior to the junction of soft and hard palate and the incision may be wound round the maxillary tuberosity to reach small extensions in the pterygopalatine fossa. Part of the hard palate bone can be removed for better exposure if the tumor, the junction of soft and hard palate extend further anteriorly. This gives good exposure of the nasopharynx but has risk of developing oro-nasal fistula which should be kept in mind (Figs 54.7 and 54.8).
- Lateral rhinotomy approach with medial maxillectomy gives good exposure and is suitable for extensions to maxillary sinus.
- Combined transpalatal in combination with Denker's modification of Caldwel-luc operation is suitable for extensions into the maxillary antrum.

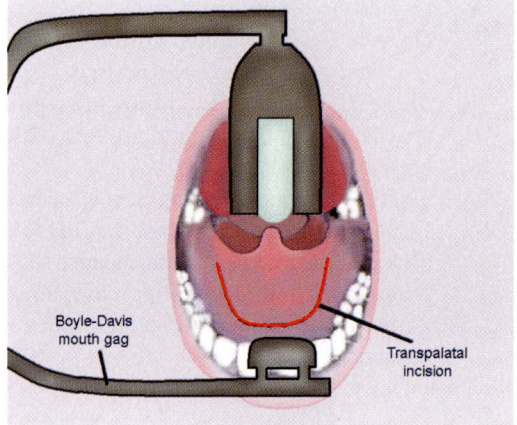

Fig. 54.7: Incision in the hard palate for Wilson's transpalatal approach

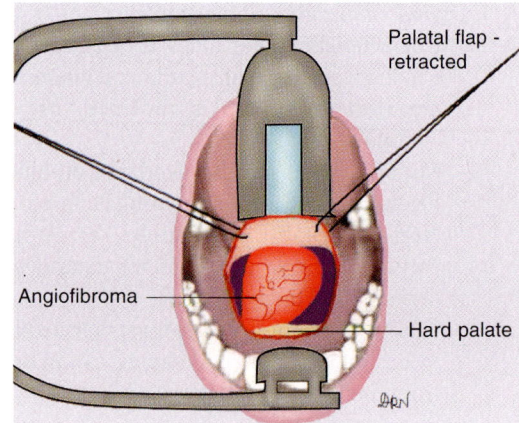

Fig. 54.8: Showing the exposure of the tumor after the palatal flap have been reflected and part of the hard palate being removed for better exposure

- *Sardana's approach:* Sublabial extension of transpalatal approach
- *Mid-facial degloving approach:* This gives good cosmetic results as it avoids facial incisions.
- Le Fort-I osteotomy approach: It is similar to mid-facial degloving approach and avoids facial incision. This gives good exposure for extra-nasopharyngeal extensions.
- Endoscopic endonasal approach for small and medium sized tumors with limited extensions to pterygopalatine fossa and sphenoid sinus.
- *Biller's approach:* Transmandibular lip-splitting approach gives excellent exposure of the infra-temporal fossa, pterygoid muscles and is suitable for very large tumors with multiple extensions including pterygopalatine fossa, infratemporal fossa and cheek. It has a disadvantage of external scar.
- Infratemporal fossa approaches for extensive tumors with intracranial extension to middle fossa (Fisch type C).
- Facial translocation approach (Janika 1997)
- Craniotomy if extensive intracranial extension is present.

Other modalities of treatment

- Radiotherapy, chemotherapy and hormonal therapy have been tried but none are curative. They are indicated in:
  - Extensive unresectable tumors
  - Tumors with extensive intracranial extensions.

Prognosis

- Depends on the stage
- Early diagnosis favor complete resection
- Prognosis good (>90%) if completely excised.

OTHER BENIGN TUMORS OF THE NASOPHARYNX

Chondroma

This is a neoplasm of cartilaginous origin. This can occur in solitary or multiple forms. It is rare in head and neck. Prevalence in nasopharynx and the first case reported was by Muller in 1970. They may arise from basi-occiput or basi-sphenoid. It is sometimes difficult to differentiate between chondroma and chondrosarcoma. Clinically it has an intact non-ulcerating mucosa.

Teratoma

They are autonomous new growths derived from pleuripotential tissue and are composed of elements of all three germinal layers. Teratoma of the nasopharynx is a well defined clinical entity and most of them are reported as a hairy polyp of the nasopharynx.

Hamartoma

The concept of hamartoma was introduced by Euger Albrecht 1904 to specify tumor-like malformations. The variant tissue of a part is present in improper proportion or is distributed with prominent excess of one particular tissue. They are commoner than teratomas. They are simple congenital malformations composed exclusively of components derived from local tissue. Hamartoma is common to a specific germinal layer as sebaceous adenoma, hemangioma, fibroma, etc.

Cavernous hemangioma (Fig. 54.1) is rare in pharynx and is extremely rare in nasopharynx. They are thin-walled with an effluent artery and efferent vein which do not communicate with the neighbouring capillaries. Trauma has been suggested by many as one of the causes. But, it may also be due to hormonal changes. But the recent view is that they are hamartomas and are mesenchymal in origin. Results are excellent with adequate surgical excision.

Craniopharyngioma

It has been accepted as a type of pituitary adenoma. They are defined as cystic tumors benign histologically, sellar or supra-sellar in position containing brownish fluid and is flaked with refractile cholesterol crystals. They can cause progressively increasing nasal obstruction as it fills the entire nasopharynx.

Choristoma

They represent a displacement of tissue in the course of development so that they appear in neighbouring organ. Some do not consider them as tumor but can be seen as misplaced analage. It can cause expansion and fill the whole of the nasopharynx and may extend to the para-pharyngeal space causing airway obstruction and stridor (Nayak et al).

NASOPHARYNGEAL CARCINOMA (NPC)

Cancer of the nasopharynx is the most confusing commonly misdiagnosed and most poorly understood disease. Recently with the development and recognition of the otolaryngology as a separate entity this condition is being studied with more interest. From retrospective studies there is evidence in the form of skull lesions (3000BC) in an Egyptian mummy that NPC is a disease which has existed for many centuries (Well 1963). Similar skull base abnormalities have been found in paravian and medieval English skeletons. Faradel in 1837 was first to report the finding of malignant tumors of nasopharynx at autopsy but the diagnosis was not supported by histological evidence of the neoplasm.

Incidence

It comprises 2% of all malignant tumors of head and neck in children and adult below the age of 30 years. But its incidence in Chinese is as high as 18% of all malignant tumors. It occurs more frequently than any other tumors of the upper respiratory tract (Ballenger 1985).

Surgical Anatomy of Nasopharynx

- 4 cm high, 4 cm wide and 3 cm in length
- Anterior—choanal orifice and posterior margin of nasal septum
- Floor—upper surface of the soft palate
- Roof and posterior wall
  - Body of the sphenoid, basiocciput
  - First two cervical vertebrae
- Lateral wall
  - Eustachian tube orifice

– **Fossa of Rossenmuller** (FOR)—This is the commonest site of origin of NPC. It is also called as pharyngeal recess.

Anatomical Relations of Pharyngeal Recess

- *Anteriorly*
  – Eustachian tube and levator palatini
- *Posteriorly*
  – Pharyngeal wall mucosa overlying pharyngobasilar fascia and retropharyngeal space
- *Medially*
  – Nasopharyngeal cavity
- *Superiorly*
  – Foramen lacerum and floor of carotid canal
- *Posterolateral*
  – Carotid canal and petrous apex, foramen ovale and spinosum.

Epidemiology of NPC

Geography and Race

- Distinctive epidemiological pattern
- Incidence—It is more common in:
  – Southern China (Kwantung province)
  – Hong Kong
  – Taiwan
  – South-East Asian races (Malay, Kadazan, Iban, Bidayuh, Indonesians and Thais)
  – Eskimos, North Africa, Tunisia.

Etiology of NPC

Various factors have been described as causative for NPC. They are:

- Environmental factors
- Geographical clustering in Southern China
- **Time Trend:** High risks among Chinese in Southern China
  – Incidence in Hong Kong, Singapore virtually remained unchanged 50 yrs
  – 2nd and 3rd generation born in USA shows decline.
- NPC constitute 16% of all malignant tumors among the Chinese

- Smoking and alcohol consumption
- Occupational
  – Exposure to nickel, chromium
  – Radioactive metal
  – Inhalation of chemical fumes
- Ingestions
  – Salted fish - Nitrosamine
  – Smoked food
- Drugs
  – Chinese herbal medicine
- Cooking habits
  – Household smoke and fumes
- Religious practice
  – Incense and joss stick smoke
- Socioeconomic status
  – Nutritional deficiencies, e.g. Vitamins A and C.

There are three main etiological factors in etiology of NPC; they are:

1. Epstein-Barr virus
2. Genetically determined susceptibility
3. Environmental factors that vary among populations. Etiological role of Epstein-Barr virus in NPC:

- More than 90% of patients having elevated antibody titres to Epstein-Barr virus in those who have NPC of the undifferentiated/ poorly differentiated forms. This was first established in 1966 based on serological studies. Later EB virus DNA was demonstrated in the neoplastic cells by nucleic acid hybridization. This virus is a Herpes virus that infects human B-lymphocytes.

- Moderate to well-differentiated NPC are devoid of Epstein-Barr virus antigen

- Thus clinically two types of NPC can be defined. Keratinzing versus non-keratinising.

- Histologically NPC has been classified by WHO before 1991 into 3 types:

  – **WHO type I:** Well differentiated squamous cell carcinoma (keratinizing type)
  – **WHO type II:** Non-keratinizing type resembling transitional cell type of the bladder.

– **WHO type III:** Undifferentiated carcinoma
  – Lymphoepithelioma
  – Anaplastic carcinoma

The new WHO classification in relation to EB virus association. This is of two types:

Type I: Keratinizing squamous cell carcinoma

Type II: Non-keratinizing carcinoma (a) Differentiated, (b) Un-differentiated

The most speific serological test is the IgA antibody response to EB virus induced viral capsid antigen (VCA) and the IgG antibody response to early antigen (EA/d). Anti VCA titres are also related to the total tumor burden. The antibody titre progressively increases with advancing tumor stage and are commonly lower in treated longer term survivors than untreaed patients.

Immunogenetics of NPC

- Prominent genetic susceptibility
  – High risk among southern Chinese population
  – Differential high risk in emigrant Chinese compared to indigenous population.
  – Family clustering of NPC in Chinese
  – Elevated risk in people having genetic admixture with Chinese
  – Low risk in other racial groups despite living in high-risk countries, e.g. Indians in Malaysia/Singapore
  – NPC is 4 times more common in first degree relatives of patients with the carcinoma than in controls. (Yu and Garbrant et al 1990)
  – In India it is more common in the north-eastern population
- **Histocompatibility Locus Antigen (HLA):** Loci of these HLA have been localized to the short arm of chromosome 6. By genomic hybridization technique, it has been demonstrated to have alterations at multiple chromosomes in NPC. The defects include deletion of regions at 1p, 3p, 14q, 16p and 16q. There is also amplification of 1q, 3q, 12p and 12q (Fang et al. 2001).

Pathology

Grossly the tumour presents in 3 forms:

- Proliferative growth causing nasal obstruction
- Ulcerative causing epistaxis
- Infiltrative which causes cranial nerve involvement.

Microscopy (Broder's Grading)

- **Grade I:** Well differentiated (cells show keratinization and obvious differentiation with <25% cells lacking differentiation)
- **Grade II:** Moderately differentiated (25–49% undifferentiated)
- **Grade III:** Poorly differentiated (50–74% undifferentiated cells)
- **Grade IV:** Anaplastic/undifferentiated (>75% cells are undifferentiated with marked anaplasia and mitotic figures).

Modes of Spread

This is divided into:

1. *Direct:* The most significant extension is upward into the intracranial cavity by infiltrating the bone at the base skull or through the foramina, especially foramen lacerum. The foramen lacerum lies close to the fossa of Rossenmuller and it easily allows the spread of tumor into the intracranial structures. This most frequent passage for intracranial spread is known as *Linconi highway* (Hara 1969). Invasion via this route without invading the surrounding sphenoid, petrosa or occiput is referred to as the *petrosphenoid route*. This allows early involvement of cavernous sinus and its contents in close proximity to foramen lacerum. Only in more advanced cases the extension can involve anteriorly along the middle cranial fossa involving the optic nerve

and the orbit posterior fossa involvement is very rare. Dura is relatively resistant to penetration and is invade late resulting in destruction of cerebral peduncle, optic tracts and temporal lobe. The tumor may also involve directly and can erode the basisphenoid, basiocciput and petrous temporal bone and sella turcica to optic chiasma and then extend to the orbit through the superior orbital fissure to cause proptosis. Lateral spread can involve the parapharyngeal space through the '*sinus of Morgagni*' and can involve both pre and post-styloid compartment. Anteriorly it may involve the nasal cavity and the paranasal sinuses and then to orbit, pterygopalatin and infratemporal fossae through sphenopalatine foramen. Inferiorly it involves the oropharynx and the soft palate.

2. *Lymphatic spread:* Lymphatic pathway is divided into median and lateral groups.

   • The median group drains the roof and posterior border of the nasopharynx into the lateral retropharyngeal node. This node may be bypassed, in which case, the first echelon node is the upper deep cervical lymph node chain located near the internal jugular vein.

   • The lateral group drains the lateral nasopharynx, including the fossa of Rosenmüller, and flows into the lateral half of the upper internal jugular chain or into the lateral retropharyngeal node. The lateral group is often a single node or several confluent nodes, termed the *Node of Rouviere*. Occasionally, the node is absent on one side and usually non-palpable. The node of Rouviere or the lateral cervical node is the most commonly involved lymph node. It usually lies below the base of the skull near the level of the atlas and may overlay the internal carotid artery. The upper cervical lymph node chain encases the internal jugular vein and receives lymph from the node of Rouviere. The last four cranial nerves may be involved due to compression by the node close to the jugular foramen (*node of Krause)* or from the upper deep cervical metastases or from the direct involvement of a deep pharyngeal recess lesion at the base skull. This causes paralysis of IX, X, XI cranial nerve (jugular foramen syndrome). The XII cranial nerve can be involved if the growth extends to involve the hypoglossal canal. The efferent pathway descends along the internal jugular vein to the lower deep cervical nodes, terminating at the junction of the internal jugular vein and subclavian vein on the right and the thoracic duct on the left.

3. *Hematogenous*

   • This is rare and occurs to bone, liver and lungs. Bone commonly affected is spine, shoulder, pelvis and skull.

Clinical Behavior and Survival

The survival rates and the aggressiveness of the tumor have been found to be inversely proportional to the age of onset. Younger the age, more aggressive is the tumor.

Clinical Features

   • Mostly seen in 5th to 7th decades but not uncommon to see in the twenties and thirties.
   • Males are affected 3 times more than females.

Symptoms

   • Bewildering array of symptoms and signs
   • 'Always a challenging problem, both from diagnostic and therapeutic standpoint, malignant lesions of the nasopharynx are perhaps most commonly misdiagnosed, most poorly understood, and most pessimistically regarded of all tumors of the upper part of the respiratory tract'.

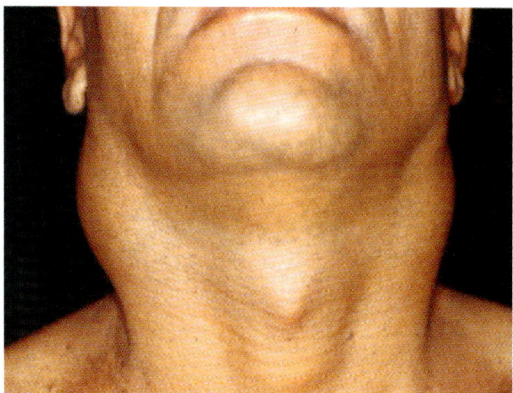

Fig. 54.9: Bilateral cervical lymphatic metastasis in nasopharyngeal carcinoma

The symptoms and signs may be described according to the part that is affected as follows:

- *Cervical*
  - Lump in the neck (60– 80%): This is most common presenting symptom for which the patient seeks advice (Fig. 54.9).
- *Nasal*
  - Nasal obstruction may be unilateral or bilateral and depends on the extent of the disease.
  - Mucoidal or blood-stained nasal discharge
  - Nasal bleeding
  - Ozaena due to tumor necrosis
  - Blood-stained saliva on hawking
- *Otological:* NPC leads to eustachian tube occlusion.
  - Block sensation of ear
  - Hearing loss
  - Otalgia may be due to otitis media or may be referred tinnitus
  - 'Adult patients of Chinese origin with unresolving unilateral serous otitis media have to be presumed to have nasopharyngeal carcinoma until proven otherwise'.
- *Ophthalmic*
  - Diplopia often due to 6th nerve involvement
  - Epiphora

- Proptosis
- Loss of corneal reflex
- Diminished vision
- *Neurological*
  - Headache may be due to dural irritation, sinus involvement, trigeminal nerve involvement or due to muscle spasm follwing invasion
  - VI-Lateral rectus palsy - Diplopia and squint
  - III, IV, VI —are commonly affected together (ophthalmoplegia)
  - V - High neck and facial pain and paraesthesia
  - IX, X & XI—Jugular foramen syndrome
  - Isolated single C.N. palsy common with nerves V & VI
- *Miscellaneous*
  - Weight loss
  - Loss of appetite
  - Trismus
  - Cachexia.

Signs

- **Pharyngeal:** Palatal swelling or bulge may be seen and the soft palate may be involved in advanced stages. Tumor may extend to the oropharynx from the nasopharynx. Postnasal examination may show a diffuse bulge or proliferative/ulcerative growth in the naso-pharynx commonly from the 'fossa of Rossenmuller'.
- **Nasal:** On anterior rhinoscopy, mass in the nose may be seen if the tumor extends into the nasal cavity. Blood-stained discharge may be noted. Mass is often friable and bleeds on touch.
- **Otological:** Tympanic membrane may show bulge with evidence of otitis media with effusion. Sometimes perforation of the drum with suppurative otitis media may be seen. Tuning fork test often reveals conductive deafness.
- **Cervical:** Enlarged palpable cervical lymph nodes are frequently found affecting the level II, III and Va nodes. Often the patient presents

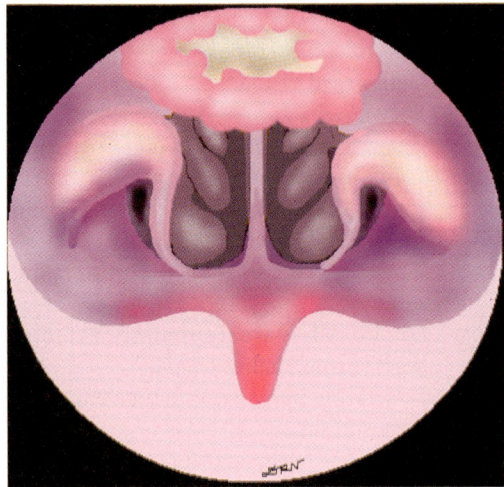

Fig. 54.10a: Carcinoma of the roof of the nasopharynx with extensive ulceration and surrounding infiltration. They can be better visualized by 120° endoscope by transnasal approach, or 45° endoscope by transoral approach.

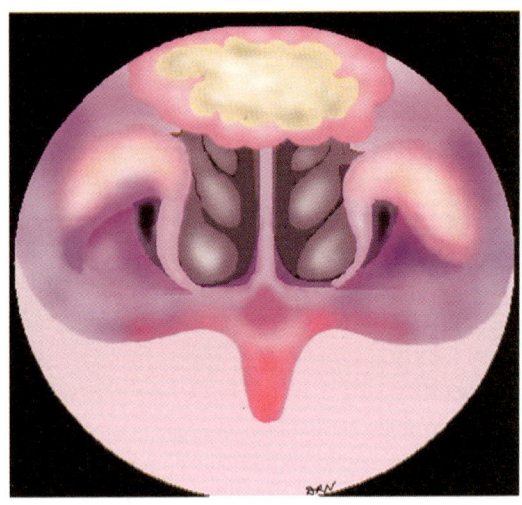

Fig 54.10b: Extensive ulcero-infilterative growth of the roof of the nasopharynx.

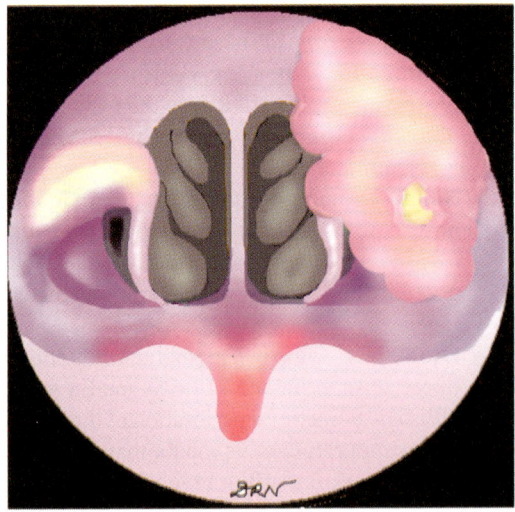

Fig. 54.10c: Undifferentiated carcinoma/lympho-epithelioma with polylobated outgrowth with little ulceration involving eustachian tubal orifice.

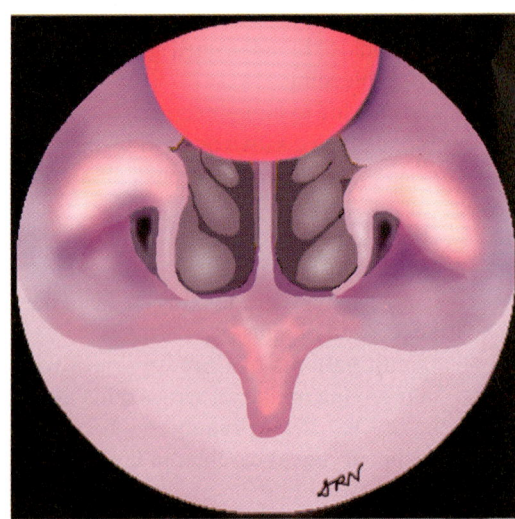

Fig. 54.10d: Lymphoma of the nasopharynx with partial obstruction of the choana

with neck swelling as the only feature. Ho's triangle is an important site for metastatic neck nodes from NPC which is situated in the posterior triangle of neck.

- Retropharyngeal group of L.N. (Rouviere) 1st lymphatic filter not palpable
- Commonest palpable node - jugulo diagastric, L2/L3/L5 level
- Contralateral lymph nodes metastasis (nasopharynx is midline structure).

- **Ophthalmological**
  - Total or partial ophthalmoplegia may be present.
  - Proptosis and decreased vision may occur if the tumor invades the orbit involving the optic nerve.
  - Epiphora can occur due to obstruction to nasolacrimal duct.

- **Neurological**
  The nerves may be compressed intra-cranially and the nerves that are more frequently involved begin with the lowest in anatomical position, i.e. V, VI, III, IV, VII and II. Intracranial involvement is more frequent in squamous cell carcinoma than in lymphoepithelioma. Loss of corneal reflex is sometimes the first sign of intracranial invasion (Lederman 1954). Extracranial nerve involvement occurs due to the carotid sheath involvement closest to the retropharyngeal nodes. This can involve the last 4 cranial nerves (IX, X, XI, XII) causing jugular foramen syndrome. Facial pain/paresthesia may be due to the V nerve involvement. Horner syndrome with ptosis, miosis, and anhydrosis occurs when the cervical sympathetic plexus coursing along the carotid is involved.

- **Trotter's triad:** This refers to decreased hearing, mandibular pain and impaired soft palate mobility. The conductive deafness is due to obstruction to the Eustachian tube orifice by the tumor. Local invasion of the soft palate may cause immobility. Paralysis of the soft palate may be due to involvement of cranial accessory nerve in the pharyngeal plexus through vagus. Pain is due to involvement of fifth cranial nerve at the foramen ovale.

- **General**
  - Loss of weight
  - Metastasis to lungs, bone, etc.
  - Trismus suggests infiltration of pterygoid muscles
  - In advanced cancers endocrine changes may be seen such as Cushing's syndrome, dermatomyositis and pseudomyasthenia gravis (Eaton-Lambert syndrome).

- **Distant Metastasis**
  - Incidence rate is about 30%
  - Sites commonly involved:
    - Skeletal—Thoracolumbar spine > 50%
    - Lung metastasis
    - Liver metastasis
  - 90% of patients die within the 1st year of diagnosis of the first distant metastasis

Investigations

- Diagnostic nasal endoscopy (DNE)
  - Inspection of the nasopharynx space (Fig. 54.11)
  - Localisation and extent of tumour
  - Biopsy under vision.
- Fine needle aspiration cytology of the neck lymph node
- CT scan (Fig. 54.12)
  - Extent of tumor
  - Neck node involvement
- Bone scan
- Skeletal metastasis-thoracolumbar region
- MRI: Gives better soft tissue delineation
- Chest X-ray for lung metastasis.

Staging of NPC (TNM Classification-AJCC 2002)

T: Primary Tumour

- T1—Tumour confined to nasopharynx

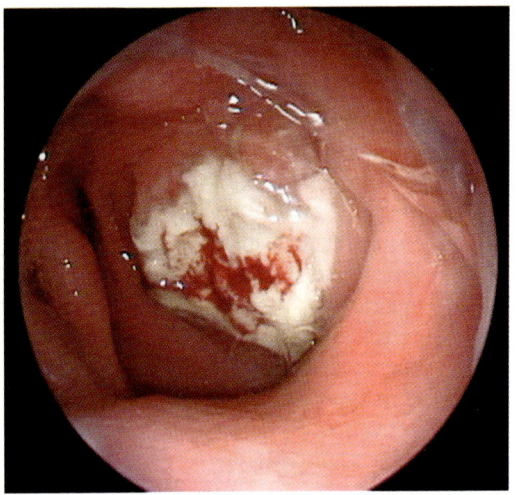

Fig. 54.11: Endoscopic picture taken using 30° nasal endoscope showing polylobated mass in the nasopharynx with ulceration

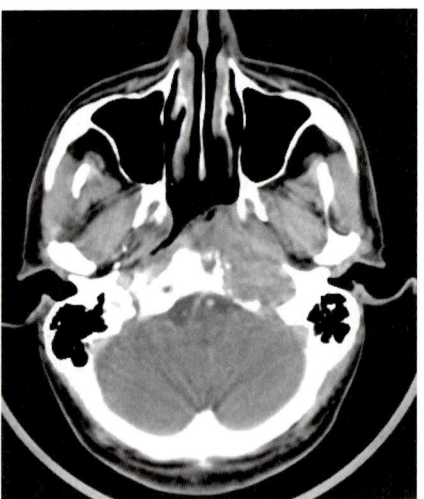

Fig. 54.12: CT scan showing destruction of the skull base in the region of the jugular foramen

- T2a—Tumour extends to oropharynx/nasal cavity without parapharyngeal spread.
- T2b—Tumor with parapharyngeal extension.
- T3—Tumor involves bony structures and/or paranasal sinuses
- T4—Tumor invasion intracranial structures and/or cranial nerves, infratemporal fossa, orbit, masticator space or hypopharynx.

N: Cervical Lymph Node Involvement

- N0—No clinically positive node
- N1—Single clinically positive homolateral node 3 cm or less in diameter
- N2—Single clinically positive homolateral node > 3 cm but < 6 cm or multiple clinically positive homolateral nodes > 6 cm in diameter
- N3—Massive homolateral node(s), bilateral nodes or contralateral node(s).

M: Distant Metastasis

- MX—Not assessed
- M0—No (known) distant metastasis
- M1—Distant metastasis present

Treatment Policy

Chemoradiotherapy

- Primary modality of treatment
- Radiotherapy: 6000 rads.
- Chemotherapy
  - Cisplatin and 5-flurouracil

Surgery has a limited role and is indicated in the following:

- Biopsy of the nasopharyngeal mucosa
- Radioresidual/recurrent primary tumor:
- Radical neck dissection for radioresistant lymph nodes.

Recurrent/residual NPC. It may be treated with:

1. Brachytherapy or 2nd course of external radiation
2. *Surgery:* The surgical approaches that can be adopted are:
   - Fisch type C approach
   - Biller's approach
   - Maxillary swing approach
     Surgery is a better option if there is brachytherapy failure or if brachytherapy is not available then a second or third

course of radiation considering the complications that can be encountered following subsequent course of radiation is considered.

3. *Chemotherapy* (palliative)
   - For distant metastasis
   - Failed radiation/surgery

Prognosis

- Early diagnosis and treatment of NPC has a good prognosis (>5years)
- Lymphoepithelioma (variant of anaplastic carcinoma) has a better survival rate.
- Patients should be followed up regularly.

POINTS TO REMEMBER

1. JNA exclusively affects adolescent males and arises around the sphenopalatine foramen.
2. Biopsy of JNA is contraindicated due to fear of fatal profuse bleeding.
3. Preoperative selective embolisation helps in reducing the intraoperative blood loss.
4. Complete excision of JNA is its treatment of choice. Surgical approach is decided by its extranasopharyngeal extension.
5. NPC has characteristic geographical distribution.
6. Fossa of Rossenmuller is the commonest site of origin of NPC.
7. Due to close proximity to skull base, surgery has a limited role in the management of NPC. Chemoradiotherapy is the treatment of choice.

Malignancy of Hypopharynx

ANATOMY OF HYPOPHARYNX

- Hypopharynx is also known as laryngo-pharynx as it is part of the pharynx that lies posterior to the larynx.
- It extends from level of floor of vallecula (hyoid bone) to lower border of cricoid cartilage
- It is made–up of 3 parts:
  - Pyriform sinus (fossa)
  - Posterior pharyngeal wall
  - Postcricoid area (Fig. 55.1).

Pyriform Fossa

This is part of the hypopharynx situated lateral to the aryepiglottic folds, one on either side. It is a 'pear' shaped fossa which is broad superiorly and narrow inferiorly called the apex. The apex lies almost at the level of the lower border of the

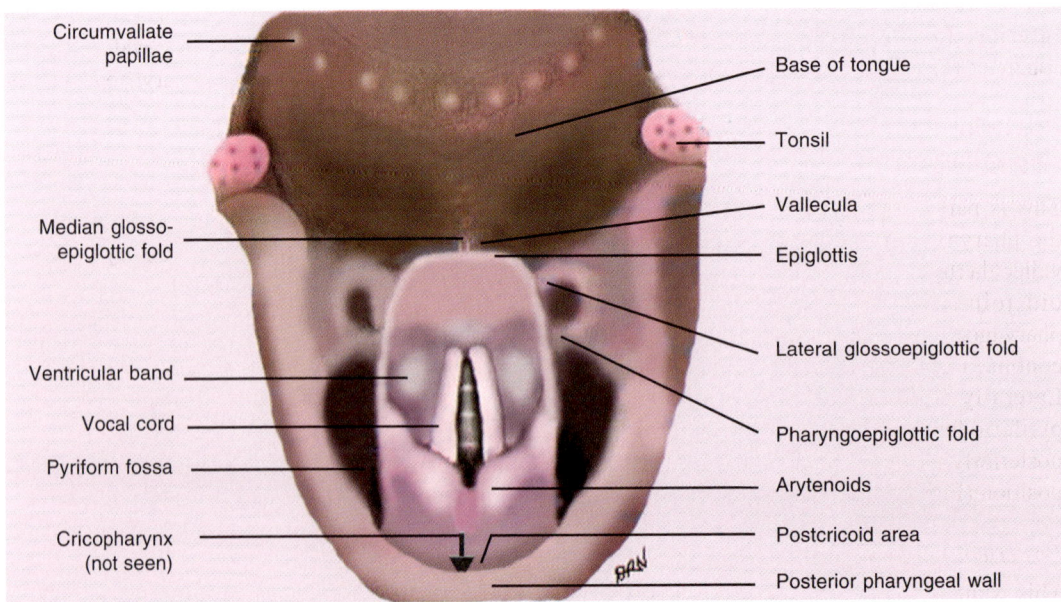

Circumvallate papillae
Base of tongue
Tonsil
Median glosso-epiglottic fold
Vallecula
Epiglottis
Lateral glossoepiglottic fold
Ventricular band
Vocal cord
Pharyngoepiglottic fold
Pyriform fossa
Arytenoids
Cricopharynx (not seen)
Postcricoid area
Posterior pharyngeal wall

Fig. 55.1: Parts of hypopharynx and larynx

cricoid where it continues with the cricopharyngeal sphincter. The pyriform fossa is membranous superiorly and cartilaginous inferiorly where it resists distension. Tumors involving lower pyriform fossa thus present early with dysphagia than the upper pyriform fossa lesions.

Boundaries of Pyriform Fossa

Medial: Aryepiglottic folds above and cricoid cartilage below.

Lateral: Thyrohyoid membrane above and thyroid cartilage below.

Anterior: Anterior mucosa of the pyriform sinus is related to the paraglottic space of the larynx. It is separated superiorly from the oropharynx by the pharyngoepiglottic fold.

Posterior: The lateral wall of this fossa continues posteriorly as the posterior pharyngeal wall. A line drawn along the vocal cords in its lateral (abducted) position as on deep inspiration is extended posteriorly. This line demarcates between the lateral wall of pyriform fossa and posterior pharyngeal wall

Superior: Level of the pharyngoepiglottic fold.

Inferior: Apex continues with cricopharyngeal sphincter (Fig. 55.2).

Posterior Pharyngeal Wall of Hypopharynx

This is part of the posterior pharyngeal wall of the pharynx from the level of the floor of the vallecula (hyoid bone) to the level of cricoarytenoid joint. Above it continues as posterior pharyngeal wall of the oropharynx and below it continues as posterior part of postcricoid area. Laterally it continues as lateral wall of the pyriform fossa, being demarcated by a line drawn posteriorly along the vocal cords in its abducted position (Figs 55.1 and 55.2).

Postcricoid Area

This is the part of the hypopharynx which is not visualized on indirect laryngoscopy. It lies

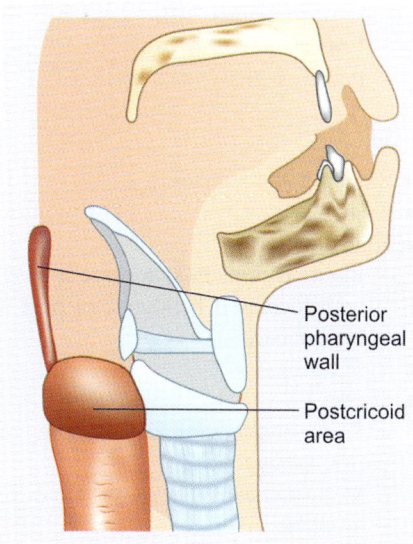

Fig. 55.2: Area of postcricoid region and posterior pharyngeal wall in relation to larynx

posterior to the cricoid cartilage and extends from the level of cricoarytenoid joint to the lower border of the cricoid cartilage where it is continuous with the cricopharyngeal sphincter. This area has an anterior wall which abuts the laminae of the cricoid cartilage and a posterior wall which is continuation of the posterior pharyngeal wall of the hypoharynx.

Types of Malignancy

- **Squamous cell carcinoma** (95%)
- Salivary neoplasms (accessory salivary glands)
- Lymphoma
- Sarcoma.

Squamous Cell Carcinoma of Hypopharynx

Incidence

- Common cause of dysphagia in elderly (50 years)
- Incidence of malignancy in different areas of hypopharynx:

– Pyriform sinus: 60%
– Postcricoid: 30%
– Posterior pharyngeal wall: 10%.

Etiology

• Smoking and alcohol
• Diet
• Nutritional
  – Plummer-Vinson syndrome is associated with increased incidence of post cricoid malignancy.
• *Age:* >50 years
• *Sex:*
  – Postcricoid malignancy is more common in females
  – Malignancy in other sites is more common in males
• Genetic predisposition has been considered. Certain 'oncogenes' have been identified making one more prone to malignancy.
• Radiation for other H&N malignancies can give rise to second primary in the hypopharynx.

Pathology

• Gross: 3 types of tumor may be seen:
  – Proliferative (exophytic) 'cauliflower-like'
  – Ulcerative (endophytic/ infiltrative)
  – Ulceroproliferative

Microscopy

Differentiated into four types:

• Well differentiated   <25%
• Moderately differentiated 25–50%
• Poorly differentiated   50–75%
• Anaplastic   >75%

Spread

• Lymphatic
• Direct
• Hematogenous (<5%)

Lymphatic spread

The lymph node involvement could be 'Obvious' or 'Occult'. The incidence of nodal metastasis depends on the site of the primary.

• Pyriform sinus
  – 60–75% (30% bilateral)
  – Jugulodigastric nodes (L2) and juguloomohyoid nodes (L3) are commonly affected.
• Postcricoid area:
  – 20% (least)
  – Paratracheal/ mediastinal and lower deep cervical nodes may be affected.

• Posterior pharyngeal wall
  – 40%
  – Retropharyngeal/ deep cervical.

Direct Spread (Fig. 55.3)

This depends on the location of the tumor in the hypopharynx. Involvement of the paraglottic space of the larynx is common which causes fixation of the vocal cords. Pyriform malignancy often involves the supraglottis and may extend above to the oropharynx crossing the pharyngoepiglottic fold. Inferiorly it may extend to the postcricoid area or the cricopharyngeal sphincter. Involvement of the laryngeal cartilages and extralaryngeal spread of the tumor of the hypopharynx is considered as advanced (T4) and

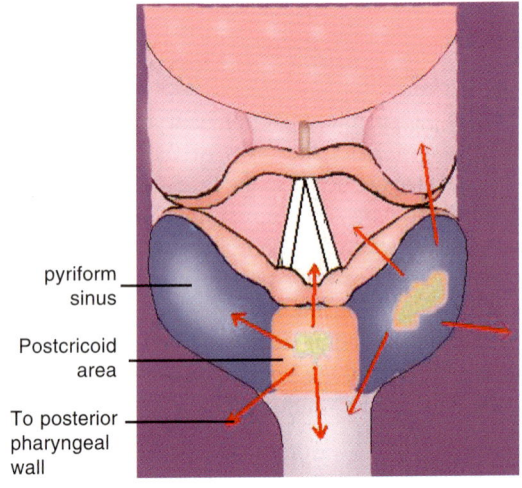

pyriform sinus

Postcricoid area

To posterior pharyngeal wall

Fig. 55.3: Mode of spread in hypopharyngeal cancer

warrants combined modality of treatment. Pyriform fossa and postcricoid tumors may extend to the thyroid gland and a total or hemi-thyroidectomy is often combined along with the laryngeal surgery.

Clinical Features

- Depends on
  - Site of involvement
  - Stage
  - Involvement of other structures
- 'Pain is a late feature'

Symptoms

- Males >50 years, females >30 years
- Progressive dysphagia more to solids is a common symptom. Thus the dictum should be 'any elderly patient or middle aged female-prolonged progressive dysphagia (>1 month) should be provisionally diagnosed as cancer throat/ esophagus and investigated'
- Feeling of lump/ FB sensation may be the initial symptom especially in upper pyriform fossa or posterior pharyngeal wall cancers.
- Discomfort during swallowing
- Neck swelling due to lymph node metastasis or extralaryngeal spread.
- Hoarseness may be seen if the vocal cord gets fixed.
- Choking spells may be encountered more at night due to spill-over of the pooled saliva in the pyriform fossa, especially during sleep.
- Aspiration
- Absolute dysphagia
- Stridor due to laryngeal involvement is not uncommon.
- Pain in the throat radiating to the ipsilateral ear (referred otalgia via the vagus nerve) is due to tumor infiltration of the nerve or due to perichondritis following cartilage involvement.

Signs

- **Indirect laryngoscopy**
  - Characteristic proliferative/ ulcerative or ulceroproliferative growth is often seen (Figs 55.4 and 55.5).
  - Pooling of saliva may be present in lower pyriform fossa or postcricoid lesions.
  - VC movement may be restricted or fixed
  - Edema of arytenoids suggest postcricoid malignancy.

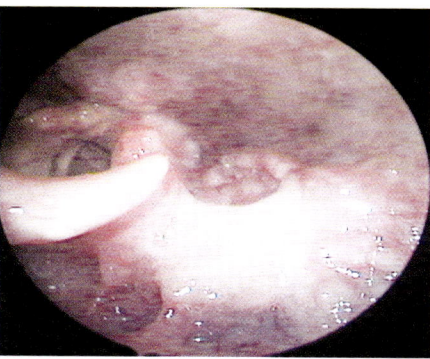

Fig. 55.4: Endoscopic picture showing ulceroproliferative growth in the left pyriform fossa extending to the pharyngoepiglottic fold and adjacent vallecula

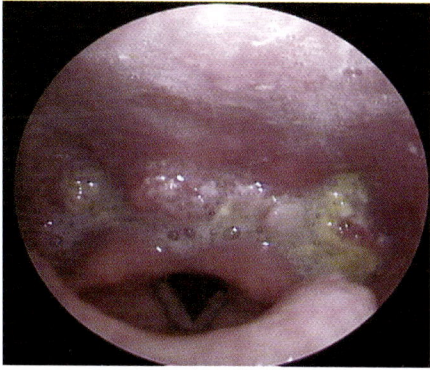

Fig. 55.5: Endoscopic picture of ulceroproliferative growth in the retroarytenoid area, pyriform fossae and adjacent posterior pharyngeal wall, in case of post-cricoid carcinoma

- **Neck**
  - Metastatic node should be looked for.
  - Laryngeal widening or 'splaying' may be present
  - Larynx is pushed forwards in post-cricoid malignancy.
  - *Laryngeal crepitus* is absent in postcricoid malignancy.
  - Look for extralaryngeal spread and laryngeal tenderness.

Investigations

- X-ray lateral/ AP view (soft tissue) (Fig. 55.6a)
  - Prevertebral widening
  - Airway patency
  - Cartilage erosion
- CXR
  - Mediastinal widening
  - Aspiration pneumonia
  - Secondaries in lungs
- Barium swallow with fluroscopy– Sensitive 90% (Fig. 55.6b).
  - Filling defects/mucosal irregularities
  - Stasis/aspiration (spill over)
- FNAC
- Flexible/rigid hypopharyngoscopy and biopsy

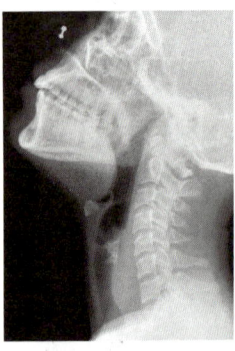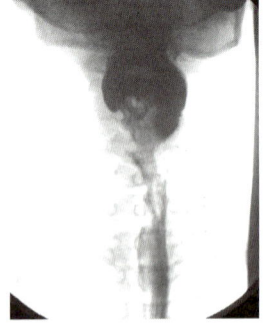

Figs 55.6a and b: (a) Plain radiograph of the neck lateral view showing prevertebral widening, (b) Barium swallow of the same patient showing the irregular filling defect in the right pyriform fossa and post cricoid area.

- CT/ MRI– To assess the extent of direct spread and involvement of nodes.

Staging

- TNM staging
  - Classified into 4 stages: I – IV
  - T 0–4: tumor size and extent
  - N 0–3: Lymph node status
  - M 0–1: Distant metastasis

Hypopharynx

T1 Tumor limited to 1 subsite of hypopharynx and 2 cm or less in greatest dimension

T2 Tumor invades more than 1 subsite of hypopharynx or an adjacent site, or measures more than 2 cm but not more than 4 cm in greatest diameter without fixation of hemilarynx

T3 Tumor measures more than 4 cm in greatest dimension or with fixation of hemilarynx

T4a Tumor invades thyroid/cricoid cartilage, hyoid bone, thyroid gland, esophagus, or central compartment soft tissue.

T4b Tumor invades prevertebral fascia, encases carotid artery, or involves mediastinal structures.

Treatment

Three modalities:

- Surgery
- Radiotherapy
- Chemotherapy
- Stage I and II: Radiation alone (to preserve voice)
- Stage III and IV: 'Combined modality'
  - Surgery+ radiotherapy
- Role of chemotherapy
  - Only 'adjuvant'
  - Cisplatin, 5 fluorouracil, methotrexate, etc.
  - May have a palliative role?

Surgery

- Tracheostomy (emergency/elective/preliminary to laryngectomy)

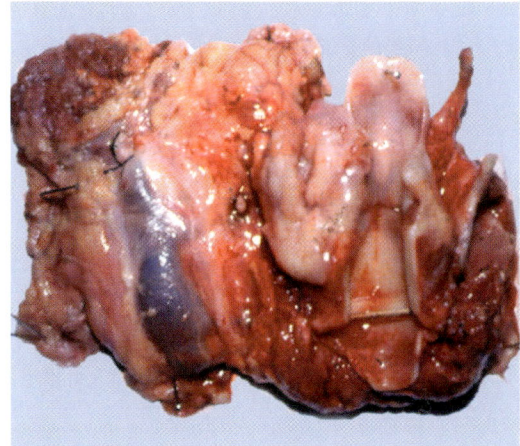

Fig. 55.7: Resected specimen after widefield total laryngectomy, partial pharyngectomy with left radical neck dissection done for cancer of the right pyriform fossa

– Total/partial laryngectomy with partial/total pharyngectomy (Fig. 55.7)
– Total laryngo-pharyngo-esophagectomy (TLPE) with gastric pull up/ colonic transposition (55.8).
– Neck dissection +/–

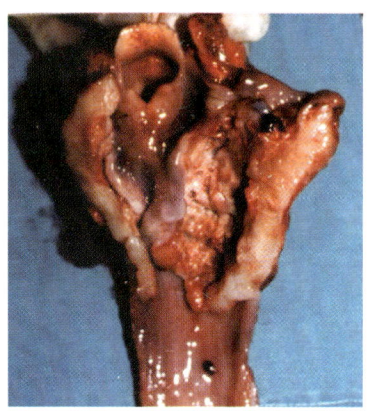

Fig. 55.8: Extent of spread of right pyriform fossa malignancy with involvement of apex

Radiotherapy
– External
– 6500 rads. over 5 weeks

Prognosis
– Good in early stages
– Stage I and II: Up to 80% 5 year survival
– Advanced and postcricoid: Poor prognosis.
– Surgery gives better quality of life by allowing early swallow.

POINTS TO REMEMBER

1. About 95% of malignancy of hypopharynx are squamous cell carcinoma.
2. Plummer-Vinson syndrome is associated with increased incidence of postcricoid malignancy.
3. Post cricoid malignancy is more common in females where as malignancy in the other site of hypopharynx is more common in males.
4. Laryngeal crepitus is absent in postcricoid malignancy.
5. Total laryngo-pharyngo-esophagectomy with gastric pull-up is one of the commonly employed surgical treatment for advanced hypopharyngeal cancer.

56

Miscellaneous Conditions of the Pharynx

GLOBUS HYSTERICUS

Definition

This term is designated to a psychosomatic condition seen commonly in females which is often associated with sensation of lump in the throat or cancerphobia.

Etiopathology

Often in the past these cases were designated as 'Globus' when no lump was seen on examination though the patient used to feel it. Sizable number of these cases are now found to have atypical reflux /acid laryngitis/reflux esophagitis which were not properly diagnosed. The term globus hystericus should be used when all these conditions have been ruled out and if the patient has a psychological background. Cancerphobia may be the predominant factor. Postnasal drip associated with chronic sinusitis could be a cause for similar complaints due to aerophagia.

Clinical Features

Symptoms

Sensation of lump in the throat is the commonest symptom for which the patient comes to see a doctor. There is no dysphagia to solid or liquid but the patient notices the lump feeling only while swallowing saliva.

Signs

Examination of the throat including indirect laryngoscopy will reveal normal pharynx and larynx in cases to true 'globus'. Reflux laryngitis may be associated with interarytenoid congestion and edema. Postnasal drip may be seen if associated with chronic sinusitis.

Differential Diagnosis

- Cricopharyngeal spasm
- Pharyngeal pouch
- Hiatus hernia
- Gastroesophageal reflux disease (GERD)
- Achalasia cardia
- Osteophytosis of the cervical vertebra
- Dysphagia Lusoria.

Diagnosis

Careful and detailed history and clinical examination should be undertaken to rule out any organic pathology. History of neoplasm in a member of the family/friends should arouse the suspicion of cancerphobia as the cause.

Investigations

- Barium swallow preferably under fluoroscopy: shows normal study
- X-ray neck– Lateral view to rule out cervical osteophytosis and prevertebral widening.

- Flexible esophagoscopy
- Manometric studies for reflux
- pH monitoring.

Treatment

- Reassurance
- Psychotherapy
- Placebo treatment may be of help.

PHARYNGEAL POUCH

Definition

It is defined as a herniation of the pharyngeal mucosa through the 'Killian's dehiscence' caused by neuromuscular incoordination of the cricopharyngeal sphincter and gives rise to dysphagia with regurgitation.

Etiopathology

Killian's dehiscence is a potential space between the thyropharyngeus, the fibers of which are oblique and the cricopharyngeus, the fibres of which are transversely placed. This area is sometimes embryologically weak leading to prolapse of the pharyngeal mucosa as a result of neuromuscular incoordination causing premature closure of the cricopharyngeal sphincter during the act of swallowing. This leads to enormous pressure on the pharyngeal mucosa above the sphincter by the food bolus. Thus the mucosa gets prolapsed through this potentially weak space (Fig. 56.1). Ownes et al (1994) has mentioned two areas of inherent weakness in the posterior pharyngeal wall including Killian's dehiscence. The other area of weakness being Laimer-Hackerman triangle between inferior constrictor muscle and the proximal end of the esophagus.

The pouch is composed of mucosa and fibrous tissue and as it grows, it tends to sag downwards behind the esophagus and in rare occasion may extend to the mediastinum. The esophageal opening may get concealed in front of the mouth of the pouch. When food gets collected in the

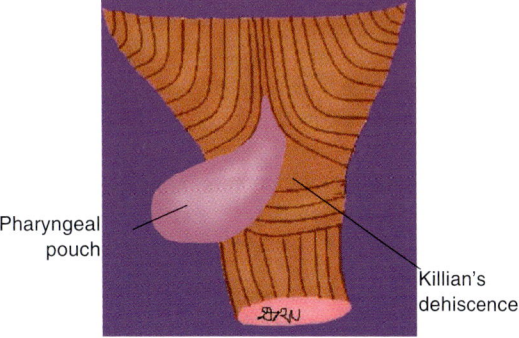

Pharyngeal pouch

Killian's dehiscence

Fig. 56.1: Pharyngeal pouch in the Killian's dehiscence

pouch it compresses the lumen of the esophagus causing dysphagia.

Clinical Features

Symptoms

- This condition is often seen in elderly.
- Dysphagia is the predominant feature and of long standing duration.
- Regurgitation of undigested food, which may be foul smelling.
- Swelling is more obvious after taking food and compression of the swelling may cause gurgling sound.
- Cough may be present due to spillover of the food over the larynx
- Chronic cases may present with emaciation due to long standing dysphagia
- Aspiration pneumonia may be seen in severe cases
- Choking spells at night due to aspiration.

Signs

- Swelling may be present commonly on the left side. It can be better elicited after taking food.
  External compression- gurgling sound may be noted.
- Indirect laryngoscopy may show intense congestion in the inter and retroarytenoid area.
- Pooling of saliva if the dysphagia is absolute.

Investigations

- X-ray neck soft tissue lateral view may show prevertebral widening at level C6 vertebra.
- Barium swallow will confirm the diagnosis (Fig. 56.2).
- Flexible esophagscopy may reveal the fundus of the pouch.

Treatment

No treatment is required if the pouch is extremely small and there is no collection of food particles. However, if the pouch is large enough to produce symptoms it should be treated surgically as there is possibility of developing carcinoma in the pouch.

Surgical treatment includes one stage resection of the pouch through the transcervical approach by separating the sternocleidomastoid muscle from the strap muscles and the pharynx. Posterior wall of the esophagus and the cricopharynx should be exposed. After retracting the great vessels, the pouch is identified. Pouch is excised and the defect is closed primarily after dividing the circular muscle fibers of the cricopharynx. Alternatively the pouch can be exposed endoscopically by introducing a Weerda's expandable laryngoscope keeping the blades on either side of the septum that lies between the two lumens (esophagus and the pouch). The intervening septum may be excised with laser till the lower extent of the pouch (Figs 56.3 and 56.4a to c).

If the pouch extends down to the mediastinum, then a mediastinal exposure along with cervical approach is necessary. Endoscopic approach is contraindicated in such cases.

Hyperkeratosis of Pharynx (Keratosis Pharyngis)

- Formation of plugs of white or yellow hard material in the tonsillar crypts and in the gland mouths of the lateral folds of the pharyngeal granulations and lingual tonsil and rarely in the clefts of the adenoids.
- Etiology is unknown.
- Plugs are composed of horny desquamated epithelium in layers about a center of inspissated mucous, bacteria, debris and often leptothrix and other fungi.

Symptoms

- Usually asymptomatic
- Patient complains of plugs protruding from tonsil and is alarmed by appearance of spots on throat.
- At times, a scratchy feeling, mild soreness or a feeling of foreign body is present.

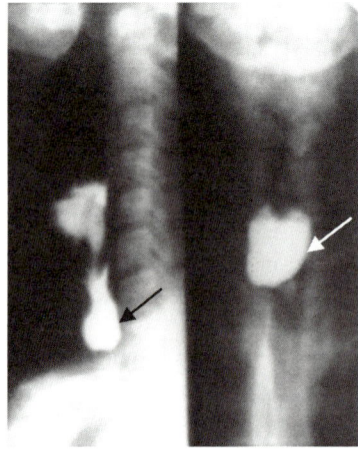

Fig. 56.2: Barium swallow showing the pharyngeal pouch

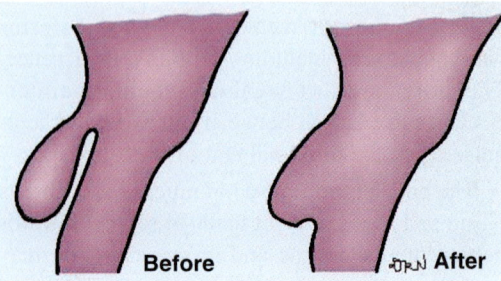

Fig. 56.3: Endoscopic resection of the septum between esophagus and pharyngeal pouch

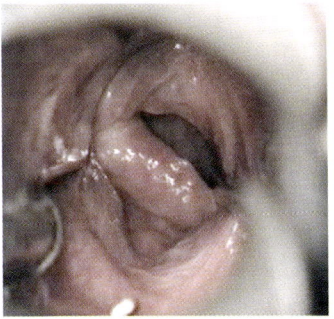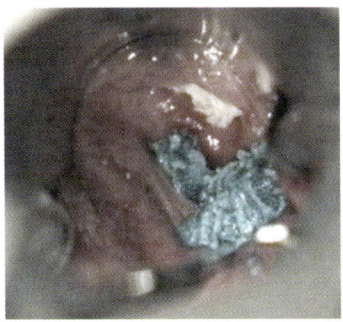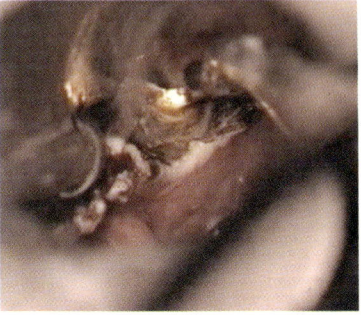

Figs. 56.4a to c: (a) Showing endoscopic view of the pharyngeal pouch, (b) Endoscopic view with green color gauge in the pharyngeal pouch and white color gauge in the esophageal lumen, (c) Endoscopic view of laser excision of the intervening septum

Signs

Examination of oral cavity will show multiple horny keratin plugs in the tonsillar crypt and posterior pharyngeal wall (Fig. 56.5).

Treatment

- Remove plugs with small ring curette.
- Widen crypts by electrocautery.
- If irritation or chronic infection is present, surgical removal of tonsils, lingual tonsils, lateral folds or granulations is indicated.

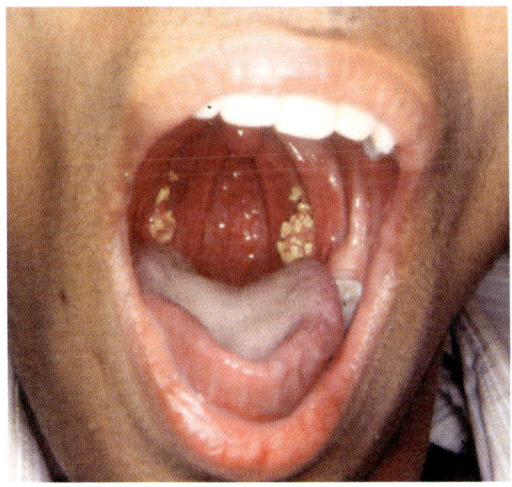

Fig. 56.5: Multiple horny Keratin plugs in the crypts of the tonsils

PLUMMER–VINSON SYNDROME (PATERSON-BROWN -KELLY SYNDROME)

Definition

This is a syndrome characterized by gradually progressive, hypochromic microcytic anemia, angular stomatitis and superficial glossitis, seen commonly in females. The other associated features are achlorhydria, koilonychia, splenomegaly and superficial pharyngoesophagitis.

Etiology

- This condition is predominantly seen in females (90%) above the age of 40.
- Iron deficiency anemia is always associated
- Typically occurs in patient with Scandinavian origin.
- Common in India.

Pathology

- Characterized by thinning of mucosa of upper digestive tract including the pharynx and esophagus and is associated with superficial pharyngeal esophagitis.
- Disappearance of rete pegs from mucosa as a result of thinning
- Submucosal fibrosis and atrophy of mucosa.
- Degeneration of esophageal musculature.
- Narrowing and web formation (86%) at the region of cricopharynx. It is a precancerous

condition and can progress to form postcricoid, upper esophagus and tongue malignancies.

- Atrophy of the gastric mucosa is commonly seen.
- Hiatus hernia may be present.

Clinical Features

Symptoms

- Dysphagia is the predominant symptom, which is initially to solids and then to liquids.
- Patient may complain of lump in the throat
- Painful mouth ulcers are common

General Examination

- Pallor
- Koilonychia
- Splenomegaly

Examination of Oral Cavity

- Angular stomatitis
- Glossitis
- Mouth ulcers

Examination of Hypopharynx and Larynx

- Pooling of saliva in pyriform fossa
- Postcricoid malignancy may be associated with, and should be suspected for if there is edema of arytenoids, retroayrtenoid area and absence of laryngeal crepitus.

Investigation

- Complete blood picture including peripheral smear shows microcytic hypochromic anemia.
- Serum iron level is reduced and iron binding capacity increased.
- *Radiological investigation*: X-ray barium swallow may show web at the level of cricopharynx
- Gastric fluid analysis often shows evidence of achlorhydria
- Upper GI endoscopy helps to confirm the web and help in detection of early cancer

Treatment

- Large doses of iron
- Vitamin supplementation
- Rigid esophagoscopy / hypophayngoscopy and excision of web if present. The excised web should be sent for histological examination. Biopsy should be taken from the suspicious site to detect early cancer. Balloon dilatation or a bougie dilatation is required to improve dysphagia
- As it is a precancerous condition and there is possibility of developing cancer of hypopharynx and tongue, a regular follow-up is mandatory.

DYSPHAGIA LUSORIA

Definition

It is the condition associated with dysphagia due to an abnormal compression of the esophagus by anomalous vessel or vascular malformations.

Common Causes

- Compression of esophagus by aortic arch.
- Double aortic arch.
- Aberrant right subclavian artery.
- Vascular ring.
- Other vascular malformation involving third and fourth arch arteries.

Clinical Features

Symptoms

- Main complaint is dysphagia.

Signs

- Laryngopharyngeal examination
  - Pooling of saliva in both pyriform fossa.

Investigation

- Barium swallow shows abnormal indentation in posterior wall of esophagus near the level of aortic arch.

Treatment is rarely necessary.

STYALGIA

(Synonym: Elongated styloid process, Eagle's syndrome).

Definition

This is the syndrome associated with pain in the upper part of the neck that may radiate to the ear, the TM joint and may be associated with odynophagia.

Etiology

- Occurs as the result of the abnormally elongated and/or angulated styloid process causing disturbance, irritation of nerve plexus around the carotid vessel.
- Impingement of styloid process may affect the glossopharyngeal nerve, trigeminal nerve and cervical sympathetic plexus.

Clinical Features

Symptoms

General

- Discomfort in the throat
- Foreign body sensation.

Neurological

- Glossopharyngeal neuralgia
- Pain radiating to the ear
- Pain radiating to the neck.

Vascular

- Compression of the carotid vessels and the surrounding plexus leading to occasional bradycardia , vasovagal attack, etc.

Local

- Pain over the tonsillar fossa.

Signs

- Pain can be elicited on palpating the tonsillar fossa and the tip of the styloid process may be felt.

Investigations

- Plain X-ray lateral view neck may show elongated styloid process.
- Orthopantomogram (OPG) is very useful investigation, as both the styloid process can be seen at the same time and can be compared and its medial angulation may be calculated (Fig. 56.6).
- 3D CT reconstruction gives the exact length and can depict accurate medial angulation. Relation of styloid process to other structures can be detected from the plain CT axial cuts. Computer plays very important role in these cases (Fig. 56.7).

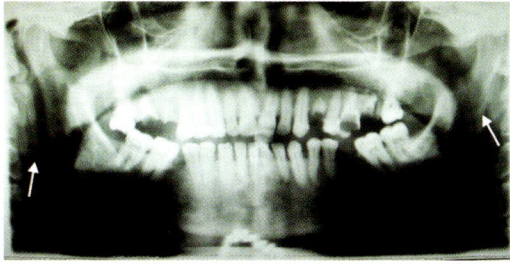

Fig. 56.6: Orthopantomogram showing elongated styloid process on both the sides (arrows)

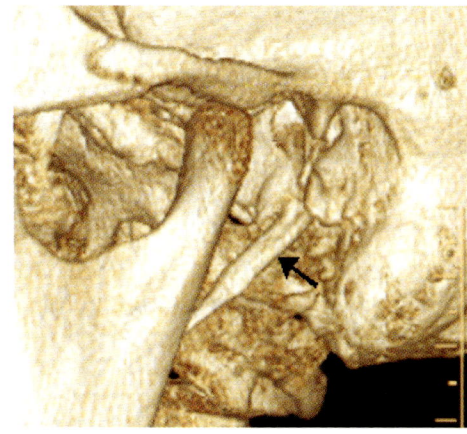

Fig. 56.7: 3D scan showing elongated styloid process (arrow)

Treatment

- *Medical*: Analgesics like combination of paracetamol and tramadol can be given to reduce the pain.
- *Treatment is mainly surgical:*
  Transoral transtonsillar approach is the treatment of choice. The procedure includes routine tonsillectomy operation, palpation of the styloid process in the tonsillar fossa, separation of superior constrictor muscle to expose the styloid process and excision of the excess styloid process. Stylohyoid ligament may have to be removed if it is calcified. Some prefer transcervical approach to excise elongated styloid process (Fig. 56.8).

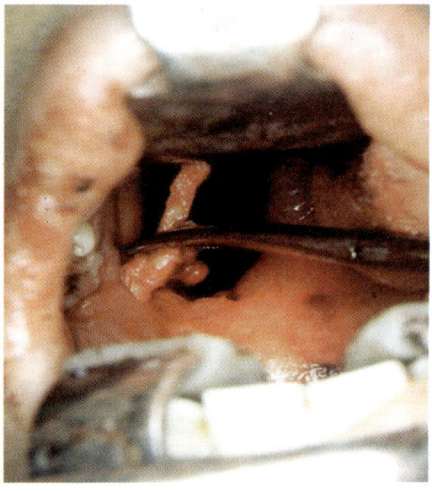

Fig. 56.8: Intraoperative photograph left elongated styloid process before excision

Vallecular Cyst (Fig. 56.9)

This is a retention cyst of the minor salivary glands in the vallecula and base of the tongue. Obstruction to the duct of these mucous glands may cause cyst formation which gradually increases in size due to continued secretion into the cyst. Initially they are asymptomatic but large cysts may cause foreign body sensation in the throat, dysphagia and a muffled hot-potato voice.

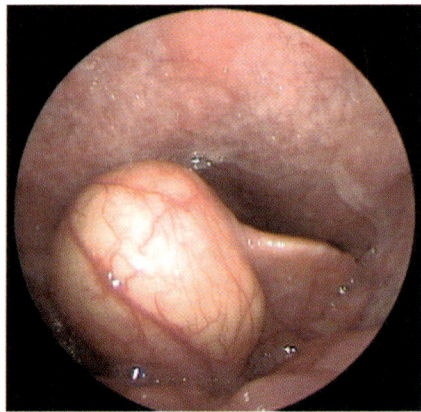

Fig. 56.9: Endoscopic view of vallecular cyst

When small, they may be incidentally found during indirect laryngoscopy. Majority of patients presenting with vallecular cysts are in the pediatric age group, most of them being infants and children. In children it may also give rise to stridor.

The differential diagnoses include internal thyroglossal duct cysts, dermoid cysts, lingual thyroid, teratomas, lymphangiomas and haemangiomas.

Treatment of choice is surgical excision or marsupialization by microlaryngoscopic approach using electrocautery or KTP-532 laser. Incomplete excision/ inadequate marsupialization lead to recurrence.

Lingual Thyroid (Fig. 56.10)

Presence of ectopic thyroid tissue in the base of the tongue is known as lingual thyroid. The thyroid gland develops for the thyroglossal diverticulum and congenital persistence of this in the region of foramen cecum (in the midline at the junction of anterior two third and posterior one third of the tongue) gives rise to lingual thyroid. In some cases it may be the only functioning thyroid gland and patient may present with features of hypothyroidism. For more details please refer to the chapter on swellings in the neck.

Clinical Features

- Patient may be asymptomatic when it is small.
- Gradually increasing foreign body feeling in the throat. Sudden increase in size may occur if there is hemorrhage into the gland.
- Increase in size may occur during periods of stress like menarche.
- Large lesions may give rise to dysphagia and hot-potato speech.

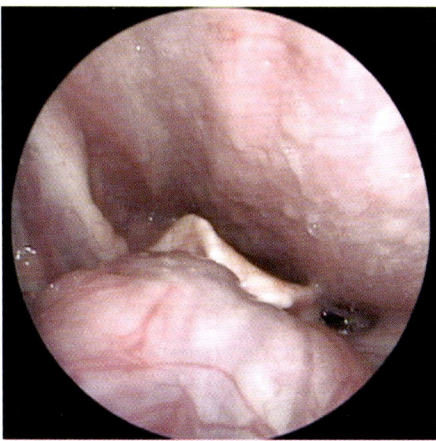

Fig. 56.10: Endoscopic view of lingual thyroid

- Examination of the base of the tongue by asking the patient to protrude the tongue or by indirect laryngoscopy shows well demarcated smooth reddish swelling in the midline.

Investigations

- Thyroid scan to ascertain the nature and presence of normal and other ectopic thyroid tissue.
- T3, T4, TSH

Treatment

- *Asymptomatic:* No treatment necessary. Wait and watch policy.
- Thyroxine supplementation if TSH is raised.
- *If symptomatic:*
  - Not the only functioning thyroid: Excision by transoral or transcervical approach.
  - *If it is only functioning thyroid*: Pedicled translocation of the lingual thyroid in the lateral cervical gutter may be done with its blood supply intact or reimplantation of the thyroid tissue may be done into the sternomastoid or rectus abdominus muscle.

POINTS TO REMEMBER

1. Globus hystericus refers to a false sensation of lump in the throat. A sizeable number of these cases are now found to have atypical reflux/laryngopharyngeal reflux esophagitis.
2. Pharyngeal pouch occurs as a result of herniation of pharyngeal mucosa through the killian's dehiscence due to neuromuscular incoordination.
3. Dysphagia lusoria occurs as a result of abnormal compression of the esophagus by an anamalous vessel.
4. Pressure of ectopic thyroid tissue in the region of base tongue is called lingual thyroid.

57

Anatomy of Esophagus

EMBRYOLOGY

At four weeks of intrauterine life, a small diverticulum appears on the floor of the foregut, at its junction with pharyngeal gut. This is called tracheobronchial diverticulum. It is separated into developing esophagus and the trachea by tracheo-esophageal septum.

Heart and lungs descend caudally as the esophagus lengthens. Muscular portion of the esophagus is formed by surrounding mesenchyme. Upper 2/3rd muscle coat is striated and supplied by vagus. Lower 1/3rd is smooth muscle and supplied by splanchnic plexus.

ANATOMY OF THE ESOPHAGUS

Esophagus is a muscular tube, 25 cms in length connecting the pharynx into stomach. Its diameter is about 20mm. It extends from the lower border of the cricoid cartilage at the level of 6th cervical vertebra to the cardiac orifice of the stomach at the side of the body of 11th thoracic vertebra.

Esophagus presents an anteroposterior flexure corresponding to cervical column. It presents two curves in coronal plane. First coronal curve just below the commencement at the lower border of cricoid cartilage (cricopharynx) it deviates to left through the cervical and thoracic parts of its course. Second coronal curve is formed as the esophagus bends to the left to cross the descending thoracic aorta. Esophagus is the narrowest region in the entire alimentary tract except appendix.

It has various *constrictions* in its course. From the upper incisor teeth, the distance at which the various constrictions exist are follows (Fig. 57.1).

1. *Cricopharyngeal sphincter*: 15cms
2. *Crossed by aortic arch*: 25cms
3. *Crossed by left main bronchus*: 27cms
4. *Hiatus or the lower esophageal sphincter (where esophagus pierces the diaphragm)*: 40cms. The cardiac end of esophagus is at 42cms.

Wall of the Esophagus

The wall of the esophagus contains 4 layers. From within outwards, they are:

1. Mucous membrane
2. Submucosa
3. Muscle coat
4. Outer fibrous layer
1. **Mucous membrane** is lined by non-keratinizing stratified squamous epithelium. The epithelium has typical basement membrane beneath which is loose connective tissue lamina propria containing a very fine network of elastic fibres and lymphoid nodules. At rest, mucous membrane is thrown

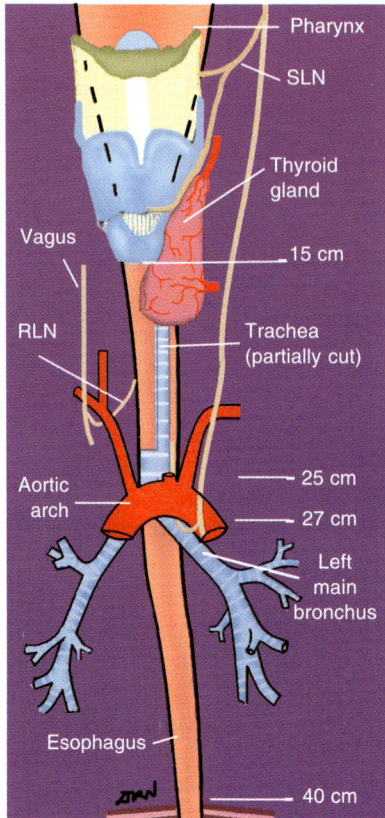

Fig. 57.1: Relation of esophagus to various structures. The trachea lies in front of esophagus (trachea is cut to show the esophagus). The thyroid gland which lies in front of trachea extends laterally on either side of esophagus. The natural constructions at various levels (Cricopharynx—15 cms, Arch of aorta—25 cms, crossed by left main bronchus—27 cms, where esophagus pierces the diaphragm—40 cms) are shown

into longitudinal fold. At the lower end of esophagus mucous membrane layer becomes thicker than in any other part of GIT.

2. **Submucosa:** It connects mucous membrane and muscular coat. It contains the larger blood vessels and the Meissner's nerve plexus and esophageal glands. They lubricate the passage of food. Other glands in abdominal part of esophagus are called as esophageal cardiac glands.

3. **Muscular coat:** It is composed of outer longitudinal and an inner circular coat.
   • *Upper third:* Muscle fibres of both coats are striated.
   • *Middle third:* Muscles show gradual transition to non-striated muscle.
   • *Lower third:* Non-striated muscle only.
4. **Fibrous layer:** It consists of external adventitia tissue. This tissue allows expansion during swallowing. Presence of this tissue makes possible the blunt finger dissection during operation from above and below without opening the chest. Example as in total laryngopharyngoesophagectomy.

Nerve Supply of Esophagus

The striated muscle in the upper third of the esophagus is supplied by the recurrent laryngeal branches of vagus. Middle to lower third receives direct branches from the vagal plexus.

Blood Supply of Esophagus

Arterial Supply
1. *Cervical part*
   1 Inferior thyroid arteries which arise from the thyrocervical trunks of the subclavian artery
   • Also a supply from the left subclavian artery
2. *Thoracic part*
   • Directly from descending thoracic aorta
   • Or from upper posterior intercostal arteries
3. *Abdominal part*
   • Left gastric branch of celiac trunk
   • Left inferior phrenic artery directly from abdominal aorta.

Venous Drainage

In the neck, veins drain into the inferior thyroid veins. In the thorax, they drain into the azygos and hemiazygos system. In the abdomen they drain into the left gastric vein.

Lower end of the esophagus is an important site for portosystemic anastomosis.

Lymphatic Drainage

Two types of networks

1. Large vessels continuous above with the lymphatics of the pharynx and below with the lymphatics of gastric mucosa.
2. Finer vessels present in muscular coat.

Drains into:

1. Cervical part: Lower deep cervical nodes and paratracheal nodes
2. Thoracic part: Into posterior mediastinal nodes and tracheobronchial nodes
3. Abdominal part: Left gastric nodes.

Esophageal Sphincters

1. Upper esophageal sphincter is formed by the cricopharyngeus part of the inferior constrictor.
2. Lower esophageal sphincter: Manometric studies demonstrate a zone of raised pressure about 3 cm in length at the esophagogastric junction extending above and below the diaphragm. The mean pressure here is approximately 8mm Hg higher than the intra gastric pressure. So regurgitation of gastric contents does not occur.

RELATION OF THE ESOPHAGUS

Cervical Part

Anterior: Trachea and recurrent laryngeal nerve
Posterior: Longus coli muscle and vertebral column
On each side: Lobe of thyroid gland and thoracic duct on left side.

Thoracic Part

Anterior
(i) Trachea
(ii) Right pulmonary artery
(iii) Left bronchus
(iv) Pericardium with left atrium
(v) Diaphragm

Posterior
(i) Vertebral column
(ii) Right posterior intercostals arteries

(iii) Thoracic duct
(iv) Azygos vein and terminal part of hemiazygos vein
(v) Thoracic aorta
(vi) Right pleural recess
(vii) Diaphragm

Right
(i) Right lung and pleura
(ii) Azygos vein
(iii) Right vagus

Left
(i) Aortic arch
(ii) Left subclavian artery
(iii) Thoracic duct
(iv) Left lung and pleura
(v) Left recurrent laryngeal nerve

Abdominal Part

This is half an inch long, enters the abdomen through esophageal opening of diaphragm at T_{10} vertebra.

Applied Anatomy

1. Lower end of esophagus is one of the sites for portocaval anastomosis.
2. Left atrial enlargement causes shallow depression on the front of the esophagus.
3. During esophagoscopy normal constrictions should be kept in mind.
4. Improper separation of the trachea from esophagus during development gives rise to tracheoesophageal fistula.
5. Neuromuscular incoordination in esophagus like achalasia cardia
6. Lower end of esophagus is also prone for peptic esophagitis and peptic ulceration— Most common site for esophageal carcinoma.

APPLIED PHYSIOLOGY

Esophagus is responsible for the third stage of deglutition. During this stage, as the food enters, the cricopharyngeal sphincter relaxes thereby allowing opening of the mouth of the esophagus and with assistance of simultaneous closure of the sphincter and elevation of the larynx facilitated by longitudinal fasciculi to the cricoid cartilage. This helps in pulling of the esophagus upwards over the bolus and food descends through gravity. This has already been described in Chapter 47.

INVESTIGATIONS FOR ESOPHAGEAL DISORDERS

I. Endoscopy of the Esophagus

No clinical examination is possible for a direct visualization of esophagus. But with the evolution of flexible endoscopy, it has been possible to have a detailed visualization of the upper gastro-intestinal tract.

Following are the various endoscopic procedures:

1. *Examination by esophageal speculum (Rigid hypopharyngoscope):* This allows examination of the upper end of the thoracic esophagus. Foreign bodies can be removed and biopsy specimen can be obtained while performing this procedure.
2. *Rigid Esophagoscope* : It is used when the whole length of the esophagus must be examined. The cricopharyngeal sphincter is identified and scope is passed through the esophagus when the cricopharyngeal sphincter is relaxed. The relation of level of arch of aorta can be identified by its pulsation. When scope is passed close to the cardiac sphincter, the stomach is recognized by its redder rugose mucosa.
3. *Flexible fibre-optic endoscopy of the esophagus*: This latest instrument can help in the examination of the entire length of esophagus and stomach. Biopsy can be taken as an out-patient procedure with ease avoiding the complications of rigid scopies. However large foreign bodies cannot be removed with this procedure.

II. Radiological Examination

1. X-ray chest and lateral view of the neck are two most important investigations required prior to any rigid endoscopy of the esophagus. In most cases, a barium swallow examination is also indicated. If these precautions are not taken, an unsuspected pharyngeal pouch may be entered and perforated or an aneurysm of the aorta may be ruptured.
2. Contrast radiography (Barium swallow) can demonstrate well the esophageal obstruction due to stricture, neoplasm and the other causes.
3. Cineradiography is very useful in the diagnosis of neuromuscular diseases of the esophagus.

III. pH Monitoring for Reflux Esophagitis

A 24 hour pH monitoring is useful to diagnose reflux esophagitis

IV. Manometric studies

Useful in diagnosis of neurological conditions of esophagus

POINTS TO REMEMBER

1. The length of the esophagus is 25 cm.
2. The natural constrictions of the esophagus that are situated at various levels from the incisors are:
   (a) Cricopharyngeal sphincter (15 cm)
   (b) Crossed by aortic arch (25 cm)
   (c) Crossed by left main bronchus (27 cm)
   (d) Hiatus or lower esophageal sphinctor at the entry through diaphragm (40 cm).
3. Esophagus is responsible for the third stage of deglutition.

Congenital Conditions of the Esophagus

The common congenital conditions of the esophagus include the following

1. Laryngo-tracheo-esophageal clefts/Congenital tracheoesophageal fistula
2. Congenital esophageal atresia
3. Congenital stricture
4. Congenital hiatus hernia
5. Congenital diverticula of the esophagus
6. Dysphagia lusoria due to vascular obstruction due to abnormally placed right subclavian artery.

Congenital Tracheoesophageal Fistula/ Laryngo-tracheo-esophageal clefts

The esophagus and the tracheobronchial tree arise from a common tube which is connected by a long laryngotracheal groove. Laryngo-tracheo-esophagial cleft or fistula results from the fusion failure of the lateral furrows that creates the tracheoesophageal septum during the 5th and the 7th week.

They are of three types:

- **Type I:** It involves a deformity that is created by a cleft of the posterior cricoid lamina (laryngeal cleft which is described under congenital anomalies of the larynx).
- **Type II:** This cleft extends partially down the length of the trachea with the adjoining

corresponding esophagus. Sometimes incomplete fusion may be associated with a upper tracheoesophageal fistula.
- **Type III:** This involves the entire length of the tracheoesophageal septum that is from the interarytenoid region till the carina.

Partial closure leads to fistula formation than a cleft.

The tracheoesophageal fistula may be associated with other abnormalities of the trachea and the esophagus. Some are associated with esophageal atresia.

There are 4 types of tracheoesophageal fistula

- *Type I fistula or complete esophageal atresia:* The upper and lower esophagus both end in blind pouches.
- *Type II fistula:* The upper esophageal segment communicates with the trachea and the lower esophageal segment ends in a blind segment.
- *Type III fistula:* The upper segment ends in a blind pouch and the lower segment communicates with the trachea. This is the most common form of tracheoesophageal fistula (82%).
- *Type IV fistula:* Both the upper and lower esophageal segments communicate with the trachea. If the esophageal lumen is intact then the fistula is called an H type fistula. H-type

fistula is not associated with atresia. This can occur at any level in the posterior wall of the larynx or the trachea.

Clinical Features

Symptoms are seen immediately after birth. Infant has barking cough with choking and cyanosis which increases on feeding. Features of broncopneumonia due to aspiration are often present. Death can occur if the abnormality is not corrected.

Investigations

1. Lateral view radiograph of the neck and thorax: This may show the communicating tract and evidence of aspiration.
2. Passing of the nasogastric tube does not reach the stomach as in most of the cases esophageal atresia is present.
3. Radio-opaque dye is best avoided as it can cause aspiration. A dye contrast media using cineradiography is useful for diagnosis of 'H' type fistula.
4. Methylene blue dye may be injected through the endotracheal tube and the esophagus can then be examined by doing an esophagoscopy.

Treatment

- Stabilization of respiratory function by either endotracheal intubation or by performing a tracheostomy.
- Tracheobronchial toilet
- Antibiotics to prevent secondary infection in associated pneumonia due to aspiration.
- Gastrostomy may be required in certain cases where fistula is absent.
- Laryngofissure and anterior tracheotomy approach is preferred for upper tracheo-esophageal fistula of type I and II.
- Type III fistula requires extensive surgical repair of the cervical and thoracic trachea

and the esophagus and may involve staged procedures like colonic or gastric transposition. Mortality rate is quite high.
- Atresia associated with tracheoesophageal fistula may necessitate closure of fistula with end-to-end anastomosis via a trans-thoracic approach.

Congenital Esophageal Stricture

This is very rare and may be present either at the cricopharygeal sphincter like a web or fold or in the thoracic esophagus as a smooth circular lumen of a pin-hole size. Dysphagia may not be evident until late adult life as the patient accommodates themselves to small swallow all their life. Barium swallow may show considerable dilatation of the esophagus above this stricture site. This is treated with boogie or balloon dilatation. Web near the stricture can be excised with laser. Lower stricture may be managed with initial gastrostomy followed by subsequent balloon dilatation which may be helpful in some cases. If not, a transcervical, transthoracic resection and reconstruction may be required.

Hiatus Hernia

This occurs as a result of obstruction of the esophagus due to pressure from the herniated stomach. Discomfort on lying down may not be evident until adult life. This is treated with surgical reduction of the hernia and repair of the diaphragm.

Congenital Shortening of the Esophagus

This occurs in association of thoracic stomach as the esophagus ends at the 7th thoracic vertebra. This causes shortening of the esophagus bringing a portion of the stomach above the level of the diaphragm into the thorax as the diaphragm develops late.

Patient can present with dysphagia due to narrowing of the lower end of the esophagus.

Discomfort due to thoracic stomach, occasional vomiting, pain in the chest due to reflux esophagitis and loss of weight are some of the characteristic symptoms.

This is treated by antireflux measures, balloon dilatation and later a trans-thoracic surgery may be done to mobilize the stomach. Anastomosis may be required between the two parts of the stomach.

POINTS TO REMEMBER

1. Laryngo-tracheo-esophageal cleft/fistula results from the fusion failure of the lateral furrows that form the tracheoesophageal septum.
2. Hiatus hernia occurs as a result of obstruction of the esophagus due to pressure from the herniated stomach.
3. Congenital shortening of the esophagus can present with dysphagia due to narrowing of the lower end of the esophagus and thoracic stomach.

59

Traumatic Conditions of the Esophagus

The traumatic conditions of the esophagus include the following:

Burns and scalds, corrosive poisoning, trauma due to introduction of boogies or instrumentation and foreign bodies. Tear and wound may occur due to injury to the chest or the neck.

Pathology

Superficial injury causes localized or diffuse esophagitis depending on the length of the esophagus involved. Deep involvement can cause necrosis of the esophageal wall or perforation. Mediastinum and the pleura may be involved with fatal consequences.

Clinical Features

Symptoms

- Pain is often severe and acute in onset. It confines to supraclavicular region if cervical esophagus is involved. The pain is retrosternal when the injury is in the thoracic region. The pain may radiate to the back of the epigastrium in such cases.
- Dysphagia is usually severe.
- Features of shock may be present and is often severe following the rupture of the esophagus into the pleural cavity.

- Dyspnea is immediate if there is associated pneumothorax or empyema. Dyspnea sometimes appear slightly delayed when the infection spreads to the mediastinum due to mediastinitis.

Signs

- Cervical cellulitis or abscess
- Surgical emphysema may be present
- Features of intrathoracic lesion, pneumothorax or mediastinitis
- Lower esophageal perforation may be associated with acute abdomen with classical cardboard rigidity due to peritonitis.

Investigations

- Plain radiograph should be taken immediately. It may show air in the neck or mediastinum or features of hydropneumothorax. Unsuspected foreign body may be demonstrated.
- *Barium swallow*: This should be done 3 to 4 days after the trauma to localize the site of the trauma.
- *Endoscopic examination*: Esophagoscopy is dangerous to locate the injury and may be done immediately along with exploratory operation in very early cases where primary

repair of the injured structure is possible. Endoscopy is contraindicated immediately following corrosive poisoning. If it has to be done in such cases the scope should not pass beyond the burn and feeding the tube may be passed without force. If no burns is found remainder of the scopy is done with flexible scope to examine the stomach for extent of the injury in the stomach and the duodenum.

Treatment

- Shock should be treated immediately
- Systemic antibiotics in full dose is given
- Later steroid therapy may be necessary to inhibit fibrosis
- Dilute alkaline fluids may be taken in small amounts in mild degrees of esophagitis without danger of perforation. Nasogastric feeding tube should be inserted without delay. Intravenous or rectal fluids are necessary if there is acute dysphagia and if there is danger of perforation. Fluid per orally should be avoided at least for 4 days. Gastrostomy is preferred to maintain nutrition if the perforation of the esophagus is diagnosed. Cervical esophagostomy is done by some surgeons and a small tube is passed into the stomach to diminish the risk of stricture. Transcervical transthoracic drainage of the mediastium or pleural cavity is necessary if the spaces are infected. External approach should be preferred for immediate repair of the tears and ruptures.

Complications

Immediate

- Para-esophageal abscess in the neck
- Mediastinitis
- Infection of the pleural cavity
- Tracheoesophageal fistula

Delayed

- Stricture of the esophagus

POINTS TO REMEMBER

1. Traumatic conditions of the esophagus can be associated with acute onset of pain.
2. Injury of cervical esophagus can cause supraclavicular pain.
3. Injury of thoracic esophagus can cause retrosternal pain which may radiate to back of the epigastrium.
4. Features of shock is suggestive of perforation of esophagus into the pleural cavity.
5. Lower esophageal perforation is associated with acute abdomen with classical cardboard rigidity due to peritonitis.

60

Neurological Conditions of the Esophagus

VARIOUS NEUROLOGICAL CONDITIONS OF THE ESOPHAGUS

- Cricopharyngeal spasm
- Achalasia cardia (Cardiospasm)
- Diffuse spasm

CRICOPHARYNGEAL SPASM (CRICOPHARYNGEAL DYSPHAGIA)

In this condition the cricopharyngeal muscle (Inferior constrictor) fails to relax during swallowing. Kirschner (1958) studied the relation of the cricopharyngeus muscle to the vagus nerve and the sympathetic trunk in dogs and found that it maintains the normal state of tonus and relaxes to receive the bolus of food and contracts to a pressure level higher than its resting state to assist in the movement of the bolus. Unilateral section of the vagus nerve at the base skull reduces the relaxation state. When both the vagus nerves are sectioned the relaxation phase is abolished causing severe dysphagia. Thus the relaxation is mediated by the parasympathetic and contraction by the sympathetic. Dysphagia can also result from sympathetic overactivity or vagal loss. Cricopharyngeal function is also influenced by the distal esophagus (Henderson 1976).

Causes

- *Reflux esophagitis:* Distal esophagitis can cause gastroesophageal motor dysphagia, peptic stricture and cricopharyngeal spasm.
- Cerebrovascular accident
- Vagal paralysis
- *Recurrent laryngeal paralysis:* This should be considered in unexplained dysphagia especially if aspiration is present.
- Bulbar paralysis
- Myasthenia gravis
- Pharyngectomy

Clinical Features

Symptoms

- Dysphagia
- Retrosternal burning
- Lump feeling in the throat (globus hystericus)
- Poor eating especially in infants and children
- Choking spells
- Aspiration
- Nasal regurgitation

Signs

- Diffuse congestion in the throat
- Pooling of saliva
- Interarytenoid congestion
- Vocal cord or palatal palsy may be present.

Investigations

- Barium swallow may show shelf–like semicircular filling defect. Stasis in the pyriform fosse may be seen.

553

- Manometric studies may help in showing the incoordination at the cricopharyngeal area.
- Endoscopy under local anesthesia may elicit the cricopharyngeal spasm.

Treatment

- Antireflux treatment as in GERD.
- Balloon dilatation may give temporary relief.
- Cricopharyngeal myotomy
  - *External:* Lateral pharyngotomy approach
  - *Internal:* Endoscopic laser assisted myotomy may be done using KTP 532 or CO_2 laser.
- Botulinium toxin and other medical treatments have been tried with limited success.

ACHALASIA CARDIA (SYNONYM: CARDIOSPASM)

Definition

It is a primary esophageal motility disorder associated with the spasm of the lower esophageal sphincter due to neuromuscular incoordination characterized by spasm of the cardiac end of the esophagus and dilatation of the lower two thirds of the esophagus.

Etiology

Exact cause is not well understood. Hurst postulated the failure of relaxation of the cardiac orifice as the cause due to degeneration of the Auerback's plexus. This theory is not widely accepted. Jackson suggested an abnormal pinch-cock action by the right crus of the diaphragm. Aerophagia may play a part in dilating the esophagus. Principal lesion is the denervation of the esophageal smooth muscles. Infection by *Trypanosoma cruzi* of the myentric plexus may be associated with megaesophagus (Chaga's disease).

Clinical Features

Symptoms

- It commonly affects both males and females

- Usually insidious in onset
- Retrosternal or epigastric fullness following meals is the main symptom
- Dysphagia is a late symptom which is more to fluids than solids.
- Regurgitation of undigested food which is frequently taken a day before may be noted
- Loss of weight.

Signs

Pooling of saliva may be seen on indirect laryngoscopy and may be associated with reflux laryngitis.

Investigations

- Barium swallow (Fig. 60.1)
  - Fusiform dilatation of the esophagus with fluid level
  - 'Pencil-tip' or 'bird's beak' smooth filling defect of the cardiac end of esophagus
  - *Hurst phenomenon*: Barium gets into the stomach like snow flakes.
  - Loss of fundal gas shadow
- Endoscopy should be done with caution if dilatation is not significant.

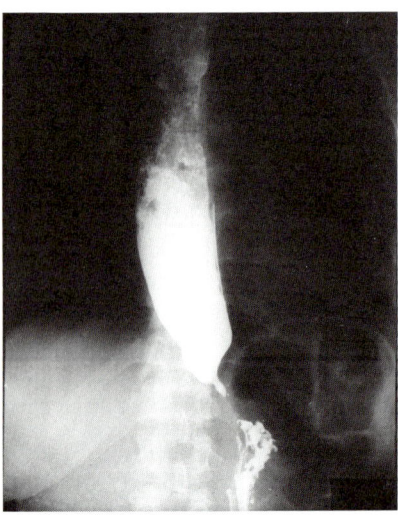

Fig. 60.1: A smooth stricture with fusiform dilatation of esophagus

- Manometric studies may be helpful.
- Prolonged Ambulatory pH Monitoring.

Treatment

Medical

Smooth muscle relaxants like isosorbide dinitrite, and calcium channel blockers, such as diltiazem, nifedipine and verapamil, have been tried.

Surgical

- Botulinum toxin type A injection has been tried to relax the lower end of the esophagus.
- Balloon dilatation or dilatation with hydrostatic bag or 'Hurst-mercury' boogies.
- Heller's cardiomyotomy (cardioplasty) is now being done thoracoscopically or laparoscopically facilitating minimally invasive procedure and less morbidity.
- Anastomosis between the stomach and esophagus may be necessary if the esophagus is grossly lengthened or kinked.

DIFFUSE ESOPHAGEAL SPASM

Definition

Diffuse esophageal spasm refers to dysphagia due to entire segment of the esophagus caused by an uncoordinated or spastic esophagus.

Etiology

The cause appears to be disruption of the complex system of nerves that coordinates the muscular activity often due to aging.

Clinical Features

- **Dysphagia:** Soft and liquid foods pass more easily than solid pieces.
- Retrosternal pain that feels like a heart attack.

Investigations

- Radiologically characteristic 'corkscrew' esophagus is seen on barium swallow.
- Manometric studies may be helpful.

Treatment

- Medications of several types may be helpful. Nifedipine, hydralazine, isoproterenol, and nitrates are the most successful ones.
- For severe cases, cutting the muscles along the entire length of the esophagus may be necessary.

Prognosis

The condition does not get progressively worse as time passes.

POINTS TO REMEMBER

1. Cricopharyngeal spasm is a condition of the cricopharyngeal muscle (Inferior constrictor) which fails to relax during swallowing. The commonest causes are reflux esophagitis, Cerebrovascular accident, vagal paralysis, etc.
2. Barium swallow may show a shelf-like semicircular filling defect in cricopharyngeal spasm.
3. Endoscopic laser assisted myotomy is the latest mode of treatment which can be done as an office procedure.
4. Achalasia cardia is a primary esophageal motility disorder associated with the spasm of the lower esophageal sphincter due to neuromuscular incoordination, the exact etiology is not known. This condition is characterized by spasm of the cardiac end of the esophagus and dilatation of the lower two third of the esophagus.
   Barium swallow shows the characteristic fusiform dilatation of the esophagus with fluid level.
5. Heller's cardiomyotomy is the treatment of choice for achalasia cardia and can now be done thoracoscopically or laparoscopically.

61

Foreign Body: Upper Digestive Tract (Pharynx/Esophagus)

The impact of the foreign body chiefly depends on its size and shape depending on which it can be located at various sites.

Etiology

- *Age:* Children and adults
- Accidental
- Altered sensorium (Reduced protective reflexes)
  - Dentures, drugs, alcohol, etc.
- *Carelessness*: Poor mastication
- Psychiatric
- Esophageal strictures.

Types

- *Sharp or blunt*: Sharp ones tend to lodge any part of the pharynx and esophagus. Blunt objects unless big in size, usually passes through the GI tract but may be lodged in the illeocaecal junction (narrowest part of the GI tract after cricopharyngeal sphincter)
- Radio-opaque or radiolucent
- Metallic
  - Coins, pins, denture wires, battery, etc.
- Bones
  - Fish, chicken, etc.
- Plastic
  - Toys, beads, etc.
- Miscellaneous
  - Wooden objects, etc.

Sites

- *Commonest site:* Cricopharynx (cricopharyngeal spincter): which corresponds to lower border of C6 vertebra
- Esophagus
  Common at the constrictions
  - 15 cm: Cricopharynx
  - 25 cm: Arch of aorta
  - 27 cm: Left bronchus
  - 40 cm: Right crus of diaphragm
- Strictures.

Fish Bones

Common sites of lodgment

- Tonsillar crypts
- Vallecula
- Base tongue
- Pyriform fossa
- Cricopharynx.

Clinical Features

Symptoms

- H/O FB ingestion is elicited usually in adults who usually come immediately and may help in localizing the site. Some objects like coin or other smooth articles may be impacted for weeks to months without producing significant symptoms.

- *Children and insane*: History of foreign body ingestion may not be present. Missing objects with which they were playing with should raise the suspicion of the foreign body.
- Discomfort/FB sensation.
- Throat/retrosternal pain is the predominant symptom.
- Dysphagia/odynophagia may be present. Some may have feeling of obstruction without obvious dysphagia.
- Drooling of saliva, excessive salivation.
- Dyspnoea.
- Hoarseness/stridor in case of laryngeal edema/large FB.

Clinical Features

Signs

- Fish bone may be visible in oropharynx
- ILS: Pooling of saliva/ FB in pyriform fossa
- *Laryngeal crepitus*: Tender and may be absent.

Investigations

- Plain X-ray lateral/ AP view soft tissue neck
  - *Radio-opaque*: Coronal position in prevertebral region
  - Radiolucent
    - Prevertebral widening
    - Anteriorly displaced airway
- Fluroscopy with thin barium swallow
  - Fine radiolucent FB get coated with barium
- *Chest X-ray:* PA view and lateral
- *In children*: X-ray neck to pelvis to rule out multiple FBs (Figs 61.1a and b).

Treatment

- Fish bone-look for it in the oropharynx and it may be removed as an out-patient procedure
- If foreign body is impacted for more than 24 hours, intravenous antibiotics, analgesics and fluids should be given. If the foreign

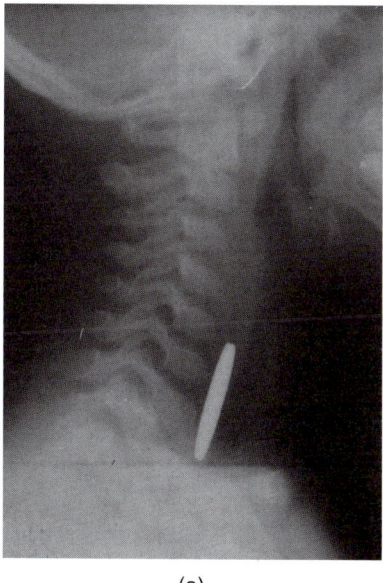
(a)

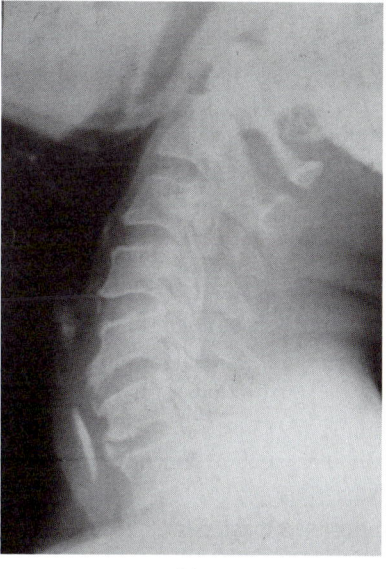
(b)

Figs 61.1a and b: (a) Lateral view X-ray neck soft tissue showing tracheal air column in front of cricopharyngeal foreign body, (b) Lateral view soft tissue neck showing small linear radio-opaque foreign body at the level of C5-C6

body is a migrating one in the cervical soft tissues, metronidazole or tinidazole should be given to prevent/treat anaerobic infection.
- Removal is preferably done under general anesthesia using rigid hypopharyngoscope/ esophagoscope using foreign body forceps (Fig. 61.2).
- Flexible esophagoscopy not preferred because:
  - Patients tend to keep swallowing during the procedure

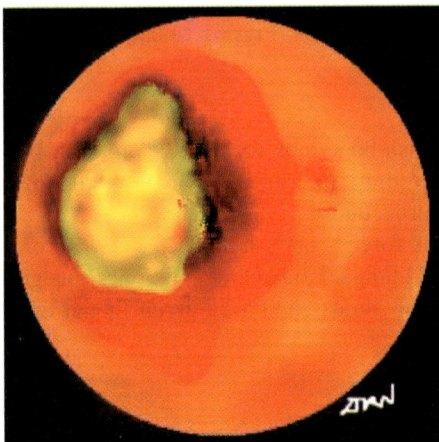

Fig. 61.2: Appearance of foreign body on esophagoscopy

- The scope does not distend the area for dis-impaction of the foreign body
- FB forceps is too small to grasp a big foreign body.

But a non-impacted blunt foreign body may be removed under flexible scopy guidance using balloon catheter.

- If the impacted FB cannot be removed endoscopically an external approach-lateral pharyngotomy/thoracotomy may be required.

Complicatons

- Fluid/electrolyte imbalance
- Esophagitis/periesophagitis
- Retropharyngeal/ parapharyngeal abscess
- Paraesophageal abscess
- Mucosal laceration
- *Esophageal perforation*:Surgical emphysema
- Mediastinits/mediastinal abscess
- Pneumothorax
- Tracheoesophageal fistula
- Esophageal stenosis
- Perforation of aorta in case of sharp foreign bodies.

POINTS TO REMEMBER

1. The commonest site of lodgement of ingested foreign body is cricopharynx.
2. Fish bone is commonly lodged in tonsillar crypts or vallecula.
3. Big foreign body like meat bone or chicken bone commonly lodges in the cricopharynx and at various constrictions of the esophagus.
4. Plain X-ray lateral and AP view of the neck and chest readily picks up radio-opaque foreign body. Prevertebral widening with a positive history should be suspected for radio-lucent foreign body.
5. Untreated impacted foreign body can cause deep neck space infection and abscess or esophageal perforation.
6. Removal of upper esophageal foreign body should be done under rigid endoscopy.

62

Neoplasms of the Esophagus

Benign neoplasms are rare which include leiomyoma, papilloma, adenoma, fibroma, etc. True dysphagia is usually absent and sensation of lump in the throat may be felt. Condition is very slowly progressive. They are usually polypoidal and may be removed endoscopically.

MALIGNANT TUMORS OF THE ESOPHAGUS

Etiology

- Smoking and alcohol
- Tobacco chewing
- Diet
- Sites of normal narrowing are susceptible sites.
- Plummer-Vinson syndrome
- Achalasia cardia
- Diverticulum
- Benign strictures
- Age: Elderly> 50 years. 75% of the cases occur in age of >50 years.
- Sex: > males (80%) but upper one-third is more in females (Plummer-Vinson syndrome).

PATHOLOGY AND MODES OF SPREAD

Types of Malignancy

- Upper one-third: Squamous cell carcinoma is the most common type.

- Lower one-third: is usually adenocarcinoma
- Middle one-third: Either but usually squamous cell ca.

Overall

- Squamous cell carcinoma: 93%
- Adenocarcinoma: 3%
- Others: Rare

Gross Appearance

Neoplasm may be infiltrative, ulcerative or proliferative. Tumor may be annular or longitudinal. Annular usually produces early obstruction. Satellite growth may be seen near the primary site.

Spread

- Direct
  - May involve the trachea/subglottis/ Left bronchus
  - Recurrent laryngeal nerve may be involved
  - Aorta/pericardium/pleura/ mediastinum/ spine
- Lymphatic
  - Cervical nodes in upper esophageal malignancy
  - Mediastinal node involvement is common

– Lower esophageal growth drain into upper abdominal nodes like coeliac nodes
- Hematogenous
  – Liver, lungs, brain, etc.

Clinical Features

Symptoms

- >50 years male, >30 years female
- Retrosternal discomfort is the earliest symptom: This is often well localized by the patient
- Insidious onset
- Patient presents with progressive dysphagia initially to solids and later to both. Sudden impaction of food should raise the suspicion of esophageal malignancy. Complete dysphagia is known as absolute dysphagia which is a late sign.
- Any patient with abnormal sensation on swallowing should be evaluated.
- Hoarseness may be due to recurrent laryngeal nerve paralysis
- Emaciation, dehydration
- Pain—Back and chest
- Aspiration and cough may be due to trcheo-esophageal fistula or the recurrent laryngeal nerve involvement.

- Hematemesis
- Stridor.

Signs

- Indirect laryngoscopy
  – Normal +/–
  – Rec. lar. N palsy +/–
  – Pooling of saliva in pyriform fossae in upper one-third growth.
- Neck
  – Supraclavicular node
  – Superior vena cava obstruction syndrome (mediastinal involvement).

Investigations

- *Barium swallow*: 'Rat tail deformity' or irregular filling defect is seen (Figs 62.1 and 62.2)
- Flexible/rigid esophagoscopy and biopsy
- Chest X-ray may show mediastinal widening or signs of aspiration
- LFT, abdominal ultrasound to rule out liver metastases
- CT/MRI gives better delineation of the extent of tumor
- Bronchoscopy to rule out tracheobronchial involvement.

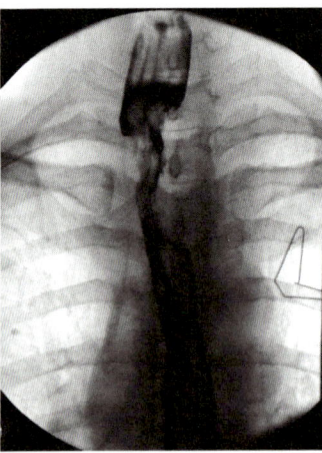

Fig. 62.1: Barium swallow showing irregular filling defect in the upper esophagus

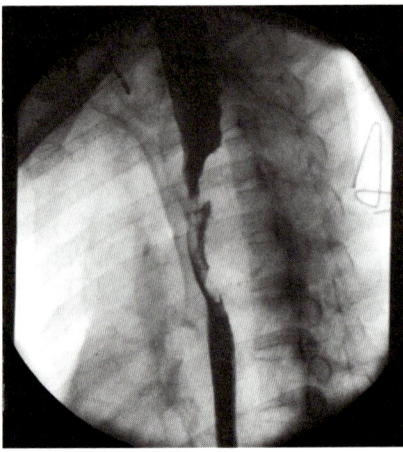

Fig. 62.2: Barium swallow showing irregular filling defect in middle one third of the esophagus

Treatment

- Squamous cell carcinoma
- Radiotherapy +/– chemotherapy
- Surgery difficult due to vital structures and mediastinal spread likely
- *Upper one-third growth*: Total laryngo-pharyngo-esophagectomy with gastric pull up/colonic transposition (Fig. 62.3)
- *Middle one-third growth*: Non-surgical management preferred with full course of radiotherapy.
- Adenocarcinoma.
  - Not radiosensitive
  - Surgery is the treatment of choice
  - Esophagogastrectomy and reconstruction.

Palliative Procedures

- Mouseau-Barbin tube
- Soutter's tube
- Ryle's tube
- Gastostomy/jejunostomy
- Pain—Morphine
- Palliative radiotherapy

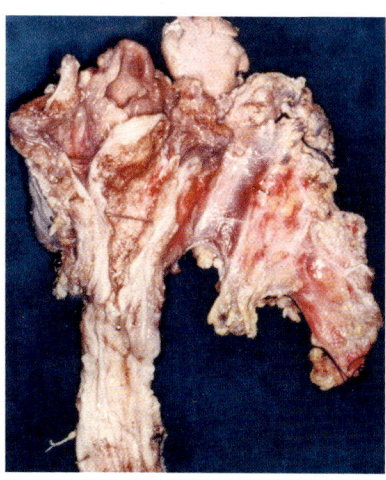

Fig. 62.3: Resected specimen of total laryngo-pharyngo-esophagectomy with right radical neck dissection which is cut open posteriorly. Arrow showing the extent of the growth into the esophagus

Prognosis

- Usually poor
- 5 year survival rate—10%
- Early stages—Prognosis better

POINTS TO REMEMBER

1. Plummer-Vinson syndrome is commonly associated with postcricoid and upper esophageal malignancy.
2. Squamous cell carcinoma commonly involves the upper and middle one-third of the esophagus.
3. Adenocarcinoma usually involves the lower one-third of the esophagus.

63

Dysphagia

Definition

Dysphagia is defined as difficulty in swallowing which results from interference or obstruction to the food passage.

The mechanism of deglutition has been described under pharynx. It includes three phases namely oral, pharyngeal and esophageal. The interference in the first phase of swallowing can be either anatomic or neuromuscular. The anatomical involvement is trauma, infection and neoplasia. The second phase involves interference in the involuntary transport mechanism of the pharynx which can be anatomic or neuromuscular. The phase three involves the lesions in the esophagus.

Odynophagia: Painful Swallow

- Patients with dysphagia may complain of:
  - Throat discomfort
  - FB sensation
  - Feel of hold up
  - Absolute difficulty in swallowing.

Stages of Deglutition

Oral stage includes mastication, salivation and movement of tongue and soft palate.

Pharyngeal stage is associated with closure of oral, nasopharyngeal isthmus and larynx, while there is simultaneous opening of cricopharynx.

Esophageal stage is associated with involuntary propulsion of bolus.

Etiology: Given in Table 63.1.

EVALUATION OF DYSPHAGIA

HISTORY

- *Age:* Child-congenital, adults-malignancy
- *Onset:* Acute-inflammatory/trauma/ neurological
- *Sex:* Female-Plummer Vinson Syndrome
- *Duration:* Less-inflammatory/malignant, more-benign tumor
- *Progression:* Same-benign/stricture, increasing-malignancy
- *Type:* Solids > liquids- usual, liquids > solids-achalasia
- *Severity:* Absolute: malignancy, aspiration-neurological
- Vomiting/choking/regurgitation: Achalasia, pouch
- H/O FB, scopy, corrosive poisoning
- Pain/fever: inflammatory
- Loss of weight/appetite: malignancy/tuberculosis
- Hoarseness: Laryngeal/hypopharyngeal cause
- Nasal regurgitation/nasal voice: Palatal palsy.

Table 63.1: Various causes of dysphagia at various levels

Site / Etiology	Oral cavity	Pharynx/Larynx	Esophagus	Central and gen. causes
• Congenital	Cleft palate, lingual thyroid	• Pharyngeal diverticulum	• TEF, atresia, diverticulum, hiatus hernia	
• Inflammatory	Stomatitis, glossitis, ulcer, sialadenitis, TMJ arthritis, Ludwig's angina, anginal, trismus, dental	• Pharyngitis, tonsillitis, lingual tonsillitis quinsy, retro-parapharyngeal abscess, TB laryngitis, acute epiglottis, etc.	• Reflux esophagitis, TB esophagitis	
• Traumatic	# maxilla/ mandible, cheek/ tongue bite, corrosive poisoning *Palsy :* Palatal/ lingual/ facial, *Spasm:* Trismus/tetanus	FB, corrosive poisoning iatrogenic trauma, road traffic accidents • Surgical following glossectomy laryngectomy, etc.	• FB, corrosive poisoning, poisoning stricture iatrogenic trauma, etc.	
• Neurological	Hypoglossal paralysis, palatal paralysis	Cricopharyngeal spasm, VC palsy (aspiration) tetanus, etc	• Achalasia cardia, motility, disorders, diffuse spasm, scleroderma amyatrophic lateral sclerosis, etc.	Bulbar paralysis, Myasthenia gravis, poliomyelitis
• Neoplastic	Papilloma, salivary tumors, oral carcinoma of tongue, jaw tumors associated with trismus	• *Benign:* Salivary tumors, papilloma, etc. • *Malignant :* Ca tonsil/ base tongue/hypopharynx/ larynx, salivary tumors, etc.	• Benign tumors, malignant: Ca esophagus/ bronchus, thyroid malignancy mediastinal tumors, thymoma, etc.	
• Miscellaneous	• Xerostomia-nutritional/ radiotherapy	Plummer-Vinson syndrome, globus hystericus	• Osteophytes, dysphagia lusoria, aneurysm, cardiac enlargement esophageal, varices, etc.	Thyro-toxicosis
• External compression			• Osteophytes, mediastinal tumors, vascular malformations aneurysm	

Clinical Examination

It includes general, and local ENT—Head and neck and systemic examination.

Investigations

- *Blood*: Plummer-Vinson syndrome, nutritional deficiency, fluid-electrolyte imbalance
- *Chest X-ray:* Mediastinum, cardiac and pulmonary status, aspiration pneumonia, secondaries
- *X-ray neck (soft tissue) AP/ lateral*: prevertebral widening, osteophytes, etc (Fig. 63.1).
- *Barium swallow/fluroscopy*: Stricture, filling defects, shouldering, dilatation, fistula, aspiration, extraluminal compression (Figs 63.2a and b)
- *CT/ MRI:* Neck/mediastinum/base skull/brain
- Manometric studies.

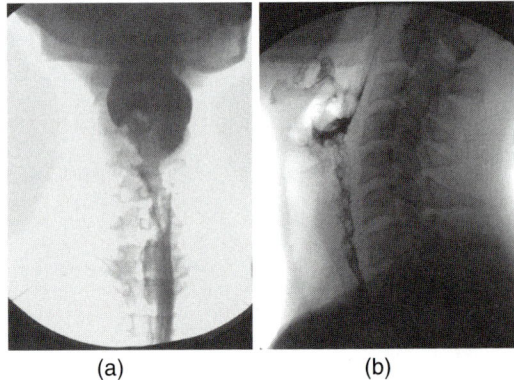

(a)   (b)

Figs 63.2a and b: (a) Contrast X-ray barium swallow showing irregular filling defect involving the apex of right pyriform fossa, cricopharynx and upper esophagus, (b) Contrast X-ray barium swallow lateral view of the same patient showing the irregular filling defect involving the cricopharynx and upper esophagus

- Peroral panendoscopy including DLS and hypopharyngoscopy, esophagoscopy, bronchoscopy and nasopharyngoscopy.
- Thyroid scan
- Angiogram

Treatment

Hydration/nutrition

- *Parenteral:* IV fluids
- Enteral feeding through Ryle's tube or through feeding gastrostomy or jejunostomy.

Treatment of the Cause

- *Medical:* Anemia, inflammation, trauma, aspiration pneumonia, etc.
- *Surgical*: Dilatation, conduits (bypass), resection, fracture reduction and fixation.

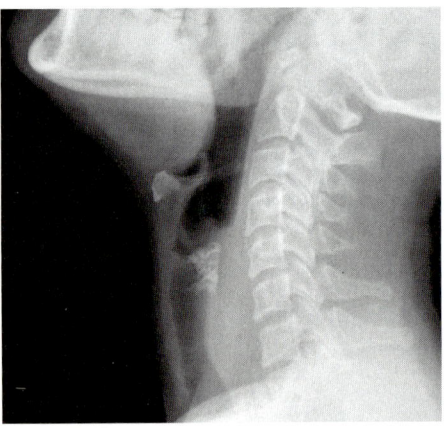

Fig. 63.1: Widening of the prevertebral space shadow

Larynx and Trachea

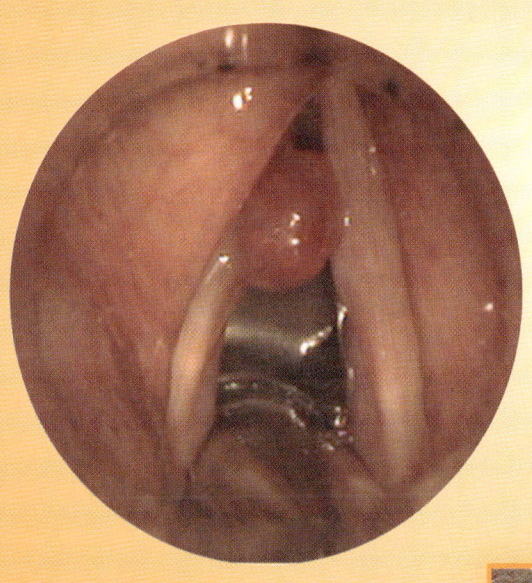

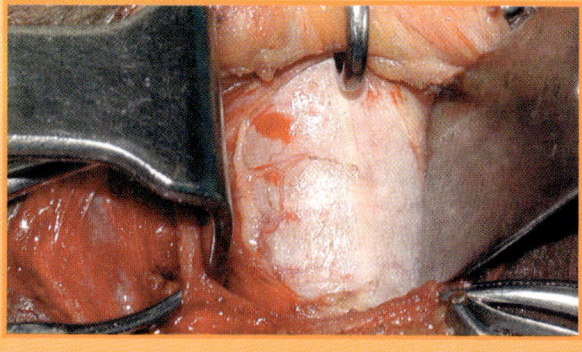

64

Anatomy of Larynx

Embryology

The ***hypobranchial eminence*** is formed in the floor of the primitive pharynx between the ventral end of the third, fourth and second arch. The ventral foregut groove becomes demarcated as the laryngotracheal sulci at the end of third week of fetal life—Fig. 64.1 also refer Chapter 66 for development of tracheobronchial tree.

Two distinct components are identified at this stage namely medial pharyngeal groove and caudal laryngotracheal sulcus (Fig. 64.2). The entire pulmonary system develops with development of the laryngeal portion which occurs initially and the lungs being formed last.

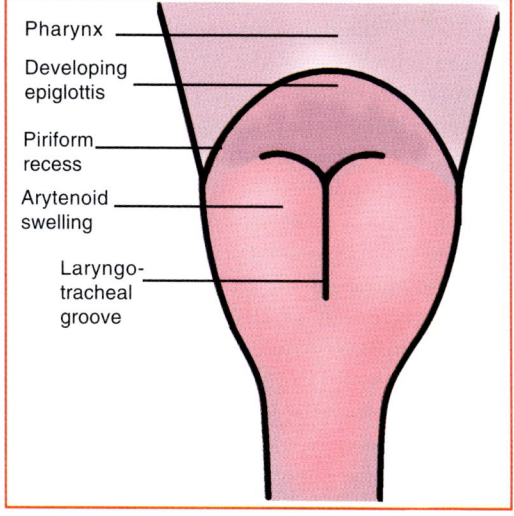

Fig. 64.2: Development of different parts of the larynx at 8 weeks

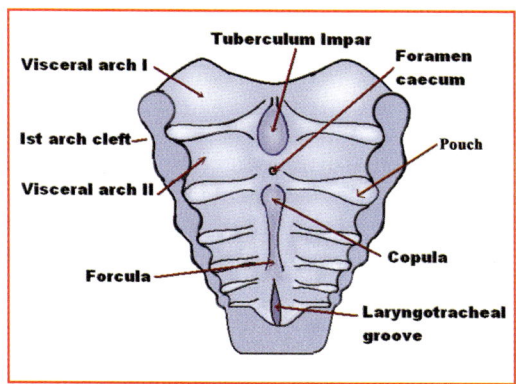

Fig. 64.1: Branchial apparatus with its various arches, clefts and pouches

The oesphagorespiratory separation occurs by a laryngotracheal septum. The structure derived caudal to the third pharyngeal arch forms the mesodermal elements of the larynx and will be innervated by superior laryngeal nerve. The tracheo-bronchial groove appears caudal to the hypobranchial eminence.

The larynx, trachea and lungs develop from this groove which arises as a diverticulum posterior to hypobranchial eminence from foregut at about 4 weeks of embryonic life. A

567

mesenchymal condensation from behind surrounds the oesophagus and respiratory tube while angiogensis is beginning in the mesenchyme. This mesenchyme is denser in the glottis than the periphery and is localized in two planes, i.e., the inner constrictor which is derived from the fifth and sixth arch and the external constrictor which is derived from the fourth arch.

The external constrictor is the analogy of the inferior constrictor and the cricothyroid muscle. The inner constrictor is analogous to all the intrinsic muscles of the larynx. The primitive respiratory groove which transforms into a laryngotracheal groove that communicates with the pharynx with the laryngeal fissure.

Two swellings develop lateral to the laryngeal fissure which forms the arytenoids and the primitive aryepiglottic fold. The hypobranchial eminence in the midline is responsible for the formation of primitive epiglottis. The hypobranchial eminence is notched rostrally and caudally denoting fusion of anterior extension of fourth arch and suggests a paired origin of epiglottis. The future laryngeal inlet is the representation of the paired arytenoid swelling and the midline eminence in the floor of the pharynx. The triangular laryngeal inlet has a midline epiglottic swelling, lateral aryepiglottic fold and arytenoid swelling. Gradually, the laryngeal lumen takes a T-shape and the laminar epithelium grows ventrally to obliterate the lumen by a solid cellular plug.

The cellular condensation is then followed by central necrosis to form two canals, i.e., anterior vestibulotracheal canal and posterior pharyngotracheal canal allowing the trachea to be separated from the oesophagus and the hypopharynx. At about 8th week, the analage of the vocal cord is formed by an epithelial and mesodermal mass between the vestibule and the upper trachea.

By 10th week, this mass splits sagittally giving rise to both pairs of vocal cords. Any incomplete or complete fusion at this stage can lead to laryngeal web or atresia respectively. The laryngeal ventricle develops as a medial and lateral fissure around the arytenoid eminence, from the 4th branchial arch and cleft.

The lateral part forms the saccule of the ventricle and as it develops the true and false cords separate. The epiglottis is the last cartilaginous tissue to develop. At 18 mm stage, hyoid cartilage is delineated. At 20 mm stage, the thyroid cartilage develops from the ventral part of the 4th branchial arch and fuses anterior to the pharyngotracheal canal.

The development is complete by 10th week by the formation of the cricothyroid joint and at 55mm stage the cricoid cartilage develops. The hyaline cartilage of the larynx develops from the branchial arch mesoderm, while the elastic cartilage develops from the mesoderm of the floor of the pharynx. Thyroid cartilage is derived from the ventral end of 4th arch.

Epiglottis and the cuneiform cartilage develops from the floor of the pharynx through the 4th arch which forms the lateral glossoepiglottic fold and may contribute to the formation of the epiglottis (Fig. 64.2). The hyoid bone is derived from the 2nd and 3rd branchial arches. Cricoid cartilage is derived from the 6th arch derivative from the two mesodermal masses that fuses anterior to the pharyngotracheal canal which fuses at the 6th week.Laryngeal musculature develops as intrinsic mesenchymal condensation within the larynx. The laryngeal cavity has its adult form in 90 mm stage.

ANATOMY OF THE LARYNX

Larynx is a midline structure situated at the meeting point of digestive and respiratory passage in the neck. It lies in front of the laryngopharynx between the level of third and sixth level of cervical vertebra. It consists of a skeletal framework composed of nine cartilages, connected to each of these by ligaments and membranes. It is lined internally by mucous membrane.

The size of the larynx is more in adults than before puberty. In adults, all the cartilages enlarge and the projection of the thyroid cartilage produces the Adam's apple. The male larynx is more prominent than the female larynx as the angle between the thyroid laminae is more acute in males. The larynx is suspended from the hyoid bone by muscles and ligaments and is not a part of the structure of the larynx.

The larynx has two joints which are moved by various intrinsic and extrinsic muscles.

FRAMEWORK OF THE LARYNX

The skeletal framework is made up of the following structures (Fig. 64.3).

- Hyoid bone
- Unpaired cartilages
  - Epiglottis
  - Thyroid cartilage
  - Cricoid cartilage
- Paired cartilages
  - Arytenoid cartilage
  - Cuneiform cartilage
  - Corniculate cartilage

Hyoid Bone

The hyoid bone comprises of a body and the lesser and greater horns on either sides. The body is the central part and is quadrilateral in shape with anterior, and posterior surface with superior and inferior borders. The superior border of the hyoid bone serves as an attachment for the hyoepiglottic and thyrohyoid membrane. Thus the hyoid bone forms the anterosuperior boundary of the pre-epiglottic space (Fig. 64.7). Vallecula lies just immediately above it. The hyoid bone is attached to the mandible and skull base by stylohyoid ligament, digastric, mylohyoid, stylohyoid, geniohyoid and hyoglossus muscles, hence helping in raising the larynx during deglutition and phonation.

Thyroid Cartilage

It is the largest hyaline cartilage in the larynx and its surface is covered by outer and inner perichondrium. It has two wings which meet

anteriorly at an angle of 90 degree and 120 degree in male and female, respectively. The angle gives the prominence to the laryngeal skeleton in males. The ala begins to ossify at the age of 25 years and mostly completes conversion into bone by 65 years of age. Medially the anterior portion of the ala is related to the glottis and the posterior portion medially forms the lateral boundary of the pyriform fossa. The point of junction of the upper portion of alae forms a V-shaped notch called the thyroid notch. On the outer surface of each lamina there is an oblique line for muscular attachment.

The superior cornu arises from the posterosuperior angle of the ala, whereas the inferior cornu arises from the posteroinferior angle of the ala. There is a small oval facet on its inner surface for articulation with cricoid cartilage (Fig. 64.3).

Cricoid Cartilage

It is thicker and stronger than thyroid cartilage which resembles a signet ring. The cartilage is narrow in front and broad behind. The ossification starts at the age of 30 and is completed by 65 years for age.

The cricoid cartilage consists of the lamina posteriorly which is flat and quadrate in shape. There is a vertical ridge in the posterior surface of the lamina which gives attachment of the upper fibres of the esophagus. There is a smooth oval

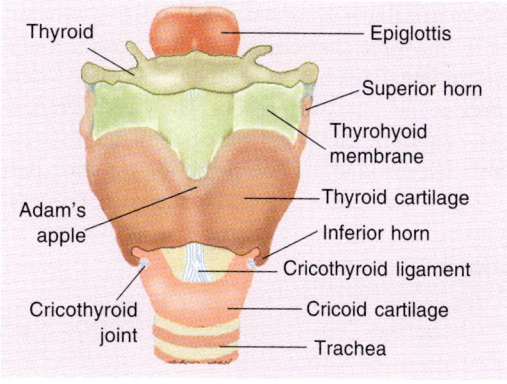

Fig. 64.3: Various structures forming the skeletal framework of the larynx

facet on each side of the upper border of lamina which gives articulation to the arytenoids cartilage.

The arch of the cricoid cartilage is situated anteriorly which is narrow in front and expands posteriorly to the lamina. The lower border of the lamina is almost straight and horizontal and there is a rounded facet at the junction of the arch and lamina on each side which gives articulation to the inferior cornu of thyroid cartilage.

Epiglottis

Arises up behind the tongue. It is a long thin leaf like sheet of elastic cartilage directed upwards and posteriorly. The free border of the epiglottis is directed upward and is broad and rounded from side to side. The anterior surface is free in the upper part but is separated from the hyoid bone and the thyrohyoid membrane by some fatty tissue in its lower part known as pre-epiglottic space (Fig. 64.7). The posterior surface is indented by several small pits containing mucous glands. The lower part of the epiglottis consists of the tubercle which is projected backwards.

Arytenoid Cartilage

They are paired three sided pyramidal hyaline cartilage and at its base it articulates with the cricoid cartilage by the cricoarytenoid joint. It is larger in males than in females. The articulating facets are flat in long axis and concave in short axis. The three surfaces are medial, posterior and anteriolateral. It has two processes—The vocal process and muscular process. The vocal ligament extends from the vocal process to the anterior commissure tendon. The posterior-superior part of conus elasticus is attached to the vocal process. Muscular process gives attachment to cricoarytenoid muscle.

Corniculate Cartilage (Cartilage of Santorini)

A pair of cartilage that articulate with arytenoids cartilage

Cuneiform Cartilage *(Cartilage of Wrisburg)*

A pair of rod-shaped cartilage that is situated just in front of Corniculate cartilage.

JOINTS OF LARYNX

They are two in number and are simple synovial joints.

Cricothyroid Joint

This joint articulates the inferior cornu of the thyroid cartilage to articular facet on the cricoid cartilage. The movements are across the transverse axis passing through the joints.

Cricoarytenoid Joint

This joint is strengthened by the capsular ligament and firm posterior cricoarytenoid ligaments. Two major movements occur in this joint.
1. Axis runs obliquely upwards giving rotation of the arytenoids helping in abduction and adduction.
2. Complex gliding and tipping motion, moving the arytenoid laterally and downwards. Cricoarytenoid ligament prevents excessive forward movement of the arytenoid.

Ligaments and Membranes of Larynx

Links the various parts of the framework
- Thyrohyoid ligament
  - Thyrohyoid membrane
  - Median and Lateral thyrohyoid ligaments
- Cricothyroid ligament
  - Medial and lateral cricothyroid ligaments
  - Conus elasticus
- Cricotracheal membrane
- Quadrangular membrane

Most of these ligaments and membranes are natural barriers of cancer spread (Fig. 64.4)

- *Quadrangular membrane:* This membrane on either sides extend from the lateral border of the epiglottis, forming a fibrous sheet of

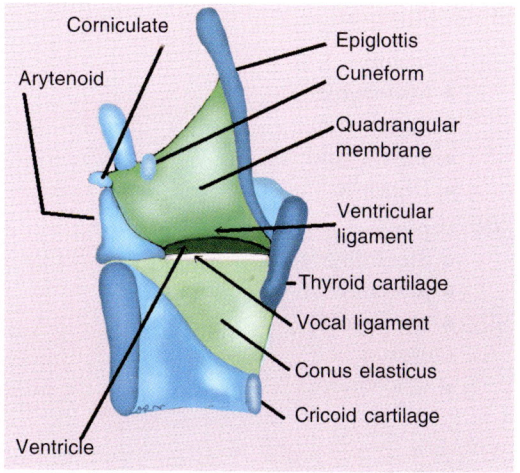

Fig. 64.4: Showing various cartilages and membranes of the larynx

tissue within the mucosa of the aryepiglottic folds superiorly and the false cords inferiorly. At the inferior level of the false cord, a condensation of fibrous tissue extends from the thyroid cartilage to the arytenoid. This fibrous scaffold supports the aryepiglottic folds and false cords, separating the supraglottic endolaryngeal structures from the pyriform sinuses.

- **Conus elasticus:** This membrane extends from the upper border of the cricoid cartilage to the vocal ligament, vocal process, and the inferior lateral portion of the arytenoid cartilage. The anterior condensation of the conus elasticus is the cricothyroid ligament, and the superior condensations bilaterally are the vocal ligaments.

- **Thyrohyoid membrane:** The membrane extends from the hyoid to the thyroid cartilage. The superior laryngeal neurovascular pedicle passes through the lateral aspect of this membrane.

- **Anterior commissure tendon (Broyle's ligament):** The anterior condensation of the vocal tendons with the internal aspect of the thyroid cartilage meshes with the thyroepiglottic ligament. This area of the thyroid cartilage is devoid of perichondrium.

- **Hyoepiglottic ligament:** This ligament extends from the epiglottis to the hyoid and serves as the roof of pre-epiglottic space. The hypoepiglottic ligament serves as a formidable barrier to invasion from the supraglottis to the tongue base.

- **Cricothyroid ligament:** This ligament is the anterior condensation of the conus elasticus connecting the cricoid and inferior border of the thyroid cartilage. Unlike the thyrohyoid membrane, the cricothyroid ligament is present only in the midline. Because the conus elasticus does not form a continuous layer between the thyroid and cricoid cartilages, no significant barrier exists to cancer extension beyond the larynx at that level.

MUSCLES OF LARYNX

Intrinsic Muscles (Fig. 64.5)

They connect the laryngeal cartilages and thus are directly involved in the various functions of the larynx. All intrinsic muscles are paired except transverse interarytenoid muscle.

- **Muscles which change size and shape of inlet of larynx:** Aryepiglottic and oblique arytenoid

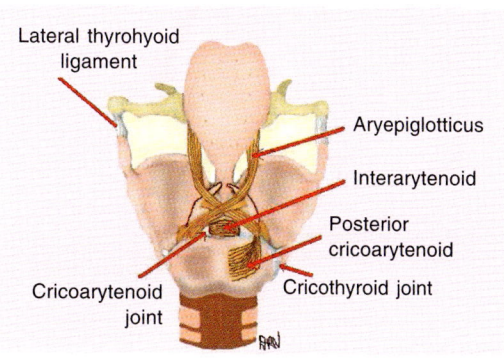

Fig. 64.5: Intrinsic muscles of the larynx

- *Muscles which move the vocal cord*
  (a) Abductors
  - *Posterior cricoarytenoid:* This is the only abductor of the vocal cords and is the most important muscle of the larynx. It arises from a depression on the posterior surface of the cricoid laminae and the fibres run upwards and laterally and get inserted to the posterior surface of muscular process of the ipsilateral arytenoids as shown in the Fig. 64.6.
  (b) Adductors
  - *Lateral cricoarytenoid:* This arises from the upper portion of the arch of the cricoid lamina and runs posteriorly to be inserted to the anterior surface of the muscular process of ipsilateral arytenoid.
  - Thyroarytenoid and interarytenoid
  - Cricothyroid (External)
  (c) Tensors (Fig. 64.6)
  - Thyroarytenoid (Vocalis)
  - Cricothyroid (External tensor)

Extrinsic Muscles

These muscles connect the laryngeal framework to the adjacent structures and move the laryngeal skeleton as a whole.

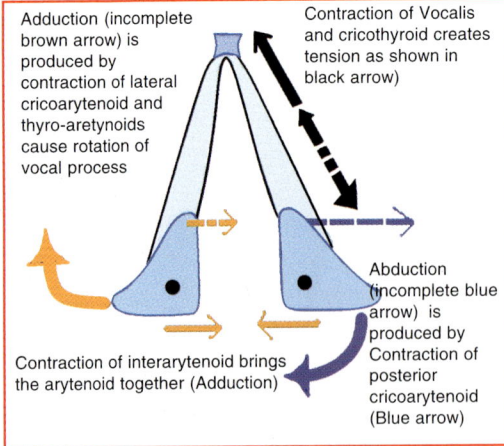

Fig. 64.6: Various intrinsic muscles of the larynx and their functions

Strap Muscles

(a) Elevators
- Mylohyoid
- Stylohyoid
- Thyrohyoid
- Digastric

(b) Depressors
- Sternothyroid
- Sternohyoid
- Omohyoid

(c) Tensor of VC
- Cricothyroid

Pharyngeal Muscles

- Inferior constrictor

INTERIOR OF THE LARYNX

The interior of the larynx is lined by respiratory epithelium except over vocal cords and parts of epiglottis which is lined by stratified squamous epithelium.

Laryngeal inlet is bounded by

1. Above and in front by the free margin of the epiglottis
2. Laterally by the aryepiglottic fold
3. Posteriorly by the interarytenoid region

DIVISIONS OF THE LARYNX

The laryngeal interior is divided by two folds into 3 parts. The two folds are the true vocal cord and the false vocal cord (ventricular band). The three parts are:

- Supraglottis
  - Vestibule
  - Ventricle
- Glottis
- Subglottis

The division of the larynx is based on the developmental analage. The parts that are derived from the 3rd and the 4th arch is the supraglottic larynx whereas the parts that are derived from the 6th arch (respiratory analage) are the glottis and the subglottis. The 5th arch disappears during the development. This embryological subdivision also creates natural barriers as the lymphatic drainage, blood and nerve supply are well compartmentalized depending on the arch of origin. The malignancy of the larynx is also restricted to laryngeal compartments in the early stage due to the natural barriers before they infiltrate into other compartments. Thus conservation laryngectomy is possible in early stages.

The supraglottic larynx includes the epiglottis, aryepiglottic folds, arytenoids, and false cords. The true vocal cords and the anterior and posterior commissures comprise the glottis. The subglottis begins below the true vocal cords and involves the remaining portion of the larynx to the inferior border of the cricoid cartilage.

Supraglottis

The wall is formed by quadrangular membrane which extends from vestibular fold ligaments to aryepiglottic folds.

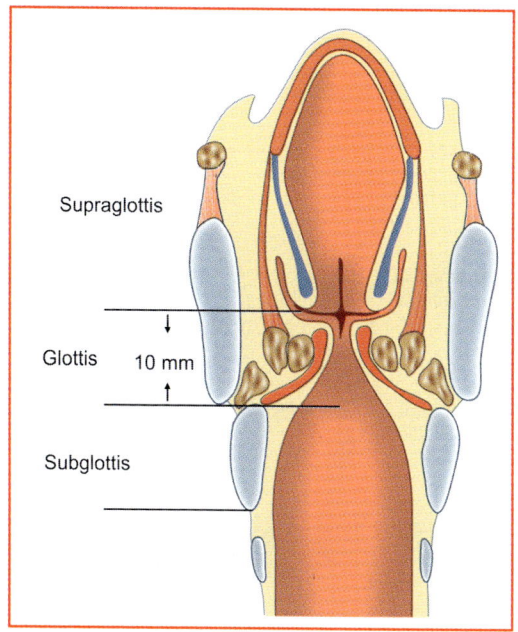

Fig. 64.7: Divisions of the larynx

The supraglottis comprises of:

1. Epiglottis
   - Suprahyoid part
   - Infrahyoid part
2. Laryngeal aspects of aryepiglottic folds
3. Arytenoids
4. Ventricular bands
5. Ventricles

The inferior limit of the supraglottis is:

1. Clinically—Imaginary horizontal plane passing through the apex of laryngeal ventricle.
2. Anatomically—Superior arcuate line where the squamous epithelium and respiratory epithelium meet.

Thus the roof of ventricle and saccule are included in supraglottis and floor belongs to glottis.

The 'Marginal zone' comprises of:

(a) Suprahyoid epiglottis and
(b) Aryepiglottic folds.

It is recognized because of:

- Aggressive clinical behavior of cancer arising in this area.
- There is lack of embryologic separation from the adjacent hypopharynx and it carries worse prognosis among laryngeal cancers.
- Mucous glands are abundant in saccule and periarytenoid area.
- Early lymphatic spreads of supraglottic cancer is because of rich vascularity and lymphatics associated with these glands

Glottis

This includes:

1. True vocal cords
2. Anterior commissure
3. Posterior commissure

The glottis extends from the lateral angle of the ventricle to the upper border of the cricoid cartilage. Lower limit of glottis is controversial and the commonly accepted level is horizontal plane passing

1 cm below the free margin of the vocal cords at the anterior commissure and 0.5 cm below the posterior commissure. Some authors feel that the lower limit of the glottis is horizontal plane 20 mm below the anterior commisure.

Lamina propria of the vocal cords consists of 3 layers. The superficial layer is composed of loose fibrous tissue that makes the **Reinke's space**. The intermediate and deep layer consist of elastic and collagenous fibers that makes the **Vocal Ligament**.

Conus elasticus is a membrane which extends from superior border to cricoid cartilage to merge with inferomedial surface of vocal ligament. It resists the extralaryngeal spread of glottic and subglottic cancers.

Subglottis

Embryologically it develops from VI arch and extends inferior to glottis to lower border of cricoid cartilage.

- This is a rare site of origin of cancers of larynx but may be involved in glottic cancers.
- Subglottic malignancy has higher incidence of extralaryngeal spread.

Reasons

1. Proximity of cricothyroid membrane
2. Rich postcricoid lymphatics.

COMPARTMENTS OF LARYNX (PRESSMAN 1956)

Reinke's Space

The mucosa over the vocal ligaments is attached loosely to the ligaments themselves. There is a submucosal space along most of the length of free edge of the true vocal cord extending from superior arcuate line to inferior arcuate line. Blood vessels and lymphatics are almost absent in Reinke's space preventing early spread of cancers.

Supraglottis Area

Lies beneath the supraglottic mucosa superficial to quadrangular membrane.

Subglottic Area

This area extends from inferior margin of the true cord to the inferior rim of cricoid.

It is a potential space filled with fibroelastic submucosal tissue between mucosa and conus elasticus.

The subglottic area does not include the vocalis muscles and is limited superiorly at anterior commisure by the anterior commisure tendon.

Cricoid Area

This potential space contains the areolar tissue medial to the internal perichondrium of the cricoid. The compartment is situated between the subglottic area and trachea.

Pre-epiglottic Space / Space of Boyer

Boundaries (Fig. 64.8)

Anterior

- Thyrohyoid membrane
- Thyroid cartilage above the thyroepiglottic ligament

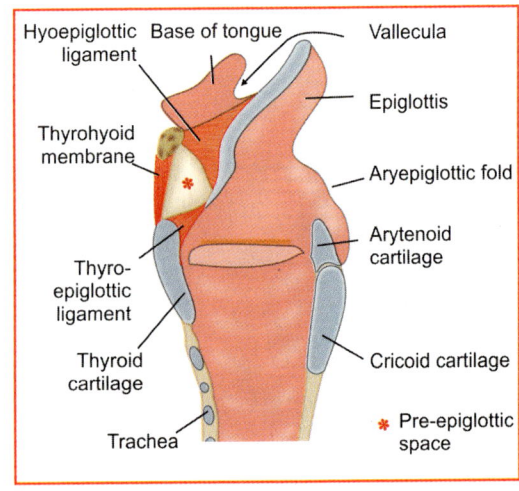

Fig. 64.8: Boundaries of the pre-epiglottic space

Superior

- Hyoepiglottic ligament
- Mucosa of the vallecula

Posterior

- Infrahyoid epiglottis
- Thyroepiglottic ligament

This space is continuous laterally with paraglottic space deep to the quadrangular membrane and superior to the ventricle.

Clinical Importance

Cancer on laryngeal surface of the infrahyoid epiglottis spreads readily into the pre-epiglottic space. (Tucker. G.F-1962)

Paraglottic Space (Figs 64.9 and 64.10)

This space is situated lateral to the ventricle and the glottis. Involvement of this space by malignancy causes fixation of the vocal cord and is considered as advanced stage of cancer.

Boundaries

- *Anterolaterally:* Thyroid cartilage and cricothyroid membrane
- *Superomedially:* Quadrangular membrane
- *Inferomedially:* Conus elasticus
- *Posteriorly:* Anterior reflection of pyriform sinus mucosa.

It blends with pre-epiglottic space anterosuperiorly.

The submucosa of the ventricle is continuous with paraglottic space which is bounded by conus elasticus inferiomedially, quadrangular membrane superomedially, thyroid ala laterally. The posterior limit of the paraglottis space is the mucosa of the pyriform sinus. Inferolaterally the paraglottic space is continuous with the cartilaginous defect between the thyroid and cricoid cartilage (cricothyroid space).

Paraglottic space has great significance in determining the spread of cancer within the larynx. Tumor involving the ventricle invades the paraglottic space and later spreads transglottically.

Vocal cord tumors which extend deeply into the thyroarytenoideus muscle invade the paraglottic space, which later on extends to subglottis and extra laryngeal spread.

Lateral supraglottic tumors can travel lateral to ventricle along the inner surface of the thyroid ala and thus spread subglottically.

The close proximity of pyriform sinus mucosa to the posterior paraglottic space makes this a potential route for spread of pyriform sinus

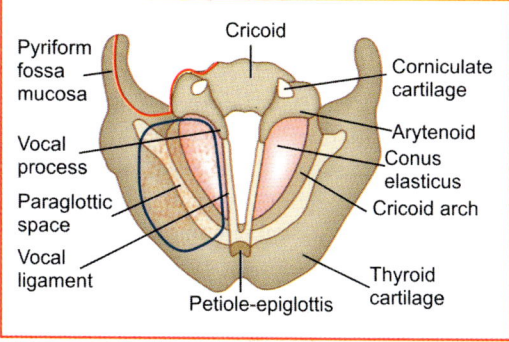

Fig. 64.9: Aerial view of the larynx showing the paraglottic space (shaded area with blue outline) and its relation to the conus elasticus (light green) and the pyriform fossa (pink line)

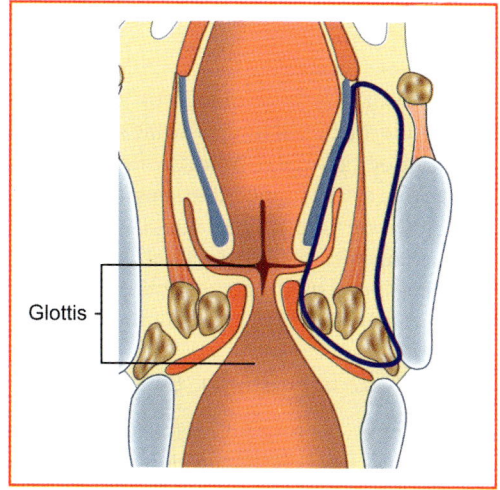

Fig. 64.10: Coronal section of the larynx showing the paraglottic space (red outline)

carcinoma into the endolarynx resulting often in fixation of hemilarynx.

Nerve Supply

Sensory
- Supraglottis and upper surface of the vocal cords: Internal branch of the superior laryngeal nerve.
- Subglottis and lower surface vocal cords: Recurrent laryngeal nerves.

Motor

> *Intrinsic*
> - *All muscles except cricothyroid*: Recurrent laryngeal nerve
> - *Cricothyroid:* External branch of superior laryngeal nerve.
>
> *Extrinsic*
> - *Ansa cervicalis*: Branch of hypoglossal.

Galen's anastomosis: Presence of anastomosis between superior and recurrent laryngeal nerve originally described by Galen as well as right and the left side has significant implication in understanding the vocal cord paralysis with special response to recovery, compensation and reinnervation.

Blood Supply

Arterial and Venous
- Superior laryngeal branch of the superior thyroid artery and it supplies the supraglottis.
- Inferior laryngeal branch of the inferior thyroid artery supplies the subglottis and the under surface of the vocal cord. This accompanies the recurrent laryngeal nerve. Some blood supply comes through the cricothyroid branch of the superior thyroid artery.

Lymphatic Drainage (Fig. 64.11)

The lymphatics of the two sides hardly communicate thus restricting the tumor spread in laryngeal cancers.

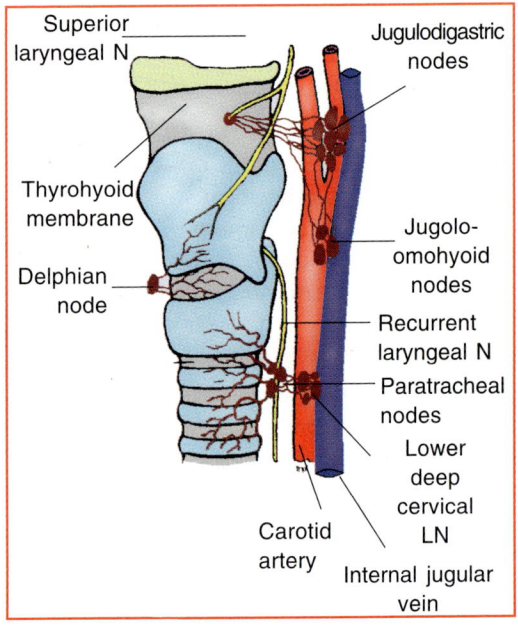

Fig. 64.11: Showing the lymphatic drainage of the larynx

- *Supraglottis:* The lymph vessels pierce the thyrohyoid membrane and drain into nodes Level II and III (Jugulodigastric and juguloomohyoid). Ventricular lymphatics also pass through the cricothyroid membrane and ipsilateral thyroid gland to the L3 and L4 lymph nodes.
- *Subglottis:* The lymphatics form three main trunks. One superficial trunk (anterior) pierces the cricothyroid membrane and drains to the Delphian (prelaryngeal) node which in turn drains into the pre and paratracheal and supraclavicular nodes. The two posterolateral trunks penetrate the cricotracheal membrane and terminate in the paratracheal node and the superior mediastinum. The nodes drain into deep cervical nodes (lower deep cervical nodes).
- *Glottis:* This is the 'Water-shed area'- with poor lymphatics. Anterior commissure drains into the prelaryngeal (Delphian node).

Physiology of Larynx

65

Larynx performs many functions and its primary function is to protect the lower respiratory tract. Phonation is also an important function of the larynx which facilitates communication. The *functions* are enumerated as follows:

- Protection of tracheobronchial tree is facilitated by:
  - 'Three-tier' sphincter action
  - Laryngeal elevation – Mylohyoid
  - Laryngeal tilting – Stylopharyngeous
  - Cricopharyngeal spincter relaxes
  - Cough reflex
  - Cessation of respiration
- *Respiration:* Reflex adjustments of the glottic apparatus plays a role in the mechanism of respiration which contributes to the regulation of acid-base balance.
- Phonation
- *To increase intrathoracic pressure:* This is done for fixation of the chest by glottic closure. This is essential for straining, climbing, etc.

Protection of the Lower Respiratory Tract

Phylogenetically this is the most primitive function of the larynx. This protective function is carried out by the closure of the laryngeal inlet that occurs during swallowing by a 'three-tier'

sphincter action. There is closure of the laryngeal vestibule by contraction of the aryepiglottic and the interarytenoid muscles. The ventricular bands approximate which constitute the second tier. The third tier is by the adduction of the vocal cords by contraction of the adductors. The epiglottis plays a negligible role in closure of the laryngeal vestibule.

The cough reflex plays an important role in expelling foreign particles entering the tracheobronchial tree.

Phonation

The phonation function of the larynx has developed with the evolution. It occurs at the time of inspiration when the vocal cords are approximated following adduction and the air escapes through causing vibration of the vocal cords (Figs 65.1 and 65.2). These vibratory tones are articulated by various structures in the oral cavity and resonated by the pharynx, nasal/ oral cavity and paranasal sinuses to produce speech.

The pitch of the voice is determined by the number of vibrations of the vocal cord per second. The length and volume are determined by the capacity of the lungs. The quality of the speech is dependent on the resonators as described. The articulars of voice include the lips, gums, teeth, tongue, palate and the jaws.

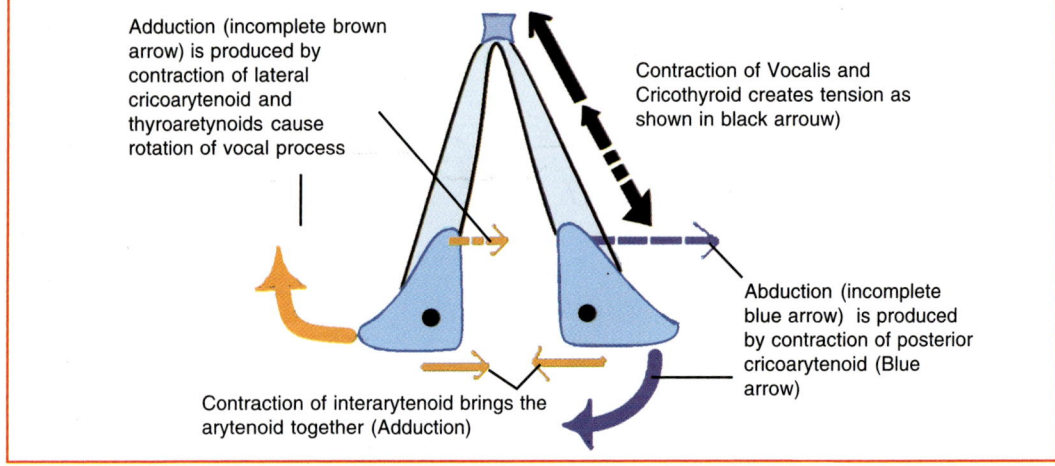

Adduction (incomplete brown arrow) is produced by contraction of lateral cricoarytenoid and thyroaretynoids cause rotation of vocal process

Contraction of Vocalis and Cricothyroid creates tension as shown in black arrouw)

Abduction (incomplete blue arrow) is produced by contraction of posterior cricoarytenoid (Blue arrow)

Contraction of interarytenoid brings the arytenoid together (Adduction)

Fig. 65.1: Showing various muscles that move the vocal cord

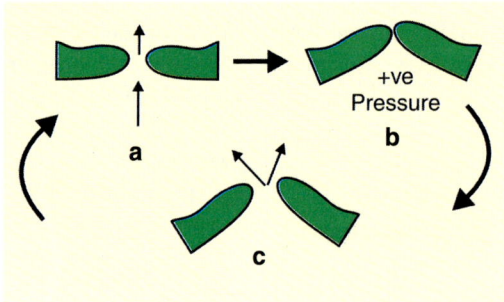

+ve Pressure

a

b

c

Fig. 65.2: The mechanism of phonation (myoelastic theory) **a.** Vocal cords in abducted position allowing expiration. **b.** Vocal cords in adducted position causing positive subglottic pressure during expiration. **c.** Sudden separation of vocal cords producing sound due to elastic recoil and vibration of cords during air escape

- *Intensity and duration* depends on the respiratory bellows and subglottic pressure build up by adduction of the cords.
- *Pitch* depends on the vibratory mass of vocal folds, laryngeal adductors and tensors (Fig. 65.1)
- *Quality (Timbre)* depends on resonators and articulators

POINTS TO REMEMBER

1. The primary function of the larynx is to protect the lower respiratory tract.
2. The phonation function of the larynx has developed with evolution.
3. The pitch of the voice is determined by the number of vibrations of the cord per second.
4. The length and volume of the speech is determined by the capacity of the lungs.

66

Anatomy and Physiology of the Tracheobronchial Tree

Development

At the beginning of the third week the tracheo-bronchial tree develops as a median groove arising from the floor of the primitive foregut and a prominent ventral keel (future laryngotracheal sulcus). At the end of third week the ventral foregut groove becomes demarcated as the tracheobronchial sulcus. The sulcus elongates in the rostrocaudal direction and is associated with an esophago-respiratory separation by a septum (tracheoesophageal septum) which unites at the luminal midline to divide system into ventral respiratory and caudal digestive system. In the beginning of fourth week the pulmonary primordium divides at the caudal end of the laryngotracheal sulcus to right and left area which forms the right and left lung bud. The pulmonary system develops from a rostral to caudal direction with the laryngeal portion forming first and the lungs forming last. The primary and secondary bronchi form around the mid of the fourth week.

Anatomy

- The trachea is a membranocartilaginous tube that extends from the lower border of the cricoid cartilage at the level of 6th cervical vertebra to the level of upper border of 5th thoracic vertebra where it divides into right and left bronchi.

- Length of the trachea is about 10 to 11.5 cm
- Width (diameter) is around 2 to 2.5 cm. Width is more in males than females and children.

Structure of the Trachea and Bronchial Tree

The trachea consists of 16 to 20 incomplete hyaline cartilaginous rings which are deficient posteriorly. The cartilaginous incomplete rings are about 4 mm in width and 1 mm thickness and are piled on one another with intervening membranous tissue made up of fibrous tissue and smooth muscles (trachealis). Deficiency of the cartilage behind makes the tube membranous and flattened posteriorly. The cartilages are in fact sandwiched between the two layers of fibrous membrane. In the intercartilaginous region, these two layers merge. Posterior part of the trachea is devoid of tracheal rings and consists of trachealis muscle fibers. The inner part of the tracheal tube is lined by ciliated columnar epithelium.

Relations of Trachea in the Neck (Fig. 66.1)

Anterior

- Strap muscles
- Isthmus of thyroid between the 2nd and 4th tracheal rings. Isthmus lies at a higher level in infants.

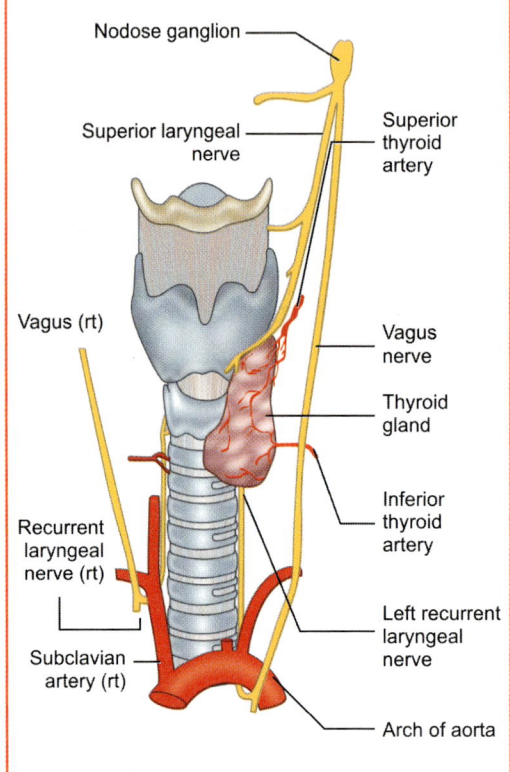

Fig. 66.1: Structure of trachea and bronchial tree

- Anastomotic vessels between the two superior thyroid arteries.
- Innominate and left brachiocephalic vein crosses in the lower neck at the upper border of the manubrium in children. In adults it is at a lower level.
- Thymus gland at the root of the neck.

Lateral

- Lobes of the thyroid gland till the level of the 6th ring
- Common carotid artery, internal jugular vein, inferior thyroid artery, vagus nerve

Posterior

- Membranous part of trachea is closely related to the esophagus

- Recurrent laryngeal nerves lie posteriorly in the tracheoesophagial groove

Relations of Trachea in the Thorax

Anterior

- Sternum
- Arch of aorta at the site of bifurcation
- Origin of innominate and left carotid arteries
- Innominate and left brachiocephalic vein cross in front of trachea.

Lateral

> *Right side*
> - Pleura
> - Right vagus
> - Innominate artery at the root of the neck.
>
> *Left side*
> - Left recurrent laryngeal nerve
> - Aortic arch
> - Left common and subclavian arteries.

Posterior

- Esophagus

Blood Supply

- *Arterial*: Inferior thyroid artery
- *Venous*: Thyroid venous plexus

Nerve Supply

- Recurrent laryngeal nerve.

Bifurcation of Trachea
(Figs 66.2 and 66.3)

The trachea bifurcates at the upper border of 5th thoracic vertebra at about 25 cm from the incisor teeth in adults. Carina is a keel like spur produced by the lowest ring of trachea at the point of separation into two main bronchi. Right main bronchus wider, short and more vertical than the left and hence foreign body bronchus frequently gets lodged here. The left bronchus is more obliquely placed and runs more posteriorly than the right.

The **right main bronchus** divides into lobar bronchi which in turn divide into segmental bronchi as follows:

1. *Right upper lobe bronchus:*
   (a) Apical
   (b) Posterior
   (c) Anterior
2. *Right middle lobe bronchus :*
   (a) Medial branch
   (b) Lateral branch
3. *Right lower lobe bronchus:*
   (a) Apical
   (b) Medial basal
   (c) Subapical
   (d) Three basal bronchi (posterior, lateral and anterior).

The **left main bronchus** is narrow, longer and more horizontal than right and unlike the right side has two lobar bronchi divide. The lobar bronchi divide into segmental bronchi as follows:

1. *Left upper lobe bronchus*
   (a) Apical
   (b) Posterior
   (c) Anterior
   (d) Lingular
2. *Left lower lobe bronchus*
   (a) Apical
   (b) Subapical

(c) Three basal bronchi
   (i) Anterior basal
   (ii) Lateral basal
   (iii) Posterior basal

Bronchopulmonary Segments

These are definite segments of the lung which is ventilated by a segmental bronchus.

Tracheobronchial Lymphatics

- Pre and paratracheal nodes
- Tracheobronchial nodes
- Hilar nodes

Physiology of Tracheobronchial Tree

The tracheobronchial tree during inspiration allows airflow from the upper airway through the larynx to the alveoli of the lungs wherein there is exchange of gases between the alveolar sacs and the capillaries. Each alveolus is ventilated by a terminal bronchiole which is about <1 mm in diameter. During expiration the direction of airflow is towards the upper airway.

Tracheobronchial tree offers a safe passage for respiration by the virtue of its protective function. This is achieved by:

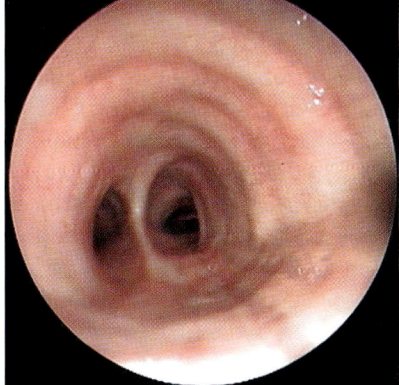

Fig. 66.2: Trachea and carina and left and right main bronchus

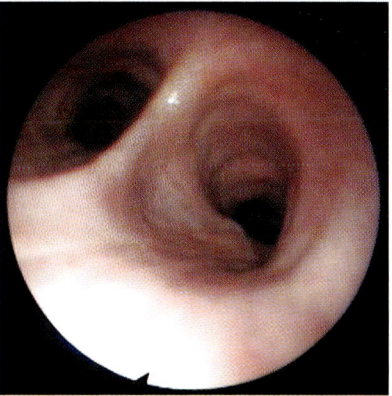

Fig. 66.3: Close-up view of trachea at carina showing the right main bronchus

1. **Mucociliary system:** The tracheobronchial tree is lined inside by respiratory epithelium (pseudostratified ciliated columnar epithelium) which is rich in mucous glands and goblet cells. There are no mucous glands in the bronchioles. The mucous blanket thus formed is transported towards the larynx by the ciliary motility. The mucous in the larynx is drained into the pharynx wherein it is swallowed. This mucous is rich in macrophages and lysosomal enzymes which can inactivate or kill the microorganisms in the inspired air.

2. **Cough reflex:** Cough is forced expiration against closed glottis. This neural reflex helps in expulsion of irritant or allergic or infected mucous into the pharynx from where it can be swallowed or spit out.

The volume of air in the tracheobronchial tree which is not directly involved in the exchanges of gases is called the dead space. The amount of airflow through this passage is regulated by the neural controls. The tracheobronchial tree being made of incomplete cartilaginous rings and fibromuscular tissue, it is able to distend or contract to certain extent thus influencing on the amount of airflow.

Mechanism of Breathing

A pressure gradient is created by the rib cage and the diaphragm to generate airflow in the respiratory passages. During inspiration air is drawn in by increasing the volume of the thoracic cavity under the action of the inspiratory muscles. During expiration the intra-alveolar pressure becomes slightly higher than atmospheric pressure resulting in gas flow towards the mouth.

Diaphragm, a muscular sheet separating the thorax from the abdomen is the main muscle generating the negative intrathoracic pressure that produces inspiration. It is supplied by the phrenic nerves (C3-5) and contraction moves the diaphragm downwards. Additional inspiratory efforts are produced by the external intercostal muscles (innervated by their intercostal nerves T1-12) and the accessory muscles of respiration (sternomastoids and scalenes), although the latter only become important during exercise or respiratory distress. During quiet breathing expiration is a passive process, relying on the elastic recoil of the lung and chest wall. Active expiration occurs when ventilation has to be increased, such as during exercise, by contraction of the muscles of the abdominal wall and the internal intercostals.

Respiration can be controlled both involuntarily and voluntarily. The mechanism by which respiration is controlled is complex. There is a group of respiratory centers located in the brainstem producing automatic breathing activity. This is then regulated mainly by input from chemoreceptors. This control can be overridden by voluntary control from the cortex. Breath-holding, panting or sighing at will are examples of this voluntary control. The main respiratory center is in the floor of the 4th ventricle, with inspiratory (dorsal) and expiratory (ventral) neurone groups. The inspiratory neurones fire automatically, but the expiratory ones are used only during forced expiration. The 2 other main centers are the apneustic center, which enhances inspiration, and the pneumotaxic centre, which terminates inspiration by inhibition of the dorsal neurone group above.

The chemoreceptors that regulate respiration are located both centrally and peripherally. Normally control is exercised by the central receptors located in the medulla, which respond to the CSF hydrogen ion concentration, in turn determined by CO_2, which diffuses freely across the blood-brain barrier from the arterial blood. The response is both quick and sensitive to small changes in arterial CO_2 ($PaCO_2$). In addition, there are peripheral chemoreceptors located in the carotid and aortic bodies most of which respond to a fall in O_2, but some also to a rise in arterial CO_2. The degree of hypoxia required to produce significant activation of the O_2 receptors is such that they are not influential under normal circumstances, but will do so if profound hypoxia (< 8kPa or 60 mmHg) occurs, for example at high altitude when breathing air (see later—Special circumstances). It also happens when the response to CO_2 is impaired, which can occur if the $PaCO_2$ is chronically elevated, leading to a blunting of the central receptor sensitivity. In this event the plasma bicarbonate (HCO_3^-) concentration will also be elevated.

Understanding of the respiratory physiology is important in understanding the pathophysiologic effects of airway obstruction and in management of airway obstruction by tracheostomy, tracheobroncial toileting, etc.

POINTS TO REMEMBER

1. Trachea develop as a median groove arising from the floor of the primitive foregut and extends from lower border of cricoid cartilage at the level of 6th cervical vertebra to the level of upper border of 5th thoracic vertebra.
2. Length of the trachea is 10–12 cms.
3. Trachea consists of 16–20 incomplete hyaline cartilagenous rings.
4. Tracheobronchial tree is lined by pseudostratified ciliated columnar epithelium.
5. Right main bronchus is wider, short and more vertical than left and hence foreign bodies frequently gets lodged here.

67

Clinical Examination of Larynx

Laryngeal examination is frequently ignored by the general physicians due to lack of expertise. A good history is also often missed. Both these two are very much essential in proper diagnosis. Treatment based on vague symptoms sometimes causes delay in the management of curable laryngeal diseases and late presentation of laryngeal cancer. A proper history and meticulous clinical examination and selected investigations of the larynx are the key to the accurate diagnosis.

The common symptoms presented by the patients with laryngeal pathology:

1. Hoarseness
2. Dysphagia
3. Pain in the throat
4. Referred otalgia
5. Cough
6. Dyspnea/ stridor.
7. Swelling of the neck.

Hoarseness

Hoarseness is the most common symptom of laryngeal disease. It is present in almost every case. A short history of hoarseness suggests inflammatory cause. A long standing history which is slowly progressive should be considered for a benign neoplastic condition. History of longer duration with rapidly progressive hoarseness and often associated with dyspnea and stridor should be suspected for laryngeal cancer. If there is sudden onset of hoarseness or aphonea with gradual improvement of voice after a period of time, we should suspect vocal cord paralysis which improves due to compensation by the healthy cord. Hoarseness following surgery or trauma can be due to recurrent laryngeal nerve paralysis.

Causes of Hoarseness

- *Congenital*
  – Web, cyst, vocal cord palsy, etc.
- *Infective*
  – Acute/ chronic laryngitis/tubercular laryngitis, etc.
  - *Trauma*
  – Inhalant– Fumes, chemicals, etc.
  – Penetrating/ blunt injury
  – Acid reflux
- *Tumors:* Benign/ malignant
- Voice abuse
- *Neurological:* Vocal cord paralysis, spastic dysphonia.
- *Miscellaneous:* Functional aphonea, endocrine cause like hypothyroidism, rheumatoid arthritis, hyperparathyroidism, leukoplakia, etc.

Dysphagia

Dysphagia or difficulty in swallowing can sometimes be associated with advanced laryngeal cancer. Tuberculosis of the larynx often presents with dysphagia and odynophagia. Feeding difficulties in children can sometimes be due to laryngeal problem. Acute supraglottitis can sometimes present with difficulty in swallowing.

Pain

Pain often suggests late stage of laryngeal cancer. Acute supraglottitis and laryngeal diphtheria secondary to the faucial diphtheria may be associated with pain and dysphonia.

Referred Otalgia

This can be associated with laryngotracheal trauma, laryngeal cancer, acute inflammatory conditions of the larynx, laryngeal tuberculosis, etc. This is due to common source of nerve supply.

Cough and Choking Spells

Chronic dry cough can be associated with chronic laryngitis. Dry cough at night with choking spells should raise the suspicion of aspiration, acid laryngitis (Laryngopharyngel reflux disease).

Dyspnea and stridor of sudden onset is commonly associated with acute supraglottitis, acute laryngo-tracheo-bronchitis, foreign body larynx, etc. If these are of insidious onset gradually progressive, malignancy should be suspected. Newborn baby infant should be suspected for congenital anomalies of the larynx.

Swelling in The Neck

Cystic swelling in the neck may be due to subhyoid bursitis, laryngocele, etc. The laryngeal framework may be pushed forwards in case of postcricoid cancer. Splaying the cartilage occurs in extra-laryngeal spread of laryngeal cancer. Perichondritis of the laryngeal cartilages can be associated with pain and swelling of the laryngeal framework. Cancer of the supraglottis is frequently associated with neck metastasis.

General history taking format has been described in detail in the previous chapters. History of the above symptoms should be taken in the following order.

Chief Complaints

The presenting symptoms should be listed in chronological order based on their duration.

History of present illness should mention detailed description of the above symptoms with respect to their onset, duration, progress, precipitating factors, etc.

Treatment History

Thyroid/cardiovascular surgeries may be associated with vocal cord paralysis.

Personal History

1. Occupation–Certain occupation is associated with laryngeal diseases due to exposure to dust, fumes, chemicals, smoke, etc. and may cause chronic laryngitis
2. Personal habits like smoking, alcohol intake, drugs, etc. may be associated with laryngeal cancer.

CLINICAL EXAMINATION OF THE LARYNX

External Examination

Inspection
1. Position and movements of the larynx should be noted
2. Splaying of laryngeal cartilages is associated with advanced laryngeal cancer.
3. Swelling in the neck may be due to neck metastasis following laryngeal cancer.
4. Look for stridor.

Palpation

Should palpate for broadening of the laryngeal skeleton, fullness of the thyrohyoid and cricothy-roid membrane, cervical metastasis, etc. Laryngeal crepitus should be elicited.

Auscultation

May be helpful in stridor and vascular swellings.

Indirect Laryngoscopy

Visualization of the larynx and the laryngopharynx using a laryngeal mirror is called indirect laryngoscopy. It is called 'indirect' as we see the mirror image of the structures.

Technique (Fig. 67.1)

The patient is asked to sit in front of the examiner. The patient faces the examiner and is seated erect at the same level as the examiner with the chest and head leaning forward. The patient is explained about the procedure and is asked to sit relaxed and is asked to protrude the tongue forwards keeping the mouth wide open. Protruded tongue is gently held with a piece of gauze piece between the left thumb and index finger as shown in the Fig. 67.2. A suitable size laryngeal mirror is gently placed against the uvula and the soft palate after proper defogging with savlon or any antifog solution. Alternatively the mirror can be gently warmed to prevent fogging.

The patient should breathe through the mouth during indirect laryngoscopy. The mirror facing downwards is tilted in different directions to visualize the various parts. If the patient has excessive gag reflex, the throat may sprayed with 10 percent xylocaine spray. To examine the vocal cord movement the patient is asked to phonate 'aa' for adduction and 'aee' to look for adduction and tension. Abduction of the cords is looked by asking the patient to take deep breath.

The structures that can be seen by indirect laryngoscopy from above downwards are:

Oropharynx

- Base of the tongue and tonsillolingual sulcus
- Lingual tonsils
- Vallecula
- Lateral and median glossoepiglottic folds.

Larynx

- Epiglottis
- Aryepiglottic folds
- Arytenoid, cuneiform and corniculate cartilages
- Pharyngoepiglottic folds
- Ventricular bands (false vocal cords)
- Vocal cords
- Interarytenoid area
- Tracheal rings through the glottic chink (Rima glottides)
- Anterior commissure may be seen in some cases but may be difficult to see if the epiglottis is overhanging.

Laryngopharynx

- Posterior pharyngeal wall
- Pyriform fossa
- Retroarytenoid area.

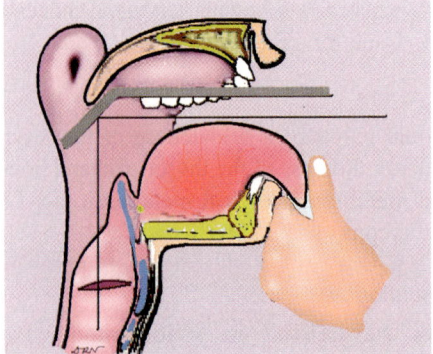

Fig. 67.1: Technique of indirect laryngoscopy

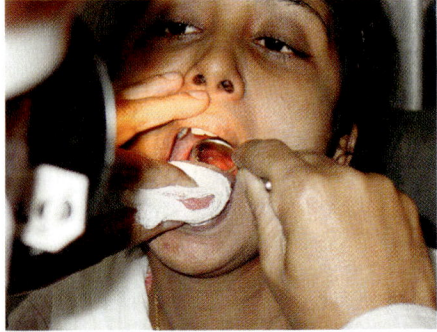

Fig. 67.2: Indirect laryngoscopy being performed by using laryngeal mirror

These sites should be evaluated for any swelling/ fullness, growth, ulcers or any mucosal changes. Look for any white patch over the vocal cords. Pooling of saliva in the pyriform fossa suggests obstruction to the esophageal/ cricopharyngeal lumen (Fig. 67.3).

Voice Assessment

The quality of the voice and any change in voice like hoarseness, breathy voice, whispering voice, hot-potato speech, etc. should be noted.

Investigations for Laryngeal Diseases

Direct Laryngoscopy

This refers to direct visualization of the larynx. There are various types of direct laryngoscopy, which include:

- Rigid laryngeal telescopy/ stroboscopy
- Flexible laryngoscopy
- Rigid direct laryngoscopy
- Negus
- Jackson's
- Anterior commisure laryngoscopy
- Microlaryngoscopy
- Conioscopy
- MacIntosh laryngoscopy used often by the anesthetists and the emergency room doctors for endotracheal intubation.

Rigid Telescopy/ Stroboscopy of the Larynx

A 70 degree, 9 mm rigid telescope may be used to visualize the larynx. This gives better and detailed visualization of the larynx than indirect laryngoscopy. This can also be used as a video-stroboscope by using flickering light source which gives more information about the vocal cord pathology. It gives a slow motion picture of the cord movement and vibrations or the cord may be studied in a freeze position. It is an important investigation procedure for voice evaluation and phonosurgery.

Flexible Fibreoptic Laryngoscopy

This is very useful procedure to visualize the larynx in uncooperative patients for indirect laryngoscopy, sensitive patients with gag reflex, comatose patients and in patients with cervical spine

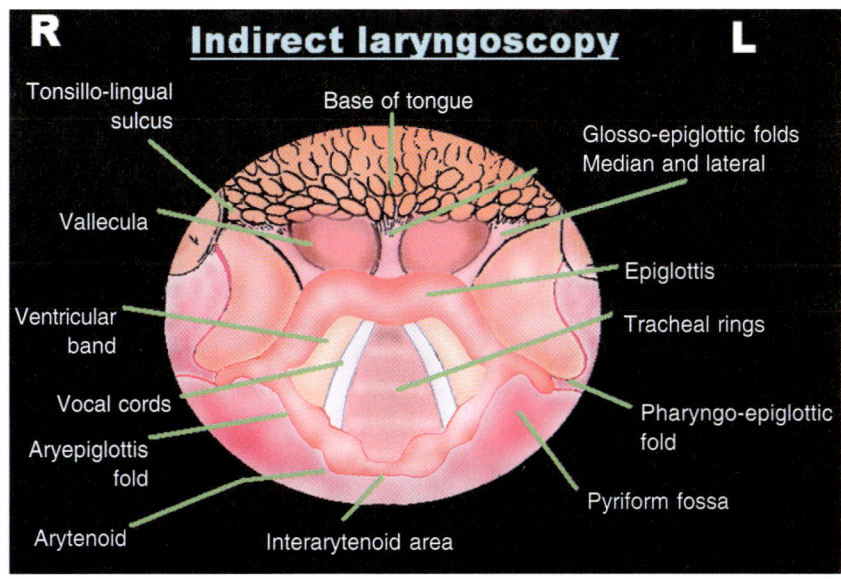

Fig. 67.3: Structures seen on indirect laryngoscopy

problems wherein rigid direct laryngoscopy may be difficult.

Rigid Direct Laryngoscopy

There are basically two types of rigid direct laryngoscopes.

- *Negus*: Proximal illuminating system
- *Jackson's*: Distal illuminating system

The distal illuminating system illuminates the target tissue better than the Negus type, but its bulb is prone to get fogged or smeared with secretions. With the advent of distal cold light system and fiber-optics, the illumination system has been improved in the Negus type and is more popular today.

Indications

Diagnostic

- Evaluation of cause of hoarseness
- Evaluation and biopsy of laryngeal mass/ulcer
- Evaluation of cause of hemoptysis
- Evaluation as a part of peroral panendoscopy in vocal cord paralysis, search for second primary or in case of a metastases of unknown origin (MUO).
- Evaluation of a case of laryngeal trauma/stenosis

Therapeutic

- Removal of laryngeal foreign body
- Treatment for laryngeal stenosis/ web
- Excision of laryngeal cysts/ papilloma/ polyp/ nodules

Technique

The procedure is done either under general anesthesia or local anesthesia.

If general anesthesia is opted, a smaller nasotracheal tube is preferred which allows better visualization of the laryngeal structures.

If local anesthesia is opted, laryngeal anesthesia may be achieved by

- 4 percent or 10 percent xylocaine spray into the throat or 4 percent xylocaine viscus may be kept in throat for few minutes.
- Internal laryngeal block by placing gauze piece soaked in 4 percent xylocaine in the pyriform fossae using a Mackenzie's forceps. This blocks the internal branch of the superior laryngeal nerve which runs submucosally in the pyriform fossa.
- External laryngeal block is given injecting 2 percent xylocaine into the thyrohyoid membrane where the superior laryngeal nerve pierces it.
- Transtracheal or criothyroid membrane – 4 percent xylocaine injection into the laryngotracheal lumen.

The patient is positioned in the Boyce's position with the neck flexed minimally and the head extended at the atlanto-occipital joint. This position is achieved by placing a small ring under the head.

The laryngoscope is introduced into the oral cavity superior to the tongue after safeguarding the teeth and the gingival using a teeth guard or a gauze piece. The various structures as mentioned under indirect laryngoscopy are sequentially examined. In addition the postcricoid area and the cricopharyngeal sphincter also may be visualized.

Complications

- Vasovagal attack and consequent cardiovascular complications especially if done under local anesthesia. Preoperative atropine is thus given to prevent it.
- Injury to the structures in the oral cavity, oropharynx and the larynx.
- Laryngeal edema and stridor may occur especially in a post-radiation case.
- Arytenoid dislocation.

Microlaryngoscopy (MLS)

This refers to direct laryngoscopy with suspensions (suspension laryngoscopy) and use of a microscope. The direct laryngoscope once introduced in the desired position, may be fixed using suspensions which holds the scope onto the operating table or on the chest of the patient. Then a microscope is focused through the scope to visualize the target structure/s. The advantages of microlaryngeal surgery are (Mnemonic-HIM):

Hands-free: Both hands are free for precise excision.

Illumination: Better illumination from the microscope, in addition through the laryngoscope.

Magnification: Magnified view of the structures in the larynx, helping in evaluation of the precise site and extent of the abnormality and also helps in precise excision with or without lasers.

Indications, technique and complications are almost similar to direct rigid laryngoscopy.

Radiological Investigations

Plain Radiographs (Fig. 67.4)

Two views are preferred for evaluation, namely AP view and lateral view. The radiographs are taken as for a soft tissue exposure and the following features may be studied:

- Size and shape of the epiglottis. Thumb sign is seen in acute epiglottitis wherein the epiglottis is grossly edematous.
- Aryepiglottic, venricular and the vocal folds. Look for any mass of edema of these folds.
- Arytenoid bulge– Look for edema.

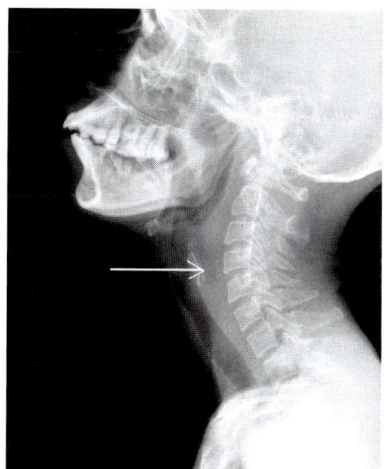

Fig. 67.4: Prevertebral widening due to postcricoid malignancy (white arrow)

- Laryngeal and tracheal airway– Subglottis is the part that is prone for obstruction in prolonged intubation or in acute laryngotracheobrionchitis. Airway obstruction or tracheal shift may be noted in laryngeal, hypopharyngeal or thyroid malignancies.
- Prevertebral widening—The pre-vertebral soft tissue shadow (anterior to the vertebral column and posterior to the tracheal air shadow) is usually less than three forth the body of the cervical vertebra. If more, it is known as pre-vertebral widening. The common causes of pre-vertebral widening are:
  - Postcricoid malignancy
  - Retropharyngeal abscess—Acute or chronic
  - Radiolucent foreign body
  - Large thyroid goiter.
- Status of the vertebral bodies like osteophytes, destruction of the vertebral bodies, collapse of the spine, reduced intervertebral space, changes of cervical spondylosis, etc.
- Any foreign body in the upper aerodigestive tract.

Barium Swallow

This helps in detecting obstruction, irregular filling defect, benign and malignant strictures involving the hypopharynx and esophagus which could be associated with laryngeal involvement (Fig. 67.5)

Laryngogram

May be done antegrade by injecting radio-opaque substance at the laryngeal inlet or may be done retrograde if the patient is having a tracheostoma by injecting radio-opaque material into the subglottis-trachea. Laryngograms are very useful in cases withy laryngotracheal stenosis to assess the site, length and amount of stenosis. This investigation is rarely being done nowadays after the availability of CT or MR imaging.

CT Scan

High resolution CT imaging (HRCT) of the larynx with contrast taken with thin slices gives detailed

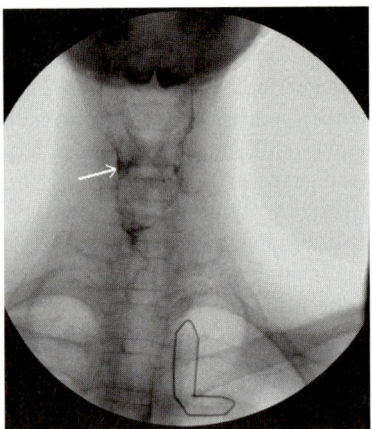

Fig. 67.5: Barium swallow radiograph showing irregular filling defect of the right pyriform fossa (white arrow) and postcricoid area

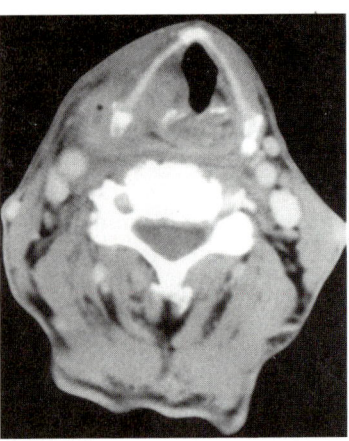

Fig. 67.6: CT scan showing laryngeal malignancy involving left glottis and paraglottic space

account of the laryngeal anatomy and the various intralaryngeal spaces (Fig. 67.6). This allows detailed evaluation of site and extent of laryngeal tumor and its relation to the laryngeal cartilages. CT also delineates the involvement of the cervical lymph nodes and the status of the carotid sheath in case of laryngeal/ hypopharyngeal malignancy.

MR Imaging

MRI scan of the neck gives better soft tissue delineation of the various structures in the neck in relation to the larynx and helps in assessment of laryngeal tumor and cervical metastases.

PET-CT

Positron emission tomography (PET scan) gives physiologic images based on the detection of radiation from the emission of positrons. Positrons are tiny particles emitted from a radioactive substance administered to the patient. The subsequent images of the human body developed with this technique are used to evaluate a variety of diseases This recent introduction to the medical field in combination with high resolution CT scan helps in early detection and more accurate assessment of laryngeal malignancy and its metastases. Hidden nasopharyngeal malignancy and other primary sites like base of tongue may be picked up in cases of metastases with occult primary.

POINTS TO REMEMBER

1. Laryngeal examination is difficult in children.
2. Hoarseness is the most common symptom of laryngeal disease.
3. Dysphagia can sometimes be associated with advanced laryngeal cancer.
4. Referred otalgia can be present in advanced laryngeal cancer due to mediation through vagus nerve.
5. Flexible fiberoptic laryngoscopy is very useful in uncooperative patients and children for examination of the larynx.
6. Stroboscopy is used for assessing vocal cord movements in slow motion.

68

Congenital Malformations of the Larynx

As the endolarynx enlarges by fusion of the epithelium and subsequent recanalization at about 10 weeks, a failure of epithelial primordium to split in the sagittal plane would result in a congenital atresia, a glottic or infraglottic laryngeal web or a subglottic stenosis.

At the time of true cord separation, lateral outpouchings extending from the arytenoids masses anteriorly forms the ventricle and the saccule. Abnormality of this process is responsible for laryngeal cysts.

Symptoms of Laryngeal Malformations

There are three modes of presentation as follows:
1. Stridor with cyanosis and restlessness.
2. Dysphonia with weak cry and hoarseness
3. Feeding difficulties due to choking associated with cyanosis and respiratory compromise

Evaluation

Owing to the smaller age group involved, evaluation of the larynx is often difficult. The evaluation is by systematic examination, beginning with anterior nares and ending with direct laryngoscopy and bronchoscopy.

Diagnosis is confirmed by direct laryngoscopy and flexible laryngoscopy.

Other Investigations

- Soft tissue X-ray of neck and chest (inspiratory and expiratory)

- Fluoroscopic examination of the laryngeal structures.
- HRCT scan imaging of the larynx

Laryngomalacia

It is a congenital malformation of the larynx associated with excessive softening of the skeletal framework of larynx. This is the commonest cause of congenital stridor in children.

Etiology

The cartilage framework of the larynx shows a consistent change in the proteoglycan content. Neonatal cartilage consists mainly of chondrotin-4-sulphate and lesser amounts of chondroitin-6-sulphate while chondroitin-6 sulphate is predominantly seen in adults thus contributing for more keratin thickening in adults. The syndrome appears to be more in lower socio-economic group with possibility of poor nutrition being an etiological factor.

Pathology

1. Excessive softness, flabbiness, or lack of consistency of laryngeal tissue
2. Thinning and hypocellularity of laryngeal cartilages
3. Wrinkled loose edematous mucosa.

Clinical Features

1. Stridor is usually the symptom that appears at or soon after birth.

2. Tubular epiglottis or 'Omega' shaped epiglottis is seen (Fig. 68.1).
3. Inlet of the larynx has a typical 'cruciate' appearance due to prolapse of laryngeal soft tissues into the vestibule during inspiration.
4. Stridor is croaking in character and mainly in inspiratory phase. It is diminished by rest and sleep, increased by exertion. Periods of quite breathing occurs intermittently.
5. It disappears between second and fifth year of life.
6. Cyanosis is rare and may occur if there is secondary infection.
7. Voice is unchanged
8. Rales and rhonchi are commonly present at the base of the imperfectly expanded lungs and can be precipitated during secondary infection. .
9. Exaggerated infantile type of larynx can be seen in direct laryngoscopy.
10. The edges of the laryngeal inlet are seen to be drawn in with inspiration sometimes associated with micrognathia.

Diagnosis

1. Careful history and examination–Inspiratory stridor with hoarseness soon after or at birth.
2. Flexible fiberoptic laryngoscopy
3. Direct laryngoscopy

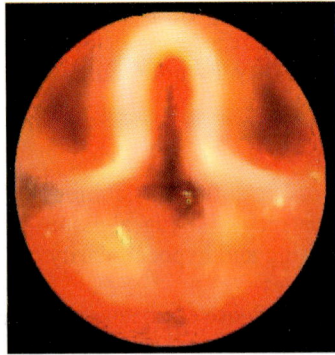

Fig. 68.1: Showing omega shaped epiglottis and classical cruciate appearance of laryngeal inlet in laryngomalacia

Differential Diagnosis

1. Congenital web
2. Papilloma
3. Laryngismus stridulus
4. Simple acute laryngitis
5. Laryngeal diphtheria
6. Cysts of larynx.

Treatment

Reassurance is required in majority of the cases. This usually subsides spontaneously by age of 2 years. Treatment of upper respiratory tract infection often relieves the stridor. Tracheostomy has to be done if necessary.

Congenital Hemangioma of the Larynx

This is usually of a cavernous type. 50 percent of patients will have cutaneous hemangioma.

Etiology

- It tends to occur anteriorly in the infraglottic area of larynx.
- Most common in females.

Symptoms

- Stridor – which is biphasic
- Dyspnea
- Cyanosis may be present
- Retraction of intercostal spaces.

Symptoms may be absent at birth and may first appear in association with upper respiratory tract infection and even persist after infection is resolved. Presence of cutaneous hemangioma, absence of symptoms in early postnatal period offers clue to the diagnosis.

Investigation

- *CT Scan or MRI Scan* reveals contrast enhancing mass in the larynx
- *Direct laryngoscopy:* This reveals asymmetric red purple mass in the region of subglottis. The mass is covered by normal epithelium. Color varies with thickness of the overlying mucosa and helpful diagnostic

maneuver is the subcutaneous injection of 1 or 2 minims of 1:1000 epinephrine causes blanching and shrinking which causes relief of symptoms and should be done during direct laryngoscopy when the changes can be clearly appreciated. Biopsy of the lesion is dangerous unless a tracheostomy is done earlier. If the symptoms are minimal the child may be periodically watched.

Treatment

When associated with stridor, this condition should be treated with antibiotics and anti-inflammatory medications. Generally, hemangioma has a period of rapid growth for 3 to 6 months after which they will regress spontaneously between the first to second years of life. If the regression doesn't take place then definitive treatment should be done. When respiratory distress is present then tracheostomy is required. Lesions can be approached by vertical tracheal incision and resection submucosally without entering the tracheal lumen for anterior tracheal wall hemangioma.

If the hemangioma is in the posterior wall, the vertical mucosal incision is made, resection is performed taking care to preserve as much of the mucosa as possible taking care not to injure the cartilage. Intralaryngeal stent can be kept in the infraglottic area for three to four weeks post-operatively to prevent stenosis.

After resection is completed, careful approximation of tracheal ring is required to prevent granulation tissue formation and stenosis. Good results can be obtained by use of KTP and CO_2 laser.

Congenital Vocal Cord Palsy

This is second most common congenital laryngeal anomaly and bilateral palsy is more frequent than unilateral. 50 percent are associated with anomaly of other systems particularly nervous and cardiac systems.

Clinical Features

Infant has a weak or hoarse cry, inspiratory stridor or difficulty with feeding.

Bilateral paralysis causes more severe obstructive symptoms. True vocal cords are invariably observed to be in the median or paramedian position. Right cord is more frequently involved.

Investigations

- Chest X-ray to rule out mediastinal and pulmonary pathology
- X-ray neck (soft tissue exposure) lateral view to rule out subglottic stenosis.
- Direct laryngoscopy is more confirmatory and should be done without anesthesia.

Treatment

- No treatment is required for unilateral paralysis.
- Most cases will spontaneously resolve within 6 months of age.
- Bilateral paralysis—Tracheostomy may be necessary in most of these cases.
- Cord lateralization procedures can be done after 5 years of age if recovery has not occurred.

Congenital Subglottic Stenosis

This is the third most common congenital laryngeal anomaly and is the most common reason for tracheostomy under 1 year of age.

Pathology

Four main pathological abnormalities can be seen namely.

1. Abnormal submucosal tissue thickness
2. Abnormal shaped cricoid cartilage
3. Cricoid cartilage with small dimension
4. A posterosuperior displacement of 1st tracheal ring.

Clinical Features

1. Symptoms become more evident in 1st week to 1st month of life.
2. 30 percent of subglottic stenosis presents as recurrent or persistent croup.
3. Male: female = 2:1

4. Stridor is the most common symptom which may be biphasic. Stridor and dysnoea becomes more severe during attacks of URTI.

Differential Diagnosis

1. Laryngeal web
2. Subglottic hemangioma

Investigations

1. Direct laryngoscopy/microlaryngoscopy (Fig. 68.2).
2. Bronchoscopy is useful to exclude associated laryngotracheal abnormalities.
3. Soft tissue X-ray of the neck show smooth symmetric narrowing of the subglottis 2 to 3 mm below the free edge of the vocal cords. If there is unilateral bulge, a subglottic hemangioma should be suspected.

Treatment

1. Tracheostomy is often necessary.
2. Subglottic dilatation.
3. Laryngotracheoplasty may be helpful in some and in successful cases patients may be decannulated.

Congenital Laryngeal Web

Etiology

The condition is due to an arrest of development (incomplete splitting). In 75 % of the cases the web is situated in the glottis.

Pathology

Web may be seen in the glottis, supraglottis or subglottis.

Two types: Thin membraneous and thick fibrous. They are mostly situated anteriorly.

Symptoms

1. Vary with the size of the web.
2. No symptoms if the web is small.
3. Hoarsness is usually present.
4. Inspiratory stridor in severe cases.
5. Dyspnea on exertion.

Signs

- In severe cases with stridor, signs of respirtory obstruction can be noted.
- *Indirect laryngoscopy:* White or pink, thick or thin membrane, attached anteriorly to both vocal cords with a sharp and curved posterior border (Fig. 68.3).

Differential Diagnosis

Aquired web of the larynx due to

1. Trauma.
2. Acute specific infection.
3. Chronic specific infection.

Treatment

- No treatment in the milder form
- Hoarseness is usually not relieved completely by operation

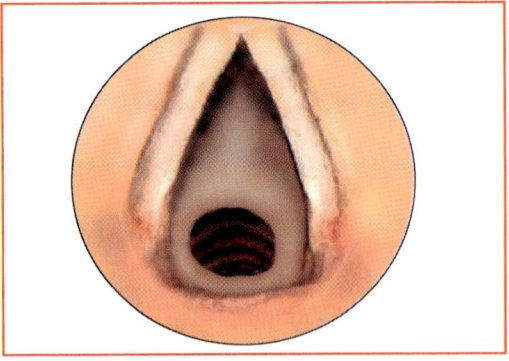

Fig. 68.2: Laryngeal examination showing subglottic stenosis

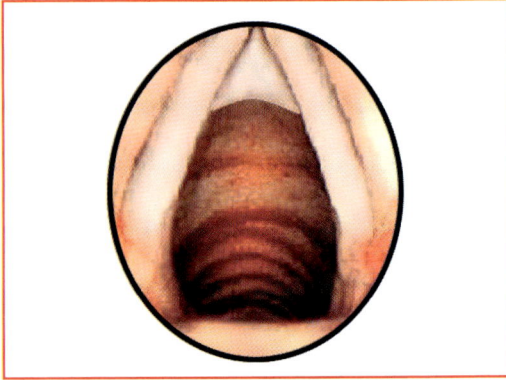

Fig. 68.3: Laryngeal web in the glottis

- Tracheostomy when stridor and dyspnea are severe
- Excision by laryngofissure may be advised later
- McKnought keel is kept after surgery to prevent synechia formation
- Small web can be excised by Micro laryngo scopy (MLS).

Tracheoesophageal Fistula and Laryngeal Cleft

Etiology

- Result from fusion failure of the lateral furrows that create the tracheoesophageal septum during the 5th to 7th week
- 30 percent of the infants had the history of prematurity or hydraminos

Clinical Features

- Persistent barking cough
- Feeding difficulty associated with choking and cyanosis
- Aspiration leading to bronchopneumonia which can be associated with wheeze and crepitations on auscultation.

Diagnosis

- Lateral X-ray soft tissue neck and chest
- A dye contrast medium using cineradiography/ fluoroscopy is diagnostic.
- Flexible laryngoscopy can also help in confirming the diagnosis as an office procedure.
- Direct rigid laryngoscopy under anasthesia to confirm in unco-operative children.

Treatment

- Tracheostomy/endotracheal intubation
- Antibiotics
- Nutrition by gastrostomy or parenteral
- Surgical repair of the cleft and fistula.

Laryngocele

An air filled dilatation of sacculus or appendix of the laryngeal ventricle.

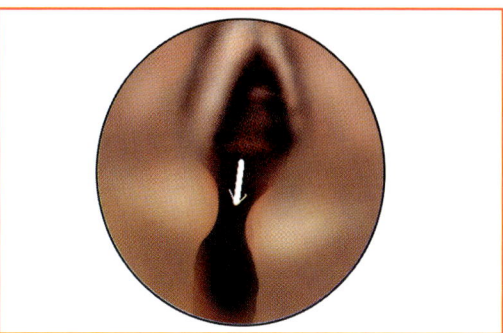

Fig. 68.4: Laryngotracheal clcft/laryngotracheo esophageal cleft

Etiology

- It occurs in person with congenitally large ventricular appendix
- The deformity is rare in adults
- Occurs commonly in males

Precipitating Factors

1. Activity which increases intralaryngeal pressure
2. Straining
3. Coughing
4. Playing wind instruments
5. Gas blowers.

Pathological Types (Figs 68.5 and 68.6)

- **External:** Cystic mass lateral to the thyrohyoid membrane.
- **Internal:** Air containing sac confined to the area of the false cord and aryepiglotic fold within the thyrohyoid membrane

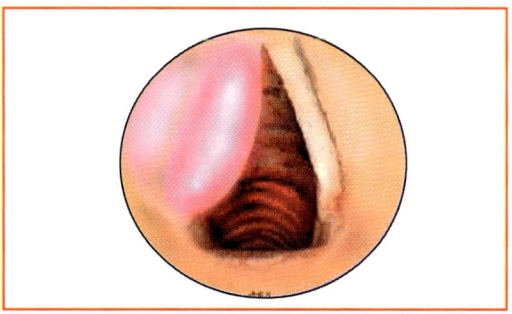

Fig. 68.5: Internal laryngocele

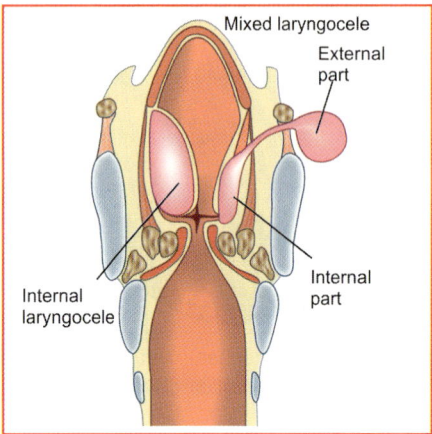

Fig. 68.6: Types of laryngocele

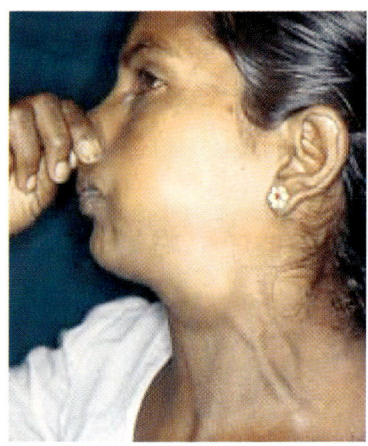

Fig. 68.7: Laryngocele swelling on valsalva maneuver

- **Both external and internal (mixed):** Combination of both.

Clinical Features

In Internal and Mixed Type
- Hoarseness
- Stridor
- Dysnoea.

In External Type
- Compressible spherical mass in the neck which increases valsalva maneuver (Fig. 68.7).
- **Bryce's sign:** Gurgling and hissing sound in the throat when the neck mass is externally compressed.
- If the sac opening is obstructed it can give rise to mucocele.

Investigations
- Soft tissue X-ray neck/ CT imaging of the larynx during Valsalva maneuver.
- Direct laryngoscopy to rule out underlying neoplasm.

Treatment
- Excision of the cyst/ marsupialization by microlaryngoscopic or external approach is done depending on internal/ external/ mixed type. External type/ mixed type should be approached transcervically with careful dissection and part of the thyroid lamina may be removed to facilitate complete removal of the intralaryngeal part of the cyst.
- Pyocele is first treated with injectable antibiotics and is later excised or marsupialized.

POINTS TO REMEMBER

1. Failure of the epithelial primodium to split in the sagittal plane results in atresia / web / stenosis of the larynx.
2. The cardinal symptoms of laryngeal malformations are stridor and cyanosis, dysphonia / hoarseness and feeding difficulties associated with choking spells.
3. Laryngomalacia is the commonest congenital malformation of the larynx followed by congenital vocal cord paralysis and congenital subglottis stenosis.
4. Tracheoesophageal cleft and fistula results from fusion failure of the lateral furrows that create the tracheoesophageal septum.

69

Inflammation of the Larynx

The inflammation of the larynx (laryngitis) can be classified as follows:

I. Acute Laryngitis

1. Acute non-specific
- Acute simple laryngitis
- Acute epiglottitis
- Acute laryngo-tracheo-bronchitis (ALTBS)

2. Acute specific
- Diphtheritic laryngitis

II. Chronic Laryngitis

1. Chronic Non-specific
- Chronic simple laryngitis (Catarrhal laryngitis)
- Chronic hyperplastic laryngitis
- Hemorrhagic laryngitis
- Vocal nodules
- Vocal polyp

2. Chronic Specific
- Tuberculosis
- Syphilis
- Leprosy
- Scleroma
- Wegener's granuloma

ACUTE NON–SPECIFIC LARYNGITIS

ACUTE SIMPLE LARYNGITIS

This is defined as an acute inflammation of the laryngeal mucosa of mild form, often occurring as a manifestation of generalized upper respiratory tract infection.

Etiology

It occurs primarily as a viral infection (Common viruses involved are influenza, rhino, adenovirus, etc.) and may be followed by secondary bacterial invasion.

Precipitating Factors

- Allergy
- Winter and early spring
- Voice abuse
- Irritants– Smoking, chemical fumes, excess alcohol, tobacco, acid reflux, etc.
- Trauma– Thermal, chemical, mechanical, etc.

Pathology

- Vasodilatation and hyperemia of laryngeal mucosa

- Generalized extracellular edema
- Sticky mucopurulent exudate
- Formation of pseudomembrane
- Superficial abrasions/ ulcerations
- Perichondritis in purulent form (*H. influenzae*)

Clinical Features

Severity is variable. In professional voice users even minimal catarrh may give rise to severe symptoms. Children can be worst affected.

Symptoms

General

- Fever +/–
- Malaise
- Toxemia is rare (mostly seen in children).

In Adults

- Hoarseness usually following Upper respiratory tract infection (URTI) or voice abuse
- Complete loss of voice in severe cases (aphonia)
- Dysphonia – Difficulty in speaking
- Pain in the throat on swallowing and speaking
- Voice fatigue (phonasthenia)
- Painful irritant dry cough

In Children

- Symptoms are more severe than in adults
- Patients may have dysphagia due to involvement of epiglottis and arytenoids
- Dyspnea and breathing difficulty may be present in very severe forms

Signs

- Raised temperature
- Husky-hoarse voice
- Generalized nasal and pharyngeal congestion
- ILS:
  - Congestion and edema of epiglottis, ventricular bands and vocal cords. This is often severe in children.

- Thick inspissated mucus / sticky secretions may be seen over the vocal cords.

Treatment

General

- Bed rest
- Avoidance of alcohol and cold weather.

Local

- Voice rest
- Tackle etiological factors, if any. Stop smoking.
- Humidification– Medicated steam inhalation (mucolytic and soothing)
- Mucolytics like Bromhexine
- Irritant and painful cough may be suppressed by linctus codiene, dextromethorphan, etc.
- NSAIDS

Systemic

If secondary infection is present and there is delayed resolution, broad spectrum antibiotics should be advised like ampicillin/amoxycillin/cephalosporins.

Prognosis

- Usually resolves in 1 to 2 weeks.
- Functional aphonia may follow especially in women.

ACUTE EPIGLOTTITIS

Synonym: Acute supraglottic laryngitis.

Definition

An acute inflammatory condition involving the supraglottis, caused by *Hemophilus influenzae*–type B, which is common in children, and may lead to fatal respiratory obstruction

Etiology

Commonly seen in pediatric age group 3 to 6 years. Most significant in children because of the configuration of supraglottic larynx which predisposes to obstruction by even a small amount of swelling of the structures around the laryngeal vestibule (inlet).

Causative Agent

- Hemophilus influenzae – type B
- Arises as a part of *Haemophilus influenzae* septicemia.

Pathology

- Severe cellulitis of the tissue of epiglottis and aryepiglottic fold.
- Congestion and edema of mucous membrane
- Thick and inspissated secretions.
- Obstruction of the laryngeal vestibule prevents effective cough and removal of secretions

Clinical Features

Rapidly progressive from milder respiratory infection to severe respiratory obstruction in a short period of time as little as half an hour. Both adults and children can be extremely ill.

Symptoms

General

- Usually starts as an URTI
- High fever (40°C)

Local

- Sore throat
- Dysphagia / odynophagia
- Muffled (Hot potato) voice
- FB sensation in the throat.
- *Breathing difficulty:* Inspiratory stridor is variably present and may be associated with expiratory rattles.

Signs

General

- Fever, toxic appearance and flushed skin, and appears lethargic
- Dribbling saliva
- On auscultation decreased air entry

Oral

- Pharynx is usually congested and pooling of saliva may be seen
- On depressing the tongue or on protrusion of tongue we may see a red and edematous epiglottis popping up—'Cherry red epiglottis'(Fig. 69.1). Examination of the throat may precipitate respiratory obstruction due to laryngospasm.
- Stridor is inspiratory and increases on supine position. Patient tends to sit up leaning forward supporting on upper limbs (Tripod sign), which relieves stridor to some extent.
- Inspiratory stridor, if severe, causes intercostal retraction, active accessory respiratory muscles and perioral cyanosis.

Diagnosis

- Diagnosis is often based on clinical presentation.
- Flexible laryngoscopy may precipitate or increase stridor
- Throat swab/ blood culture
- Radiological investigation like X-ray lateral view neck (soft tissue exposure) shows:
  - 'Thumb sign'–Grossly edematous epiglottis
  - Narrowed supraglottic airway
- TC/DC–Leucocytosis.

DD of Pyrexial Stridor in Children

- Acute epiglottitis

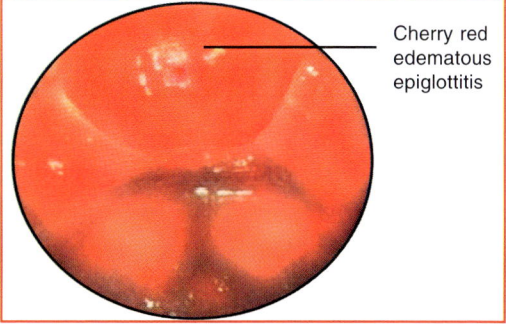

Cherry red edematous epiglottitis

Fig. 69.1: Features of acute epiglottitis

- Acute laryngo-tracheo-bronchitis
- Laryngeal diphtheria
- Angioneurotic edema
- Laryngeal edema secondary to retropharyngeal abscess, acute tonsillitis, etc.

Treatment

- Hospitalize preferably in ICU
- IV fluids
- IV antibiotics-ampicillin and chloram phenicol (50 mg/kg/day-q6h) combined or single agents such as ceftriaxone (75 mg/kg/day-q12h) or cefotaxime (50-100 mg/kg/day-q6h) - response seen in 24 to 48 hours
- O_2 administration-venturi-mechanical ventilation
- Humidifier tents
- If stridor is present, IV steroids (hydrocortisone) is given. Role of steroids and racemic epinephrine is controversial
- Intubation/ tracheostomy to secure airway, if no response to steroids.

Complications

Mortality may be as high as 5 to 10 percent owing to difficulties in maintaining the airway early in the illness:

- Otitis media
- Adenoids
- Meningitis
- Pericarditis
- Pneumonia.

ACUTE LARYNGO-TRACHEO-BRONCHITIS

Definition

This is defined as an acute inflammatory disease of the larynx and lower respiratory tract predominantly involving subglottis, trachea and tracheobronchial tree.

Etiology

- Seen in children below 5 years

- Causative agent:
  - Myxovirus/Para-influenza virus type-1 (frequently), influenza virus type A and B.
  - Secondary bacterial invasion (*Hemophilus influenzae*, pneumococcus, *hemolytic streptococci*).

Pathogenesis

See flow chart 69.1.

Pathology

May lead to fatal respiratory obstruction due to subglottic edema and crust formation.

Mechanical obstruction is due to

1. Narrow subglottis due to mucosal edema
2. Edema and swelling of conus elasticus
3. Mucosal edema involving tracheobronchial tree
   Secretional obstruction due to intense inflammatory reaction

Symptoms

- Pediatric age group (>3 months to 3 years)
- Initial presentation as an URTI
- Acute, rapidly progressive symptoms
- Restlessness and refusal to take food
- Patient looks anxious.

Signs

- Marked fever, toxic with increased pulse rate
- Cry may be weak
- Croupy cough–'Seal's bark' is most prominent at night
- Inspiratory/ biphasic stridor (incidence of stridor is less compared to acute epiglottitis) Severe infection causes increase in stridor with indrawing of supraclavicular area
- Air hunger, hypoxia and cyanosis may be present in severe stridor.

Flow chart 69.1: Pathological events that takes place in acute laryngo-tracheo-bronchitis

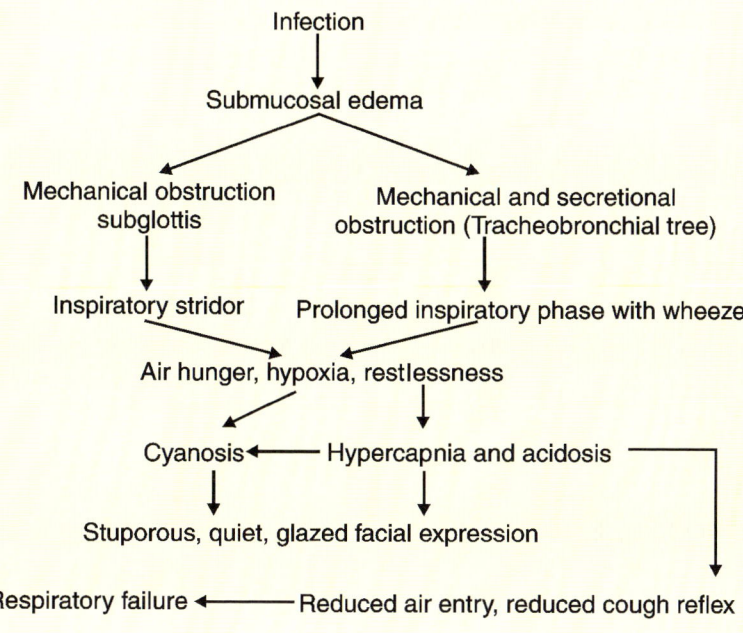

Investigations

- X-ray neck AP view: Steeple sign
- X-ray lateral view neck (soft tissue exposure) shows subglottic narrowing
- X-ray chest– Pneumonic patches can be seen
- Flexible laryngobronchoscopy should be done with caution
  - Subglottic edema can be seen
  - Crusting in the tracheobronchial tree

Treatment

- Immediate hospitalization, preferably in Intensive Care Unit
- IV fluids and antibiotics
- Humidification– To soften the crusts and liquefy thick mucous
- Mucolytics– Bromhexine
- O_2 administration
- IV Steroids are given to relieve stridor
- Tracheotomy preferred over intubation as it avoids subglottic trauma and favors effective tracheobronchial toilet however both are effective.

Prognosis

- Self-limiting condition usually
- With supportive care, prognosis is good.

ACUTE SPECIFIC LARYNGITIS

Laryngeal Diphtheria

Laryngeal diphtheria is often seen secondary to faucial diphtheria. Primary laryngeal diphtheria is rare.

Etiology

- Causative agent–*Corynebacterium diphtheriae*

- Children below ten years are commonly affected
- The incidence has been drastically reduced following immunization.

Pathology

The features of faucial diphtheria are already described under the chapter *Pharynx*. If the laryngeal disease is due to an extension of faucial diphtheria, the toxic features will be same. The laryngeal involvement produces superficial necrosis of the epithelium of the larynx. The membrane may be seen anywhere in the larynx. It commonly forms over vocal cords and the laryngeal vestibule. It may spread over to the subglottis and the trachea. In primary laryngeal diphtheria the absorption of the endotoxin is less and the patient presents with laryngeal obstruction and stridor.

Clinical Features

Symptoms

- In the pre-antibiotic era, patients presented with true croup
- Onset is insidious
- Hoarseness of voice is the first symptom
- Croupy cough (hoarse) is the initial feature
- Stridor is the prominent feature when the false membrane involves the laryngeal inlet and vocal cord.
- Later the cough becomes weak and muffled.

Signs

- Stridor is the most common feature which is inspiratory and is often accompanied by cyanosis and recession of chest wall.
- Membrane can be seen over the vocal cords and the laryngeal vestibule.
- Cervical lymphadenitis is usually present in association with faucial diphtheria.

Diagnosis

Any form of membranous pharyngitis or laryngitis should be suspected for laryngeal diphtheria.

Treatment

- Prophylaxis is the most important and the successful method of therapy.
- Antitoxin should be given empirically if there is reasonable suspicion of the disease. It is given in one dose of 20000 to 100000 units, ½ intramuscularly and ½ intravenously
- Penicillin is the drug of choice, but it will not alter the course of the disease. It is used to eliminate the carrier state.
- Tracheotomy is indicated if there are symptoms of respiratory obstruction. Bronchoscopy is done prior to that, to remove membrane from the trachea and the bronchus.

Complication

- Myocarditis
- Neuritis

CHRONIC NON-SPECIFIC LARYNGITIS

Definition

It refers to chronic inflammatory changes in the larynx that frequently occurs as a result of persistent single or multiple sources of irritants/infection that the larynx is exposed to.

Etiology

The sources of irritants/infections that can cause chronic inflammation are as follows:

- *Infective (non-specific bacterial or viral)*
  - Local sepsis associated with non-specific bacterial infections like chronic sinusitis, tonsillitis, orodental sepsis, etc.
- *Reactive*
  - Allergy
  - Exposure to irritants—Chemicals, smoke, fumes, etc.
  - Reflux laryngitis
  - Voice abuse
  - Cigarette smoking– Produces inflammatory changes of laryngeal mucosa and can lead to hyperkeratosis and leukoplakia.

– Chronic cough
– Mouth breathing
– Alcohol.

Pathogenesis

Persistent irritation of the laryngeal mucosa can lead to localized or diffuse inflammatory changes depending on the nature of irritants like voice abuse causes localized changes at the junction of anterior one-third and posterior two-thirds of the vocal cords whereas smoking can cause diffuse inflammatory change.

The pathological changes that occur due to the basic effects of the laryngeal irritants are:

• Persistent hyperemia and vasodilatation.
• Submucosal hemorrhage and interstitial edema which may be localized or diffused due to acute laryngitis/hyperkinetic use of voice.
• Production of inflammatory exudates associated with infiltration of mononuclear cells.
• Hyperplasia of the epithelium which may be diffuse or localized.
• Invasion of fibroblast into the injury site of the lamina propria with subepithelial hyalinization.
• Thickening and deformity of affected laryngeal structure.
• Squamous metaplasia occurs in the respiratory epithelium of the supraglottic larynx.
• The stratified squamous epithelium of the glottis may under go thickening due to acanthosis, keratosis and parakeratosis and the term laryngeal keratosis is used.
• In small number of cases the chronic mucosal changes may be complicated by submucosal hemorrhages as described earlier due to hyperkinetic phonation and the term hemorrhagic laryngitis have been applied to this condition.
• Irritation or trauma due to hyperkinetic voice/voice abuse can lead to inflammatory changes causing localized forms like vocal polyp, singer's nodules, contact ulcer, etc.

Pathology

The pathological changes that can occur may be localized or diffuse.

The diffuse form can be of the following types:

1. Chronic simple laryngitis
2. Hemorrhagic laryngitis
3. Laryngeal keratosis
4. Laryngeal sicca
5. Pachydermia laryngitis (Acid laryngitis).

The localized form affecting the larynx is:

1. Vocal nodule
2. Vocal polyp.

CHRONIC DIFFUSE LARYNGITIS

Types

• Chronic simple laryngitis
• Chronic hypertrophic laryngitis
• Chronic hemorrhagic laryngitis.

Definition

Chronic inflammation of laryngeal mucosa usually consequent to recurrent acute laryngitis due to persistent exposure to irritating factors leading to permanent mucosal changes like glandular hypertrophy, keratosis and subepithelial hemorrhage.

Etiology

Same as described under chronic nonspecific laryngitis.

• Infective
  – Septic focus could be in the nose, PNS, nasopharynx, oral cavity, salivary glands, tonsils, hypopharynx, tracheobronchial tree, etc.
• Reactive
  – Allergy
  – Environmental irritants
  – Reflux
  – Voice abuse
  – Chronic cough

Symptoms

• Hoarseness is the most notable symptom associated with roughening of voice, variation in pitch (usually lower) and breaks in tone. Hoarseness is usually worse early in the day and improves as the day progresses.

- Raw sensation in the throat, vocal fatigue, dysphonia, phonasthesia and complete aphonia are present in severe cases.
- Pain in the throat while speaking/ swallowing (muscle spasm)
- Sticky sensation in the throat and feel of need to clear throat often

Signs

- Diffuse hyperemia of the cords. The true vocal cord looses the pearly white luster and appears pink or dull red (Fig. 69.2).
- Small engorged blood vessels may be seen on the surface of the true vocal cord, running parallel to the margins.
- The margins of the true vocal cords appear rounded and when the patient phonates, the pattern of vibration is asynchronous and the cord appear flabby.
- Sticky secretions over the vocal cords can be seen.
- In advanced cases mucosal surface may appear thickened, granular due to glandular hypertrophy and polypoidal changes in the true and false cord and later it can be diffuse and the term hypertrophic or hyperplastic laryngitis is used.

- In further advanced cases heaping of epithelium with keratosis of the stratified epithelium of true cord can occur leading to keratosis of larynx which is discussed separately.
- In small number of cases as described under the pathogenesis, hemorrhage can occur as a complication due to voice abuse leading to submucosal hemorrhage, causing hemorrhagic laryngitis. Indirect laryngoscopy may show hemorrhagic polyp in association with features of chronic laryngitis (Fig. 69.3).

Investigations

- To rule out septic focus–based on clinical suspicion, e.g.: X-ray PNS, CXR, nasal endoscopy, etc.
- To rule out a reactive cause, e.g.: Reflux (GERD), allergy, etc.
- Throat swab for culture and sensitivity
- *Flexible laryngoscopy*
- *Microlaryngoscopy*—Supravital staining (Ex: Tolulidine blue) and biopsy to rule out malignancy
- Speech assessment and recording

Treatment

Medical

   1. Elimination of irritants
- Stop smoking, alcohol, exposure to irritants

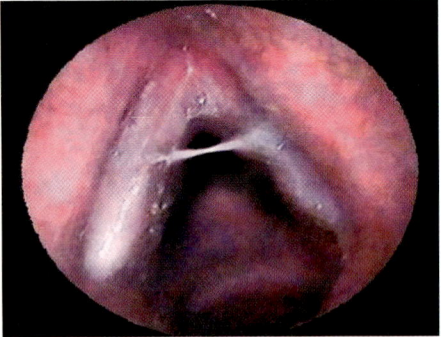

Fig. 69.2: Indirect laryngoscopy showing diffuse congestion of the vocal cords with mucoid strands between them

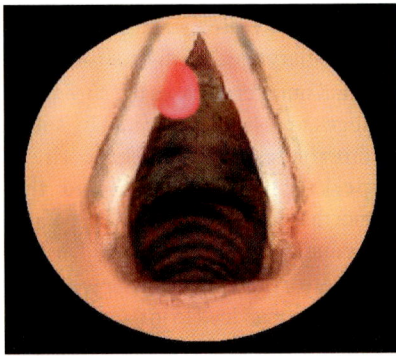

Fig. 69.3: Hemorrhagic polyp of the vocal cord

- Treat the cause of infective focus including sinus and pulmonary infection, tonsillitis, etc.
- Treatment of allergy, GERD
2. Vocal hygiene and speech therapy
3. Complete voice rest during acute episode
4. Use of antibiotic treatment may rarely be necessary
5. Steam inhalation, humidifies, soothing
6. Steroid in form of topical inhalers helps in reducing mucosal edema
7. Expectorants – Mucolytic like bromhexine, ambroxyl, etc.
8. High fluid intake.

Surgical

- Microlaryngoscopy (MLS) is done to confirm the diagnosis. Stripping of the vocal cords is the treatment of choice in refractory cases.
- ***Supravital staining*** may be useful to rule out malignancy if suspected. Biopsy should be done in such cases
- ***Stripping of the cords*** is done one cord at a time to prevent adhesion. Injury to the anterior commissure should be avoided.
- Hemorrhagic polyp can be excised under microlaryngoscopy. Care should be taken to preserve mucosa as much as possible. Sub mucosal microdissection of the polyp can help in this regard.

KERATOSIS LARYNX

Definition

This is a clinical terminology used to describe a group of epithelial lesions in which an abnormality of epithelium and changes of growth and maturation is noted. The changes that can be seen are acanthosis, keratosis, hyperkeratosis, cellular atypia, dyskeratosis and malignant dyskeratosis. The term leukoplakia is used clinically when there is a flat white plaque like lesion seen over the superior mucosal surface of the vocal cord. These changes may be associated with or may undergo malignant transformation to carcinoma-in-situ.

Papillary keratosis refers to a less commonly found keratosis and is associated with irregular peeling of the epithelium associated with a warty verrucous type of lesion. The lesion may appear slightly reddish sometimes. The lesion tends to be more localized than leukoplakia.

Etiology

- Exact etiology is still less understood.
- The condition is seen more commonly in elderly males.
- Persistent exposure to tobacco and several other carcinogens can cause mucosal thickening and in advanced cases heaping of epithelium with keratosis of the stratified squamous epithelium of true cord can occur.

Pathology

Gross: The lesions appear as small discrete irregular patch which may be localized raised white patch or extensive white sheet occupying the whole length of the vocal cord. Sometimes it may have a verrucous (warty) appearance and more so in cases of papillary keratosis. This is a more aggressive form of lesion.

Histopathology

1. Thickening of the stratum corneum associated with thickening of the mucosa.
2. Submucosal edema
3. Hyperplasia and hyperkeratosis
4. Change of cellular morphology with association of dysplasia, parakeratosis and acanthosis.
5. Dysplasia with cellular atypia, malignant dyskeratosis and anaplasia with evidence of carcinoma-in-situ.
6. Papillary keratosis frequently shows epithelial atypia (malignant dyskeratosis), pseudo-epitheliomatous hyperplasia and subepithelial inflammation. Subepithelial inflammation is suggestive of a more aggressive type of alteration which may involve the basal cell layer causing blurring

of the basement membrane and is associated with diagnostic confusion.

Keratosis with or without cellular atypia occurs frequently in association with carcinoma. Patient with laryngeal keratosis showing atypia have a more likelihood of developing invasive carcinoma.

Clinical Features

Symptoms

- Hoarseness
- Feeling of need to clear the throat frequently
- Sticky feeling in the throat.

Signs (Fig. 69.4)

Thick raised white area on the vocal cords may be seen with mobile cords in indirect laryngoscopy.

Investigation

Microlaryngoscopy and supravital staining with Toluidine blue is useful in detecting the suspicious sites. More representative biopsy can be taken from that site.

Treatment

- Microlaryngoscopy and stripping of the involved vocal cord should be done. Entire specimen should be subjected for serial section biopsy.

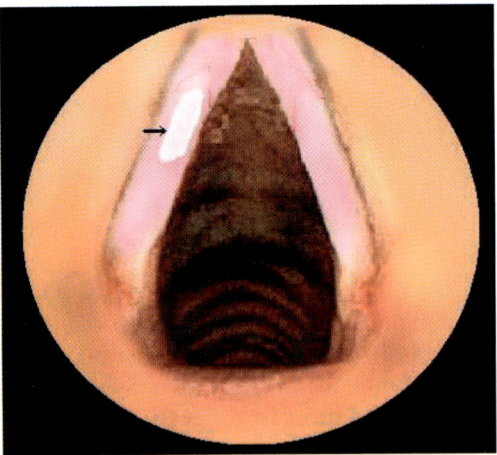

Fig. 69.4: White patch on the right vocal cord

- Avoidance of the etiological factors.
- Chemoprevention for malignancy by antioxidants and beta-carotine has been tried recently.

PACHYDERMIA LARYNGITIS

Definition

A chronic inflammatory condition of the larynx that affects the posterior part of the larynx, associated with epithelial and subepithelial hyperplasia.

Etiology

Exact etiology is not known. The various factors that are blamed for are

- Laryngopharyngeal reflux
- Tobacco addiction
- Excessive intake of alcohol.

Pathology

This often involves the posterior aspect of the vocal cord and the interarytenoid region. In the past it was described as hyperkeratotic papilloma. If the area involved had thickened epithelium with changes of acanthosis, parakeratosis and keratosis. The epithelium maturation is orderly and there is absence of cellular atypia and dyskeratosis.

Clinical Features

Symptoms

- Hoarseness is the main symptom.
- Dry cough may be associated.

Signs

Indirect laryngoscopy reveals a white mass of tissue over the interarytenoid region which often extends to the region of vocal process. Usually it has a raised smooth nodular appearance. Sometimes it may have a white verrucous appearance.

Investigation

Microlaryngoscopy, supra-vital staining and biopsy may be required. Often this condition is benign.

Treatment

Microlaryngoscopy and excision is the treatment of choice if the lesions prevent approximation of the vocal cords and cause persistent hoarseness. Biopsy and histopathological evaluation is a must.

GASTRO-ESOPHAGEAL REFLUX DISEASE (GERD)

Synonym: Laryngopharyngeal reflux

Definition

It is defined as a condition where the reflux material escapes esophagus and enters the laryngopharynx causing laryngeal and pharyngeal symptoms.

Pathology

Of all the causes of laryngeal inflammation, GERD is the most common and underdiagnosed cause. 10 to 15 percent of patients with laryngeal complaints have a GERD related cause. It affects both children and adults and can cause acute, chronic and recurrent laryngitis with or without granuloma formation.

The term globus pharynges described earlier may be one of the common misdiagnosed conditions in the past where psychological factors are blamed for overlooking the underlying reflux problem.

Clinical Features

Symptoms

The common symptoms of GERD like heartburn or regurgitation are commonly not associated with laryngopharyngeal reflux. Rather the patients' complaint more about vague throat pain, discomfort in throat, hoarseness, sensation of foreign body in the throat, chronic throat clearing and cough. In the past the term atypical reflux was used to describe this condition by the gastro-enterologists.

Patients may complain of laryngospasm, choking spells, dysphonia, vocal fatigue, voice breaks, excessive mucous in the throat, etc. Symptoms similar to globus hystericus, like mass in the throat feeling, rarely dysphagia may be present due to cricopharyngeal spasm.

Patients with postnasal drip due to chronic rhinosinusitis may lead to frequent swallowing and aerophagia and may predispose to GERD.

Signs

Posterior Laryngitis

Inflammation involves the arytenoids and the inter-arytenoid area. The mucosa over the arytenoids and interarytenoid area are grossly congested, edematous and may have a velvety appearance. Later edema involving Reinke's space may be seen with associated mucosal thickening without significant erythema. In advanced disease the mucosa becomes granular associated with diffuse erythema and is often friable. Discrete granuloma may be seen in the vocal process.

Complications of Laryngopharyngeal Reflux

- Chronic persistent laryngitis
- Subglottic stenosis
- Posterior glottic stenosis
- Prone for intubation trauma as the posterior mucosa is friable in advanced disease especially in the region of vocal process.
- Contact ulcer/ granuloma
- Arytenoid fixation
- Paroxysmal laryngospasm
- Childhood asthma
- Carcinoma of the larynx

Investigations

24 hour double pH monitoring of the pharynx and esophagus.

Technique

Lower probe is inserted and kept 5 cm above the lower esophageal sphincter and the upper probe is kept at the hypopharynx behind the laryngeal inlet. The monitoring results are highly sensitive and specific for laryngopharyngel reflux and the treatment can be customized by using this technique. The second pharyngeal probe is invaluable in reflux laryngitis as it is placed above the cricopharynx and just behind the larynx.

- Rigid laryngoscopy/stroboscopy of the larynx may help to identify mucosal changes better.
- Endoscopic evaluation of the esophagus and biopsy will suggest esophagitis which are commonly not associated in laryngopharyngeal reflux. Pattern of reflux can be studied in upright position when awake and in supine position (noctural). It is often positive in upright position than in supine position in laryngopharyngeal reflux.
- Radionucleotide studies for reflux are more useful in children.
- Chest X-ray and barium swallow may be helpful in ruling out other conditions which may be missed otherwise.

Treatment

Three levels of treatment are recognized.

Level I

1. *Modification of diet*: Sufficient gap between food and sleep, avoid alcohol, smoking, coffee, tea, soda, and other food that causes exacerbations.
2. *Modification in lifestyle*: Reduce weight, head end elevation of the bed, avoiding of tight fitting garments and belt, etc.
3. Medications (Fig. 69.5)
   - *Liquid antacids*: Given 4 times daily including 3 to 4 teaspoonful, one hour after each meal and at bed-time.

Level II

1. Same as level I treatment
2. Ranitidine 150 mg twice a day or an equivalent dose of another H2 blocker
3. Prokinetic agents used as adjuvants like Cisapride, Mosapride, etc.
4. *Failure of above medication*: The dose of ranitidine or other H2 blocker may be increased. (Ranitidine 150–300 mg 4 times a day).

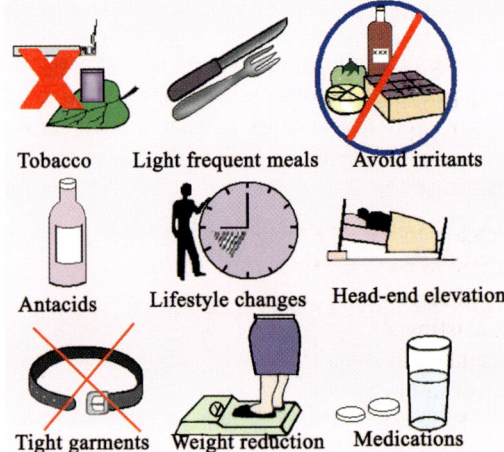

Fig. 69.5: Various forms of prevention and treatment of GERD

Level III

1. Same as level I minus antacids
2. *Medical treatment:*
   (a) Omeprazole at morning and at 5.00 P.M. for a period of 6 months. This is not recommended in children.
   (b) Obese patients may require larger dose.
3. *Surgical treatment:* Indicated if medical treatment fails. Fundoplication is the treatment of choice.

SINGER'S NODULES

Synonym: Vocal nodules

Definition

It is a localized form of chronic laryngitis characterized by deposition of inflammatory tissue due to organization of edematous or hemorrhagic fluid at the junction of the anterior third and posterior two thirds of the true vocal cords in the subepith- elial space.

Etiological Factors

- Persistent vocal abuse
  - Hyperkinetic phonation
  - Teachers, hawkers, jugglers, etc.

- Professional singers
- Nervous hyperkinetic individuals
- Common in males under 20 years of age.
- Chronic cough
- GERD

Pathogenesis

Voice with high pitch is an important factor for it is rare to be seen in people with base tones.

The peculiar anatomy of the true vocal cord consisting of the subepithelial potential space (Reinke's space) on its free margin is the main factor in the genesis of the vocal nodules.

Hyperkinetic voice or vocal abuse leads to change in the vibratory pattern of the vocal cord and sometimes excessive vibration at the junction of anterior one third and posterior two thirds of the true vocal cords, bilaterally. This leads to sub-epithelial hemorrhage and/or inflammatory edema which get collected within the potential space. This infiltration of edema fluid/blood gets organized and subsequent progressive inflam- matory changes occur thereafter.

Recent development of videostroboscopy can identify this change in the vibratory pattern of the vocal cord and early identification of localized abnormalities.

Pathology

Early nodules appear soft and reddish covered with normal squamous epithelium. The underlying stroma may be edematous. Sometimes there may be increased vascularity, dilated blood vessels and hemorrhage. More mature nodules will be more firm and contain areas undergoing fibrosis and hyalinization and appears pale. Mature nodules are seen commonly in professional singers. Surface epithelium may show keratosis, acanthosis and parakeratosis or histopathological examination.

Clinical Features

Symptoms

Hoarseness is the cardinal symptom. It may appear suddenly after an episode of straining of the voice especially in professional singers with faulty voice (who sing above their natural range) and in public speakers. Often it appears slowly and insidiously over as period of months as seen in teachers. Vocal fatigue is commonly noticed.

Signs

Small pin-head sized pale, fibrous nodules can be seen involving both vocal cords at the junction of anterior one third and posterior two thirds at its free edges. Early developing nodule may have congestion.

Investigations

Videostroboscopy and Microlaryngoscopy (MLS) (Fig. 69.6a).

Treatment

- Voice rest is very important and may cure early extremely small nodules
- Steroid inhalers in the form of Fluticasone propionate are helpful in the early stages.
- *Speech therapy* helps to re-educate proper use of voice. It is the corrective or rehabili-tative treatment of physical deficits or cognitive disorders resulting in difficulty with verbal communication. This includes both the speech and language. The common treatment range from physical strengthening exercises instructive or repetitive practice and to the use of audiovisual aid.

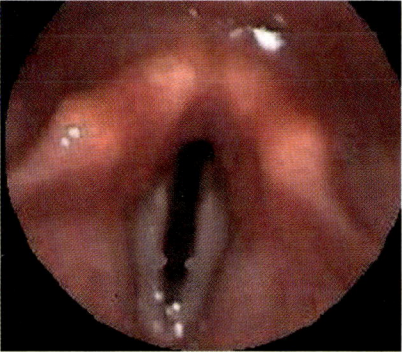

Fig. 69.6a: Vocal nodule

- ***Surgical treatment:*** Microlaryngoscopy and precise excision of the bigger nodules which do not respond to medical treatment. Care should be taken to preserve mucosa. Laser should be avoided as it can cause damage to the membranous cords with permanent hoarseness.

VOCAL CORD POLYP

Definition

A disorder of voice abuse commonly seen in professional voice users, characterized by hoarseness and presence of a sessile or pedunculated mass (localized or diffuse) usually arising from one of the vocal cords.

Localized Type

This is most common benign lesion of the larynx and it is usually confined to the middle of the membranous vocal cord.

Etiology

It is similar to vocal nodule. It is usually secondary to trauma due to vocal abuse. Single episode of vocal strain also may cause the polyp. It sometimes occur following acute respiratory tract infection.

Pathology

The lesion is localized to the area of true vocal cord within the Reinke's space. It contains varying amount of edematous stroma, dilated blood vessels, fibrous tissue and area of hemorrhage.

Early polyp represents an exaggeration of early polypoidal stage of vocal nodules and tends to be more vascular. Fibrosis and fibrinoid and hyaline degeneration occurs in the stroma as the lesion matures.

Clinical Features (Fig. 69.6b)

- Hoarseness is the main complaint
- Sometimes sticky sensation in the throat
- Constant attempt to clear the throat.

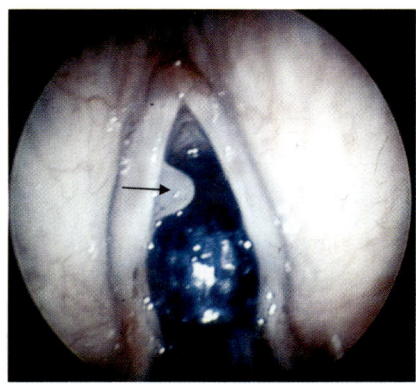

Fig. 69.6b: Vocal polyp arising from right vocal cord as shown in black arrow

- ILS may reveal a solitary polypoidal mass which may be pedunculated or sessile. A pedunculated polyp is better visible on phonation. The color vary from bright reddish purple to pale translucent depending on its maturity

Treatment

- Microlaryngeal excision (Figs 69.7 to 69.9)
- Speech therapy

DIFFUSE VOCAL POLYPOSIS

Synonym

Reinke's edema, localized hypertrophic laryngitis (Fig. 69.10 and 69.11)

Etiology

- Vocal abuse especially hyperkinetic use of voice is the main cause
- Untreated hypothyroidism
- Smoking
- Females are more affected in middle age.

Pathology

The margin of the true vocal cords is diffusely involved with collection of edematous tissue masses. The edema is confined to the Reinke's

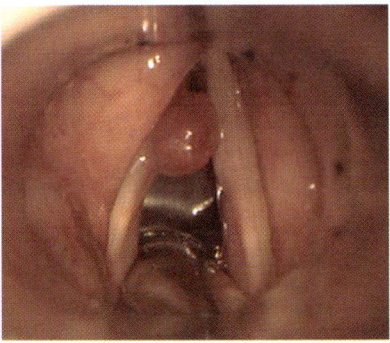

Fig. 69.7: Microlaryngoscopy showing hemorrhagic polyp of the left vocal cord

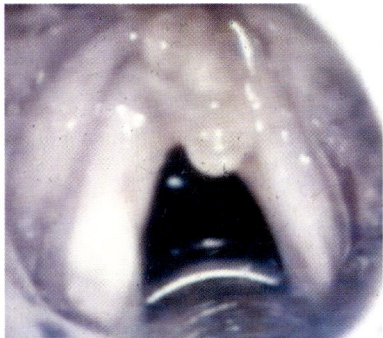

Fig. 69.8: Microlaryngoscopy showing multiple hyaline polyp at the anterior commissure

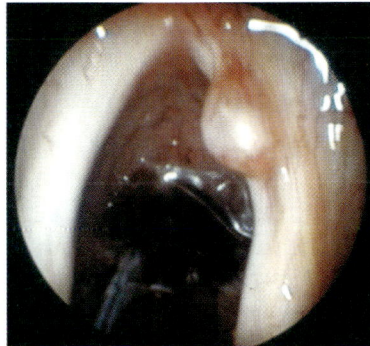

Fig. 69.9: Microlaryngoscopy showing intracordal cyst of the right vocal cord

space. The space is usually widened and gets filled with mucoid material devoid of cells, fibrous tissue and blood vessels.

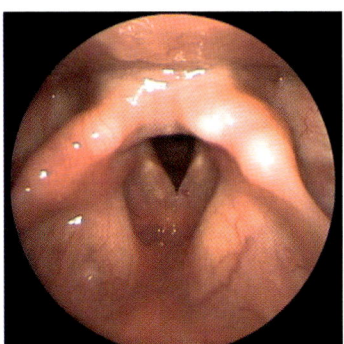

Fig. 69.10: 45° Laryngeal telescopy showing Reinke's edema

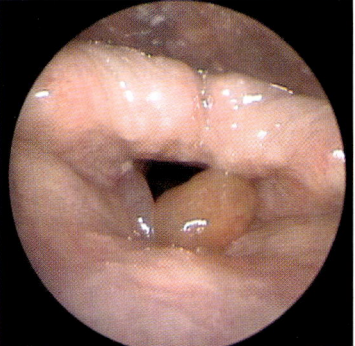

Fig. 69.11: 45° Laryngeal telescopy showing gross bilateral diffuse vocal cord polyposis

Clinical Features

Symptoms

- Severe hoarseness is the main clinical feature
- Aphonia may occur intermittently
- The voice is low pitched and tends to be monotonous which makes singing impossible.

Signs

Indirect laryngoscopy shows symmetrical pale sausage like masses hanging from each membranous cord. This frequently obliterates the anterior glottis so that the only airway is present between the arytenoids. The masses are translucent, grayish pink and may appear bright red if associated with acute inflammation.

Treatment

- Microlaryngoscopic stripping of the vocal cord.
- This should be done in two stages, one cord at a time, to prevent anterior glottic web formation.

Contact Ulcer

The thin layer of mucosa and perichondrium overlying the cartilaginous process makes it prone for ulceration from a variety of insults. The common causes are vocal abuse, coughing, GERD, endotracheal intubation. Because of the shape of the larynx endotracheal tube frequently lies in the posterior commissure causing contact with the vocal process leading to ulceration and granuloma formation. Granuloma of the vocal process is 5 times more common than the contact ulcer.

Pathology

Once the vocal cord mucosa is acutely damaged it becomes more prone for continuous trauma such as throat clearing, cough and reflux leading to ulceration. The attempt of healing of the ulcer is frequently prevented by secondary infection, reflux and persistent trauma that results in granuloma formation.

Clinical Features

- Hoarseness and foreign body sensation

Signs

Indirect laryngoscopy shows the granuloma at the vocal process of one side and may be associated with contact ulcer on the vocal process of the opposite side.

Treatment

Microlaryngeal excision of the granuloma may be necessary when suspected for malignancy or the granuloma has formed into a fibroepithelial mass or if there is associated laryngeal obstruc- tion. The medical therapy is directed towards treating the cause which include

- Voice modification to prevent continual vocal process trauma
- Anti-reflux treatment–Pantoprazole/omeprazole, etc.
- Steroid inhalation may be useful.

CHRONIC SPECIFIC LARYNGITIS

TUBERCULAR LARYNGITIS

- 95 percent of the cases are secondary to pulmonary TB and is due to direct implantation of the tubercle bacilli from the sputum.
- 5 percent of cases are primary tuberculosis of the larynx

Pathology

The posterior parts of the larynx are more affected which includes arytenoids, interarytenoid space, posterior part of the vocal cord and sometimes the laryngeal surface of the epiglottis. These sites are commonly exposed to the sputum impaction following cough as seen in pulmonary tuberculosis.

Clinicopathological Stages

- *Catarrhal stage or stage of inflammation:* This is associated with diffuse inflammation with resultant hyperemia, edema and infiltration of non-specific cellular exudates.
- *Granulomatous stage:* This is associated with the formation of tuberculous granuloma in the subepithelial tissue. The avascular tubercles has a characteristic central caseation which is surrounded by the epithelioid cells and Langhan's type of giant cells. Gradually fibrous tissue replaces the tubercle depending on the host resistance. The tubercles may coalesce to form

yellowish grey nodule. These tubercles stimulate hyperplasia of the epithelium and subepithelium and frequently causes thickening of the interarytenoid area resembling pachydermia. Edema may be quite marked secondary to lymphatic obstruction by the granuloma. This pseudo-edema commonly affects the epiglottis and the tissue overlying the arytenoids.

- **Ulcerative stage:** (Fig. 69.12) The epithelial surface of the yellowish nodule may be lost which results in ulceration and secondary infection. This process often occurs first in the vocal process and epiglottis because of the thinness of the mucosa covering the avascular cartilage. As the inflammation progresses the cartilage may develop perichondritis which ultimately get destroyed.
- **Stage of cicatrization:** Healing of the lesion is associated with fibrosis and encapsulation and replacement of the tubercles. In very advanced lesions healing may endup with fibrous stenosis and may fix the cricoarytenoid joint.

Clinical Features

Symptoms

- Patient is often a known case of or gives history suggestive of pulmonary tuberculosis.
- Weak voice due to myositis
- Hoarseness which is often chronic
- **Odynophagia** is usually to liquids and is due to exposed nerve endings following ulcerations and perichondritis
- Pain on speaking
- Phonesthenia/dysphonia/aphonia
- Hemoptysis is present in advanced cases associated with ulceration and destruction of the epiglottis, arytenoids and surrounding soft tissue.
- Stridor is a late feature commonly due to stenosis.

Signs (Figs 69.12 and 69.13)

- Unilateral congestion

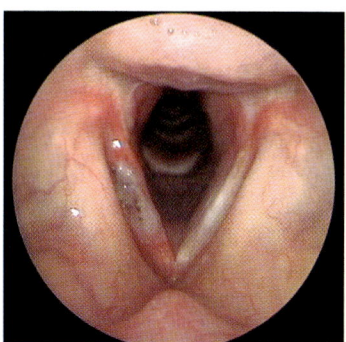

Fig. 69.12: Unilateral congestion and ulceration of the right vocal cord (45° telescopic picture)

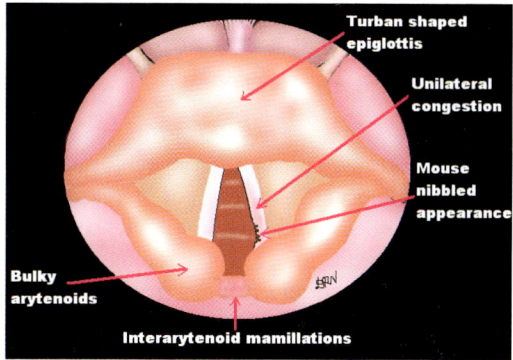

Fig. 69.13: Characteristic feature of tubercular laryngitis

- Bowing of the cords due to myositis
- Multiple tubercles in pale background (pallor)
- Posterior commissure mamillations
- Mouse nibbled appearance of the vocal cords (Fig. 69.13).
- Tuberculoma may appear as a tumor resembling malignancy
- Turban epiglottis
- Stenosed/ deformed larynx

Investigations

- As for pulmonary TB
- Sputum for AFB, Chest x-ray, Mantoux test, etc.
- X-ray lateral view neck to assess airway patency

- Direct laryngoscopy (MLS) and biopsy
- TB can coexist with carcinoma of the larynx

Treatment

- Anti-tubercular treatment includes ethambutol (15 to 25 mg/kg in divided doses), rifampicin (450 mg OD) and INH (300 mg OD) and pyrazinamide (650 mg)
- Anti-inflammatory gargles
- Laryngeal sprays
- NSAIDS
- Tracheostomy, if patient has stridor
  Laryngeal reconstruction, only after the active infection resolves (Laryngoplasty).

LUPUS OF THE LARYNX

This is a distinguished and indolent form of tuberculosis caused by atypical tuberculosis bacilli and probably occurs as a result of increased host resistance or decreased bacterial virulence. There is tendency for the tubercle undergoing caseation and is more associated with fibrosis of the surrounding tissue. It commonly affects the anterior part of the larynx including the aryepiglottic fold and the laryngeal surface of the epiglottis. Its stages include:

- Nodular
- Ulcerative and
- Cicatrization

The disease is relatively painless and is free of symptoms often. Scattered yellowish pink discrete nodules on the epiglottis and the aryepiglottic fold may be seen in the early stage. Later the lesion may ulcerate and subsequently results in perichondritis and cartilage destruction. There is tendency for spontaneous healing with associated resultant scarring of the lesion. There may be persistent swelling of the false vocal cord. The lesion should be suspected when it is associated with facial, nasal and pharyngeal lesions.

Treatment

Anti-tubercular treatment

LEPROSY OF THE LARYNX

This is caused by *Mycobacterium Leprae* and occurs after prolonged exposure. The disease is transferred in younger patients. Commonly the lepromatous type affects the larynx. There will be associated lesions in the skin as anesthetic patch. The stages include

- Catarrhal (infiltration)
- Nodular (granulomatous)
- Ulcerative
- Cicatrization

Clinical Features

Muffled voice is the common symptom in the early stage due to involvement of the supraglottic structures. Hoarseness and dyspnea in the later stage. Pain and odynophagia is often absent as the lesions are often anesthetic. Classical features of leprosy may be seen in other parts of the body.

Signs

The lesions appear dull grey in color. There may be associated ulcerations of the supraglottic larynx and areas of healing and scarring. After fibrosis, the epiglottis appears as *'a hook over a button hole'* due to laryngeal stenosis. The cervical nodes may be enlarged and mimics malignancy.

Investigations

- FNAC
- Biopsy from the cutaneous lesions.

Treatment

- Dapsone, clofazimine and rifampicin are often given in combination
- Steroid/ Tracheostomy for laryngeal stenosis

Prognosis

Lepromatous type has poor prognosis.

SCLEROMA OF THE LARYNX

This commonly affects the subglottic region. It is caused by *Klebsiella rhinoscleromatis*. Etiopathology is described under rhinoscleroma.

The condition tends to spread to the trachea and bronchus

Clinical Features

Symptoms

Hoarseness, cough and increasingly progressive dyspnea

Signs

Swelling of the subglottis may be seen which can be appreciated as pale pinkish swelling on either side of the vocal cord.

Differential Diagnosis

- Malignancy of the larynx
- Syphilitic lesions
- Laryngeal leprosy
- Laryngeal tuberculosis.

Treatment

- Same as rhinoscleroma of the nose.
- Laryngeal obstruction and stridor will need tracheostomy

SYPHILITIC LARYNGITIS

Definition

This is a chronic granulomatous condition caused by a spirochete *Treponema Pallidum* which can be seen as congenital or acquired forms.

Types

Congenital form is extremely rare and can be seen in two stages.

- **Early form:** It presents within first few months after birth with laryngeal obstruction due to associated perichondritis causing laryngeal edema. Classical signs like infantile snuffles (as described under rhinology), hepatosplenomegaly, etc. may be seen.
- **Late form:** This occurs usually between 2 to 10 years of age and is commonly asso-

ciated with laryngeal mucosal hyperplasia and granulations. Ulcerations in the vocal cords may be seen. Laryngeal stenosis and stridor can occur due to destruction of the cartilage and may need a tracheostomy. Other stigmata (e.g., interstitial keratitis, nerve deafness, anterior bowing of shins, frontal bossing, mulberry molars, Hutchinson teeth, saddle nose, rhagades, or Clutton joints) may be seen.

ACQUIRED SYPHILIS

Secondary mucosal patches are very rare in the larynx. It commonly presents in the tertiary stage.

Clinicopathological stages of tertiary syphilis of the larynx

Stage of Infiltration

This resembles chronic hyperplastic laryngitis and later it may appear nodular simulating carcinoma or tuberculosis of the larynx.

Granulomatous Stage

The lesion is called 'Gumma' which commonly affects the epiglottis and sometimes the ventricular band. The lesion appears as a diffuse swelling associated with a dark red hue with areas of ***wash-leather ulceration.***

Stage of Ulceration

This can be superficial ulcers involving epiglottis or arytenoids or a deep punched out ulcer involving the epiglottis as a result of gumma. Perichondritis and necrosis of the part of the cartilage may occur. The resultant necrosis and scarring can result in atrophic changes.

Stage of Cicatrisation

Healing of the necrosed area associated with inflammatory changes and granulations lead to formation of scar tissue and adhesions. The ultimate result is a laryngeal stenosis.

Clinical Features

Symptoms

- Hoarseness
- Dyspnea
- Stridor

Signs

As described under the stages.

Diagnosis

Syphilis can mimic other diseases including malignancy. Serological tests confirms the diagnosis.

Investigations

Demonstration of *T. pallidum* by darkfield microscopy, fluorescent antibody, or other specific stains in specimens from lesions is commonly done. Serological tests including VDRL. Wassermann reaction, TPI, TPHA, etc. help in confirming the diagnosis.

Biopsy is helpful in confirming and ruling out other conditions.

Treatment

Medical

The gold standard for treatment of syphilis is consecutive daily intramuscular injections with procaine penicillin for a period of 10 days. Benzathine penicillin 1.8 gm/4ml syringe for I.M. injection as a single injection will adequately treat primary and secondary syphilis. Alternatively Doxycycline 300 mg daily for 21 days may be given to those allergic to penicillin.

Surgical

Tracheostomy may be necessary if there is airway obstruction. Definitive laryngoplasty procedure is done after the active infection is controlled.

PERICHONDRITIS OF THE LARYNX

This is an inflammatory condition of the perichondrium of the larynx.

Etiology

It can be due to acute or chronic infection, chronic inflammatory condition, traumatic causes like road traffic accidents, cut throat injuries, high tracheostomy or cricothyroidotomy, post radiotherapy, etc.

Perichondritis following secondary infection of laryngeal cancer is not uncommon.

Pathology

If it is not identified and treated early, perichondrial infection can lead to accumulation of exudates and subperichondrial abscess formation, causing separation of the perichondrium from the cartilage and consequent local necrosis.

Clinical features

Fever, malaise rigors occur following perichondritis

Local symptoms include pain over the laryngeal skeleton often radiating to the ears, widening of the laryngeal framework, swelling of the neck and if the abscess bursts there may be associated fistula. Cough, hoarseness and dysphagia are also common advanced features. Dyspnea and stridor can occur following mucosal edema or laryngeal stenosis. The abscess may sometimes burst into the larynx causing aspiration.

Treatment

- Absolute bed rest
- Broad spectrum systemic antibiotics
- 2 percent laryngeal xylocaine spray with adrenaline may be useful in reducing pain and edema
- Tracheostomy may be needed if there is stridor due to laryngeal edema/ stenosis

- Incision and drainage of the abscess is done if present
- Stenosis may be corrected later by laryngofissure approach
- Rarely a narrowfield may be necessary if there is aspiration associated with laryngeal stenosis.

Laryngismus Stridulus

It is a non infective spasmodic condition of the larynx and affects commonly the young children

Etiology

- Commonly seen in boys at around 4 years of life.
- More common in winter.
- Dietary deficiency of calcium is said to be one of the causes

- Flabby soft tissues of the larynx is also one of the factor.

Pathology

- Laryngeal spasm usually occurs as a result of tetany following calcium deficiency due to vitamin D or parathyroid deficiency.
- The flabby soft tissue of the larynx is passively sucked inwards during inspiration.

Clinical features

Symptoms include 'crowing stridor', cyanosis and carpopedal spasm.

Treatment

The condition usually recovers spontaneously. Dietary supplementation of vitamin D and calcium is advocated. Nasal obstruction if present should be treated to prevent precipitation of attack.

POINTS TO REMEMBER

1. Acute epiglottitis (supraglottic laryngitis) is caused by *Haemophilus influenzae type B*. Clinically 'cherry red edematous epiglottis' and radiologically 'thumb sign' on X-ray lateral view of the neck are the characteristic features.
2. Acute laryngotracheobronchitis can cause fatal airway obstruction which can be mechanical due to narrowing of the lumen and secretional due to inflammatory reaction.
3. Odynophagia is a characteristic presentation of laryngeal tuberculosis.
4. Turban larynx, mouse nibbled appearance of vocal cords, posterior commissure mammilations are few of the characteristic features of tubercular laryngitis.
5. Gumma is a feature of tertiary syphilis which has a wash leather appearance.
6. Laryngeal leprosy is characterized by hook-like epiglottis on a botton hole laryngeal inlet.
7. Laryngopharngeal reflux can cause laryngeal keratosis which is a premalignant condition.
8. Reflux laryngitis can be prevented by lifestyle changes, dietary restrictions, excercise and medication.
9. Hyperkinetic voice users like teachers, singers, hawkers, etc. are prone to develop vocal nodules or polyp.
10. Vocal nodules are always bilateral and occurs at the junction of anterior one-third and posterior two-thirds of the vocal cords.
11. Vocal polyp is often solitary and may occur at the junction of anterior one-third and posterior two-thirds of the vocal cords or at the anterior commissure of the larynx.
12. Precise microlaryngeal excision of the nodules/polyp is the surgical treatment of choice if speech therapy fails.

70

Laryngotracheal Trauma

Increasing incidence of road traffic accident has made the larynx susceptible for direct trauma. Also, more and more cases are being diagnosed as more patients survive due to better intensive care. But the commonest cause of internal laryngeal trauma is iatrogenic due to prolonged intubation or a high tracheostomy. Laryngotracheal trauma if not diagnosed early and treated properly can lead to laryngotracheal stenosis.

Etiology

External

This is usually mechanical trauma which could be blunt or penetrating.

Common causes include the following
- *Road Traffic Accident (RTA):* This is the commonest cause of external laryngotracheal injury.
- Assaults
- Strangulation, hanging
- Sports injuries
- Accidental fall, whiplash injuries
- *'Cut-throat'* wounds
- Occupational trauma
- Gun shot wounds, etc.

Internal

(a) Iatrogenic
  (i) Traumatic intubation
  (ii) ***Prolonged endotracheal intubation***

  (iii) Traumatic instrumentation- scopies
  (iv) High tracheostomy
(b) Swallowed foreign body like pin, glass, etc.
(c) Chemical injury
  (i) Corrosive poisoning
  (ii) Inhalation of fumes
(d) Thermal injury – Burns and scalds
(e) Radiation to head and neck region

Pathology

1. Extralaryngotracheal
   - Hematoma
   - Surgical emphysema
   - Open wounds
   - Injury to vessels and nerves
   - Incised and penetrating wounds of the larynx.
2. Injury to laryngotracheal framework
   - Fracture of hyoid
   - Injury to thyroid cartilage
   - Injury of cricoid cartilage
   - Injury to trachea
   - Laryngotracheal separation
   - Thyrohyoid membrane separation.
3. Intralaryngotracheal
   - Mucosal edema, tears, hematoma
   - Avulsion of epiglottis
   - Cricoarytenoid joint disarticulation,
   - VC palsy
   - Disruption of the vocal cords

Factors determining degree of Laryngotracheal trauma

1. Age
   (a) >40 years– Calcified cartilages   fracture
   (b) <40 years– Recoil
2. Type of trauma:
   (a) Blunt
   (b) Penetrating
3. *Position of mandible during trauma*: Flexion of head during trauma, brings the mandible anterior to the larynx, thus protecting it.
4. *Force of impact*: Serverity of injury is directly proportional to the force of impact.
5. Angle of impact
   (a) *Force is from the front*: Larynx pressed against the cervical vertebrae and causes more damage.
   (b) *Lateral force*: Larynx moves to certain extent and the damage is less.

Ossification of the laryngeal cartilages occurs after 40 years of age. If age is more than 40 years, the cartilage fracture occurs in multiple areas and incidence of obstructed airway is high. If the age is less than 40 years of age, the commonest site of fracture is in the mid-line and elastic recoil tends to bring the fracture site forwards reducing the incidence of airway obstruction (Figs 70.1 to 70.2a to c).

Clinical Features

Symptoms

- Respiratory distress (Stridor)— This could be immediate/ early or delayed
- Hoarseness/aphonia
- Pain in the throat on swallowing, speaking, touch, coughing
- Otalgia
- Aspiration
- Hemoptysis
- Swelling or open wound
- Cough

Signs

External

- Bruises/abrasions/ swelling

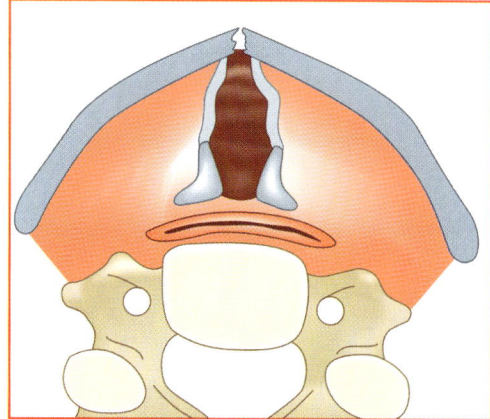

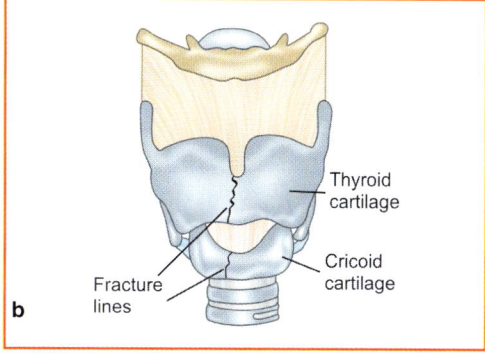

Figs 70.1a and b: Fracture of the thyroid and cricoid cartilage in a patient less than 40 years of age

- Surgical emphysema
- Tenderness on 'Springing' of bone/cartilage
- Flattening of the thyroid prominence suggests thyroid cartilage fracture (Fig. 70.3).
- Step deformity may be present in fracture of laryngeal cartilages
- Open wound with/without larynx/trachea exposed (Fig. 70.4).
- Stridor.

Internal (ILS/ Scopy)

- Edema/ hematoma/ mucosal tears
- Airway obstruction
- Dislocation of cricoarytenoid joint
- VC palsy
- Falling back of epiglottis, avulsion
- Disrupted vocal cord or ventricular bands

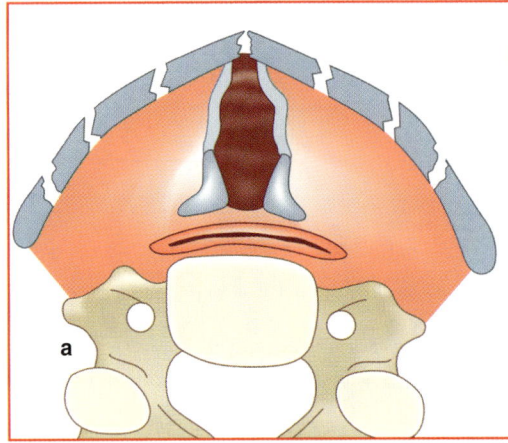

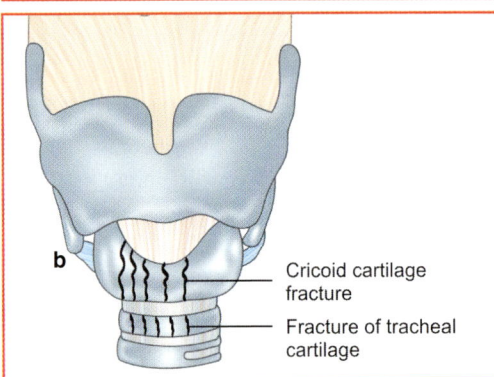

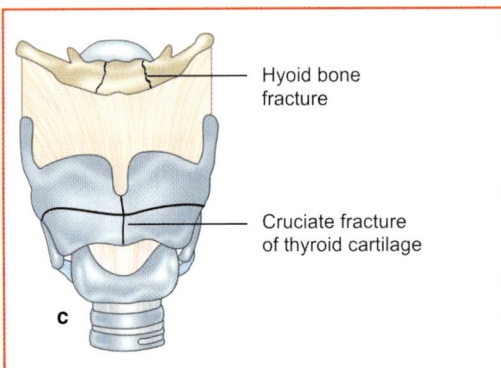

Figs 70.2a to c: Multiple fracture of the cricoid cartilage in a patient more than 40 years of age

- Exposed cartilage and laryngotracheal lumen (Fig. 70.4).
- Asymmetrical laryngeal inlet and laryngotracheal lumen (Fig. 70.4).

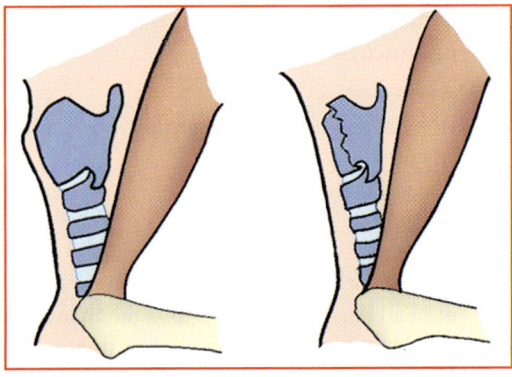

Fig. 70.3: Flattening of laryngeal prominence

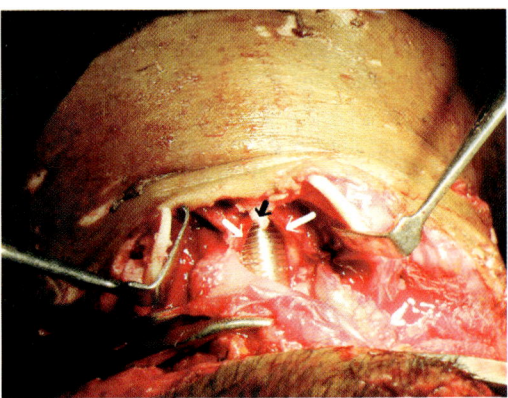

Fig. 70.4: Deep laceration of the neck following road traffic accident with fracture of the thyroid cartilage (fragments retracted by retractors) and laryngeal lumen opened exposing the vocal cords (white arrows) and petiole of the epiglottis (black arrow)

Management

First aid – **ABCDE**

- **A**irway management
- **B**reathing – assisted ventilation if required
- **C**irculation – Blood volume replacement
- **D**isability assessment
- **E**xpose entire body to detect polytrauma.

Airway Management

This can be achieved by

- Jaw thrust–chin lift

- Oral airway
- Lateral position to prevent aspiration if there is bleeding into the pharynx.
- Bolus parenteral steroids to tackle laryngeal edema
- O_2 administration
- Intubation/tracheostomy
- Open larynx/trachea, intubate through the wound
- Arrest bleeding and its aspiration
- Treat polytrauma
- Management of shock and blood loss
- Antibiotics, anti-inflammatory, tetanus toxiod, etc. may be given.

Investigations

- X-ray neck AP/ lateral
  - Look for fracture lines, surgical emphysema, airway patency, spine injury, etc.
- Chest X-ray
  - Look for aspiration pneumonia/polytrauma
- CT scan/tomograms are helpful in assessment of
  - Extent of laryngotracheal injury
  - Airway patency
- Direct laryngoscopy or microlaryngoscopy is often done after a tracheostomy
  - Assessment of laryngotracheal injury and airway
  - Drain hematoma
  - Stenting/keel placement.

Treatment

Medical

- Antibiotics
- Steroids– Prevents scarring and LTS
- Anti-inflammatory drugs
- Voice rest
- Observe for delayed onset stridor
- Humidification
- Supportive measures.

Surgical

- Tracheostomy/Cricothyroidotomy
- Surgical exploration by laryngofissure approach.
- Open reduction is best done before fibrosis sets in (<10 days)
- Internal fixation of fracture segments
- Suturing of tears
- Debridement
- Repositioning of epiglottis/ arytenoids
- Repair of laryngotracheal separation
- Stenting/silastic keel placement
- Laryngectomy.

Complications

- Perichondritis
- Abscess
- VC paralysis
- Granuloma
- Laryngotracheal stenosis.

Laryngotracheal Stenosis

Etiology

- Laryngotracheal trauma
- Iatrogenic
  - Prolonged intubation
  - High tracheostomy
  - Cricothyroidotomy
- Corrosive poisoning
- Chronic granulomatous conditions
- Post–RT for laryngeal malignancy.

Pathology

- Fibrosis following
  - Mechanical trauma
  - Ischemic necrosis (ET tube/cuff)
  - Inflammatory process (chronic Infections)
- Adhesions (Glottic web).

Clinical Features

- Depends on the site and extent of stenosis
  - Hoarseness

- Difficulty in clearing secretions
- Dysphonia
- Stridor
- Difficult decannulation
- Indirect Laryngoscopy (ILS)
  - Narrowing, web, etc. may be seen.

Investigations

The investigations are done to assess the site, length and severity of the laryngotracheal stenosis and thus in planning management strategies.

- X-ray neck– AP/ lateral
- Laryngeal tomograms
- Laryngogram
- CT scan/ MRI
- Endoscopy- flexible/ rigid

Treatment Options

- Tracheostomy
- Dilatation and stenting
- Laryngotracheoplasty with or without stenting/ keel insertion
- Laser excision of web/ stenosis
- Segmental resection of stenotic trachea and end to end anastomosis (<4 cm) may be done.
- 'Laryngeal drop': The larynx is detached from the suprahyoid attachments enabling segmental resection of trachea and end to end anastomosis.

Prognosis

- Depends on the site and extent
- Generally poor prognosis
- Decannulation rate—Approximately 50 percent
- Functional gain– only in 25 percent.

Prevention

- In case of laryngotracheal trauma, actively investigate, explore and treat
- Avoid prolonged intubation
  - If >3 to 5 days intubation is necessary, change over to a tracheostomy
- If patient needs intubation
  - Prefer a smaller size endotracheal tube to prevent subglottic stenosis.
  - Cuff management– Deflate cuff every hour for 5 to 10 minutes if possible. Avoid over-inflation of the cuff.
  - Use endotracheal tubes with low pressure high volume cuffs
  - Or use endotracheal tubes with double cuffs wherein one may be inflated for some time then the other.
- First tracheal ring spared in tracheostomy
- Prevent laryngotracheal trauma in road traffic accident by use of
  - Seat belt
  - Inflatable bags
  - Collapsible steering wheel
  - Crumpable body
  - Engine in front and high seating.

POINTS TO REMEMBER

1. RTA is the commonest cause of external laryngotracheal injury.
2. Iatrogenic causes like prolonged endotracheal intubation and high tracheostomy are the most common preventable causes of internal laryngotracheal injury.
3. Multiple fractures of the laryngeal skeleton are seen commonly in patients above 40 years of age due to ossification of the cartilages.
4. Untreated or inadequately treated laryngotracheal trauma gives rise to laryngotracheal stenosis.
5. Laryngotracheal stenosis is preventable but extremely difficult to treat successfully.

Neurological Conditions of the Larynx

71

Applied Neuroanatomy

The laryngeal sensory and motor innervation is from the vagus nerve. The vagus nerve has two nuclei–nucleus ambiguous and dorsal nucleus.

Nucleus ambiguous is situated in the medulla and gives origin to special efferent fibers for the motor supply of the pharynx and larynx. The outgoing fibers run laterally and give rise to IX, X and XI cranial nerves. The fibers going to the accessory nerve (cranial part) are finally distributed entirely to the vagus nerve at the jugular foramen. This cranial part of accessory nerve shares the supply of laryngeal muscles with the vagus.

The *dorsal nucleus of vagus* is an autonomic nucleus serving only a general efferent visceral function. The outgoing fibers run anterolaterally and are joined by those of nucleus ambiguous before coming to the lateral surface of medulla as a series of rootlets. These fibers all go to form a part of the tenth nerve trunk which supplies smooth muscles and glands of trachea and bronchi, heart and abdominal viscera.

This nerve also carries taste fibers from the pharynx (particularly vallecula and epiglottis) other than supplied by the VII and XI cranial nerve to the tractus solitaries.

The auricular branch of vagus (Arnold's nerve) is the only somatic afferent part of the vagus nerve which ends in the descending tract of the fifth cranial nerve.

As the vagus descends in the jugular foramen, it widens to form the superior ganglion where the sensory components of the sensory nerve fibers reside. As it exits the *jugular foramen,* it widens again to form the 'nodose ganglion'. The cell bodies contain the visceral afferents from the pharynx and the larynx.

The superior laryngeal nerve exits the vagus nerve at the inferior border of the 'nodose ganglion' and passes medial to the internal and external carotid artery (*see* Fig. 66.1). It then passes inferior to a point slightly superomedial to the superior thyroid artery. About two cm from the nodose ganglion the nerve divides into external and internal branches. The internal branch travels medially along the superior laryngeal branch of the superior thyroid artery and pierces the thyrohyoid membrane about 1 cm anterior to the superior cornu and 1 cm above the ala of the thyroid cartilage.

The nerve then runs submucosally in the lateral wall of the pyriform fossa. It supplies sensory fibers to the larynx above the level of the glottis and to the laryngopharynx. The *nerve of Galen* is a small branch which arises from the internal laryngeal nerve to anastomose with the posterior branch of the recurrent nerve to form 'Ansa Galeni', which has a sensory function. The external branch runs along the posterior aspect of the superior thyroid artery and proceeds inferiorly along the oblique line of the thyroid cartilage. As

623

it reaches the inferior constrictor muscle it sends a branch to it and then passes deep to the sternothyroid muscle to reach the cricothyroid muscle. In the region of the superior pole of the thyroid gland the nerve is often slightly above the superior thyroid artery and may be injured during thyroid surgery or may be ligated with the superior thyroid artery. The interarytenoid muscle innervation is controversial and is said to have double innervation from the superior and the recurrent nerves and also bilateral innervation.

The pharyngeal branch travels between the internal and external carotid arteries and enters the pharynx at the upper border of the middle constrictor muscle and joins the pharyngeal plexus. It supplies all the muscles of the pharynx and soft palate except the stylopharyngeus and tensor palatini. These include the three constrictor muscles, levator veli palatini, salpingopharyngeus, palatopharyngeus and palatoglossal muscles.

As the vagus nerve leaves the nodose ganglion inferiorly to the neck lateral to the internal carotid artery the vagus nerve stays slightly anterior in position in relation to the common carotid artery in the lower neck. Since the recurrent laryngeal nerve is derived from the 6th branchial arch, the nerve is displaced by the arteries of the preceeding arch to finally lie low in the neck. In the right side it traverses below the subclavian artery after emerging from the vagus.

In the left side it winds round the arch of aorta after emerging from the vagus in the neck. This displacement of the nerve by the preceding branchial arch arteries necessitates change in direction and the course of the recurrent laryngeal nerve.

The right recurrent nerve stays lateral to the tracheoesophageal groove in the fat plane of the neck and comes close to the groove as it crosses the branches of the inferior thyroid artery. This may cause injury to the nerve during the thyroid and other neck surgery.

The left recurrent nerve has a longer course from its origin at the anterior surface of arch of aorta to the interspace between the origins of the left common carotid artery and subclavian artery. The nerve loops under the aorta distal to the ligamentum arteriosum and then enters the neck and lies deeper in the tracheo-esophageal groove. Rest of the course of both recurrent laryngeal nerves are similar as they reach the suspensory ligament of the thyroid gland and lie either medial lateral or from within. The nerve divides sometimes before entering the larynx through the 'Killian-Jamieson' area under the cricopharyngeus muscle posterior to the cricothyroid joint. Then the nerve divides further to supply the intrinsic muscles of the larynx.

VOCAL CORD PARALYSIS

It is a sign of disease and not a diagnosis. It can be a lesion at any point from the cerebral cortex to the neuromuscular junction. The type of vocal cord paralysis depends on the site of lesion.

1. Vagal trunk above the nodose ganglion-Combined abductor paralysis (Cadaveric position)
2. Vagus nerve below the nodose ganglion/Recurrent laryngeal nerve-Recurrent laryngeal nerve paralysis (Paramedian cord position)
3. Superior laryngeal nerve alone-Superior laryngeal nerve paralysis (Bowing of the cord)

Causes of Vocal Cord Paralysis

Central Causes (10% of all vocal cord paralysis)

- *Cortical causes* are rare and causes include cerebral concussion, congenital cerebral paralysis, encephalitis, diffuse arterial sclerosis, etc. Usually it causes spastic paralysis.
- *Corticobulbar causes:* Basilar artery occlusion or insufficiency causing incomplete paralysis produces spastic in-coordination.
- *Bulbar causes:* This occurs due to vascular insufficiency or occlusion of vertebral, PICA, AICA and lateral medullary branches.

Less common causes include bulbar polio-mellitus, progressive bulbar paralysis, multiple sclerosis, glioma, etc. It produces flaccid type of paralysis.

Peripheral causes (accounts to 90% of all vocal cord paralysis)

It can be high or low vagal paralysis as mentioned above.

The causes include

- *Surgery:* Thyroid surgery, neck dissection, tracheostomy, parathyroid surgery, esophageal surgery, brainstem surgery, thoracotomy, mediastinal surgeries, etc. may cause vocal cord paralysis. Depending on the type and site of surgery, it can be unilateral or bilateral. Bilateral paralysis is common in total thyroidectomy/esophageal or tracheal surgery and surgery at the brainstem.
- *Trauma:* External blunt injury, penetrating wound of the neck, as a complication of prolonged endotracheal intubation, base of skull fracture, birth trauma, etc.
- *Inflammatory:* Meningitis, diphtheria, leprosy, tuberculosis, syphilis, viral neuritis, acute polyneuritis, relapsing polyneuritis, Gullian Barre syndrome, post-radiation neuritis, osteomyelitis of the temporal bone, etc.
- *Neoplasm:* Thyroid malignancy, neoplasm of the upper lobe of the lung (pancoast tumor), cancer of the cervical and the thoracic esophagus, laryngeal neoplasm, nasopharyngeal cancer etc. Lymphoma of the superior mediastinun, glomus jugulare, neck metastases, lymphomas of the neck, glomus vagale or Schwannoma excision can also cause paralysis.
- *Neurological causes:* Stroke (CVA), brain abscess, meningomyelocele, Arnold Chiari malformation, etc.
- *Systemic causes associated with peripheral neuropathy:* Diabetes mellitus, collagen vascular diseases, alcoholic neuropathy, neuritis due to poisoning or toxicity like organophosphorous, lead, arsenic poisoning, etc.
- *Metabolic causes:* Hypokalemia and hypo-calcemia. Kernicterus also may give rise to nerve paralysis.
- *Idiopathic* (about 20 to 25% of the laryngeal paralysis)

The common causes of vocal cord paralysis are malignant disease (35%), surgical trauma (30%) and idiopathic (25%). In our experience bilateral vocal cord paralysis is most commonly due to thyroid disease.

Paralysis of peripheral origin can be divided into two groups:

- High vagal paralysis
- Low vagal paralysis

High vagal paralysis is due to lesion at or proximal to the nodose ganglion. Therefore all the nerves supplying to half of the larynx are involved causing combined paralysis. Sometimes other cranial nerves may be involved due to tumor involvement at the base of the skull commonly due to nasopharyngeal carcinoma

Low vagal paralysis: Here the nerve to cricothyroid is intact and the fibers to the recurrent laryngeal nerve are damaged. This is more common than the high vagal paralysis and occurs twice as frequently on the left side than the right because of its longer course. Neuritis is a common cause of isolated recurrent nerve paralysis following upper respiratory infection caused by influenza A or B virus. Infectious mononucleosis also should be considered for isolated recurrent laryngeal nerve paralysis.

Causes of High Vagal Lesion

Intracranial lesions

- Arnold Chiari malformations
- Stroke (CVA)
- Meningitis
- Tuberculoma
- Tumors
- Meningomyelocele

- Demyelinating diseases
- Head injury.

Skull Base Lesions

- Nasopharyngeal carcinoma
- Glomus jugulare
- Metastatic node of Krause
- Skull base osteomyelitis
- Surgery of skull base

Cervical Causes

- Malignant tumor of parapharyngeal space
- Lymphoma
- Glomus vagale
- Neurilemmoma of vagus nerve
- Extracalvarial meningioma
- Surgery of parapharyngeal tumors.

Position of the Vocal Cord in Vocal Cord Paralysis

Lot of controversy has been raised in the past regarding the position of the vocal cord. **Semon's law (1881)** states that the sequence of position of the vocal cords, associated with a slowly progressive organic lesion of the centers, trunks of motor laryngeal nerve the fibers supplying the abductors of the vocal cords becomes involved much earlier than the adductors. This means partial lesion of the cord will leave the cords in paramedian than a cadaveric position. Either the Semon's law or the site of the lesion decides the position of the cord absolutely but both are useful guides. On the basis of this increased susceptibility of the abductor fibers to injury, four stages of paralysis are recognized.

1. Isolated abductor paralysis
2. Median and paramedian position is due to spasm of adductor muscles.
3. Cadaveric position when all the muscles innervated by the recurrent laryngeal nerve are paralyzed
4. Stage of compensation by the normal vocal cord.

It is now recognized that this sequence of events is rarely associate with isolated recurrent laryngeal nerve paralysis.

Wagner and Grossman explained the median and paramedian position of the vocal cord after recurrent laryngeal nerve paralysis on the basis of continued function of the cricothyroid muscle which is tensor of the vocal cords and an adductor of the arytenoids. This explanation supported experimentally and is generally accepted.

Negus has supported the Semon's theory on the basis of the phylogenetic development of the laryngeal sphincter and the respiratory function of the larynx. Semon's observations of the greater vulnerability of the abductor function are in fact a clinical sign of insipient recurrent laryngeal nerve paralysis.

It can be explained by the fact that the posterior cricoarytenoid is the sole abductor of the vocal cord which operated at a considerable mechanical advantage. Therefore when paralysis is developing weakness may produce the clinical picture of abductor paralysis. Semon's theory is difficult to refute and impossible to prove.

In summary there can be no fixed laws governing the position assumed by the paralyzed vocal cords.

The factors determining the position of the vocal cord are

1. Continued function or paralysis of the cricothyroid muscles.
2. The degree of fibrosis of the denervated musculature.
3. Persistent tonus associated with the autonomic nerve supply
4. Fibrosis and ankylosis of the cricoarytenoid joint.
5. Function of the interarytenoid muscle.
6. Tension of the conus elasticus.

The difference between Paralized and Fixed vocal cord are discussed under Table 71.1.

Clinically five positions of the vocal cord are recognized (Fig. 71.1)

- *Median*: Cords touching the midline
- *Paramedian position*: 1.5 mm from midline
- *Intermediate (Cadaveric position)*: 3.5 mm from the midline

Table 71.1: Differences between fixed and paralyzed vocal cord (Watkinson et al)

Paralyzed vocal cord	Fixed vocal cord
• No swelling	• May have some obvious swelling around the cricoarytenoid joint
• Aryepiglottic fold is paralyzed and sags forward and inward with its cartilage of Wrisberg.	• Aryepiglottic fold may occupy some usual position and may be unaltered in appearance unless involved by the growth
• The arytenoids cartilage on paralyzed side is pushed aside by the sound and over-abducted healthy cord during phonation. (As the paralyzed cord in time gets fixed from disuse, this diagnostic point has a greater positive than negative value).	• Active arytenoid cartilage approaches but does not displace that on the affected side. Any excursion of movement is incomplete.
• The cord is fixed is midline or paramedian position.	• If the cord is quite immobile, its fixation may not correspond in position with any recognized form of laryngeal palsy.
• If the interarytenoid muscle retains any power and twitches the arytenoids cartilage on the paralyzed side slightly inwards, it shows the passive mobility of articulation and is a reliable means of excluding joint disease.	• Jerky movements of the cord
• If the position of the cord is at first median and then paramedian then it is a nerve lesion.	
• Presence of central or peripheral lesion that can produce paralysis.	• Absence of other neurological symptoms and signs.
• By pressing the arytenoid cartilage with a large probe with recent paralysis, absence of fixation can be proved.	• No change of position by manipulation
• Purely a neurological condition	• Fixation may be due to mass effect, involvement of muscles, joint or the nerve as in case of malignancy or arthritis.

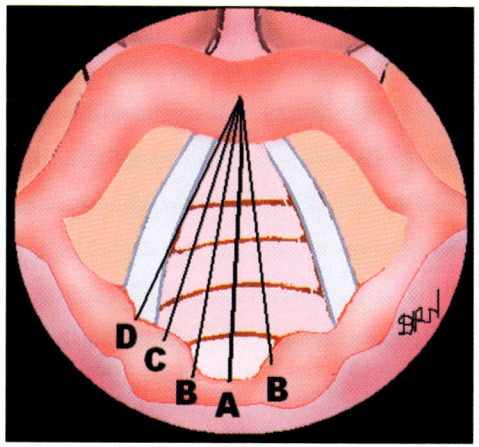

Fig. 71.1: Showing various cord positions in different types of vocal cord paralysis. (**A.** Median, **B.** Paramedian, **C.** Cadaveric, **D.** Full abduction)

- *Slightly abducted*: 7 mm from midline
- *Fully abducted*: 9 mm from midline.

The investigations for vocal cord palsy are done with objectives to:

1. Find out the cause of the vocal cord palsy like chest X-ray to rule out lung/ mediastinal pathology, CT scan of the skull and skull base with particular interest to jugular foramen, nasopharynx and the CP angle. Per-oral panendoscopy under general anesthesia helps in ruling out malignant disease in upper aero-digestive tract.
2. Find the result of palsy like chest X-ray and pulmonary function tests for aspiration.
3. Confirm and document the type and degree of palsy by stroboscopy, ultrahigh speed cinematography, glottography, speech and acoustic analysis.
4. Find the progress of palsy, whether recovering or increasing by EMG and speech analysis.

Objectives of treatment of vocal cord paralysis

The treatment comprises of:

1. Management of the etiology
2. Definitive treatment for the palsy which may be non-surgical or surgical.

EVALUATION AND MANAGEMENT OF DIFFERENT TYPES OF VOCAL CORD PARALYSIS

SUPERIOR LARYNGEAL NERVE PARALYSIS

This is a rare paralysis to occur in isolation. Common causes include thyroid surgery, neck dissection, trauma including penetrating injury, neuritis of viral origin.

Clinical Features of Unilateral Superior Laryngeal Nerve Paralysis

Symptoms

Weakness or alteration of the voice is the prominent feature which occurs due to loss of tension. The voice becomes monotonic. There will be anesthesia of the supraglottis which may cause aspiration in elderly patients. Compensation may occur early by the other cord leading to quick recovery and the condition may be overlooked unless the patient is a professional singer who will be unable to raise the pitch of the voice.

Signs

On indirect laryngoscopy:

- Oblique laryngeal inlet.
- Bowing of the affected cord during phonation. Cords appear bulky.
- Aspiration may be noted at the time of examination.
- Posterior commisure tends to deviate towards the paralyzed side

Clinical Features of Bilateral Superior Laryngeal Nerve Paralysis

Symptoms

1. Cough and choking spells due to aspiration
2. Breathy voice with inability to raise the pitch due to loss of cord tension
3. Short phonation time due to air wasting
4. The symptoms become more persistent in compared to unilateral paralysis.
5. Dysphonia
6. Phonesthenia
7. Spontaneous improvement to some extent related to the duration

Signs

1. Examination features are similar to unilateral superior laryngeal nerve paralysis but the changes are seen bilaterally.
2. Severe aspiration

Investigation

- Videostroboscopy helps in detecting the subtle functional defects in the vocal cords. Psychogenic causes may be identified by asking the patient to sniff or whistle.

- CT/ MRI scan from the skull base to neck
- Spiral CT is helpful if lung cancer is suspected and also helps in diagnosing mediastinal conditions causing the paralysis.
- Chest X-ray if patient cannot afford a CT
- Endoscopy which may consist of naso-pharyngoscopy using angles nasal or nasopharyngeal telescopes
- Rigid telescopy of the larynx.
- Ultrahigh speed cinematography, glotto-graphy, speech and acoustic analysis.

Treatment

1. Speech therapy is useful in unilateral abductor paralysis and post operatively.
2. If aspiration is present, surgery is the main treatment.
3. Teflon/ collagen injection into the vocal cords under operating microscope.
4. Arytenoid adduction procedure may be helpful to lengthen the vocal cord on the affected side.

RECURRENT LARYNGEAL NERVE PARALYSIS

Isolated paralysis of this nerve is due to a lesion/injury between the nodose ganglions to its termination in the larynx.

Clinical features depend on acute or chronic cause.

Acute paralysis is often due to trauma but sometimes it is due to neuritis of viral origin. Chronic progressive is due to slowly advancing lesion anywhere during its course or advancing bulbar lesion.

Clinical Features of Unilateral Recurrent Laryngeal Nerve Paralysis

Symptoms

Severe voice disturbance including hoarseness or temporary aphonia due to lack of compensation by the normal cord may occur. Later the voice improves over a period of time as the paralysis cord moves to paramedian position and the compensation by the normal cord. In some cases

the voice returns to normal. Sometimes the cord may stay in the intermediate position resulting in incomplete compensation. This could be due to retrograde degeneration of the nucleus ambiguous causing superior laryngeal nerve paralysis, in addition.

Signs

Indirect laryngoscopy shows

- Cord in paramedian or median position.
- Shallow pyriform fossa
- The arytenoid falls forwards
- Paralyzed vocal cord is at a lower level
- Cartilage of Wrisberg lean forwards
- Thickness of the cords may be affected
- Cricoarytenoid joint may be affected by thickness and contracture.

Causes of Recurrent Laryngeal Paralysis

1. *Trauma:* Blunt or penetrating injury to the neck like cut throat injury to the neck
2. Iatrogenic causes
   - *Surgical trauma* like thyroid surgery, cervico-esophageal surgery, bilateral neck dissection cndio thoracic surgery
   - Prolonged *endotracheal intubation*
3. *Neoplasm:* Malignancy of the thyroid gland, esophagus, larynx, hypopharynx and trachea
4. *Miscellaneous causes:* Parkinson's disease.

Clinical Features of Bilateral Recurrent Laryngeal Nerve Paralysis (Fig.71.2)

This is usually of acute onset. The most common cause of this is direct surgical trauma.

Initially the cords lie in intermediate or paramedian position causing severe dysphonia and hoarseness. As the cord gradually comes to the midline, voice improves and patient develops inspiratory stridor and dyspnea which increases on exertion. Patient may come to emergency with acute airway obstruction if associated with URTI requiring tracheostomy. Elderly patients may have problem of aspiration.

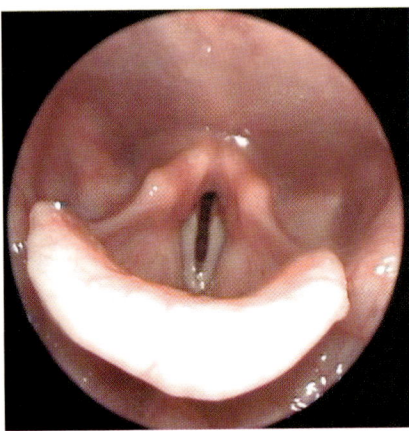

Fig. 71.2: Showing both cords in paramedian position due to bilateral abductor paralysis

Investigation

- CT/MR imaging from skull base till the superior mediastinum.
- Chest x-ray to rule out mediastinal lesion and features of aspiration pneumonia.
- Spiral CT is helpful if lung cancer is suspected and also helps in diagnosing mediastinal conditions causing the paralysis.
- Direct layngoscopy
- Tracheostomy may be needed
- Panendoscopy may be required if the cause is idiopathic.
- Ultrahigh speed cinematography, glottography, speech and acoustic analysis.

Treatment

The treatment comprises of:

1. Management of the etiology
2. Definitive treatment for the palsy which may be non-surgical or surgical.

Non-surgical Treatment

This includes wait and watch policy, speech therapy and medical treatment. In cases of congenital palsy, over 50 percent recover spontaneously and surgery is indicated only if recovery does not occur.

1. ***Unilateral vocal cord paralysis:*** Surgery is usually reserved until 6 to 12 months have elapsed or when patient has a troublesome aspiration or weak cough. Various surgical techniques are described in various types of palsy. In unilateral RLN palsy, the common techniques employed include:
   a. Intracordal injection of Teflon, collagen or gelfoam, etc.
   b. Medialization procedures include ***Static procedures*** (like augmentation, medialization laryngoplasty and arytenoid rotation) and ***Dynamic procedures*** (like nerve-muscle pedicle transfer with branch of ansa hypoglossi-anterior belly of omohyoid to lateral thyroarytenoid muscle or an ansa-recurrent laryngeal nerve anastomosis).

2. ***Bilateral vocal cord paralysis:*** Various surgical procedures are available to improve the airway of the patient which includes tracheostomy, arytenoidectomy and lateralization procedures. Whatever procedure is undertaken the voice is usually made worse to a greater or lesser extent. The immediate management is to do a tracheostomy to establish the airway. Among the lateralization procedures at present, endoscopic procedures are more popular which include endoscopic lateral fixation of the vocal cords to the thyroid cartilage or temporarily to the skin after cauterization of the lateral aspect of the vocal cord (Figs 71.3a and b). More recently CO_2/ KTP-532 laser arytenoidectomy/ laser posterior cordotomy have been advocated, but long term results are yet to be established.

COMBINED LARYNGEAL PARALYSIS

Paralysis of both superior and recurrent laryngeal nerves is known as combined paralysis. When it affects one side of the larynx, then all the muscles larynx on that side are affected except interarytenoid muscle. This commonly occurs following a high vagal lesion which may either be affected in the jugular foramen or by a bulbar lesion but also can occur following thyroid surgery where both the nerves can be injured.

Common causes have been highlighted under *'causes of high vagal lesions'*.

Clinical Features

Symptoms

Hoarseness is persistent due to an incompetent glottis. Patient may complain of aphonia. Aspiration is seen initially and persists till the patient adapts. Sometimes aspiration may persist. Clinical features are same as unilateral recurrent laryngeal paralysis.

Signs

The affected vocal cord is oblique. Manipulation test and determination of cricothyroid space may be done but is not conclusive in unilateral paralysis. Vocal cord is seen in a position between phonation and quiet respiration and is called as intermediate or cadaveric position.

Bilateral combined paralysis is extremely rare where the patients may have severe aspiration, hoarseness, dyspnea and stridor (in upper respiratory infections).

Investigations

EMG studies are very helpful in knowing the cricothyroid muscle function. Other investigations are as described earlier.

Treatment

Immediate treatment includes voice therapy and physiotherapy.

Surgical Treatment

- Aspiration is treated by cricopharyngeal myotomy or tracheostomy.
- Medialization thyroplasty (as in unilateral RLN paralysis) is ultimately required to improve voice and relieve aspiration and is done under local anesthesia.

THE TECHNIQUE OF MEDIALIZATION THYROPLASTY (ISSHIKI TYPE I) INCLUDES (Figs 71.4 and 71.5)

1. Horizontal skin incision preferably given on one side extending till the midline at the level of lower border of thyroid cartilage laterally till the anterior border of sternocliedomastoid muscle.

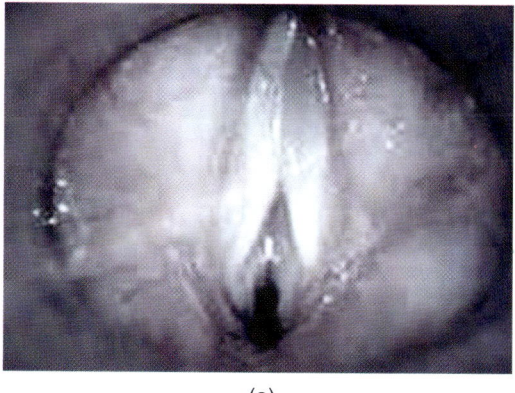
(a)

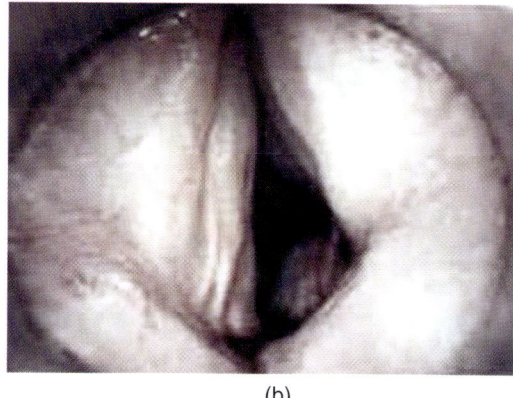
(b)

Figs 71.3a and b: Pre and post operative pictures of endoscopic vocal cord lateralization with permanent lateral fixation technique

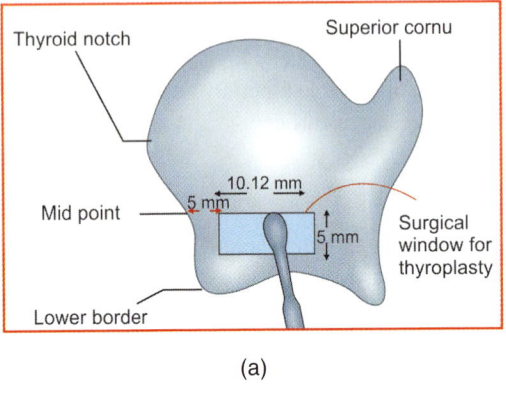

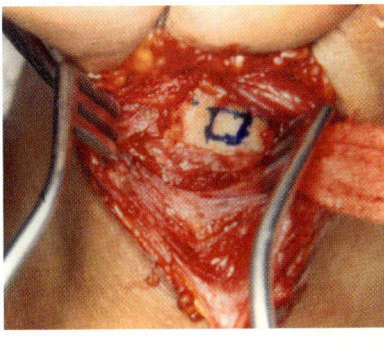

(a)

(b)

Figs 71.4a and b: Surgical window being made on the thyroid ala

2. Subplatysmal skin flap elevation is done till the upper border of the thyroid cartilage and the thyroid notch is exposed.
3. Midpoint between the thyroid notch and the lower border of the thyroid cartilage in the midline is determined using calipers. A window is then created of a size of about 5 mm in width and 10 to 12 mm in length in the transverse plane after elevating a perichondrial flap on the outer surface. Care is taken not to injure the inner perichondrium.
4. A silastic block is designed appropriately to fit into the window for proper medialization. The amount of medialization is monitored with flexible laryngoscope and on table voice analysis.

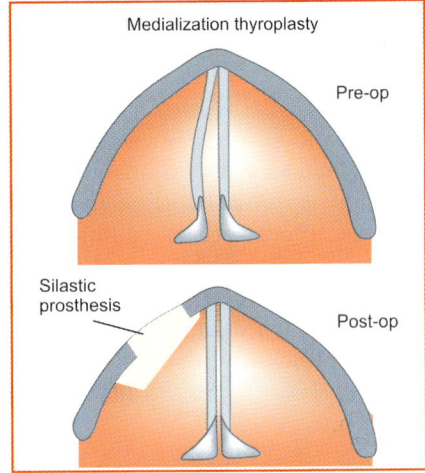

Fig. 71.5: Silastic prosthesis being fit into the surgical window created for medialization

72

Functional and Other Voice Disorders of the Larynx

DYSPHONIA PLICA VENTRICULARIS

(*Synonym*: **False cord voice**)

Definition

This is a condition where the voice is produced by the apposition of false vocal cords during phonation.

Etiology

Exact etiology is not known. It is commonly associated with psychogenic conditions and vocal cord disabilities. Vocal cord disability may include compensation for inadequate function, central nervous system diseases, and functional in-coordination of laryngeal musculature. Other associated causes may be vocal cord paralysis, fixation, surgical excision, neoplastic diseases.

Symptoms

Voice is harsh, low-pitched with a crackling and rumbling sound.

Patient often complains of disturbed phonation. Sometimes the voice may be good with minor hoarseness particularly when the ventricular band compensates. Diplophonia (double voice) may be seen due to voice production by both folds.

Signs

Indirect laryngoscopy shows apposition of ventricular folds during phonation. Ventricular band is hypertrophied and reddened. Vocal cord may be hidden by the false cords (Figs 72.1a,b).

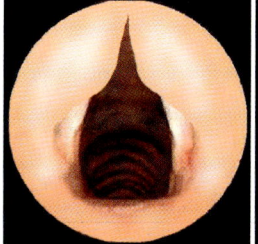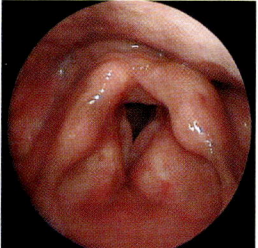

Figs 72.1a and b: (a) Hypertrophy of the false cord hiding the view of the vocal cords, (b) Video-endoscopic picture showing gross hypertrophy and congestion of the ventricular band

Investigations

Videostroboscopy is helpful.

Treatment

- *Speech therapy* should be started immediately.
- Psychotherapy is helpful.
- Laser excision of false cord may be done in difficult cases.

FUNCTIONAL APHONIA

Definition

This is a condition associated with an abrupt onset of loss of voice following emotional crisis giving rise to functional paralysis of adductors during phonation.

Etiology

It is associated with psychological conditions including emotionally unstable individuals like young females.

Symptoms

Aphonia is often sudden and complete. Sometimes the patient may speak in a faint whisper. It is typically seen in young females who might have undergone some psychological trauma. Though the patient is not able to phonate, laughing, crying or coughing are not affected.

Signs

Indirect laryngoscopy shows failure of vocal cords to appose on phonation. Occasionally the vocal cords may appose closely without any production of sound. Sometime the pharyngeal reflexes are found to be insensitive. Cough is normal when the glottis is able to close normally.

Treatment

Persuasion may lead to resolution but relapses are not uncommon. Speech therapy and psychotherapy is helpful in early recovery and prevention of relapses.

Sulcus Vocalis

A groove parallel to vocal fold margin occurs as a result of congenital or development cause. It may be unilateral or bilateral and usually associated with a weak voice. Indirect laryngoscopy may show inability of vocal folds to adduct along its entire length. Speech therapy may be helpful and rarely thyroplasty (type I) may be necessary. In bilateral cases endoscopic collagen injection is helpful.

STUTTERING

(Synonym: **Stammering)**

It is one of the most enigmatic speech disorders encountered by otolaryngologists' and speech pathologists.

Clinical Features

It is a disturbance of rhythm and fluency of speech. There is a disruption in the frequency of verbal expression and is characterized by involuntary, audible silent utterance of short speech elements like sounds, syllables and words. This disruption is not readily controllable. Sometimes they may be accompanied by accessory activities involving the speech apparatus. It occurs commonly in the preschool years and is commonly seen in boys than in girls.

The speech has the following features:

- Hesitation
- Repetition
- Blocks
- Prolongations.

Treatment

It can be successfully treated by speech therapy. Stigmatization should be avoided and speech counseling is very important. The treatment should always be conducted by individuals who have training and experience in the areas of speech language pathology and clinical psychology.

Lisping

- Functional speech disorder
- Difficulty in learning to make specific speech sound/s
- Cause—Probably due to habitual incorrect pronunciation (Developmental)

- Problems saying 's', 'z', 'r', 'l' and 'th' are common
- Difficulty in achieving the correct tongue position
- When a person lisps, their tongue either protrudes between (interdental lisp), or touches their front teeth (dentalized lisp)
- Treatment is by speech therapy.

SPASTIC DYSPHONIA

It is a condition associated with a harsh and soft voice alternatively, as a result of severe vocal disability, with excessive adduction of vocal cords during phonation. Exact etiology is not known. The patient may have strained, cricking or choked vocal attacks. Squeezed voice appears to be accompanied by spasm of entire pulmonary system. Laughing, singing appears to be less affected. The stressed vowels are broken into two portions and the voice fluctuates in its intensity. High sedation or high alcohol intake may produce temporary voice improvement.

Indirect laryngoscopy: Excessive adduction of vocal cords may be seen on phonation. Stroboscopy is helpful in the diagnosis of this condition after a careful history. They respond poorly to psychotherapy and speech therapy. Some advocate sectioning of the recurrent laryngeal nerve to reduce spasm. This is done after temporary paralysis by injection of lignocaine to know the outcome of the nerve sectioning. Botulinum toxin injection into the laryngeal muscles has been tried in the treatment of spastic dysphonia.

PHONASTHENIA

It is a condition associated with a functional weakness of voice although the patient has a normal vocal organ.

Etiology

Caused primarily by faulty usage of voice. Commonly seen in emotionally labile individuals.

Symptoms

Patient may complain unpleasant sensation around neck, throat and the larynx. These patients talk more. Professionals like doctors, teachers are more prone. Voice may be weak.

Signs

Indirect laryngoscopic examination reveals slight reddening of vocal cord margins. There may be tenderness around the strap muscles of the neck.

Treatment

Speech therapy, removal of the causative factor. Psychological counseling may be helpful including vocal hygiene.

PUBOPHONIA

Synonyms: *Puberphonia, functional falsetto voice, mutational falsetto voice*

Definition

A functional voice disorder of pitch control wherein adolescent male's voice fails to descend to a normal adult pitch level at puberty.

Etiology

- Emotional stress
- Personality disorder—Patients are thin, effeminate, shy, insecure and usually dominated and protected by mother.
- Psychosocial changes during puberty.

Pathology

Cricothyroid is the main tensor responsible for the falsetto voice. There is hyperkinetic function and spasm of cricothyroid muscle.

Symptoms

Adolescent male continues to have a high pitch which he had during his childhood. Normally at puberty due to structural changes in the larynx pitch of the voice breaks to a lower pitch. If this does not occur, it is called puberphonia.

Social stigma and consequent psychological impact may be present.

Signs

Glottis is oval or elliptical slit. Sometimes the vocal process partially closes to produce a triangle posteriorly and is called **mutational triangle**. This is seen normally during puberty but its persistence is abnormal. True cords may be hyperemic and slightly edematous.

Investigations

Stroboscopy can confirm the vocal cord pathology, particularly the mutational triangle. Radiology of neck shows narrowing of cricothyroid space.

Treatment

Vocal rehabilitation and re-education often resolves the pitch disorder. Psychological counseling may be beneficial.

LARYNGEAL VERTIGO

A rare condition characterized by attacks of vertigo with temporary unconsciousness following spasm of vocal cord leading to glottic closure.

Etiology

This commonly occurs in males and the patients may complain of cough due to laryngeal paresthesia. Other contributing factors are chronic bronchitis or chronic pulmonary disease. Emotional instability is seen in most of the cases.

Pathophysiology

There is sharp decrease in cardiac output causing cerebral ischemia as a result of spasm of the vocal cord following cough. This causes excessive complete emptying of lung air with a resultant sub-atmospheric pressure that traps blood in the lungs. Thus the temporary ischemia resulting from decreased cardiac output causes loss of consciousness.

Clinical Features

- High sharp inspiratory stridor following spasm
- Pale and cyanotic followed by experiencing dizziness and light headedness or momentary loss of consciousness.
- Tremors, convulsions, urinary incontinence is absent unlike epilepsy.
- Recovery is rapid.

Treatment

No treatment is required in majority of the cases. The underlying pathological conditions that precipitate the problem should be treated.

RHINOLALIA

This is a condition associated with nasal intonation of speech which may be hyponasal or hypernasal and is also known as 'nasal speech'.

There are two types of rhinolalia, namely:
- Rhinolalia clausa
- Rhinolalia aperta

- ***Rhinolalia clausa (Hyponasal speech):*** There is reduction in nasal resonance in speech due to obstruction in the nose/nasopharynx.
  - Blocked nose/nasopharynx: Examples- rhinitis, polyp, mass in nose, nasopharynx, adenoid hypertrophy, etc.

- ***Rhinolalia aperta (Hypernasal speech):*** There is increased airflow into the nose causing increased nasal resonance.
  - Cleft palate, submucous cleft palate, velopharyngeal insufficiency, palatal palsy, palatal fistula, post-adenoidectomy, habitual hypernasality, etc.

VOCAL HYGIENE

It is a habit that maintains proper functioning of the vocal cords. Faulty vocal habits can cause persistent psychological and organic lesions of the vocal cords. The common psychological conditions that can occur due to faulty vocal habits are functional aphonia, spastic dysphonia, etc. and organic lesions include vocal nodules, vocal polyp, etc. It is very important for a professional voice user. The common vocal habits that can be taken care of are

- Mouth breathing can cause exposure of the larynx to environmental factors like allergen, humidity. Cold weather can give rise to drying effect and can affect voice functioning.
- Exposure to smoke and dust should to be avoided.
- Vigorous exercise can cause noisy and breathy voice which should be avoided.
- Spicy food can be a factor. Care should be taken to avoid laryngeal trauma.
- While speaking one should not strain facial and laryngeal musculature.
- If having any functional or organic voice problem, one should stop singing, talking and give appropriate voice rest for two weeks

for the recovery of vocal cord damage. Whispering voice should be strictly avoided. Reduction of professional activity like acting, singing and talking improves the condition drastically.

- Professional voice users should avoid speaking during an attack of upper respiratory tract infection.
- Should not speak in a noisy voice without voice amplification and should not strain the voice or raise the voice in such a situation.
- Should not do forced coughing, throat clearing as they can cause voice strain,
- Should not scream loudly.
- Alcohol, aspirin and medications with drying potential like antihistaminic should be avoided.
- Professional voice users and singers should use their own speech range.
- Habitual breath holding or improper glottic valving during exercise should be avoided.
- Gastroesophageal reflux should be controlled by lifestyle changes as described in the chapter 'laryngitis'.
- Increased fluid intake to optimize laryngeal hydration
- Voice rest is the mainstay of treatment in all voice disorders and should be strictly followed.

73

Neoplasms of the Larynx

True benign neoplastic tumors of the larynx other than squamous papilloma are rare. Benign tumors like hemangioma/ lympangioma are congenital in origin and are described under congenital lesions of the larynx. Malignant neoplasm of the larynx is most commonly seen in elderly patients. Cigarette smoking is the principal risk factor. Squamous cell carcinoma is the most common type of malignancy of the larynx.

Classification (Table 73.1)

PAPILLOMA OF THE LARYNX

80 per cent of all benign tumor of the larynx is papilloma. It is the most common laryngeal tumor in children.

Table 73.1: Classification

Benign	Malignant
• Papilloma	• Squamous cell carcinoma
• Hemangioma	• Adenocarcinoma
• Glomus	• Carcinosarcoma
• Chondroma	• Small cell carcinoma
• Fibroma	• Chondrosarcoma
• Lymphangioma	
• Adenoma	

Definition

Papillomas are of epithelial origin that consists of fronds of connective tissue covered by a well differentiated squamous epithelial covering with no invasion of stroma or submucosal tissues.

Types

- Juvenile laryngeal papillomatosis (Children)
- Solitary laryngeal papilloma (Adults)

JUVENILE LARYNGEAL PAPILLOMATOSIS (JLP)

Synonym: Recurrent respiratory papillomatosis (RRP)

Definition

Benign neoplasms of the larynx are commonly seen in children and are characterized by presence of multiple warty lesions on the larynx which may give rise to fatal respiratory obstruction and are considered to be a representation of an abnormal tissue response to a viral agent *(Abramson et al)*.

Incidence

- Most common benign tumor of the larynx in infancy and childhood
- Approximately 1500 new cases reported annually
- Higher incidence in children whose mother has genital warts.

Etiology

- Human papilloma virus 6 and 11 which is tissue specific and targets stratified squamous epithelium of the oropharynx, larynx and anogenital region. Virus like particles resembling human papilloma virus has been found in excised lesions. HPV 6, 11 and 16 have been demonstrated by southern blotting in situ hybridization and immunocytochemistry .
- Genetic predisposition
- 80 to 90 percent of cases present before 3 years of age
- May get infected during birth if mother has genital condylomata (Genital warts)—50 percent of cases have mothers with this!
- But delivery by cesarian section does not prevent it. Probably is spreads transplacentally or due to postnatal infection

Pathology

- *Gross:* Multiple pinkish white warty lesions on the supraglottis and vocal cords– May obstruct the airway
- Can occur anywhere in the respiratory tract but common glottis and supraglottis
- *Microscopy:* Finger–like projections of epithelial tumor cells with central fibrovascular core.

Symptoms

- *Hoarseness:* 'Any child with hoarseness of more than 1 month duration should be diagnosed as JLP until otherwise proved'
- 'Asthma-like' features
- Stridor.

Signs

- Hoarse voice/ harsh weak cry
- ILS: May resemble like multiple small grapes and has a warty appearance (Fig. 73.1). It often obscures the laryngeal lumen because of size and bulk
- Inspiratory/ biphasic stridor +/–

Investigations

- X-ray lateral/ AP view of the neck—Look for the patency of the airway
- Chest X-ray
- Flexible/ rigid laryngoscopy
- Microlaryngoscopy and excision—Biopsy
- Bronchoscopy to rule out tracheobronchial lesions.

Treatment

- Various methods of treatment are described
- Microlaryngoscopy and excision with microcautery are the common methods of treatment
- Microlaryngoscopic KTP-532 /CO_2 laser vaporization is presently the treatment of choice with no touch technique. This can cause less trauma to the surrounding tissue.
- Avoid trauma to the larynx, adjacent areas and lower respiratory tract as seeding into raw areas may result in recurrence.
- As recurrence rates very high child may need such procedures repeatedly to clear the airway
- Spontaneous regression may occur after puberty

Other Methods of Treatment

Inconsistent success reported

- Cryosurgery

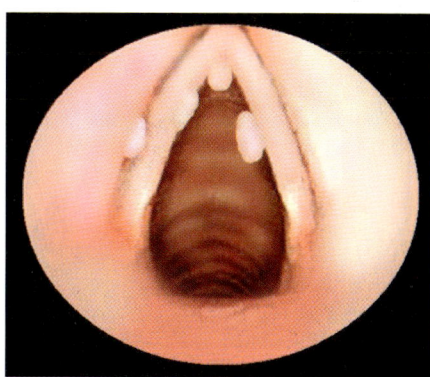

Fig. 73.1: Multiple papillomas in the larynx

- Ultrasonic destruction
- MLS and application of podophyllin
- *Interferon therapy:* Large trials are currently in progress in various medical centers.
- Autogenous vaccines
- Long-term antibiotics have been tried
- Antiviral treatment.

If stridor is present

- Tracheostomy is done only if endotracheal intubation is not possible
- Tracheostomy should be avoided because recurrence in the tracheostoma site can occur and is more difficult to treat

Prognosis

- It is often aggressive and resistant to treatment and has high recurrence rates. Multiple surgical excisions are often needed.
- Death due to respiratory obstruction
- Its recurrence decreases after puberty hence, if child survives till puberty, prognosis is good
- Unlike adult papilloma, it has no malignant potential, unless it is irradiated.

SOLITARY PAPILLOMA

This occurs in adults. Their behavior is less aggressive than juvenile papillomatosis. The recurrence rate is less compared to the juvenile papilloma. Interval between occurrence and recurrence is long.

Etiology

- Human papilloma virus.

Pathology

- Although considered premalignant, papillary carcinoma has been reported in adults. Most pathologists doubt that they result from malignant degeneration but rather are malignant from the onset (Yoder and Batsakis 1980)
- Recurrences frequently exhibit dysplasia.

Clinical Presentation

It is similar to vocal polyp. On indirect laryngoscopy is appears as white to pinkish red and has a glistening mulberry nodule. It may be pedunculated or sessile. It bleeds easily upon removal. It commonly occurs in the free edge of the membranous vocal cord or the anterior commisure.

Treatment

- Microlaryngoscopy and KTP-532 /CO_2 laser assisted excision/ vaporization.
- *It is treated as a* **premalignant condition**
- **DD:** Verrucous carcinoma
- Prognosis is good if completely excised. Recurrence rates are very low compared to juvenile papillomatosis.

PAPILLOMA OF THE LARYNX (HIGHLIGHTS)

- Hallmark of juvenile papilloma is its multiple nature and notorious propensity to recur. Human papilloma virus is believed to be the causative agent.
- They regress after puberty.
- KTP-532 /CO_2 laser vaporization is the treatment of choice.
- Theater personnel should be protected from inhaling the fumes during laser surgery as it may contain the viral particles.

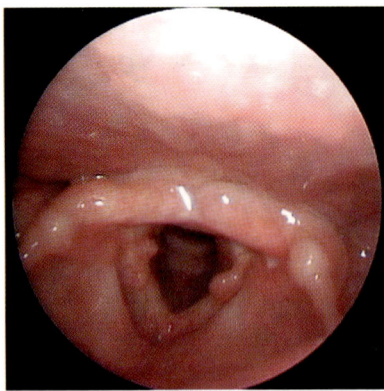

Fig. 73.2: Showing multiple papillomas in the larynx (Telescopic picture)

- Tracheostomy should be avoided at all costs unless absolutely indicated.
- Effort should be made to avoid recurrence in trachea and bronchi.
- Adult papilloma is solitary, pedunculated/sessile warty lesions pinkish in appearance and is seen in the anterior commisure or free margin of the vocal cord. Recurrences frequently exhibit dysplasia
- Most patients with carcinoma larynx arising from a papilloma have received irradiation.

FIBROMA OF THE LARYNX

They are small pedunculated lesions that usually arise from the true vocal cords.

Etiopathology

They are probably not true neoplasm but rather a representation of localized fibrous overgrowth of the tissue.

Symptoms

Hoarseness is the only symptom.

Signs

On indirect laryngoscopy they appear as a small pedunculated nodular mass seen commonly in the anterior one thirds of the larynx.

Treatment is microlaryngoscopic excision.

Prognosis

Clinical course is benign and prognosis is good.

LARYNGEAL CANCER

It is basically a disease of the elderly and represents 2.3 percent of all malignant tumors in males and 0.4 percent of all malignant tumors in females excluding basal and squamous cell carcinoma of the skin.

Peak incidence is 6th to 7th decade. But a number of cases have been reported in less than 20 years of age.

SQUAMOUS CELL CARCINOMA OF THE LARYNX

- 95 to 98 percent of malignant lesions of the larynx
- 70 percent occur in glottis
  - Glottic tumors present early with hoarseness
  - Glottis has poor lymphatic drainage
  - Hence early treatment can give cure rate of 90 to 95 percent
- 'Adult with hoarseness of more than a month not responding to treatment should be diagnosed as carcinoma of the larynx until otherwise proved'.

Incidence

- Incidence is high in age group of 40 to 70 years (recent trends—More and more younger people are being affected).
- Male/Female ratio is 10:1 (recent trends– Increasing incidence in females which is probably due to smoking/ alcohol).
- More in Indians (Supraglottic laryngeal tumors are more common in Indians compared to the same in world population).

Etiology

Mnemonic TARGET

- **T**obacco
  - *Carcinogens*: Benzopyrene. Less than 5 percent of laryngeal carcinomas occur in non-smokers.
- *Alcohol*: Synergistic with tobacco
  - Commonly in supraglottic ca.
- **R**adiation
- **G**enetic– Familial tendency
- **E**nvironmental/occupational: Asbestos, petroleum, mustard gas, petroleum products, wood products, painters, construction workers, metal and plastic workers, etc. have

been related but none as high as smoking and alcohol.

- *Tumors*: Solitary papilloma, leukoplakia, erythroplakia, etc.
- *Others:*
  - Dietary factors are also postulated. Salt preserved meat and high dietary fat are said to be associated with higher risk for carcinoma of the larynx (Freudenheim et al, 1992). Green leafy vegetables contain antioxidants and may have a protective role.
  - Gastroesophageal reflux disease has been blamed for a significant risk factor by several studies (Olson, 1991, El-Serag et al, 2001).

Pathology

- Gross
  - Proliferative—Exophytic (usually well differentiated)
  - Ulcerative—Endophytic (usually poorly differentiated)
  - Ulceroproliferative
- Glottic malignancy are usually well differentiated squmous cell carcinoma.

SITES OF LARYNX AND INCIDENCE OF MALIGNANCY (Fig. 73.3)

Supraglottis

Extends from the free border of the epiglottis till the laryngeal ventricles including the false cords.

Glottis

Extends from the floor of the ventricle to about 10 mm inferior to the free border of the true cords (this has been recently extended to almost 20 mm).

Subglottis

Extends from more than 10 mm from the free border of the vocal cord to the lower border of the cricoid cartilage.

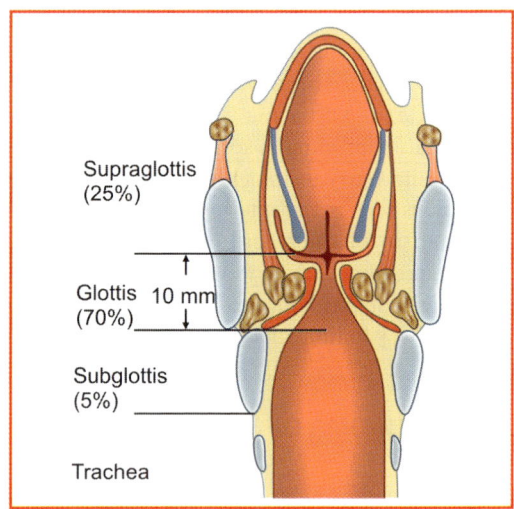

Fig. 73.3: Incidence of cancer larynx in various sites

Supraglottic Carcinoma

Sites

- Epiglottis
- Ventricular band
- Aryepiglottic fold (marginal zone)
- Ventricle

Spread (Fig. 73.4)

(a) *Local:* This is facilitated by numerous mucus glands in the supraglottic region. Numerous pits in the cartilage of the epiglottis facilitate its spread to the pre-epiglottic space. Behavior of the tumor depends on its site as shown in Fig. 73.3.

Lesions arising from the laryngeal surface of the epiglottis spread superficially to involve whole of the epiglottis in addition to the pre-epiglottic space. Inferiorly it can involve the petiole of the epiglottis and the anterior commisure. Supraglottic cancer tends to remain above the laryngeal ventricle. Hyoepiglottic ligament serves as a barrier to tumor spread from the epiglottis.

Lesions from the false vocal cord may involve epiglottis, aryepiglottic folds and the arytenoid cartilages. If the paraglottic space

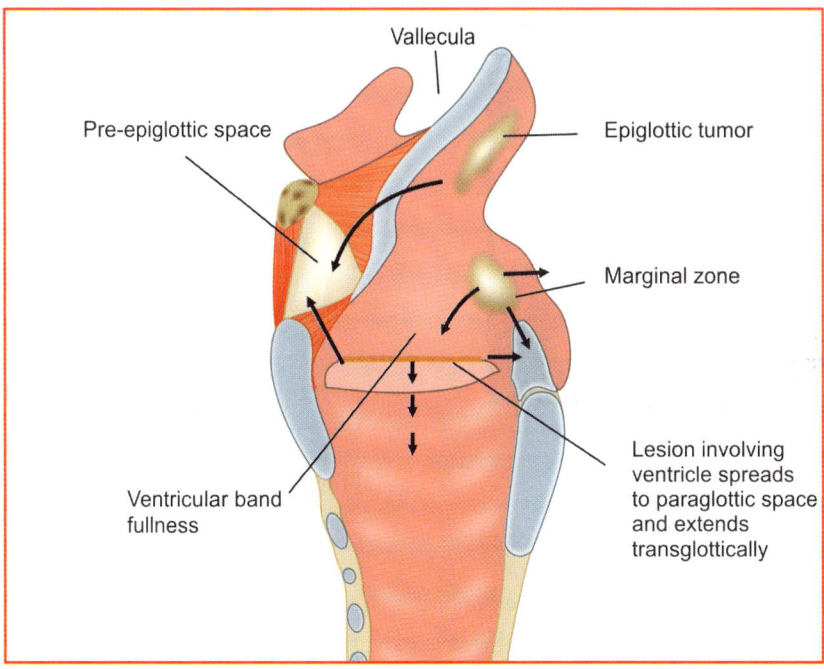

Fig. 73.4: Mode of local spread in supraglottic carcinoma

is involved the tumor can spread easily superiorly and inferiorly. The anterior commisure tendon serves as a barrier to inferior spread of supraglottic tumors.

Primary tumors of the ventricle are rare and the surface of the lesion is usually not visible and presents as a fullness of the ventricular band as shown in the Figs 73.5 and 73.6 These tumors spread to the paraglottic space and become transglottic early.

Aryepiglottic fold leisons exhibit biological behavior similar to the pyriform sinus and are called marginal zone lesions. Growth arising from this area is more proliferative than fungative with small ulcerations with heaped up margins.

(b) *Lymphatic spread:* They drain via the thyrohyoid membrane to the jugulodigastic (L2) and jugulomohyoid (L3). Incidence of cervical metastasis is very high with 20 to 40 percent of clinically, no neck can have occult metastasis.

Symptoms of Supraglottic Cancer

- Muffled voice ('Hot potato speech') rather than a true hoarseness is the initial symptom.

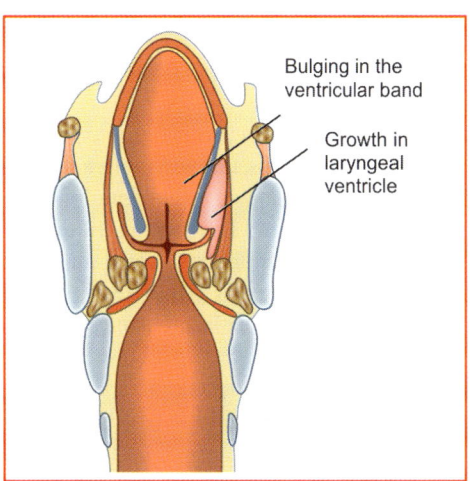

Fig. 73.5: Showing growth in the laryngeal ventricle presenting as ventricular band fullness

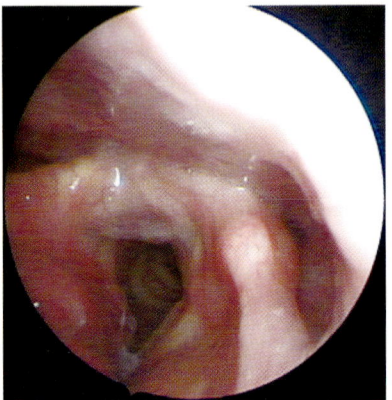

Fig. 73.6: Telescopic picture showing malignancy of the right ventricle with fullness of the ventricular band

Presence of hoarseness is late when the glottis is involved. The symptoms are sometimes are not obvious until the tumor extends to the hypopharynx, vallecula or the base of the tongue.
- FB sensation/lump in the throat
- Dysphagia
- Pain throat and referred otalgia (through vagus) are late features.
- Neck swelling (L2, L3 levels)
- Aspiration
- Stridor.

Signs

Indirect Laryngoscopy
- Proliferative/ ulcerative growth is seen in the supraglottis. Growth is often fungating with heaped up edges with multiple areas of ulceration. Infiltrating tumor with spreading peripheries. Usual appearance of the larynx is distorted by bulky ulcerated lesions which may erode the epiglottis.
- Glottis may be obscured
- Vocal cord mobility may be restricted or fixed
- Extralaryngeal spread may be present. Fullness of ventricular band is seen if tumor is arising in ventricle (Fig 73.5).

Neck
- 40 percent present with cervical metastasis (Jugulodigastic/Jugulo-omo- hyoid lymph nodes), may be bilateral
- Splaying of larynx (widening) may be present
- Laryngeal cartilage may be tender
- Extralaryngeal spread

Glottic Cancer

This is the most common type of laryngeal cancer accounting for about 50 to 75 percent of all laryngeal cancers (Templar 1987). Its symptoms appear early as the lesion interferes with voice and this calls for early medical attention. It often involves the anterior part of the vocal cord. Lymphatic spread occurs only in advanced stage.

Sites
- Membranous cord
- Anterior commisure
- Posterior commisure.

Spread
- **(a)** *Local:* It spreads in the beginning in the Reinke's space, which is a potential space between the vocal ligament and margin of the true vocal cord. It can extend anteriorly to the anterior commisure and can extend to opposite cord. Posterior commisure involvement is rare. Advanced lesions involve the vocalis muscle and the vocal ligament. It can extend to the ventricle and supraglottis above and/or subglottis below without cord fixation (T2). Growth extending posteriorly can involve the rim of vocal process and then the arytenoid cartilages and the crico-arytenoid joint. It can finally cause vocal cord fixation due to involvement of the deep laryngeal muscles (T3).
- **(b)** *Lymph node metastasis* is rare and can involve the 'Delphian node' due to anterior commisure. If the tumor involves the laryngeal cartilage, and escapes the confinement of the larynx, it is considered advanced (T4).

A transglottic tumor is defined as the malignant tumor involves the paraglottic space. It extends supraglottis above and subglottic below by more than 10 mm. These tumors have a high incidence with the laryngeal cartilage invasion with extra-laryngeal spread. (Lamb 1983).

Clinical Features of Glottic Tumors

Symptoms

- Persistent hoarseness which is progressive is cardinal feature of glottic cancer.
- Cough may occur due to aspiration
- Hemoptysis is rare and it is an advanced symptom which occurs if subglottis is involved.
- Dyspnea and stridor are due to advanced lesions causing impaired mobility of both cords and fixation of both cords. Very rarely it may be due to a large bulky lesion that occupies most of the subglottis.

Signs

Indirect Laryngoscopy

- Slight irregular thickening or roughening is seen on the vocal cord in the early stages (Fig. 73.7). This is surrounded by area of hyperemia. The characteristic lesion has a whitish cauliflower appearance. Sometimes there may be whitish area of superficial ulceration. Area surrounding by hyperkeratosis may be present. Glottic lesions tend to be proliferative rather than ulcerative and often seen in the membraneous cord in its free edge. It may extend to the anterior commissure and other vocal cord (Fig. 73.8).
- Glottic chink may be compromised
- Mobility of cords may be restricted or fixed.

Neck: Look for:

- Laryngeal splaying
- Laryngeal tenderness

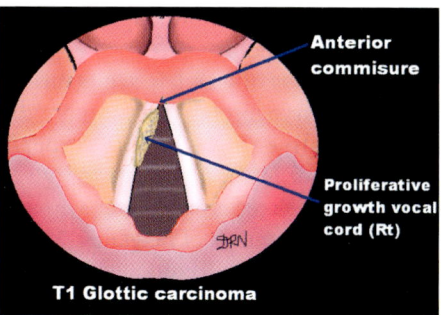

Fig. 73.7: Showing early proliferative tumor of the right vocal cord

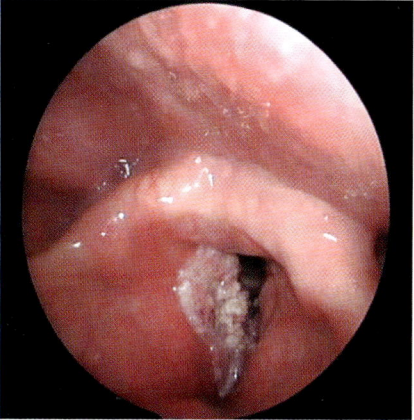

Fig. 73.8: Endoscopic picture of verrucous carcinoma of the glottis

- Extralaryngeal spread
- Lymph nodes metastases are rare. It occurs if the growth extends to the anterior or posterior commissure or if it involves the supraglottis/subglottis or laryngeal cartilages.

Subglottic Cancer

- Primary subglottic tumors are rare (1 to 5%).
- 80 percent of the cases are diagnosed as T3, T4 at the time of initial diagnosis. They often present with large tumors associated with cord fixation, impending airway obstruction.

- Patients present with cough, hemoptysis, dyspnea or stridor.
- Hoarseness is often a late symptom.
- Indirect laryngoscopy shows more diffuse proliferative growth with superficial ulcerations in the subglottis (Fig. 73.9). Surrounding area is raised over a broad area. They are generally not fungating. More than 30 percent have fixed vocal cords on presentation (Table 73.2).
- Cervical metastasis—Through the cricothyroid membrane to the paratracheal nodes. Incidence of metastasis is high.
- It has a very poor prognosis.

Investigations

- Plain X-ray
  - *AP/ Lateral*: Assess the patency of the laryngeal airway and the extent of mass in the larynx.
- *Chest X-ray*: To rule out pulmonary metastasis, signs of aspiration pneumonia, second primary (bronchogenic), pulmonary status for surgical intervention, coexistent pulmonary tuberculosis, mediastinal widening, etc.
- Laryngogram/tomogram

- *CT scan*: Helps in assessment of the extent of the growth, tumor volume and laryngeal cartilage/ extralaryngeal spread or involvement of cervical/ mediastinal lymph nodes (Fig 73.10).
- *FNAC:* Of the clinically suspected metastatic node to confirm metastases.
- *Microlaryngoscopy with biopsy:* Histopathological confirmation is mandatory before radical treatment. Supravital staining (toluidine blue) helps in taking a more representative biopsy especially if the lesion is small and suspicious.

TNM Staging

- Stage I, II: Good prognosis
- Stage III, IV: Poor prognosis

T staging for cancer of the larynx (AJCC 2002):

- TX Primary tumor cannot be assessed
- T0 No evidence of primary tumor
- Tis Carcinoma in situ

Supraglottis

- T1 Tumor limited to one subsite of supraglottis with normal vocal cord mobility.
- T2 Tumor invades mucosa of more than one adjacent subsite of supraglottis or glottis or

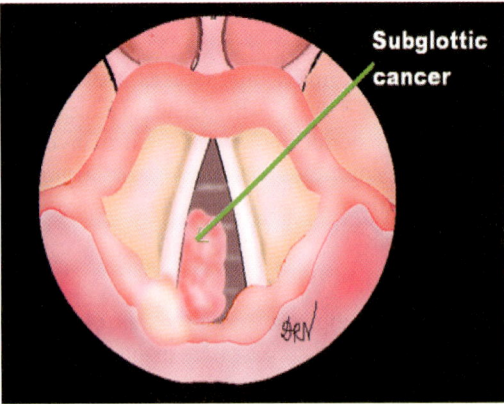

Fig. 73.9: Showing proliferative mass in the subglottis

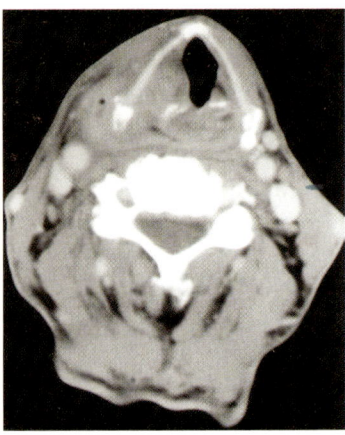

Fig. 73.10: Axial CT scan showing involvement of right paraglottic space by malignant growth

Table 73.2: Difference between fixed and paralyzed vocal cord (Watkinson et al)

Fixed vocal cord	Paralyzed vocal cord
• May have some obvious swelling around the cricoarytenoid joint	• No swelling
• Aryepiglottic fold may occupy some usual position and may be unaltered in appearance unless involved by the growth	• Aryepiglottic fold is paralyzed and sags forward and inward with its cartilage of Wrisberg.
• Active arytenoid cartilage approaches but does not displace that on the affected side. Any excursion of movement is incomplete.	• The arytenoids cartilage on paralyzed side is pushed aside by the sound and over-abducted healthy cord during phonation. (As the paralyzed cord in time gets fixed from disuse, this diagnostic point has a greater positive than negative value).
• If the cord is quite immobile, its fixation may not correspond in position with any recognized form of laryngeal palsy.	• The cord is fixed in midline or paramedian position.
• Jerky movements of the cord	• If the interarytenoid muscle retains any power and twitches the arytenoids cartilage on the paralyzed side slightly inwards, it shows that the passive mobility of articulation and is a reliable means of excluding joint disease.
	• If the position of the cord is at first median and then paramedian then it is a nerve lesion.
• Absence of other neurological symptoms and signs.	• Presence of central or peripheral lesion that can produce paralysis.
• No change of position by manipulation	• By pressing the arytenoid cartilage with a large probe with recent paralysis, absence of fixation can be proved.
• Fixation may be due to mass effect, involvement of muscles, joint or the nerve as in case of malignancy or arthritis.	• Purely a neurological condition

region outside the supraglottis (e.g. mucosa of base of tongue, vallecula, medial wall of pyriform sinus) without fixation of the larynx
• T3 Tumor limited to larynx with vocal cord fixation and/or invades any of the following: postcricoid area, preepiglottic tissues, paraglottic space, and/or minor thyroid cartilage erosion (e.g. inner cortex)
• T4a Tumor invades through the thyroid cartilage and/or invades tissues beyond the larynx (e.g. trachea, soft tissues of neck including deep extrinsic muscle of the tongue, strap muscles, thyroid, or esophagus)
• T4b Tumor invades prevertebral space, encases carotid artery, or invades mediastinal structures

Glottis

• T1 Tumor limited to the vocal cord(s) (may involve anterior or posterior commissure) with normal mobility
• T1a Tumor limited to one vocal cord

- T1b Tumor involves both vocal cords
- T2 Tumor extends to supraglottis and/or subglottis, or with impaired vocal cord mobility
- T3 Tumor limited to larynx with vocal cord fixation
- T4a Tumor invades cricoid or thyroid cartilage and/or invades tissues beyond the larynx (e.g. trachea, soft tissues of neck including deep extrinsic muscles of the tongue, strap muscles, thyroid, or esophagus)
- T4b Tumor invades prevertebral space, encases carotid artery or invades mediastinal structures

Subglottis

- T1 Tumor limited to the subglottis
- T2 Tumor extends to vocal cord(s) with normal or impaired mobility
- T3 Tumor limited to larynx with vocal cord fixation
- T4a Tumor invades cricoid or thyroid cartilage and/or invades tissues beyond the larynx (e.g. trachea, soft tissues of neck including deep extrinsic muscles of the tongue, strap muscles, thyroid, or esophagus)
- T4b Tumor invades prevertebral space, encases carotid artery, or involves mediastinal structures

Treatment

- Modalities of treatment for laryngeal cancer are:
  - Surgery
  - Radiotherapy
  - Chemotherapy
- If patient has stridor with severe dyspnea, tracheostomy is done to relieve obstruction before the definitive treatment is planned. This is best avoided as it can give rise to stomal recurrence.

Treatment Depends on the Stage of Tumor

- *Stage I & II*: **Organ preservation** techniques are employed.
  - Radiotherapy or Conservation laryngectomy or laser excision.
- *Stage III & IV*: **Combined modality** of treatment with
  - Surgery (total laryngectomy with neck dissection) followed by radical radiotherapy or
  - Radical radiotherapy followed by surgery for salvage.

Radiotherapy

- *Curative:* 6500 grays/30 fraction/ 5 to 6 weeks.
- *Palliative:* Less radiation

Surgery

- Total laryngectomy/ near total laryngectomy (with partial pharyngectomy if paraglottic space is involved) are often done. **Near total laryngectomy** leaves one functioning arytenoid and healthy subglottic mucosa which is used to reconstruct a dynamic shunt connecting the trachea that can produce aspiration free voice. Search for speech therapists is not important in such cases to rehabilitate the voice.
- **Conservation laryngectomy** or laser excision is employed in early stages (Figs 73.11a and b)
- Modified neck dissection/ functional/ selective neck dissection is done to tackle lymph node and lymph bearing structures.

Chemotherapy

- Neoadjuvant chemotherapy/concomitant radiotherapy (simultaneous radiotherapy and chemotherapy) has been tried with curative intension with **organ preservation.**
- Chemotherapy alone—Palliative

Speech Rehabilitation after Laryngectomy

- **Esophageal speech:** This is instituted by 3rd to 6th week postoperatively. Speech therapists play a crucial role in rehabilitation by this method. The technique of swallowing the air to produce voice can be learnt who takes time to master this method. Unmotivated patients do not persevere learning to talk by this method should be encouraged for tracheoesophageal puncture and voice for speech rehabilitation.

- **Electronic larynx:** Patients who cannot develop after extensive efforts including tracheo-esophageal puncture may use electronic (artificial) larynx.

- **Surgical voice restoration:** Surgically shunts are created between the trachea and the esophagus to shunt the air into the neopharynx to produce voice. Most popular method is tracheoesophageal puncture with **Blom-Singer's prosthesis**. Details are described under surgeries of the pharynx and larynx.

Verrucous Carcinoma (Fig. 73.8)

This is a rare tumor in the larynx and is more frequently seen on the oral cavity. It was first described by Ackermann in 1948. It is relatively non-aggressive tumor which seldom metastasis in the neck. It often involves the supraglottis or the glottis. It appears as fungating, papillomatous, saggy grayish white neoplasm. They are histologically characterized by well differentiated keratinizing squamous epithelium arranged in compressed invaginating folds. It has a warty papillary surface. Cleft between the adjacent capillary folds can be traced to the depth of the tumor. Infiltration is on a broad base with pushing margins against the stroma containing prominent inflammatory reaction. Usual pattern of squamous cell carcinoma is absent. Treatment is wide excision with normal tissue. Depending on the extent of the growth cordectomy or excision or hemilaryngectomy may be done and in advanced malignancy total laryngectomy may be done. Hybrid variety may have foci of poorly differentiated non-verrucous carcinoma. Radiotherapy is generally contraindicated for the fear of anaplastic transformation.

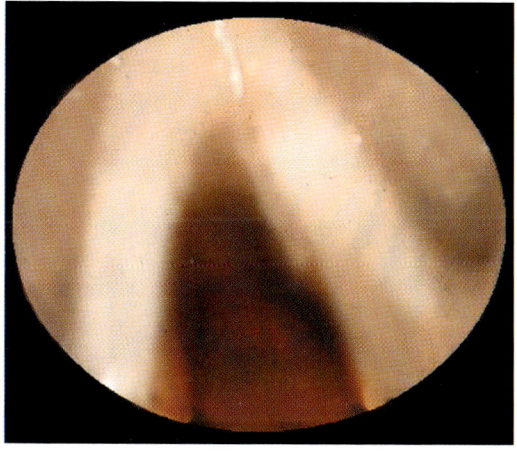
A

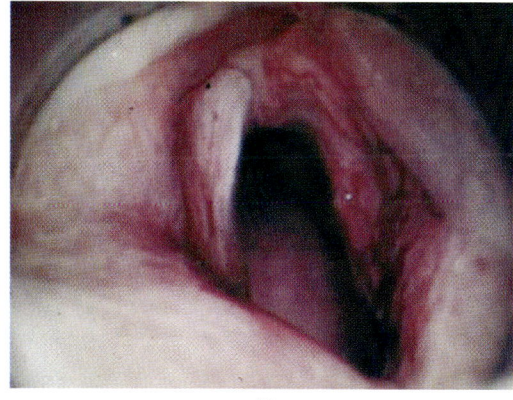
B

Figs 73.11a and b: (a) Showing early glottic malignancy. (b) Showing endoscopic view of larynx in the same patient following conservation laryngectomy and laryngoplasty

74

Foreign Body in the Airway

FOREIGN BODY IN THE LARYNX

Incidence

- Rare
- Usually sharp foreign body gets impacted (Fig. 74.1)
- Large foreign body like boluses of food are always fatal.

Symptoms

- Dyspnea
- Violent cough
- Hoarseness or aphonia
- Stridor.

Complications

Perichondritis and stenosis of larynx.

Treatment

Heimlich maneuver can be done by performing abdominal thrusts involves a rescuer standing behind a patient and using their hands to exerts pressure on the bottom of the diaphragm as a first aid. If still chocking persists or unable to remove patient has to undergo

1. Removal by direct laryngoscope
2. Laryngofissure
3. Tracheostomy or laryngotomy
4. Systemic antibiotics.

FOREIGN BODY IN TRACHEA AND BRONCHI

- This can lodge anywhere after in the tracheo-bronchial tree after passing the larynx
- Most commonly in the right bronchus because it is more wide and more in line with the trachea.

Etiology

- *Age:* More common in children (1 to 4 years)
- *Accidental:* Sudden deep inspiration during swallowing due to fright/ shock/ laughter/ sneezing, etc.

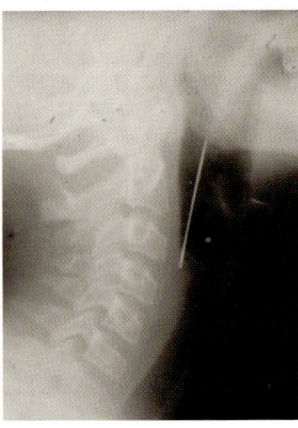

Fig. 74.1: Soft tissue X-ray neck lateral view showing linear long radiao-opaque foreign body with an eye in the lower end (needle)

- *Altered sensorium (reduced protective reflexes):* Alcoholics, drugs, head injury, epileptic fits, anesthesia, etc.
- Psychiatric patients

Types of Foreign Body (Table 74.1)

1. Vegetative foreign body
2. Non-vegetative foreign body

Site of Impaction

- Depends on the size and shape
  - *Large FB*: Larynx/ trachea
  - *Small/ thin FB*: Trachea/ bronchus
- Bronchial FB is more common in the right side because it is
  - More in line with trachea
  - More wide
  - *Right lungs larger*: Bigger air intake during inspiration causing suction effect.

Pathogenesis

No obstruction

- Tend to become chronic
- Vegetable foreign body can produce tracheitis, bronchitis, pneumonia
- Non-vegetable foreign body can cause granuloma formation which in turn can give rise to hemoptysis and pneumonia.
  - Consolidation on chest X-ray.

Partial obstruction
  - *Foreign body in the larynx:* Hoarseness or stridor.
  - *Tracheobronchial foreign body:* Partial obstruction in the bronchus produces 'Valvular obstruction' allowing air into the lungs during inspiration but traps air in the lungs due to expiratory obstruction. This gives rise to emphysema, emphysematous bullae and if they rupture it causes pneumothorax (Fig. 74.2).

Complete obstruction
  - *Larynx and trachea*: Choking, cyanosis, death.
  - *Bronchial*: Collapse of the lung (Fig. 74.3).

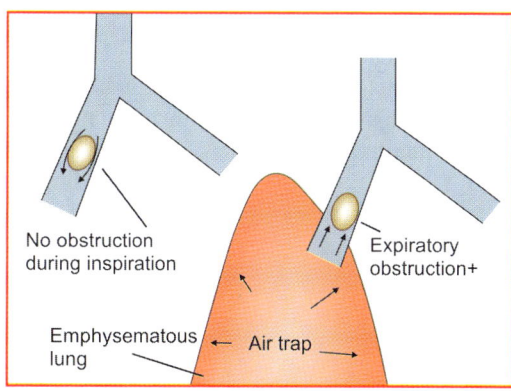

Fig. 74.2: Partial obstruction

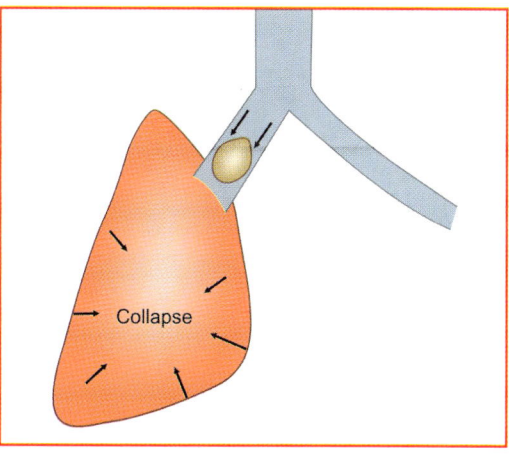

Fig. 74.3: Atelectastis due to complete obstruction

Table 74.1: Types of foreign body	
Vegetable	*Non-vegetable*
• More toxic	• Less irritant
• Hygroscopic: Foreign body swells and symptoms may increase later	• May become a chronic FB
	• Granuloma-hemoptysis
• Examples: Seeds, peas, nuts, wooden pieces, fruits	• Examples: Plastic pieces- toys/ buttons, metals-pins, marbles, etc.

Clinical Features

Symptoms

Initial symptoms

- Bouts of cough and dyspnea
- Blood stained expectoration (latent period).

General symptoms

1. Cough with or without dyspnea
2. Expectoration
3. Asthmatic wheeze is common.

Signs

- Signs of hypoxemia
  - Rapid pulse – Tachypnea
  - Tachycardia – Cyanosis
- Stridor
- Auscultation
  - Unilateral in bronchial foregin body
  - Clicks, wheeze, etc. during particular phase of respiration
  - Features of collapse/ emphysema/ abscess/ pneumothorax, etc.

Differential Diagnosis of Chronic Foreign Body

- Pulmonary tuberculosis
- Acute tracheobronchitis
- Pneumonia
- Bronchiectasis with lung abscess

Investigations

1. Soft tissue X-Ray neck (AP, Lateral) and chest x-ray

- Opaque objects can be seen (Fig 74.4)
- Translucent object when suspected shows :
  1. Atelectasis
  2. Obstructive emphysema
  3. Mediastinal shift
  4. Consolidation of the lung
  5. Abnormal position of the diaphragm
2. Bronchoscopy

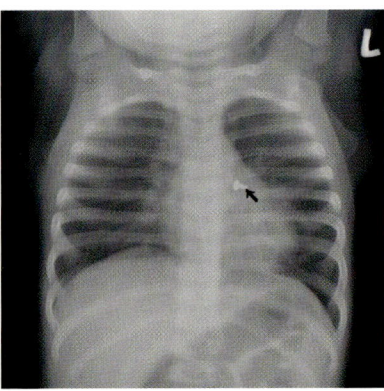

Fig. 74.4: Foreign body in the left bronchus (arrow)

Treatment

Heimlich maneuver can be done for tracheal foreign bodies.

1. Removal through the rigid bronchoscope. Flexible bronchoscope has a limited role in removal of foreign body bronchus. If the foreign body is bigger than the lumen of the rigid bronchoscope, the foreign body is held with a suitable foreign body grasping forceps and is removed along with the scope. If the foreign body cannot be removed with a forceps basketting or removal with a Fogarty catheter may be tried.
2. Tracheostomy
3. *Removal by thoracotomy*: This approach is rarely indicated and is used as a last resort. Penetrating foreign body or impacted foreign body in the segmental bronchiole may have to be removed with this approach.

Complications

Lung complications
  - Consolidation
  - Collapse
  - Emphysema
  - Emphysematous bullae
  - Pneumothorax
  - Hemoptysis

POINTS TO REMEMBER

1. Foreign body commonly lodges in right bronchus.
2. Vegetable foreign body causes more reaction.
3. Partial bronchial obstruction causes emphysema.
4. Total bronchial obstruction causes collapse.
5. Bouts of cough and dyspnea are presenting symptom.
6. X-ray neck AP/lateral and chest X-ray can show opaque foreign body.
7. Foreign body in the bronchus is removed by rigid/flexible bronchoscopy.

Stridor

Definition

Stridor is an abnormal, harsh, high-pitched, turbulent musical breathing sound caused by partial obstruction in the larynx/ tracheobronchial tree and is usually associated with dyspnea. Stridor indicates an emergency and should always be evaluated immediately.

OTHER TYPES OF NOISY BREATHING

Stertor

Harsh, low-pitched turbulent sound during respiration due to partial obstruction proximal to the larynx and may be associated with dyspnea. Some consider it as part of stridor.

Snoring

Same as stertor which occurs only during sleep.

> **Stridor: Things to know**
> - Types
> - Pitch
> - Site of obstruction
> - Severity
> - Causes

Types of Stridor
- Inspiratory (croup)
  - Glottic lesions
  - Supraglottic lesions
  - Hypopharyngeal lesions involving supraglottis / glottis
- *Expiratory (wheeze)*: Seen in lesions involving
  - Distal trachea
  - Bronchi
- *Biphasic*: See in lesions of
  - Subglottis
  - Proximal trachea.

Severity of Stridor
- Mild
  - Only on unaccustomed exertion
  - Deep breathing.
- Moderate
  - On minimal exertion
  - Not able to do day-to-day activities.
- Severe
  - Even at rest
  - Accessory muscles are active
  - Recession of intercostal spaces is present
  - Features of hypoxemia like tachycardia, tachypnea, cyanosis, irritability and restlessness.

Pitch
  - Low pitch–Indicates proximal obstruction
  - High pitch–Indicates distal obstruction

Site of Obstruction

This can be clinically assessed by the following.

- Type of stridor, Example: Inspiratory– Site of obstruction is supraglottis/ glottis
- Pitch of stridor: Example High pitch indicates distal obstruction.
- Associated symptoms: Examples:
  - Hoarseness: Larynx
  - Dysphagia/ FB sensation in throat: Hypopharynx
  - Hot-potato voice: Supraglottic/oro-pharynx.

Etiology in Children (Flow chart 75.1)

Congenital

- Proximal to larynx
  - *Nose:* Choanal atresia
  - *Tongue:* Macroglossia, hemangioma, lymphangioma, lingual thyroid, etc.
  - *Mandible:* Micrognathia.
- Laryngeal
  - *Supraglottic:* **Laryngomalacia**, cysts, tumors
  - Glottic: Webs, palsy, cyst
  - Subglottic: Stenosis, tumors

- Tracheobronchial
  - Vascular loops
  - Tracheoesophageal fistula
  - Mediastinal congenital tumors
  - Atresia, stenosis.

Acquired

Infective

- Acute epiglottitis
- Acute laryngo-tracheo-bronchitis
- Laryngeal diphtheria
- Laryngeal edema secondary to quinsy, acute tonsillitis, Ludwig's angina, retro/parapharyngeal abscess, etc.

Traumatic

- FB in upper aerodigestive tract
- Thermal
- Chemical
- Physical– (Machanical trauma like road traffic accident) RTA
- Radiation

Tumors

- Juvenile laryngeal papillomatosis
- Chondroma
- Thymoma
- Cystic hygroma

Flow chart 75.1: Etiology of stridor in children

Flow chart showing:

Stridor in children

CONGENITAL
Laryngeal causes
Laryngomalacia
Vocal cord paralysis
Subglottic stenosis
Subglottic hemangioma
Laryngeal web
Laryngocele
Mucocele of the ventricle

Extralaryngeal causes
Tracheomalacia
Cri-du-chat syndrome
Pierre Robin syndrome
Lingual thyroid
Vascular ring over trachea

ACQUIRED

INFECTIVE
Acute epiglottitis
Acute laryngo-tracheobronchitis
Laryngeal diphtheria
Edema of the larynx

NON-INFECTIVE
Neurological
Bilateral vocal cord paralysis
Neonatal tetany
Trauma
Birth injury
Foreign body
Tumors
Juvenile papilloma

Others
- *Neurological:* Bilateral vocal cord palsy
- *Allergy:* Angioneurotic edema
- Laryngismus stridulus
- Tetany
- Tetanus.

Etiology in Adults

- *Trauma:* Laryngotracheal trauma, laryngo-tracheal stenosis – RTA/ Iatrogenic, FB
- *Tumor:* Larynx, pharynx, trachea, bronchus, esophagus, thyroid, any neck/ mediastinal mass: Examples
  - Carcinoma larynx
  - Carcinoma hypopharynx
- *Infection:* TB laryngitis, neck space infections
- *Allergy:* Angioneurotic edema
- *Neurological:* Bilateral abductor palsy
  - Post-thyroidectomy/ Cardiothoracic surgery

Evaluation of a Case with Stridor

First priority is to secure the airway if it is an emergency. Detailed evaluation includes:

- Detailed history
- Clinical examination
- Investigations.

Investigations

Radiography
- *Plain X-ray neck AP/ lateral:* Look for soft tissue mass in the larynx/ hypopharynx, airway patency, prevertebral widening, etc.
- *Chest X-ray—PA/ lateral:* For assessment of pulmonary status, mediastinal widening, secondaries in the lungs, features of aspiration pneumonia, etc.
- Barium swallow with valsalva and under fluoroscopy to look for any filling defect in the postcricoid area and esophagus.
- CT scan/ MRI- neck/ mediastinum

Endoscopy
- Rigid/ flexible Laryngoscope—Caution: Can give rise to laryngospasm

- Rigid/ flexible Bronchoscope– after securing airway.

Treatment

- Conservative
- Intubation
- Cricothyroidotomy
- Tracheostomy.

Conservative

- Antibiotics– Parenteral
- Steroids–Parenteral and high dose. Example Hydrocortisone, IV 100 to 200 mg bolus dose.
- Humidification
- Mucolytics like bromhexine
- O_2 administration
- IV fluids
- *Positioning:* If tongue falls back, lateral position or use of oropharyngeal airway may be useful. In laryngomalacia, stridor may reduce in prone position.
- Bronchodilators may be given if there is bronchospasm
- No sedation till the airway is secured.

Intubation (Table 75.1)

A suitable size endotracheal tube is introduced into trachea through oral cavity orotracheal or through the nose (naso-tracheal) using MacIntosh larynmgoscope.

Tracheostomy (Table 75.2)

Discussed in the next chapter.

Cricothyroidotomy

Open the cricothyroid membrane in the midline by a:

- Large bore needle or stab incision and O_2 administration by catheter
- Tracheostomy to be performed at the earliest.

Complication: Subglottic stenosis.

Other methods of airway management:

- Transtracheal O_2 administration using a large gauge Gelco needle, which is introduced percutaneously into the trachea.
- Minitracheostomy
- Percutaneous tracheostomy.

Table 75.1: Advantages and disadvantages of intubation	
Advantages	*Disadvantages*
Easy and quick in some cases	Difficult intubation should be suspected in cases with trismus, mandibular fracture and oropharyngeal supraglottic tumors. Prolonged intubation can cause stenosis of subglottis trachea. Morbidity is more RT feeds: Patients cannot take oral feeds Difficult to maintain the patency of the tube Tracheobronchial toileting is difficult Airway resistance and deadspace is increased

Table 75.2: Advantages and disadvantages of tracheostomy	
Advantages	*Disadvantages*
• By passes proximal obstruction • Can be maintained for prolonged periods • Maintainance easy • Morbidity: Less • Airway resistance reduced • Dead space reduced • Tracheobronchial toilet better • Oral feeds can be given as swallow is not affected.	• More time to secure airway • Surgical procedure • Major in children • Difficult in children • Expertise is necessary • Complications of surgery may occur

For details on tracheostomy, please refer to the Chapter 'Tracheostomy'.

POINTS TO REMEMBER

1. Stridor is an abnormal harsh, high pitched turbulent musical breathing sound that occurs due to partial obstruction in the larynx and tracheobronchial tree.
2. Stridor indicates an emergency and should be evaluated and addressed immediately.
3. Stridor of glottic origin is always inspiratory.
4. Subglottic and proximal trachea can cause biphasic stridor.
5. Laryngomalacia is the most common congenital laryngeal condition causing stridor.

76

Tracheostomy

Definition

- *Tracheostomy*: Surgical procedure wherein a stoma (window) is created connecting anterior wall of trachea to the exterior.
- *Tracheotomy*: Opening the trachea
- *Laryngotomy*: (Cricothyroidotomy/coniotomy) Opening the larynx at the cricothyroid membrane

History

- Rig Veda: 2000 BC
- Sushruta: 1000 to 600 BC
- First successful tracheostomy was reportedly done by Brasovala in the 1546 AD
- Fabricus in 1600 introduced the use of a tube
- 1799: George Washington died of an upper airway blockage on which a tracheostomy could have been performed. Though his physician knew of the procedure, he was not willing to perform his first on his first president.
- Chevalier Jackson standardized the technique in 1932.

Functions of Tracheostomy

1. Relief from upper airway obstruction as it acts as a *Bypass*
2. Reduces the airway resistance which in turn reduces the force required to move the air facilitating more effective alveolar ventilation, provided the tracheostomy tube is large enough (7 size).
3. Decrease the dead space in the tracheobronchial tree which is normally 70 to 100 ml.
4. Enables the patient to swallow without reflex apnea. This is important in COPD patients.
5. Helps in better tracheobronchial toilet and provides access for medication and humidification to the tracheobronchial tree.
6. Aspiration can be prevented by cuffed tracheostomy tube
7. It provides airway for general anesthesia for various surgical procedures.
8. Prolonged assisted ventilation
9. Decrease the power of cough and thus preventing peripheral displacement of secretions by the high intrathoracic pressure.

Physiologic Alterations following Tracheostomy

1. Humidification and warming of the inspired air is affected as it bypasses the upper respiratory tract.
2. Phonation is not possible unless the stoma is temporarily occluded diverting air to the larynx.
3. Loss of olfaction.
4. Ciliary activity and tracheal mucosal integrity can be affected.

5. Tracheostomized patients are prone to atelectasis due to drying of the secretions and pulmonary infections as a result of loss of normal filtering mechanism provided by the respiratory mucosa.

6. Swallowing and coughing mechanism may be affected as the subglottic pressure cannot be built up.

Indications for Tracheostomy

- Obstructive indications
- Non-obstructive indications

Obstructive indications (Table 76.1)

Non-obstructive indications

- Assisted ventilation
- Assist tracheobronchial toilet
- Aspiration
- Anesthesia
- Alaryngeal

1. **Assisted ventilation:** Tracheostomy helps in assisting ventilation in case of alveolar hypoventilation which could be due to various causes at various levels.
   - *Higher center, comatosed*: Head injury, CVA, encephalitis, etc.
   - *Respiratory center*: Bulbar paralysis, barbiturate poisoning, OP poisoning, drug intoxications
   - *Anterior horn cells/nerves*: Polio, poly-neuritis, cervical spine injury
   - *Myoneural junction*: Tetanus
   - *Respiratory muscles*: Myasthenia gravis
   - *Chest wall*: # ribs, pain
   - *Lungs*: COPD, status asthmaticus, collapse, emphysema, pneumothorax, etc.

2. Protection of lower respiratory tract from aspiration: Aspiration could be due to various causes like:
   (a) Bilateral combined paralysis of the vocal cord
   (b) Unconscious patient
   (c) As a complication following laryngeal conservation surgery like supraglottic laryngectomy
   (d) Tracheoesophageal fistula

3. Assist tracheobronchial toilet, insufflations, humidification, especially in cases with COPD.

4. It provides airway for general anesthesia for major head and neck and maxillofacial surger-ies when obstruction is anticipated or to avoid the endotracheal tube in the nose and the throat.

5. Permanent tracheostomy following total or near-total laryngectomy for providing airway.

Indications for Tracheostomy in Children

Local Causes

- **Laryngeal:** Congenital subglottic stenosis, laryngeal web causing obstruction, hemangioma of the subglottis, acute epiglottitis, acute laryngotracheobronchitis, laryngomalacia, subglottic edema, foreign body in the larynx, etc.

- **Above the larynx:** Micrognathia, Pierre-Robin syndrome, hamartoma and teratoma of the nasopharynx and the pharynx, meningo-encephalocele,

- **Below the larynx:** Tracheomalacia, tracheal hemangioma, cystic hygroma compressing the trachea, etc.

Systemic Causes

Arnold-chiari malformations, VSD, ASD, Fallot's tetrology, congenital myopathies, congenital multiple neurofibromatosis, anoxic encephalo-pathy, bulbar poliomyelitis

Technique

Position

- Place a sand bag under and between the shoulders to achieve a position of extension of neck and extension of head at the atlanto-occipital joint. This helps in bringing the trachea forwards (Fig. 76.1).

Anesthesia

- Local or general anesthesia may be given.

Table 76.1: Obstructive indications for tracheostomy

Obstructive indications	Oral	Pharyngeal	Laryngeal	Tracheobronchial	Mediastinal/extraluminal
Congenital	Macroglossia, micrognathia, congenital tumors	Macroglossia, Micrognathia, Congenital tumors, Lingual thyroid	Laryngomalacia, stenosis, web, cyst, congenital tumors	Atresia, tracheo-esophageal fistula	Abnormal vessels, mediastinal tumors
Inflammation	Ludwigs angina	Acute tonsillitis, quinsy, OSAS	Acute epiglottitis, ALTBS, diphtheria, laryngeal edema	ALTBS	Mediastinitis, pneumomediastinum, retro/parapharyngeal abscess
Traumatic	# mandible, edema tongue, hematoma, corrosive poisoning	Hematoma, corrosive poisoning, FB	FB, LTT, LTS, corrosive poisoning	FB	Hematoma, pneumomediastinum
Neoplasm	Ca. tongue	Ca. base tongue, tonsils, hypopharynx	Ca. larynx, juvenile laryngeal papillomatosis	Ca. trachea, bronchus	Thyroid malignancy, Mediastinal tumors, Lymphoma
Neurological	Unconscious	Cricopharyngeal spasm-aspiration Pharyngeal pouch	Bilateral abductor palsy-post thyroidectomy and CTS, aspiration and secretional obstruction		

Key to abbreviations:
ALTBS : Acute Laryngotracheal Bronchitis
FB : Foreign Body
LTS : Laryngotracheal Stenosis
LTT : Laryngotracheal Trauma
CTS : Cardiothoracic Surgery
Ca : Carcinoma

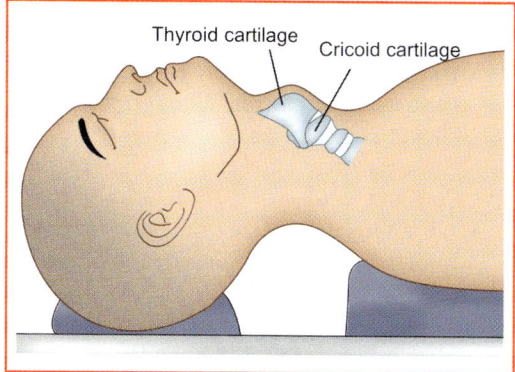

Fig. 76.1: Positioning of the patient in tracheostomy

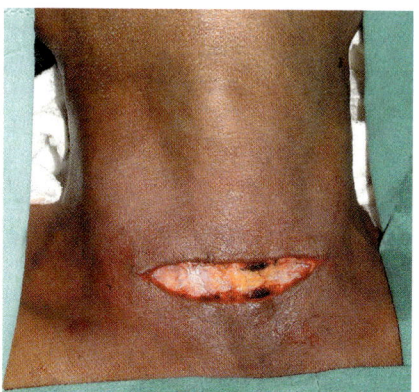

Fig. 76.2: Horizontal skin incision along the skin crease two fingers above the sternal notch

- If local anesthesia is contemplated, the area of infiltration of 2 percent lignocaine is between the cricoid and the suprasternal notch and between the two sternomastoid muscles. In emergency tracheostomy when there is associated emphysema, infiltration is done till the laryngeal prominence (Adam's apple) favoring a midline incision.

Incision

- Emergency tracheostomy: In acute emergency situations, a vertical incision in the midline from cricoid to suprasternal notch is made. Other landmark to be kept in mind is the thyroid notch which helps us to stay in the midline.
- In elective or semi-emergency cases a transverse incision is preferred along the skin crease approximately two fingers from the sternal notch or at the midpoint between cricoid and suprasternal notch (Fig. 76.2).

Dissection of Deeper Layers

All the deeper layers are dissected vertically in the midline to reduce bleeding using Mayo's scissors. The layers encountered are:

1. Superficial fascia with its fatty and membranous layers is first dissected. The anterior communicating vein may be encountered which can be cauterized or ligated. The use of diathermy and bipolar cautery helps in preventing the bleeding during the procedure.
2. Investing layer of deep cervical fascia is divided and retracted laterally
3. Strap muscles are separated in the midline and are retracted using Langenbeck's retractor (small size). Alternatively a double hook retractor may be used (Fig. 76.3).
4. Pretracheal layer covering isthmus of thyroid is divided to expose the isthmus of the thyroid gland (Fig. 76.4).

Isthmus of Thyroid

This may be dealt in one of the following three methods:

1. Retract the isthmus upwards using blunt single hook tracheal retractor (Isthmus hook).
2. Divide the isthmus between clamps and later suture the stumps
3. Expose trachea either below or above the isthmus

   The inferior thyroid veins may supply the isthmus and may have to be retracted or ligated.

Exposure of Trachea

- Pretracheal layer covering trachea should be dissected and retracted to expose the trachea

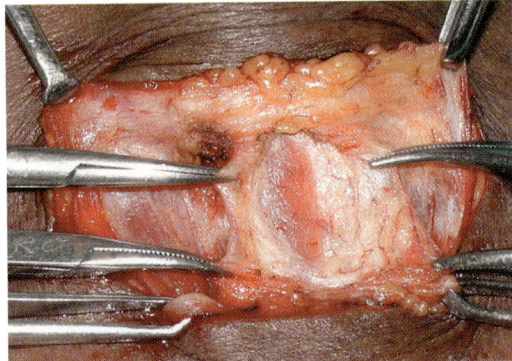

Fig. 76.3: Showing the skin flap being retracted and strap muscles being exposed after dividing investing layer of deep cervical fascia

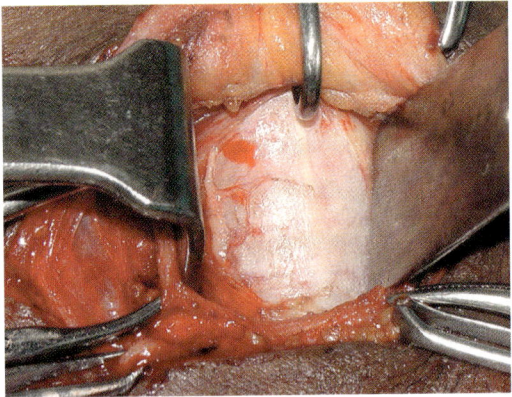

Fig. 76.4: Note that the isthmus of the thyroid gland is being retracted using a single hook blunt tracheal retractor to expose the pre-tracheal fascia and the trachea. Strap muscles have been retracted laterally

- Palpate for cricoid cartilage and it may be stabilized using the sharp single hook tracheal retractor (cricoid hook)
- Inject 4 percent lignocaine into the trachea which will anesthetize the tracheal mucosa and also help in confirming that we are on the airway.

Opening the Trachea

- The trachea is slit opened vertically or horizontally in children. In children the

cartilage should not be removed. In adults a window is often created between 3th to 5th tracheal rings by removing part of the cartilage. The horizontal cut on the trachea should not be given too laterally as it may cause recurrent laryngeal nerve injury (Figs. 76.5 and 76.6).

- An appropriate size tracheostomy tube (preferably cuffed) is inserted and inflated (Fig. 76.7).
- The tube is stabilized in position using straps after flexing the neck. The collar of the tube may be sutured to skin especially if the tube

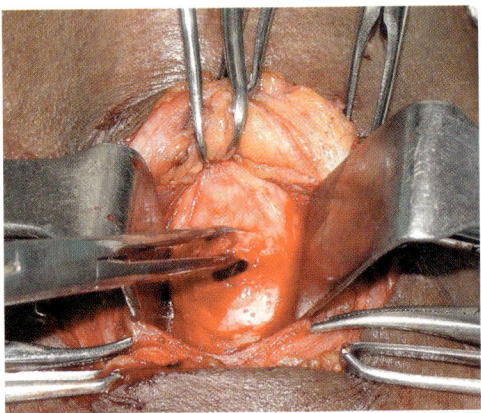

Fig. 76.5: Note that the trachea is opened while the cricoid is fixed with a sharp tracheal hook and the thyroid isthmus is being retracted with the blunt hook

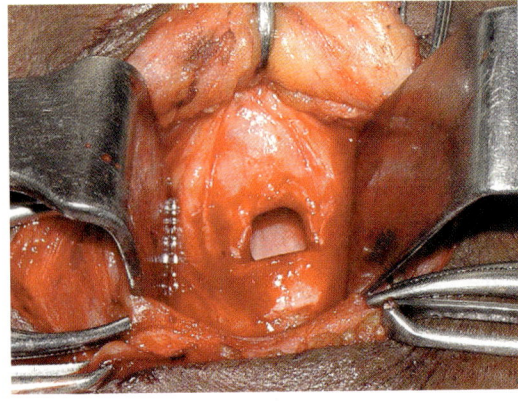

Fig. 76.6: Anterior tracheal wall being opened after removing a piece of cartilage

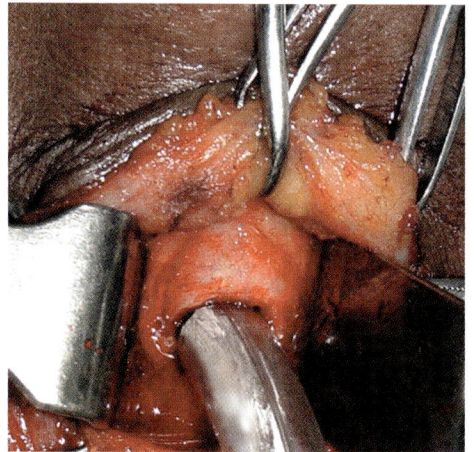

Fig. 76.7: Insertion of portex tracheostomy tube

is connected to ventilator to prevent traction and dislodgement of the tube.

- Wound closure is not done to prevent surgical emphysema.
- Assisted ventilation may be initially necessary to prevent apnea.

Postoperative Care

- 'Aseptic precautions', 'Barrier nursing'
- Tube position and patency should be checked in regular intervals
- Cuff management– Cuff should be deflated for 5 minutes every hour if possible to prevent tracheal stenosis.
- First change of tube should be done only after the tract has formed (3 days). In emergency situations within <72 hours after the procedure, the neck should be extended, another tube should be kept ready and then using tracheal dilator, the tube is changed quickly.

- Subsequently the tube should be changed once 7 days to prevent formation of granulations in the stoma.
- Wound should be dressed to prevent maceration from secretions and skin erosion from tube straps
- Tracheobronchial toilet is done regularly using suction tube with 'Y' connector.
- Antibiotics, mucolytics, analgesics and other supportive care

Types of Tracheostomy (Table 76.2)

Tracheostomy tubes

Metallic

- Jackson's (Fig. 76.8a)
- Fuller's (Fig. 76.8b)

Plastic (Portex)

- Cuffed (Fig. 76.9)
- Non-cuffed
- Single cannula
- Double cannula

Complications of Tracheostomy

Immediate (ABCDE)

- **A**pnea or aspiration
- **B**leeding
- **C**ollapse of the lungs
- **D**amage to adjacent structures like larynx, esophagus, thyroid, vessels, recurrent laryngeal nerves, etc.
- **E**mbolism – 'air'.

Table 76.2: Types of tracheostomy				
Timing	**Duration**	**Site**	**Technique**	**Age**
• Elective	• Temporary	• High	• Anterior wall-skin	• Adult
• Emergency	• Permanent	• Mid	-Slit/ window/ 'U' or 'H' flap	• Pediatric
• Semi-emergency	-Tracheal fenestration	• Low	• End-skin	
	-Postlaryngectomy			

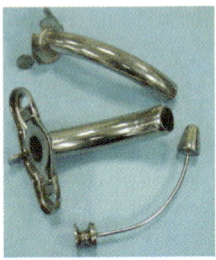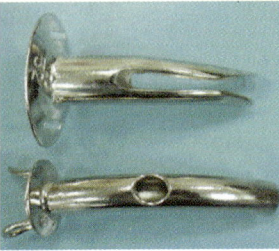

Figs 76.8a and b: Metallic tracheostomy tubes (a) Jackson's type with inner and outer tubes and obturator, (b) Fuller's bivalved tracheostomy tube

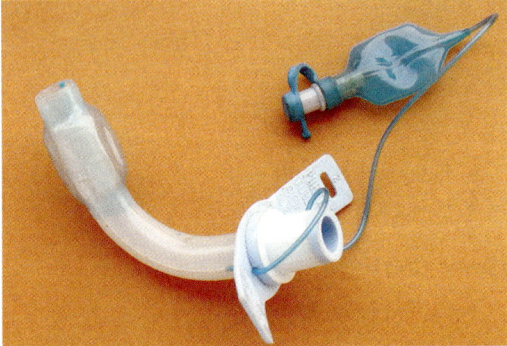

Fig. 76.9: Portex cuffed tracheostomy tube

Apnea may occur once the tube is in position in emergency tracheostomy for prolonged obstruction. This is due to sudden wash-out of the accumulated carbon dioxide which was stimulating the respiratory center.

Intermediate

- Tube obstruction
- Tube displacement
- Tracheal erosion
- Surgical emphysema
- Wound infection
- Tracheitis, tracheobronchitis, lung infections
- Granulation tissue, bleeding
- Dysphagia– Subglottic pressure, pain, cuff.

Late

- Difficult decannulation
- Tracheomalacia

- Tracheocutaneous fistula
- Tracheoesophageal fistula (especially if both inflated cuff + nasogastric tube is present)
- Tracheoarterial/venous fistula
- Laryngotracheal stenosis
- Scar
- Foreign body (Part of the tracheostomy tube may get separated and dislodged into tracheobronchial tree).

Decanulation

This is a process of weaning the patient off the tracheostomy tube. Before decanulation any proximal obstruction should be ruled out by taking X-ray of the neck, AP and lateral view, chest X-ray to visualize the tracheal lumen below and above the tracheostoma. Direct or indirect laryngoscopy and occasionally a tracheobronch-oscopy may be required to rule out proximal obstruction. In children arterial blood gas analysis may be required.

A Fuller's tube tracheostomy is inserted or a fenestra is created in a plastic tracheostomy tube which is inserted and corked using a rubber cork. Observe the patient for 48 hours. If the patient is able to tolerate corking for 48 hours or more, then the tube is removed and the wound is strapped or sutured.

Other Methods of Airway Management

1. Endotracheal intubation
2. *Minitracheostomy/ cricothyroidotomy*: The skin and the cricothyroid membrane is opened by a one cm stab incision and a 4 mm endotracheal tube is passed for ventilation. This should be followed by a regular tracheostomy as infection can occur to the cricoid cartilage causing subglottic stenosis.
3. *Percutaneous tracheostomy*: This was first described by Toye et al in 1969. It is a safe alternative to standard tracheostomy and is a rapid procedure associated with less bleeding. A one cm transverse skin incision between the first and third tracheal ring is made

followed by dissection of the pretracheal tissues using a curved artery forceps. Once the trachea is reached a 14 gauge IV canula with needle is passed into the trachea below the 2nd tracheal ring and its position is confirmed by aspiration. The needle is removed and a Slendiger guide wire is inserted through the canula. The canula is then removed and 30F Teflon dilator is passed over the wire followed by 20F. Once a suitable stoma is created after dilating, a tracheostomy tube is advanced and the guide wire with the dilator is removed.

POINTS TO REMEMBER

1. First successful tracheostomy was reported by Brasovala in 1546 AD.
2. Fabricius in 16th century introduced the use of tracheostomy tube.
3. Chevalier Jackson stadardized the technique of tracheostomy in 1932.
4. Tracheostomy decreases the dead space of the airway.
5. It protects the lower respiratory tracts from aspiration.
6. Fuller's tracheostomy tube is commonly used for decannulation and phonation.
7. The inner metallic tracheostomy tube is longer than the outer tracheostomy tube to prevent clogging of the outer tube.
8. Portex cuffed tracheostomy tube is used for preventing aspiration and for positive pressure ventilation.

77

Common Surgical Procedures of the Pharynx and Larynx

The common surgical procedures of the pharynx and larynx include the following:

- Tonsillectomy
- Adenoidectomy
- Direct laryngoscopy
- Rigid hypopharyngoscopy
- Rigid esophagoscopy
- Microlaryngoscopy
- Rigid bronchoscopy
- Uvulo-palato-pharyngo-plasty (UPPP)
- Laser assisted uvulo-palato-plasty (LAUP)
- Oncological surgeries
  - Total laryngectomy
  - Total laryngectomy with partial pharyngectomy
  - Total laryngo-pharyngo-esophagectomy (TLPE)
  - Conservation laryngectomy
  - Commando operation.

ADENOIDECTOMY AND TONSILLECTOMY

This has been dealt with in detail in the chapter 'Diseases of the Waldeyer's ring'.

DIRECT LARYNGOSCOPY (DLS)

History

1854 - Manuel Garcia, Professor of singing made first attempt to see his own vocal cords by aid of two mirrors. He is recognized as Father of Laryngology.

1895 - Kirstein demonstrated examination of larynx without reflecting mirrors.

1907 - Chevalier Jackson published his first book on endoscopy.

1932 - Negus introduced twin light system tubes.

Types of Direct Laryngoscopy

According to Robert Leroux direct laryngoscopy is classified as:

- **Direct Heterostatic:** Where the scope is held by the examiner.
- **Direct Autostatic:** Involves autofixation of laryngoscope and hands of examiner are free for operative procedure. It is also called as Suspension Laryngoscopy.

Indications for DLS

Diagnostic

- To take biopsy for histopathological examination.
- To know the site and extent of tumor.
- In cases of cervical metastasis of unknown origin, to rule out primary in the larynx.
- Assessing laryngeal trauma, e.g. tracheal fractures or separation.
- In infants and children with noisy breathing.
- To examine hidden areas like anterior commissure, subglottis, ventricles, laryngeal surface of epiglottis.

- Vocal cord palsy of unknown cause.
- To see mobility of arytenoids with probe and diagnose cricoarytenoid joint fixation.
- In patients with hoarseness of voice when larynx is not seen properly with indirect laryngoscopy, which may be due to excessive gag reflex or over hanging epiglottis.
- As a prerequisite for bronchoscopy and esophagoscopy.

Therapeutic

- Removal of benign lesions like vocal polyp, vocal nodule, laryngeal web, cyst, papilloma (Ideally microlaryngoscopy is done for these cases).
- To remove foreign bodies in the larynx/pharynx.
- Dilatation of laryngeal stricture.
- Injection of teflon paste in vocal cords for vocal cord palsy.

Prognostic

To assess the results after surgery or radiotherapy.

Contraindications

- Cervical spine diseases like caries, dislocation, fracture, unstable spine where further manipulations can lead to quadriplegia.
- Trismus and temporomandibular joint ankylosis.
- Severe stridor, which may get aggravated.
- Aneurysm of aorta
- Acute corrosive poisoning.

Prerequisite

- Indirect laryngoscopy should be done prior to DLS and its findings should be drawn and labeled.

Investigations

- *X-ray neck (AP and lateral view)*: To know
  - Patency of airway
  - Tracheal shift

- Status of laryngeal skeleton
- Prevertebral soft tissue enlargement suggesting postcricoid growth
- Radio-opaque foreign body
- *X-ray chest*: Look for lung secondaries, pulmonary status and mediastinal widening.
- Barium swallow to rule out hypopharyngeal tumor and cricopharyngeal stricture.
- *CT scan of neck*: To know
  - Extent of laryngeal tumor especially in transglottic and subglottic tumors.
  - Site and extent of tracheal stenosis.
  - Details of soft tissue and skeletal damage in case of laryngeal trauma.
  - Relationship of mass to the great vessels of neck.
  - Evaluation of vascular, inflammatory and neoplastic lesions.
- Tomography and laryngography
  - Demonstrates pathophysiological changes.
- MRI gives information of vascular, inflammatory and neoplastic lesions.
- Non-specific investigations
  - Complete blood picture
  - Prothrombin time, activated partial thromboplastin time, bleeding time and clotting time
  - ELISA for HIV/HbsAg
  - Random blood sugar, renal function test, liver function test
  - Urine for sugar/proteins and microscopy.

Preoperative Preparation

- Preoperatively any caries, loose or capped tooth should be managed.
- Patient should be nil per oral for 4 to 6 hours.
- Premedication with atropine half hour before procedure, to reduce pharyngeal secretions intraoperatively and to prevent sinus bradycardia.
- Hypertension and diabetes should be evaluated and managed preoperatively.

Anesthesia

Newborns and children: No anesthesia is required.

Most important here is well organized and efficient team work. If required xylocaine can be used topically in children above the age of 8 years.

Jackson described few contraindications in children for GA

- Acute laryngotracheobronchitis
- Diphtheria
- Extreme dyspnea.

Adults

1. Topical

It is given in sitting position in cooperative patients. First 10 percent xylocaine spray followed by xylocaine suspension gargles followed by dropping few drops of xylocaine in larynx with help of ILS mirror. Alternatively local anesthesia can be given by holding xylocaine soaked swabs in pyriform fossae with help of laryngeal forceps (Meckenzie').

2. Local

It is achieved by superior laryngeal nerve block by injecting 1 to 2 cc of xylocaine with adrenaline 1 cm below greater cornua of hyoid on either side of neck.

3. General

It is by using small endotracheal tubes, e.g. Coplans tube.

General anesthesia is preferred because of unhurried examination.

Occasionally large tumors obstructing the airway makes intubation difficult. In such cases tracheostomy is done under local anesthesia, preliminary to direct laryngoscopy.

Position

- In past sitting position of mouret was used in adults
- Now-a-days, Boyce lying down position is used where neck is flexed and head is extended at atlanto-occipital joint with the help of pillow under shoulder and head ring under head.

Technique

In Adults

- Patient's upper lip is retracted by 1st and 2nd finger of surgeon
- Teeth are protected with gauge piece or by a teeth guard
- Lubricated endoscope is held in left hand and passed along right side of mouth
- When posterior third of tongue is reached scope is directed in midline and uvula is looked for which is the First Landmark.
- Endotracheal tube may be followed by lifting the epiglottis by lifting dorsum of tongue which is the Second Most Important Landmark.
- Teeth are never used as fulcrum.
- Beak of scope is passed beneath the epiglottis and lifted .This is called **Engagement of epiglottis**.
- Scope is advanced about 1 cm and now larynx is exposed and examined.
- Thyroid cartilage can be pressed from external surface by an assistant in case of difficulty in seeing anterior commissure and subglottis.
- Hypopharynx can be seen when scope is slided laterally on either sides.
- Head should always be in midline.
- Anterior commissure scope is used to see the hidden areas.

In Newborns and Children

- Here the technique of DLS is much simpler than in adults.
- All the structures are flexible and there is little muscular resistance. Smaller scopes are used here.
- As it is done without any anesthesia, child's head is held in proper position by an assistant who uses his right index finger as a bite block.
- Further technique is similar to as described in adults.

- Gentleness is fundamental and familiarity with the technique is mandatory.

AUTOSTATIC LARYNGOSCOPY

Autostatic laryngoscopy is also called as **Suspension Laryngoscopy.**

Suspension laryngoscope was conceived by Gustave Killian.

Advantages

- Both the hands of surgeon are free for surgical procedure.
- Tumors of large size and impacted foreign bodies can be easily removed.
- Electrocoagulation and hemostasis with sutures can be done.
- Microscope can be attached with scope for magnification and precision.

Technique

- Anesthesia: General anesthesia either small endotracheal intubation, jet ventilation or apneic technique can be used.
- Suspension apparatus is set up and patient is positioned.
- Suspension laryngoscope is introduced along the base of tongue.
- Laryngeal surface of epiglottis is engaged with tip of tongue spatula.
- Slight traction is made on suspension unit and by means of thumbscrew mouth gag, the jaws are spread open and tongue is fixed.
- After the structures are exposed, it is attached to the horizontal base of gallows by means of hooks.
- Difficulty in this procedure is to maintain the tongue in midline and exposure of anterior commissure.

HYPOPHARYNGOSCOPY

- After every direct laryngoscopy, examination of hypopharynx and upper esophagus should be done.

- The scopes used here for this are in various lengths such as
  - Jackson's hypopharyngoscope 30 cm in length
  - Negus esophageal speculum 22 cm in length.

Indications for Hypopharyngoscopy

Diagnostic

- In case of dysphagia to know the cause and extent of lesion and for taking biopsy.
- In cases presenting with neck mass of unknown primary to rule out primary in the hypopharynx / upper esophagus.

Therapeutic

- Removal of foreign body in the hypopharynx/ upper esophagus.
- Dilatation of stricture in the hypopharynx/ upper esophagus.
- Inserting Ryle's tube (nasogastric tube) in case of absolute dysphagia due to hypo-pharyngeal/upper esophageal malignancy or stricture, by rail-roading technique.

Contraindications: Same as DLS.

Prognostic

To assess the results after surgery or radiotherapy

Technique

- Scope is held in right hand like a pen, supported by thumb and other fingers of left hand.
- Inserted from right side of mouth, over the tongue and passed along the pyriform fossae one at a time, examining its medial and lateral walls and apex.
- Tip is passed along apex to reach postcricoid region and advanced till cricopharyngeal sphincter is visualized (approximately 15 cm from upper incisor teeth).
- Upper part of esophagus can be examined by gently sliding the scope further down when the sphincter is relaxed.

- It is essential in all the scopies to keep looking into scope while it is withdrawn.

Postoperative Method

- It is important to write and draw accurate findings immediately.
- In uncomplicated scopies clear fluids followed by soft diet is allowed when patient fully recovers from anesthesia.
- If possibility of perforation or tear of pharynx or esophagus is there, then:
  - Patient is kept nil per oral (NPO) for 6 to 12 hrs
  - TPR/BP monitoring.
  - Observe for neck pain radiating to back
  - Observe for air emphysema in neck.
- If bleeding from biopsy site, patient is kept in lateral position and watched for breathing difficulty.
- If procedure has taken long time with too much of laryngeal manipulations, steroid injections in 2 or 3 doses for 24 hrs are advised, to reduce laryngeal edema.
- Voice rest is advised for few days, when surgery is done to improve voice.

Complications

- Laryngospasm due to blood or secretions or irritation or edema of larynx by passage of endoscopes.
  Steroid injections are advised and patient is kept in recovery area with facilities of resuscitation or reintubation.
- Perforation of pharynx or esophagus–If signs and symptoms suggest perforation, it should be treated surgically or medically by keeping the patient nil per oral.
- Missing teeth–Loose teeth may break and get dislodged. Radiography chest is done and if the tooth has entered the bronchial tree, it is removed by bronchoscopy.
- Bleeding from lips, gums due to trauma.
- Damage to cervical spine if spine is already diseased.
- Anesthetic complications like cardiac or respiratory arrest due to vagal stimulation.

MICROLARYNGOSCOPY

Microlaryngoscopy is a procedure for viewing and recording of anatomical structures of the larynx and their functions using special instruments for exposure and lighting (Fig. 77.1).

Classical microlaryngeal technique has the following instruments:

1. Operating microscope: Provides magnification and illumination
2. Microlaryngoscope
3. Chest support
4. Microsurgical instruments
5. Laser – CO_2 / KTP-532 along with micromanipulator

History

- Bozzini, Babingston, Histon—Indirect laryngoscopy (ILS)
- Kinstein, Killian—Direct laryngoscopy (DLS)
- Chevalier Jackson– Distal illumination
- Yankauer developed Laryngoscope for Binocular vision
- Kleinsasser combined microscope/ magnifying glass to laryngoscope with Riecker-type chest support (Fig. 77.1).

Advantages of Microlaryngoscopy

- Magnification and precision

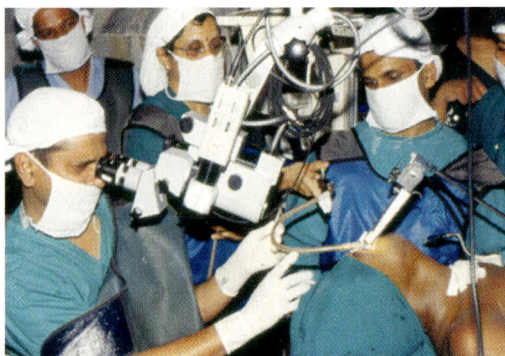

Fig. 77.1: Microlaryngoscopy being performed

- Black metal finish which prevents glare and reflection
- Binocular vision
- Both hands are free
- Diagnostic and therapeutic
- Excellent views of:
  - Anterior commissure
  - Ventricular bands
  - Vocal cords
  - Laryngeal surface of epiglottis
  - Subglottis
- Can check the mobility of the Cricoarytenoid joint
- Allows injection of Teflon-Gelfoam
- Supravital staining
- Documentation
- Biopsy
- Can be coupled with Laser using special delivery systems.

Instruments

(a) Laryngoscopes

Requirements of Laryngoscopes

1. Wide proximal end for binocular vision
2. Easy entry of equipments
3. Safe use of Laser
4. Distal end of suitable size for exposure of Larynx
5. Suitable for anesthesia.

In Adults

The scopes used are

1. Kleinsasser
2. Jako
3. Dedo
4. Nagashima
5. Lindholm laryngoscope
6. Benjamin slime line binocular laryngoscope
7. Weerdra's/Steiner's distensible laryngoscope specially for laser use.

In patients in whom there is difficulty to visualize using standard scopes, the following can be used.

- Holinger–Anterior commissure laryngoscope
- Split expanding type.

In Children

1. Storz slotted pediatric laryngoscope
2. Jackson pediatric laryngoscope
3. Holinger pediatric laryngoscope
4. Tucker-Benjamin pediatric laryngoscope.

(b) Chest Support

To keep the laryngoscope in position, it has a mechanism to fit its handle and the chest ring. The chest ring may be fixed to:

1. Mayo stand
2. Mustard stand.
3. Chest of the patient supported with folded towel. This evenly distributes the force.

(c) Operating Microscope

Standard operating microscope is used with the magnification of 400 mm objective. The magnification provided is 10X. This can be connected to the camera (Fig. 77.1).

(d) Light Source

- Halogen light source 250 watt lamp
- Xenon light.

(e) Microsurgical Instruments for Larynx

They have reinforced shaft that are 18 cm long. They have:

- Firm action
- Positive feel.

Types

1. Straight grasping forceps.
2. Grasping forceps to the right and left.
3. Cup forceps straight, angled and upwards.
4. Microlaryngeal scissors.
5. Diathermy with suction.
6. High pressure syringe gun for injecting Teflon or Gelfoam.
7. Injection canula 19 FG, 20 cm beveled at 45 degrees.

Indications

Adults

1. Persistent hoarseness.
2. Stridor.
3. Foreign body sensation in the throat.
4. Difficulty in swallowing with hoarseness.
5. Biopsy from a suspected neoplasm.
6. Removal of benign lesions:
   – Vocal nodule
   – Vocal cord polyp
   – Granulomas
   – Reinke`s edema
   – Organized hematoma.
7. Laser treatment of
   – Multiple papillomas
   – Mucosal dysplasia
   – Early malignancy.
8. For determining the extent of the lesion.
9. Assessment of laryngeal trauma following prolonged intubation.
10. Treatment of congenital and acquired webs.
11. Vocal cord medialization
12. Vocal cord lateralization
13. Tracheal stenosis for stenting by Ultraflex or T-tube
14. Assessment of subglottic obstruction.

In Children

1. Diagnostic examination to determine the cause of stridor.
2. Investigation of atypical or recurrent croup.
3. Intubation to relieve acute inflammatory airway obstruction by croup or acute epiglottis.
4. Foreign body removal.
5. Laser treatment of laryngeal papillomas, hemangiomas or lymphangiomas.
6. Treatment of congenital or acquired web or stenosis.
7. Preoperative and postoperative assessment of Tracheoesopahgeal fistula.
8. Diagnosis and repair of minor posterior laryngeal cleft.

Investigations

1. Rigid telescopy.

2. X-Ray of the neck; AP and Lateral view.
3. Barium swallow in cases of patients with dysphagia.
4. Non-specific investigations.
   – Complete blood picture with absolute eosinophil count
   – Bleeding parameters
   – ELISA for HIV/HBSAg
   – Urine for routine examination
   – Liver and renal function tests
   – Chest X-ray
   – Cardiology evaluation for elderly patients
   – Pulmonary function test for patients with history of asthma.

Preoperative Preparations

1. Antibiotics.
2. Sedation.
3. Injectable steroids if the patient is in stridor or breathing difficulty.
4. Consent for surgery.
5. Consent for tracheostomy.
6. Adequate hydration in case of children.

Precautions

In children and neonates it is **vital to**

- conserve body heat
- maintain adequate hydration.

In case of pre-existing airway obstruction in neonates and children, irritation and edema due to inflammation and trauma can cause rapid swelling in the subglottic space. This can be avoided by:

1. Gentle handling
2. Judicious use of drugs, which depress the respiratory system.
3. Prudent selection of instruments.
4. Optimal humidification of air.
5. Adequate hydration.
6. Aspiration of blood and secretions during and after completion of examination.
7. Adequate facilities in the recovery room for recognition and treatment of potential complications.

Anesthesia

Ideal Anesthesia is the one, which is safe and pleasant to the patient, simple to monitor, control secretions, allow the surgeon to work unhindered in a completely relaxed patient and also which allows observation of the dynamics of the larynx at the end of the procedure.

Types of anesthesia are

- Endotracheal intubation with small tube preferably
  - 5 to 5.5 mm in females
  - 5.5 to 6 mm in males.
- Usually microlaryngoscope tube is used.

In case of laser, a laser friendly tube is used.

Following paralysis, anesthesia is maintained with

- Jet ventilation or
- Apneic technique or
- Specialized endotracheal tube
- IV short acting barbiturates with paralytic agent (Succinyl choline/Atracurium).

Operative Technique

After intubation the patient is positioned and draped.

Position (Sniffing the morning air position).

Head should be well extended on the atlas and neck flexed. It may be achieved by placing a pillow under the shoulders and partly under the head of the supine patient. Plumping the pillow beneath the occiput further flexes the neck and the head extends over the upper pillow edge. Final adjustments may be made by lifting the headpiece of the table.

Teeth are protected with thick gauge or teeth guard lubricated with xylocaine jelly. Laryngoscope is passed held in right hand, left hand is used to hook the upper incisor and maxillary area. Thumb of the left hand pushes the scope forwards. The right hand lifts the whole tongue base and the epiglottis. The laryngoscope follows the endotracheal tube till the vocal cords are visualized. Once adequate position is attained it is fixed with the help of a chest support. In some cases external pressure/ manipulation on larynx may be required by the assistant. The scope tip ideally should go beyond the ventricular band to visualize and fix the true cords.

In case of longer operating time, mayo stand is used to support both the elbows of the surgeon.

During the procedure any risk of bleeding may require cottonoids soaked in xylocaine and adrenaline. Excess use of diathermy can cause scarring and post-op edema.

Abnormal positions of the vocal cords can also be noted. Mobility of the cords can also be checked. Benign lesions are excised. While excising it is important to preserve the Reinke's space which, if not preserved can cause voice abnormalities later. In case of suspected malignant growth tissues are taken for biopsy after assessing the extent of the lesion.

Laryngeal ventricle can be visualized by

- Retracting the ventricular band with a right angled microlaryngeal probe
- Angled endoscope can also be used for same purpose, biopsy can be taken under visualization.

Examination of subglottis can be done by

- Introducing the tip of scope beyond the vocal cords
- The under surface of vocal cords can be visualized by everting it with the use of a ball probe or a suction tip by pressing on its lateral aspect
- 30 and 70 angled endoscopes can be used
- Small angled mirrors also can be utilized for inspection.

In case of bilateral benign lesions close to anterior commissure, only one cord should be dealt with at a time, lest adhesions may develop between the cords. Excision of benign lesions should be precise and injury to underlying vocal ligament should be avoided.

Postoperative care

1. Nil per orally for 5 hours.
2. Antibiotics if indicated.

3. If bleeding is suspected, patient to be nursed in left lateral position.
4. Injectable steroids–A dose of hydrocortisone 100 mg. is given, then continued with dexamethasone 6th hourly for 24 to 48 hours.
5. Analgesics
6. Serratiopeptidase
7. Voice rest–Patient is advised so that he should not whisper nor shout.
8. Steam inhalation with tincture benzoin 8th hourly.
9. Steroid inhaler like budesonide, beclamethasone can be prescribed after excision of benign laryngeal lesions to prevent postoperative edema.
10. Temperature, BP and respiration to be monitored.
11. X-Ray chest, in patients who underwent the procedure under jet ventilation to look for pneumothorax.

Complications

On Table

1. Bradycardia, syncope, cardiac arrest or arrhythmias.
2. Fracture or dislocation of the tooth.
3. Minor lacerations in the soft palate or epiglottis.
4. Bleeding

Immediate Post-op

1. Bleeding from the operative site usually following major procedures like arytenoidectomy or cordectomy.
2. Breathing difficulty as a result of edema, can be managed by steroids. In some cases reintubation and in rare cases may require tracheostomy.
3. As a result of jet ventilation which depend on positive pressure ventilation, can lead to pneumothorax formation.

Late Complications

1. Granulomas.
2. Scars.

3. Adhesions.
4. Recurrence of the primary lesion.

Contraindications

1. Medical contraindications.
2. Fracture of cervical spine.
3. Aneurysms of vertebral artery, arch of aorta.
4. Temporomandibular joint (TMJ) fixation
5. Fracture of mandible.

Expect difficult microlaryngoscopy in cases of

1. Patients with burns contracture of neck.
2. Patients with swelling floor of the mouth.
3. Macroglossia.
4. Prominent unstable tooth.
5. Restricted mouth opening.
6. Limitation of cervical spine movements.
7. Cervical osteophytes.
8. Large mass in the neck.
9. Obese patients with short neck.

RIGID ESOPHAGOSCOPY

History

In early 19th century Manuel Garcia , singing teacher in London first reported visualization of larynx with mirrors and reflected sunlight.

In 1868 Adolph Kussmaul looked into esophagus with reflected light after studying technique of sword swallower.

Indications

Diagnostic Indications

- Difficulty in swallowing/obstructive dysphagia, which may be acute, or chronic, or acute on chronic.
  - Acute due to ingestion of foreign body
  - Chronic may represent local oesophageal disease such as stenosis, malignancy, hypopharyngeal pouch, achalasia cardia, or general diseases such as scleroderma, neuropathy, brainstem pathology.
  - Acute on chronic due to lodgement of

foreign body on underlying pathology such as malignancy.

- Painful swallowing
- High lesions in hypopharynx and eso-phagus, e.g.: postcricoid malignancy.
- Lower lesions such as esophagitis
- Lump or sticky sensation in throat
- Vocal cord paralysis
- Retrosternal pain, heartburn, hematemesis, and other evidence of gastrointestinal tract bleeding.
- GERD (Gastro Esophageal Reflex Disease)
- Regurgitation
- Vomiting
- Suspected foreign body
- Caustic ingestion.

Radiographic evidence of intrinsic or extrinsic esophageal obstruction such as esophageal stenosis, vascular anomalies, tracheooesophageal fistula, esophageal diverticulum.

To look for second synchronous primary carcinoma in patients with squamous cell carcinoma in the respiratory tract or other parts of GI tract as part of pan endoscopy.

Therapeutic Indications

- Foreign bodies
- Achalasia
- Pulsion diverticula
- Stenosis
- Dilatation of strictures caused by congenital webs, infectious process, esophagitis, trauma.
- Insertion of indwelling tubes [Atkinson, Celestin, Souttar] in palliative treatment of carcinoma. Insertion of stents to overcome an obstructive lesions or in the treatment of tracheo oesophageal fistula.
- Brachytherapy
- Dohlmans upper esophagoscopy with bivalved esophageal speculum for treatment of hypopharyngeal pouch.

Advantages of Rigid Technique

- Better visualization of pharynx and upper sphincter

- Larger deeper biopsies
- Easier removal of foreign bodies
- Direct visualization during dilatation is permitted
- Ability to use endoscopic laser techniques.
- Endoscope is more durable, cheaper and easier to maintain.

Advantages of Flexible Technique

- General anesthesia is not needed
- Allows concurrent examination of stomach and duodenum
- Closer examination of mucosal lesions
- Endoscopic photography and videotaping permitted
- More flexibility in difficult anatomy conditions.

Contraindications

Absolute

- Gross spinal abnormalities like kypho-scoliosis or spinal rigidity due to ankylosing spondylitis.
- Spontaneous perforation of esophagus–Mallory–Weiss syndrome
- Massive bleeding from esophageal varices within 24 to 48 hours in whom bleeding appears to have ceased.
- General condition of patient like severe heart disease or extreme old age.
- Acute corrosive esophageal burns (contro-versial).

Relative

- Bleeding diathesis
- Perforation due to previous esophagoscopy.

Preoperative Evaluation

History regarding medical illness, previous endoscopic procedures, medications which interfere with coagulation.

To rule out bleeding abnormalities via: BT, CT, PT, APTT, Platelet Count.

For procedures which involve removal of tissue, antiplatelet drugs (NSAIDS) should be stopped for 2 to 3 days, aspirin for 7 to 10 days.

Anticoagulants as long as 2 weeks in patients who are to be treated with electrocoagulation for polypectomy.

Patient Preparation

- Barium swallow
- Written consent
- Nil Per Oral for solids for at least 6 to 8 hours, Nil Per Oral for liquids for up to 4 hours.
- Antibiotic prophylaxis in patients with pre existing heart condition.

Anesthesia

Premedication via sedative, narcotic, cholinergic agents.

Local anesthesia for flexible esophagoscopy. Spraying the pharynx and pyriform fossa.

Alternatively

- 2 ml anesthetic sprayed between vocal cords
- Superior laryngeal nerve block or larynx via cricothyroid membrane.
- General anesthesia for rigid esophagoscopy.
- Intraoperative monitoring for excessive sedation.
- Cardiopulmonary resuscitation PR equipment must be available.

Procedure

- Scope is held in fingers and thumb of right hand.
- Left hand is used for retraction of lips and protection of the teeth.
- Lead or plastic splint protects the upper teeth.
- Scope is introduced into the right side of mouth under the upper surface of right side of the tongue till right side of larynx or endotracheal tube is visualized.

Passage through Cricopharynx

Head is extended at atlanto-occipital joint. Scope is passed from right pyriform fossa towards midline and once it is behind larynx advanced downwards applying gentle pressure with tip of esophagoscope to open the cricopharyngeal sphincter.

Even after this if sphincter fails to open, anesthetists are asked to give a muscle relaxant if not given previously, to deflate the cuff of endotracheal tube. Alternatively few drops of 4 percent xylocaine can be instilled through the scope.

Gum elastic bougie can be used as a guide.

Passage through Esophagus

Scope is passed downwards and to the left.

Lumen should always be in the center of the field of vision. Secretions are to be sucked out. Neck is further extended as instrument descends.

Tip of the scope should be in the direction of left anterior superior iliac spine as scope is negotiated towards gastroesophageal junction.

In case of difficulty in negotiating the thoracic esophagus head of the patient is dropped down from edge of the table with support or the chest is raised to straighten the thoracic spine.

Flexible Esophagoscopy

Patient sits facing the surgeon or lies in left lateral decubitus position. Index and third finger of left hand are placed on the back of patients tongue. Forward traction allows endoscope entry into hypopharynx. Voluntary swallowing allows instrument to pass into cervical esophagus. Mouth piece is installed between patient's teeth.

Complications and Treatment

1. **Bleeding** can be tackled endoscopically, therapy using electrocoagulation/ diathermy or by applying haemostatic clips. Hemodynamic stabilization of patient.
2. **Perforation**—most vulnerable areas are hypo pharynx just above cricopharyngeus muscle, cervical esophagus proximal to gastro esophageal junction. It manifests within first 24 hours.
3. Cardiopulmonary complications.

Cervical Esophagus and Hypopharynx Perforation

Signs and Symptoms

- Steady pain and tenderness in neck
- Swelling and subcutaneous crepitus in neck
- X-ray shows subcutaneous emphysema
- Water miscible contrast media is given to detect the exact site of perforation.

Treatment

Nil per oral, antibiotics, Ryle's tube insertion under fluoroscopic guidance.

Exploration and drainage of the para esophageal area.

If not infected, repair can be done by left lateral pharyngotomy approach.

Thoracic Esophagus Perforation

This is the most serious type of esophageal perforation as it can give rise to fatal consequences.

Signs and Symptoms

- High fever
- Tachycardia
- Hypotension
- Pain in chest radiating to back
- Tenderness on sternal pressure
- Subcutaneous emphysema in the neck
- Radiographs show mediastinal widening shifting and emphysema / pneumomediastinum
- Unilateral or bilateral pleural effusion
- Water miscible contrast–exact point of perforation.

Treatment

- Nil per oral, insertion of chest tube if there is empyema or pneumothorax thoracotomy and drainage of mediastinum if early, esophagus may be repaired or definitive therapy with esophagectomy and cervico esophago gastric-anastomosis to be carried out.
- Stenting can also be done.

Perforation of Abdominal Esophagus

This is rare. Patient usually presents with features of peritonitis. Exploration and repair is done by laparotomy. It is seen in cases of dilatation of achalasia cardia, or in cases of malignancy.

RIGID BRONCHOSCOPY

History

Gustave Killian, father of bronchoscopy demonstrated endoscopic feasibility of removal of foreign bodies from tracheobronchial tree.

Chevalier Jackson introduced distally lighted bronchoscopes.

Application of the principles that **Lamm** developed in 1930 in the transmission of an image through a coherent bundle of small flexible glass threads developed flexible endoscopes.

Development of **Hopkin's** rod lens system has lead to wider viewing and greater magnification.

Indications

Bronchoscopy is a primary method of investigating the problem in patients with diseases of respiratory system.

Along with history and physical examination and imaging it is indicated in patients with respiratory diseases that are not self-limiting and are not of short duration.

Diagnostic Indications

- Unexplained chronic cough
- Change of cough in a smoker
- Sputum production
  - Sputum cytology less commonly used, as bronchoscopic examination is more definitive in localizing the pathology and diagnosis.
  - Can be obtained in a sterile fashion to assess for opportunistic infections in immuno compromised patients.
  - Stridor.

Abnormal radiographic findings—segmental, lobar/pulmonary atelectasis, compensatory or obstructive emphysema, local parenchymal densities/pleural effusion/radiopaque foreign bodies.

- Unresolved pneumonia
- Diffuse lung disease
- Shortness of breath of a non cardiac cause.
- Hemoptysis
- Suspected foreign body—Pediatric airway obstruction.
- Paralysis of a vocal cord
- Mass in neck thought to be of metastatic carcinoma.
- Auscultatory evidence of tracheal, mediastinal and pulmonary parenchymal disease.
- Esophageal and thyroid neoplasms secondarily invading tracheobronchial tree.
- To look for synchronous primary carcinoma in patients with squamous cell carcinoma in URTI and upper alimentary tract.
- Bronchoalveolar lavage

Therapeutic Indications

- Atelectasis: For aspiration of tracheobronchial secretions that cannot be handled by the patient.
- Lung abscess–Drainage of lung abscess, passage of brushes and biopsy forceps into abscess cavity can promote bronchial drainage.
- Foreign body and broncholiths
- Stricture excision with laser
- Removal of benign endobronchial neoplasms such as papillomas, osteochondromas/lipomas, and neurofibromas.
- Dilatation of bronchial stenosis
- Aspiration in bronchiectasis
- Lung lavage in asthma, cystic fibrosis and alveolar proteinases.

Other Indications

- Prolonged intubation
- Difficult intubation
- Bronchography
- Gastric aspiration
- Lobar gas sampling.

- Massive hemoptysis should be assessed with rigid bronchoscopy immediately (600 ml in 24 hours).

Airway control with rapid and repeated suctioning is readily accomplished, major bronchus can be packed with epinephrine-soaked pledget.

- When using laser photoablation, rigid bronchoscopes permit photoablation and rapid debridement of obstructing lesion.
- While simultaneously maintaining control of airway.
- Placement of endobronchial stents.
- Inhalation of caustic fumes or smoke–It is a safe way of assessing damage to tracheobronchial tree,
- Surveillance biopsy in lung transplant recipients (controversial) to rule out acute rejection and silent CMV pneumonia.
- Interventional techniques—YAG and CO_2 laser bronchoscopy.
- Placement of radioactive brachytherapy.

Contraindications

- Absolute contraindication—Inability to adequately oxygenate the patient during procedure.
- Coagulopathy or bleeding diathesis that cannot be corrected.
- Rigid bronchoscopy—Aneurysm, marked kyphosis.
- It should not be performed in patient with bilateral vocal cord paralysis, as the passage of bronchoscope through the glottis can lead to edema causing life-threatening airway obstruction.
- Patients having uremia and pulmonary hypertension.
- Recent MI or unstable angina.
- Respiratory failure requiring mechanical ventilation.
- Obstruction of superior vena cava.
- Lack of patient cooperation.
- Bronchoscopy should be avoided in acute respiratory infection particularly in children because of the possibility of producing edema of the respiratory tract.
- Cardiac arrhythmias

- Despite the relatively low risk the benefits of performing the bronchoscopy must be weighed against the potential for complication in each patient.

Autofluorescence Bronchoscopy

Using a helium-cadmium laser for illumination, in vivo, spectroscopy with an optical multichannel analyzer is performed during bronchoscopic examination.

Areas of severe dysplasia and carcinoma can be easily recognized by their decrease in autofluorescence intensity. Whereas, normal tissues autofluorescence predominantly in short (green) wavelengths of the visible spectrum. Preferential horizontal diffusion of longer wavelength fluorescent light from adjacent normal submucosa causes the premalignant and malignant epithelium to appear red.

Anesthesia

Rigid Bronchoscopy (Table 77.1)

- Performed under general anesthesia using the ventilation port on the side of the bronchoscope.
- Loss of tidal volume can be minimized by packing the hypopharynx with gauze or by compression of the supraglottic area by the fingers of the assistant.
- Method is safe for procedures lasting not more than 20 minutes.
- Jet ventilation.

Flexible Bronchoscopy (Table 77.1)

- Topical anesthesia is preferred but general anesthesia may be considered particularly for prolonged examination.
- Required to identify carcinoma in situ with normal chest radiograph.
- Most commonly used are lidocaine [2% and 4%]
- Tetracaine [0.5%, 1%, and 2%].

Through nasotracheal route, nasopharynx is anesthetized using an atomized topical agent", flexible bronchoscope passed through the nares to a level just proximal to false vocal cords, when larynx is in clear view additional anesthetic is administered directly onto vocal cords and into trachea.

Bronchoscope is then passed through glottis and topical anesthesia instilled further down the tracheobronchial tree.

Other Methods

- Topical anesthesia sprayed into hypopharynx with atomizer.
- 5 ml 4% lidocaine injected transtracheally through cricothyroid membrane, care is taken to confirm the position of the needle.
- Supplemental 2 percent lidocaine is then instilled into tracheobronchial tree while advancing the bronchoscope.

Bronchoscopy Procedure

Position of the Patient

- Cervical spine flexed and head extended
- Eyes protected
- Surgeon's left hand steadies/protects and controls the upper jaw.
- Bronchoscope introduced through the right side of mouth.
- Lifting and following the tongue to the epiglottis.
- Bronchoscope steadied by the thumb, index and third finger of the left hand at the level of the teeth while 4th and 5th fingers rest on teeth or hard palate.
- Proximal end manipulated by right hand.

Identification of Glottis

- Tip of epiglottis elevated.
- Using left thumb as fulcrum bronchoscope is brought to a more horizontal level revealing posterior aspect of glottis.

Passing through the Glottis

- Scope is passed towards glottis and rotated 90 degree with tip to the right.
- View centered on the left vocal cord.
- Instrument is advanced towards this until

Table 77.1: Advantages and disadvantages of rigid and flexible bronchoscopy

Rigid bronchoscopy	Flexible bronchoscopy
Advantages	**Advantages**
• Foreign body removal as it allows good exposure and airway control	• Patient comfort
• Massive hemoptysis	• Segmental visualization
• Infant endoscopy	• Segmental biopsy
• Dilate strictures	• Peripheral biopsy
• Tracheal obstruction	• Transbronchial needle aspiration
• Laser bronchoscopy.	• Bedside aspiration of retained secretions
Disadvantages	• Patients on ventilator
• General anesthesia	• Can bypass small stenosis and distortion
• Cannot visualize upper lobe and distal segments for biopsy.	• Photography
• Peripheral biopsy of upper lobe cannot be taken.	• Increased cancer diagnosis
	• Brachytherapy
	Disadvantages
	• Small channel
	• Breakdown
	• Sterilization

beak passes through the vertical axis of glottis.

- Gentle twisting movement allows further advancement.
- Head is further extended.
- Scope is advanced viewing the tracheal walls until sharp outline of normal carina is seen.

Entry to Left Main Bronchus

- Scope is positioned in right angle of mouth.
- Head is rotated to right.
- Orifice of left upper lobe of bronchus is viewed.
- Next, left lower lobe of bronchus is also viewed.

Entry into Right Main Bronchus

Head and neck moved to left and right bronchus is viewed.

Flexible Bronchoscopy

- Patient is placed in semirecumbent position.

- Operator stands to the right facing the patient.
- Right hand controls instrument housing.
- Left hand inserts the fiber bundle.
- Procedure can be done through open bronchoscope, tracheoscope, tracheostomy tube, nasal or oral ET tube, nose or mouth.
- When passed through the nose, instrument is passed between MT and IT into nasopharynx.
- Tip is deflected down into oropharynx giving good view of larynx.
- After LA tip is advanced through glottis into upper trachea.
- In the first phase vocal cord mobility is assessed.
- Walls of tracheobronchial tree are visualized.

Monitoring during Procedure

- Level of consciousness
- Blood pressure

- Heart rate/rhythm/and change in cardiac status
- Lavage volumes delivered and retrieved.

Foreign Body Removal

Entrance of foreign body into tracheobronchial tree produces severe spasmodic cough often accompanied by cyanosis.

- Coughing lasts for 30 minutes and subsides as it comes to rest.
- Auscultation–Expiratory wheeze and other signs of bronchial obstruction.
- It may produce bypass valve, an expiratory check or one way valve or inspiratory check or stop valve.
- Radiography–Inspiratory or expiratory PA view of chest.
- Endoscopic retrieval–30 min as there after endobronchial and subglottic edema occurs.
- Maximum manipulation for 50 to 60 min.
- If still unsuccessful wait for 24 to 48 hrs before retrying.
- Both flexible and rigid bronchoscopes can be used for foreign body retrieval if it is lodged in distal airway or in upper lobe bronchi.

In patient with foreign body indwelling for more than 24 hrs, adequate attention to hydration and febrile reaction should be given.

Complications and Treatment

Hypoxemia most severe in patients with underlying lung disease–Patient should receive O_2 before and during procedure.

Bronchospasm–Most severe in asthmatics should be premedicated with corticosteroids and bronchodilators.

Laryngospasm–Consequence of inadequate topical anesthesia therefore adequate topical anesthesia should be applied on the vocal cords.

Pneumothorax common in patients undergoing transbronchial lung biopsy — to perform procedure under fluoroscopic control to prevent lung perforation.

Bleeding

- Topical epinephrine solution 1:100000 instilled into segmental bronchus.
- Wedging the scope in the segmental bronchus to tamponade the lumen by clot.
- Laryngospasm/ subglottic edema and bronchospasm, compromise the airway in pediatric patients—humidification of supplemental oxygen and administration of systemic corticosteroids.

Most other complications occur due to premedication and topical anesthesia—to be used cautiously.

UVULO-PALATO-PHARYNGO-PLASTY (UPPP)

This is the procedure of choice for the treatment of snoring and obstructive sleep apnea as uvulopalatal obstruction is its predominant cause. Recently it has been replaced by laser assisted uvulopalatoplasty. This procedure includes tonsillectomy, resection of the uvula, part of the soft palate and the redundant palatoglossal and palatopharyngeal folds.

The remnant anterior and the posterior pillars are sutured. In children adenoidectomy is also done. UPPP is more effective in snoring than in sleep apnea. Additional procedures may be required like genial/ mandibular or combined mandibular-maxillary advancement depending on the site of obstruction.

LASER ASSISTED UVULOPALATOPLASTY

This has replaced the Uuvulopalatoplasty (UPP) as it is less morbid and more effective. It is done using KTP-532 laser or CO_2 laser. The uvula and triangular areas on either side of the base of the uvula is resected using laser and a new uvula may be created by shortening the residual uvula. The upper and lower cut edges of the soft palate are sutured using 4-0 Vicryl® sutures. This improves

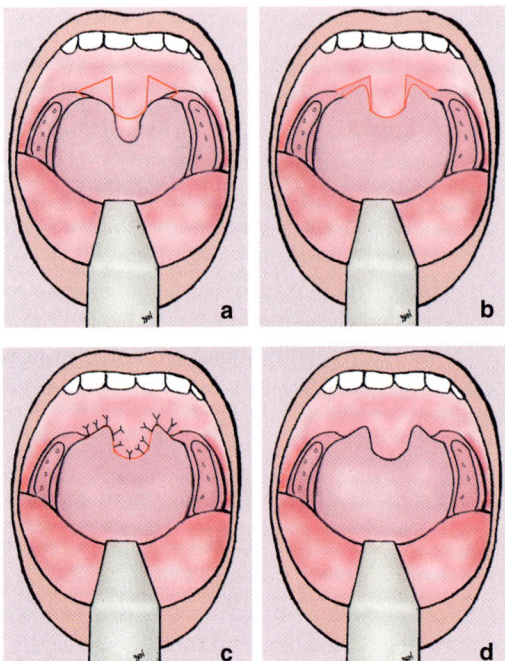

Figs 77.2a to d: (a) Incision, (b) Areas resected with laser (c) Resected edges sutured, (d) After healing

the symptoms of sleep apnea as well as snoring (Figs. 77.2a to d).

LARYNGECTOMY

It is a surgical procedure involving partial or complete resection of laryngeal structures including the skeletal framework. Depending on the type and extent of resection it is classified into various types.

Types

1. **Total Laryngectomy**
   - Widefield laryngectomy
   - Narrow-field laryngectomy.
2. **Conservation (partial) laryngectomy** (Figs 77.3 a to e)
   Vertical partial laryngectomy
   - Laryngofissure and cordectomy
   - Vertical hemilaryngectomy

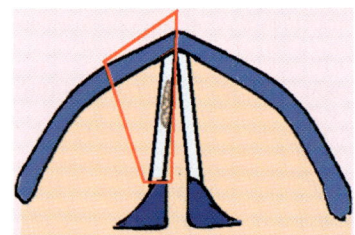

Fig. 77.3a: Vertical partial hemilaryngectomy

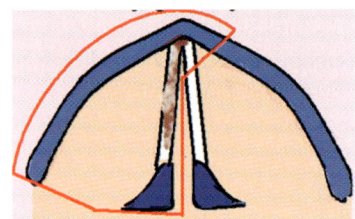

Fig. 77.3b: Extended frontolateral partial laryngectomy

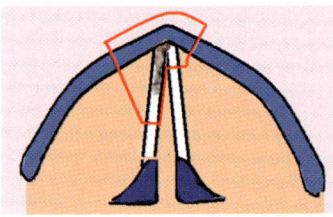

Fig. 77.3c: Frontolateral partial laryngectomy

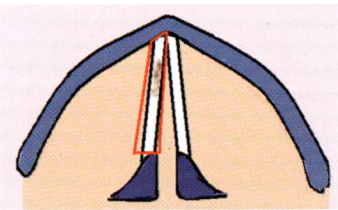

Fig. 77.3d: Cordectomy

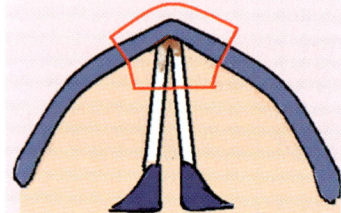

Fig. 77.3e: Frontal partial laryngectomy

– Extended vertical hemilaryngectomy
– Frontolateral vertical partial laryngectomy
– Extended frontolateral vertical partial laryngectomy
– Posterolateral vertical partial laryngectomy
– Frontal vertical partial laryngectomy
– Lateral vertical partial laryngectomy
Horizontal partial laryngectomy
– Supraglottic laryngectomy
– Extended supraglottic laryngectomy
Supracricoid partial laryngectomy
Endoscopic laser assisted procedures
3. *Near total laryngectomy*
4. *Cricohyoidopexy*
5. *Cricoepiglottopexy*

Widefield Laryngectomy

This is the treatment of choice for treating the cancer of the larynx when total laryngectomy is contemplated. Narrow-field laryngectomy is not done as an oncosurgery but may be done for severe aspiration or laryngeal trauma.

Widefield laryngectomy is now conventionally known as total laryngectomy and comprises of en-block resection of entire laryngeal skeleton including hyoid to the 3rd tracheal ring, strap muscles and level 4 and 6 nodes. Ideally a lateral neck dissection including the level 2, 3 and 4 with the level 6 nodes (central compartment) are resected along with the larynx for an N0 neck the steps of which are described below. For a positive neck node a modified or radical neck dissection should be done as described in the chapter 'neck dissections'.

Technique of Widefield Laryngectomy
(Figs 77.4 to 77.9)

1. Modified Sorenson's incision–A 'U' shaped incision is given from one mastoid process to the other running downwards along the posterior border of the sternocliedomastoid muscle and wound round to the opposite side

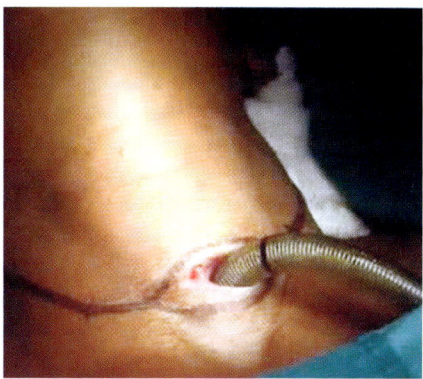

Fig. 77.4: Photograph showing the modified Sorenson's incision incorporating the tracheostoma for total laryngectomy

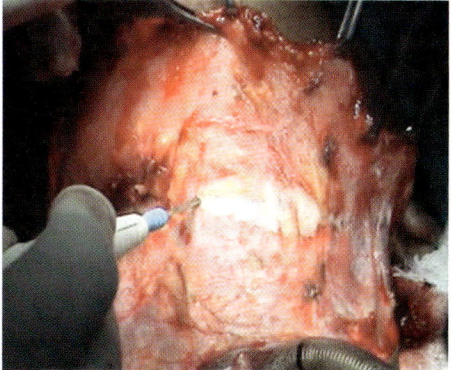

Fig. 77.5: Intraoperative photograph showing subplatysmal flap elevation till the level of hyoid bone

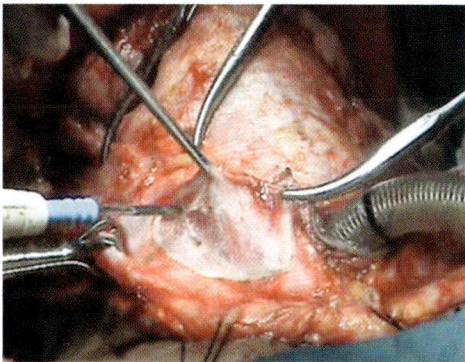

Fig. 77.6: Intraoperative photograph showing dissection and separation of the investing layer of the deep cervical fascia from the sternocleidomastoid muscle

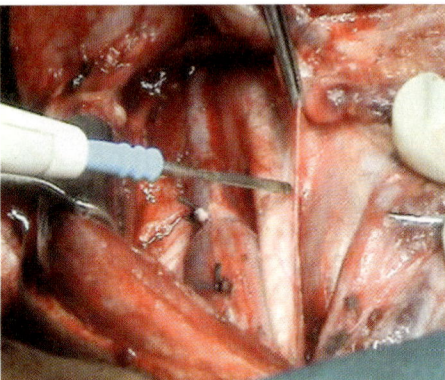

Fig. 77.7: Intraoperative photograph showing clearance of the carotid sheath and the nodes associated as part of the lateral neck dissection. The internal jugular vein and the carotid artery may be appreciated

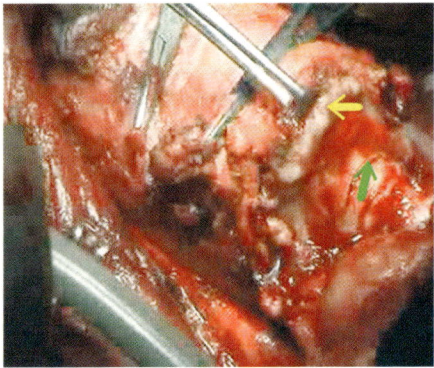

Fig. 77.8: Intraoperative photograph showing separation of the superior attachments of the hyoid bone (yellow arrow) and opening of the vallecula (green arrow) to expose the laryngeal inlet

at about 2 fingers from the suprasternal notch. If the patient has a tracheostomy, the site of tracheostoma should be included.

2. Subplatysmal flap elevation till the level just above the hyoid bone.

3. The dissection starts at the anterior border of the sternocleidomastoid muscle with separation of the investing layer of deep cervical fascia on both the sides of the muscle.

4. The omohyoid muscle is transected.

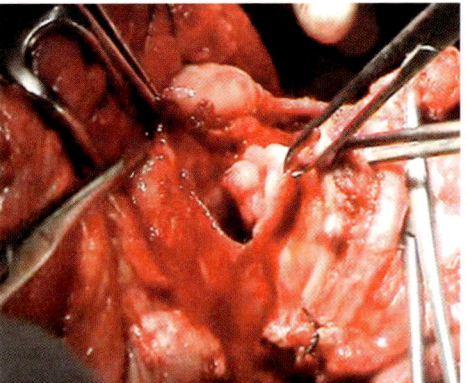

Fig. 77.9: Intraoperative photograph showing the laryngeal tumor being exposed by incising the vallecular mucosa

5. Interjugular dissection is carried out to clear the level 2, 3 and 4 nodes by separating them from the carotid sheath including the internal jugular vein and carotid vessels to include them with the laryngeal specimen. The middle thyroid vein and common facial veins are divided.

6. The superior and inferior thyroid vessels are divided between ligatures. While doing so the parathyroid may be preserved if possible on the contralateral side to that of the primary lesion.

7. The strap muscles are divided at its lower end to expose the trachea. The recurrent laryngeal nerve is identified in the tracheoesophageal groove and is divided. The inferior thyroid veins are ligated and divided.

8. At this point a fresh beveled tracheostoma is created and the endotracheal tube is reinserted through this.

9. The release of the constrictor muscles is done on the contralateral side after rotating the thyroid lamina.

10. The hyoid bone is skeletonized and the suprahyoid strap muscles are detached from the hyoid bone.

11. The vallecular mucosa is exposed and is opened to expose the larynx.

12. The mucosal cut is extended towards the

pyriform fossa till the postcricoid area is exposed (Fig 77.9).

13. The postcricoid mucosa is separated to expose to detach the pharyngeal mucosa from the larynx.
14. The trachea is now separated from the esophagus till the tracheostoma and the specimen is delivered (Fig. 77.10).
15. The pharyngeal defect is sutured primarily in layers after inserting a nasogastric tube. The mucosal layer is sutured by continuous, interlocking, extramucosally using 3-0 vicryl® sutures. The muscular layer is sutured by interrupted 3-0 vicryl® sutures and then the constrictor muscles are also sutured.
16. The permanent tracheostoma is created
17. Neck incision is closed in layers after placing drain tubes.

Indications of Widefield Laryngectomy

- T3 and T4 cancer of the larynx.
- T3 and T4 cancer of the pyriform fossa, along with partial pharyngectomy.
- T3 and T4 cancer of the postcricoid and posterior pharyngeal wall, where in it is done along with total pharyngectomy/total pharyngoesophagectomy.

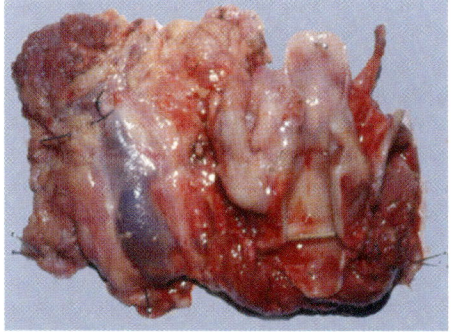

Fig. 77.10: Resected specimen of total laryngectomy with partial pharyngectomy and radical neck dissection on the left side in a case of carcinoma of the left pyriform fossa

Complications of Widefield Laryngectomy

Local

- Wound infection and dehiscence
- *Pharyngocutaneous fistula:* This can occur due to improper pharyngeal mucosal closure, postirradiated neck, secondary infection, early feeding and poor nutritional status.
- *Carotid blowout:* This usually occurs due to pharyngocutaneous fistula and wound dehiscence and is common in postirradiated neck if the tumor is involved the adventitia.
- *Chylous fistula:* This is due to injury to the thoracic duct during surgery.
- *Trachea-stomal stenosis:* This may be due to improper technique of stomal reconstruction or due to secondary infection.
- *Pharyngeal stenosis:* Inadequate pharyngeal mucosa due to extensive resection.
- Stomal recurrence can occur due to preoperative tracheostomy, subglottic extension without proper dissection of paratracheal node or without mediastinal dissection and inadequate excision of the lower margin or due to second malignancy in the trachea.

Systemic

- Cardiovascular complications
- Lower respiratory infection and pneumonia
- Fluid and electrolyte imbalance
- Anemia
- Acute renal failure
- Septicemia.

TRACHEO-ESOPHAGEAL PUNCTURE FOR SURGICAL VOICE REHABILITATION

Introduction

Even though total laryngectomy has considerably improved, the prognosis of patients with laryngeal and hypopharyngeal cancer in terms of life expectancy and disease free status, the loss of speech following this surgery constitutes a severe blow to the patient's functional and psychological well-being. The restoration of speech is a major priority in the rehabilitation of laryngectomies.

The methods of speech restoration have been described in the past with the use of electronic larynx, (Figs 77.11a and b) esophageal speech and also use of surgical procedures like Asai's technique. At present, the technique preferred is the surgical voice restoration (SVR) by tracheoesophageal puncture and use of Blom-Singer's prosthesis. (Figs 77.12 and 77.16) High success rate in the acquisition of speech and simplicity of this procedure have been the reason for its preference.

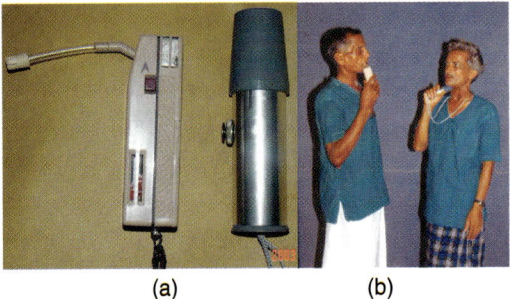

(a)   (b)

Figs 77.11a and b: Different types of electronic larynx and their use

Principle

Generation of Speech basically requires

1. Respiration (bellows)
2. Phonation (voice generator)
3. Articulation (articulators)

Selection of Cases

1. Carcinoma of larynx/hypopharynx being adequately treated by uncompromised extirpative cancer surgery with or without pre or postoperative radical radiotherapy. A residual or recurrent disease especially at the stoma precludes surgical voice restoration by blom-Singer's prosthesis.
2. A minimum of three weeks of time is needed for healing a newly reconstructed pharynx before voicing through the TEP Prosthesis (Hamaker et al, 1985).

3. *Stomal size:* Inadequate tracheostoma requires stomoplasty or dilatation with a stomal vent. Otherwise the prosthesis insertion becomes difficult and it may cause airway obstruction.

4. *Hypertonicity of Pharyngo-esophageal segment:* This can be ruled out by esophageal insufflation test. This test described by Blom, Singer and Hamaker (1985), is performed with a disposable system consisting of a special 30 cms. long no. 14 FG latex catheter; imprinted with an adapter. The patient's nostrils are anesthetized with local xylocaine spray and then the catheter is introduced into the esophagus, transnasally until the 22 cm marker resides at the nostril. Proximal end of the catheter is then attached to the adapter, which is inserted into the trac-heostoma housing. Now, the patient has to do light finger occlusion of the stoma and attempt phonation on exhalation. If the patient is able to sustain phonation with or without interruption of 10 to 15 seconds, and count fluently from 1 to 15, that is interpreted as a successful response, and he is considered not to have pharyngoesophage al (PE) segment spasm, and thus is a suitable candidate for TEP.

   The failed candidate requires cricopharyngeal constrictor myotomy (Blom-Singer 1980, Goldstein et al, 1984) or a pharyngeal plexus neurectomy (Singer, Blom, Hamaker 1986) to reduce the tonicity of the PE segment.

5. A well counseled patient who is adequately motivated and educated regarding the use and maintenance of the prosthesis.

Instruments

A. For tracheoesohageal puncture
B. Prosthesis

For Tracheoesophageal puncture (TEP)

TEP can be done either primarily along with laryngectomy or as a single stage procedure.

Secondary TEP which is widely favored, needs the following instruments:

1. Jelco cannula 14 FG size.
2. Stainless steel malleable wire can be inserted into the 14 FG jelco cannula
3. Rigid adult size hypopharyngoscope and esophagoscope with proximal cold light system and fiber optic light carrier.
4. Red rubber catheters – 14 FG size.
5. Crocodile jaw forceps of suitable lengths for use along with the rigid scopes
6. Artery forceps.
7. Suction cannulae, tubing and suction apparatus.
8. Preferable flexometallic endotracheal tubes for intubation for anesthesia.

Prosthesis are available in two forms (Fig. 77.12)

- Duckbilled valve (slit valve)
- Low pressure valve (circular valve)

The duck billed prosthesis is a 3 cm long hollow silicon tube with flanges on either side, which retain the prosthesis. The outer diameter is 5.4 mm (16 FG). At the proximal end (esophageal end) is a razor thin slit paralleling along the axis of the tube. It opens as a duckbill with positive air pressure, thus permitting airflow into the esophagus. It remains closed during swallowing and performs as a competent one-way valve. The tracheal end (distal end) includes a portion the inferior surface measuring 3.5 × 7 mm for exhaled air entry. This end is opened to permit cleaning and to decrease the mechanical resistance to airflow at the stoma. The prosthesis is retained in the tracheoesophageal party wall with retention collar and adhesive. Total airway resistance offered by this valve ranges from 106.5 to 117.5 cms of water/LPS. The opposition offered to the airflow by human larynx is in the range of 35 to 43 cms of water/LPS.

The low-pressure valve prosthesis is especially designed to reduce the airway resistance inherent in the duckbill prosthesis. This consists of a hinge type circular valve recessed within the hollow tip of the prosthesis to protect the opening movement of the valve from restriction by tissue contact. In the commercially available low-pressure valves, the tip has been reduced from 8 mm to 2 mm, to minimize the potential obstruction when used in patients with narrow esophageal lumen, and the diameter increased from 5.3 mm to 6.6 mm to enhance airflow. Also, the thickness of the retention collar has been substantially increased to eliminate the prosthesis extrusion.

The use of tracheostoma valve avoids the necessity for the manual occlusion of the stoma enabling " hands free speech". This consists of an airflow sensitive curved latex diaphragm, which remains fully open during normal respiration and closes with slight increase in expiratory flow for speech. Decreasing expiratory airflow allows the diaphragm to return to the open position.

HRA Voice Prosthesis (Fig. 77.13)

This modification of Blom Singer prosthesis introduced in 1993 by 'Hazarika, Rajashekhar and Ajit is an indigenous prosthesis made of silicone, which has multiple bellows in the body and is very economical. This is commercially available as HRA prosthesis (Hazarika-Rajashekhar-Ajit

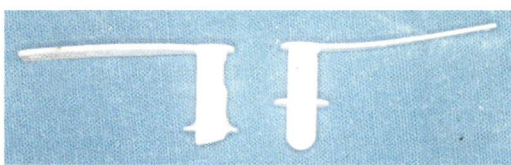

Fig. 77.12: Duckbilled valve and low pressure valve

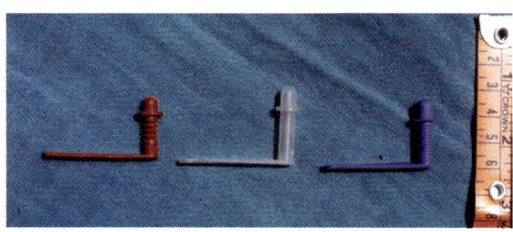

Fig. 77.13: HRA prosthesis of various sizes

prosthesis) (Fig. 77.13) and its use has shown good results without any incidence of salivary leakage.

Procedure

Primary TEP

After total laryngectomy/ total laryngectomy with partial pharyngectomy, primary TEP is done as follows:

(a) A hemostat is inserted into the esophagus and a stab wound is made 1 cm below the cut edge of the trachea through which a nasogastric tube is passed.

(b) Primary pharyngeal reconstruction is done in a vertical straight line using vicryl.

(b) A long vertical myotomy is made to divide all the three constrictor muscles on the posterior surface of the pharynx.

(d) The reconstructed neopharynx is anchored to the prevertebral fascia to prevent excessive displacement postoperatively.

(e) The tracheostoma is fashioned and repaired by Hamaker's technique.

(f) After 10th postoperative day, if there is no fistula, the nasogastric tube is removed and the patient fitted with prosthesis.

Secondary TEP

Steps

(a) Supine position suitable for rigid scopy.

(b) Flexometallic intubation for general anesthesia is preferred as it facilitates working around the stoma. Following hyperventilation, the tube can be removed for short periods, if necessary, without any problem.

(c) A hypopharyngoscope is passed up to the level of the stoma and here the scope is rotated to bring the larger beveled end of the scope towards the stoma. This will give an enhanced light glow on the posterior tracheal wall to guide the needle to avoid injury to the posterior wall of the oesophagus.

(d) An ordinary thin stainless steel wire is passed through a 14 FG Jelco cannula with needle so that the distal end of the wire is slightly bent and can be inserted through the tracheooesopha- geal partition wall, 5 mm below the mucocutaneous junction the midline, into the hypopharyngoscope. Distal end of the wire is pushed further and retrieved through the scope and secured at the oral end.

(e) The needle is withdrawn and the wire is attached to a straight urethral catheter 14 FG. The puncture site may be dilated with a right-angled hemostat. The catheter is drawn into the pharyngoesophagus. The distal end of the catheter is then pushed down into the esophageal lumen and is retained there for 48 hrs, which will act as a stent for the puncture.

(f) After 48 hrs, the stent is removed and the prosthesis is inserted immediately, after measuring the transverse diameter of the anterior esophageal wall and the tracheostoma. A stenosed neopharynx will need dilatation with bougies before TEP (Figs 77.14 and 77.15).

Advantages of TEP over other methods

1. Safer, simple and easy to perform.
2. High rate of success. Even 100 percent success rate can be achieved in expert hands.

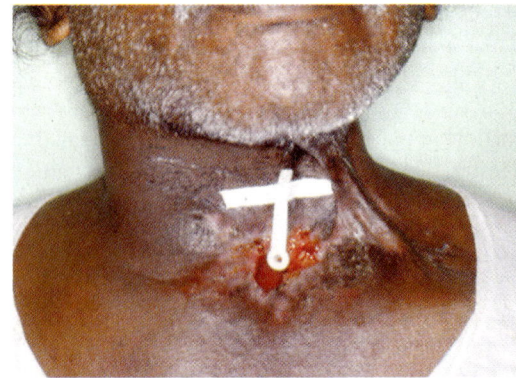

Fig. 77.14: Patient is wearing a Blom-Singer prosthesis after a tracheoesophageal puncture

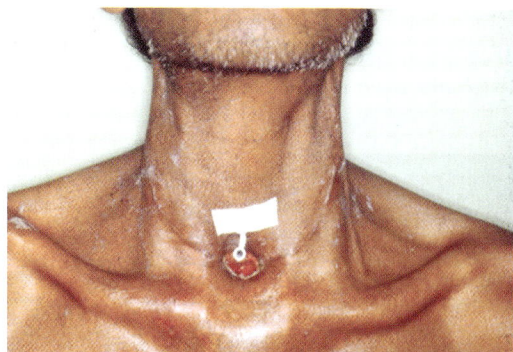

Fig. 77.15: Patient is wearing a Blom-Singer prosthesis after a tracheogastric puncture

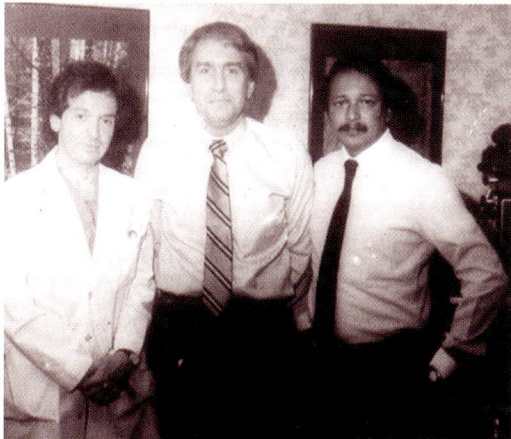

Fig 77.16: Shown in the photograph are from left to right Blom, Singer & Senior author (In 1986 senior author performed TEP first time in India)

3. This technique eliminates the need for skin/ mucosa lined, multi-staged shunt construction and the complicated air bypass devices.
4. It can be performed months or even years after a laryngectomy.
5. It is cost-effective in terms of short hospital stay, rapid return to occupation and avoidance of prolonged speech services.
6. Aspiration is very uncommon.
7. Avoids repeated belching, which is obvious in esophageal speech.

Disadvantages

1. Need for finger occlusion of the stoma. This can be avoided by use of tracheostomy valve.
2. Prosthesis has to be cleaned and changed daily.
3. Cost of B.S. prosthesis is quite high. This is substantially reduced by the use of equally efficient indigenous HRA voice prosthesis.

COMMANDO OPERATION

(**CO**mbined **MA**ndibulectomy, **N**eck **D**issection and **O**ropharyngeal malignancy resection)

This refers to composite en - bloc radical resection of the tumor in the oropharynx/ oral cavity, with a healthy margin of normal tissue, along with the modified or radical neck dissection and mandibulectomy (marginal/segmental/ hemimandibulectomy) (Fig. 77.17).

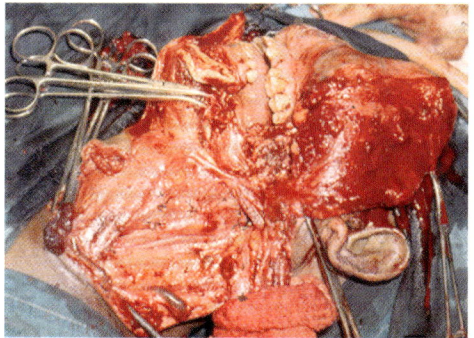

Fig. 77.17: Composite resection of the tumor involving the oral cavity along with hemimandibu- lectomy and radical neck dissection (Commando operation)

The mandible is removed usually due to its involvement though some authors remove even uninvolved mandible to accommodate the myocutaneous flap which is used for reconstruction. Neck dissection is often indicated in oropharyngeal, floor of the mouth, retromolar trigone and tongue malignancies as these areas are rich in lymphatics and neck metastases are very common. As the surgery is quite extensive some authors called it as 'commando' operation. This procedure leaves large mucosal surgical defects which can be reconstructed by various pedicled or free myocutaneous flaps which could be osteointegrated if necessary (Fig. 77.18).

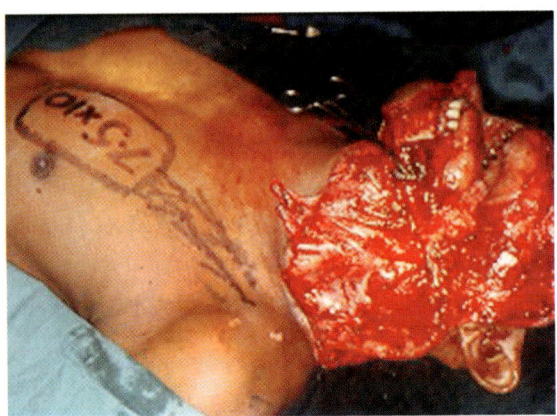

Fig. 77.18: Preparation for pectoralis major myocutaneous flap for the reconstruction of the defect

POINTS TO REMEMBER

1. Microlaryngoscopy has distinct advantages like precise assessment and excision aided by better illumination, magnification and binocular vision. In addition, the surgeons both hands are free for instrumentation.

2. Rigid esophagoscopy and hypopharyngoscopy are more advantageous than flexible scopy for therapeutic indications like foreign body removal, stricture dilatation, etc.

3. Flexible bronchoscopy is best avoided in the case of compromised laryngeal airway due to the risk of fatal laryngospasm and worsening of stridor.

4. General anesthesia for rigid bronchoscopy can be given either by jet ventilation or by ventilation through the bronchoscope using apneic technique.

5. Early glottic cancers can be resected by conservation laryngectomy or using KTP-532 laser, thus preserving the functions of the larynx.

6. Widefield laryngectomy is the treatment of choice in advanced laryngeal malignancies which is followed by radical radiotherapy. Surgical voice restoration is best done by TEP and Blom-Singer prosthesis.

Head and Neck

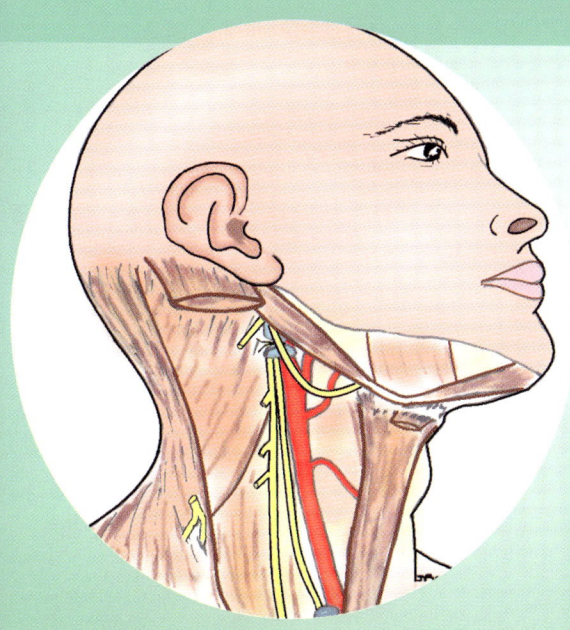

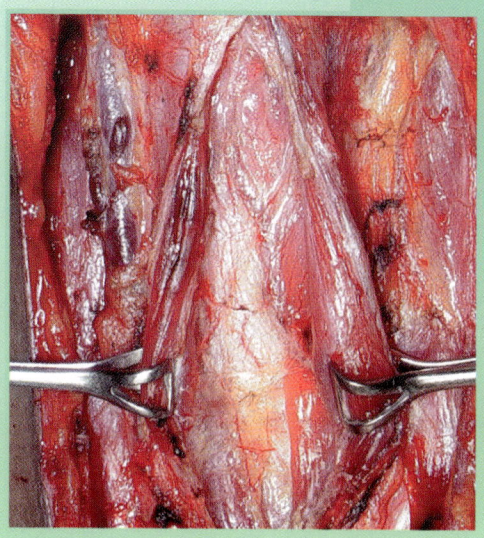

78

Anatomy of the Neck

Anatomical Division

The neck is divided into two triangles, the anterior and the posterior. These triangles are three-dimensional in shape and change with position of the neck. These triangles are divided further as follows (Figs 78.1 and 78.2).

The anterior triangle is bounded by the sternocleidomastoid muscle, the mandible and the midline of the neck. The anterior triangle is further divided into submandibular, submental and the carotid triangle which together makes the **supra-omohyoid triangle**. Part of the anterior triangle between superior belly of omohyoid muscle, sternocleidomastoid muscle and midline is called musculovisceral triangle which contains strap muscles covering the trachea and the thyroid gland.

The posterior triangle is bounded by the trapezius muscle, the middle third of the clavicle and the posterior border of the sterno-cleidomastoid muscle. This triangle is further divided into occipital and supraclavicular (subclavian) triangle by the inferior belly of the omohyoid muscle.

Fascial Compartments

The neck is covered by both superficial and deep cervical fascia. These fascial coverings produce various compartments of the neck. These fascial compartments are very important for surgeons, as they help in identifying proper planes of dissection. They also help in limiting the spread of infection.

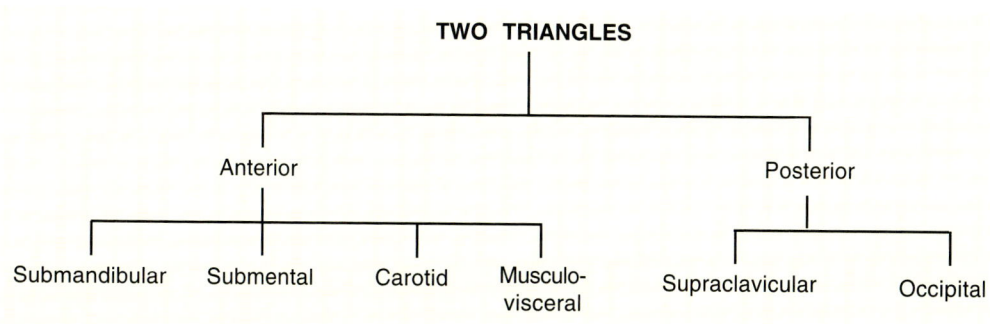

Fig. 78.1: Triangles of the neck

693

1. **Superficial fascia:** It is a single layer of fibro-fatty tissue that covers the subcutaneous tissue and the platysma.
2. **Deep cervical fascia:** It is a more extensive and important layer, which lies deep to the platysma. It has three layers:
   (a) **Superficial (Investing) layer:** This layer invests whole of the neck and splits to surround two muscles, the trapezius muscle posteriorly and the sterno-cleidomastoid muscle laterally, and two glands, i.e. parotid and submandibular salivary glands.
   (b) **The Visceral (pretracheal) layer:** It surrounds the middle compartment of the neck and covers the trachea and the thyroid gland.
   (c) **The internal layer (prevertebral fascia):** This surrounds the deep muscles of the neck.

See chapter 'Deep neck space infections' under section pharynx for more details.

Lymphatics

There are approximately 75 nodes on each side of the neck. Most of the nodes present in deep jugular and spinal accessory chain. The deep jugular chain extends from the base of the skull to the clavicle. Metastatic nodes frequently involve the deep jugular chain. The deep jugular (cervical) chain can be further divided into the following groups:

- Superior (upper) deep cervical
- Middle deep cervical
- Inferior (lower) deep cervical.

The other groups of nodes are:

- Submental
- Submandibular
- Superficial cervical
- Retropharyngeal
- Paratracheal
- Spinal accessory
- Anterior scalene
- Supraclavicular.

The various groups of lymph nodes of the neck receive their lymphatic drainage as follows:

1. **Superior deep jugular nodes:** These groups of lymph nodes drain from the soft palate, tonsils, tonsillar pillars, base of the tongue, supraglottic larynx and pyriform fossa.
2. **Middle deep cervical nodes:** They drain from supraglottis, pyriform sinus (apex) and post cricoid region.
3. **Lower deep cervical nodes:** They receive lymphatics from thyroid, trachea, and cervical esophagus.
4. **Submental nodes:** They drain the skin of the chin, mid portion of the lower lip, tip of the tongue, anterior oral cavity and nasal vestibule.
5. **Submandibular nodes:** They drain the lower oral cavity, upper lip, lateral lower lip, anterior nasal cavity and skin of the mid face.
6. **Superficial cervical nodes:** They drain the parotid gland and retroauricular area.
7. **Retropharyngeal nodes:** They drain the nasopharynx, posterior nasal cavity, paranasal sinus, posterior pharyngeal wall and hypopharynx.
8. **Paratracheal nodes:** They drain the lower larynx, hypopharynx, cervical esophagus, upper trachea and thyroid gland.
9. **Anterior Scalene (Virchow) nodes:** They drain the infraclavicular area and are situated in the lower neck in relation to the thoracic duct.

Oncological Classification

Level I (L1): Lies in the submandibular and the submental triangles.
- Ia: Submental
- Ib: Submandibular.

Level II (L2) Jugulodigastric nodes: Nodes of the upper jugular chain (jugulodigastric) in the retromandibular area in relation to the upper third of the sternocleidomastoid muscle.
- IIa: Jugulodigastric: Anterior to upper third of sternocleidomastoid muscle.

- IIb: Jugulodigastric: Deep to upper third of sternocleidomastoid muscle which lies in close relation to the spinal accessory nerve.

Level III (L3) Jugulo-omohyoid nodes: They are mid-jugular group along the middle third of the jugular vein from carotid bifurcation above to omohyoid muscle below and between the anterior and posterior border of the sternocleidomastoid muscle.

Level IV (L4) Lower deep cervical nodes: They lie between the omohyoid muscle and the clavicle.

Level V (L5) Posterior triangle nodes:

- Va: Those superior to the cricoid cartilage
- Vb: Those inferior to the cricoid cartilage.

Level VI (L6): Central compartment with paravisceral nodes like pre and para tracheal and laryngeal nodes. They are the nodes medial to the carotid from the level of hyoid to suprasternal notch.

Level VII (L7) Superior mediastinal nodes: Ultrasound of the neck is an inexpensive yet invaluable investigation in the assessment of the neck nodes.

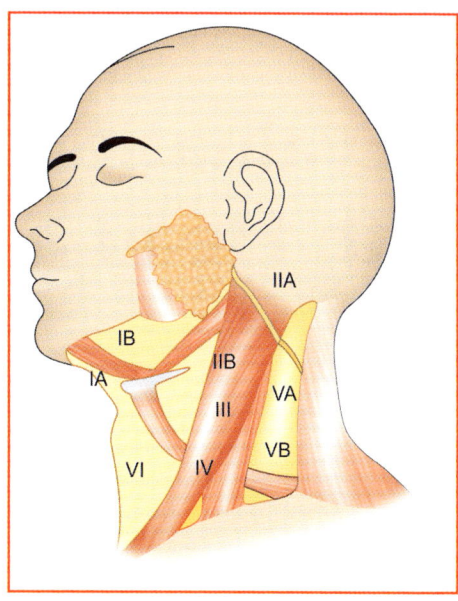

Fig. 78.2: Anatomical divisions of the neck

POINTS TO REMEMBER

1. Neck is divided into anterior and posterior triangles.
2. Anterior triangle consists of submandibular submental, carotid and musculovisceral triangles.
3. Fascial compartment helps in identifying proper plane for neck dissection.
4. There are approximately 75 nodes on each side of the neck.
5. Neck nodes are oncologically classified into various levels (L_1–L_7) depending on locations.

79

Evaluation of the Patient with Head and Neck Cancer

History Taking

A detailed history is taken to evaluate the following common symptoms. History taking for head and neck cancer is no different from that of other medical and surgical illnesses. The patient with head and neck cancer are usually over 45 years of age and they may have various personal habits like tobacco chewing or smoking with years of abuse to the affected epithelium. These factors should be carefully noted as they may cause cancer and it is also important for subsequent rehabilitation. A careful history generates a complete differential diagnosis which helps in ensuring all possible diagnosis before concluding into a definitive diagnosis and management planning. Various benign conditions have already been discussed in the related chapters. Since cancer evaluation and management needs a different approach, this chapter will highlight essentials of management in such cases with particular reference to the neck.

The patients may come with the following symptoms:

- **Hoarseness:** This is an early symptom in the glottic cancers. Hypopharyngeal malignancy may produce hoarseness due to direct involvement of the supraglottis or due to the involvement of the recurrent nerve.
- **Obstruction:** Obstruction of the food passage can cause foreign body feeling,

lump in the throat, dysphagia or odyno-phagia. Obstruction to the airway produces stridor.

- **Pain:** Pain in the affected site or referred otalgia is usually a late feature and this suggests deep infiltration and due to involvement of the nerves.

In the larynx, pain may also suggest involvement of the laryngeal cartilages and consequent perichondritis.

- **Bleeding:** Patient with cancer in the throat may present with history of spitting of blood on violent attempt to clear the throat.
- **Presence of a mass/ulcer** in oral malignancies
- Swelling in the neck due to cervical nodal metastasis.

General Examination

This should include looking of status of nutrition and hydration, body weight in addition to pallor, icterus, cyanosis, clubbing, pedal edema, generalized lympadenopathy, etc. Generalized lymphadenopathy may be seen in lymphoma and granulomatous conditions. Other systems should also be examined as they may have a bearing in the management of the patient. Examination of the respiratory, cardiovascular and the nervous system should be done.

Clinical Examination

The individual primary site evaluation has been covered under the respective chapters and should be examined for ulcers or swelling. Malignant ulcers are irregular in size and shape and rodent ulcers are common in the upper part of the face. Tumors due to squamous cell carcinoma have an everted edge. Floor is covered with slough and unhealthy granulations. Base of the ulcer is where the floor rest and is often indurated in squamous cell carcinoma. This is best palpated to determine its actual extent, depth and tenderness. Its fixity to the underlying or surrounding structures should be evaluated by palpation. Bleeding on touch indicates friable nature of the ulcer. The site and extent of the primary tumor should be carefully documented as text and diagrammatic representations. Second opinion by the colleagues helps in better assessment as it eliminates bias and even this should be well documented. This helps in better planning of the management strategy and also in comparison during the follow up period

GENERAL POINTS TO BE REMEMBERED

1. The most common neck mass is a **reactive** node, and these are most often secondary to bacterial or viral infections of ear, nose, sinuses, teeth, tonsil or skin and soft tissues of the head and neck.

2. Most neck masses in children are **benign.**

3. Most neck masses in adults are **malignant.**

4. The rule of 7 is a useful guide:
   a. A mass present for 7 days is inflammatory.
   b. Present for 7 months is malignant.
   c. Present for 7 years is congenital/benign

5. Multiple lumps are almost invariably lymph nodes.

6. FNAC (Fine Needle Aspiration Cytology) is a very useful diagnostic tool for benign and malignant lumps.

7. Malignant lumps should be staged accurately and managed along with the primary.

of the patient. The clinical examination of only neck is being briefly discussed below. For detailed account please refer to the same authors' book entitled 'Clinical and operative methods in ENT-Head and neck'.

Examination of the Neck

In head and neck cancer, neck may be involved by the neck nodes or by the primary tumor itself due to direct spread. But this rarely produces symptoms until they are quite large.

Attitude of the Neck

The position of the head and the neck may be altered due to muscle spasm or pain in advanced malignancies.

Examination of Neck Mass

It is mandatory before the examination of the neck with neck mass to include the systematic and complete examination of the head and neck area which should include the inspection of the skin of face and scalp and the mucosal surface of the entire upper aerodigestive tract. Palpation of the neck mass along with examination of the nose, pharynx, larynx, thyroid and salivary gland is a vital part of a thorough examination of the head and neck before examining for the lymphatic system of the head and neck (Figs 79.1 to 79.4).

Examination of Lymph Nodes of the Neck

The neck nodes are systematically examined based on the triangles they belong to and are noted based on their oncological nodal levels as per the TNM classification. The examiner should inspect the neck from the front and then should stand behind the patient to palpate the nodes. The clothing should be separated to expose the neck and shoulders completely. The neck should be flexed slightly to relax the neck muscles. The index finger is placed on both mastoid process and then the palpation started downwards till the fingers meet at the clavicle. To palpate the nodes

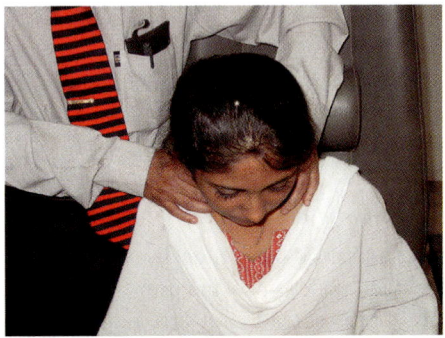

Fig. 79.1: Palpation of the neck from behind with the neck flexed, for examining the lymph nodes deep to the anterior border of trapezius from the mastoid process to the level of clavicle

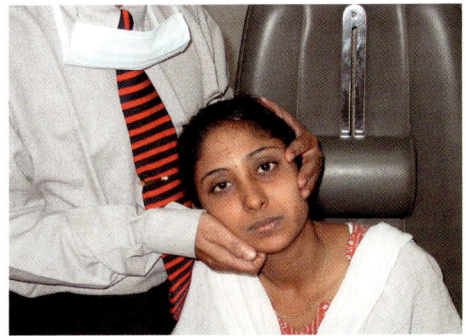

Fig. 79.2: Palpation of the neck by flexing and tilting the neck laterally to relax the muscles for examining the level I neck nodes

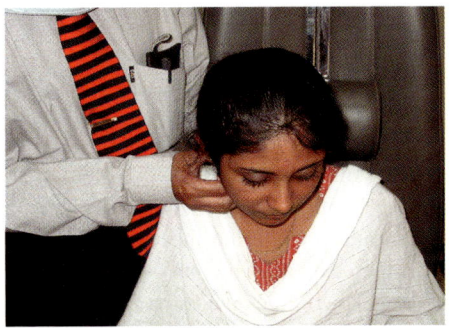

Fig. 79.3: Correct method of palpation of the level II, III and IV nodes in the neck

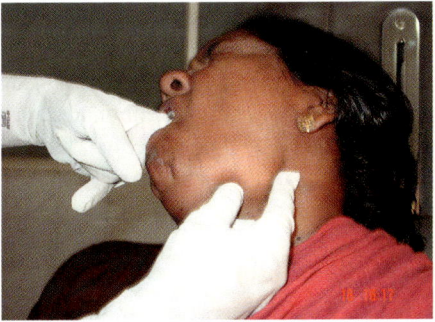

Fig. 79.4: Bimanual (bi-digital) palpation to differentiate submandibular salivary gland from the submandibular lymph node.

under the trapezius muscle, fingers should be inserted under its anterior border while the thumb is pressing from the back of the muscle to make the node prominent for palpation. After reaching the clavicle the posterior triangle nodes should be palpated between the skin and the muscles of the floor of the triangle.

To palpate the jugular chain the neck is slightly flexed laterally and the fingers are placed in front and medial to the sternocleidomastoid muscle with the thumb behind. The examination should proceed to palpate between level 2 and 4. Level 6 nodes should be looked for at the suprasternal notch (Fig. 79.5). Then the submandibular triangle is examined to palpate the submandibular salivary gland and the nodes including the submental

nodes (level 1). The reliability of the neck examination depends on the ability and the experience of the examiner, post-radiotherapy status, post surgery status, fat and thick muscular neck, etc.

The nodal levels should be mentioned diagrammatically and the possible draining sites should be kept in mind. Following parameters should be noted:

- Number of nodes
- Ipsilateral/contralateral/bilateral
- Site
- Size
- Surface
- Consistency

- Mobility/Fixity in relation to underlying structures in transverse and vertical planes
- Skin involvement
- Distal carotid pulsations.

Metastatic nodes are those palpable and present in the draining area of the primary tumor. They are obviously malignant if they are hard in consistency and if fixed to the underlying structures suggesting advanced neck disease.

Classification of the Neck Nodes

Cervical nodes are classified based on the nodal groups to standardize the clinical observation. They are classified into seven levels (Level 1 to 7). For more details please refer to the Oncological classification mentioned in the previous chapter.

Position and Status of the Normal Landmarks

- Tracheal shift
- Laryngeal framework may be pushed forwards in a postcricoid carcinoma

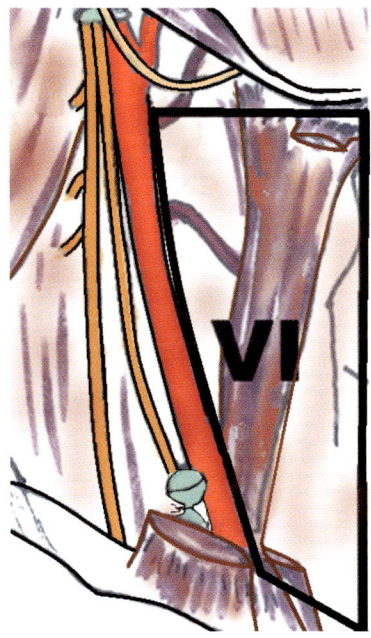

Fig. 79.5: Level 6 (paravisceral nodes)

- Large cervical node may displace the larynx laterally
- Splaying of the thyroid cartilage (widening) may be seen in advanced laryngeal and laryngopharyngeal malignancy (Fig. 79.6)

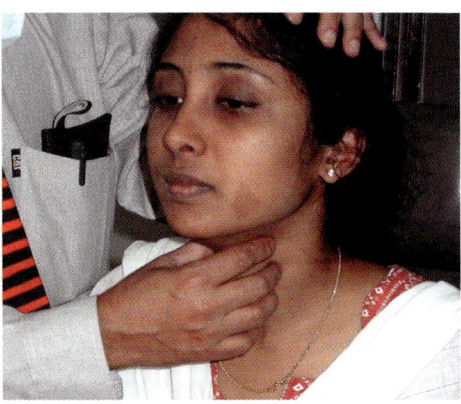

Fig. 79.6: Showing laryngeal crepitus being elicited

- Laryngeal crepitus—The grating sensation on moving the laryngeal cartilages side to side against the cervical vertebrae is lost in a postcricoid malignancy (**Bocca's sign**).
- Laryngeal cartilage tenderness indicates cartilage involvement.
- Swelling in the thyrohyoid or the cricothyroid or the cricotracheal membrane area suggests extralaryngeal spread of tumor.

Superior Mediastinal Obstruction

May show the following features due to superior venacaval obstruction:

1. Thoracic vein distention
2. Neck vein distention
3. Facial edema
4. Tachypnea
5. Plethora of the face and cyanosis
6. Edema of upper extremities

Investigations

Detailed account has been given in the respective chapters.

1. Radiological
   (a) Plain X-ray
   (b) CT Scan
   (c) Angiography
   (d) Sialography
   (e) Radioisotopic scanning
   (f) Ultrasound.
2. Endoscopy and biopsy
3. FNAC.

N STAGING FOR ALL HEAD & NECK SITES
UICC 1997 (Except the Nasopharynx & Thyroid)

- **Nx:** Regional lymph nodes cannot be assessed
- **N0:** No regional lymph node metastasis
- **N1:** Metastasis in a single ipsilateral lymph node, 3 cm or less in greatest dimension
- **N2:** Metastasis in a single ipsilateral lymph node, more than 3 cm but not more than 6 cm in greatest dimension; or in multiple ipsilateral lymph nodes, none more than 6 cm in greatest dimension; or in bilateral or contralateral lymph nodes, none more than 6 cm in greatest dimension
- **N2a:** Metastasis in a single ipsilateral lymph node more than 3 cm but not more than 6 cm in greatest dimension
- **N2b:** Metastasis in multiple ipsilateral lymph nodes, none more than 6 cm in greatest dimension
- **N2c:** Metastasis in bilateral or contralateral lymph nodes, none more than 6 cm in greatest dimension
- **N3:** Metastasis in lymph node more than 6 cm in greatest dimension

80

Classification of Neck Swelling

Swellings in the neck frequently cause diagnostic dilemma. Most neck masses of specific cause occur in specific age group at specific locations.

According to incidence of various causes, three main age groups need to be considered including pediatric (< 15 years), young adult (16 – 40 years) and elderly (≥ 40 years) which can be classified as follows (Table 80.1).

Most of the patient with neck swelling may ask for medical advice with following complaints:

- Lump/swelling in the neck associated with
  - Pain in the neck (Inflammatory).
  - Fever with chills in acute infection and evening rise of temperature (Tuberculosis).
  - Loss of appetite (T.B./Malignancy)

Patient may also have undergone medical or surgical treatment

A detail ENT-Head and Neck examination is the key to the diagnosis and should include the following:

- Surgeon should perform prior examination of all mucosal surfaces of upper aero-digestive tracts.
- Systemic examination of all mucosal and sub-mucosal areas is the key to diagnose the etiology of neck mass.

Capability to perform examination and diagnose, distinguishes the otolaryngologist as specialist for head and neck surgery.

ENT–Head and Neck Examination

Inspection: The following features should be noted in the case of a neck swelling/lymph node enlargement.

Table 80.1: Showing various causes of neck swelling according to the order of its incidence

< 15 Age	16–40 Age	> 40 Age
1. Inflammatory	1. Inflammatory	1. Neoplasia • Malignant • Benign
2. Congenital/Developmental	2. Congenital/Developmental	2. Inflammatory
3. Neoplasia • Malignant • Benign	3. Neoplasia • Benign • Malignant	3. Trauma
4. Trauma	4. Trauma	4. Congenital/developmental

Table 80.2: Classical location of few neck swellings

Swelling	Location
Branchial cyst	Upper part of neck posterior half deep to sternomastoid
Dermoid cyst	Midline
Sternomastoid	Along sternomastoid tumor muscle

1. **Number:** Lymph node swelling is multiple where as the other swellings are single.
2. **Location:** Location is typical for each swelling (Table 80.2).
3. **Movement on swallowing:**
   - Goiter
   - Thyroglossal cyst
   - Subhyoid bursitis
4. **Expansible on coughing :** Laryngocele
5. **Movement on protrusion of tongue:** Thyroglossal cysts.

Palpation

1. *Size and shape*: Round and regular in benign swellings
2. *Surface:* Smooth and regular in benign
3. *Irregular and nodular:* Malignant.
4. *Margins*: Well defined in benign swelling, ill defined in malignant
5. *Vascular pulsation*
   - Carotid body tumor
   - Aneurysms
6. *Consistency*
   - Hard to firm lymph node—Malignant
   - Matted—Tubercular
   - Cystic—Cold abscess
7. *Involvement to neighboring structures*
   - Hypoglossal nerve—Tongue deviates to effected side, on protrusion.
   - Recurrent laryngeal nerve—Vocal cord palsy.
   - Jugular veins—Venous engorgement of head and neck.
   - Involvement of deep muscles of the neck can cause fixity of the node/swelling in either transverse/vertical directions or both.

Auscultation: Bruit is felt in:
- Aneurysm
- Carotid body tumor

Movements of the Neck
Movement of the cervical spine is restricted in cold abscess.

Investigations for Neck swelling (Table 80.3)

Causes of congenital neck masses (Table 80.4)

Causes of midline and lateral neck swelling (Table 80.5)

Following lesion can occur anywhere in neck
- Sebaceous cyst
- Lipoma
- Neurofibroma
- Hemangioma

Based on onset the Swelling of neck can be classified as:

1. Acute swelling
2. Chronic swelling.

Acute Swelling

1. Ludwig's angina
2. Furuncle
3. Carbuncle
4. Acute lymphadenitis.

Chronic Swelling

1. Cystic
2. Solid
3. Pulsatile.

Cystic Swellings (see chapter 81)

- Branchial cyst
- Thyroglossal cyst
- Dermoid cyst
- Cystic hygroma
- Sebaceous cyst
- Cystic adenoma of thyroid gland
- Cold abscess
- Abscess of lymph nodes
- Plunging ranula

Table 80.3: Showing various investigations and their objectives in the evaluation of neck swellings

Investigations	Purpose and comments
Endoscopy and biopsy	Primary tumor as source of metastatic node
Radionuclide scan	1. Thyroid gland
	2. Salivary gland
Ultrasonography	• Solid and cystic masses
	• Vascular lesion
Arteriography	• Vascular lesions
	• Tumors fixed to carotid artery
Sialography	• Diffuse sialadenitis
	• Locate the mass In/outside the gland
Plain radiography	Rarely helps in differentiating neck mass –Useful
	• Tracheal shift
	• Bony erosion
	• Calcification in mass
CT scan	Most informative use – But cost limits the use
MRI scan	Much the same as CT. But T_2 weighted images – Useful for soft tissue involvement of tumor
Fine needle aspiration cytology	Most useful as initial invasive diagnostic procedure
Open biopsy	Done if diagnosis is not evident
Skin test	Chronic/Granulomatous inflammatory lesion
Culture and sensitivity	For inflammatory tissue at open biopsy

Table 80.4: Few examples of midline and lateral neck masses

Midline and anterior neck masses	Lateral neck masses	Entire neck
Thyroglossal cyst	Branchial cyst	Hemangiomas
Thymic cyst	Laryngocele	Lymphangioma
Dermoid cyst		
Plunging ranula		
Teratoma of neck		

- Pharyngeal pouch
- Laryngocele
- Retention cyst of salivary gland

Solid Swellings (see chapter 82)

- Lymph node swelling
- Swelling arising from thyroid
- Swelling arising from salivary gland
- Branchiogenic carcinoma
- Sternomastoid tumor

- Carotid body tumor
- Cervical rib.

Pulsatile Swellings (see chapter 81)

- Aneurysm of carotid artery
- Aneurysm of subclavian artery
- Carotid body tumor
- Lymph node swelling in proximity to carotid artery (Transmitted pulsation)
- Few primary toxic goiter

Midline swelling	Lateral swelling		
	Submandibular/ Digastric triangle	Carotid triangle	Posterior triangle
Submental lymph nodes	Enlarged lymph node	Lymph node swelling	Enlarged supraclavicular L. node
Thyroid gland enlargement	Enlargement of submandibular salivary gland	Thyroid swelling	Cystic hygroma
Thyroglossal cyst	Deep/plunging ranula	Branchial cyst	Pharyngeal pouch
Sublingual dermoid	Extension of growth from Jaw	Sternomastoid tumor in newborn	Subclavian aneurysm
Lipoma Ludwigs angina Subhyoid bursitis Retrosternal goiter Thymic swelling Bony swellings arising from manubrium sterni	Sjögren's syndrome	Laryngocele	Cervical rib Cervical tumor Lipoma Cold abscess

Table 80.5: Causes of midline and lateral neck swelling

POINTS TO REMEMBER

1. Neck swelling in a child is often congenital or inflammatory.
2. Acute painful neck swelling could be due to acute lymphadenitis, acute sialadenitis or due to deep neck space infections like Ludwig's angina and parapharyngeal abscess.
3. In an adult more than 40 years of age, a neck swelling may be of malignant nature.
4. A metastatic node in the neck is often due to primary in the upper aerodigestive tract.
5. A clinically obvious metastatic node is hard in consistency and may be fixed to the underlying structures.
6. Tubercular lymph node is often multiple and matted.
7. Pulsatile neck swelling may be due to carotid/subclavian artery aneurysm or due to a carotid body tumour.
8. Cystic swelling in the neck may be branchial or thyroglossal cyst.
9. Ultrasonography of the neck is an invaluable tool in assessment of cervical lymph nodes and other swellings and helps in differentiating solid from cystic masses. It also helps in assessment of the relation of the neck mass to the carotid artery and the internal jugular vein.

For detailed account on Clinical examination methodology please refer to the same authors' book entitled 'Clinical Operative methods in ENT and Head & Neck Surgery'.

Cystic Lesions of the Head and Neck

81

CYSTIC LESION OF JAW

Dental Cyst

This arises due to inflammatory change in the tooth root membrane due to injury or disease. It has already been discussed under chapter 'Benign tumors of nose and PNS'.

Dentigerous Cyst

Cyst arising from an expansion of tooth follicle associated with an unerupted tooth, presenting as a slow growing swelling involving the lower or upper tooth. (Discussed under chapter 'Benign tumors of nose and PNS').

CYSTS OF THE FLOOR OF THE MOUTH

RANULA

It is a mucous retention cyst of the sublingual salivary gland and is seen as a brilliantly translucent cystic mass in the floor of the mouth.

Etiology

It occurs as a result of obstruction of the secretary duct of the sublingual salivary gland.

Clinical Features

Patients present with swelling in the region of floor of the mouth, bluish in color. The swelling may cause dysarthria and difficulty in chewing. It may also interfere with deglutition. In case of plunging ranula, patient may also present with a neck swelling in the submandibular/ submental swelling (more details given later in this chapter). The swelling is brilliantly positive for transillumination and is fluctuant (Fig. 81.1).

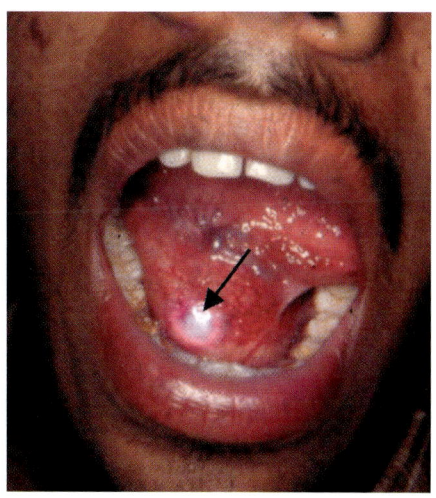

Fig. 81.1: A ranula (arrow) in the floor of the mouth

Treatment

Marsupialization is treatment of choice. Excision may be associated with recurrence if the cyst ruptures because of its thin wall.

DERMOID CYST

The cyst is seen anteriorly and medially in the oral cavity in the region of the floor of the mouth. The cyst is opaque and is seen posterior or lateral to the frenulum. Superficial dermoid appears white.

Etiology

It originates from varied germinal epithelium trapped during embryonic fusion.

Pathology

The swelling is superior to the mylohyoid muscle.

Clinical Features

It appears as a slow growing cystic painless swelling in the floor of the mouth. Fluctuation is positive and transillumination test is negative. It is noticed commonly in young adulthood and is rare in infants. It is difficult sometimes to differentiate dermoid cysts from ranula if the lesion is deep and posterior.

Treatment

No treatment is required if the cyst is not large enough to interfere with eating and speaking. Treatment should be complete excision as recurrence can occur.

CYSTS PRESENTING AS LATERAL NECK MASS

BRANCHIAL CYST OR FISTULA

Definition

It occurs as a result of an abnormal development of primitive ectodermal pharyngeal pouches and/or the endoderm of the embryonic cervical sinus.

It is of two types
- Above the hyoid bone
- Below the hyoid bone.

Applied Embryology

Branchial apparatus was first described by Baer in 1827. Branchial apparatus begins to develop during the second week of gestation. By beginning of 4th week there are 4 well defined pairs of branchial arches separated by branchial clefts (Fig. 46.1).

First Branchial Arch Anomalies

They are much less common. They form less than 1 percent of all branchiogenic anomalies. 1st branchial anomalies usually appear on the face or are related to the auricle.

Second Branchial Anomalies

They are most common type. They can present as cyst, sinus, or fistula.

Etiological Factors

Age and sex: Defects of the branchial tract are usually found in the young people and predominantly in females. Though congenital it does not usually present before puberty. Most patients are between the age of 20 to 25 years or even later because fluid which it contains takes time to accumulate.

Pathology

The cysts is usually lined by stratified squamous epithelium and:
- Contains lymphoid tissue, so it is prone to infection.
- Contents are viscid, mucoid, cheesy material contains cholesterol crystals.

True branchial cyst is above the hyoid bone. Defects below the hyoid bone may be located at any level in the neck including the nasopharynx.

The tracts or cysts extends below the anterior portion of the sternomastoid and carotid vessels and the posterior belly of the digastric muscle. It arches behind the stylopharyngeus muscle and ends in the tonsillar fossa.

Clinical Features

Symptoms (Fig. 81.2)

- Painless swelling in upper and lateral part of neck.
- If infected it becomes painful
- Sometimes it is difficult to differentiate from acute lymphadenitis, chronic lymphadenitis, tubercular lymphadenitis (cold abscess).

Signs

- Swelling is usually oval in shape but may be round and soft in consistency and cannot be reduced or compressed.
- Fluctuation test—Positive
- Transillumination may be negative
- It is commonly seen in the upper and lateral portion of the neck deep to the upper third of anterior border of the sternomastoid muscle and beneath the angle of mandible.
- An infected cyst can present like an abscess and if it ruptures or is drained it can result in fistula formation.
- The fistula is associated with intermittent or continuous discharge.

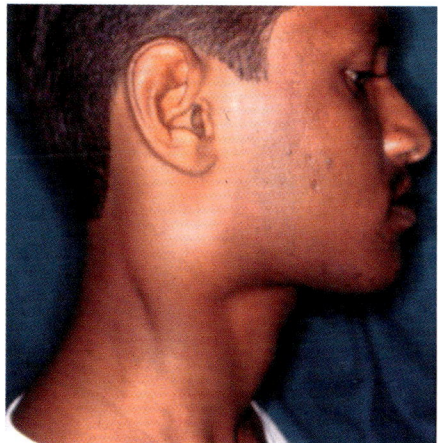

Fig. 81.2: Branchial cyst of the right upper neck

Investigations

- Contrast X-ray (Fistulogram)
- Fine needle aspiration cytology— Cholesterol crystals (+)

Cysts that contain Cholesterol Crystals

- Branchial cyst
- Dental cyst
- Dentigerous cyst
- Cystic hygroma (rare)
- Thyroglossal cyst (rare).

Differential Diagnosis

1. ***Submandibular Salivary Gland Swelling***
   - Submandibular triangle
   - Usually solid.

2. ***Plunging Ranula***
   - Present in floor of mouth
   - Cross fluctuation—Present
   - Brilliantly translucent swelling.

3. ***Cervical Dermoid***
   - Usually midline swelling
   - Rare in submandibular triangle
   - No cholesterol crystals in aspirates.

4. ***Cystic Hygroma***
   - Seen since birth
   - Translucent swelling
   - Present in posterior triangle
   - Attain large size.

5. ***Cervical Lymph Node***
   - Solid swelling
   - Transmitted pulsations (+).

Complications

- Recurrent infection
- Acquired branchial fistula.

Treatment

Complete excision of the cyst or fistula from the neck to the pharynx is the treatment of choice.

Steps of Surgery

1. Incision made parallel to skin crease (Langer's line)
2. Step ladder incision for exposure of cyst/fistula.
3. Methylene blue can be injected in the cyst to aid in surgery.
4. Some amount of fluid may be aspirated to have grasping over the wall.
5. Care is taken not to leave any portion of cyst.
6. Hypoglossal nerve, glossopharyngeal nerve and carotid artery lie deep to cyst and they should be protected.

Laryngocele

It is an air filled dilatation of sacculus or appendix of the laryngeal ventricle that occurs in person with congenitally large ventricular appendix. It presents as a neck mass if the cystic mass is situated lateral to the thyrohyoid membrane (external type).

This is discussed under the chapter 'congenital diseases of larynx'.

Lymphangioma and Cystic Hygroma

Lymphangioma results from abnormal development of the lymphatic system with obstruction of lymphatic drainage from the affected area causing multicentric endothelial lining spaces. Cystic hygromas are large lympangiomas found most commonly in children.

Etiology

Cervical cystic hygroma may appear before 30th week of gestation and are associated with chromosomal abnormalities.

Pathology

- Cystic swelling which contain multiple locules of clear lymph.
- Sequestration of a portion of the jugular sac from lymphatic system which fails to join the regular lymphatic system gives rise to cystic hygroma.

Sites of Cystic Hygroma

- Posterior triangle of neck is commonest site. The swelling gradually extends upward to the ear and down towards lower neck.
- Cheek
- Tongue
- Base of tongue
- Supraglottic larynx
- Mediastinum

Clinical Features

Symptoms (Fig. 81.3)

- Commonly seen in infancy and early childhood
- Presents with painless, slowly progressive lump or swelling commonly in the lateral aspect of the neck

Signs

- Swelling often seen in the lower third of neck in posterior triangle
- Size varies extremely, usually round in shape with smooth indistinct margin, with a smooth and lobulated surface.
- Swelling is often soft and cystic in consistency and it may increase in size on coughing (cough impulse)
- Transillumination test is brilliantly positive

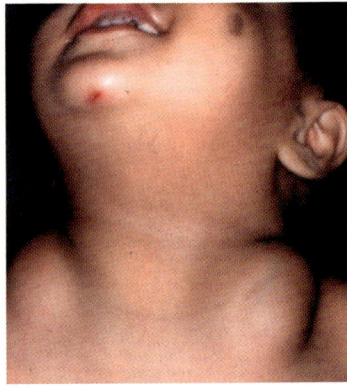

Fig. 81.3: Cystic hygroma of the neck

Complications

- Stridor may be seen due to tracheal shift and compression or supraglottic involvement. Tracheostomy is required in such cases.
- Hemorrhage can cause painful enlargement of cystic hygroma with evidence of acute blood loss.
- Infection of the cystic locules can cause pain and rapid increase in size.

Investigations

MRI/ CT imaging to assess the exact extent of the lesion and its relation to the vital structures in the neck/ mediastinum and the skull base. Invasion of the lesion to local structures and the airway can also be assessed.

Treatment

Medical treatment

Injection of sclerosing agents like absolute alcohol, Picibanil (OK-432 which contains penicillin and streptococci) and/or steroids may be tried.

Surgical treatment

Tracheostomy has to be done if airway obstruction is present. This may be difficult if there is tracheal shift or if the tumor is anterior to the trachea causing compression. Hence it is better done after endotracheal intubation, if possible. Surgical excise is preferably carried out at the same sitting.

Excision is the mainstay of treatment and it may be delayed until child is 3 to 4 years if there is no airway obstruction. During resection care must be taken to resect the extensions of cyst through muscle plane. A cystic hygroma of the neck may require an extensive neck dissection and a median sternotomy to excise a mediastinal component. Care should be taken to preserve neurovascular structures.

Complications resulting from excision of a cystic hygroma include damage to a neurovascular structure, chylous fistula, chylothorax, and hemorrhage

Dangers of Incomplete Removal

- Recurrence
- Chyle leak—Continuous fluid and electrolyte loss through open cyst
- Wound infection.

CYSTS PRESENTING AS MIDLINE NECK MASS

THYROGLOSSAL CYST (Fig. 81.4)

Cystic swelling developed in the remnant of thyroglossal tract is called *Thyroglossal cyst*. It is the commonest retention cyst below the level of the hyoid and is the most common congenital neck mass.

Pathology

- Lymphoid tissue is present outside the epithelial lining and hence it is prone for infection.
- May form anywhere in the midline of the neck along the tract of the vestigial thyroglossal

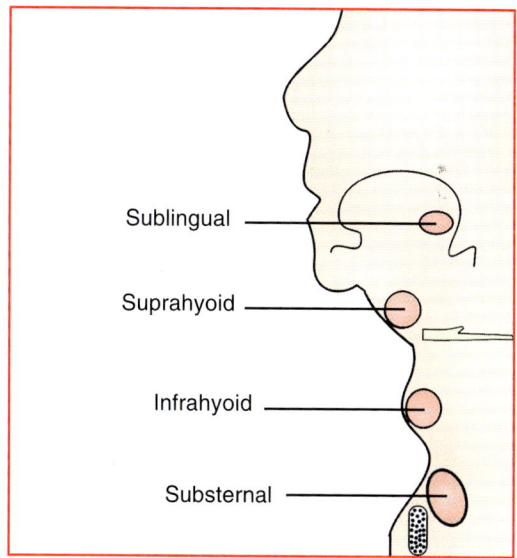

Fig. 81.4: Showing various sites of thyroglossal cyst

duct, from the base of the tongue to the region of the thyroid gland. It most commonly occurs in the subhyoid area and can be rarely seen in the retrosternal area.

- Thyroglossal fistula is formed due to secondary infection resulting in rupture of the cyst on the surface of the neck in the midline and sometimes due to incision and drainage for suspecting it to be an abscess.

Clinical Features

Symptoms

- Midline swelling seen in the anterior aspect of the neck
- Painless if not infected
- May suddenly increase in size following infection.
- Infected cyst may rupture leading to formation of discharging thyroglossal fistula.

Signs (Fig. 81.5)

- Cyst can occur anywhere from foramen cecum to the isthmus of thyroid gland but most frequently it is seen in:
  1. Subhyoid region
  2. In region of thyroid cartilage
  3. Suprahyoid position

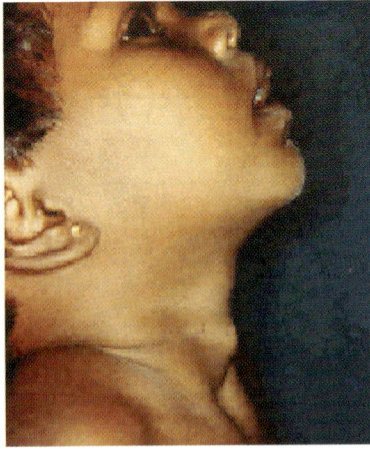

Fig. 81.5: Thyroglossal cyst

4. At the level of cricoid cartilage
5. Beneath the foramen cecum.

- Cystic Swelling or fistula in the midline moves with deglutition and protrusion of the tongue as the tract extends superiorly till the foramen cecum of the tongue.
- The discharge from the fistula may be mucoid and sometimes it may be watery or milky. The discharge is purulent if the cyst is infected.
- *'Hood sign':* The skin above the fistulous opening is pulled upwards by the thyroglossal tract and this gives rise to puckering of the skin resembling a hood of a snake.

Investigations

- Thyroid scan to rule out an ectopic thyroid
- Fistulogram is done if it is associated with fistula, which helps in identifying the extent of the tract.

Differential Diagnosis

- Dermoid cyst
- Pyramidal lobe hyperplasia
- Thymic cyst
- Subhyoid bursitis.

Treatment

- Excision of the entire tract from the neck to the foramen cecum is necessary.
- Preliminary injection of the methylene blue into the tract helps in identification of the tract before surgery
- Sistrunk procedure is recommended for complete removal, which includes complete resection of the cyst along with all the abnormal tissue, body of the hyoid bone and the fibrous cord extending to the foramen cecum.

Prognosis

The patient should be followed up as papillary carcinoma as well as Hurthle cell adenoma has been reported to be arising from thyroglossal duct cyst.

SUBLINGUAL DERMOID CYST

This is a thin walled cyst lined by squamous epithelium and contains cheesy material. These cysts are always in midline.

Types

1. Midline variety
   - Sublingual
   - Cervical.
2. Lateral variety
   - Sublingual
   - Cervical.

   Lateral variety cysts usually derives from 2nd branchial cleft.

Clinical Features

Present usually in the ages of 10 to 15 years and present equally in both sexes.

Symptoms

Patient presents with painless swelling under the tongue. Sometimes sudden increase in size may become painful.

Signs

Sublingual type

Median variety is usually sublingual type and appears as a midline swelling in floor of mouth with a smooth surface.

Cervical type

- Gives rise to double chin appearance
- Does not move with protrusion of tongue

Differential Diagnosis

- *Ranula:* Brilliant translucent midline swelling
- *Suprahyoid thyroglossal cyst:* Moves up with protrusion of tongue
- Submental lymph node.

Treatment

- Total excision is treatment of choice.
- Supramylohyoid variety is approached through floor of mouth.
- Inframylohyoid variety is approached through the neck by curved incision along the Langer's line.

SUBHYOID BURSAL CYST

It occurs due to enlargement of subhyoid bursa as a result of accumulation of inflammatory fluid within it and is located below the hyoid; in front of thyrohyoid membrane

Diagnosis

- Pain with swelling just below hyoid
- Swelling is oval in parallel to long axis of hyoid bone.
- The cyst moves up during swallowing.

Treatment

Complete excision of cyst along the Langer's lines.

Swelling which moves up with deglutition

1. Thyroid swelling
2. Ectopic thyroid
3. Enlarged pretracheal lymph node
4. Thyroglossal cyst
5. Subhyoid bursal cyst
6. Laryngocele.

Deep Plunging Ranula

This is a ranula with cervical extension. Ranula is an extravasation cyst arising from damaged sublingual gland.

Course

It passes beyond the floor of mouth along posterior border of myelohyoid muscle to appear in submandibular region.

Clinical Features

Symptoms

1. Painless midline swelling in the submandibular region
2. Secondary infection can cause pain and sudden increase in size.
3. Rupture of the cyst may occur due to trauma or infection of the cyst.
4. Dysarthria and dysphagia may be present

Signs (Fig. 81.6)

- Bidigital palpation may elicit cross fluctuation.
- Cyst is brilliantly translucent

Differential Diagnosis

- Sublingual dermoid
- Submandibular salivary gland swelling

Treatment

Treatment of choice is excision of the cyst by a transcervical approach in continuity with sublingual gland of origin. Careful dissection is necessary to prevent rupture of the cyst during surgery.

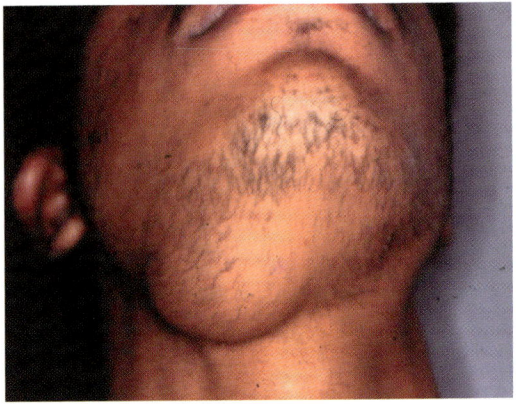

Fig. 81.6: Plunging ranula presenting as a neck swelling

Thymic Cyst

During 6th week of fetal life III pharyngeal pouch gives rise to thymus gland and during 9th week, thymus descends below the clavicles. Thymic remnant may persist as cords of cysts along path of migration from angle of mandible to midline of neck and may present as a swelling in lower neck. Excision of the cyst is done for cosmetic or mechanical reason.

POINTS TO REMEMBER

1. Though branchial cyst is congenital, the swelling usually appears after puberty.
2. Branchial cyst is commonly seen over upper one third of anterior border of sternomastoid muscle.
3. Ranula is a retention cyst of sublingual salivary gland and is seen in the floor of the mouth as a bluish thin walled cyst. Plunging ranula presents as a neck swelling in the submandibular region as the cyst extends into the neck posterior to the mylohyoid muscle.
4. Cystic hygroma is a lymphangiomatous swelling present since birth and is commonly seen in the posterior triangle.
5. Most common site of thyroglossal cyst is subhyoid region.

82

Solid Swellings in the Neck

The common solid neck swellings include the following:

- Lymph node swelling
- Swelling arising from thyroid
- Swelling arising from salivary gland
- Carotid body tumor
- Branchiogenic carcinoma
- Sternomastoid tumor
- Cervical rib.

LYMPH NODE SWELLING

Most common solid neck swelling is of the cervical lymph nodes. Cervical lymph node enlargement or cervical lymphadenopathy can be due to various causes like:

Inflammatory

- Acute non-specific lymphadenitis—viral or bacterial
- Acute specific lymphadenitis like infectious mononucleosis
- Chronic nonspecific lymphadenitis commonly due to adenotonsillar or orodental sepsis
- Chronic specific lymphadenitis like tuberculosis, syphilis, leprosy, etc.

Neoplastic

- **Primary:** Lymphoma
- **Secondary:** Metastatic cervical node from squamous cell carcinoma of head and neck

or adenocarcinoma from the aerodigestive tract or from papillary carcinoma of the thyroid.

As part of Systemic Conditions

- Leukemia
- Storage diseases like Niemann-Pick disease, sphingomyelin
- Drug reactions—Examples: Mephenytoin, pyrimethamine, phenylbutazone, allopurinol, and isoniazid
- Langerhans cell histiocytosis
- Epstein-Barr virus (EBV)—Associated lymphoproliferative disease
- Autoimmune etiologies include juvenile rheumatoid arthritis
- Sarcoidosis and graft verses host disease

In India tubercular lymphadenitis is a very common condition and hence is discussed in more detail.

TUBERCULAR LYMPHADENITIS

Definition

It is a chronic infection of the lymph nodes due to *Mycobacterium tuberculae* and is characterized by presence of matted lymph nodes in the neck.

Portals of Entry of Infection

- Pharyngeal lymphoid tissue like tonsils 'Bovine type'

713

- Secondary to pulmonary tuberculosis
- Hematogenous-rare

Recently there has been an increase in its incidence due to AIDS.

Pathological Stages (Fig. 82.1)

1. **Stage of adenitis:** The nodes are enlarged but discrete
2. **Stage of periadenitis:** causing matting of the nodes.
3. **Stage of cold abscess formation:** This is due to central caseation within the node (Fig. 82.2).
4. **Stage of collar-stud abscess formation:** The cold abscess ruptures out of the deep fascia into the subcutaneous plane to give rise to dumb-bell shaped abscess cavity.
5. **Stage of tubercular sinus:** The abscess ruptures through the skin causing fistula or sinus with undermined edges.

Clinical Features

- Lateral neck swelling/s
- Often multiple/ bilateral
- Initially it is painless and gradually increases in size
- Non-healing discharging ulcer
- Systemic symptoms of tuberculosis may be present like evening rise in temperature, night sweats, weight loss, etc. may be present.

Signs (Figs 82.3 and 82.4)

- Pallor and/or clubbing may be present.
- Fever more in the evenings may be present.
- Multiple matted nodes that are not freely mobile.
- Skin involvement in the form of congestion, edema or ulcer/ sinus may be seen.
- Fluctuant abscess may be palpated.
- Ulcer if present has characteristic undermining edges.

Investigations

- FNAC
- Biopsy

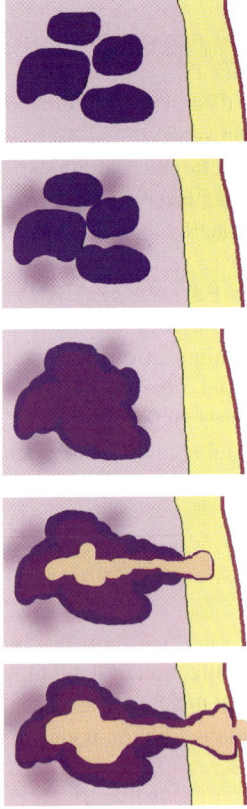

Fig. 82.1: Various stages of tubercular lymphadenitis

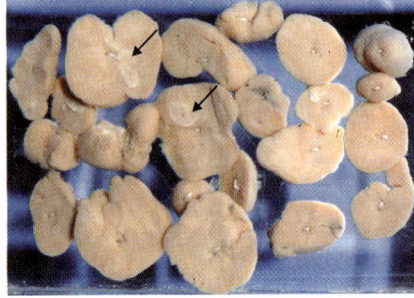

Fig. 82.2: Resected lymph nodes showing caseation necrosis within the nodes

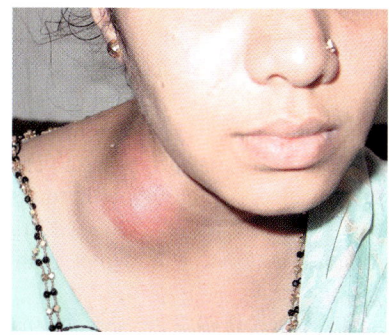

Fig. 82.3: Photograph showing collar-stud abscess in the neck

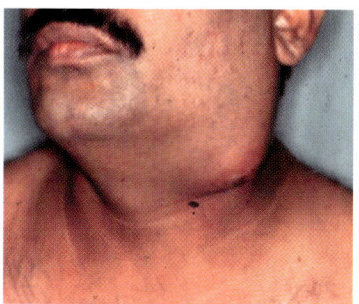

Fig. 82.4: Clinical photograph showing a case of tubercular lymphadenitis with matted nodes

- Full blood picture including hemoglobin, total and differential counts and ESR.
- Chest X-ray to rule out pulmonary focus
- Mantoux test.

Treatment

- Anti-tubercular treatment: Ethambutol, rifampicin, isoniazid and pyrizanamide is preferred for a period of 9 to 12 months.
- Surgical excision if residual nodes are present.

ECTOPIC THYROID

Definition

Ectopic thyroid is defined as a developmental anomaly associated with change of location of the thyroid tissue from its normal site which can occur anywhere between foramen cecum to the lower neck.

Embryogenesis

Primitive thyroid gland begins as a diverticulum of endodermal origin from the foramen cecum that is situated between the tuberculum impar and copula at about 4 weeks of fetal life. This thyroglossal diverticulum descends caudally adjacent to the primitive hyoid bone as a duct called thyroglossal duct. This duct reaches its final position in the midline of the neck and subsequently develops into the thyroid gland. Then the duct gradually atrophies. Persistence of the duct anywhere in the line of descent due to failure to obliterate completely gives rise to ectopic thyroid. Rarely the duct may descend even inferiorly to give rise to substernal thyroid. A partially descended thyroglossal diverticulum also can give rise to ectopic thyroid tissue where a normal thyroid tissue may be absent.

Clinical Features

The most common locations of the ectopic thyroid is shown in the diagram (Fig. 82.5). They include:

- Lingual (Fig. 82.6)
- Sublingual
- Prelaryngeal
- Normal
- Substernal

Symptoms vary with the site of the ectopic thyroid. Lingual thyroid is described under chapter 'Miscellaneous conditions of the pharynx'. Sublingual and prelaryngeal thyroid frequently present as a neck mass above and below the hyoid bone respectively. Lingual thyroid presents as a swelling in the base tongue and can cause difficulty in deglutition and if excessively enlarged can cause airway obstruction. Sublingual thyroid may grow more posteriorly pushing the epiglottis backwards and can present as a swelling in the valleculae which may extend laterally to the level of the pharyn-

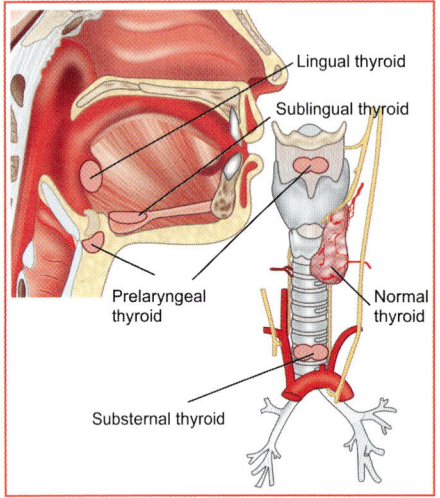

Fig. 82.5: Showing various sites of ectopic thyroid

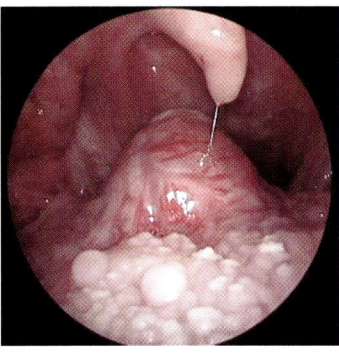

Fig. 82.6: Endoscopic picture showing lingual thyroid

goepiglottic folds. Substernal ectopic thyroid can present with features of superior mediastinal syndrome. The ectopic thyroid may increase in size due to hemorrhage into the thyroid or during the periods of stress like pregnancy.

Investigations

- Thyroid scan
- T3, T4, TSH estimation
- Ultrasound of the neck
- CT/ MRI scan may be helpful especially in retrosternal and sublingual thyroids.

Treatment

Asymptomatic cases may be observed periodically as these cases may present with sudden increase in size due to hemorrhage and it may give rise to dyspnea, dysphagia, change of voice, etc. Features of hypo/hyperthyroidism also may be seen in some cases. Malignant transformation may occur. In symptomatic cases surgery is indicated.

All ectopic thyroids can be approached trans-cervically, however retrosternal thyroid may require sternotomy/ thoracotomy especially if there is mediastinal extension. Attempts have been made to implant the ectopic thyroid tissue if they are the only functioning thyroid tissue, in the neck. However such cases should be kept on a regular follow-up as there may be malignant transformation. Regular hormonal assessment and thyroxin supplementation is required if indicated.

CAROTID BODY TUMOR

This is a paraganglioma of the chemoreceptor cells (glomus bodies) seen in the carotid bulb. This is vascular tumor with more surface vasculature than glomus vagale and is often deeply embedded in the vessel wall making its resection difficult. It is more common in high altitude area like Peru, Colarado, Tibet and Mexico.

Etiology

High altitude area where there is chronic hypoxia which leads to carotid body hyperplasia. It is an autosomal dominant disease with family history in 10 percent of the cases.

Pathology

It arises from the chemoreceptor cell on the medial aspect of the carotid bulb. Histologically it is similar to the normal carotid body cells. It is often hormonally inactive though they may have pheochromocytoma-like features.

Clinical Features

Symptoms

- Slow painless swelling or lump in the neck and commonly present as a parapharyngeal mass.
- Dysphagia and change in voice may be present in cases with advanced disease.

Signs

- Tonsil may be pushed medially
- Neck swelling is firm, rubbery, pulsatile synchronizing with the arterial pulsations
- Bruit is often present
- Size may decrease with carotid compression

Investigations

CT/MR imaging

Digital subtraction angiography: Lyre's sign showing widening of angle between the internal and external carotid arteries.

24 hours urine for Vanellyl Mandelic Acid (VMA)

Treatment

Small or medium sized tumor can be surgically removed relatively easily than a large tumor. Trans-cervical approach is the preferred approach. The incision preferred is a long one from mastoid tip to the clavicle on the side of the tumor so that the entire length of the carotid sheath can be exposed. Tumor close to the skull base makes tumor resection difficult and in such case a transcervical transmandibular approach gives better exposure. The carotid artery may have to be resected and a vascular reconstruction is necessary in such cases.

Extensive tumor with metastasis or in high risk patients or in those who refuse surgery, radiotherapy may be indicated.

Diseases of thyroid and salivary glands are discussed in detail in the respective chapters and hence are not included here.

POINTS TO REMEMBER

1. Enlarged lymph nodes are most common solid swellings of the neck.
2. In children, solid neck swelling is usually due to chronic non-specific lymphadenitis and is often secondary to adenotonsillar disease.
3. Tubercular lymphadenitis is characterized by multiple lymph nodes with matting.
4. In adults, solid neck swelling could be due to metastasis into the lymph node from a primary squamous cell carcinoma arising in the upper aerodigestive tract.
5. Ectopic thyroid can present anywhere between foramen cecum (base of the tongue) to the lower neck.
6. Ectopic thyroids can be only functioning thyroid and hence excision can give rise to hypothyroidism. Only symptomatic ectopic thyroids should be surgically treated and attempt should be made to reimplant the thyroid tissue or relocate the ectopic thyroid.
7. Carotid body tumor are more common among people living in high altitude areas.
8. Carotid body tumors are highly vascular and are closely related to the carotid artery. Hence, its excision should be done only by surgeon with expertise in microvascular anastomosis.
9. Digital subtraction angiography is an invaluable tool in a case of carotid body tumor as it helps in assessing the feeding vessels, its relation to the carotid arteries and also the collateral circulation of the brain.
10. Disease of thyroid and salivary glands also may present as solid neck swellings.
11. Malignancy arising from a branchial cyst is known as branchiogenic carcinoma.

Thyroid Neoplasm

Introduction

In general thyroid swellings are recognized by its position, shape and the fact that it moves up with deglutition. Goiter (in Latin; Gutter =Throat) means any enlargement of the thyroid irrespective of its pathology.

Virtually any disease of the thyroid gland can present as goiter. The spectrum varies from simple goiter to malignancy. Diagnosis of a malignancy in such patients remains challenging and often unaccomplished task. In spite of its limitations clinical judgment remains an important and cost effective initial step and various diagnostic procedures have been developed and they further assist in detecting malignancy in suspicious cases.

Surgical Anatomy

Thyroid gland (Greek = Shield like) is roughly butterfly in shape and is the largest endocrine gland. Normally it is not visible outside unless it is enlarged. It contains two lateral lobes connected by isthmus. In the adult, the thyroid gland is located deep to the cervical strap muscles extending from the middle of the thyroid cartilage to the fourth or fifth tracheal rings. Position varies with the length of the neck. Isthmus overlies second and third tracheal rings.

Thyroid is covered by true and false capsules. The true capsule is a peripheral condensation of the connective tissue. False capsule is formed by pretracheal fascia, which forms the posterior suspensory (Berry) ligament. It attaches the posteromedial aspect of the thyroid lobe to the cricoid cartilage and the first and second tracheal rings. Because of this attachment only thyroid swellings moves up with deglutition.

Surgical Implications

1. Dense capillary plexus is present deep to the true capsule, so to avoid hemorrhage gland is removed along with true capsule.
2. The recurrent laryngeal nerve (RLN) passes deep to the Berry's ligament or between the main ligament and the lateral leaf, or rarely above the ligament.
3. The RLN, when it does branch extra-laryngeally, often branches proximal to the ligament.
4. Deep to the ligament or along its inferior edge a branch of inferior thyroid artery crosses and if it bleeds the surgeon is often tempted to clamp indiscriminately which can give rise to recurrent laryngeal nerve injury.

Blood Supply

The thyroid is a highly vascular organ, with a normal flow rate of 5 ml/g per minute. Knowledge of its blood supply facilitates any related surgical procedure and minimizes hemorrhage.

Arterial

- Two pairs of arteries (superior and inferior thyroid arteries)
- An inconstant artery (arteria thyroidea ima)

Venous Drainage

- Three pairs of veins (superior, middle and inferior thyroid veins)
- An inconsistent vein (Kocher's vein).

The **superior thyroid artery** is the first branch of the external carotid artery, arising from its lower anterior part (just below the tip of the greater horn of the hyoid bone), turning caudal to the apex of the corresponding lobe of the thyroid, and dividing into glandular branches. As the superior thyroid artery reaches the upper pole of the lateral lobe, it trifurcates. The superior laryngeal artery enters the larynx with the internal branch of the superior laryngeal nerve.

The **superior thyroid vein** accompanies the superior thyroid artery and ends in the internal jugular vein. On the anterior surface of the thyroid gland are prominent connections between the superior and the inferior thyroid veins.

A **middle thyroid vein**, which has no corresponding artery, is often present; this vein leaves the gland in its midportion to follow the outer border of the omohyoid muscle, cross the common carotid artery, and terminate in the internal jugular vein.

The **inferior thyroid artery** is a branch of the thyrocervical trunk, which is the first branch of the subclavian artery. It ascends along the anterior border of the anterior scalenus muscle and, opposite the cricoid cartilage, turns medially, traversing deep to the common carotid artery and to the middle of the posterior border of the corresponding lobe of the thyroid. It then curves medially and downward and descends to the lower half of the lobe.

The inferior thyroid artery provides the major blood supply to the upper half of the trachea, usually through three branches, of which the first and lowermost is the largest. The branch near the lower pole of the thyroid gland is the third and uppermost and is the smallest. Division of that branch during surgical removal of the thyroid should not impair tracheal vascularization.

As the inferior thyroid artery passes medially behind the gland, it crosses the recurrent laryngeal nerves in front, behind, or on both sides of them.

Usually, the inferior thyroid artery closely approximates the middle cervical sympathetic ganglion

The **inferior thyroid veins** originate on the anterior surface of the gland and descend anterior to the trachea. Both may terminate in the left innominate vein or the left may end in the left and the right in the right innominate vein. Both inferior thyroid veins may have numerous connections and form a plexus in front of the trachea beneath the isthmus.

In 10 percent of cases, a fifth artery normally present in the embryo (the **thyroidea ima**) arises form the aortic arch or innominate artery or lower common carotid artery and reaches the inferior border of the isthmus after running upward on the anterior surface of the trachea.

In very rare cases, a fourth thyroid vein (of **Kocher**) may emerge between the middle and inferior thyroid veins and drains into internal jugular vein (Fig. 83.1).

Nerve Supply

The principal innervation of the thyroid and parathyroid is derived from the sympathetic and parasympathetic divisions of the autonomic nervous system. The sympathetic fibers descend from the superior, middle, inferior sympathetic ganglia of the sympathetic trunk, and enter with the blood vessels.

The parasympathetic fibers are derived from the vagus nerve and reach the gland via branches of the laryngeal nerves. The specific role of the autonomic nervous system in relation to glandular secretion is not clearly understood, but it is postulated that most of the effect is on blood vessels and perfusion rate of the glands.

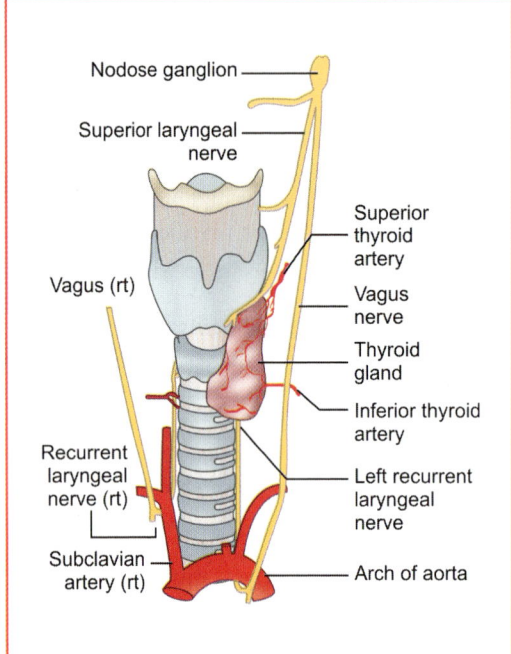

Fig. 83.1: Showing anatomy of the recurrent laryngeal and superior laryngeal nerves

Nerves related to Thyroid Gland

The relationship of the thyroid gland to the recurrent laryngeal nerve, the external laryngeal nerve, and the cervical sympathetic systems is of major surgical importance. Embryologically, the recurrent laryngeal nerve (inferior laryngeal nerves) originates from the vagus nerves near the fourth branchial arches. These arches later become the aortic arch on the left and the subclavian artery on the right, and as these structures descend in the upper thorax, they 'pull' the recurrent laryngeal nerves with them.

Recurrent Laryngeal Nerve

On the right side, the RLN leaves the vagus nerve as the latter crosses the first portion of the subclavian artery, the recurrent laryngeal nerve then turns upward and medially, it lies in a triangle bounded laterally by the carotid sheath, medially

by the trachea and esophagus and superiorly by the inferior pole of thyroid gland (Beahr's Recurrent laryngeal nerve triangle).

Most often but not always, travels upward in the groove between the trachea and the esophagus. The RLN may run laterally in this visceral compartment and the right is more likely than the left to lie lateral to the traditional tracheo-esophageal groove position.

Right RLN is more vulnerable to injury during surgery on the thyroid gland because of its more anterior and lateral position at the inferior pole of the thyroid gland, rather than being protected in the TE groove.

On the left side, the recurrent laryngeal nerve turns under the arch of the aorta and ascends into the neck, most often in the tracheoesophageal groove. At the level of the inferior border of the thyroid lobe, the left recurrent laryngeal nerve, like its counterpart, may be in front of, behind, or between the terminal branches of the inferior thyroid artery.

The extralaryngeal division of RLN has been described in 35 percent to 80 percent of anatomic dissections. The typical division includes an anterior (motor) and a posterior (sensory) division but patterns with two to eight branches were described.

The RLN enters the larynx through the Killian-Jamieson area posterior to the cricothyroid joint (Inferior cornu of the thyroid cartilage).

A few patients (0.3 to 0.8 percent) have a 'nonrecurrent' laryngeal nerve on the right side, originating from the cervical trunk of the vagus at the level of the thyroid cartilage and passing directly into the cricothyroid membrane. The vast majority of these occur on the right side in conjunction with an anomalous retroesophageal subclavian artery. Rare cases of left nonrecurrent laryngeal nerves have been reported associated with transposition of great vessels.

Superior Laryngeal Nerve (SLN)

The nerve divides at the level of hyoid bone into a large internal laryngeal nerve and a small external laryngeal nerve. The latter descends on the fascia of the inferior constrictor muscle and courses below the oblique attachment of the sternothyroid muscle, which is on the thyroid cartilage to innervate the cricothyroid muscle. Several investigators identified the variable branching pattern of the SLN particularly the external branch and its relationship to the superior thyroid vascular pedicle.

Lymphatic Drainage

The lymphatic drainage of the thyroid gland is mainly by lymphatic vessels that accompany the arterial blood supply.

The superior border of the isthmus, the medial surface of the lateral lobes, and the ventral and dorsal surfaces of the upper part of the lateral lobes drain into the superior lymphatic channels that empty into the upper deep cervical nodes either directly or through the prelaryngeal nodes (Delphian node).

The inferior channels drain most of the isthmus and lower portions of the lateral lobes into the lower deep cervical nodes and into the pretracheal and paratracheal nodes. However, a portion of the lymphatic drainage of the lateral lobes proceeds to the retropharyngeal and retroesophageal areas where local metastatic disease can occasionally be seen.

However, it must be noted that in the thyroid the lymphatics form a plexus through which lymph may pass in any direction.

Classification of Thyroid Swellings (Goiter)

1. **Physiological**
   (a) Puberty
   (b) Pregnancy
   (c) Lactation.
2. **Non-toxic:** This could be diffuse or solitary nodule or multinodular goiter
   (a) Endemic
      (i) Iodine deficiency
      (ii) Iodine excess
      (iii) Dietary goitrogens

(b) Sporadic
   (i) Dietary goitrogens
   (ii) Congenital defect of hormone synthesis
   (iii) Iodine deficiency
   (iv) Compensatory hypertrophy following subtotal thyroidectomy.
3. **Toxic**
   (a) Primary (Grave's disease)
   (b) Secondary (multinodular goiter turning toxic).
4. **Neoplasm**
   (a) Benign
      – Adenoma
   (b) Malignant
      – Well differentiated
      – Papillary carcinoma: Low grade, high grade, Hurthle cell carcinoma
      – Follicular carcinoma.
   (c) Medullary carcinoma
   (d) Undifferentiated/ Anaplastic carcinoma
   (e) Lymphoma
   (f) Metastatic carcinoma
   (g) Sarcoma
5. **Autoimmune**
   (a) Hashimoto's thyroiditis
   (b) Reidel's thyroiditis.

In this chapter we discuss only about thyroid neoplasm as it is more relevant in head and neck surgery.

Benign Neoplasm

Benign enlargement of the thyroid gland is common. Colloid goiter and adenomatous goiter with multiple nodules of varying size are commonly encountered. Solitary nodules occur in 5 percent of the population. A solitary nodule can be defined as a discrete mass greater than or equal to 1 cm in diameter discovered by palpation of the thyroid gland and otherwise the thyroid is normal in size and consistency. The most common cause of solitary thyroid nodule in children and adolescents is follicular adenoma. Malignancy is reported in 25 percent of cold nodules.

Adenoma

This is the most common benign thyroid neoplasm presenting as a solitary thyroid nodule. It can also present as a dominant nodule in a multi-nodular goiter. It is more common in middle aged females. They rarely become toxic. It may become functioning nodule and may be autonomous. Histopathologically it can be follicular, microfollicular, Hurthle cell type and very rarely papillary. Low grade papillary carcinoma should be ruled out in papillary adenomas.

DIAGNOSIS OF MALIGNANCY IN A NODULAR ENLARGEMENT OF THE THYROID

Clinical Evaluation

When a patient presents with a thyroid nodule, clinical evaluation starts with a thorough history and a comprehensive head and neck examination. There are important factors in the history and physical examination that lead the surgeon to suspect malignancy.

History

Age: Thyroid is the only endocrine organ wherein malignant tumors occur in children, young age, middle age and old ages. A thyroid nodule is more likely to be malignant at age extremes (age younger than 20 or older than 60). Children may also develop thyroid nodules, with a greater risk (approximately 30%) of malignancy than adults. After the age of 60, the incidence of carcinoma in thyroid nodule rises.

Gender: Thyroid cancers are more common in females.

Neck mass: Thyroid cancer most commonly presents as an asymptomatic, solitary nodule within the thyroid gland. Unfortunately, this is also a very common presentation for nonmalignant diseases of the thyroid gland.

Duration of the thyroid mass: Rapidly progressive mass could be anaplastic carcinoma or lymphoma, rather than well differentiated thyroid carcinoma (WDTC).

Pain is present in the thyroid region most often in patients with anaplastic carcinoma but is not a typical symptom of malignant thyroid disease. Hoarseness usually results from infiltration of the recurrent laryngeal or vagus nerve.

Dyspnea and stridor may result from distortion, compression, or invasion of the trachea by the tumor.

Dysphagia is usually a late phenomenon, due to malignant infiltration of the gullet rather than due to simple displacement by huge goiters.

A history of childhood exposure to radiation suggests the likelihood of a malignancy, usually of the papillary type. However, benign disease is three to four times more likely to be found in radiation-exposed patients with thyroid nodules.

A positive family history for thyroid carcinoma suggests the possibility of medullary carcinoma, although most cases of medullary thyroid carcinoma occur sporadically. Papillary carcinoma may occasionally exhibit a familial pattern as well.

A history of previous thyroid disease should also be investigated.

Symptoms of hypothyroidism or hyperthyroidism may be important clues to underlying undiagnosed thyroid disease. Patients with a history of Hashimoto's thyroiditis have an 80 times higher incidence of thyroid lymphoma than other patients. A nodule in a patient with a history of Graves' disease has a much higher risk for harboring carcinoma than the solitary nodule in a patient without a history of thyroid disease.

In areas where dietary iodine deficiency is prevalent, follicular carcinoma is the most common thyroid malignancy. Among groups with high dietary iodine content (for example, Fishermen), papillary carcinoma occurs with greater frequency than in the general population. This apparent paradox has not been explained.

It is rare to see a thyroid cancer that is hormonally active (except medullary). In this respect, thyroid gland malignancies differ from those of the other endocrine glands, since the latter usually exhibit overt symptoms and signs of hormonal activity. The syndrome of coexisting medullary carcinoma, parathyroid disease, and pheochromo-cytoma (Multiple endocrine neoplasia – MEN) may produce symptoms related to the excessive production of catecholamine and symptoms identical to those of the carcinoid syndrome (diarrhea, flushing and asthma).

Metastatic deposits of thyroid cancer may be responsible for a multitude of symptoms. The finding of pulmonary metastasis in a patient with a goiter or thyroid mass suspected of being cancerous increases the accuracy of the clinical diagnosis. Pulmonary metastasis may present as chest pain, cough, or dyspnea. Bone metastasis may be manifested by bone pain or pathologic fractures. In the rare instance of functioning metastasis, there are symptoms of thyrotoxicosis even after removal of the entire gland.

Signs: On physical examination, the characteristics of the nodule itself, as well as the remainder of the thyroid gland, are important to note and can raise or lower one's index of suspicion for carcinoma. The size of the nodule should be estimated as the risk for malignancy is increased with larger nodules (greater than 1.5 cm). The presence of other nodules in the gland makes a benign diagnosis such as multinodular goiter more likely, but does not exclude the possibility for malignancy.

Incidence of malignancy in a solitary nodule is approximately 10 percent and if it is truly solitary during investigations then it raises upto 20 percent. Incidence of malignancy in case of multinodular goiter (MNG) is around 5 percent.

Attempts to draw conclusions about the nature of the swelling from its **consistency** are generally unrewarding, for by no means every cancer possess the hardness of a squamous cancer, and in any case the interposition of numerous soft tissue layers between the fingers and the neoplasm makes interpretation of the consistency difficult (Fig. 83.2).

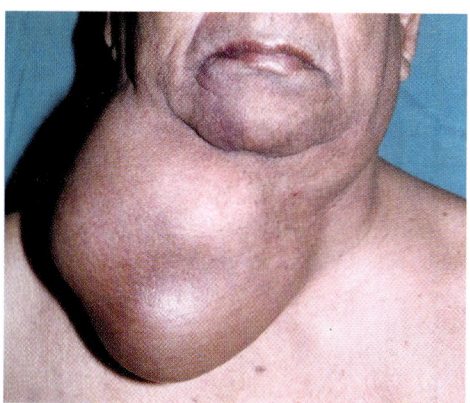

Fig. 83.2: Showing large thyroid swelling in the case of well differentiated thyroid carcinoma

Fixity due to extrathyroidal spread is an important criterion for diagnosing malignancy, although present in many patients with thyroiditis (especially Riedel's fibrous thyroiditis) and when a large benign goiter becomes wedged in the thoracic inlet.

Displacement of the trachea doesn't signify malignancy, since any large goiter do this. Bur compression and narrowing leading to stridor, especially on lying down, should arouse the suspicion of malignancy.

Encroachment on the carotid sheath may render it impossible to detect the carotid artery pulse, this sign, was described by Sir James Berry (1960) and is known as Berry's sign.

Invasion or compression of vessels of the neck is a relatively infrequent finding. However, obstruction of the veins may occur, precipitating venous congestion and edema of the head and neck. In a patient with a large cervical goiter, the examiner may precipitate suffusion of the patient's face, giddiness, or syncopal episodes by having the patient raise his hands above his head – this is known as Pemberton's sign. Involvement of the cervical sympathetic nerve is manifested as Horner's syndrome.

Assessment of vocal cord mobility should be carried out on every patient with a thyroid mass to rule out recurrent laryngeal nerve involvement by tumor, and to document any impairment of vocal cord motion before surgery.

Careful assessment of the upper aerodigestive tract should be carried out because metastasis or direct spread of squamous cell carcinoma of the head and neck may be present near or even within the parenchyma of the thyroid gland.

The remainder of the neck should be palpated for the presence of adenopathy, paying particular attention to the paratracheal region. The presence of a discrete, firm, non-tender lymph node in conjunction with a thyroid nodule suggests malignancy.

Lymphatic metastasis from WDTC, particularly papillary carcinoma, is not uncommon, and, in many patients, may be the initial sign of presentat- ion. In the presence of a seemingly normal thyroid gland, a lateral neck mass with biopsy-proven thyroid tissue was previously misconceived to represent an embryologic rest of thyroid tissue and erroneously termed "lateral aberrant thyroid". This presentation is now considered to be a metastatic WDTC from an occult primary within the thyroid gland until proven otherwise.

Flow chart 83.1: Management of solitary nodule of thyroid. RAI—Radioactive iodine, FNAC—Fine needle aspiration cytology, TSH—Thyroid stimulating hormone

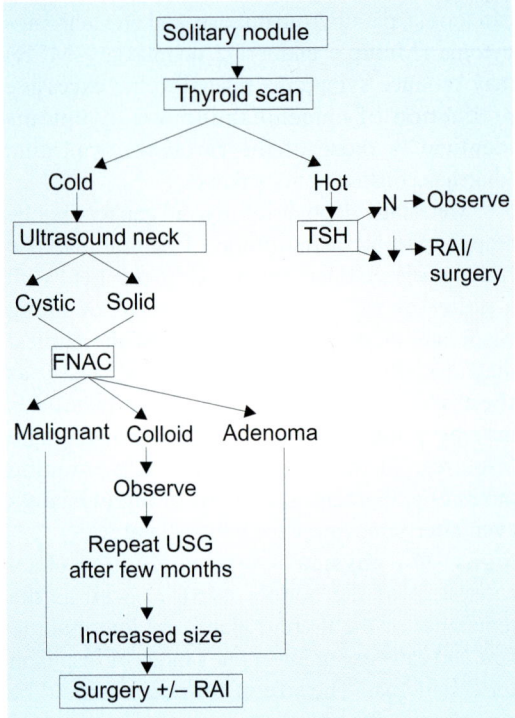

INVESTIGATIVE PROCEDURES

Laboratory Evaluation

In general, thyroid malignancy is unaccompanied by functional derangement. However, exceptions do occur. A more accurate assay is the free T4 level, which correlates better with the activity of thyroid hormones in the body. A more useful assay is the high-sensitivity thyrotropin assay (TSH). This assay is the only test that is necessary to detect abnormalities in thyroid function. This will pick up thyroid function abnormally before fluctuations in T4 can be detected. Most patients with thyroid nodules are euthyroid, and thus thyrotropin will most often be normal. When an abnormal thyrotropin result is identified, levels of T4 and T3 should be obtained.

A thyroglobulin level can also be obtained. The best use of this test is in the follow-up of patients with thyroid cancer after thyroidectomy with postoperative radioiodine ablation in the treatment of WDTC.

Many factors exist that may produce falsely elevated or decreased levels. It is produced by both benign and to a lesser extent malignant thyroid tissue.

Although not used routinely, calcitonin level should be considered in high-risk patients, such as patients with familial medullary thyroid carcinoma or multiple endocrine neoplasia. This can be done for screening, diagnosis, and follow-up of the disease. It is routine to measure the basal and pentagastrin-stimulated serum calcitonin levels in all patients who are suspected of having medullary thyroid carcinoma (MTC). Also serum and urinary catecholamines, serum calcium and parathormone should be obtained in appropriate cases.

Soft Tissue Radiographs

1. Neck – Soft tissue radiographs of the neck may be useful in defining the malignant potential of a thyroid mass.
   - 'Stippled polymorphous calcifications'– Papillary carcinoma
   - Dense polymorphous calcification – Amyloid formed by medullary carcinoma
   - Displacement of the trachea.
2. Chest radiograph:
   - Tracheal lumen narrowing.
   - Tracheal deviation
   - Pulmonary metastases

Radioisotope Imaging

Thyroid scintigraphy was the mainstay in the evaluation of the thyroid nodule before the widespread use of FNACB. In 1939, Hamilton and Soley demonstrated that malignant thyroid tissue concentrated much less radioactive iodine than normal tissue.

In 1951, Dobyns and Maloof first classified thyroid nodules as cold (non-functioning), warm (normal) or hot (hyperfunctioning). They implied that cold lesions were suspicious of malignancy.

The most commonly used isotopes nowadays are Technetium (Tc–99 m), Radioiodine (I–123) and Thallium (T1–201)

The choice of radioisotope is dependent on the preference of the clinician and radiologist, because they provide similar information (Table 83.1).

Limitations
- Nodules <1 cm cannot be detected reliably by either scan, as they are below the discriminating power of scintigraphic devices.
- Do not delineate the nodules at the thyroid's periphery or isthmus adequately.
- Artifacts may distort a normal thyroid gland, resulting in an abnormal scan.
- A cold area may be caused by an asymmetrical gland, agenesis of the contralateral lobe or a tortuous carotid artery.
- The main limitation regardless of the isotope used is that it will not differentiate between a benign and malignant nodule.

Although malignant nodules are more likely to be cold or warm by scan, most nodules fall into these two categories. Furthermore, the finding of a hot nodule substantially reduces the likelihood of cancer but does not exclude it.

Although scintigraphy does not offer any additional diagnostic value, it is a powerful adjunct test to more accepted modalities, such as FNACC and ultrasound.

Indications
- Identification of a functional solitary thyroid nodule when initial serum thyrotropin is decreased.
- If an FNACC is reported as 'follicular neoplasm' or 'suspicious', the finding of a 'hot' nodule may decrease the suspicion of a malignancy.
- Detecting neck metastasis

Table 83.1: Differences between technetium-99 and iodine-123 scans	
Technetium–99	*Iodine –123*
Can be performed immediately after the administration.	Performed 24 hours after administration
Shorter scanning time (20–30 minutes).	Scanning time can run 4 to 6 hours
Imaging resolution is better.	More physiological

Recently, Thallium-201 scan has proved to be an a useful diagnostic tool to differentiate between benign and malignant thyroid nodules. Three mCi of thallium-201 is used to image the thyroid gland and the nodule uptake was categorized into low, intermediate, and high uptake. Higher the uptake will increase the risk of malignancy.

Ultrasound

Introduced in 1965, ultrasonography now is used extensively to study the thyroid. It measures the size of the gland and documents the number, dimensions and physical character of thyroid nodules.

Conventional gray scale or B-mode ultrasonography is the technique used most commonly. Modern ultrasound is performed with high frequency transducers (7–13 MHz), can detect solid nodules of 3 to 4 mm and cystic nodules of 2 mm in diameter. When routinely used for solitary nodules, it can discover coexisting nodules in approximately 50 percent of patients.

The procedure is simple, painless, reproducible, nonradioactive test and requires no patient preparations. Recommendations for ultrasound are;

- Non-palpable or difficult to palpate nodules for US-guided FNAC.
- Follow-up imaging for solitary nodules that are managed medically or by observation.
- Non-diagnostic fine needle aspirate (as an adjunct to repeat FNAC).

It classifies nodules as solid, cystic or mixed lesions with more than 90 percent accuracy. Purely cystic nodules are uncommon (~1%), with partially cystic lesions accounting for up to 20 percent of nodules. Cystic lesions were reported to carry a lower risk of malignancy (0.5%–3%). The discovery of a purely cystic nodule should not discourage a needle aspiration for cytological analysis, however.

Predominantly solid nodules carry a higher risk of malignancy (~10%). No one specific ultrasonographic criterion distinguishes malignant from benign thyroid disease.

Most malignant nodules are hypoechoic compared with the remainder of the gland, perhaps because of their low grade necrosis or disordered architecture. In contrast most benign lesions are hyperechoic and often have a 'halo' sign or rim of sonolucence.

Ultrasound Features Suggesting Malignancy

1. Absent 'halo' sign
2. Solid or hypoechogenicity
3. Heterogeneous echo structure
4. Irregular margin
5. Fine calcifications
6. Extraglandular extension

Computed Tomography and Magnetic Resonance Imaging (Table 83.2)

The indications and the efficacy of the above investigations has been admirably summarized by Friedman et al (1988) who suggested their use for the following six primary purposes.

1. The nodule occurs in a diffusely enlarged gland that makes palpation difficult.
2. Determining the exact location and degree of invasiveness of large cancers.
3. Evaluating substernal or retrotracheal extension of thyroid tumors.
4. Detecting regional metastases.
5. Detecting cervical lymphadenopathy preoperatively
6. Detecting local recurrent disease.

A few studies (Tancredi et al 2001) investigated the use of MRI to study the nodules in different functional status.

Positron Emission Tomography

It evaluates areas of increased metabolic activity by assessing the uptake and use of a labeled glucose analog, and may have some usefulness in whole body scans to detect

- Metastatic disease in patients with known thyroid cancer, particularly medullary thyroid cancer.

Table 83.2: Differences between CT and MR imaging in evaluation of thyroid

CT Scan	MRI
The inherent high iodine content of the thyroid gland will increase the brightness of the gland on CT scan even without contrast material.	Demonstrates exquisite soft tissue details and vascular anatomy.
The iodinated contrast use with CT offers excellent anatomic detail of the thyroid gland, and is superior to MRI in evaluating metastatic adenopathy.	Avoids the use of iodinated contrast and ionizing radiation, yet provides excellent anatomic detail of the thyroid gland, adjacent critical structures, and cervical lymph nodes.
Less expensive than MRI	More expensive than CT and US
Contrast CT interferes with subsequent thyroid uptake scans for 4 to 8 weeks	The possible use of contrast (gadolinium) without interfering with nuclear scintigraphy.

- In identifying residual or recurrent WDTC that does not concentrate radioactive iodine.

Fine Needle Aspiration

Fine needle aspiration is the 'gold standard' in the evaluation of thyroid nodule. There are many reasons for this.

1. Most nodules are benign, and surgical excision is not required in most cases. Even when scintigraphy was part of the routine evaluation, most 'cold' nodules were histologically benign. With the wide acceptance of FNAC, there has been a decrease in the number of thyroidectomies performed and an increase in the yield of malignancies in excised glands.
2. FNAC is a safe and quick procedure with few complications and it does not involve radiation exposure.
3. FNAC decreases the overall cost of care.

Technique

The choice of smearing technique or biological preparation is based on preference and convenience. Air-dried smears and wet smears can be obtained concurrently, as they are complementary.

Ancillary tests to improve the accuracy of FNAC include immunohistochemistry, ploidy studies, molecular markers, and more recently, reverse transcription- PCR (RT-PCR), to detect thyroglobulin mRNA and thyrotropin receptor mRNA.

Reports of cytology are standardized, and the current guidelines were discussed and reported by the Papanicolaou Society in 1997. The four recognized categories of FNAC are malignant, benign, suspicious, and insufficient.

The "malignant" category includes have unequivocal typical cytologic characteristics of a malignant neoplasm. This category includes papillary, medullary, poorly differentiated or undifferentiated thyroid cancers, lymphomas, and metastatic non-thyroid cancers.

"Benign" reports include hyperplastic colloid nodule in 90 percent of the cases and chronic inflammatory lesions (Hashimoto's thyroiditis, subacute lymphocytic thyroiditis, De Quervain's thyroiditis) in the other 10 percent.

The category of "suspicious" lesions on FNAC is due to the inability to unequivocally detect cytologic features of either benign or malignant neoplasm. The most common cause of categorizing an FNAC aspirate as "suspicious" is the inability to differentiate a follicular adenoma from a well-differentiated follicular carcinoma. Some of the other possible cause is as follows.

- Hurthle cell neoplasm

- Follicular variant of papillary carcinoma
- Low-grade papillary carcinoma
- Hyalinizing trabecular adenoma
- Hashimoto's thyroiditis with metaplasia
- Any cancer with suboptimal sampling
- Adenomatous goiter with microfollicular structure predominance.

Complications of FNAC

- Pain
- Hematoma
- Entry into trachea
- Transient thyroid swelling
- Cystic degeneration
- Transient bradycardia
- Transient vocal cord paralysis
- Formation of calcification
- Necrosis of nodule
- Capsular pseudoinvasion
- Fibrosis
- Transient thyrotoxicosis
- Elevation of thyroglobulin level.

The main goal of FNAC is to accurately predict which nodule is cancerous. Numerous studies cited the following data. Sensitivity is 65 percent to 100 percent and specificity is 70 percent to 100 percent. Overall accuracy is estimated at 92 percent to 95 percent. An ultrasound guided FNAC is the best in accuracy.

ETIOPATHOLOGY OF THYROID NEOPLASMS

Papillary Thyroid Carcinoma (PTC)

PTC occurs more frequently in women than in men (3:1) with the peak incidence occurring in the third and fourth decades of life. Exposure to ionizing radiation is known to increase the likelihood of developing PTC. Grossly, PTC appears as 'an invasive neoplasm of ill-defined margins, firm in consistency with a whitish color and a granular cut surface'. Large tumors may undergo cystic degeneration and may therefore grossly resemble a benign thyroid cyst.

Papillary thyroid carcinoma is characterized histologically by the presence of papillae with a fibrovascular stalk and an overlying neoplastic epithelium. The cells that comprise the neoplastic epithelium possess unique nuclear features that have diagnostic importance. The nuclei are comparatively large with prominent nucleoli surrounded by a large, clear nucleoplasm, giving an 'Orphan Annie eye' appearance. Laminated calcifications called psammoma bodies are seen in 40 percent to 50 percent of PTC specimens. These structures are highly suggestive of PTC when present, although they have been seen to occur in other malignant as well as certain benign thyroid diseases.

Histologic variants of PTC, each of which possesses a somewhat variable clinical course are

1. The follicular variant of PTC has a follicular growth pattern whereas the nuclear features and the clinical course resemble those of PTC.
2. The encapsulated variant is surrounded by a fibrous capsule and has a prognosis that is more favorable than typical PTC.
3. Unfavorable histological variants are diffuse sclerosing, tall cell and columnar cell variants.
4. Occult PTC, or papillary thyroid microcarcinoma, is defined as an intrathyroidal lesion measuring 1.5 cm or less. These lesions are often discovered incidentally at autopsy or after thyroidectomy for other reasons and are associated with a very favorable prognosis.

Extrathyroidal spread is seen in 14 percent of PTC cases at primary surgery. The presence of extrathyroidal spread is one factor that increases the risk for recurrent disease. Other factors include advanced age at presentation, large primary size, less than bilateral thyroid surgery, absence of postoperative radioactive iodine ablation, and the presence of regional lymph node metastasis.

Papillary thyroid carcinoma is well known for being a lymphotropic malignancy and multicentric involvement of the thyroid gland. Some debate exists as whether this multicentric tendency represents intrathyroidal lymphatic spread or true multifocal malignant transformation. The lymphotropic nature of PTC is further demonstrated through the tendency to spread to regional cervical lymph nodes. Numerous large series have demonstrated that approximately 35 percent of individuals with PTC will have clinical cervical lymph node involvement at presentation. Distant metastasis occurs less frequently with PTC than with other forms of thyroid malignancy. When present, the lungs and bones are most frequently involved.

Prognostic factors in Papillary Carcinoma

- Better in people less than 40 years despite nodal metastasis
- Better in females
- Better if < 0.5cm in diameter
- Poor prognosis if nodal involvement is present in >40 years of age
- No extrathyroid spread.

Follicular Thyroid Carcinoma (FTC)

FTC seems to occur with somewhat greater frequency in patients with a low iodine intake and in older females (3:1 female to male ratio). The peak incidence of FTC occurs in the fifth decade of life. Ionizing radiation exposure is also considered a risk factor for FTC, although most radiation-induced thyroid cancers are PTC. Unlike PTC, which has no benign precursor, follicular lesions can occur as benign adenomas on one extreme or poorly differentiated FTC on the other extreme with a spectrum of intermediate histologic appearances.

Histologic findings of FTC have considerable overlap with benign follicular adenoma. Follicular thyroid carcinoma tends to demonstrate microfollicular arrays that are hypercellular and lack the presence of considerable colloid. As cellularity decreases, colloid increases and the size of follicular arrays increases, the likelihood of a follicular lesion being benign increases. However, the only way to distinguish FTC from follicular adenoma with certainty is with identification of capsular or vascular invasion upon pathologic evaluation of the entire gland.

Follicular thyroid carcinoma can be broadly divided into minimally invasive or widely invasive forms with differing prognoses and clinical behavior. Minimally invasive FTC, also referred to as encapsulated FTC, behaves clinically as a follicular adenoma but will demonstrate the presence of focal capsular invasion upon complete pathologic analysis of the gland after extirpation. Widely invasive FTC lesions behave more aggressively with a tendency toward becoming locally invasive and distantly metastasizing. As the size of follicular thyroid lesions increases, the likelihood of capsular invasion and the rate of malignancy increase such that 30 percent of all follicular lesions larger than 3 cm will contain carcinoma.

Follicular Ca spreads either hematogenously or through direct extension. This tendency causes FTC to lack the multicentric nature of thyroid involvement seen in PTC.

The main prognostic factors for FTC have been identified through several studies. These factors include age older than 45 years at presentation, presence of extrathyroidal extension, size of tumor larger than 4 cm, high-grade (more poorly differentiated) histology, and presence of distant metastatic disease. Factors such as gender, regional nodal metastasis, and multifocality appear to have no influence on survival. Individuals who are 45 years or older at presentation and possess one or more of the other listed risk factors fall into a high-risk group with decreased survival. These patients will generally require more aggressive treatment than those patients who are younger than 45 years at presentation and who possess none of the other listed risk factors.

Hurthle Cell Carcinoma (HCC)

HCC is considered a subtype of FTC. The optimum management strategy for HCC remains a subject of some debate because of the paucity of cases seen. Patients with HCC tend to be diagnosed at a slightly greater age than those with non-Hurthle cell FTC with the peak incidence seemingly occurring in the sixth decade of life. Hurthle cell carcinoma, like FTC, demonstrates a female gender predilection, although not as pronounced (1:2 male to female ratio).

Histologically, diagnosis depends on identification of capsular or vascular invasion.

Hurthle cell carcinoma is less likely to metastasize to regional lymph nodes than PTC but more likely than FTC. HCC has a higher incidence of distant metastasis than both PTC and FTC. In general, HCC is thought to be more aggressive in nature than non-Hurthle cell FTC with a reduced 10-year survival.

Medullary Thyroid Carcinoma (MTC)

Medullary thyroid carcinoma originates from the calcitonin-producing parafollicular C cells of the thyroid. MTC can present as

1. Sporadic MTC represents approximately 75 percent to 80 percent of all MTC. The peak incidence of sporadic MTC occurs in the fourth decade of life and, is not associated with concomitant endocrine disease.

2. Hereditary MTC accounts for the remaining 20 percent to 25 percent of MTC. These neoplasms typically affect a younger demographic group and are associated with multifocal thyroid disease as well as multiple endocrine neoplasia (MEN) syndromes 2A (Sipple syndrome) and 2B.

3. Familial medullary thyroid carcinoma syndrome, shares the hereditary predisposition and multifocal disease tendency of the MEN syndromes but not the tendency toward concomitant endocrinopathy. Inheritance is autosomal dominant and early parafollicular C-cell hyperplasia and elevated blood calcitonin levels are seen in all 3 familial forms.

In both MEN syndromes, pheochromocytoma will develop in approximately 50 percent of individuals. Hyperparathyroidism will occur in 10 percent to 30 percent of individuals with MEN 2A but can also occur, much less frequently, in MEN 2B. Distinct clinical features of MEN 2B include Marfanoid habitus, seen in up to 90 percent of individuals, and extensive ganglioneuromatosis involving mucosal membranes (particularly of the tongue, lips, conjunctivae, and intestine).

RET proto-oncogene screening has now supplanted calcitonin family screening as a means of early detection.

The gross appearance of MTC is a solid, well-circumscribed though non-encapsulated tumor with a gray cut surface. Most lesions are located in the mid-to-upper posterior portion of the thyroid gland because of the greater concentration of C cells in these area. Histologically, MTC consists of eosinophilic cells that can vary in shape between round cells to spindle-shaped cells. Cells are typically arranged in solid sheets or nests and are separated by abundant vascular stroma and amyloid. Medullary thyroid carcinoma can mimic the architecture and morphology of other thyroid neoplasms; therefore, the tissue diagnosis often lies in immunohistochemical staining for the presence of calcitonin.

Medullary thyroid carcinoma has a tendency toward early regional lymph node metastasis with more than 50 percent of individuals having pathologically positive lymph nodes at the time of initial surgery. When individuals with MTC are detected through familial screening, the likelihood of having nodal metastasis is greatly reduced and 10-year survival increased. Distant metastasis can occur and tends to involve the lungs, liver, bones, and adrenal glands.

Prognosis for MTC has shown overall 10-year survival to be as high as 80 percent. This is owed to increased early detection of the various familial forms of MTC. Within hereditary MTC, survival is greatest among individuals with familial MTC syndrome and worst among those with MEN 2B. Good prognostic factors for MTC include young age, familial subtype, absence of extracapsular spread of tumor, and female gender.

Anaplastic Thyroid Carcinoma

Anaplastic thyroid carcinoma (ATC), or undifferentiated thyroid carcinoma, is one of the most aggressive forms of cancer seen in human beings and is uniformly fatal with an average survival measured in terms of months. ATC occurs within an older demographic group, typically presenting in the seventh decade of life. Females are affected more often than males.

Thirty percent of individuals with ATC will have a personal history of pre-existing multinodular goiter and 20 percent will have a history of previously treated WDTC, thereby supporting the idea that ATC may arise through dedifferentiation of pre-existing thyroid neoplasms.

At presentation, these lesions are typically seen to invade locally into the larynx, trachea, and cervical musculature. Hoarseness resulting from recurrent laryngeal nerve invasion is common as is cervical lymphadenopathy and distant metastasis.

Histologically, ATC exhibits many mitotic figures within markedly pleomorphic cells. Necrosis and vascular invasion are readily seen in nearly all cases.

Lymphoma

Primary thyroid lymphoma typically occurs in the sixth decade of life with a female predominance ranging from 4:1 to 8:1. It typically presents as a rapidly enlarging, non tender mass with or without associated hoarseness, dysphagia, or breathing difficulty. In 80 percent of case, it will arise in the setting of pre-existing Hashimoto thyroiditis, which increases an individual's risk for primary thyroid lymphoma by 70-fold.

The majority of thyroid lymphomas are non-Hodgkin B-cell type.

Extrathyroidal spread of disease is the main prognostic factor in primary thyroid lymphoma. Stage 1 disease is limited to the thyroid and is associated with a 5-year survival of 86 percent. In individuals with extrathyroidal spread, 5-year survival is reduced to 38 percent and in those with disseminated metastasis, 5-year survival is a dismal 5 percent.

Metastatic Carcinoma

Metastatic carcinoma within the thyroid gland most frequently arises from malignant melanoma, kidney, breast, lung, and colon cancer. Metastatic lesions to the thyroid are seen in 2 percent to 4 percent of individuals who die of cancer and are important to recognize, as surgical excision is not beneficial in these cases.

TREATMENT OF THYROID NEOPLASMS

1. Well Differentiated Carcinomas

(a) Thyroidectomy

Surgical resection is the mainstay of treatment of patients with WDTC and it ranges from total thyroidectomy or near-total thyroidectomy to lobectomy, with or without isthmusectomy.

Arguments in favor of total or near-total thyroidectomy include

- The relatively high risk (particularly with papillary) for contralateral malignancy
- Enhanced postoperative I-131 ablation
- Better postoperative surveillance by palpation and thyroid scans
- The ability for following thyroglobulin levels as an indicator of early recurrence of disease.
- Near-total thyroidectomy results in a decreased likelihood of recurrence and mortality.

The argument against routine total or near-total thyroidectomy.

- In early stage tumors there is increased risk of bilateral recurrent laryngeal nerve injury that results in airway obstruction
- The increased risk of permanent hypocalcemia are not justified by an improvement in disease control or survival rates

A small papillary carcinoma identified in a younger patient with no evidence of metastasis or extrathyroidal extension probably merits nothing more than an ipsilateral lobectomy. Such patient has a low-risk of tumor recurrence or distant metastasis that probably does not justify the need for adjuvant radioactive iodine or the added risk of total thyroidectomy. In contrast, patients older than 45 years with larger tumors (greater than 4 cm), and with evidence of extrathyroidal extension or metastasis are at a high-risk of tumor recurrence and should be treated with total thyroidectomy and adjuvant postoperative radioactive iodine.

(b) Neck Dissection

Although papillary carcinomas harbor occult nodal metastasis in as many as 90 percent of elective neck dissection specimens, the impact of such finding on survival is debatable. Therefore, the role for elective neck dissection remains controversial. In general, most thyroid surgeons recommend intraoperative inspection of the central compartment of the neck (paratracheal region, Delphian node, upper mediastinal nodes) for any evidence of metastatic adenopathy at the time of the thyroidectomy. If suspicious nodes are identified, a thorough lymphadenectomy of these regions is recommended. If, on palpation of the jugular chain, malignant adenopathy is identified, a modified radical neck dissection or a selective neck dissection that spares level I is generally performed.

(c) Adjuvant Treatment

Adjuvant therapy for patients with WDTC most often includes

1. Postoperative iodine–131 treatment
2. Thyroid hormone suppression

The advantages of postoperative radioactive iodine treatment include the treatment of microscopic metastases and the ablation of residual thyroid tissue. Ablation of the remainder of the thyroid tissue facilitates optimal follow-up because subsequent radioiodine total body scans will not be hindered by residual activity in the neck, and the absence of thyroglobulin production by normal thyroid tissue allows for sensitive detection of recurrence.

These results strongly suggested that postoperative ablation is indicated in:

1. Patients with tumors greater than 1.0 cm to 1.5 cm at the time of resection. The need for ablation in younger patients with smaller lesions confined to the thyroid gland remains controversial.
2. Patients with other negative prognostic factors such as extrathyroidal extension, metastasis, and unfavorable histologic features.

The main disadvantages of radioactive iodine treatment include the risks of radiation toxicity and the need for thyroid hormone withdrawal. To achieve optimal uptake of the radioactive iodine, the patient is withdrawn from thyroid hormone replacement therapy for about 6 weeks. This induces a profound hypothyroidism with serum thyrotropin levels ideally more than $30\mu U/mL$. Many patients poorly tolerate this degree of hypothyroidism. Fortunately, recombinant human thyrotropin has become available and obviates the need for thyroid hormone withdrawal.

The role of *external radiation therapy* (XRT) in patients with WDTC remains to be completely defined. External beam radiation therapy has been most commonly used in the treatment of:

• Unresectable tumor that is locally invasive into the visceral compartments or deep muscles of the neck
• Recurrent tumor that failed I–131 therapy.

Chemotherapy has a limited role in the treatment of patients with WDTC and is reserved for the palliative management of patients with inoperable, advanced disease that does not concentrate I–131. Doxorubicin used either alone or in combination with Cisplatinum demonstrated modest response rates in patients with inoperable disease that was radioiodine insensitive. Higher response rates were reported with combined low-dose doxorubicin and XRT.

2. Medullary Thyroid Carcinoma

Total thyroidectomy with central compartment neck dissection has become a standard therapy for sporadic and hereditary types. In patients with MEN and pheochromocytoma treatment is first directed to pheochromocytoma to avoid the possible hazardous effects of hormonally active pheochromocytoma on surgery.

The high incidence of multifocality, the lack of effective adjuvant therapies, and the observation that patients with completely resected disease do better than those with residual disease or with disease that cannot be resected are justifications for aggressive surgical treatment. Familial medullary thyroid cancer is almost always multifocal and bilateral; 67 percent sporadic cases have bilateral disease. Cervical metastases, clinically or pathologically are observed at the time of presentation in up to 75 percent of cases.

Both thyroid lobes and the isthmus are resected with central compartment neck dissection. The lateral neck is inspected and palpated: for the positive neck, a comprehensive neck dissection is indicated removing levels II through V in addition to the central compartment. The surgeon should also be aware of the incidence of metastatic superior mediastinal nodes. On some occasion nodal disease does low down in the superior mediastinum requiring a superior mediastinal dissection through a sternotomy.

During thyroidectomy every attempt is made to find and preserve the parathyroid glands, because of only small incidence of hyper-parathyroidism. Use of a handheld gamma probe to help localize the parathyroids intraoperatively after injecting the patient with 99Tc sestamibi has been tried.

An invasive medullary carcinoma may require resection of a part or a sleeve of trachea or a part of pharyngeal musculature; rarely does it require a laryngectomy.

Radiation therapy is used as an adjuvant for patients with extensive soft tissue invasion or those with significant extracapsular extension in positive nodes after removal of all gross disease. It may also be considered for palliative control of inoperable disease.

Preoperative serum calcitonin and CEA should be assessed in every patient. Following surgical treatment the patients are best monitored with a regular measurement of basal and pentagastrin-stimulated serum calcitonin levels. Calcitonin and CEA levels should usually be assessed for baseline levels approximately 4 weeks after surgery. A persistent or re-elevating level may indicate loco-regional failure or metastatic disease. Comprehensive radiographic evaluation and reoperation, whether cervical or mediastinal dissection, is still the best treatment for locoregional recurrence.

Patients presenting, on initial presentation, with metastatic disease should undergo comprehensive thyroidectomy as well as neck dissection(s) for metastatic regional disease for the long-term control of local/regional processes. The extent of surgery should be individualized based on the knowledge of the natural history of the neoplasm and the expected outcome in each patient. Although there are ongoing clinical trials, no single agent or combination chemotherapy has been shown to be beneficial in the control of metastatic disease.

Future directions include the use of gene therapy, treatments that target inactivation or destruction of RET, and 131–iodine Metaiodo benzyl guanidine (MIBG) for the treatment of advanced and metastatic disease.

3. Lymphoma

Surgery is advocated for patients with localized MALT lymphomas, where complete excision is possible. Radiation was advocated for patients with local lymphomas, but a combination of chemotherapy and radiation are recommended for patient with DCBCL and more advanced staged lymphoma. CHOP (cyclophosphamide, adriamycin, vincristine, prednisone) or CHOP-like regimens have been the most successful.

4. Anaplastic Carcinoma

Anaplastic carcinoma can only rarely be completely surgically resected because of the extensive invasiveness; should attempt to remove as much local disease as possible to reduce airway compression without the sacrifice of vital structure be made. Complete thyroid resection is associated with longer survival rates than biopsy alone. Radical neck dissection, however, offers no survival advantage over a less aggressive surgical approach. Although anaplastic carcinoma is considered a radioresistant tumor, combined modality protocols of surgery, radiation, and chemotherapy, especially using altered radiation fractionation schemes, offer the longest survival rates.

5. Sarcoma

The treatment for sarcomas involving the thyroid gland is total thyroidectomy with excision of any locally involved tissue along with neck dissection for involved cervical lymph nodes. Postoperative radiotherapy is indicated for aggressive disease, which includes extracapsular spread, high mitotic count, abundant nuclear pleomorphism, or surgically unresectable disease. Adjuvant chemotherapy was recommended for aggressive subtypes of sarcoma, such as the follicular dendritic cell sarcoma.

STEPS OF TOTAL THYROIDECTOMY

1. *Anesthesia:* General anesthesia, hypotensive anesthesia is preferable.
2. *Position:* Extension of the head and neck with sand bag between the shoulders and a ring below the head.
3. *Incision:* Transverse incision 2 fingers above the clavicle along the skin crease. It may be extended posteriorly to about 2.5 cm from the anterior border of the sternocleido-mastoid muscle. The incision can be extended further posterosuperiorly to convert

to a hockey stick for unilateral or modified apron flap for bilateral neck dissection, if required (Fig. 83.3)

4. *Subplatysmal flap elevation* is done till the level of the hyoid bone above and suprasternal notch below.
5. The strap muscles are separated in the midline and in cases where neck dissection has to be done or in case of revision surgery, a lateral approach from the anterior border of sternomastoid muscle may be preferred (Fig. 83.4).
6. After separating the sternothyroid and the sternohyoid muscles from the thyroid lobe they are retracted or if found involved a portion of the muscles may be resected (Fig. 83.5).
7. The middle thyroid vein is identified and divided between sutures which facilitate dissection in the deeper plane.
8. Care is taken to identify and separate the caramel colored parathyroid gland from the thyroid gland if it is found to be uninvolved by the tumor. Following the inferior thyroid artery helps in identification of the parathyroid and it should be preserved along its blood supply.
9. Blunt dissection is continued further laterally towards the carotids. The recurrent laryngeal nerve is identified in the tracheoesophageal

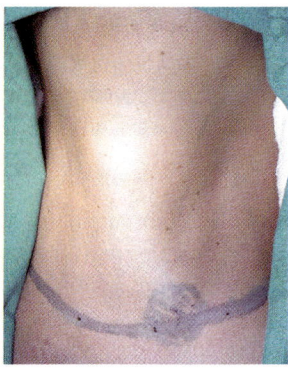

Fig. 83.3: Showing transverse cervical incision for thyroid surgery

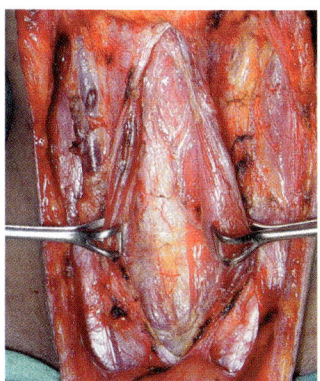

Fig. 83.4: Showing separation of strap muscles in the midline exposing thyroid gland

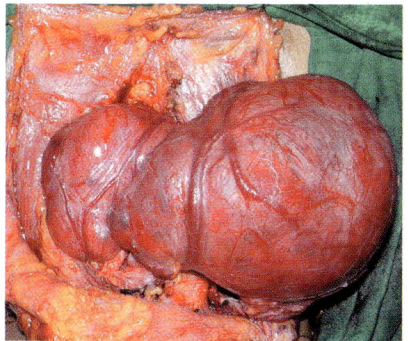

Fig. 83.5: Showing complete exposure of the thyroid gland

groove inferior to the gland. The nerve can be detected crossing the inferior thyroid artery and its branches. Occasionally a non-recurrent laryngeal nerve may be present directly from the vagus especially on the right side. The recurrent nerve is traced superiorly and care is taken to preserve all the branches of the nerve. The inferior thyroid artery is ligated after preserving its branches to the parathyroid gland (Fig. 83.6).

10. The Berry ligament is divided with preservation of the recurrent laryngeal nerve as it enters the larynx.

11. The superior pole is made free and the superior laryngeal nerve is looked for by identifying the superior thyroid artery. It runs

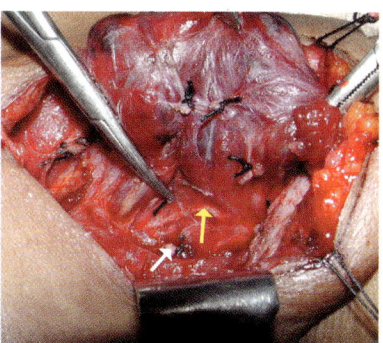

Fig. 83.6: Intraoperative photograph showing the recurrent laryngeal nerve (yellow arrow) and the ligated stump of the inferior thyroid artery (white arrow)

medial to the artery and may run across the superior pole. Care is taken to separate the superior laryngeal nerve before ligating and cutting the superior thyroid vessels. Some surgeons prefer to ligate the superior pole first but there is danger if injuring the nerve especially if it is non-recurrent.

12. The lobe is separated from the trachea medially along with the isthmus. Inferior thyroid veins are ligated and cut in the process.

13. Similar procedure is followed in the opposite side and the total thyroidectomy specimen is delivered (Fig. 83.7)

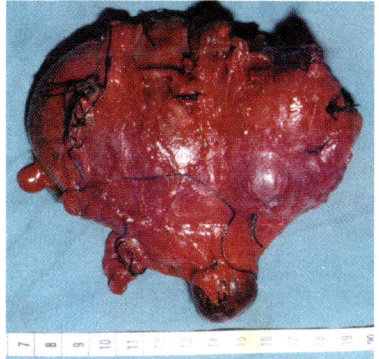

Fig. 83.7: Showing resected specimen following total thyroidectomy

14. Some prefer to, preserve a part of the thyroid gland at the superior pole that is not grossly involved and is called near total thyroidectomy.

15. In malignant thyroid disease some prefer removal of central compartment nodes also (level 6) while dissecting the thyroid gland especially in papillary and medullary carcinoma. If found to be grossly involved a modified neck dissection (level 2 to 5) is removed after preservation of the internal jugular vein, sternocleidomastoid muscle and the spinal accessory nerve (Fig. 83.8).

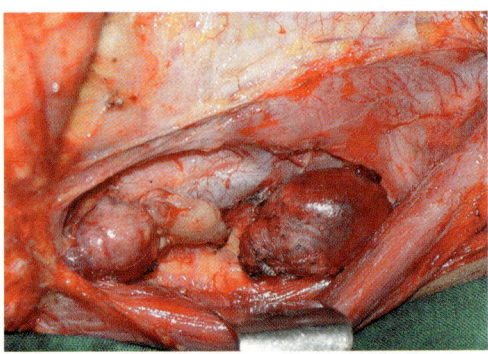

Fig. 83.8: Photograph showing neck dissection in progress and a lateral to medial approach is taken for thyroidectomy

Complications of Thyroid Surgery

- Hemorrhage and hematoma formation
- Recurrent laryngeal nerve injury
- Superior laryngeal nerve injury
- Pneumothorax
- Chylous fistula
- Hypoparathyroidism
- Hypothyroidism
- Seroma
- Fluid-electrolyte imbalance and metabolic derangement.

POINTS TO REMEMBER

1. Recurrent laryngeal triangle is bounded medially by the trachea and esophagus, laterally by carotid sheath and superiorly by the inferior pole of thyroid gland.
2. Adenoma is the most common benign thyroid neoplasm.
3. Thyroid malignancy with positive family history is more likely to be medullary carcinoma.
4. Patients with Hashimoto's thyroiditis are more prone to develop thyroid lymphoma.
5. Papillary carcinoma is most common thyroid malignancy.
6. Follicular carcinoma commonly occurs in goiter associated with dietary iodine deficiency.
7. Serum thyroglobuline is the marker for follow up of patients with thyroid cancer after thyroidectomy.
8. Absent carotid pulsation in thyroid malignancy is due to encroachment of carotid sheath and is known as Berry's sign.
9. Ultrasound guided FNAC is a gold standard in evaluation of thyroid nodule.

Diseases of the Salivary Gland

84

Anatomy

Salivary glands are exocrine glands situated in relation to oral cavity and oropharynx that secret saliva. About 1500 cc of saliva is secreted per day. Salivary glands are classified as follows:

Paired Major Glands

- Parotid glands
- Submandibular glands
- Sublingual glands

Minor Salivary Glands

- They are present scattered in the upper aero digestive tract

Development

They are simple tubular or tubuloacinar glands and they arise from the pharyngeal ectoderm. Initially there is proliferation and budding of the epithelium as a solid cord which later canalizes and branches repeatedly to form the ductal system into the surrounding mesenchyme. Terminal parts of this duct system develop into secretory acini.

The common developmental anomalies include Aplasia, hypoplasia and ectopic salivary tissue.

Parotid Gland

This is the largest salivary gland which has the shape of an inverted three sided pyramid, and is flattened side to side. The gland derives its name from *para*-around and *otic* -ear, i.e. around the ear. The gland is well encapsulated. The gland is divided into a larger superficial lobe and a smaller deep lobe by the neurovascular plane consisting of the facial nerve and superficial and transverse temporal arteries and veins.

The parotid secretions are serous in nature. Stensen's duct is the main duct of the gland which opens into the vestibule of the mouth, opposite the upper second molar tooth.

Lymphatic vessels drain into:

1. Superficial group lying under the external parotid fascia
2. 15 to 20 lymphoid follicles embedded in the gland superficial to facial nerve and the deep lobe may contain 1 to 2 follicles.

They ultimately drain into the jugulodigastric group of lymph nodes.

Submandibular Salivary Gland

It has a superficial part which is situated in the submandibular triangle and a deep part that is situated in the floor of the mouth.

Wharton's duct, the main duct of the submandibular salivary gland arises from the deep lobe of the gland and opens into the floor of the mouth on either side of the frenulum of the tongue. It is a mixed gland with both serous and mucous secretion.

Lymphatic vessels drain into the nodes present on the outer aspect of the gland and a few into the nodes in relation to the facial vessels.

Sublingual Salivary Gland

This gland is situated in the floor of the mouth. It has no specific duct system. As many as 20 ducts may emerge from this gland of which half drain directly into the oral cavity and the remainder into the submandibular duct. Lymphatic drain into the submandibular and submental lymph nodes.

Minor Salivary Glands

They are numerous and are seen mainly in the mucosal fold, mucosa of the palate, cheek, tongue, nasopharynx, supraglottic larynx.

PHYSIOLOGY

Function of Saliva

1. Glycoprotein and mucoprotein content act as a lubricant for food and protects mucous membrane from trauma during mastication.
2. Keep mucous constantly moist and helps in maintaining oral hygiene. It also has bacteriostatic function by lysozymes.
3. Buffering function protects dental enamel.
4. Salivary amylase helps in early carbohydrate digestion
5. Maintenance of water balance through antidiuretic hormone.
6. Acts as a solvent and effective spreading agent to facilitate taste sensation.

INFLAMMATORY CONDITIONS

MUMPS

Definition

It is a contagious disease of viral origin, characterized by acute non-suppurative enlargement of one or both the parotid glands, associated with involvement of other organs. Average incubation period is 17 days.

Etiology

Mumps is caused by the paramyxovirus. It mainly spreads through saliva.

Symptoms

- Fever up to 103 degree F
- Malaise
- Headache
- Acute painful swelling in the parotid region
- Trismus
- Difficulty in swallowing
- Referred otalgia.

Signs

- Swelling and tenderness of the parotid glands.
- Duct orifice is congested.

Treatment

- Analgesics
- Antibiotics
- Antipyretics
- Plenty of fluids.

Complications

- Orchitis
- Oophoritis
- High frequency deafness (unilateral)
- Encephalitis
- Meningitis
- Pancreatitis
- Myocarditis
- Facial neuritis
- Arthritis.

NON-SUPPURATIVE PAROTITIS

Etiology

- Debilitated patients
- Dehydrated adults-hospitalized
- Premature baby.

Clinical Features

- Acute onset of pain and tenderness locally
- Erythema of the overlying skin
- Gland is hard to palpate and massage over the gland will produce purulent discharge from the Stenson's duct.

Treatment

- Hydration
- Antibiotics

ABSCESS OF THE PAROTID GLAND

Etiology

- Acute suppurative parotitis
- Trauma with secondary infection
- Common in elderly patients.

Symptoms

General

- Malaise
- Fever
- Headache.

Local

- Painful swelling of the parotid region
- Trismus and odynophagia.

Signs (Fig. 84.1)

- Swelling over the parotid gland with tenderness.
- Progressive edema, induration, sepsis, fluctuation is less often apparent.

Treatment

- Parenteral antibiotics
- Incision and drainage
- Iodoform gauze packing.

CHRONIC SIALADENITIS (Fig. 84.2)

Definition

Recurrent salivary gland enlargement associated with pain, tenderness, and frank suppuration from the duct.

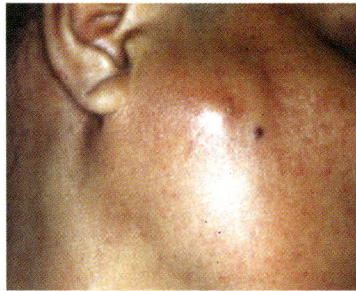

Fig. 84.1: Showing parotid swelling in acute parotitis

Clinical Features (Figs 84.3 and 84.4)

- Pain
- Tenderness
- Purulent discharge from the Stenson's duct or Wharton's duct
- Gradual localized swelling can simulate tumor.

Investigations

- Sialography
- Ductal dilatation and sacculation.

Treatment

- Good hydration
- Antibiotics
- Therapeutic sialography
- Surgery–Superficial parotidectomy or submandibular gland excision.
- Sialoendoscopic dilatation of stricture

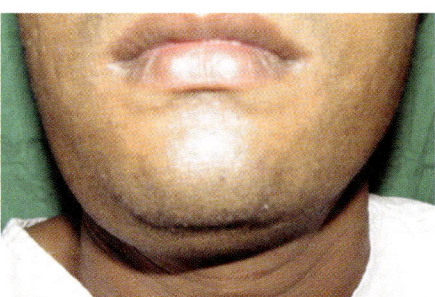

Fig. 84.2: Chronic sialadenitis

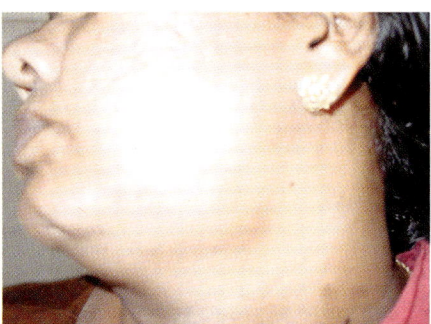

Fig 84.3: Showing submandibular sialoadenitis secondary to ductal caliculus

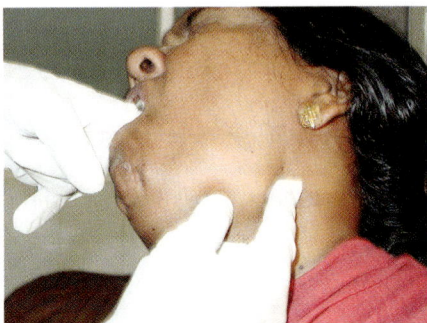

Fig. 84.4: Bidigital palpation of submandibular salivary gland

SIALOLITHIASIS (SALIVARY GLAND CALCULUS)

Sites

- 70 percent to 80 percent seen in submandibular salivary duct/gland because of the tortuous course of the duct and thicker mucinous secretions.
- Commonest sites include duct / hilum of the gland.

Etiology

- Not known.
- Duct is more favorable site because:
  1. Wide and large in diameter
  2. Secretion pass against gravity
  3. Submandibular secretions are alkaline
  4. Subjected to repeated trauma.

Compositions

- Similar to tartar.
- Organic matrix with inorganic crystalline body carbohydrate and phosphates of calcium and magnesium.

Symptoms: **Pain and swelling.**

Signs

- Tenderness over the affected gland.
- Purulent material can be expressed from the duct.

Investigations

- X-ray occlusal view (Figs 84.5 to 84.7)
- Radio-opaque mass in the duct
- 90 percent of the calculi are radio opaque.

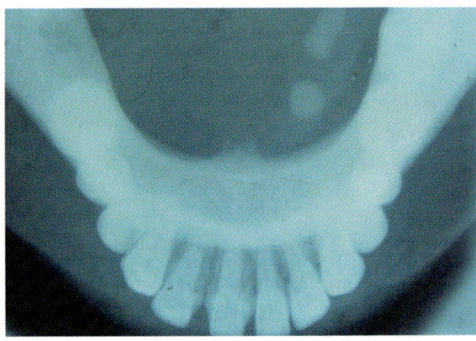

Fig. 84.5 X-ray occlusal view showing stone in duct

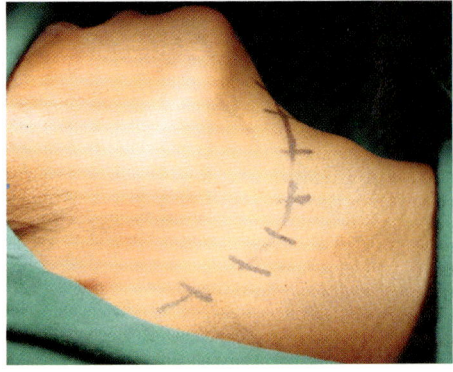

Fig. 84.6: Incision line given before surgery

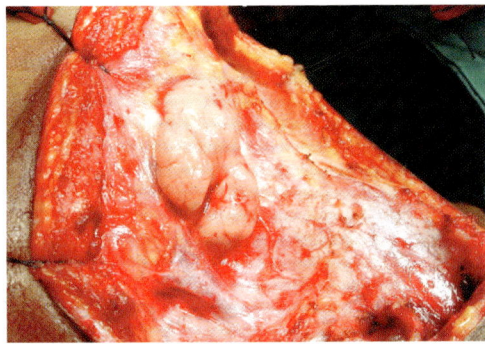

Fig. 84.7: Exposure of submandibular salivary gland

Treatment

- Ductal sialolithiasis can be approached transorally
- For the calculi deep in the gland a submandibular gland excision is required (Figs 84.8 and 84.9).

Recently sialoendoscopic lithotripsy is being used.

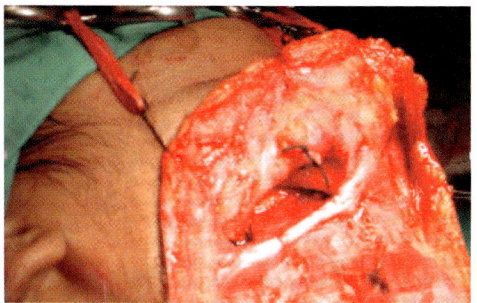

Fig. 84.8: Showing submandibular triangle after excision of submandibular salivary gland

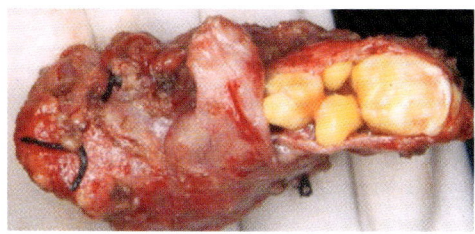

Fig. 84.9: Excised submandibular salivary gland specimen showing sialolithiasis in the duct

RANULA

Definition

This is defined as a retention cyst arising from sublingual salivary glands and presents as swelling in the floor of the mouth and if extending beyond the mylohyoid muscle it presents as a swelling in the submandibular region.

Etiology

- Degenerative process of the salivary gland, obstruction to the duct.
- Retention cyst – Mechanical obstruction of the orifice of the duct located on one side of the frenulum.

Clinical Features

Present as a translucent swelling in the floor of the mouth. Painless and sometimes extends through mylohyoid muscle to present as a swelling in the submental region or submandibular region called as plunging ranula.

Treatment

- Marsupialization is the treatment of simple ranula.
- Complete excision is required for plunging ranula to prevent recurrence.

TUMORS OF THE SALIVARY GLAND

Most of the salivary tumors present as a painless swelling in the region of the gland. 80 percent of salivary tumors occur in the parotid gland. 80 percent of parotid tumors are benign and 80 percent of benign parotid tumors are pleomorphic adenomas. Congenital tumor like hemangioma and lymphangioma may be seen in the parotid region (Fig. 84.10)

50 percent of the submandibular, sublingual, minor salivary glands are malignant.

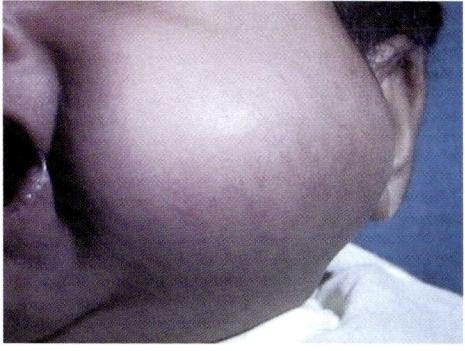

Fig. 84.10: Showing hemangioma of the parotid region and lips in an infant

A parotid mass is more likely to be malignant if it is associated with facial paralysis or if there is rapid enlargement of the parotid swelling. Dumb bell shaped tumor of the parotid involves parapharyngeal space. Classification of salivary tumors are mentioned in Table 84.1.

BENIGN TUMORS

PLEOMORPHIC ADENOMA (BENIGN MIXED TUMOR)

This is the most common benign salivary gland tumor and is characterized by the proliferation of epithelial and myoepithelial cells of the ducts and an increase in its stromal components. Patient presents with painless, slow growing swelling and commonly involves the superficial lobe of the parotid gland.

Pathology Gross

Grossly the tumor is typically encapsulated but under microscope pseudopodia-like projection of tumor cells outside the capsular surface is seen in higher magnification. Hence adequate wide excision should be done to prevent recurrence.

Histopathology

Tumor contains cells of both epithelial and mesenchymal elements. Mesenchymal stroma is thought to originate from the myoepithelial cells which may vary from scanty to abundant. The stroma within the same tumor may have myxoid,

Table 84.1: Classification of salivary tumors

Benign	Malignant
₂ **Pleomorphic adenoma**	₂ **Mucoepidermoid carcinoma**
₂ **Warthin Tumor (adenolymphoma)**	₂ **Adenoid cystic carcinoma**
• Myoepithelial adenoma	• Adenocarcinoma
• Basal cell adenoma	• Squamous cell carcinoma
• Oncocytoma (oncocytic adenoma)	• Undifferentiated carcinoma
• Canalicular adenoma	• Acinic cell carcinoma
• Sebaceous adenoma and sebaceous lymphadenoma	• Polymorphous low-grade adenocarcinoma
• Ductal papilloma	• Clear cell carcinoma
• Inverted ductal papilloma	• Basal cell adenocarcinoma
• Intraductal papilloma	• Sebaceous carcinoma and sebaceous lymphadenocarcinoma
• Sialadenoma papilliferum	• Papillary cystadenocarcinoma
• Cystadenoma	• Low grade cribriform cystadenocarcinoma
• Papillary cystadenoma	• Mucinous adenocarcinoma
• Mucinous cystadenoma	• Oncocytic carcinoma
• Sialoblastoma	• Salivary duct carcinoma
• Keratocytoma	• Adenocarcinoma, not otherwise specified
• Lymphadenoma	• Malignant myoepithelioma (myoepithelial carcinoma
• Soft tissue tumors	
• Hematopoeitic	• Small cell undifferentiated carcinoma
• Secondary tumors	• Large cell undifferentiated carcinoma
• Salivary cysts	• Lymphoepithelial carcinoma

chondroid, fibroid or osteoid appearance and hence it is called mixed tumors.

Clinical Features

Symptoms

- Painless swelling in the parotid region. It can also occur in the other salivary glands.
- Deep lobe tumors may give rise to throat symptoms like foreign body feeling in the throat, dysphagia, etc.

Signs (Fig. 84.11)

- Smooth, non-tender, lobular, firm, mobile swelling in the parotid
- Facial nerve is clinically normal
- Skin is not adhered to the underlying swelling.

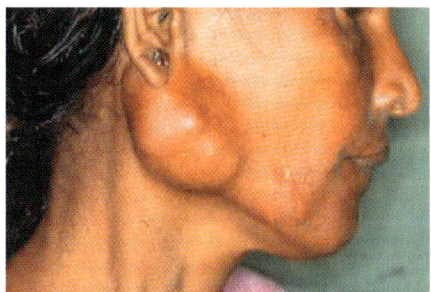

Fig. 84.11: Showing smooth lobular mass in the right parotid gland

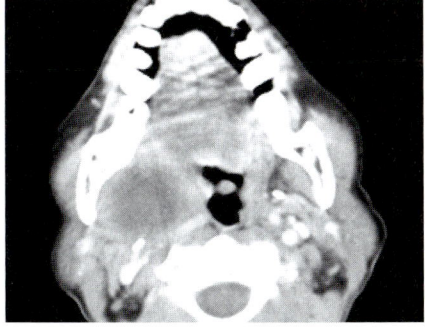

Fig. 84.12: Showing the round cystic mass in the left parapharyngeal space arising from the deep lobe of the parotid gland

- Deep lobe tumors involving the parapharyngeal space can cause swelling in the lateral pharyngeal wall with tonsil being pushed medially.

Investigations (Fig. 84.12)

- FNAC
- Sialogram
- CT/MRI scans especially for the deep lobe tumors. Deep lobe tumors may be seen as oval or dumb-bell lesions.
- CT sialogram may be helpful in differentiating inflammatory from neoplastic conditions.

Treatment (Figs 84.13 and 84.14)

- Superficial parotidectomy is the treatment of choice. Enucleation of the tumor should not be done as the recurrence rates are high. The facial nerve should be identified and spared. Deep lobe tumor can be excised by transcervical, transmandibular approach.
- If it occurs in submandibular salivary gland, the gland should be excised completely.

Prognosis

Inadequate excision causes recurrence. Malignant transformation can occur in 2 to 10 percent of the

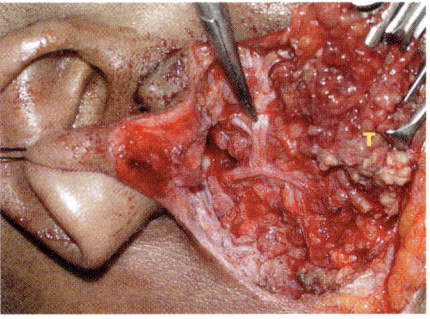

Fig. 84.13: Facial nerve being dissected to separate the superficial lobe with the tumor from the deep lobe. The artery forceps point towards the upper division of the facial nerve and 'T' is the tumor in the superficial lobe of the parotid gland

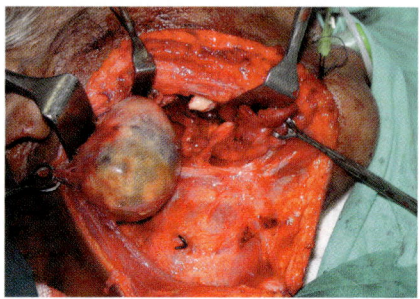

Fig. 84.14: Photograph showing deep lobe tumor being dissected out of the right parapharyngeal space by a transcervical, transmandibular approach (angle mandibulotomy)

these tumors and is called 'carcinoma expleomorphic adenoma'

WARTHIN TUMOR (CYSTADENOMA LYMPHOMATOSUM, ADENOLYMPHOMA)

This exclusively occurs in the parotid gland and is more common in males with male to female ratio being 26:1. This is the second most common benign tumor. Patient presents with a painless slow growing swelling most commonly in the tail of the parotid gland. It is often well defined and superficially placed. Incidence of bilateral and multicentric lesion is 10 percent.

Etiology

The most popular etiologic theory suggests that it arises from the salivary ducts that are trapped within the intraparotid lymph nodes.

Pathology

The tumor is made of double layered epithelium with tubulopapillary cystic pattern within the lymphoid tissue. Epithelial cells similar to that of oncocytes are seen.

Clinical Features

- More common in males, in their 6th and 7th decades

- Painless, slow growing, soft/ cystic/ firm mass
- Acute pain and increase in size may occur
- Rarely patients may complain of pain in the ear and tinnitus
- Facial nerve is unaffected.
- Malignant transformation can occur in 0.3 percent of cases.

Investigations

- Technetium scan (Tc99m) shows a 'hot nodule' in the gland.
- FNAC may be useful in the diagnosis.

Treatment

Complete surgical excision after preserving the facial nerve.

MALIGNANT TUMORS

MUCOEPIDERMOID CARCINOMA

This is the most common malignant salivary gland tumor. Half of all mucoepidermoid carcinomas occur in the parotid gland.

Pathology

Site of origin: Excretory and intercalated ducts of the salivary gland. It contains both mucous secreting and epidermoid cells. The ratio between the Epidermoid cells and the mucous secreting cells varies.

The histological grading is as follows.

- *Low grade:* Prominent cystic structures with mature cellular elements.
- *High grade:* Sheets of solid cells associated with atypia and is more aggressive.

High grade tumors have high rate of regional metastasis.

Clinical Features

Low grade: Slowly growing tumors that rarely metastasize.

High grade are aggressive and nodal metastasis is around 40 percent and 30 percent may have distant metastases. TNM staging is mentioned in Table 84.2.

Investigation

- CT/MR imaging
- Ultrasonography
- Sialogram– This is helpful investigation to differentiate inflammatory from neoplastic conditions
- Technetium scanning is useful to rule out Warthin tumor and oncocytoma.
- FNAC

Treatment

- *Low grade:* Wide excision/superficial parotidectomy. Attempts should be made to preserve the facial nerve, unless involved directly.
- *High grade:* Wide surgical margins required. Facial nerve resection is required as passes

---

Table 84.2: T Staging for tumors of the major salivary glands (AJCC 2002)

- **TX** Primary tumor cannot be assessed
- **T0** No evidence of primary tumor
- **T1** Tumor 2 cm or less in greatest dimension without extraparenchymal extension*
- **T2** Tumor more than 2 cm but not more than 4 cm in greatest dimension without extra-parenchymal extension*
- **T3** Tumor more than 4 cm and/or tumor having extraparenchymal extension*
- **T4a** Tumor invades skin, mandible, ear canal, and/or facial nerve
- **T4b** Tumor invades skull base and/or pterygoid plates and/or encases carotid artery

Extraparenchymal extension is clinical or macroscopic evidence of invasion of soft tissues. Microscopic evidence alone does not constitute extraparenchymal extension for classification purposes.

---

through the tumor. Block dissection of the neck followed by postoperative radiotherapy.

Prognosis

- *Low grade:* 5 year survival rates 80 to 90 percent and they rarely recur after complete surgical resection.
- *High grade:* Local recurrence is around 60 percent after surgical resection.

ADENOID CYSTIC CARCINOMA

It is the second most common malignant salivary neoplasm. It commonly involves the submandibular and minor salivary glands and is uncommon in the parotid gland. .

Clinical Features

It arises as a slowly progressive swelling the affected salivary gland and is associated with pain. Perineural involvement is frequent. Regional and distant metastases occurs in 40 percent and can occur along the perineural lymphatics.

Treatment

- Wide excision with neck dissection
- Adjuvant radiotherapy with neutron irradiation is being tried.

Acinic Cell Tumor

This is rare and accounts for 1 percent of all salivary gland tumors. 95 percent of these tumors are seen in parotid. They present as painless, slow growing superficial mass and occasionally lead to rapid growth involving the facial nerve. This is known to metastasize. Superficial parotidectomy is the treatment of choice.

Diagnostic Techniques for Salivary Neoplasm

- Fine needle aspiration cytology
- Sialography
- CT/ MRI
- Technetium scan
- Frozen section biopsy

85

Parapharyngeal Tumors

Anatomy of the Parapharyngeal Space

Parapharyngeal space lies deep in the pharynx extending from base of the skull to the level of the hyoid bone. It is bounded medially by the fascia of the pharynx laterally by the pterygoid muscle and the sheath of the parotid gland. Mandible and masseter muscle lie anteriorly (Figs 85.1 and 85.2a).

The stylomandibular canal which is bounded by the base of the skull above and the styloid process and stylomandibular ligament posteriorly is also closely related to the peripharyngeal space (Figs 85.2b and 85.3).

It is divided into the prestyloid and poststyloid compartment. The space contains not only fascia and muscles but also the bifurcation of the carotid artery, internal and external carotid artery, 9th, 10th, and 12th cranial nerve and cervical sympathetic nerve. The tumors arising from the prestyloid compartment commonly are salivary gland tumors whereas, the postsyloid compartment tumors are of neurogenic origin.

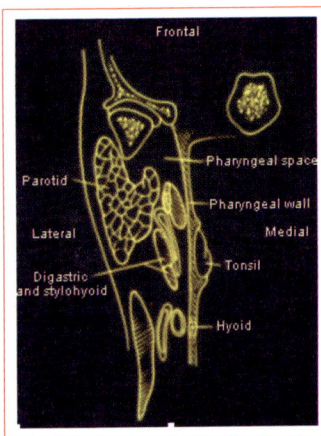

Fig. 85.1: Showing the relation of deep lobe of the parotid to the parapharyngeal space

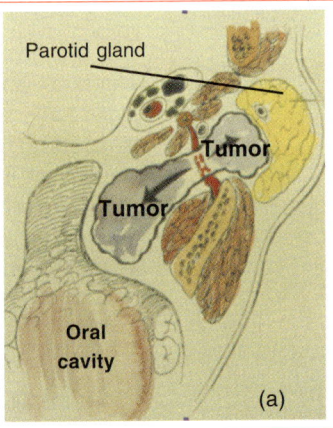

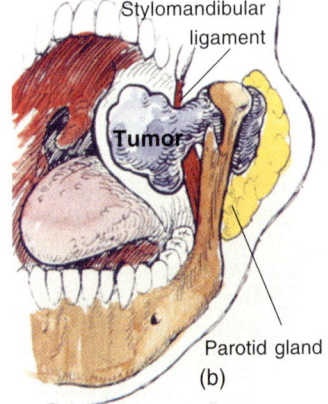

Figs 85.2a and b: Showing dumb-bell tumor arising from the deep lobe of the parotid gland and is being constricted by the stylomandibular ligament

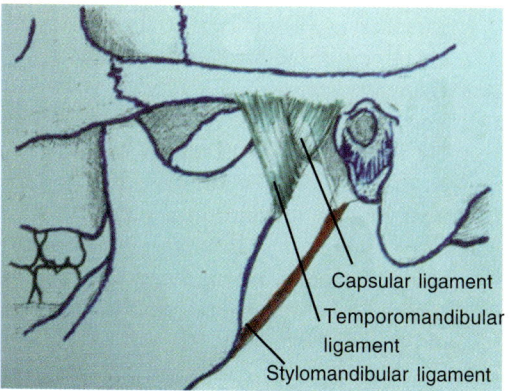

Fig. 85.3: Stylomandibular ligament

Common Tumors in the Parapharyngeal Space

Benign Tumors

- Schwannoma or Neurilemoma (Figs 85.4 and 85.5)
- Pleomorphic adenoma
- Warthin's tumor
- Paraganglioma
- Meningioma
- Osteolipoma
- Chondroid chordoma.

Malignant Tumors

- Malignant schwannoma
- Mucoepidermoid carcinoma
- Synovial sarcoma
- Mesenchymal chondrosarcoma
- Malignant fibrous histiocytoma.

Clinical Features

Symptoms

1. They often present as a painless swelling or a lump in the lateral neck.
2. The neck swelling may not be obvious but there may be a swelling in the lateral pharyngeal wall/oral cavity.
3. Dysphonia
4. Dysphagia
5. Trismus
6. Nasal obstruction
7. Aural fullness.

Signs

- Neck swelling which is often firm.
- Vascular tumors may be pulsatile and bruit may be present.
- Prestyloid compartment tumor is often due to deep lobe of parotid and can present as a mass or bulge in the tonsillar fossa and adjacent soft palate or lateral pharyngeal wall. Poststyloid compartment tumors commonly present as a neck mass with a bulge in the lateral pharyngeal wall. The common poststyloid tumors are neurogenic like schwanoma of the vagus or hypoglossal nerve or rarely it may arise from the carotids (features of carotid body tumors are described under solid tumors of the neck) or the sympathetic chain.

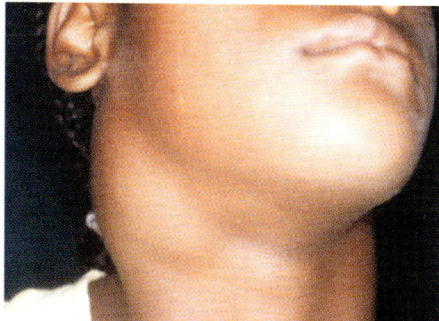

Fig. 85.4: Benign neurilemoma

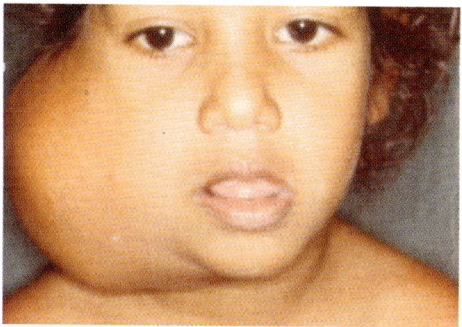

Fig. 85.5: Schwannoma

- Consequently neurological signs like vagal palsy, hypoglossal palsy or features of Horner's syndrome may be seen.

Investigations

- CT/ MR imaging is the main investigation of choice. This gives the exact location and extent of the tumor and its relation to the carotids and the internal jugular vein.
- DSA–Clinically vascular mass or contrast enhancing mass on CT could be carotid body tumor or glomus vagale and needs a digital subtraction angiography to identify the feeding arteries and the extent of contralateral blood supply to the brain.
- 24 hours VMA to rule out secreting paraganglioma.
- FNAC in non-vascular mass.
- Rigid telescopy of the larynx.

Treatment

Surgical resection is the treatment of choice. The common approaches to the parapharyngeal space tumors are:

- *Transcervical:* This is the most commonly employed approach. This is suitable for parapharyngeal tumors which lie towards the lower part of the parapharyngeal space.
- *Transcervical, transmandibular approach:* This is opted if the tumor is high up towards the base of the skull and it gives better exposure. This is suitable for tumors involving the jugular foramen (Fig. 85.6).
- *Cervicoparotid approach:* Preferred in parotid tumors involving the parapharyngeal space like dumb-bell tumors and oval tumors of the deep lobe.

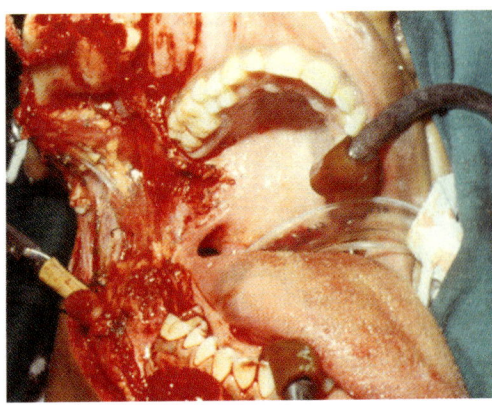

Fig. 85.6: Biller's approach

POINTS TO REMEMBER

1. Most common prestyloid compartment tumor is pleomorphic adenoma arising from the deep lobe of the parotid gland.
2. Most common poststyloid compartments are of neurogenic origin.
3. C.T. imaging, FNAC are the most important investigation.
4. Mandibulotomy is often required for large parapharyngeal tumors.

86

Neck Dissection in Head and Neck Malignancy

'Neck dissection or cervical lymphadenectomy is a systematic en block removal of the lymph nodes and lymph-bearing structures including the surrounding fibrofatty tissue from the various compartments of the neck'

—**Cummings.**

Neck dissection or block dissection of the neck is an oncologically sound procedure as it encompasses systematic removal of all the draining lymph nodes from the primary site including its lymphatic vessels situated in the lymph bearing structures.

Various triangles of the neck are covered by the deep cervical fascia. The investing layer of the deep cervical fascia encompasses the muscles in the neck resulting in the formation of various compartments. This compartmentalization of the neck helps in removal of fibrofatty tissue containing the lymphatics which are engulfed by the cervical fascia. Any partial removal of structures like lymph node breaches the compartment and if node is malignant the surgery causes seeding of the tumor into the surrounding compartments thus facilitating its spread. Hence a neck dissection should encompass the fibrofatty tissue of the entire compartment.

A suprahyoid dissection for removal of a group of nodes is not an oncologically sound procedure in comparison to supraomohyoid neck dissection, as in the former, only part of the compartment is dealt with.

For the same reason a lymph node biopsy for suspected metastatic node should be condemned. Fine needle aspiration cytology (FNAC) is a sensitive test for metastatic squamous cell carcinoma in the lymph node and should be the investigation of choice in such cases for tissue diagnosis.

In case of a negative FNAC from the cervical lymph node and no primary malignancy detected by all endoscopic and radiological investigations, a lymph node biopsy is done under frozen section control. If this is positive a radical or modified neck dissection should be proceeded with.

Historical Perspectives

1847 - **Warren** first attempted to remove metastatic cancer in the neck.

1880 - **Kocher** described the resection of tongue combined with removal of regional lymphatics via submandibular approach.

1906 - **George Crile** gave the first description of a standardized anatomic dissection of the cervical lymphatics.

1951 - **Hayes Martin** advocated radical neck dissection as the only acceptable procedure for cervical lymph node metastasis.

1966 - **Bocca** of Italy and **Ballantyne** of USA advocated functional neck dissection. They were supported by Pignataro and Jesse.

1972 - **Lindberg** advocated selective neck dissection.

1994 - **Spiro, Strong and Shah** advocated limited neck dissection.

TYPES OF NECK DISSECTION

Neck dissection can be classified into various types depending on the lymph nodes and lymph bearing structures removed.

1. Radical neck dissection
2. Modified neck dissection
3. Extended radical neck dissection
4. Selective neck dissection
5. Limited neck dissection.

Limited neck dissection is done when one or two levels of nodes are dissected (central compartment including pre and paratracheal nodes (level 6) or mediastinal node dissection (level 7). This is not done as an isolated procedure for a squamous cell carcinoma of the head and neck but may be done for thyroid cancer like papillary and follicular thyroid carcinoma where the central compartment dissection is done routinely for N0 neck. Mediastinal neck dissection along with central compartment dissection is done in advanced cancer of thyroid. This may however be done with other forms of neck dissection for squamous cell carcinoma, for example in subglottic malignancy or stomal recurrence.

RADICAL NECK DISSECTION

This is defined as a surgery for metastatic cervical lymph node and consists of en-block resection of all the lymph nodes [Levels 1-5] and all the lymph bearing structures from mandible to clavicle and from anterior border of trapezius to midline (Fig. 86.1).

Indications

1. Metastatic lymph node in the neck from a known primary squamous cell carcinoma in

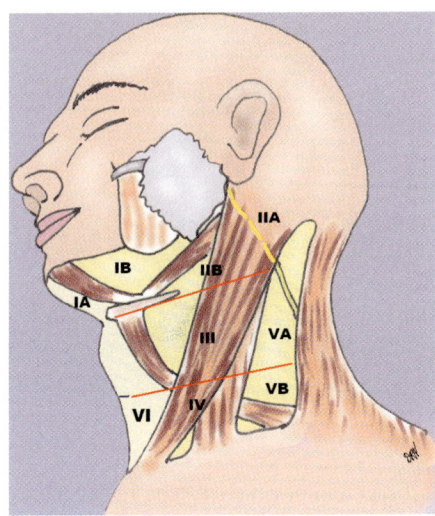

Fig. 86.1: Various lymph node levels in the neck

the upper aerodigestive tract, which is clinically palpable or detected radiologically.
2. Metastasis of unknown origin (MUO)

Technique

Anesthesia: General anesthesia: Airway is maintained by endotracheal intubation or if airway is compromised by a tracheostomy.

Position: Supine with neck extended and head rotated to the contralateral side.

Steps of Surgery

1. *Incision:* The incision that can be used is modified Gluck-Sorenson's or bilateral hockey stick or bilateral Macfee's incision for bilateral neck dissection and unilateral hockey stick incision, inverted hockey incision, etc. may be used for unilateral neck dissection.
2. *Subplatysmal flap elevation:* The skin including the subcutaneous tissue and platysma is elevated exposing the area of the neck from clavicle to angle of mandible and anterior border of the trapezius and midline.

The following structures should be exposed: Mastoid tip with attachment of the sternocleidomastoid muscle, hyoid bone, submandibular salivary gland, tail of the parotid gland and clavicular and sternal heads of the sternocleidomastoid muscle. The marginal mandibular nerve should be identified and preserved (Fig. 86.2).

3. The dissection starts from below. The sternal and clavicular heads of the sternomastoid muscle are divided (Fig. 86.3).

4. The dissection is carried further along the clavicle till the anterior border of the trapezius is reached.

5. The external jugular vein is divided between ligatures.

6. After dissecting the fibrofatty tissue in the supraclavicular area, the omohyoid muscle is divided and dissected along the fat plane. On the left side care is taken to identify and not to injure the thoracic duct while dissecting to expose the internal jugular vein (Fig. 86.4).

7. The internal jugular vein is isolated and divided between transfixation sutures. The vagus nerve should be identified and spared before ligation of the internal jugular vein (Fig. 86.5).

8. Then the dissection is carried out posteriorly from the prevertebral fascia to dissect out the fascia and the fat. The phrenic nerve is identified. Transverse cervical artery crosses the phrenic nerve and should be spared.

9. The dissection in then carried on to identify the brachial plexus in the supraclavicular area in posterior triangle. The fibrofatty tissue is dissected out from the trapezius border and

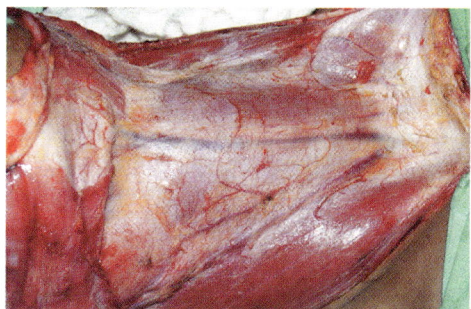

Fig. 86.2: Exposure of the neck by modified Gluck-Sorenson's incision

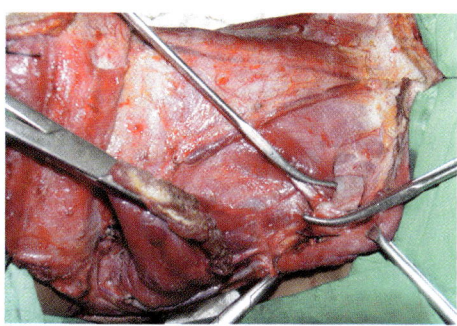

Fig. 86.4: Division of inferior belly of omohyoid and exposure of lower end of internal jugular vein

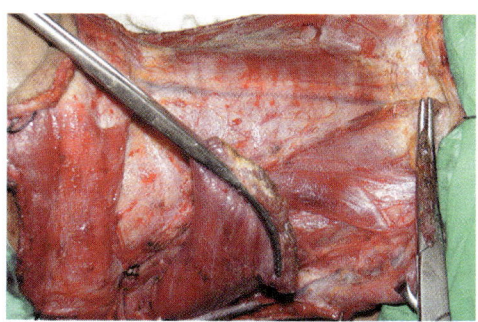

Fig. 86.3: Division of sternal and clavicular heads of sternocleidomastoid muscle

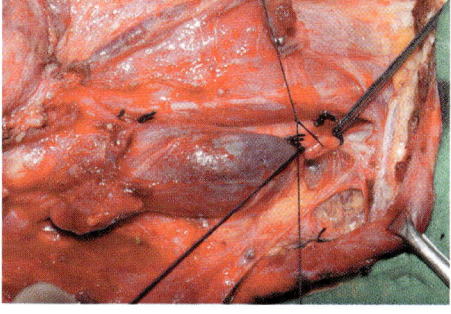

Fig. 86.5: Ligation of the lower end of internal jugular vein

from its deep pocket and dissected further superficial to the deep fascia. The spinal accessory nerve is identified and divided but it is preserved in a modified neck dissection. Cervical C3, C4 are divided carefully across the nerve roots and rest of the phrenic nerve is preserved.

10. Carotid dissection is done and the specimen is dissected upwards till the carotid bifurcation is reached. The superior thyroid artery is identified and ligated. Dissection is continued towards the tail of the parotid and the mastoid (Fig. 86.6).

11. The hypoglossal nerve is identified as it crosses the external and internal carotid artery above the carotid bifurcation and is preserved in its entire course.

12. The sternocleidomastoid muscle is divided from the mastoid tip. The posterior belly of the digastric is seen and preserved which lies lateral to the internal jugular vein and the internal carotid artery.

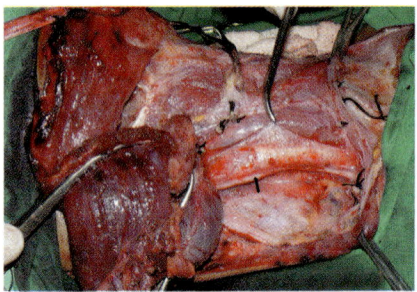

Fig. 86.6: Exposure of the carotid artery as the radical neck dissection is continued upwards

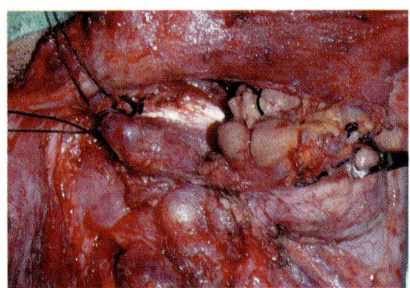

Fig. 86.7: Dissection of the submandibular triangle

13. The tail of the parotid is divided and carried towards the angle of the mandible. Sharp dissection is then carried out towards the base of the skull and the hypoglossal nerve is identified, internal jugular vein is identified and divided between transfixation sutures.

14. Structures lateral to the hypoglossal nerve are divided. Facial artery and the common facial vein are identified and ligated. Submandibular salivary gland and the fibrofatty tissue are dissected anteriorly and the facial vein and artery is again ligated at the margin of the mandible on the masseter muscle (Fig. 86.7).

15. The entire specimen is dissected anteriorly and connected to the main specimen of the primary tumor, if any, after ligating and dividing the submandibular duct and dissecting the submental triangle (Figs 86.8 and 86.9).

Structures Removed in Radical Neck Dissection

1. Lymph node level 1 to 5
2. Spinal accessory nerve
3. Internal and external jugular vein
4. Sternocleidomastoid and omohyoid muscle
5. Cervical plexus- sensory branches
6. Submandibular salivary gland
7. Tail of the parotid gland

Contraindications of RND

1. Uncontrollable cancer of the primary site
2. Evidence of distant metastases
3. Life expectancy is less than 3 months

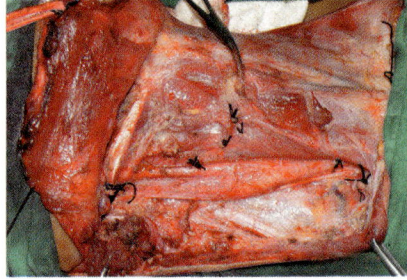

Fig. 86.8: Completion of radical neck dissection for a metastatic node with unknown primary

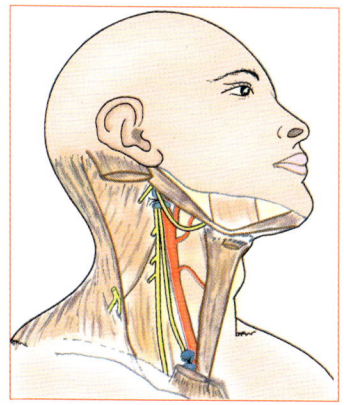

Fig. 86.9: Structures preserved following completion of radical neck dissection

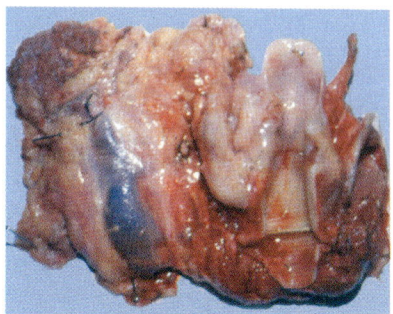

Fig. 86.10: Specimen showing en block resection of the radical neck dissection with total laryngectomy

4. Patient is unfit for major surgery
5. Mass fixed to the cervical plexus, brachial plexus and trachea
6. Unresectable nodes unchanged by radiotherapy and chemotherapy.

Modified Neck Dissection

This is defined as a surgical procedure for a metastatic cervical node with radical clearance of the all the disease (nodes level 1 to 5) without sacrificing some of the lymph bearing structures that is resected in the radical neck dissection, with an intent to preserve their function.

Rationale

Lymph nodes of the neck lie in specific facial plane which can be carefully dissected with preservation of one or more important structures like spinal accessory nerve, sternocleidomastoid muscle, and internal jugular vein.

Types

Type I: Spinal accessory nerve is preserved. Internal jugular vein and the sternocleidomastoid muscle are resected.
Type II: Spinal accessory and the IJV are preserved. Sternocleidomastoid muscle is resected.
Type III (functional neck dissection): All three vital structures spinal accessory, IJV and the sternocleidomastoid muscle are preserved.

In all these three types lymph nodes level 1 to 5 is resected en bloc.

EXTENDED RADICAL NECK DISSECTION

This is a surgical procedure more than a radical neck dissection when the disease extends superiorly to the skull base and inferiorly to the mediastinum.

Indications

Extension of the cervical disease to involve the skull base and extension of laryngopharyngeal cancer to the superior mediastinum.

Contraindications

- Same as RND and in addition
- Extension to skull base with erosion of the posterolateral wall of sphenoid sinus, cavernous sinus, foramen lacerum and vertebral bodies.

Selective Neck Dissection

This is a type of neck dissection where lymph nodes and the lymph bearing structures are removed within a specific facial compartment for a preferably N0 neck (no clinically palpable or otherwise detected cervical nodal disease). This is also called staging neck dissection and the nodes are sent for frozen section biopsy. If they turn positive for malignancy, a radical or modified neck dissection is done.

Types

- Supraomohyoid neck dissection
- Extended suprahyoid neck dissection
- Lateral neck dissection
- Posterolateral neck dissection.

SUPRAOMOHYOID NECK DISSECTION

This is a type of neck dissection comprising of en-block resection of level 1 to 3 lymph nodes with submandibular salivary gland.

Indications

- Oral and oropharyngeal malignancy with N0 neck or N1 located in the first echelon lymph node in the neck.
- For cancer of the floor of the mouth, tongue bilateral dissection is done
- Squamous cell carcinoma of the skin and the midface.

EXTENDED SUPRAHYOID NECK DISSECTION

This is a type of neck dissection comprising of en-block resection of level 1 to 4 lymph nodes along with submandibular salivary gland.

Indications

Same as supraomohyoid neck dissection. Now-a-days some surgeons prefer to include level 4 unlike conventional suprahyoid neck dissection

LATERAL NECK DISSECTION

This is a type of neck dissection comprising of enbloc resection of level 2 to 4 lymph nodes and is done for laryngeal, laryngopharyngeal or cervical esophageal disease with N0 neck. This is often done bilaterally.

POSTEROLATERAL NECK DISSECTION

This is a type of neck dissection comprising of en-bloc resection of level 2 to 5 lymph nodes and is done for laryngeal, laryngopharyngeal or cervical esophageal disease with N0 neck.

CENTRAL COMPARTMENT NECK DISSECTION (LEVEL VI)

This is done in conjunction with total thyroidectomy for well differentiated carcinoma of the thyroid gland.

Superior Mediastinal Neck Dissection (Level VII)

This is done in conjunction with total thyroidectomy for well differentiated carcinoma of the thyroid gland. However it may be done with other neck dissections for advanced laryngeal carcinoma with subglottic extension, postcricoid and upper esophageal malignancy or for a stomal recurrence.

POINTS TO REMEMBER

1. Neck dissection is a systematic enblock removal of the lymph nodes and lymph bearing structures including fibro-fatty tissue from various compartments of the neck.
2. George Gile gave the first description of a standardized anatomic dissection of cervical lymphatics.
3. Radical neck dissection includes en bloc resection of all the lymph nodes from level-1 to level 5 and all the lymph bearing structures from mandible to clavicle and from anterior border of trapezius to midline along with sternocleido mastoid muscle, internal jugular vein and accessory nerve.

Anesthesia in ENT: Head and Neck Surgery

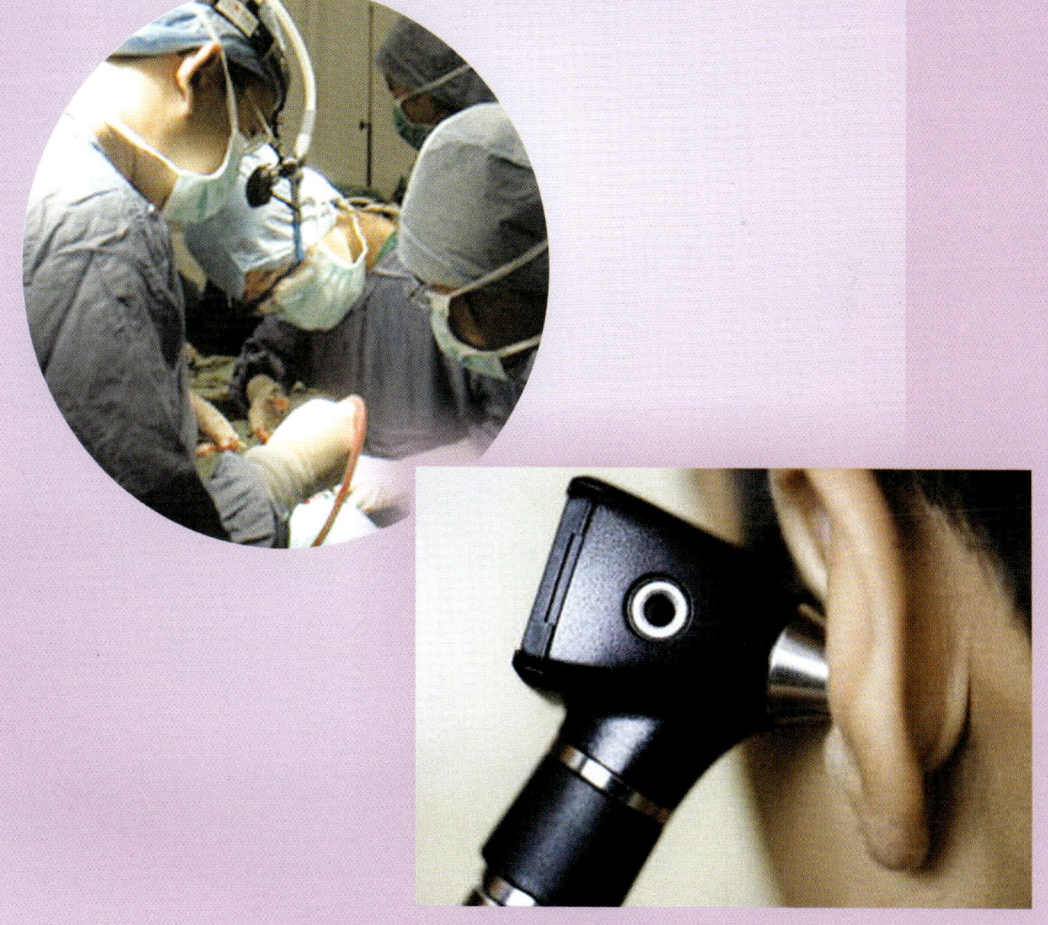

87

Local Anesthesia in ENT

INTRODUCTION

Pain is one of the most commonly experienced symptoms in surgery and is a major concern to the surgeon. It is often spoken of as a protective mechanism, since it is usually manifested when an environmental change occurs that causes injury to responsive tissue. One of the methods of pain control is to block the pathway of painful impulses.

In regional anesthesia (regional, local anesthesia), the pathway is blocked by depositing a suitable chemical agent extraneurally in proximity to the nerve or nerves to be blocked.

Classification

Regional anesthesia can be divided into component parts depending on the areas to be anesthetized, and the technique employed into:

1. Nerve block
2. Field block
3. Local infiltration
4. Topical analgesia.

1. **Nerve block:** It consists of depositing a suitable local anesthetic solution within close proximity to a main nerve trunk, thus preventing afferent impulses from traveling centrally beyond that point.
2. **Field block:** It consists of depositing a solution in proximity to the larger terminal nerve branches, so that the area to be anesthetized is walled off or circumscribed to prevent central passage of afferent impulses.
3. **Local infiltration:** Small nerve terminals in the area of surgery are flooded with local anesthetic solution rendering them insensible to pain or preventing them from becoming stimulated and creating the impulse.
4. **Topical analgesia:** Topical analgesia renders the free nerve endings inaccessible structures (intact mucous membrane/abraded skin) incapable of stimulation by the application of a suitable solution directly to the surface of the area.

Factors in Selecting the Method of Induction

- Area to be anesthetized
- Profoundness required
- Duration of anesthesia
- Age of the patient
- Condition of patient
- Hemostasis if needed.

Advantages with Regional Anesthesia

- Patient remains awake and cooperative.
- There is little distortion of normal physiology and the method can therefore be used to advantage on poor risk patients.

- Functional assessment like hearing gain following ear surgery can be done on the operation table itself.
- There is low incidence of morbidity.
- The patient may leave the office unescorted.
- No additional trained personal is necessary.
- There is no additional expense to the patient.

Disadvantage/Contraindication

- The patient refuses regional anesthesia because of fear or apprehension.
- Infection rules out the use of regional anesthesia.
- Patient is allergic to various local anesthetics.
- Patient is mentally deficient and is unable to cooperate.
- Major and prolonged surgeries make regional anesthesia unfeasible.
- Extremes of age where patient may not cooperate.
- Anomalies make regional analgesia difficult or impossible.

Ideal Local Anesthetic

- Adequate potency
- Short latency
- Good penetration
- Good diffusion
- Low toxicity
- Controllable duration of action with complete reversibility.
- Water solubility
- Soluble in solution
- Non-irritant, non-antigenic and should not interfere with wound-healing.

Mechanism of Action of Local Anesthesia

Local anesthetics are drugs that irreversibly block the initiation and propagation of nerve action potentials distal to point of application by virtue of:

(a) **Hydrophobic bonding:** Drug base is absorbed by the cell membrane, therby hindering sodium access.
(b) **Lipid solubility:** Drug base dissolves in the phospholipids of cell membrane causing swelling which tends to obstruct the ion channels through membrane.

Drugs

Local anesthetics are divided into
1. Aminoesters, e.g. Cocaine, procaine, tetracaine (Drug name has single 'i')
2. Aminoamides, e.g. Lidocaine, bupivacaine, mepivacaine, prilocaine (Drug name has double 'i').

Lignocaine

- Lignocaine is aminocyl amide
- Heat stable
- Metabolized in liver excreted in urine
- Rapid onset of action, good diffusion
- Duration of action about 1 hour can be increased to 2 to 3 hours by addition of vaso-constrictor.
- Maximum dose in 3 mg/kg for 0.5 percent (200 mg), 7 mg/kg when adrenaline is added (max. dose 500 mg).
- Surface anesthesia 2 to 4 is used. 2 percent available for viscous form of oral analgesia 4 percent hand operated sprays, pressured 10 percent aerosol spray, 2 to 5 percent gels and ointment for lubricating tubes and instruments.
- Onset of action is rapid but of short duration (20 min).

VASOCONSTRICTORS

Aim

- Reduces tissue bleeding
- Delays the rate of absorption
- Prolongs the action of anesthetic
- Reduces toxic effects.

Drugs

- Adrenaline
- Felypressin
- Phenylephrine hydrochloride.

Adrenaline

Commonly used vasoconstrictor. Add adrenaline to the anesthetic solution immediately before use.

Dose of adrenaline by injection should not exceed 0.01 mg/kg, with a total maximum of 0.5 mg (0.5 ml of 1:1000 solution) in a healthy adult.

Adverse Effects

Anxiety, vertigo, pallor, palpitations, increase in systolic blood pressure, tachyarrhythmia. Do not infiltrate tissues, which are supplied by end arteries. Its use is contraindicated in IHD, severe hypertension, thyrotoxicosis, halothane and patients on MAOI drugs.

LOCAL ANESTHETIC TECHNIQUES

NOSE AND PARANASAL SINUSES

Topical Anesthesia

4 percent lignocaine with adrenaline is used for minor surgery to the nose, removal of polyps, local electrocautery and antral puncture.

Procedure

Nasal cavities are sprayed with anesthetic. Nose is carefully packed with ribbon gauze/cottonoids soaked in LA solution for 10 min. Cottonoid is inserted at an angle of 20 degrees to the floor of the nose until bone is felt at a depth of 6 to 7 cms, now lying adjacent to sphenopalatine foramen. Second applicator is inserted along anterior border of nasal cavity until anterior end of cribriform plate about 5 cms deep.

Field Block

Sites for injection of local anesthetic are:
- Above nasal bones and beneath skin of dorsum to block infratrochlear nerve.
- Into infraorbital foramen bilaterally to block infraorbital nerve.
- Greater palatine nerve at incisive foramen.
- Nasal tip and base of columella.

ANTERIOR ETHMOIDAL NERVE BLOCK

Technique

Anterior ethmoidal nerve and infratrochlear nerves can be blocked together at their origin from nasociliary nerve in the upper half of the medial wall of the orbit 2.5 cms from the orbital margin. A 5 cms needle with a marker 2.5 cms from the tip is inserted 1 cm above the inner canthus and directed horizontally backwards. At a depth of 2.5 cms the tip lies close to anterior ethmoidal nerve where it enters its foramen, 1 ml is injected and 1 ml is injected as the needle is slowly withdrawn.

Procedures that can be performed are:
1. External dacryocystorhinostomy.
2. Ligation of anterior and posterior ethmoidal arteries can be performed using Lynch incision for epistaxis.

NERVE BLOCKS FOR HEAD AND NECK SURGERY

Trigeminal Nerve Block

Trigeminal nerve divides into ophthalmic, maxillary and mandibular nerves which supply the eye, forehead, midface, upper and the lower jaw.

Clinical Applications

Blockade of II and III divisions of the trigeminal nerve is useful in diagnosis and management of pain syndromes and surgical procedures.

Maxillary Nerve Block

Nerves anesthetized are

Entire maxillary nerve and all its subdivisions peripheral to the site of injection.

Areas anesthetized are
- Anterior temporal and zygomatic regions
- Lower eyelid
- Side of nose
- Anterior cheek

- Upper lip
- Maxillary teeth
- Maxillary alveolar bone and overlying structures
- Hard and soft palate
- Tonsil
- Part of the pharynx
- Nasal septum and floor of the nose
- Posterior lateral mucosa and turbinate bones.

Technique

Maxillary nerve is blocked as it exits the skull through foramen rotundum and crosses the pterygopalatine or infratemporal fossa between the skull and the upper jaw.

The coronoid notch of the mandible is located and with the patients mouth closed, a 22 gauge, 8 cm needle is inserted at the inferior edge of the coronoid notch perpendicular to skin entry sit. Needle contacts lateral pterygoid plate at a depth of about 5 cm. It is then withdrawn and redirected anteriorly and superiorly to walk off the plate and is advanced approximately 0.5 cm into pterygopalatine fossa. 3 to 5 ml of the solution is injected.

Mandibular Nerve Block

Nerves anesthetized are

- Mandibular nerve and its subdivisions
- Inferior alveolar nerve
- Buccinator nerve
- Lingual nerve
- Mental nerve
- Incisive nerve.

Areas anesthetized are

- Temporal region
- Auricle of the ear (tragus, root of the helix)
- External auditory meatus
- TM joint
- Salivary glands
- Anterior two-thirds of the tongue
- Floor of the mouth
- Mandible
- Lower teeth, gingival and buccal mucosa
- Lower portion of the face.

Technique

The mandibular nerve, i.e. third division, leaves the cranium through the foramen ovale and innervates the skin of the lower jaw and the skin anterior and superior to the ear by its posterior division. The mandibular nerve is blocked via the same entry site as the maxillary nerve. The needle is advanced along the inferior margin of the coronoid notch until the bone of the lateral pterygoid plate is contacted (about 5 cm). The needle is withdrawn and is redirected to walk off the posterior border of the pterygoid plate, should not be inserted farther than 0.5 cm past the plate.

Side Effects and Complications

- Hematoma formation
- Temporary blindness
- Pharynx may be entered, increasing the risk of contaminating the infratemporal fossa.
- Brainstem anesthesia.

Clinical Applications

- Blockade used for diagnosis and therapeutic purposes such as trigeminal neuralgia and tics.
- Used for surgical procedures where anesthesis of entire distribution of the maxillary nerve is required.

Supraorbital and Supratrochlear Nerve Block

Nerves anesthetized are supraorbital nerve and supratrochlear nerve.
Areas anesthetized are whole forehead, upper eyelids.

Technique

The supraorbital notch can be easily palpated. This landmark lies on a vertical line with the pupil (when the eye is looking directly forward), the infraorbital foramen, and the mental foramen. A 25 gauge, 2 cm needle is inserted immediately superior to the supraorbital notch, and 2 to 4 ml of local anesthetic solution is injected. The supratrochlear nerve can be blocked by extending the supraorbital injection site medially with an additional 2 to 4 ml of solution.

Infraorbital Nerve Block

Nerves anesthetized are
- Infraorbital nerve
- Inferior palpebal, lateral nasal and superior labial nerves
- Anterior and middle superior alveolar nerves.

Areas anesthetized are
- Upper lip, portions of the side of the nose, lower eyelids
- Labial alveolar plate and overlying tissues
- Incisors and bicuspids on the side injected
- Sometimes maxillary molars and their buccal supporting structures.

Technique

The infraorbital notch lies on the line connecting the supraorbital and mental foramina and the pupil of the eye. The nerve can be blocked by advancing a 25 gauge, 3 cm needle laterally and cephalad toward the foramen from a point 1 cm inferior.

Mental Nerve Block

Nerves anesthetized: Mental nerve
Areas anesthetized are:
- Lower lip
- Mucous membrane in the mucolabial fold anterior to the mental foramen.

Technique

The mental foramen lies on the vertical line connecting the supraorbital notch, pupil of the eye with the infraorbital foramina, if continued downwards to the mandible. The foramen is palpated in the mandible, and a 25 guage, 3 cm needle is inserted inferomedially and 1 ml of anesthetic solution is injected.

Inferior Alveolar Nerve Block

Nerves Anesthetized

Inferior alveolar nerve and its subdivisions namely the mental nerve and incisive nerve.

Areas anesthetized are:
- Body of the mandible and inferior portion of the ramus
- Mandibular teeth
- Mucous membrane and underlying tissues anterior to first mandibular molar.

Technique
- (Right side) Operator stands to the right and front of the patient.
- Patient is instructed to occlude the teeth
- Operator retracts patient's lips exposing the maxillary and mandibular teeth.
- Syringe is aligned parallel to the occlusal and sagittal planes, but positioned at the mucogingival junction of the maxillary molars.
- Needle penetrates mucosa just medial to the ramus and is inserted approximately 1½ inches.
- Aspirate and inject the anesthetic.

Lingual Nerve Block

Nerves anesthetized: Lingual nerve
Areas anesthetized: Anterior two-thirds of the tongue and the floor of the oral cavity, mucosa and periosteum on the lingual side of the mandible.

Technique
Same as inferior alveolar nerve block

Buccinator Nerve Block

Nerves anesthetized: Buccinator nerve
Areas anesthetized: Buccal mucous membrane and mucoperiosteum of the mandibular area.

Technique
- A 1 inch 25 gauge needle is inserted onto the buccal mucosa just distal to the third molar and 0.5 ml of solution is deposited.
- Insert the needle and deposit the solution directly into retromolar trigone.

Cervical Plexus Block

The cervical plexus is derived from the C1, C2, C3 and C4 spinal nerves and supplies branches to the prevertebral muscles, strap muscles of the neck, and phrenic nerve. It supplies the musculature of the neck segmentally and the cutaneous sensation of the skin between the trigeminally innervated face and the T2 dermatome of the trunk. Blockade of the superficial cervical plexus results in anesthesia of only the cutaneous nerves.

Clinical Applications

Surgical procedures lymph node dissections, plastic repairs, and carotid endarterectomy. Bilateral blocks for tracheostomy and thyroidectomy.

Superficial Cervical Plexus Block

Technique

The superficial cervical plexus is blocked at the midpoint of the posterior border of the sternocleidomastoid muscle. A skin wheal is made at this point, and a 22 gauge, 4 cm needle is advanced, it is an injection of 5 ml of solution along the posterior border and medial surface of the sternocleidomastoid muscles. It is possible to block the accessory nerve with this injection.

Deep Cervical Plexus Block

Technique

The deep cervical plexus block is a paravertebral block of the C2 to C4 spinal nerves as they emerge from their foramina in the cervical vertebrae. The traditional approach uses three separate injections at C2, C3 and C4. The patient lies supine with the neck slightly extended and the head turned away from the side to be blocked. A line is drawn connecting the tip of the mastoid process and the Chassaignac tubercle (i.e. transverse process of C6); a second line is drawn 1 cm posterior to this first line. After skin wheals are raised over the transverse processes of C2, C3 and C4, three 22 guage, 5 cm needles are advanced perpendicular to the skin entry site with a slight caudal

angulation. The transverse process is contacted at a depth of 1.5 to 3 cm. 3 to 4 ml of solution is injected. This block can also be performed with a single injection of 10 to 12 ml, at the C4 transverse process. Cephalad spread of the local anesthetic usually anesthetizes the C2 and C3 nerves.

Side Effects and Complications

- Intravascular injection.
- Blockade of the phrenic and superior laryngeal nerve.
- Spread of local anesthetic solution into the epidural and subarachnoid spaces.

Local Anesthesia of the Airway

Clinical applications

- To facilitate diagnostic laryngoscopy
- Bronchoscopy
- Placement of a tracheal tube in patients
- Blocks of the superior laryngeal nerves bilaterally, along with translaryngeal injection of local anesthetic, provide anesthesia of the airway from the infraglottic area to the epiglottis, provides satisfactory analgesia for endoscopic procedures.

Superior Laryngeal Nerve Block

Nerve anesthetized is superior laryngeal nerve. **Areas anesthetized** from inferior aspect of epiglottis to vocal cords.

Technique

The patient is placed supine with the neck extended. The hyoid bone is displaced laterally toward the side to be blocked, and a 25 gauge, 2.5 cm needle is walked off the greater cornu of the hyoid bone inferiorly and is advanced 2 to 3 mm. As the needle passes through the thyrohyoid membrane, a slight loss of resistance is felt, and 3 ml of local anesthetic solution is injected superficial and deep to this structure. The block is then repeated on the opposite side. This technique produces anesthesia from the inferior aspect of the epiglottic to the vocal cords.

Translaryngeal Block

Nerve anesthetized is recurrent laryngeal nerve.
Areas anesthetized: Subglottis and trachea.

Technique

With the patient in the supine position, the cricothyroid membrane is located, and a 20 gauge or smaller, 3 to 5 cm plastic catheter over a needle is introduced in the midline. The inner steel cannula is withdrawn with the plastic catheter held firmly in place; aspiration of air confirms correct catheter placement. Between 3 and 5 ml of 4 percent lidocaine solution is injected rapidly, usually resulting in a vigorous cough, which aids in the spread of the solution within the trachea.

Glossopharyngeal Nerve Block

Nerve anesthetized is glossopharyngeal nerve.
Areas anesthetized: Posterior one-third of the tongue, the pharynx, and the superior surface of the epiglottis.

Technique

It can be blocked intraorally by injecting 5 ml of local anesthetic into the base of each posterior tonsillar pillar. An angled 22 gauge, 9 cm needle, which can be formed by bending the distal 1 cm of a spinal needle with its stylet remove, is employed for this block.

Side Effects and Complications

1. Rapid uptake of local anesthetics
2. Local anesthetic toxicity.
3. Abolish the airway reflexes.

Local Anesthesia for Ear Surgeries

Local anesthesia is useful for brief procedures. The delicate nature of surgery and the use of operating microscope necessitates that the patient stays absolutely still during surgery.

The advantages of LA are that an awake patient will be able to evaluate a hearing change (e.g. following stapedotomy) and a dry operating field can be maintained.

Anesthesia for myringotomy can be obtained by application of 2.5 percent lignocaine and 2.5 prilocaine (EMLA) cream.

For permeatal operations 0.5 ml of 1 percent lignocaine just medial to bony and cartilaginous meatus are injected superiorly, inferiorly, posteriorly and anteriorly at the same depth. Two further injections superiorly and inferiorly 5 mm lateral to the margin of the TM are given.

Auriculotemporal nerve can be blocked by injecting 1–2 ml lignocaine just anterior to meatus.

Greater auricular nerve is anesthetized behind the pinna. A weal is raised in front of the lower anterior border of the mastoid process. A 7 cm needle is inserted and directed upwards and 2 to 3 ml anesthetic solution placed between mastoid process and meatus.

Anesthesia within tympanic cavity can be obtained by placing 4 to 6 drops of 4 percent lignocaine.

All the procedures involving the pinna, external auditory canal, tympanic membrane, and the middle ear can be done.

POINTS TO REMEMBER

1. Amides group of local anesthesia are lidocaine, bupivacaine, mepivacaine and prilocaine (mnemonic has two 'i').
2. Maximum dose of lignocaine required without adrenaline is 200 mg. (3 mg/kg) and with adrenaline is 50 mg (7 mg/kg).
3. Nerve blocks are useful in diagnosis and management of various neurologies, in addition to finding local anesthesia for surgical procedures.

88

General Anesthesia for Major ENT—Head and Neck Surgery

Prerequisites for a Good General Anesthesia

1. Perfect control of airway
2. Good reliable venous access
3. Careful monitoring of vital functions.

Monitoring should include pulse oximetry, ECG display, end tidal carbon dioxide concentration, inspired and expired oxygen and anesthetic vapor concentration, and blood pressure measurement with radial artery canulation. Urinary catheter is needed to measure urinary output.

Air embolism though rare is a potential complication. Condition is detected by observation of the end tidal carbon dioxide concentration which would fall rapidly should this mishap occur. Aspiration of air from central venous catheter, external cardiac massage can be done. Treatment consists of jugular veins. Patient is placed in left lateral head down position and ventilated with 100 percent oxygen.

Major Head and Neck Surgeries

The otolaryngologist and the anesthetist share the common airway of the patient, which could even be obstructed. Careful assessment of airway patency and possible difficulties in intubation during induction is necessary. Care must be taken not to traumatize the neoplastic area with consequent hemorrhage and possible tumor spread. A smaller tube than usual may be indicated. Inhalational agents with muscle relaxants and controlled ventilation are often employed for long surgeries. A few minutes before dividing the trachea the patient is ventilated with 100 percent oxygen and an inhalational agent. After tracheal division the oral tube is removed and a sterile cuffed tracheostomy tube or a special preformed armored laryngectomy tube is inserted by the surgeon. The tube position may change (may go in deep into one bronchus) during the course of a prolonged surgery and the anesthetist should be able to detect the same in time.

In a case of difficult airway for endotracheal intubation like mass in the throat, trismus, short neck, obese patient, etc. a **tracheostomy** may have to be done as a preliminary procedure. With the advances in the airway management techniques, it can be avoided in most cases by an experienced anesthetist. **Fiberoptic bronchoscopy guided endotracheal intubation,** specially designed laryngoscopes coupled with fiberoptic telescope aided endotracheal intubation, **retrograde intubation using guide wires,** etc. are few of the advanced techniques.

Controlled ventilation is used throughout. Deliberate lowering of blood pressure is to be avoided. Blood loss has to be replaced. When the trachea becomes unsupported after mobilization of the esophagus, the fragile posterior wall may rupture at the site of the tracheostomy cuff, making the inflation of the lungs difficult. Manual ventilation of the lungs with 100 percent oxygen until the stomach is drawn into the neck up to tamponade the lead may cope with the situation.

Flexometallic endotracheal tubes allow frequent change in position without the fear of kinking of the airway tube. **Laser surgery** warrants use of specially designed laser tubes which helps in avoiding intraoperative anesthetic burns.

Laryngeal laser surgeries are best done using jet ventilation wherein the anesthetic has is pumped into the airway under high pressure without intubating the patient, provided there is a patent laryngeal and tracheobronchial airway. It is also useful in rigid bronchoscopy.

If a chylous injury and lead is suspected during neck dissection, the site of leak may be better seen by asking the anesthetist to give sustained positive pressure ventilation.

Mediastinal surgeries or lower neck surgeries or transhiatal gastric or colonic mobilization may cause pleural injuries and consequent pneumothorax. The anesthetist should anticipate and act in the time in such cases.

Blood loss in a head and neck surgery may be more and enough blood or plasma expanders should be arranged to replace the loss.

Tracheal Surgery

Airway management may necessitate a multi-stage approach, each step being planned before surgery, with the nature, site and the extent of the obstructed segment and the repair planned.

Small bore non-cuffed orotracheal tube and controlled ventilation is a suitable technique. In very tight stenosis the ordinary tracheal tube is positioned just proximal to the stenosis.

If surgical access is interfered the tube is with drawn in the proximal segment of the trachea and a catheter passed down the orotracheal tube to the distal segment. When the stenosis is very low, two tubes may be passed one down each bronchus. As soon as the anastomosis is completed the catheter withdrawn and ventilation continued through the tracheal tube. Anesthesia during the period of the tracheal anastomosis is usually with intravenous drugs.

Skull Base Surgery

Skull base surgery requires an experienced neuroanesthetist. Intraoperative monitoring of the nerves needs a nerve stimulator or a nerve monitor. Muscle relaxants should be avoided in such cases. Facial nerve stimulator or monitor is routinely used in lateral skull base and parotid surgeries. In some intracranial procedures mannitol may have to be given or may require a CSF drain to reduce intracranial pressure, especially when there is need for dural retraction.

Controlled Hypotension

The efficacy of the ENT surgery especially that of microear and endosopic sinus surgery can be enhanced by achieving a bloodless field. A reduction in the blood pressure with the aim to provide bloodless operative field, and to limit the volume of blood loss, without endangering in any way the life of well-being of the patient is controlled hypotension.

Venous oozing is an important component of bleeding and can be controlled by careful positioning of the patient, securing the airway and ensuring a complete absence of coughing or straining. Infection and resistance of the autonomic system and the hormonal control may resist attempts at lowering blood pressure.

A significant impairment of the lung function, cerebrovascular, cardiovascular, long-standing diabetics, hypertensives, anemia, and pregnancy are contraindication to this technique. Deliberate hypotension in the elderly is avoided if possible.

Techniques

Reducing the cardiac output or the peripheral vascular resistance reduces blood pressure or the combination of both.

1. Positioning the patient head end up decreases arterial and venous pressure at the

operative site and pool blood in the lower parts of the body decreases the venous return to the heart and cardiac output.

2. Inhalational agents reduce blood pressure by depressing the myocardium and vaso-dilatation.

3. Drugs are used to lower blood pressure, e.g. trimethaphan camsylate, sodium nitro-prusside, nitroglycerine, labetalol.

Monitoring during Hypotensive Anesthesia

1. Blood pressure
2. Arterial oxygen saturation
3. ECG
4. Carbon dioxide tension
5. Blood loss
6. Temperature.

Recent Advances
and Related Topics

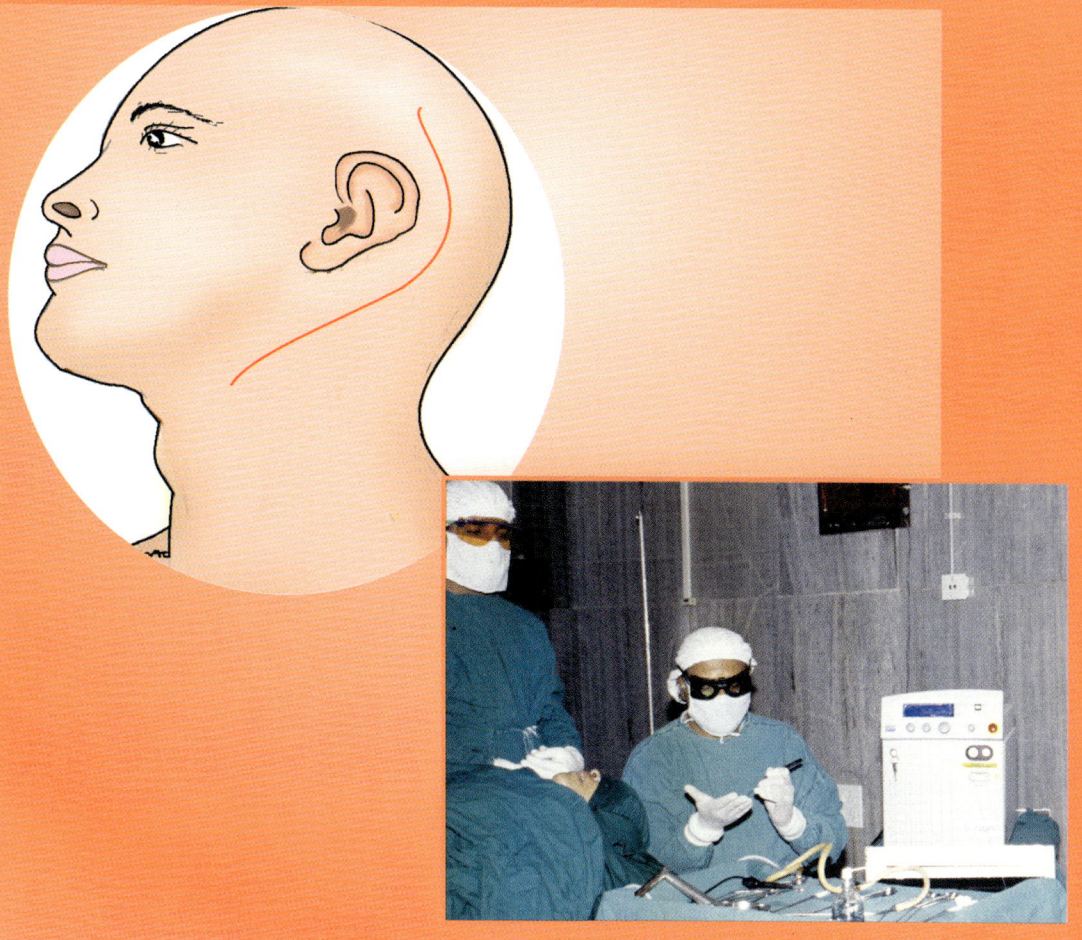

89

Radiological Advances in ENT

- Computerized Axial Tomography imaging (CAT scan)
- Virtual endoscopy
- 3D CT reconstruction
- Magnetic resonance imaging (MRI)
- Digital subtraction angiography (DSA)
- Image guided procedures
- PET scan.

Computerized Axial Tomography Imaging (CAT scan)

This uses special X-ray equipment to obtain image data from different angles around the body and then uses computer processing of the information to show a cross-section of body tissues and organs. This scan gives 2-dimentional images in various planes like axial, coronal and sagittal planes and a 3-D reconstruction may also be done. Use of high resolution CT (HRCT) scans give images as thin slices (1.5mm). A spiral scan can usually be obtained during a single breath hold allowing scanning in 10 seconds or less. Such speed is beneficial in all patients especially in elderly, pediatric or critically ill patients and population in whom the duration of scan can be a problematic. **The multi-detector CT** also allows applications like CT angiography to be more successful. With conventional CT, small lesions may go undetected because lesions may be missed by unequal spacing between scans. The speed of spiral scanning increases the rate of lesion detection.

HRCT with contrast is very useful in proper assessment of various conditions of Otolaryngology-Head and Neck surgery. HRCT of temporal bone in thin slices help in assessment of the middle and the inner ear structures, internal auditory canal, cerebellopontine angle (Fig. 89.6a) and facial canal, etc. 20° high resolution coronal cuts of the temporal bone helps to see even minute structures like the stapes. Tumors of the base of the skull, larynx, laryngopharynx, parapharyngeal and retropharyngeal spaces and pterygopalatine and infratemporal fosse, etc. can be better delineated by HRCT.

Image guided fine needle aspiration cytology and also image guided surgical procedures like image guided endoscopic sinus surgery are being performed today to increase its efficacy and safety.

Virtual Endoscopy

This is done by computerized reconstruction of the spiral HRCT images taken in different planes, by using sophisticated computer software. An experience radiologist is able to perform non-invasive laryngoscopy and tracheobronchoscopy using this technology as there is air-soft tissue interface. Thus the tumors and stenosis in these regions can be well assessed (Fig. 89.1).

3D Reconstruction

It is the recent advance in computer hardware and image processing software which has made it possible to reconstruct 3D images.

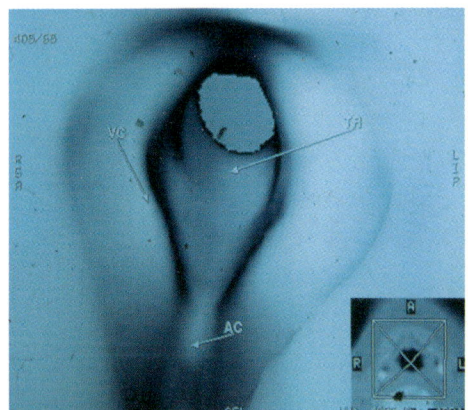

Fig. 89.1: Virtual endoscopic picture showing the normal vocal cords (VC), anterior commissure (AC) and the subglottictracheal lumen (TR)

3D views provide key information about the morphology that was not apparent in conventional images. It helps in detecting abnormal soft tissue and bony morphology and facilitates in surgical planning. It also allows good comparison of the pre and postoperative status (Fig. 89.2 and 89.3).

Applications of 3-D reconstruction in ENT-Head and Neck Surgery:

1. **Head and neck tumors:**
   - In larynx, evaluation of extent of invasion helps in surgical planning for conservation procedures.
   - In mandible, minimal invasion of tumor allows for marginal recession with preservation of rest of the mandible. It gives information about inner cortex and outer cortex as they relate to entire height of mandible (Fig. 89.2).
2. **Temporal bone:**
   - A 3-D reconstruction of temporal bone CT might be useful for education and increasing understanding of the anatomical structures of temporal bone (Fig. 89.3).
3. **Paranasal sinuses and ostiomeatal complex:**
   - 3D images give better anatomical visualization of the paranasal sinuses and

the ostiomeatal complex which helps in better treatment planning and in avoiding complications of endoscopic sinus surgery.

4. **Facial trauma**
   - 3D CT scan shows the direction and extent of the fractures along with their spatial relationships (Fig. 89.2).

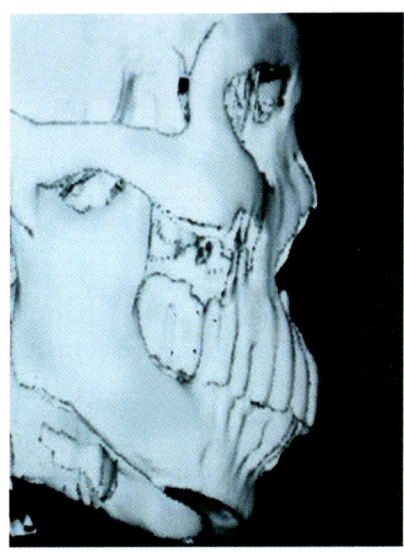

Fig. 89.2: 3D CT reconstruction image showing the maxilla, mandible, zygomatic arch and the temporal and infratemporal fossae

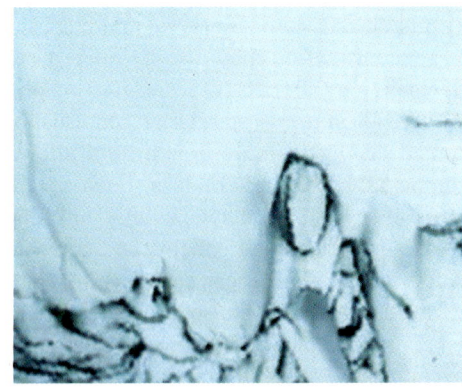

Fig. 89.3: 3D reconstruction of the temporal bone showing the mastoid process and the external auditory canal

Limitations

- Loss reconstruction times (2–7 hours)
- Decreased resolution for the fine detail in comparison with the 2D images (resolution with the 3D images was not as good as that of 2D images.

MRI

MRI is an imaging modality capable of producing cross section images of the human body in any plane without exposing the patient to ionization radiation and the images are obtained by the inter-action of hydrogen nuclei or protons of human body.

The unit of MRI is 'Tesla'. It is a unit of magnetic strength that is related to G (magnetic field strength of earth). The magnetic strength of Tesla is 10,000 G. Clinical MRI units usually operate at magnetic field strength of between 0.3 and 1.5 T.

Two types of images are obtained: T1 and T2.

- T1 weighting is a function of how quickly the stimulated nuclei return to their base state after the stimulating radiofrequency is turned off. T1 image have relatively short imaging and produce clear images.
- T2 relates to the loss of phase coherence of the nuclei after the stimulating sequences are turned off. T2 images take longer time to produce and tend to be less sharp than T1.

Different structures are shown differently in an MRI

- Fat has short T1 and produce very bright image (hyperdense in T1 and hypodense in T2)
- Solid structure such as cortical bone, enamel and fibrous tissue is hypodense show dark images in T1 and T2 scan.
- Muscle shows an intermediate signal in T1 and long signal in T2.
- The cortical bone appear black because of their sparsity of mobile hydrogenations.

Medullary cavity is bright (hyperdense) because of signals from fat content.

- Air in paranasal sinuses because of lack of hydrogen atoms appears dark in all MRI scans.
- For all malignant tumors in head and neck except for melanotic tumor. T1 scans are hypointense (dark) and appear as hyper-intense image in T2 scans. Melanotic tumors appear hyperintense on, T1 and hypointense in T2.

T1 weighted images: T1 weighted imaging is fundamental in head and neck sequences because:

- It provides excellent soft tissue contrast with a superior display of anatomy
- Minimizing motion artifacts
- Fat has high signal intensity and provides natural contrast in head and neck.
- Air, rapid blood flow, bone and fluid filled structures (example: CSF and vitreous) are low signal intensity on T1w
- Most head and neck mass lesions will show a low to intermediate signal intensity on T1.
- The retained mucous or mass lesion is low to intermediate signal intensity on T1.

T2 images

- Most head and neck masses are of higher signal intensity on T2 compared to their low to intermediate signal intensity on T1w1.
- CSF and vitreous shows high signal intensity (bright) in T2. T2 are most useful for highlighting pathologic lesions.
- Bone, rapid vascular flow, calcium, hemosiderin and air containing sinuses are black.
- Inflammatory sinus disease and normal airway mucosa appears bright
- To quickly identify a T2: CSF, vitreous and nasal mucosa are white. Fat is low to intermediate in signal (Fig. 89.4, Table 89.1).

Advantages of MRI

1. Its ability to differentiate soft tissue more easily than they can be differentiated on CT.

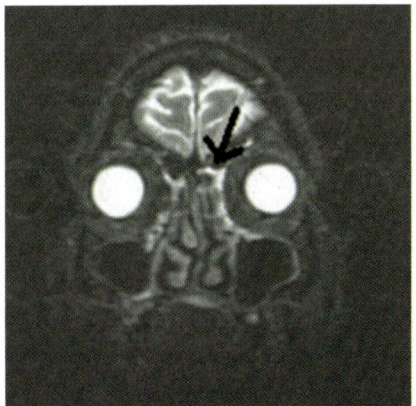

Fig. 89.4: MRI showing the site of CSF rhinorrhea leak in the anterior skull base

2. Axial, coronal, sagittal and even oblique images can be produced.
3. No radiation hazards in MRI
4. MRI can often define the margin of the tumors. As tumor extends intracranially, the relationship of the tumors to the brain can usually be better defined with MRI than CT.

Disadvantages of MRI

1. Scanning time is 45 to 90 minutes. So difficult for sick patient.

2. Motion artifacts are more frequently encountered with MRI than CT.
3. Cortical bone gives no signal in MRI
4. Absolute contraindication to MRI include patient with cochlear implants, cardiac pacemakers and intracranial aneurysm clips.
5. Generally ocular prostheses and ossicular implants are safe.
6. Unfortunately MRI is expensive than CT.
7. Neither cortical bone nor air gives signal. So ossicles and the mastoid septations are invisible on MRI.

Recent Advances in MRI

- To reduce imaging time and motion artifacts, a technique called **fast spinechoimaging** is introduced.
- Fat suppression methods:
  1. The advantage of fat suppression is reduction or elimination of chemical shift artifacts by removing fat signals from the image while preserving water signal.
  2. Some of more common clinically available methods of fat suppression are :
     (a) STIR (short T1 inversion recovery)
     (b) SPIR (shift selective presaturation)
     (c) Chemical shift selective presaturation

Table 89.1: Difference betweenT1 and T2 weighed images	
T1 Weighed images	*T2 Weighed images*
• T1 is a function of how quickly the stimulated nuclei return to their base state after stimulating radiofrequency is turned off.	• T2 relates to the loss of phase coherence of the nuclei after the stimulating sequence is turned off.
• It take shorter time to produce image	• It take longer time to produce image
• Fat has high signal intensity so produces bright image	• Fat is low to intermediate intensity so produces dark images
• CSF and vitrous are low signal intensity (dark)	• CSF and vitrous are high signal intesity (bright)
• Most head and neck masses shows low to intermediate signal intensity	• Most head and neck masses shows high signal intensity
• In PNS bones are black in color	• In PNS bones are black in color

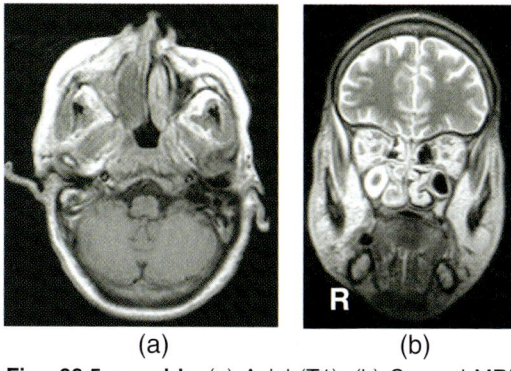

(a)   (b)

Figs 89.5 a and b: (a) Axial (T1), (b) Coronal MRI (T2) scan showing haziness of Rt. maxillary sinus confirming the pathology in fungal sinusitis

Common applications of MRI in ENT-Head and Neck Surgery

- Evaluation of regional and intracranial complications
- In the detection of neoplasm and its extent of infiltration to the various structures
- Improved display of anatomical relationship between the intra and extra-orbital compartment.
- Helpful in the evaluation of fungal sinusitis which shows low signal on T_1 images (Figs 89.5a and b).
- It is also useful in the evaluation of mucocele and encephalocele and CSF rhinorrhea.
- MRI is superior in the evaluation of acoustic neuroma. Even intracanalicular tumors are picked up by MRI (89.6a and b).
- MRI and CT are considered complimentary in the evaluation of the neck masses.

Digital Subtraction Angiography (DSA)

DSA is a powerful technique for the visualization of blood vessels in the human body.

In DSA sequence of X-ray projection images is taken to show the passage of a bolus of injected contrast material through one or more vessel of interest. The adjacent non-contrast structures are subtracted digitally using computer software to delineate the vessels and its branches as well. Thus it remains the **gold standard** for assessment of vascular evaluation.

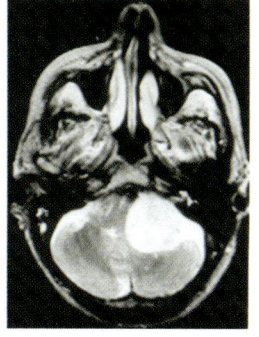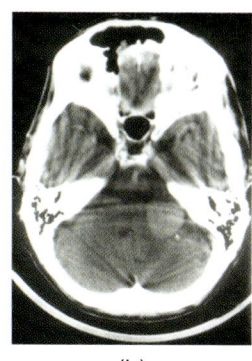

(a)   (b)

Figs 89.6a and b: (a) MRI, (b) CT scan, of same patient showing acoustic neuroma on the right side. MRI (T2) showing clear declination of accoustic neuromal.

In otolaryngology—head and neck, it delineates the vascular mass (tumor blush) and the feeding vessels as in juvenile angiofibroma, glomus tumors, etc. It also gives the information regarding the vascular tumor and its contralateral or intracranial blood supply, if any. Status of collateral circulation of the brain is also assessed and is invaluable in vascular surgery of the neck.

Carotid angiogram is obtained by introducing the cannula into the femoral artery, aorta and then into the carotid or by directly introducing the cannula into the common carotid artery in the neck.

The feeding vessel of the tumor can be selectively embolized 24 to 48 hours before surgery (Figs 89.7a and b) with gel foam/polyvinyl alcohol particles or tantalum powder, to reduce the intra-operative blood loss. This is also useful in case of refractory epistaxsis.

Contraindications of DSA

- Atherosclerotic disease
- Allergic to contrast
- Anomalous anastomosis of ECA and ICA

Complications

- Stroke 0.7 to 2 percent
- Blindness
- Facial palsy.

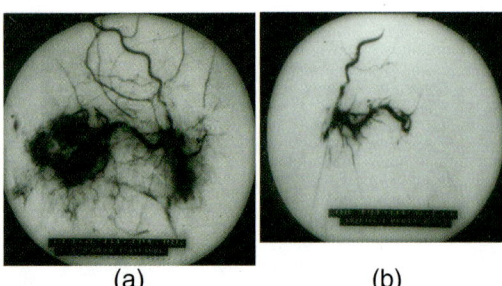

(a)   (b)

Figs 89.7a and b: (a) Figure showing DSA done for juvenile nasopharyngeal angiofibroma receiving blood supply from the internal maxillary artery (a) Pre-embolization, (b) Post-embolization

Position Emission Tomography with CT Scan (PET-CT)

Definition

It is a unique non-invasive method of measuring regional biochemical physiological process in vivo and provides three dimensional image or map of functional processes in the body.

PET gives information about the characteristics of cancer tissue and assess in distinguishing malignant from benign or therapy induced changes. PET with CT scan imaging is superior and it enables doctors to more accurately detect cancer and pinpoint its exact location in the body. **The highly sensitive PET scan picks up the metabolic signal of actively growing cancer cells in the body, and the CT scan provides a detailed picture of the internal anatomy that reveals the size and shape of abnormal cancerous growths.** Alone, each test has its limitations but when the results of the scans are fused together they provide the most complete information on cancer location and metabolism.

The combined PET/CT scan allows the tests to be performed simultaneously which leave less room for error in interpreting test results and it also helps in getting an accurate picture of the location and extent of malignant tumor.

Technique

- Preferably done in the fasting state.
- Injection of tracer.
- Local concentration of tracers is measured to obtain the scan. Areas of high and low tracer concentration are visualized as **hot spots** and **photopenic areas** respectively.

Tracers for PET

Radionuclides used in PET scanning are typically isotopes with short half life. These radionuceotides are incorporated into compounds normally used by the body such as glucose, water or ammonia and is then injected into the body to trace where they become distributed. Such labelled compounds are known as radiotracers

The commonly used tracers are:

- 18F Fluorodeoxyglucose (FDG): This is the most common tracer used in oncology.
- Carbon-11 Methionine (MET)

Factors which decrease the FDG uptake in tumor cells:

1. Hyperglycemia
2. Muscular activity such as speaking and chewing during the FDP uptake period

Most head and neck tumors are squamous cell carcinomas which do not express insulin sensitive glucose transport sites and are thus best studied in fasting state.

Sensitivity in Head and Neck malignancy

- PET-CT was reported to reveal 97 percent of all primary tumors, while 77 percent of them were found on MRI.
- The sensitivity was 88 percent in laryngeal malignancy
- PET-CT images may reveal a sensitivity of 100 percent for primary tumors
- However potentially better depiction of tumor margins with PET and disclosure of additional tumor deposits may be highly valuable for local management

Sensitivity in lymph node metastasis by PET-CT

- PET-CT may be able to detect malignant spread in normal sized lymph node

- PET may be able to differentiate the metastatic lymph nodes from the normal nodes.
- Sensitivity and specificity in detecting LN metastasis was significantly higher for PET-CT than MRI

Drawbacks of PET Scan

1. PET does not seem to be able to distinguish squamous cell carcinoma from other histological types of malignancies of head and neck such as anaplastic carcinoma and Non-Hodgkin's lymphoma.
2. Since PET has no tumor specific substance the uptake in benign lesions with increase glucose metabolism can cause false positive results.
3. There is no reliable way to differentiate between the uptake in malignant and in inflammatory cells in human PET studies.

Response to Radiotherapy

PET is useful in assessing the response to radiotherapy in head and neck cancers. But inflammatory changes such a reactive lymph node and post-radiotherapy edematous laryngeal tissue can take up FDG and MET. Hence it is better to do PET scan 4 months after radiotherapy to find any recurrence.

In detecting recurrence following irradiation of head and neck malignancy, PET-CT is superior to PET or MRI or CT alone. However, if one has to be chosen, it should be PET.

Disadvantages

- Lack of anatomic information resulting in poor lesion localization.
- Poor spatial resolution (Maximum spatial resolution of PET in 5 to 6 mm)
- PET is incapable of showing microscopic disease.

POINTS TO REMEMBER

1. HRCT with contrast is very useful in proper assessment of various conditions in otolaryngology—head and neck surgery.
2. HRCT in thin slice help in assessment of middle ear, inner ear structures, carebellopontine angle lesion and facial canal.
3. 3-D views provide key information about the morphology that was not apparent in conventional images.
4. MRI is an imaging modality capable of producing cross section images of the human body in any plane, without exposing the patient to ionization radiation.

90

Radionucleotide Imaging

Radionucleotide scan is a type of functional imaging and provides information about how an organ or part of the body works. Radioisotopes are administered to the body which then emits gamma radiation. These radioisotopes are incorporated into the part of the body that is to be imaged and during this process information is gained about the structure and function of that particular organ. Common radioisotopes include Gallium 67, Technetium 99, Thallium 201 and radioactive iodine.

Radioactive isotopes, such as I^{123} or Tc^{99} may be taken up by the thyroid, and are used to visualize the functional anatomy of the thyroid. Regions of the thyroid that are functioning and actively incorporating the isotope will be detected with a gamma camera, rectilinear scanner or scintiscan, forming an image of the thyroid that reflects the ability of specific regions of the thyroid to trap the isotope. The images may be processed by a computer to give 2 or 3 dimensional images with color and extra clarity. Regions of the thyroid that are not functioning normally, or are filled with fluid, will not take up the isotope, and will appear as 'cold' or hypo-functioning regions on the thyroid scan. Imaging studies should be avoided in pregnant women or in women who may be uncertain as to whether they are pregnant. When doubt arises, a **pregnancy test** is recommended prior to the scan.

Quantification of the amount of iodine that a thyroid gland can take up may be obtained from an **iodine uptake test**. This test does not give a picture of the thyroid, but involves ascertaining the percentage of radioactive iodine localized to the thyroid after a small amount of the isotope is administered. In most centers, the amount of radioactive iodine taken up is assessed a few hours after it is administered, and again 24 hours later. This test is commonly obtained to differentiate various forms of hyperthyroidism, such as Grave's disease versus thyroiditis.

A form of radionucleotide scanning called SPECT (single photon emission computed tomography) scan has better resolution than standard radionucleotide scanning. Like CT scanning SPECT scanning uses a rotating camera to create 3D cross sectional images or slices of the body.

Mononuclear antibodies are antibodies used to stick to specific types of cancer cells but not normal variants of the same tissue. A radioisotope can be attached to the monoclonal antibody and given into the vein until it circulates around the body to the tumor site where it attaches to proteins on the surface. This causes the tumor to light up when viewed through a special scanner.

Indications

1. Technetium-99 is used for whole body bone scans for bone metastases. It is often used in assessment of thyroid function and metastasis in a case of papillary carcinoma. **Technetium**

Sestamibi scan is helpful in localization of parathyroid glands.

2. Gallium 67 scans help in detecting cancer in the lungs, lymph nodes or bone marrow.
3. Thallium 201 scans are used in the study of heart disease, the effectiveness of treatment for brain or lung tumors as well as for the detection of lymphomas, thyroid and breast cancers.
4. Radioactive iodine can be used to detect and treat thyroid cancers and some neuroendocrine tumors.
5. In malignant otitis externa, repeated gallium scanning helps in ascertaining effect of the treatment and its prognosis.

Technique

Preparation depends on the type of radionucleotide scan planned. Nuclear scans are not recommended for pregnant women or during lactation.

The radioactive material is given by mouth or injection into a vein a few minutes or several hours before the test. For a bone scan the dose is injected two hours before the test. The patient is then asked to drink several glasses of water to flush out any of the radioactive material that is not absorbed by the bones. For Gallium scans the injection is given a few days before imaging.

The differences in the thyroid scan in normal and abnormal conditions are given in Table 90.1.

Table 90.1: Thyroid scan	
Normal:	A normal thyroid scan shows a small butterfly-shaped thyroid gland about 2 in.(5.1 cm) long and 2 in.(5.1 cm) wide with an even distribution of radioactive tracer.
Abnormal:	An abnormal thyroid scan shows a thyroid gland that is smaller or larger than normal. It can also show areas in the thyroid gland where the activity is less than expected (**cold nodules**) or more than expected (**hot nodules**). Cold nodules may be associated with **thyroid cancer.**
	A whole-body scan will show iodine absorption (uptake) in bone or other tissue after the thyroid gland has been removed for cancer.

91

Radiation Therapy (RT) in Head and Neck Cancers

Radiation therapy refers to treatment of cancer with ionizing radiation. Ionizing radiation releases sufficient energy in a localized area to break a chemical bond. It deposits its energy in the core of the cell, i.e. the nucleus and breaks them.

Mechanism

$$H_2O \rightarrow H_2O + e^-$$
$$H_2O \rightarrow H + OH^-$$

H and OH are called as free radicals. These free radicals and oxidizing agent combine with the genes and break them.

Effects of Radiation

The above reactions affect the cell in a number of ways. *It causes:*

- Early death of the cell
- Prevent or delay cell division
- A permanent modification which is passed on to daughter cells

Somatic effects are due to damage to ordinary cells and it affects only irradiated person. Hereditary effects are due to damage to cells in reproductive organs, i.e., the gonads.

Radiation therapy is more effective during G-2 and M (mitotic phase) of the cell cycle since it is more radiosensitive (Fig. 91.1).

Sources of Radiation

The penetration power of the radiation depends on its particular source. The greater the energy of radiations, deeper do they penetrate. *The sources of radiation are:*

- Kilovoltage machines
- Cobalt 60 machines
- Linear accelerator, betatron or microtron
- Radioactive material
1. **Kilovoltage machines:** They produce X-rays of 50 to 400 kV. They were the earliest machines and can be divided into superficial or orthovoltage machines.

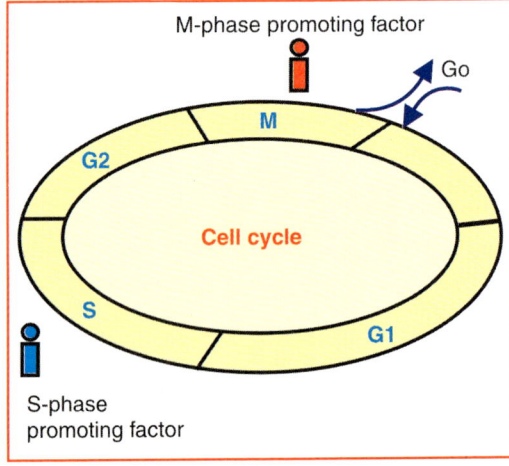

Fig. 91.1: Various phases of cell cycle

2. **Cobalt 60 machines:** It is the commonly used source for head and neck cancer and uses radioactive cobalt, which produces gamma rays of 1.17 and 1.33 MeV. The source has to be changed every 5 years since that is its natural decay time.

3. **Linear accelerator, betatron or micro-tron:** They are the megavoltage machines which work on electricity and produce radiation of 4 to 25 MV. They can produce both photon or electron beams.

4. **Radioactive material:** Earlier radium was used in the form of needles. It is replaced by safer *radionucleotides* like Cesium 137 [pellets], Iridium 192 [wire], Gold 198 and Iodine 125 [seeds or grains].

Unit of Radiation

Earlier rad [radiation absorbed dose] was used and is replaced by international unit of Gray. (1 Gy = 100 rads or 100 cGy).

Types of Radiation

- Orthovoltage
- Supervoltage [photon beams]
- Electron beams
- Neutrons
- Protons
- Hyperbaric oxygen
- hyperfractionation
- Hyperthermia
- Brachytherapy

Orthovoltage

This is the basic form of RT and is rarely used now-a-days. It produces X-rays with energy below one MeV.

Electron beams

This is the second most common form of radiation. The electron beam is characterized by a rapid dose buildup and sharp dose fall of with very little scatter. It is produced by linear accelerator.

Uses

- It is used to boost up the radiation dose to the target area avoiding radiation to vital structures. Example: Spinal cord.
- It can be given to areas of bone and cartilage without a risk of osteoradionecrosis and cartilage necrosis
- Useful for primary skin tumors round the cartilage of nose or the pinna. Also useful for anteriorly placed tumors of frontal sinus or ethmoid sinus, widespread superficial tumor of scalp.

Super Voltage

- More frequently used in head and neck cancer
- Photon beams are considered as super-voltage radiations
- Both X-rays and gamma rays fall into photon beams category
- X-rays are produced when high energy electrons bombard a metallic target
- Gamma rays are produced by Cobalt 60.

Advantages

- Skin sparing
- Greater penetration
- Relatively homogenous dose distribution

Disadvantages

- Size of isotope source is small
- There is lack of sharp edge to the beam
- It is not helpful in treatment of high radiation sensitivity areas like spinal cord and lens

Linear accelerators between 4MeV and 10MeV are appropriate energies for treatment of tumors in head and neck region.

Neutrons

- These are very heavy uncharged particles and produce a beam of high energy transfer with a low O_2 enhancement ratio. Its use is under investigation

Hyperbaric Oxygen

Conventional irradiation has been used with hyperbaric oxygen to be effective against the anoxic cells. Advanced cancer is frequently associated with central necrotic core with anoxic cells.

Hyperfraction

- The basis of hyperfractionation is to gain in tumor response relative to tissue damage. It enhances the therapeutic response of the tumor sparing the late reacting tissues.
- Traditionally patients are irradiated on weekly basis with 200 cGy per day.
- This treatment will enable the normal cells to repair after the radiation.
- It may enhance the therapeutic index if the malignant cells repair less between the fractions.
- Tumor is considered as an acutely responding tissue; by manipulating the time/dose relationship of radiation a gain in tumor response relative to tissue damage could be achieved.
- In hyperfractionation the irradiation by the traditional dose is broken into smaller fractions over the same time.
- The same dose if given over a shorter period is called as accelerated fractionation.

Advantages

- Prevents repopulation of the tumors
- Short hospital stay
- Course is completed in 12 days with 36 fractions rather than over the standard 6 to 7 weeks.

Hyperthermia

- It is used on the basis that the tumor cells respond well to high temperature.
- Anoxic cells seem to be preferentially more sensitive to raised temperature.
- It is being used with low dose interstitial brachytherapy.

Brachytherapy

- It is near beam radiotherapy and entails either endocavitary or interstitial therapy.
- It gives a very high dose to target tissue.

Radioactive substance like iridium, cesium and cobalt are used. Iridium wires and gold grains are also used to implant in the tumor bed.

Treatment with implant is selected

- For accessible tumors
- Well demarcated tumors
- Limited risk of regional LN metastases

Advantages

- Interstitial therapy is used in the management of small tumors of the anterior two third of the tongue.
- Cesium needles are used after assessing the tumor by biopsy and staging.
- It should be well planned, so that the radiation to the tissues is homogenous
- Needles are placed according to the plan under general anesthesia.
- The dose is approximately 70 cGy which takes 5 to 7 days.
- The patient is nursed in a protected room with lead screens for the protection of the nursing staff.

Disadvantages

- Poor penetration
- Used only to treat very superficial tumors.

Application of Radiotherapy

Curative Radiotherapy

Small lesions can be cured by radiotherapy alone. The advantage is that the function of the organ is preserved.

Example: Early lesions of the glottis and nasopharynx. Dose is 6500 to 7500 cGY

Palliative Radiotherapy

- When cancer is too advanced and total disease control is not anticipated.

- Presence of distant metastases
- Condition of the patient is too poor to undergo surgery
- Poor nutrition
- Systemic disorders like heart, lung, kidney diseases
- To control pain, bleeding and obstruction to air and food channels.

Palliative dose is based on the extent of the cancer and the tolerance of the normal tissues in the treated area.

If RT alone is selected, it may be delivered with the external beam irradiation or interstitial implant or combination of both.

Combined Therapy

RT can be combined with surgery and chemotherapy. RT can be given before and after the surgery. RT failures usually result from an inability to irradiate bulky masses. Surgical failures usually result from inability to eradicate microscopic extension. The two modalities of treatment are complimentary to each other.

Surgery is used to remove gross masses that are too large to eradicate by radiation, and RT is used to eradicate microscopic extensions of tumor that cannot be excised.

Preoperative Radiotherapy

Advantages

- Reduces the bulk making the inoperable to easily resectable
- Oxygenation of the tumor is not hampered and the response of the RT is better
- Lymphatics are blocked by RT and dissemination of the tumor cells is less during the surgery
- Eliminates occult metastases in regional laryngeal nodes
- Treatment portals are usually smaller than would be required for postoperative radiotherpy.

Disadvantages

- Reduces the vitality of the tissues hence delays healing process

- Incidence of flap necrosis, fistula formation and carotid blowouts in posoperative period is more.
- Dose is comparatively less than the post operative dose because of delayed wound healing.
- Dose of 45 cGy is given in 4 to 5 weeks. Adequate to eradicate subclinical disease in appox. 90 percent of the individuals.

Postoperative Radiotherapy

Advantages

- More effective, as bulk of the tumor has been removed by surgery.
- The anatomical extent of the tumor can be determined by the surgery, making it easier to define RT portals.
- The surgical planes are intact and it is technically better to resect.
- Greater dose can be given than preoperative RT.
- Morbidity of treatmet is less.
- Markedly reduces the risk of the recurrence in the surgical field
- Incidence of osteo/chondroradionecrosis is much reduced.

Disadvantages

- Surgery hampers the blood supply to tissues causing hypoxia which is not a good indicator of RT
- Microscopic spread of tumor cells by the surgical procedure
- Results are poor if the postoperative RT is delayed beyond 6 weeks.

Postoperative RT is recommended in stage III, IV tumors and when margins are positive, bone or cartilage is invaded, LN shows extracapsular invasion and neck nodes are multiple and the size of the node is > 3 cm.

Radioprotectors and Radiosensitizers

Radioprotectors: These are the compounds which protect the normal tissue from the radiation and increase the effectiveness of radiation on the tumor cells. It should be a stable compound without life threatening or permanent toxicity. They have the scavenging action and protect the cell membrane lipids by scavenging the radiation produced peroxy radicals.

Examples: Vitamin E, vitamin C, B-carotene, N-butanol.

Radiosensitization: It is a process that enhances tumor cell kill for a given radiation dose.

Radiosensitizers: These are the drugs which modify the cellular events that take place during radiochemical process.

Examples: Metronidazole, misonidazole, nitromidazole and incorporation of pyramidine analogs into DNA in rapidly dividing tumors.

IMRT (Intensity Modulated Radiation Therapy)

IMRT is a newer method of delivering radiation to target structures that differs from traditional methods of radiation delivery. The basis of IMRT is the use of intensity-modulated beams that can provide two or more intensity levels for any single-beam direction and any single-source position. This means that the intensity of the radiation beam in a given treatment fields is varied via multiple multi-leaf blocking arrangements called segments. Intensity modulation combined with multiple fields (radiation beam angles) or arcs allows for conformal radiotherapy (i.e. high radiation isodose lines conform to the target volume and spare normal tissues). IMRT treatment plans are able to generate concave dose distributions and dose gradients with narrower margins than those allowed using traditional methods. This fact makes IMRT especially suitable for treating complex treatment volumes and avoiding close proximity organs at risk (OAR) that may be dose limiting.

The high dose volume that tailors to the 3D configuration of the tumor along with the ability to spare the nearby normal tissues allows the option of tumor dose escalation. The head and neck region is an ideal target for this new technology. The results do confirm that IMRT does decrease xerostomia compared with conventional radiotherapy (Lee, et al. 2007).

Care of the Patient during Radiotherapy

- **Nutrition:** Diet rich in proteins and vitamins should be given and if necessary nasogastric tube can be used.
- **Care of the oral cavity and teeth:** Dental prophylaxis is done to prevent/ reduce mucositis, xerostomia and osteoradio-necrosis of the mandible. Application of milk of magnesia to the area of mucositis has a dual role as it gives protective coating and neutralizes the pH and prevents caries, xylocaine gel may be used to reduce pain.
- **Care of the skin:** To prevent or reduce the skin reactions of RT. Avoid wetting or shaving the area and exposure to sunlight. Topical antibiotic cream can be used for moist desquamation and topical steroid creams to relieve itching and pain
- **Care against infection:** Topical application of nystatin and clotrimazole

Complications of RT for Head and Neck Cancer

A. *Acute Effects*
- Mucositis of the oral cavity, pharynx and larynx
- Conjunctivitis
- Xerostomia
- Sialadenitis
- Radiation dermatitis.

B. *Late Effects*
- Non-healing ulcers following trauma, etc.
- Chronic sialadenitis
- Dental caries
- Temporomandibular joint dysfunction and trismus
- Osteoradionecrosis and chondronecrosis
- Radiation dermatitis
- Xerophthalmia
- Middle ear effusion and/or sensorineural hearing loss
- Radiation myelitis
- Reduced pulmonary function and cough reflex
- Chronic sinusitis and fungal sinusitis
- *Radiation induced neoplasia:* Papillary carcinoma of thyroid.

92

Chemotherapy in Head and Neck Cancers

Definition

It is defined as the use of chemical compounds in treatment of neoplastic diseases so as to destroy offending cancer cells without damaging the host.

Surgery and radiotherapy form the standard treatment for most of the head and neck cancers and role of chemotherapy is mainly as combination therapy or for palliation.

Chemotherapeutic Trials

Efficacy of a particular drug or drug combination is assessed by conducting clinical trials which is done in three phases.

Phase 1: To determine toxic effects of a new drug and to establish its highest dose that can be safely administered.

Phase 2: To see if the drug has enough activity so that it can be used in a comparative trial.

Phase 3: To compare two or more chemotherapeutic agents.

Parameters are evaluated:

- Response to the treatment which could be complete or partial or no response
- *Survival of the patient:* Duration of survival with or without disease
- Toxicity of the drug.

Cell Cycle

Almost all chemotherapeutic agents act by disrupting some aspect of cell growth cycle (Fig. 92.1).

Cell divides by progressing through a sequence of steps called cell cycle and its various phases are:

G1: Preparation for DNA synthesis (presynthesis)

S: Synthesis of DNA occurs

G2: Preparation for mitosis

M: Division of parent cell into 2 daughter cells occurs (mitosis)

At times the cell may go into resting phase or G0 phase.

Time gap between DNA synthesis and cell division is Gap number two-G2. In this phase, proteins essential for mitosis are synthesized.

Almost all chemotherapeutic agents act on one or more phases of the cell cycle, and may be classified as Phase specific and Phase non-specific.

Phase Specific Agents

These are effective only during a specific phase. *For example:*

- Methotrexate, cytosine arabinoside, 5-fluorouracil, 6-Mercaptopurine, hydroxyurea, etc. act on S-phase
- Bleomycin acts on G2 phase
- Vincristine and vinblastine act on M phase
- L-Asparaginase acts on G1 phase

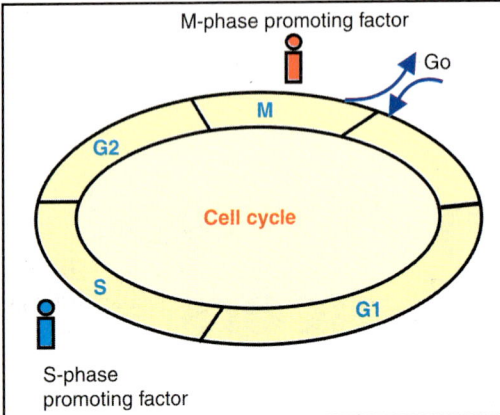

Fig. 92.1: Showing various phases of the cell cycle

Phase Non-specific Agents

These do not act on a specific phase and are independent of cell cycle phases. For example: Cisplatinum, cyclophosphamide, dacarbazine, steroid hormones, nitrogen mustard, etc.

Classification of Chemotherapeutic Drugs

1. Alkylating Agents

(a) *Nitrogen mustards*
- Cyclophosphamide
- Mechlorethamine
- Melphalan
- Uracil mustard
- Chlorambucil

(b) *Alkyl sulfonates*
- Busulfan
- Ethylenimines
- Triethylene thiophosphoramide (Thio-TEPA)
- Triethylenemelamine.

2. Antimetabolites

(a) *Folic acid antagonists*
- Methotrexate

(b) *Purine antagonists*
- 6-Mercaptopurine
- Azathioprine

(c) *Pyrimidine antagonists*
- 5-Fluorouracil
- Cytosine arabinoside
- Fluorodeoxyuridine

3. Cytotoxic Antibiotics
- Actinomycin-D
- Mitomycin-C
- Adriamycin
- Bleomycin
- Rubidomycin
- Mithramycin

4. Antimitotic Plant Products
- Vincristine
- Vinblastine
- Taxol

5. Radioactive Isotopes
- Radioiodine
- Radiogold
- Radiophosphorous

6. Hormones and Hormone Antagonists
- Androgens
- Estrogens
- Progestins
- Corticosteroids
- Tamoxifen
- Flutamide
- GnRH analogs

7. Miscellaneous
- Procarbazine
- L-asparaginase
- Streptozotocin
- Cis-platinum

8. Biological Response Modifiers
- Interferon and levamisole

Chemotherapy for Head and Neck Cancers

Majority of the malignancies encountered in the head and neck region are squamous cell carcinoma. Next most common histological type is the salivary gland tumors. Among lymphomas, Non-Hodgkin's lymphoma is seen in head and neck mostly in the Waldeyer's ring. Hodgkin's lymphoma is rare. Although melanomas and sarcomas are also seen, they are very rare.

In this chapter chemotherapy for only squamous cell carcinoma in the head and neck is dealt with, though it has a major role in the management of the non-Hodgkin's lymphoma also.

Various types of chemotherapeutic modalities are available in the treatment of squamous cell carcinomas. *These are*

1. Single agent therapy
2. Combination chemotherapy
3. Combined modality therapy

1. Single Agent Chemotherapy

One-third of the patients respond to single agents, out of which less than 5 percent have complete response and majority are partial responders.

Duration of response is 2 to 4 months and median survival time is approximately 6 months. Hence single agent chemotherapy is not adopted often. Following are the single agents that may be used in the treatment of squamous cell carcinomas of head and neck.

- Methotrexate
- Cis-platinum
- Carboplatin
- Cyclophosphamide
- Bleomycin
- 5-Flurouracil
- Adriamycin
- Vinca alkaloids.

2. Combination Chemotherapy

Combination chemotherapy was introduced with the aim to improve the response rate and the survival time.

But after many trials, it is found that although combination therapy improves the response rate, there is not much improvement in the survival time as compared to the single agents like methotrexate and cisplatin. Also toxicity is more with combination therapy.

Cisplatin and 5-fluorouracil combination is the most common drug regimen used for palliation as well as combined modality therapy in head and neck cancers. Cisplatin based regimens are the most effective combinations for the treatment of nasopharyngeal carcinomas.

3. Combined Modality Therapy

Although surgery and radiotherapy form the mainstay of the treatment of cancers of head and neck, majority of the advanced cases present with recurrences. Prevention and treatment of recurrences only with chemotherapy is not satisfactory. Hence 3 approaches of combined modality therapy are undertaken.

(a) Induction or Neoadjuvant chemotherapy
(b) Concomitant chemoradiation
(c) Adjuvant chemotherapy

(a) *Induction chemotherapy:* Chemotherapy is given before surgery or radiation. After surgery and/or radiotherapy blood supply of the tumor gets compromised, so more efficient drug delivery will occur if it is given as initial therapy.

At this time the patients are in best possible medical condition and as a result there is increased patient compliance, decreased tumor burden and decreased metastatic potential.

Response to induction chemotherapy predicts the response to radiation. It does not increase the surgical/radiotherapy complications rates and allows organ preservation and improved quality of life. Neoadjuvant chemotherapy followed by radiotherapy was found to be successful in the preservation of voice without decrease in the survival time according to VA larynx study.

Overall response rate is 60 to 90 percent and complete response rate 20 to 50 percent.

(b) *Concomitant Chemoradiation:* Radiotherapy and chemotherapy are used simultaneously in patients with unresectable disease to improve loco-regional control. Combination of two is said to result in additive/synergistic effect. Single agents or multiple agents are used along with radiation.

Major drawback is severe toxicity when multi-drugs are used. Therefore, split-course radiation is preferred that is alternate chemotherapy and radiotherapy are given to increase the tumor cell kill and decrease the tissue toxicity.

'Concomitant Chemoradiotherapy Boost' is a new approach to chemoradiotherapy in which after the standard radiotherapy to the primary tumor and the neck, radiation fields are narrowed to cover only the sites of gross disease. The reduced radiation fields are referred to as 'Boost fields' as the gross disease is treated at a higher radiation dose. Addition of concomitant chemotherapy gives additive effect to radiotherapy and allows better tumor control during accelerated repopulation. Lastly, as the chemotherapy is given in the last 2 weeks of radiation, it does not produce major toxicity that would interrupt radiotherapy.

(c) Adjuvant chemotherapy: It is the course of chemotherapy given after surgery or radiotherapy to decrease the metastatic burden of the disease. Although complete regression may occur during chemotherapy, the goal of this secondary treatment is palliation and rarely has long-term benefits. Its advantages over induction chemotherapy are:

- Surgery is not delayed.
- Induction chemotherapy can blur the tumor margins which can hamper in getting the clearance during resection.
- Induction treatment, if successful will reduce the symptoms and may lead to refusal of surgery by the patient.
- After surgical debulking there will be decrease in the population of drug resistant malignant cells.

Adjuvant chemotherapy decreases the rate of distant metastasis and is effective in treatment of micrometastasis but its role is reserved for high risk patients only.

(d) Intra-arterial Chemotherapy: Impaired drug delivery into the region invaded by cancer cells, leads to poor response to chemothe- rapy. This can be overcome by intra-arterial chemotherapy. Commonly used drugs are cisplatin, methotrexate, bleomycin or 5-fluorouracil.

Though it enhances the tumor drug exposure and decreases the systemic exposure of the drug, the major drawbacks are

- Catheter related complications
- Air/plaque emboli
- Sepsis
- Immobility of the patients.

Intra-arterial chemotherapy is tried in advanced paranasal sinus and salivary tumors. For paranasal sinus tumors cannulation of superficial temporal artery and infusion of 5-fluorouracil only or cisplatin+ bleomycin followed by intravenous 5-fluorouracil followed by surgery and radio- therapy has been tried and claimed to be effective.

Major Contributions of Chemotherapy in Head and Neck

- Chemotherapy is efficacious for the treatment of recurrent head and neck squamous cancers when given in combination with other modalities. Chemotherapy alone does not have a significant role.
- Chemoradiotherapy is the treatment of choice for nasopharyngeal carcinoma.
- Chemotherapy has a major role in the treatment of intermediate grade Non Hodgkin's Lymphomas.
- Organ preservation is a new challenge in the field of head and neck cancer and induction chemotherapy has shown positive results in case of carcinoma of the larynx.
- Role of chemotherapy in soft tissue sarcomas is only for recurrences except rhabdo-myosarcoma.
- Thyroid cancer is ablated with radioiodine if the primary tumor is inoperable or when there is residual/recurrent postoperative thyroid cancer or metastatic nodes.

Some Common Chemotherapeutic Agents

1. Methotrexate

This is a folic acid analog and it acts on S-phase of cell cycle. It inhibits dihydro-folate-reductase

(DHFR) and thus decreases synthesis of tetrahydrofolic acid. This gives rise to decrease synthesis of thymine and purine thereby decreasing DNA synthesis.

Alternate source of tetrahydrofolate is provided by leucovorin. Leucovorin gets converted into tetrahydrofolate coenzyme and thus increases purine synthesis. Leucovorin rescues cells from methotrexate toxicity, but cancer cells cannot be rescued from the lethal effects of methotrexate as they lack the transport sites for leucovorin.

Dose

- Mild: 40 to 60 mg/m^2 weekly
- Moderate: 250 to 500 mg/m^2 weekly
- High: 5 to 10 gm/m^2 weekly

Mode of Administration is IV/IM/SC/Oral

Moderate and high doses of methotrexate are followed by leucovorin rescue starting at 24 hours and continued till plasma methotrexate level is less than 10 to 8 mol/L

Toxicity

- Mild stomatitis and myelosuppression
- Confluent mucositis
- Pancytopenia
- Abnormal LFT
- Exfoliative maculopapular rash
- Renal dysfunction, i.e. due to precipitation of methotrexate in acidic urine in high doses.

Advantages

Used as standard drug to which other drugs are compared and is relatively non-toxic and inexpensive. Average response rate is 30 percent.

2. Cis-Platinum

This is an inorganic metal compound, a bifunctional alkylating agent which binds to DNA and causes inter and intra-strand cross linking.

Dose and Mode of Administration
It is given intravenously with a dose of 80 to 120 mg/m^2 every 3 to 4 weeks with mannitol diuresis, or is given as 24 hour continuous infusion.

Toxicity

- *Renal dysfunction:* It increases serum creatinine levels therefore increased hydration and diuresis is required.
- Ototoxicity occurs in the frequency of 4000 to 8000Hz and is dose related and cumulative
- Nausea and vomiting
- Hematological
  - Neutropenia
  - Thrombocytopenia
  - Anemia
  - Acute hemolytic anemia
- Hypomagnesemia
- Peripheral neuropathy is sensory more than motor

Advantages

- Rapid response
- Given only once in 3 to 4 weeks
- Response rate 30 percent
- Duration of response 4 months

Disadvantages

- High toxicity and requires hospitalization

3. Carboplatin

This is a derivative of cisplatin and has same mechanism of action as that of cisplatin.

Dose and Mode of administration: 400 mg/m^2 can be safely given in patients with creatinine clearance of 60 mg/ml.

Toxicity

- Myelosuppression
- Rarely neuro/oto/renal toxicity.

Due to its mild toxic effects it can be given on OPD basis, but it is not as effective as Cis-platinum. Its response rate is 24 percent.

4. Taxanes

- Paclitaxel (Taxol)
- Docetaxel (Taxotere).

These drugs act on G2 phase. They bind to beta subunit of tubulin and inhibits microtubule depolymerization causing cell cycle arrest.

Dose

- Paclitaxel: 135 to 250 mg/m^2 over 3 to 24 hours every 3 weeks
- Docetaxel: 60 to 100 mg/m^2 bolus every 3 weeks.

Toxicity

Neutropenia and infection. Growth factors GM-CSF, G-CSF shorten the neutropenic duration, therefore decrease the risk of infection. Its response rate is 30 to 40 percent.

5. Cyclophosphamide

This acts by cross-linking of DNA strands

Dose: 50 to 1500 mg/m^2 3 to 4 weekly IV

Toxicity

- Bone marrow suppression
- Nausea and vomiting
- Alopecia and ridging of nails
- Azospermia and cessation of menses
- Acute hemorrhagic cystitis
- Bladder cancer– rare.

6. Bleomycin

This is an antineoplastic antibiotic. It binds to DNA and generates O$_2$ free radicals which cause DNA strands to breakup.

Dose: 10 to 20 units/m^2 once or twice a week IM/IV, or 10 units/m^2/24 hours, continuous infusion over 5 to 7 days.

If creatinine clearance is 15 to 30 ml/min. dose is reduced by 50 percent, if creatinine clearance is less than 15 ml/min, dose is reduced by 75 percent.

Toxicity

- *Fever with chills* is seen in half of the patients within 24 hours.
- Anaphylactic reaction is rare.
- Alopecia
- Erythema, thickening and hyperpigmentation of skin
- Stomatitis.
- *Pulmonary toxicity*: Pneumonitis, dry cough and rales are more common in elderly, or if dose more than 200 units or in case of previous lung irradiation. If dose not reduced, pulmonary fibrosis and restrictive lung disease may occur.

7. 5-Fluorouracil

It competes with enzyme thymidylate synthetase by displacing uracil and thus inhibits the formation of thymidine causing decrease in DNA synthesis.

Dose

- 10 to 15 mg/kg/week IV OR
- 400 to 500 mg/m^2 daily for 5 days IV as a loading dose, followed by 400 to 500 mg/m^2 weekly IV. OR
- 1 gm/m^2/day as continuous infusion for 5 days and repeated 3 to 4 weekly.

Better response rate observed with continuous infusion.

Toxicity

- Myelosuppression
- Nausea, vomiting, diarrhea
- Alopecia, hyperpigmentation, maculo- papular rash.

Advantages

- Frequently used with Cisplatin in combination. Response rate is 15 percent.

8. Adriamycin

This is an anthracycline derivative. It intercalates between nucleotide pairs in DNA and thereby interferes with nucleic acid synthesis.

Dose

- 60 to 90 mg/m^2 IV every 3 weeks OR
- 20 to 30 mg/m^2 daily for 3 days, repeated every 3 weeks.

Toxicity

- Red urine for 1 to 2 days
- Severe necrosis of skin and subcutaneous tissue if given SC.
- Alopecia, nausea, vomiting, diarrhea

- Radiation recall in patients with H/O previous radiotherapy.
- Myelosuppression
- Cardiac toxicity– cardiomyopathy leading to CCF in 10 percent patients if cumulative dose is more than 550 mg/m^2.

9. Vinca Alkaloids (Vincristine and Vinblastine)

They disrupt microtubular spindle formation and thereby cause mitotic arrest.

Dose

- Vincristine (oncovin) 1 to 1.5 mg/m^2 once or twice a month IV.
- Vinblastine (velban) 5 mg/m^2 weekly IV.

Toxicity

1. **Vincristine**
   - Neurotoxicity—it causes sensory, motor and peripheral neuropathy.
   - Hoarseness and it increases if the drug is not stopped.
   - Constipation
   - Alopecia

2. **Vinblastine**
   - Myelosuppression
   - Myalgia
   - Alopecia.

Targeted chemotherapy: Improved understanding of the molecular biology of cancer cells has fundamentally changed the search for new therapies for malignant disease. The genetic changes resulted from are mediated by two effects:

A. Enhancement of the activity of the genes that stimulate cell growth, survival and spread
B. Reduction of action of the genes that repress these processes.

There are two classes of genes which mediate these effects:

1. *Oncogenes:* They are derived from mutated normal cellular genes (protooncogenes) that encodes protein which controls the cell proliferation survival and spread.
2. Tumor suppressor genes and normal cellular genes which inhibit cell proliferation and survival. They control cell cycle progression and apoptosis. Mutation of these genes can give rise to familial cancer syndrome.

The therapies are mainly targeted against the following properties of cancer cells (Hanahan, et al, 2000)

a. Growth factor independence
b. Ability to recruit a dedicated blood supply
c. Avoidance of apoptosis
d. insensitivity to antigrowth signals
e. Reactivation of telomerase
f. Ability to invade adjacent normal tissues and metastasize to distant sites.

The first major success in this approach was the development of anti-EGFR monoclonal antibody cetuximab.

Cetuximab: It is a human-murine chimeric monoclonal antibody against EGFR (epidermal growth factor receptor). EGFR (c-ErbB-1) is one of the 4 c-ErbB receptor of the transmembrane type I receptor tyrosine kinase family.

Head and neck cancer cells very frequently (> 90%) usurp normal EGFR-mediated signaling pathways, mainly by 3 mechanisms:

1. They manufacture and release growth factors which stimulate own or neighbouring receptors (autocrine/paracrine signaling respectively).
2. After the receptor number/structure/function making them more likely to send a growth signal.
3. Deregulate the signaling pathways so that they are permanently turned on (constitutively active).

Overexpression of the receptor without gene amplification appears to be the dominant process in squamous cell cancer or head and neck. Cetuximab targets these receptors and has shown antiproliferative effect, direct cytotoxicity anti-angiogenic actions and potentiation of cytotoxic effects of chemo- and radiotherapy.

In advanced head and neck cancer cetuximab with radical radiotherapy has improved overall survival.

Cetuximab (400 mg/m^2 initially, 250 mg/m^2 per week), cisplatin (100 mg/m^2) plus 5-FU (1 gm/m^2/day for 4 days) was given as palliative therapy in a phase III study and has proven to prolong median overall survival when compared to the group receiving only chemotherapy without cetuximab.

The disadvantages are statis in resistant phase of cell cycle, promote tumor hypoxia, enhance normal tissue toxicity and off-target systemic toxicity.

Similar EGFR antibodies which have entered clinical trials are zalutumumab and panitumumab.

Other Drugs

Gefitinib—low molecular weight tyrosine kinase inhibitor (TKI), specific for EGFR. Prevents receptor autophosphorylation on the intracellular domain (150–800 mg/m^2).

Lapatinib: Oral dual TKI acts against both EGFR (c-ErbB-1, HER-1) and c-ErbB-2 (HER-2/neu). 1500 mg/day with chemoradiation in locally advanced SCC of Head and Neck.

Bevacizumab—humanized MAB to VEGFR ligand (vascular endothelial growth factor). Acts as an antiangiogenic agent.

Seliciclib-cyclin—dependent kinase inhibitor and enhances apoptosis.

These agents are likely to be apart of combination regimens in the future.

93

Tumor Biology of Head and Neck Cancers

A malignant neoplasm has several phenotypic attributes such as excessive growth, local invasiveness and the ability to form distant metastasis. These characteristics are acquired in a stepwise fashion called tumor progression. There are hundreds of cancer associated genes that have been discovered in the past two decades. Each of the cancer genes has specific function. Its de-regulation help the cancer gene to contribute in the origin and progression of malignancy.

Hallmarks of Cancer

1. Tumor has a capacity to proliferate with internal stimuli usually as a consequence of oncogene activation.
2. Tumors may not respond to molecules that are inhibitory to the proliferation of normal cells such as transforming growth factor.
3. Tumors may be resistant to programmed cell death (apoptosis) as a consequence of inactivation of p53 or other changes.
4. Tumor may fail to repair DNA damage caused by carcinogens or unregulated cellular proliferation.
5. Tumor cells have unrestricted proliferatve capacity associated with maintenance of telomers length and function (immor-talization).
6. Tumors are not able to grow without formation of vascular supply, which is induced by various growth factors, the most important being vascular endothelial growth factor (sustained angiogenesis). Angio-genesis helps the tumor (cancer) to sustain growth at the cost of normal tissue.
7. Tumor metastasis is the cause of vast majority of cancer deaths and depends on process that is intrinsic to the cell or is initiated by signals from the tissue environment (Flow chart 93.1).

Multiple mutations are involved in the progression of cancer from normal mucosa to invasive carcinoma as shown in Flow chart 93.2.

Knowledge of tumor biology helps in understanding the genesis and the progress of cancer. This knowledge is vital for developing newer therapeutic strategies that can help in preventing the cancer at the molecular and genetic level. Certain chemotherapeutic agents have been under trial to arrest the progression by targeting sustained angiogenesis of the tumor, more research is needed in future to eradicate the cancer.

Field Cancerisation

Slaughter, first described the concept of 'Field carcinogenesis' or 'condemned mucosa' in 1953. He hypothesized that because of constant carcinogenesis pressure, the entire upper aerodigestive tract is at the increased risk of developing multiple primary tumors. However recently, an alternative hypothesis has been postulated that multiple lesions may form due to

Flow chart 93.1: Showing invasion growth and metastasis of malignant tumor

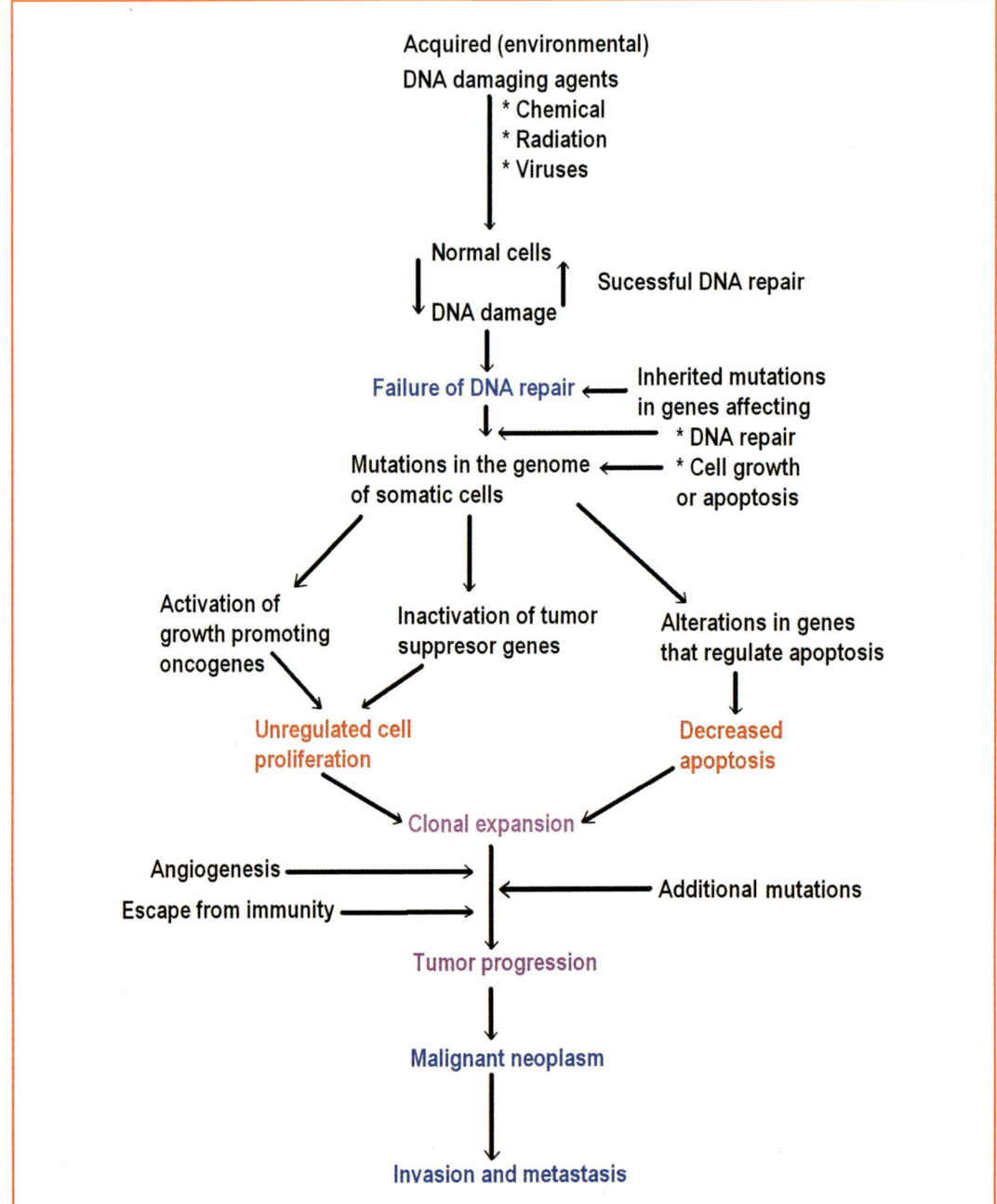

Flow chart 93.2: Cancer progression

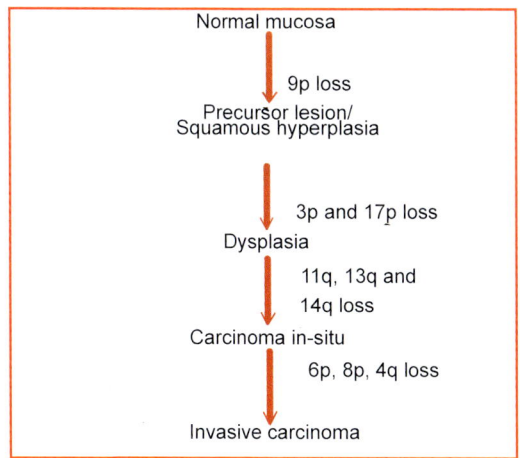

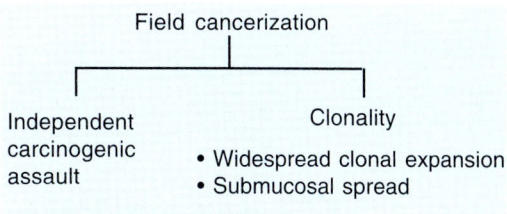

process of intraepithelial migration. Evidence exists for both the hypothesis.

The conclusion drawn from various studies indicate that the mucosa of the head and neck had undergone a change, perhaps due to carcinogen exposure, and was therefore more susceptible to the development of multiple foci of malignant transformation.

Gene Therapy

Rapidly expanding field of gene therapy is found on the ability to introduce genetic material into the body in order to treat disease or alter an ongoing pathologic process.

Various techniques have been developed for targeting cancer cells namely:

- Gene therapy, monoclonal antibodies
- Antibody toxin conjugates
- Small molecule inhibitors
- Antisense molecules
- Tumor vaccines.

The goal of gene therapy is to introduce new genetic material into cancer cells that selectively kills them without causing toxicity to the surrounding cells. This task can be accomplished by:

- Replacing tumor suppressor genes that have been lost or mutated
- Selectively inserting genes that produce cytotoxic substances
- Modifying the immune system to destroy the tumor cells

Corrective gene therapy attempts to block oncogenes or replace tumour suppressor genes. The archetypal tumour suppressor gene in HNSCC and most other forms of cancer is p53. Alteration to p53 results in continued propagation of the damaged cell line. Replacement of p53 results in reduced HNSCC growth and increased radiochemo-sensitivity.

The virus that is commonly used for gene therapy through a unique viral enzyme-thymidine kinase is Herpes simplex virus. Most gene therapy agents are administered intra-tumorally.

The major barrier in successful gene therapy is producing a vector that selectively infects all tumor cells.

POINTS TO REMEMBER

1. Tumor progression refers to phenotypic attributes of a malignant neoplasm such as excessive growth, local invasiveness and ability to form distant metastasis.
2. The goal of gene therapy is to introduce new genetic material into cancer cells that selectively kills them without causing toxicity to the surrounding cells.

94

Biomaterials in ENT

Definition

Biomaterials are synthetic or treated materials employed to replace or augment tissues and organs. An implant is a device that is placed into a surgically or naturally formed cavity of the human body if it is intended to remain there for thirty days or more.

Properties of an Ideal Biomaterial

1. It should not be physically modified by soft tissue.
2. Should not be capable of inciting an inflammatory or foreign body reaction.
3. Should not be capable of producing a state of allergy or hypersensitivity.
4. Should be chemically inert
5. Should be non-carcinogenic
6. Should be capable of resisting strain.
7. Should be capable of fabrication in the form desired.
8. Should be capable of sterilization

Biomaterials used in Otorhinolaryngology

Classification (Table 94.1)

1. Metallic
2. Non-metallic
   - Polymers
   - Ceramics

Metals

Stainless steel, cobalt-chromium alloy and titanium are the three classes of metal alloys currently used to construct surgical implants. They share the qualities of strength, biocompatibility and corrosion resistance. Stainless steel is an alloy containing carbon and 11 to 30 percent chromium which confers high degree of corrosion resistance. Titanium is used as "commercially pure" (CP) or as Ti-6A1-4V alloy with 6 percent aluminium and 4 percent vanadium, these factors increasing the strength by 4 times. Cobalt-Chromium alloy contains cobalt as the majority and chromium 27–30 percent which provides excellent corrosion resistance. Other implants are made up of platinum, tantalum and gold.

Physical Characteristics

There are certain definitions which are helpful in describing the physical characteristics.

1. *Yield strength:* Amount of load per unit area required to permanently deform the implant.
2. *Elastic modulus:* Load per unit area required to produce a certain change in shape.
3. *Tensile strength:* Load per unit area required to fracture a sample of the material.
4. *Ductility:* Ability of the material to withstand plastic deformations.

Stainless steel has got moderate yield and tensile, high ductility and good resistance to

Table 94.1: Classification of biomaterials		
Metallic	*Non-metallic: Polymers*	*Non-metallic: Ceramics*
Stainless steel Titanium Platinum Tantalum Gold Silver Cobalt Chromium Vitalium	1. Solids • Polyethylene • Polytetrafluoroethylene (Teflon) • Polydimethylxylothene (silastic) • Polydimethylsiloxane (silicon) 2. Porous • Polytetraflouroethylene carbon fiber composite – Proplast 1 (Fig. 94.2 a) • Polytetrafluoroethylene aluminium oxide composite – Proplast 2. • High density polyethylene plastipore. • Ultrahigh molecular weight polyethylene – Polymer	1. Bioinert • Aluminium oxide ceramics – Frialit® 2. Bioactive • Calcium silicate glass (cerevital, bioglass, Macor ceramics) 3. Biodegradable and biorestorable • Hydroxyapatite • Tricalcium phosphate ceramics

corrosion. Its manufacturing is easy and inexpensive.

Cobalt chromium alloy has much more corrosion resistance and exhibits excellent strength, but is very expensive and mining is extremely difficult.

Titanium has the highest corrosion resistance, high biocompatibility and low imaging density which enables it to be placed in the field of radiation and imaging without risk. It also possesses the property of osseointegration, that is, when implanted in bone, the bone will grow in intimate proximity to the implant, leading to a permanent solid implantation.

Fabrication of titanium is very difficult and expensive. Platinum and gold are highly malleable, but very expensive.

Uses

1. Stainless steel
   • Bone plates, wires and pins in maxillo-facial surgeries.
   • Pistons
   – Classic stapes prosthesis
   – Mc Gee type
   – House type wire loop
   – Fisch type, etc.
   • Middle ear ventilation tubes
2. Titanium
   • Bone plates in maxillofacial surgeries
   • Pistons and ossicular replacement prosthesis
3. Platinum
   • Pistons e.g.: Richards platinum fluoro-plastic pistons.
4. Tantalum
   • Keels in anterior glottic webs
5. Gold (Fig 94.1)
   • Eyelid weights, tympanoplasty (Fig. 94.2b).

Disadvantages

1. Hypersensitivity reactions.
2. Considerable risk of infection and great deal of wound reaction.
3. High extrusion rates.

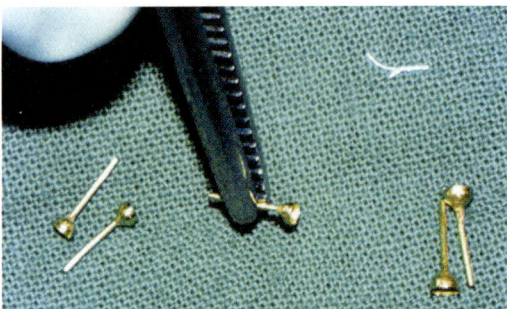

Fig. 94.1: Showing indigenous gold prosthesis

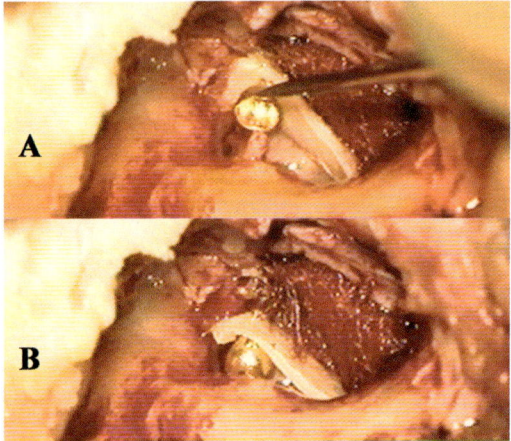

Fig. 94.2: Intraoperative photograph showing usage of gold prosthesis mounted on a piece of cartilage

Effect of Imaging and Radiation Therapy

While imaging, the implant should be identified and should not induce distortion that would lead to difficulties in identification of surrounding structures. The presence of the implant should not prevent a patient from undergoing any particular study. They produce greater attenuation with X-ray beam and produce artifacts with X-rays, CT and MRI scans. Titanium is preferred in such cases as it does not posses any magnetic properties.

Effect of Radiation Therapy

The reflected radiation is high and thus increases the radiation dose when metal implants are present in the field of radiation. Attenuation behind the metal implant is also high. It is best to use titanium in such cases to decrease the effect maximally. Also, the radiation portals can be planned tangentially to the implants, thus further decreasing its profile in relation to the beam.

Polymers

Solids (Polyethylene, Teflon, Silastic)
They are used alone or in combination with metals, especially in middle ear surgery.

   Polyethylene is no longer used, due to its high reaction time, also as a stapes prosthesis, it interrupts blood supply to incus by exerting pressure on it, leading to the necrosis of incus. It also penetrates the vein graft and slips into the inner ear in stapes surgery, leading to vertigo and sensorineural hearing loss.

Teflon

Uses

1. It is the most common material used in stapes surgery. It is well tolerated in the middle ear as it is not reactive with tissue. The disadvantage is that as there is no tissue in growth, it slips out of place if it is too short (Fig 94.3).
2. It is used in rhinoplasty as injection to the nasal dorsum or as solid dorsal implant, but no follow up results are found in the literature.
3. In atrophic rhinitis, submucosal injection of powdered Teflon in 50 percent glycerine paste

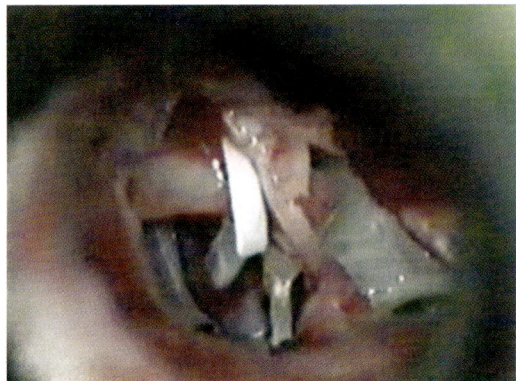

Fig. 94.3: Teflon piston in stapedotomy operation

into the lateral wall of the nasal cavity is used. Also Teflon strips are inserted into the floor and septum after raising the mucoperichondrial flaps in Wilsons operation.

4. In vocal cord paralysis Teflon paste is used which have equal weight of Teflon and glycerine per each millimeter. The goal is to mobilize the paralyzed vocal cord to the midline to maintain the adequate glottic closure.

Advantages

1. Low tissue reactivity
2. Lack of carcinogenicity

Disadvantages

1. Malpositioning
2. Teflon cannot maintain the normal vibratory characteristics of the vocal cord.
3. Granuloma formation
4. Over injection into the subglottis can lead to airway obstruction.

Silastic/Silicone

Silastic is the polymer of silicone and is used as an alternative for silicon in ENT Surgeries.

Types of Silicones

They can be watery or oily liquids or can be rubbery materials. The rubbery or elastomeric silicones are available in the form of sponge, blocks of varying hardness, adhesives and gels. Silicon adhesives are known as silastics (Fig. 94.4).

Uses

1. Chin and cheek augmentation
2. Augmentation rhinoplasty
3. Middle ear ventilation tubes
4. As a silastic sheets in middle ear surgery between the promontory and the TM to prevent adhesions and to allow regeneration of normal mucosa over denuded areas, also

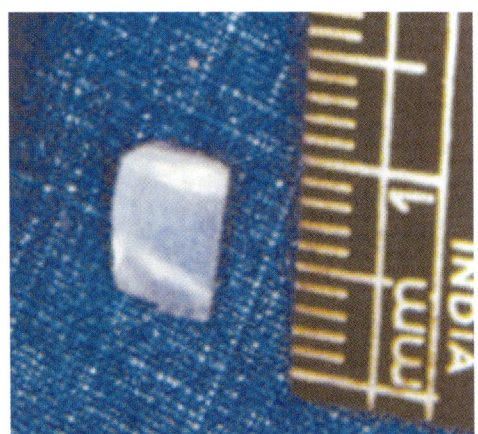

Fig. 94.4: Fashioning of silastic sheet

in an attempt to prevent fixation following ossiculoplasty.

5. As an obturator in nasal septal perforations
6. As insulatory material for electrodes in cochlear implant devices.
7. As tubes or rods in laryngeal or tracheal stenosis and phonosmogus.
8. As silastic endolymphatic shunt tubes in Menieres disease.
9. Silicon balloons in tissue expansion by injecting sterile saline into the balloon over a period of few weeks. By this method, skin suitable for advancement or rotation to fill the traumatic or surgical defects is produced.
10. Silicon is used in the manufacturing of ear, nose and ocular prosthesis. Silicon is used because it is easy to tint and duplicates the texture of skin very well.
11. Used in the manufacture of cuffed tracheostomy tubes, and voice prosthesis (Fig. 94.5).

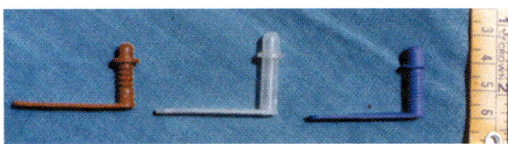

Fig. 94.5: Voice prosthesis made of silicon for TEP

Advantages

1. Heat stable
2. Time stable
3. Versatility
4. No adherence
5. Minimal tissue reaction
6. Not altered by the body.

Disadvantages

1. Tissue reaction and scar formation is seen around the silicon implant.
2. Unless reinforced, silicon is not a suitable agent to replace major stress bearing areas, nor is it suitable where there is a need for hard tissue.
3. Silastic sheet though it is inert in the middle ear, curls up after sometime, and high extrusion rate is seen, also there is associated foreign body reaction.
4. Silicon is potentially carcinogenic.
5. Silicon is said to have a role in the etiology of scleroderma, but it is controversial.
6. Silastic is vapor permeable, so while using as an electrode incochlear implants, ceramic or titanium sealed cases should be used.

Porous (Proplast, Plastipore, Polycel)

Proplast is a resilient black sponge manufactured from polytetrafluoroethylene (Teflon) and vitreous carbon. The pore size ranges from 100 micrometer to 500 micrometer and the pores occupy 75 percent of the volume and are readily infiltrated by fibrous tissue. It is malleable and can be trimmed with a knife.

Plastipore is a high molecular weight white spongy material with pores ranging from 20 to 30 micrometer in diameter, with pores forming 35 percent of its volume.

Another form of high density polyethylene sponge made of porous ultra high molecular weight polyethylene is ***polycel.***

Proplast can be readily shaped and prosthesis created to suit specific clinical circumstances.

Plastipore has gained wide use because of its ready commercial availability and its application in middle ear surgery. Polycel prosthesis with malleable stainless steel cores are available as implants.

Uses

1. TORP and PORP (Fig 94.6)
2. Reconstruction of posterior bony wall
3. Obliteration of mastoid cavity
4. Augmentation rhinoplasty
5. Maxillofacial surgery

Advantages

1. They allow tissue ingrowth, leading to stabilization of the prosthesis.
2. Readily commercially available.
3. Highly biocompatible
4. Decreased incidence of cholesteatoma
5. No degradation is seen
6. Can be readily shaped and prosthesis can be created
7. Good hearing results have been reported after middle ear surgery

Disadvantages

Extrusion is seen when in contact with mobile tympanic membrane and can be prevented by placement of cartilage between the prosthesis and the TM.

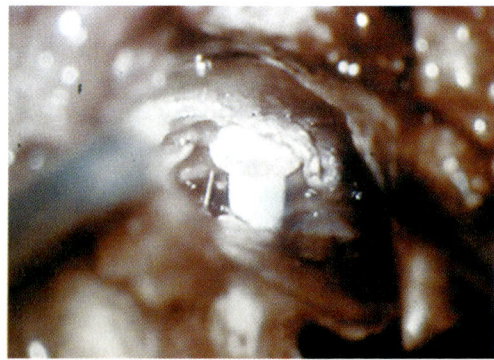

Fig. 94.6: Intraoperative photograph showing usage of plasticpore sheet's prosthesis

Ceramics

The most recent material for implantation is the ceramic material. *They are of three types:*

1. **Bioinert:** Non-degradable ceramics
   - Aluminium oxide (Frialit).
2. **Bioactive:** Calcium silicate glass ceramics (Ceravital, bioglass used in ossiculoplasty.)
3. **Biodegradable and bioresorbable**
   - Hydroxyapatite
   - Tricalcium phosphate ceramics
   - B-whitlockite.

Uses

- TORP and PORP
- Posterior canal wall and outer attic wall reconstruction
- Mastoid cavity obliteration
- Maxillofacial surgery

Hybrid prosthesis using hydroxyapatite with plastipore and silastic have been tried as middle ear prosthesis to reduce the disadvantages and to increase the advantages of both.

Advantages

1. Very stable since they are based on metal with high oxidation potential.
2. When used in ossiculoplasty, they have additional advantages over other ossicular prosthesis not leading to bony fixation in the attic or oval window.
3. Glass ceramics develop direct bond between themselves and lining tissues.
4. Hydroxyapatite demonstrates good ingrowth of tissue without giant cell formation or encapsulation.
5. Calcium phosphates are very compatible with the body, especially bony tissues.
6. No special storage is required.
7. No interposition graft is required.

Disadvantages

- Aluminium oxide as it is bioinert will have less integration and stability than the other implants.

- Aluminium oxide and glass ceramics are hard and so difficult to shape.
- Biodegradable and bioactive ceramics disappear faster than new bone formation.
- Not useful for large bony defect repair.

Injectable Collagen

This material in the form of highly purified bovine collagen has been used to correct skin irregularities such as scars and wrinkles. It is easy to use and has very few side effects. It is structurally similar to the natural collagen.

Uses

- Skin irregularities like scars and wrinklers
- Vocal cord augmentation to improve glottic insufficiency.

Disadvantages

Delayed hypersensitivity has been reported in few patients. Long-term results are not available yet.

Acrylic Resins

They are resilient plastics formed by joining multiple methyl methacrylate molecules.

Uses

- Maxillofacial prosthesis
- Stents in tracheal and laryngotracheal stenosis
- In nasal surgeries (septoplasty) to prevent synechiae formation and it also acts like a stent.

Advantages

- It may be used to provide any shade and degree of translucency. Latex is a tripolymer of acrylate, soft and inexpensive and has good blending.
- Its color and properties remain stable under normal intraoral conditions.
- Processing is easy

Disadvantages

- Special storage techniques with specific temperature and time required.
- Volumetric shrinkage (i.e. monomer - polymer). The greater the shrinkage, greater the discrepancy.
- Infection is a common problem
- Allergic reactions.

Tissue Glues

Ancient Egyptians and Indian tribes used glues made of honey and barley gruel to glue tissues together. Various types of tissue glues are present. The first to be synthesized was cyanoacrylate in 1949. The others are:

- Mecrylate - COAPT-1
- Bucrylate - COAPT
- Eubucrylate - Histo Acryl
- Tissuecol - Fibrin glue
- Tissued - Fibrin glue

Ideal Tissue Glue

It should

- Have shelf stability
- Polymerize in the presence of moisture
- Provide adequate working time
- Spread easily and be wettable
- Produce minimal heat on application
- Form a strong and flexible bond
- Be biodegradable and easy to apply
- Be non-carcinogenic.

Cyanoacrylate and Variants

Advantages

1. Has bactericidal and bacteriostatic properties.
2. Is less biodegradable and so may be seen at the site of implantation for many years.

Disadvantages

1. They have alkyl groups on their side chains, and larger the alkyl chain, less the toxic effect. Histotoxicity occurs by heat inactivation of cellular enzyme systems during polymerization. It can also occur as a result of direct toxic effect of dehydration products like formaldehyde and alkyl cyanoacetate.
2. Fungi and spores may continue to survive under a layer of adhesive, so adequate sterilization has to be ensured.
3. Cyanoacrylates are found to be neurotoxic, so it should not be used at the anastomotic site of nerve grafting.
4. Produce inflammatory reactions including foreign body reactions and osteitis in the middle ear.

Uses

- Tympanoplasty, skin closure
- Fixation of cartilage grafts as in otoplasty and rhinoplasty
- As a spray to provide protective and adhesive dressings in patients undergoing procedures in the oral cavity.
- In CSF leaks
- To repair injuries to the apical pleura

Fibrin Glue

This is made by the combination of concentrated human fibrinogen and Factor XIII with the thrombin calcium chloride solution.

Advantages

- Low cost and no inflammatory reaction
- No storage problems
- High glueing potency
- Non-toxic to the middle ear

Disadvantages

- Potential risk of transmission of viral infection like HIV, Hepatitis BB infection. Patients own blood can be used to prevent this.
- As a result of biodegradability, there is some risk of late ossicular displacement.

Uses

1. Tympanoplasty

2. Mastoid obliteration
3. Posterior canal wall reconstruction
4. To stabilize muscle and fascial grafts following translabyrinthine removal of acoustic neuroma.
5. In skin grafts, and are particularly useful in tangential abrasions of face where skin flaps are lifted by trauma, thus avoiding shrinkage of skin flaps and development of hypertrophic scars.
6. To control bleeding in the tonsillar bed after tonsillectomy.
7. As an adjunct in pharyngeal closure after laryngectomy and in esophageal closure.
8. Fixation of skin and implants in otoplasty and rhinoplasty.
9. In suturing facial nerve graft.

Robotic Surgery in ENT—Head and Neck Surgery

Recent advancements in robotics technology have allowed more complex surgical procedures to be performed using minimally invasive approaches. It has several advantages over standard surgical approaches, including more rapid recovery, lower rate of postoperative infection, decreased pain, better postoperative immune function, and cosmetic results. The first robotic surgical system developed was the Puma 560, which was used in 1985 to perform neurosurgical biopsies with increased precision. The da Vinci Surgical Robot (Intuitive Surgical Inc., Sunnyvale, CA, USA), has been approved by FDA and actively marketed system, for Transoral Robotic Surgery—TORS and includes a surgeons console, a surgical cart and a vision cart. It was first developed by Weinstein and O' Malley, who have assessed the feasibility of this technique using the da Vinci Robotic System. This technology uses a powered device that functions under programmable computerized control and may be used to manipulate instruments and perform surgical tasks.

O'Mallery Jr. et al., (2006). initiated the TORS studied in canine and cadaveric models and applied the technique to clinical practice. head and neck and several airway procedures have been associated with a large surgical incisions and extensive surgical dissection along with a large surgical incisions and extensive surgical dissection along with associated mortality and morbidity. However, with minimally invasive approaches.

However, with minimally invasive approaches, the improved video imaging, endoscopic technology, and instrumentation has provided the surgeon with multiple endoscopic access points while increasing surgeon capabilities.

Advantages

1. Enhanced visualization (three-dimensional visualization and tenfold magnification)
2. Elimination of Physiologic Tremors and Scale Motion
3. Multiarticulated instruments have 7 degrees of freedom, which improves dexterity, allowing maneuverability that approaches that of open surgery.
4. Fatigue reduction
5. Restore Proper Hand-Eye Coordination—this system eliminates the "fulcrum effect" of endoscopic surgery.
6. Telesurgery is possible
7. Training—provides some interesting tools and opportunities for teaching.

Disadvantages

1. Absence of Tactile and Haptic Sensation
2. Equipment Size and Weight
3. Cost of the Device
4. New technology with unproven benefit.

95

HIV Manifestations in Otorhinolaryngology

Acquired immunodeficiency syndrome (AIDS) first came to medical attention in the early 1980s. Earlier cases were found by retrospective analysis to have occurred in 1978 in the USA and in the late 1970s in equatorial Africa. The first case of AIDS was registered in India in the year 1986. In the 1990s, AIDS has become an epidemic.

The causative agent of AIDS is the human immunodeficiency virus type I (HIV I) a T-lympho cyte virus. It is a retrovirus containing reverse transcriptase that transcribes viral RNA into DNA. It attacks the CD4 receptors found on T-helper cells, macrophages, central nervous system (CNS) cells of monocytic origins, and other antigen-presenting cells. As a result, a T-cell immunodeficiency occurs and the host becomes susceptible to many opportunistic infections and secondary cancers. Normal CD4 lymphocyte count is 600 to 1500 cell/mm^3. Its count less than 500 cell/mm^3 indicates poor immune system. Strictly speaking, the term AIDS refers only to the last stage of the HIV infection. AIDS can be called our modern pandemic, affecting both industrialized and developing countries.

Its magnitude has increased over 100-fold since AIDS was first discovered. India has over 5.2 million people currently HIV-infected (2005) with only South Africa ahead in terms of those living with the disease and 72,000 new cases were reported in the year 2005. In 1986, India discovered its first case of HIV/AIDS. Globally, 39.4 million people are infected (2005). It is estimated that by the end of the century, 8 to 10 million people are likely to be infected with HIV in the South-East Asia region.

However, India remains a low prevalence country with overall HIV prevalence of 0.91 percent, i.e. less than 1 percent population. There are focal epidemics in the country (NACO) as found in Tamil Nadu and other states.

Modes of Transmission

1. *Sexual contact*—Homosexual or hetero-sexual
2. Through sharp instruments like needles, syringe, knife, etc.
3. Blood and its products
4. Mother to infant during birth and through breast milk.

Opportunistic Infections in AIDS

- Pneumocystis carinii pneumonia
- Tuberculosis
- *Candida albicans*
- *Cryptococcus neoformans*
- Mycobacterium species (avium and kansasii)
- *Toxoplasma gondii*
- Cytomegalovirus
- Herpes zoster
- Histoplasmosis
- Herpes simplex

- Coccidioidomycosis
- Papovavirus
- *Streptococcus pneumonia*
- *H. influenzae*

Secondary Cancers in AIDS

1. Kaposi's sarcoma
2. B-cell lymphoma.

Manifestations of AIDS in Otorhinolaryngology

Different studies have indicated that more than 40 percent of patients with HIV present initially with otolaryngological manifestations. These can be classified into:

- Opportunistic infections
- Secondary cancers and
- Direct effects of HIV infections.

EXTERNAL EAR

Otitis Externa

In immunocompromised patients like AIDS malignant otitis externa is seen with predominant causative organism being Pseudomonas. Cases have been reported in adult AIDS patients caused by *Aspergillus fumigatus*. Aggressive antibiotic therapy is necessary.

Aspergillosis is treated by IV amphotericin B followed by oral itraconazole.

Kaposi's Sarcoma of the Ear

It is the most common manifestation of AIDS. It is 300 times more common in patients with AIDS. Kaposi's sarcoma of the auricle is seen exclusively in AIDS patients. It can involve external auditory canal, tympanic membrane and middle ear resulting in conductive hearing loss. Clinically appears as red purple plaques or nodules.

Localized cutaneous lesions requires surgical extirpation, intralesional vinblastine, bleomycin, radiation therapy or interferon-Alpha.

Systemic Treatment for Kaposy's Sarcoma

Bleomycin, vincristine and liposomal doxorubicin for extensive disease or when other treatment fails. Zidovudine should be included in the treatment to reduce the extent of immunosuppression and thereby improve prognosis.

MIDDLE EAR

Serous Otitis Media

It is seen in adult and pediatric AIDS population. It occurs in up to 80 percent of cases. This is presumably due to poor eustachian tube function secondary to recurrent viral infections, adenoidal hypertrophy from HIV, nasopharyngeal tumors or viral induced allergy.

A careful nasopharyngeal examination should be done to rule out nasopharyngeal tumors. These patients usually present with nasal obstruction associated with thick mucoidal discharge and hearing loss. SOM is usually seen in these patients.

Treatment

Adenoidectomy, to rule out B-cell lymphoma and KS. An early myringotomy and grommet insertion is recommended.

Acute Otitis Media

It is seen in both adult and pediatric AIDS patients. Recurrent otitis media and chronic sinusitis are seen in pediatric age-group. The common causative agents are by *Str. pneumoniae, H. influenzae* and *Moraxella catarrhalis*.

Treatment

Ampicillin or amoxicillin. Failure may be due to beta-lactamase organisms for which clavulinic acid may be needed.

Tympanocentesis may be required if patients do not respond to antibiotics, and also in toxic patients before initiation of therapy. Myringotomy and drainage or myringotomy with grommet insertion is necessary to treat recurrent OM.

Mastoiditis

This has been reported by several authors and is caused by *Str. pneumoniae*, Aspergillus (rare), and *Mycobacterium tuberculosis* (rare).

Chronic Otitis Media

This often caused by *Pn.carinii*. It may be seen in asymptomatic HIV patients or patients with severe AIDS. Patients complain of otalgia, otorrhea and hearing loss. An aural polyp is seen frequently in external auditory canal or middle ear. Audiogram demonstrates conductive or mixed hearing loss.

The biopsy of the polyp demonstrates a typical *Pn.carinii* cyst when stained with *Grocott-Gomori* methanamine silver nitrate. Spread through (a) Eustachian tube from asymptomatically colonized nasopharynx, (b) hematogenous, (c) EAC.

Treatment

Trimethoprim-sulfamethoxazole up to three weeks.

INNER EAR

SN Hearing Loss

Its frequency in AIDS ranges from 21 to 49 percent. The commonest pathological changes are caused by HIV agent itself. The exact site of involvement is uncertain and may be cochlear or central lesion or both. CMV is the commonest secondary virus and toxoplasmosis is a frequent cause of abscess formation. Neurosyphilis, TB, meningitis, HIV drug-regime side effects or radiotherapy are known to causes SN hearing loss.

Cryptococcal Meningitis

It has a subacute onset and hearing loss due to this is seen in 30 percent of patients. It causes infiltration of the cochlear and vestibular nerves and scarpa's ganglion with cryptococcal organisms and macrophages resulting in early necrosis of the nerve.

Diagnosis is by demonstration of organism in CSF by India ink preparation, positive cultures for cryptococcus or detection of cryptococcus antigens which are positive in more than 90 percent of case. It should be obtained in all AIDS patients with c/o new onset headache.

Treatment

Amphotericin B and 5-flourocystosine.

Syphilis

It is a severe disease in HIV patients. It causes acceleration of the HIV infection through activation and destruction of helper T-cells. Otosyphilis and neurosyphilis may follow the primary infection at an accelerated rate. It may also re-activate latent syphilis. Otosyphilis may present in any stage of HIV infection. Manifestations are shortened from typical 15–30 years to 2–5 years. Diagnosis is by clinical history, uni or bilateral SN low frequency hearing loss. VDRL is an indirect test. The most specific test is fluorescent treponemal antibody absorption test which remains positive for life.

Treatment

24 million units of penicillin (IV) for three weeks.

Neurosyphilis

12 to 24 million units penicillin (IV) for 10 days followed by benzathine penicillin G 2.4 million units IM per week for three weeks. Steroid therapy is C/I as patient is immunocompromised.

Other Causes of Hearing Loss

- Progressive multifocal leukoencephalopathy (PML)—Papavovirus systemic lymphoma with CNS involvement—Predilection for meninges.
- Primary CNS involvement - encephalopathy followed by cranial neuropathy.
- Kaposi sarcoma metastatic to central nervous system
- Incidental acoustic neuromas
- Direct infection of CNS by HIV

AIDS encephalopathy or subacute encephalitis is the most common neurologic manifestation of AIDS.

Evaluation of Hearing Loss

PTA, speech audiometry, impedance, acoustic reflex, ABR to evaluate retrocochlear pathology, serologic test for syphilis, CSF for glucose, protein, VDRL cytology, cryptococcal antigen detection.

CT or MRI should be done to evaluate CNS for possible infection or malignancy.

Conductive Hearing Loss

Less common, causes are KS, granulomas and otitis media.

Vertigo

Commonly seen in AIDS encephalopathy or AIDS dementia complex. HIV is directly responsible for clinical and histologic changes seen in CNS (Brainstem and hypothalamus).

May be a side effect of pharmaceutical agents, i.e. acyclovir, amphotericin B, flucytosine, pentamidine, aminoglycosides, AZT, pyrimethamine and trimethoprimsulfamethaxozole.

KS metastatic to the CNS is likely to cause vertigo and balance disturbances.

Facial Nerve

30 percent of AIDS patients present with neurologic complications. It may result from direct HIV infection of CNS, opportunistic infections, primary or secondary CNS tumors or autoimmunity.

It may result from direct infection of the facial nerve or ganglion by the HIV. HIV has been isolated from CSF and neural tissue at all stages of HIV infection.

Usually, there is a complete or near complete recovery from idiopathic peripheral facial nerve palsy associated with HIV infection.

Most frequent CNS pathology associated is toxoplasmosis.

Bell's palsy (idiopathic) is the most common diagnosis for VII nerve palsy associated with HIV infection.

Primary infection or reactivation of herpes infection in the immunocompromised patient may explain the relative increased incidence of Bell's palsy in AIDS.

Herpes zoster infection is 7 times more common in HIV positive patients.

Clinical Features

Pain, herpetic vesicles of EAC and concha along with sensory distribution of VII nerve and peripheral facial palsy.

Treatment

High dose acyclovir and steroids is controversial.

NASAL MANIFESTATIONS

Cutaneous Lesions

1. **Kaposi's sarcoma** of nasal skin is the first indication of disease progression of asymptomatic HIV to AIDS. It can become widely disseminated. Pigmented irregular lesions (macular or nodular, blue to dark brown or red) located on the mucous membrane or the skin of nose.
2. **Herpes zoster** in the distribution of V cranial nerve. This is due to reactivation of varicella-zoster virus in the trigeminal ganglion. Characteristic vesicular eruptions along sensory distribution of V nerve may be seen.

   A related condition is giant herpetic ulcer of the nose and face. Characteristically originates in the vestibule and extends to surrounding facial skin.

   Treatment

   Acyclovir prevents post-herpetic neuralgia.
3. **Seborrhic dermatitis** is a seborrhea like rash classically involving the NL folds as a

red eruption with a greasy scale. It can involve eyebrows, nasal and malar regions, postauricular region, forehead and back. Malar rash resembles the butterfly pattern in SLE.

Treatment

Topical steroids and oral and topical ketaconazole.

Nasal Obstruction

This may be due to adenoidal hypertrophy, allergic rhinitis, polyposis, chronic sinusitis, neoplasms involving the nose or PNS.

Adenoid Hypertrophy

It is common in HIV infected population. Patients present with lymphadenopathy and proliferation of adenoids lingual and faucial tonsils.

Adenoidal hypertrophy in an adult patient even in an otherwise asymptomatic patient should raise the possibility of underlying HIV infection as a result of polyclonal B cell activation, Epstein Barr virus or cytomegalovirus.

Nasal obstruction is the most common complaint. On examination thick mucoidal discharge is found in the nasal cavity. It may be associated with features of otitis media with effusion.

Adenoidectomy should be performed in all symptomatic HIV patients to rule out lymphoma, and it also provides symptomatic relief of nasal obstruction.

Allergic Rhinitis

Depressed cellular immunity manifested by decreased total lymphocyte count and helper T cell counts. Decrease in IgG subclass has been noticed in some AIDS patients who predispose them to recurrent infections. An increase in the IgE levels has been noticed in certain AIDS patients that can be associated with IgE mediated allergic symptoms (conjunctivitis and rhinitis) and recrudescence of asthma.

Sinusitis

Prevalence of rhinosinusitis in AIDS is 20 to 68 percent. The entire spectrum from acute to chronic sinusitis with mucosal changes may be seen. The most common organisms involved are *Str. pneumoniae, H.influenzae. Staphylococcus aureus* and *pseudomonas aeruginosa* usually cause chronic sinusitis. Fungal sinusitis is caused by *Pseudoallescheria boydii, Alternaria alternate,* Aspergillus, Crytoccus, and Candida. Sinusitis can be caused by *Legionella pneumoniae, acanthamoeba castellani* and cytomegalovirus.

Patients usually present with thick mucopurulent postnasal discharge associated with features of pneumonias and bronchospasm, other symptoms include fever, headache, nasal congestion, periorbital pain or pain over the canine fossa.

CT scan is necessary to know the extent of the disease.

Treatment

It includes antibiotic and decongestant.

Amoxicillin with clavulenic acid or cephalosporin can be tried. It should be continued for minimum three weeks.

In cases resistant to therapy or signs of impending complications are present, hospital admission with IV antibiotics or surgical drainage is imperative.

Mucolytics and decongestants may be prescribed for symptomatic relief and to facilitate drainage.

Patients with CD4 count less than 200 are resistant to standard therapy. In these, antibiotic therapy should include coverage of *Staph. aureus* and *Ps. aeruginosa.* Ciprofloxacin with metrogyl for 5 to 6 weeks is the recommended therapy.

If medical therapy fails, repeat antral irrigation is helpful. Endoscopic sinus surgery is often recommended to enhance drainage as well as obtain culture material to rule out fungal, mycobacterial and other opportunistic infections.

Atrophic rhinitis has also been seen in some patients with AIDS. On examination, foul smelling, greenish discharge with crusts is ITP can cause epistaxis.

NEOPLASMS

The commonest tumors are Kaposi's sarcoma and Non-Hodgkin's lymphoma.

Presenting symptoms are nasal obstruction, intermittent epistaxis, rhinorrhea. Diagnosis is made on clinical history, characteristic appearance and may be confirmed by excision biopsy.

Treatment

- Localized—Intralesional vinblastine or low dose radiotherapy, cryotherapy and argon laser therapy also tried.
- Widely disseminated chemo and radio-therapy used, but prognosis is poor.

Lymphoma

Systemic high-grade B cell lymphoma is usually associated with AIDS. Nose, PNS, nasopharynx and oral cavity commonly involved.

Clinical Features

Bleeding, nasal obstruction, rhinorrhea, mass effect on face orbit or surrounding structures.

Diagnosis

Needle aspiration, tissue biopsy. LP necessary before institution of therapy as it has the propensity for CNS and bone marrow involvement.

Treatment

Systemic chemotherapy. Radiotherapy rarely employed except in cases of functional impairment. Prognosis is very poor.

AIRWAY MANIFESTATIONS

Although upper as well as lower airways involved, lower involvement is much more common.

Upper Airway

Infections

Bacterial tracheal infections most commonly attributable to *H. influenzae* and *Str. pneumoniae*. Viral tracheitis can also occur. Fungal infections of the upper airway are rare.

Neoplasia

Kaposi sarcoma is the most common tumor encountered. Stridor is the initial symptom. Fiberoptic bronchoscopy is important for diagnosis because of characteristic violaceous lesion of upper airway.

Biopsy contraindicated due to (a) Large pieces of tissue required which are not obtainable; (b) Hemorrhage.

Lower Airway

- Pulmonary infections are attributable to opportunistic pathogens and community acquired pathogens.
- *Pneumocystii carinii* pneumonia is most common pulmonary disease in HIV infected patients. It is the initial manifestation in more than 65 percent of HIV infected patients.
- Its clinical characteristics are subtle and long term with nonspecific respiratory symptoms such as chest or sternal discomfort, cough, dyspnea on exertion and fever.
- Chest X-ray shows diffuse bilateral alveolar or interstitial infiltrates.
- Diagnosis is by collecting induced sputum using hypertonic sodium chloride nebulization and staining with toluidine blue or with immunofluorescent technique. Sensitivity is almost 90 percent.
- Bronchoalveolar lavage and transbronchial biopsy can be done.
- Sensitivity is 95 percent.

Other Bacteria which cause Pulmonary Infection

Str. Pneumoniae, H.influenzae, Moraxella catarrhalis, Staphylococcus aureus, Ps. Aeruginosa, Legionella pneumoniae.

Mycobacterium tuberculosis, Mycobacterium avium intracellulare, Cytomegalovirus, Cryptococcus (most common fungal pathogen), Cryptosporidia.

ORAL MANIFESTATIONS

Oral Candidiasis

Most common intraoral fungal infection. Presence of oral candidiasis in an otherwise healthy individual may be an early sign of immunosuppression. Its prevalence is 30 percent to 90 percent in HIV positive patients. Can occur in various forms, i.e.

1. **Pseudomembranous infection (thrush):** The lesion appears on the mucosa as a creamy plaque which wipes off easily leaving a bleeding surface.
2. **Atrophic or erythematous form:** It appears as red patches, involved areas are tender on touching with tongue blade.
3. **Hyperplastic form:** Thick heaped white plaques which resemble leukoplakia and cannot be wiped off. Commonest site is buccal mucosa.

Angular cheilitis is another form of oral candidiasis in which there is fissuring, cracking erythema, or ulceration at the corner of mouth.

Diagnosis

KOH preparations of the surface scrapings

- Show characteristic mycelia, spores and hyphae.
- Biopsy and staining with periodic acid Schiff
- Cultures on Sabouraud's dextrose agar

Treatment

Topical and systemic antifungals (ketaconazole, fluconazole. Amphotericin B is used in severe cases).

Hairy Leukoplasia

White, hairy, slightly raised lesions of the lateral border of tongue, bilateral, that does not improve with therapy for oral candidiasis. It is a good indicator that the patient may progress to full blown AIDS. It is also seen in the floor of mouth, pharynx, buccal mucosa. Biopsy demonstrates ballooning prickle cell layer in the epithelium, shows hyperkeratosis, parakeratosis and acanthosis in the epithelial layer. Probably caused by EB virus. Treatment is with acyclovir (high doses), AZT, sulfa drugs.

Herpes Simplex

Seen in 9 percent of AIDS population. Most common manifestation is herpes labialis. It affects palate, lips, perioral and gingival area. Only responds to local or systemic acyclovir in initial stages.

CMV, V. zoster, human papilloma virus also cause oral lesions.

Gingivitis and Periodontal Disease

Rapid progression to necrosis of periodontal soft tissue, bone exposure and sequestration of alveolar bone. Acute necrotizing ulcerative gingivitis (ANUG). Causative organism may be Gram –ve anaerobic bacteria and candida.

Treatment

Periodontal care, good oral hygiene and antibiotic in case of ANUG.

Other Oral Bacterial Lesions

M. tuberculosis, E. coli, K.pneumonia, M. avium intracellulare.

ORAL NEOPLASMS

Kaposi's Sarcoma

Can occur on any mucosal surface, hard palate being the commonest.

Lymphoma

NHL is the second most common AIDS associated tumor in the oral cavity. Tonsil is commonly involved.

Squamous Cell Carcinoma

Tongue is commonly involved.

IDIOPATHIC ORAL LESIONS

Recurrent Aphthous Ulcerations

- In 20 percent of immunocompromised patients. Minor <6 mm, major >6 mm in diameter.
- Well circumscribed, erythamatous border. May appear in successive crops.
- Large lesions require biopsy to rule out lymphoma or carcinoma.

Treatment: Topical steroids.

Xerostomia

Fairly frequent. Cause unknown (?CMV).

Treatment

Frequent oral saline rinses, sugarless gum, salivary substitutes, bethanechol as a sialagogue.

Thrombocytopenia

Occurs with a typical oral ecchymosis, petechiae and spontaneous gingival bleeding.

Vocal Cord Edema

- Either due to previous radiation therapy or due to obstruction from KS.
- Recurrent laryngeal nerve paralysis due to CMV infection can occur.

Oral Mucosal Hyperpigmentation

Cause unknown.

NECK MASSES

HIV Lymphadenopathy

PGL or persistant generalized lymphadenopathy involving two or more extrainguinal sites for more than three months. Is one of the earliest sign of HIV infection. Occurs long before the other symptoms. Lymph nodes are soft, symmetric, 1 to 5 cm. Sites posterior triangle, Waldeyers ring, pre and post auricular, submandibular, submental and supraclavicular.

Routine biopsy not helpful.

Infections
Mycobacterium tuberculosis

Frequently extrapulmonary (50 to 60 percent), most commonly the cervical nodes and bone marrow. Lymph nodes are firm and nontender (10 percent tender and inflamed). In HIV PPD test of more than 5 mm is taken as positive.

Mycobacterium avium complex (MAC)

Frequently seen in end stage HIV disease as a disseminate infection. Response to ATT is poor.

Clofazimine and ciprofloxacin have been found to be useful recently.

Other Infections

Toxoplasmosis, cryptococcus, histoplasmosis, Cocciodomycosis, *P. carinii.*

Parotid Diseases

Enlargement seen in 30 percent of HIV positive children.

The lymphoepithelial cyst is unique to HIV. They are minimally tender, progressive. B/L and associated with GCL. CT and MRI helps in diagnosis. Have a benign course. Surgery limited to only diagnostic difficulties and deforming lesions. Tetracycline instillation after aspiration has been proved to be very successful.

Neoplasms

Kaposi's sarcoma, lymphoma, squamous cell carcinoma are the commonest cervical neoplasms seen.

Pediatric AIDS

1. Cervical adenopathy
2. Parotid gland enlargement

3. Otitis media
4. Sinusitis
5. Recurrent adenotonsillitis (OSAS)
6. Mucocutaneous candidiasis
7. Recurrent viral (URT) infections
8. Thrombocytopenia.

Occupational Risks

The center for disease control (CDC) has estimated that 0.15 percent of surgeons carry the HIV. More risk is from cutaneous puncture rather than contact with mucous membrane or skin. Even skin puncture with a contaminated hypodermic needle transmits disease in only one in 250 instances (0.4 percent).

Universal Precautions

Personal Protection

The concept of universal precautions includes the triad of personal barrier protection, environmental disinfection and engineering mechanisms. Blood is the predominant source of infection. In the head and neck region universal precautions do not apply to sweat, saliva, sputum, nasal secretions, tears and vomitus unless they contain visible blood.

(a) Double gloves, mask, protective eye wear, gowns and shoe cover should be used while handling body fluids.

(b) Special precautions while handling sharp instruments and needles
(c) Thos with cuts or dermatitis should refrain from handling contaminated material
(d) Use staples rather than sutures and large monofilament rather than wire
(e) Substitute scissors, laser and cutting cautery for scalpel.
(f) Do not hold tissue or needle in your fingers when suturing.
(g) Exchange sharps through *neutral area* or pass by the blunt end.
(h) Discard sharps into puncture resistant containers or embed into foam rubber.

Legal issues in AIDS

1. Mass screening discouraged as it would interfere with the doctor patient relationship and encourage a false sense of security.
2. Informed consent is necessary and should include the assurance that medical care will not be denied if testing is declined.
3. Confidentiality should be maintained.
4. discrimination of HIV positive patients is illegal.
5. Risks, benefits and alternatives to blood transfusion should be explained and informed consent should be taken prior to transfusion

POINTS TO REMEMBER

1. HIV is caused by "T lymphocyte virus".
2. Otolaryngological manifestation of HIV are classified into (a) opportunistic infection (b) secondary cancers (c) direct effect of HIV infection.

Lasers in Otolaryngology

96

Introduction

Laser is an acronym that means light amplification by the stimulated emission of radiation. The use of laser in otolaryngology is becoming very popular and most of the otolaryngologists regard it as the best surgical tool for precise cutting without any significant blood loss. Since the first clinical application of Ruby laser in ablation of retinal tumor by T H Maiman on 16th May 1960, various other lasers have also been tried in the field of otolaryngology. In 1965, Kumar Patel introduced the first continuous wave CO_2 laser and the same has been clinically applied by the American optical corporation in 1967. In 1990, Center for Advanced Technology (CAT), India, in Indore, developed an indigenous CO_2 laser for medical use. At present, lasers like argon laser, KTP/532 laser, Nd:YAG laser, Ho:YAG laser are also becoming popular along with the CO_2 laser.

The use of laser in the surgical field is undoubtedly very effective but optimal delivery system of each laser has to be considered to get the maximum benefit especially in the head and neck. Endoscopic delivery system and microscope-laser assembly system are very important in ENT and was first introduced by Jacko in 1972. At present fiberoptic delivery system of KTP/532 laser has definite advantages over other lasers (Fig. 96.1).

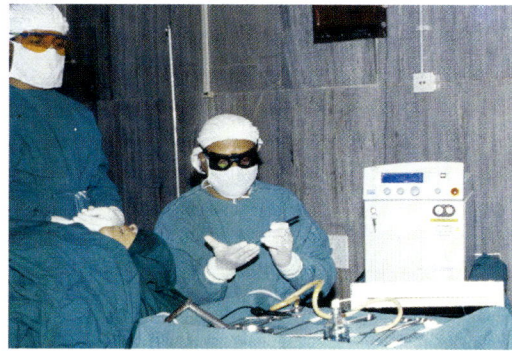

Fig. 96.1: Laser endoscopic surgery in progress with KTP/532 laser machine

Laser Biophysics for Otolaryngologists

A laser is an electro-optical device containing a lasing medium that usually comprises gas or crystal. The atoms of this lasing medium typically exist in nature at several different energy levels across the electromagnetic spectrum. When stimulated by an extrinsic energy source, these atoms emit electromagnetic radiation or photon in a narrow intense beam. Simply speaking, laser emits organised light rather than the random pattern light emitted from the common light bulb. The laser beam is an intense collimated (parallel) beam of pure monochromatic (single wavelength) light in which all light waves are of the same length and travel in the same direction (no divergence). The collimated beam can be focussed to the smallest possible spot by a lens or concave mirror producing extremely high densities. This high concentration of energy is called LASER and is used for laser tissue ablation. The wavelength of each laser may vary and have a varied effect on tissue. Shorter the wavelength, more the penetration. For CO_2 laser with wavelength 10600 nm, the depth of penetration is about 10th of a mm. Nd: YAG laser can go deeper about a mm, whereas KTP/532 can go still deeper, KTP 532 nm and Argon 488 to 514 nm wavelength fall under the visible zone of spectrum while Nd:YAG 1060 nm and CO_2 10600 nm fall under the invisible zone and require another visible source like Helium-Neon (Fig. 96.2).

Above 100°C lasers cause vaporization, carbonization, disintegration and destruction of laser irradiated tissue with smoke and gas generation. This thermal effect is used in surgery for welding, coagulation, cutting, evaporation and laser thermia.

Tissue Effect of Laser

In the center of the laser crater (wound), the volume of tissue is vapourised and few flakes of debris are noted. Immediately next to this there will be a zone of thermal necrosis less than 100 um wide. Next to this zone is a volume of thermal conductivity and repair of 300 to 500 um wide, where small vessels, nerves and lymphatics are sealed and called the zone of coagulation (Fig. 96.3). This minimal operative trauma combined

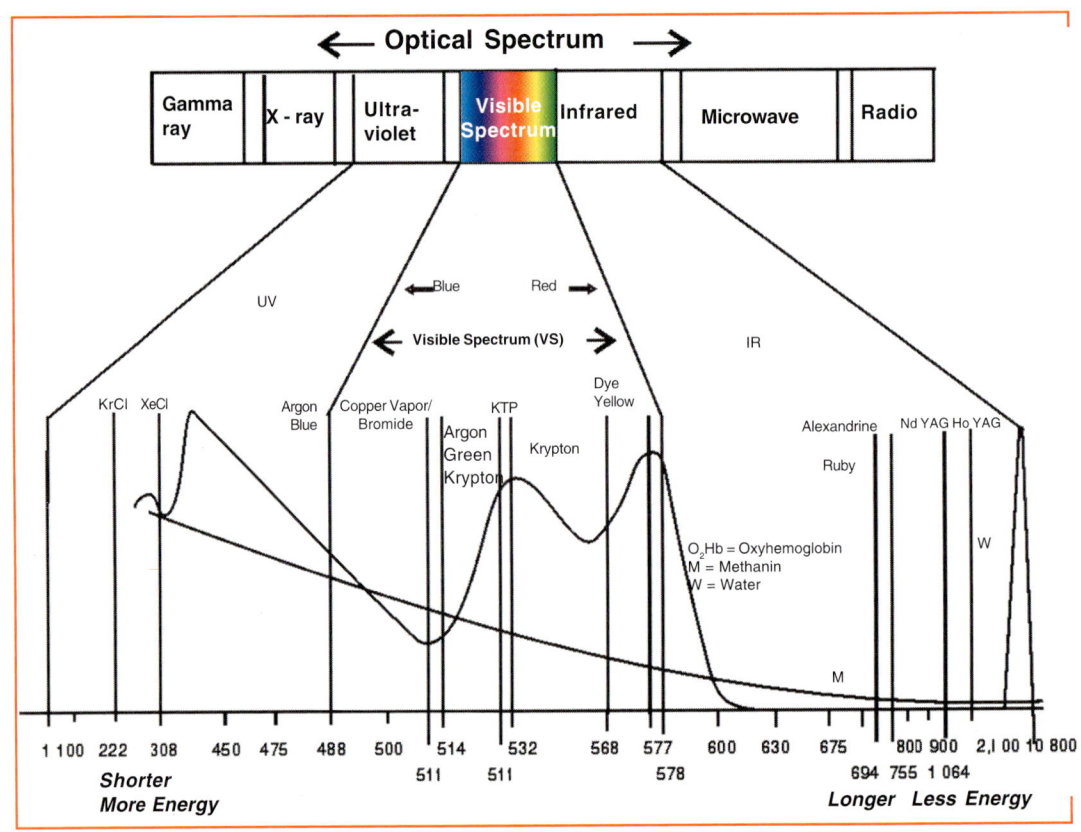

Fig. 96.2: The electromagnetic spectrum with absorbtion rates

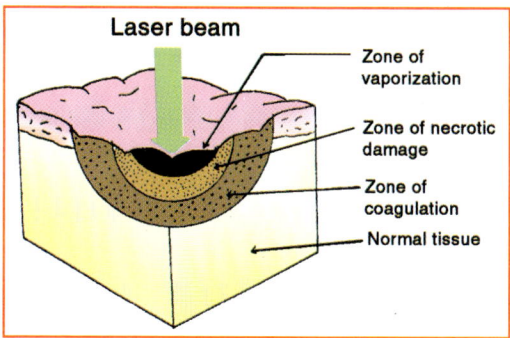

Fig. 96.3: Reaction of tissue to laser

with the vascular and nerve sealing account for notable abscence of bleeding, postoperative pain edema and spread of cells via lymphatics.

The actual tissue effect produced by radiant energy vary with specific wavelength of the laser used. Low levels of all laser energy has biostimulatory effect andat higher levels becomes inhibitory ultimately having thermal effect on the tissue. The tissue effect can broadly be divided into thermal effect and non-thermal effect.

Thermal Effect

- The laser energy is absorbed by the chromophores within the body tissue and is converted into heat. With heat above 60 to 65° C, the cell proteins undergoes denaturation due to coagulation of tissue proteins caused by randomization of protein chains.
- There is contraction of collagen fibers in the vessel wall and perivascular tissue leading to hemostatic effect
- Heat at 100° C causes drying, shrinkage and permanent damage to the tissues.
- Intracellular water absorbs laser energy resulting in chemical change in the cell. This is used for photodynamic therapy for malignant tumors, i.e. red dye laser 632.
- Photomechanical—The short pulses of high intensity lasers are used to disrupt the cellular architecture, i.e. in lithotripsy (dye laser).
- Laser induced fluorescence is used extensively for detection of cancer.

Non-thermal Effects of Laser

- Biostimulation—Low level laser energy is bio stimulative and used in sports injuries and rheumatism. Low level lasers like helium and nitrogen laser have been used in cases of acute and chronic inflammations in ENT.
- Photochemical—Radiation energy of laser can stimulate or react with specific molecules within a cell to focus them.

Types of Lasers used in Otolaryngology

Six types of lasers are currently in use in Otolaryngology—Head and Neck surgery and many more are waiting clinical trial. The characteristic potential of the clinical application of a particular surgical laser is determined by its light emission paradigm, i.e. pulse character, wavelength and absorption characteristics in tissues. To get the maximal benefit with minimal effort from the laser, the surgeon should consider the properties of each wavelength for different types of surgery.

The following are the commonest lasers:

Argon

Argon laser produces a visible blue-green light with wavelength of 488 to 514 nm. Radiant energy from an argon laser is poorly absorbed by water and can pass through aqueous tissues of the cornea, lens and vitreous humour. It is effectively absorbed by melanin pigment and hemoglobin. This is mainly used for photocoagulation such as port wine stain, hemangioma, telangiectasia and photocoagulation of retina. This laser operates in continuous mode and can be delivered through optical fibers. It is also used for stapedectomy, lysis of middle ear adhesions, spot welding of graft in tympanoplasty operation.

KTP/532 (Fig. 96.4)

(Potassium titanyl phosphate)—KTP/532 is an optically pumped solid state laser that produces a visible 532 nm beam with an emerald green color. KTP/532 laser is transmitted through a flexible

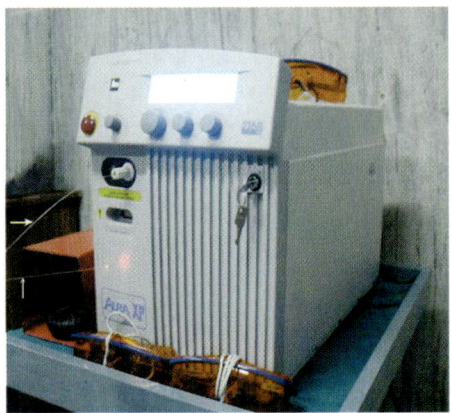

Fig. 96.4: KTP 532 laser machine

fiberoptic delivery system which can be used in association with a micromanipulator attached to an operating microscope or free hand in association with various hand-held delivery probes having several different tip angles. These hand-held probes facilitate use of KTP/532 laser for benign and malignant tumors of the oral cavity, nose, functional endoscopic sinus surgery, otologic application and microlaryngeal application. The hand-held KTP/532 laser applications delude tonsillectomy, turbinectomy, stapedotomy, excision if acoustic tumor and excision of both benign and malignant tumors. KTP/532 laser is typically available as i unit and delivered between 0.5 to 15 watts with fiber iiameters of 200, 300, 400, and 600 microns. Because of the visible green light of KTP/532 laser, chance of damaging the retina is high. So, safety measures should be properly followed by the personel in the operating room

CO_2 Laser

CO_2 laser has a wavelength in the far infrared region) of electromagnetic field of 10600 nm. Ninety percent of energy is absorbed into the tissues with the penetration depth of 0.1 mm. It controls the blood vessels up to 0.5 mm in diameter and mostly delivered to the target tissues through an articulated arm or by a hand piece for macroscopic surgeries. CO_2 laser is very widely used in the field of otolaryngology.

Nd:YAG Laser

It has the wavelength in the far infrared region of electromagnetic field at 1060 nm. Fifty percent of its energy is absorbed in the tissues and has a penetration of 4 mm into the tissue. It is delivered through optical fibers like KTP. It controls the blood vessels up to 1.5 mm in diameter. The hemostasis is better than CO_2 laser. It is mostly used in otolaryngology for excision of obstructive tracheobronchial and esophageal lesions, photocoagulation of vascular and lymphatic malformations of head and neck.

Ho:YAG Laser

It has a wavelength of 2100 nm and can be delivered by optical fibers. It has a short penetration depth. It can be used selectively in otolaryngology, i.e. facial nerve decompression, endoscopic sinus surgery. It ablates the bone easily.

Safety Measures

Proper education and training is essential for the safe operation of laser in any setting. It is a recommendation from the American society for laser in medicine and surgery and a requirement by the ANSIZ 136.3 standard, both users and operators of surgical laser should have appropriate education and training for the particular laser system they use.

In brief, laser should be used with extreme caution. Designated operation room for this procedure should be named as "Laser control area" which should be accessible only to selected persons. All the personnel should have protective glasses. The patient's eyes should be protected with a saline soaked eye pad. Room should be locked during the procedure.

The machine should be electrical and laser safety proof and should have key control emission warning, remote interlock system, aiming beam emergency, shock absorber switch and warning levels and inflammable materials should be removed from the operating room. Surgical instrument should be energized black finish and OT walls should be rough, non-reflecting.

Laser has six associated hazards. They are electrical shock, fire, eye injury, skin injury, plume (vapourized cell contents) and chemical hazards.

Anesthetic Precautions

Laser microlaryngeal surgeries may lead to anesthetic tube fire. To avoid this the following technique may be recommended:

- Jet ventilation with no endotracheal tube.
- Protected endotracheal tube wrapped with aluminium foil.
- Nasopharyngeal airway with spontaneous respiration.
- Use of complete laser proof flexometallic tube or catheter. Norton-devos tubes are more popular.
- Tracheostomy and direct tracheal intubation to avoid laryngeal accident.
- Halothane is the safest anesthetic gas.

The Laser as a Surgical Tool

Lasers were introduced as a surgical tool in the late 1960's. In otolaryngology almost all the lesions can be tackled with laser. The scalpel is able to produce only one action, i.e. cutting, the electrosurgical instrument can cut and coagulate whereas lasers can cut, coagulate and vapourize.

Indications for Laser Surgery in ENT

1. *Otologic application:* CO_2 or KTP/532 can be used in stapedotomy, ossicular sclupturing, lysis of adhesions, granulation tissue, control of bleeding.
2. *Nasal application:* Inferior turbinoplasty, epistaxis due to hereditary hemorrhagic

telangiectasia, endoscopic sinus surgery. KTP/532 laser is the preferred laser for nasal surgery. Diode laser is preferred for endoscopic transnasal dacryocysto-rhinostomy (DCR).

3. *Laryngeal application:* Benign lesions of the larynx including laryngeal papillo- malosis, subglottic stenosis, laryngotracheal stenosis, etc.

   Malignant lesions can be excised effectively, in their early stages with CO_2 and KTP/532 laser.
4. *Bronchoscopic application:* Stenosis, granulosis tissue webs. Both CO_2 and KTP/532 are effective. Vascular tumor like bronchial adenoma, obstructing carcinoma can be better treated by KTP/532 and Nd:YAG laser.
5. *Oral cavity aplication:* Used to excise lesions of the floor of the mouth, buccal or labial mucosa and lateral tongue. KTP/532 and Nd:YAG are comonly used for vascular lesions also.

Photodynamic Therapy (PDT): It is uses a combination of laser light of a specific wavelength and a light-sensitive drug to destroy cancer cells. It is a noninvasive treatment modality.

The light-sensitive drug (the photosensitising agent) is given intravenously. The drug circulated in the bloodstream is taken up by cancer cells more than by healthy cells in the body. It does not do anything until it is exposed to laser light of a particular wavelength. When a laser is shone onto the cancer, the drug is triggered to interact with oxygen, which then destroys the cancer cells.

PDT may be used to treat early cancer of the head and neck for cure is usually given as part of research trials. PDT can be used to treat advanced cancer as a palliative measure.

97

Cryosurgery and Powered Instrumentation

CRYOSURGERY

Cryosurgery is a branch of surgical techniques that makes use of local freezing for controlled destruction or excision of living tissues. Kryos has been derived from Greek work meaning cold. It was first described by Cooper in 1961, who used liquid Nitrogen at -196°C with the help of a hollow metal probe. Rand in 1964 did trans-sphenoidal hypophysectomy using cryoprobe. Von Leden in 1967 successfully treated recurrent tonsillitis by using cryosurgery. Recently the popularity of cryotherapy has reduced because of the availability of better tools like laser and radiofrequency.

Types of Therapy

Open Method

Direct application of refrigerating chemicals: Example: CO_2 snow and nitrogen spray.

Closed System

Using cryoprobe: A cryoprobe is based on Joule Thompson effect, i.e. rapid expansion of compressed gas through a small hole produces cooling. This employs liquid nitrogen, nitrous oxide or carbon dioxide used through a cryoprobe.

Pathophysiology

The low temperature applied through the cryoprobe causes intracellular ice crystal formation. This leads to:

- Intracellular dehydration associated with change in intracellular pH and increase in concentration of electrolytes, urea, etc.
- Denaturation of the lipoproteins in the cell membrane causing disruption of the nuclear and cell membranes
- Destruction within ice-sphere occurs by:
  - Thermal shock with arrest of respiratory function of the cell
  - Ischemic infarction
  - *Cryoimmunology:* Cryoinjury results in autoimmune response due to release of new antigens following destruction of tumor tissue.

Indications

- Cryoassisted tonsillectomy
- Adenoidectomy
- Lingual tonsillar ablation
- Inferior turbinate reduction in vasomotor rhinitis
- Epistaxis
- Excision of rhinosporidiosis
- *Neoplastic conditions*
  - Benign tumors of the oral cavity like papilloma
  - Tumors of the nasal cavity and nasopharynx including angiofibroma
  - Malignant tumors like carcinoma of the middle ear/mastoid, early cancer of the pinna, debulking of the tumor in head and neck.

Advantages

- Useful in poor risk patients and can be applied without anesthesia or under local anesthesia
- Useful in patients with bleeding coagulopathies
- Can be used in multiple cancers, palliation of recurrent cancers
- Minimal post-treatment discomfort or pain
- Minimal scarring and hence can be used in patients with keloid tendency
- Out-patient procedure

Disadvantages

- No tissue available for biopsy in case of small lesion
- Not possible to assess the margin of tumor
- No control on depth of freezing
- Anesthesia of the part is required when the lesion is close to the nerve.

POWERED INSTRUMENTATION

Following powered instrumentations have offered more effective surgical tools in the field of otolaryngological surgeries. They have made the surgeries more easy and bloodless with quick recovery and less hospitalization for the patients.

1. Microdebrider
2. Coblation
3. Harmonic scalpel

4. Temperature controlled radiofrequency ablation.

Microdebrider

Synonyms: Vacuum rotary dissector, soft tissue shavers, hummers.

The System (Figs 97.1 and 97.2)

The microdebrider is a powered rotary shaving device with continuous suction. It is made up of a cannula connected to a hand piece, which in turn is connected to a motor with foot control and a suction device. The cannula is made up of two parts, an outer blunt tip with a lateral port and an oscillating inner cannula with a similar lateral port has serrated blade which cuts and extracts soft tissue as it is suctioned through the side port of the cannula. The blunt tip of the outer cannula protects vital structures and only the soft tissues that are sucked into the lateral port is cut and extracted. Hence this device is built for safety. The inner cannula with the cutting blade rotates either continuously in one direction or with oscillatory movements. The oscillating mode yields better cutting and faster removal of soft tissue with minimal pulling effect compared to the continuous mode. The speed of oscillation can be controlled and the maximum speed is at least 3000 rpm. The blades with serrated edges cut more aggressively as they grip the tissues. The ones with smooth edges are less aggressive.

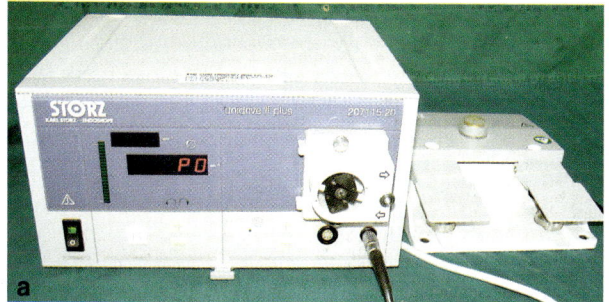
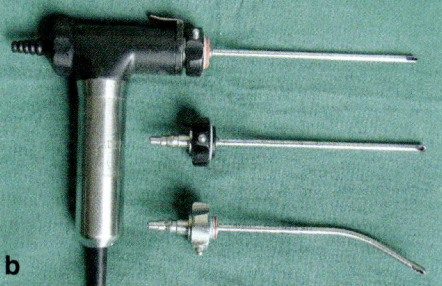

Figs 97.1a and b: (a) Stortz shavers system and foot control, (b) handpiece

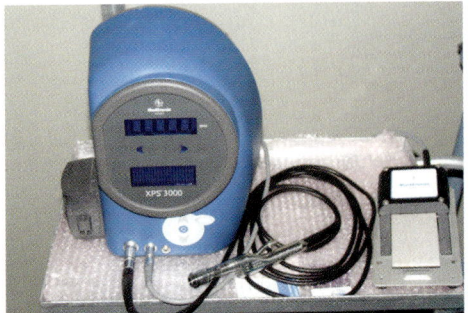

Fig. 97.2: Zomed shavers system with handpiece and foot control

The microdebrider system was developed by Urban 1969 as 'Vacuum rotary dissector' and was used for acoustic neuroma surgery. Setliff (1994) is credited with the introduction of tissue shavers for use in FESS and other otolaryngologic procedures.

Advantages

- It greatly increases cutting precision. Thus it is very useful in endoscopic sinus surgeries.
- Safe cutting instrument as only sucked in tissue gets cut and extracted
- Facilitates the removal of blood and debris from the surgical field thus enhancing visibility of the structures. Thus the surgeries can become safer.
- Specially designed malleable cannulae allow access to remote structures endoscopically.
- The hand pieces are generally small, light and ergonomic
- Decreases surgical time
- Faster postoperative healing and minimal hospitalization.
- The equipment may also be used with other optional hand piece and devices for oscillating saw or bone cutting burs with protection of the burr shaft. They are useful in endoscopic dacryocystorhinostomy,

endoscopic management of choanal atresia, endoscopic septoplasty or rhinoplasty and optic nerve decompression.

- Specially designed cannulae may be used in endoscopic adenoidectomy and laryngeal or pharyngeal procedures.

Disadvantages

- The cannulae tend to get frequently clogged and require frequent removal for unclogging.
- Blade heating may cause thermal damage of the structures and this is minimized by irrigation.
- Difficulty in obtaining tissue for biopsy. Suction traps may be used to collect the extracted tissue.
- Postoperative bleeding may be more
- Cannulae are disposable or may be used only in few cases as it looses its sharpness. The cost of the cannulae is high.

Coblation

Coblation (cold ablation) is also referred to as an electrodissociation procedure. It is a direct extension of standard electrosurgical techniques which employs an oscillating electrical current to disrupt the surrounding tissue. The electrodes at the tip of the coblation probe serve as a source if radio-frequency energy which is conducted through conductive medium (normal saline or gel). This is used to deliver the electrical energy. Radio-frequency excites the saline solution creating a field of Na^+ ions that are able to dissociate the tissue molecular bonds. Due to steady flow of saline from the probe, the system generates relatively low tissue temperature of 40 to 70° C compared to that of standard electrosurgery (400 to 600° C) thus sparing the healthy tissue. It also allows hemostasis through the coagulation option.

Indications

- Tonsillectomy
- Inferior turbinoplasty
- Palatoplasty

Harmonic Scalpel

This is similar to an electrocautery in that the ultimate result is a denatured protein coagulum that tamponade the blood vessels but coagulation is achieved through ultrasonic vibration unlike electro-cautery and laser where denaturation occurs due to heating of the tissue.

The blade vibrates at 55.5 kHz over a distance of 80 micrometers. The lateral zone of injury is very less as compared to monopolar electro-cautery. It can seal the blood vessels like arteries of 3.8 mm diameter and veins of up to 9 mm diameter. It consists of a hand-piece, a generator and a blade.

Indications

- Tonsillectomy
- Thyroid surgery
- Excision of cancer of the tongue, soft palate, etc.
- Submandibular sialadenectomy
- Parotidectomy
- Inferior turbinoplasty
- Rhinophyma

Temperature Controlled Radiofrequency Ablation (TCRFA)

This is an electrical device and consists of a radiofrequency control unit that delivers variable energy levels at controlled temperatures and is delivered through interchangeable hand-held probes.

It delivers specific amount of low temperature and low voltage energy in the form of radiofrequency to a specific site. The energy thus released agitates tissue ions by the inherent changes in the electrical flow with an alternating current. The tissue heats up due to resistance at a temperature of 60 to 90°C. In contrast laser and electrocautery produces temperature of 750°C.

The ultimate goal of TCRFA is tissue reduction that occurs in 2 stages.
1. Contraction of area of fibrosis
2. Resorption which occurs over several months further reducing the volume of the tissue.

Indications

Used in sleep apnea and snoring for procedures like palatoplasty, inferior turbinoplasty, reduction of tonsillar tissue and reduction of base of the tongue.

POINTS TO REMEMBER

1. Cryosurgery uses local freezing for control destruction or excision of tissues.
2. Powered instrumentation are new and more effective surgical tools like microdebridor, coblation and harmonic scalpel.
3. Coblation is an electrodissociation procedure and employs oscillating electrical current to disrupt the tissues.

98

Skull Base Surgery

Skull base is that portion of the cranium tying inferiorly and anteriorly to the neuroaxis, through which passes the 12 cranial nerves, major arterial and venous channels supplying the central nervous system. The skull base is composed of frontal and ethomoid bone anteriorly, occipital bone posteriorly, sphenoid and paired temporal bones in between. The following are the common discrete areas in the skull base of pathological importance.

1. Cerebellopontine angle.
2. Jugular foramen.
3. Area of petrous apex.
4. Superior orbital fissure.
5. Inferior surface of temporal bone.
6. Other selected regions.
   - Cavernous sinus
   - Pituitary.

The various pathological conditions commonly encountered are :

1. Infection.
2. Benign space occupying lesion (Glomus. Neuroma)
3. Primary and metastatic malignant neoplasm.
4. Vascular abnormalities.
5. Congenital defects.
6. Traumatic lesions.

Although there were a significant advancements in the related specialities in the past twenty five years to tackle the conditions involving the skull base effectively, most of the conditions involving lateral skull base were considered Inaccessible until recently, because of their dose relations to the great vessels and major cranial nerves passing in this part of the skull base. With the development of infra-temporal fossa approach to the lateral skull base by Ugo Fisch (1977, 1979, 1984) there was a major breakthrough in the subsequent development of surgical expertise and microsurgical techniques for adequate management of these lesions. The pioneers who brought the revolution in the surgical techniques of skull base are: William House (1961); Glasscock (1978). Fisch (1977, 1978, 1982); Biller et al (1981); Smith et al (1954) and Sekhar et al (1987). Hazarika et al (1990, 1992, 1993) popularized the skull base surgery in India.

The lesions involving lateral skull base is more difficult to approach for their dose relation to the neurovascular bundle consisting of great vessels and various cranial nerves, which necessitates thorough anatomical knowledge and expertise to tackle these tumors. Since lateral skull base lesions are more frequently encountered by the oto-laryngology-Head and Neck Surgeons, the present chapter will discuss about the Principles of Lateral Skull Base Approaches. (Fisch Approach). Approach to anterior skull base and anterior craniofacial resection are discussed under the Chapter 40 and Chapter 45 (Fig. 98.1).

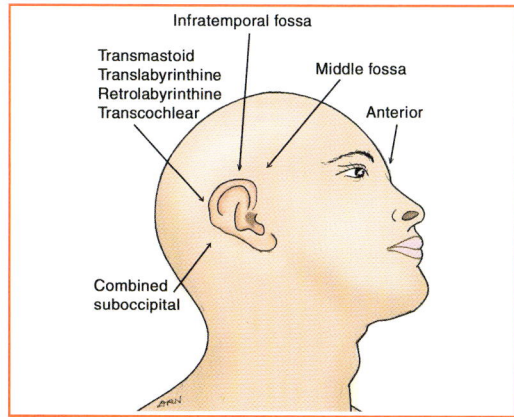

Fig. 98.1: Types of skull base approaches

Principles of Lateral Skull Base Approaches

Lateral Skull Base Approach can be further divided into:

1. Extended lateral approach (Sekhar).
2. Infratemporal fossa approach (Fisch Approach).

INFRATEMPORAL FOSSA APPROACH (FISCH'S APPROACH)

Infratemporal approach may be extended into three types depending on the extent of the disease.

Type A Approach

- Access to the temporal bone in its infralabyrinthine and apical compartments mostly employed for glomus tumors.
- Type B access to the Clivus.
- Type C access to parasellar region and nasopharynx.

Steps of Surgery for Type A: (Figs 98.2 and 98.3)

1. S-shaped skin incision as shown in the Fig. 98.2 involves wide undermining of the anterior skin edge.
2. Elevation of periosteal flap, based on the posterior aspect of the membranous canal wall.

3. Transection of external auditory canal at the bony cartilaginous junction and blind sac closure and sealing with periosteal flap in the inner aspect.
4. Identification of the facial nerve trunk distal to stylomastoid foramen along the axis formed by the bisection of a line drawn between the pointer of tragal cartilage and mastoid tip.
5. Identification of IX to XII cranial nerves, carotid and its branches and internal jugular vein in the neck is followed by ligation of tumor feeding arteries like ascending pharyngeal, occipital and external carotid artery.
6. Removal of the remaining skin of the bony external auditory canal tympanic membrane.
7. Subtotal petrosectomy by performing an extended radical mastoidectomy along with complete excenteration of petrous aircell system and contained mucosa.
8. Permanent anterior transposition of the facial nerve in the newly performed fallopian canal in the anterior attic wall.
9. Permanent obliteration of eustachian tube.
10. Double ligation of sigmoid sinus after skeletonizing it completely in the glenoid fossa.
11. Insertion of infratemporal fossa retractor and further exposure of internal carotid artery by removal of styloid process and tympanic bone covering carotid foramen.

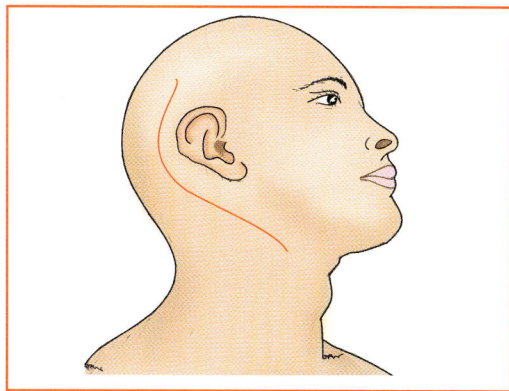

Fig. 98.2: Showing incision for type A approach

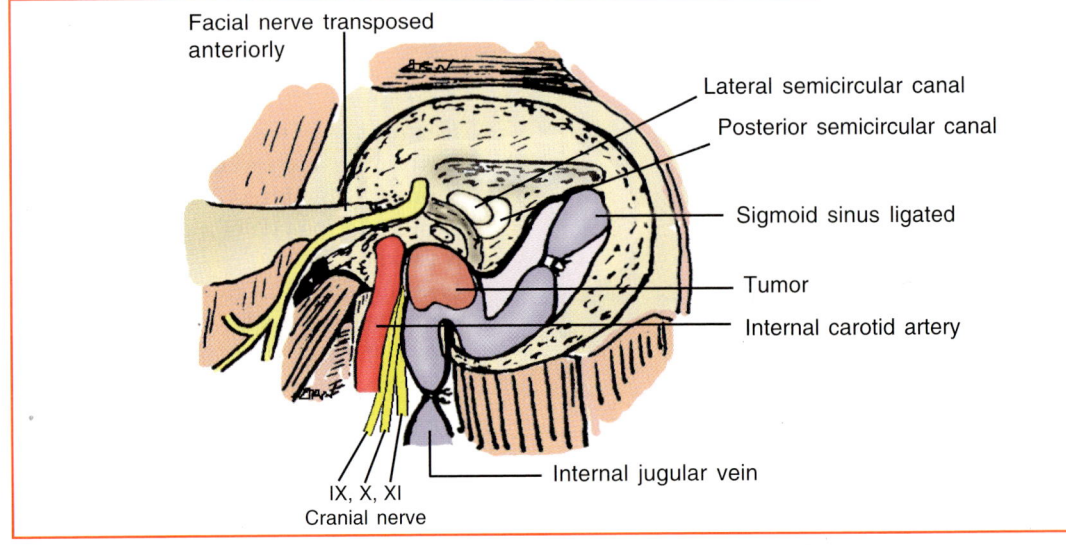

Facial nerve transposed anteriorly

Lateral semicircular canal

Posterior semicircular canal

Sigmoid sinus ligated

Tumor

Internal carotid artery

Internal jugular vein

IX, X, XI Cranial nerve

Fig. 98.3: Fisch Infratemporal fossa approach type - A

12. Mobilization of tumor poles anteriorly from carotid artery, superiorly from otic capsule, posteriorly from sigmoid sinus.

13. Separation of cranial nerves DC. X, XI from tumor surface if not infiltrated. Nerves are sacrificed if infiltrated.

14. Intracranial intradural extension upto 2 cm can be removed.

15. Any extension larger than 2 cm. is left in situ for later neurosurgical removal.

Type B Approach

Type B approach provides access to the greater part of the clivus except for a small posterior area around the margin of the foramen magnum, which can be reached more easily by the type A approach. The Surgical steps include: (Figs 98.3 and 98.5)

1. C shaped skin incision in the post-auricular region as shown in the (Fig. 98.4).

2. Elevation of the skin flap and blind sac closure of the external auditory canal.

3. Identification of the facial nerve in the retromandibular fossa and dissection peripherally upto second division.

4. Division of the zygomatic arch and mobilization with the attached masseter muscle and the temporalis muscle freed from their bony origin.

5. Subtotal petrosectomy as in type A.

6. Drilling of the glenoid fossa and disarticulation of TM joint

7. Retraction of mandibular condyle and drilling of the tympanic bone lateral and anterior to the internal carotid artery.

8. Detachment of cartilaginous portion of the eustachian tube from the infratemporal horizontal portion and exposure of the foramen lacerum.

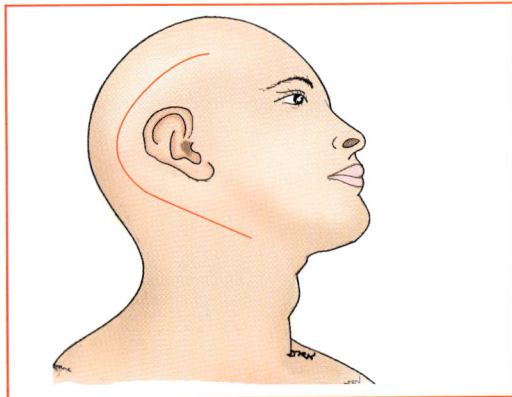

Fig. 98.4: Incision for type B and C approach

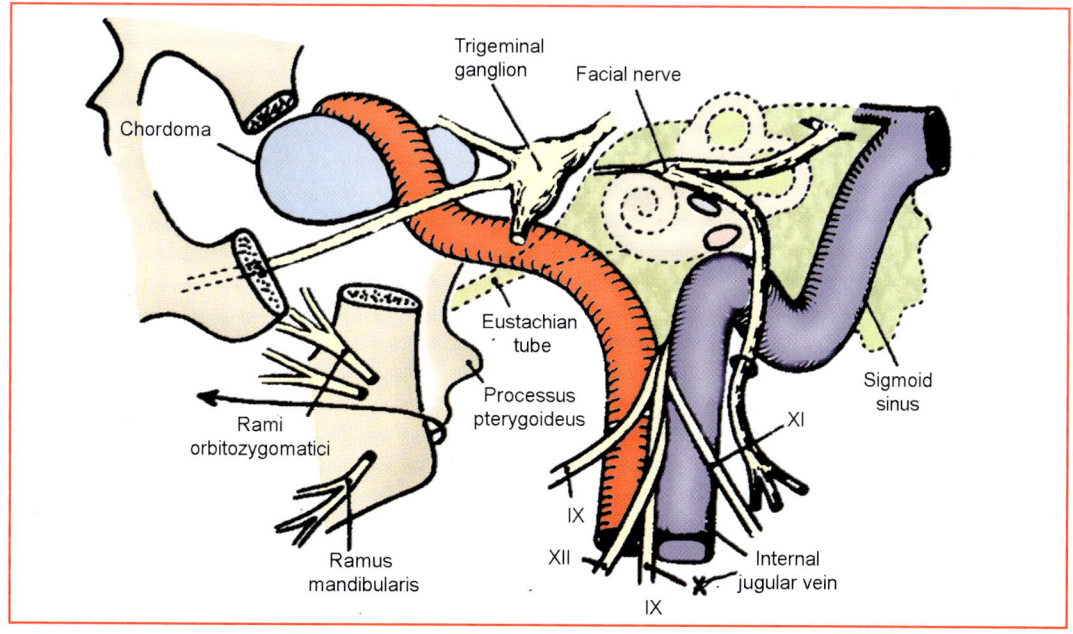

Fig. 98.5: Fisch infratemporal fossa approach type -B

9. Division of mandibular nerve and middle meningeal artery after coagulation.
10. Drilling of the eroded bone until firm bone or dura is reached.
11. Mobilization of internal carotid artery from the carotid foramen to the horizontal portion.
12. Separation of the tumor mass from the adventia of internal carotid artery under direct vision and removal of tumor.
13. Closure of the wound after wiring of the zygomatic arch.

Type C Approach

An anterior extension of the type B approach and permits access to the lesions of the nasopharynx, pterygo maxillary fossa, the eustachian tube, parasellar region, sphenoid sinus and the maxillary sinus.

Surgical Steps

1. Initial steps as in type B.

2. Zygomatic arch is divided as far forward as possible and can include lateral orbital margin if necessary.
3. Detachment of the upper head of the lateral pterygoid muscle to expose lateral pterygoid plate.
4. Removal of both the pterygoid plates and sectioning of maxillary division anterior to foramen rotundum.
5. Following of the internal carotid artery as far as cavernous sinus.
6. Entering of pterygomaxillary fossa and division of vidian nerve.
7. Exposure of the maxillary sinus, nasopharynx and sphenoid sinus.
8. Removal of the tumor after separation of the vital structures.
9. Malignant lesions should be removed en block along with eustachian tube, the levator and tensor palati muscles, pharyngobasilar fascia and the pterygoid muscles.

Instruments
and Radiology

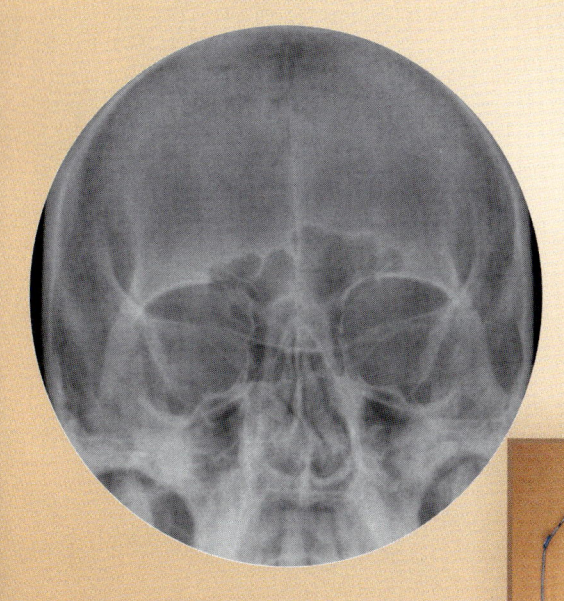

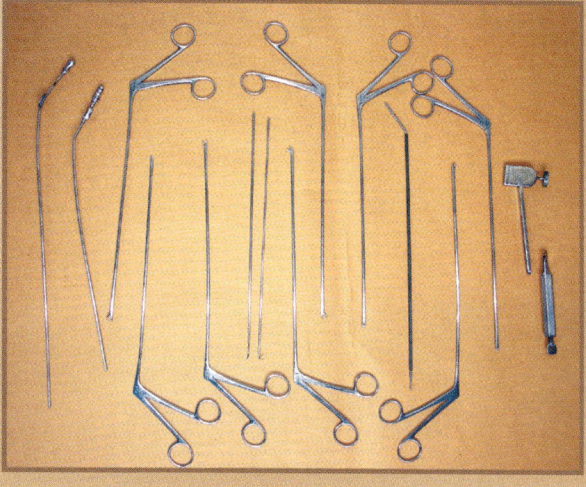

99

Instruments

- Instruments for nose and PNS
- Instruments in oral cavity and throat
- Instruments used in tonsillectomy and adenoidectomy
- Tracheostomy instruments
- Instruments used in examination and surgery of ear
- Instruments to perform oral endoscopy
- Basic surgical instruments for neck surgery
- General surgical instruments for head and neck surgery
- Instrument/implant for laryngotracheal stenosis

INSTRUMENTS FOR NOSE AND PNS

1. Nasal Speculums:
   A. Thudicum's
   B. Pilcher's
   C. Vienna
   D. Cardiff or Owen's
   E. Killian's (Long Bladed Self-Retaining)
   F. Alexander's
2. St. Clair Thomson posterior rhinoscopic mirror
3. Nasal Dressing Forceps:
   A. Tilley's
   B. Hartmann's
   C. Cawthorne's
   D. Jensen's (Bayonet shaped thumbforceps)
   E. Angular spring dressing forceps.

4. Tilley-Lichwitz' antral trocar and cannula
5. Higginson's rubber syringe
6. Tilley's antral harpoon
7. Myle's Nasoantral perforator
8. Tilley's antral burr
9. Walsham's forceps
10. Asche's septum forceps
11. Freer's double ended elevator
12. Killian's nasal gouge
13. Ballinger's swivel knife
14. Mallet (Heerman)
15. Turbinectomy scissors (Heymann)
16. Luc's nasal forceps
17. Irwin Moore's nasal forceps
18. Takahashi nasal forceps.
19. Suction tubes (Figs 99.1a to c)
    (a) Frazier's suction tube angular straight
    (b) vEcken nasal suction tube curved
    (c) vEcken antrum canula
    (d) Bannon suction tube picture (Fig. 99.1d).

    Uses: Used for all types of nasal surgeries to keep the operating field clean and bloodless. Also sucks away all the secretions.

20. Nasal Endoscope (Hopkins): 30 degree, 0 degree (Fig. 99.2)

    Uses: Nasal endoscopes are used to visualize the interior of the nasal cavity and the osteomeatal complex in middle meatus to identify the abnormalities and to treat them by doing endoscopic sinus surgery.

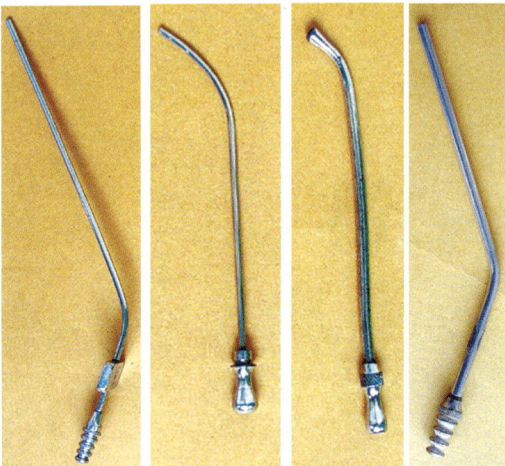

Fig. 99.1: (a) Frazier's suction tube angular straight (b) vEcken nasal suction tube curved (c) vEcken antrum cannula (d) Bannon suction tube picture

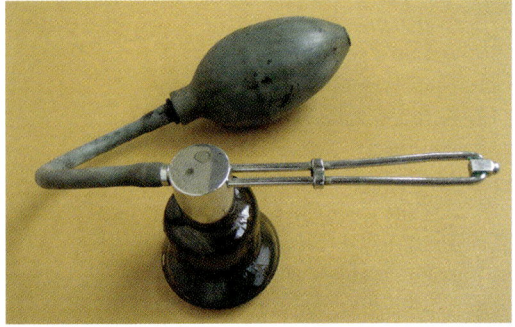

Fig. 99.3: Automizer for nasal medication and surface anesthesia

The steps of the surgery are:
a. Infundibulotomy /Uncinectomy
b. Middle meatal antrostomy and anterior ethmoidectomy
c. Clearance of the frontal recess
d. Posterior ethmoidectomy
e. Sphenoidotomy.

21. Atomizer (OHM's) (Fig. 99.3)

Uses: To spray surface anesthetic drugs like lignocaine into the nasal cavity before any local procedure. It can be used to spray with

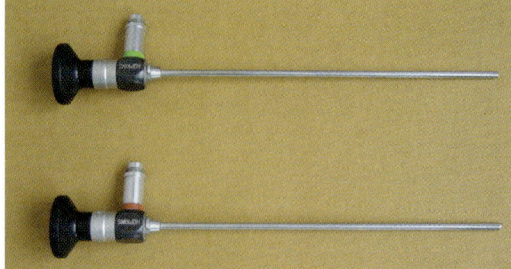

Fig. 99.2: Hopkin's nasal endoscope

decongestant for proper clinical examination especially in the nose.

NASAL SPECULUMS

Thudicum's Nasal Speculum

Thuidcum's nasal speculum is made up of stainless steel (Fig. 99.4).

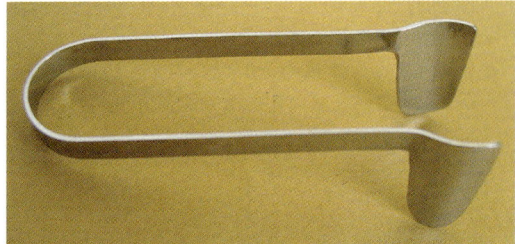

Fig. 99.4: Thudicum's nasal speculum

Parts

A U-shaped holding part with curved blunt blades directed at right angles to the U handle.

Method of holding: It is held over the hooked index finger of the non-dominant hand. Blades are closed by compression between middle and ring finger.

Uses

Diagnostic

Anterior rhinoscopy to observe:
- Nasal septum
- Little's area

- Lateral wall of the nose
- Floor of the nose

Therapeutic
- Removal of foreign bodies
- Antral wash
- For initial step of polypectomy, SMR and septoplasty.

Vienna Nasal Speculum (Fig. 99.5)

Parts: Handle, blades and a cross action joint.

Uses: Same as that of Thudicum's nasal speculum, but it is more handy.

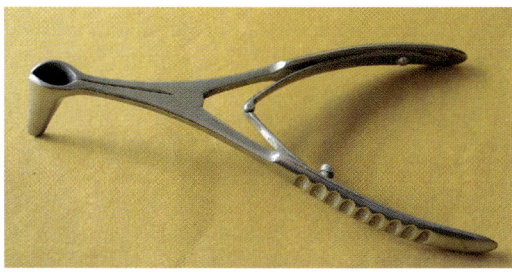

Fig. 99.5: Vienna's nasal speculum

Pilcher's Nasal Speculum (Fig. 99.6)

Parts: Designed as that of Vienna's but of smaller size.

Uses: Anterior rhinoscopic examination of children and also in adults.

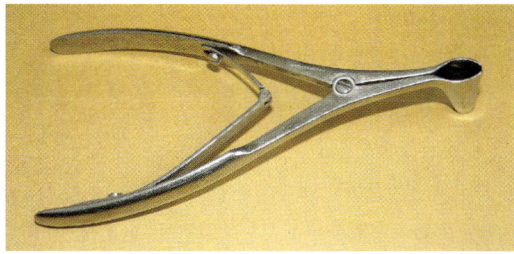

Fig. 99.6: Pilcher's nasal speculum

Killian's Long Bladed Self retaining Nasal Speculum (Fig. 99.7)

It is similar to Vienna's type but has got long nasal blades and a screw for self-retaining. Used only

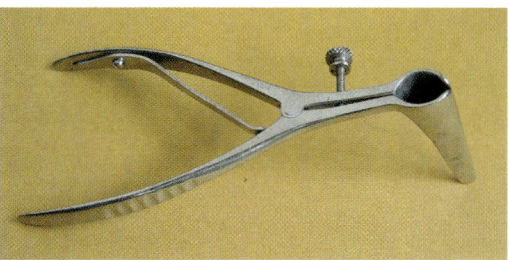

Fig. 99.7: Killian's long bladed self retaining nasal speculum

after anesthetizing patients nasal mucosa otherwise procedures will be painful.

Uses

Diagnostic to examine the deeper structures of the nasal cavity including middle meatus.

Therapeutic
1. Use in SMR and septoplasty to retract the mucoperiosteum
2. Polypectomy
3. Foreign body removal
4. Anterior nasal packing
5. Excision of rhinosporidiosis.

Advantages
- Self retaining mechanism.
- Blades are adjustable and fixed in particular position with the help of screw, during the operation causing less strain to surgeons hand.

St. Clair Thomson's Posterior Rhinoscopic Mirror (Fig. 99.8)

Parts: Handle, curved shaft, and a mirror at an angle.

Method of Posterior Rhinoscopy

Ask the patient to take nose breathing and depress the tongue with a tongue blade. Hold the instrument like a pen and gently pass behind the soft palate. The following parts are visualized.

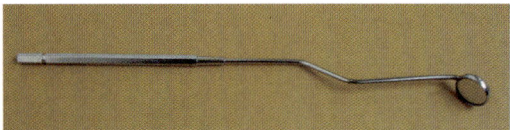

Fig. 99.8: St. Clair Thomson's posterior rhinoscopic mirror

Posterior ends of septum and turbinates, meati, choanae, nasopharynx and eustachian tube orifices.

Uses

Diagnostic

- To examine the postnasal space to rule out inflammatory and neoplastic diseases.
- To look for any residual disease after surgical excision.

Therapeutic: Occasionally used as an adjunct in tumor surgery like excision of rhinosporidiosis, angiofibroma.

Tilley's Nasal Dressing Forceps
(Fig. 99.9)

Parts

Two ring shaped finger grip handles and two long slender blades with transverse serrations at flat straight tip.

It has a bend, so that hand of the surgeon does not obscure the view of nasal cavities.

Uses

- For nasal packing
- Removal of foreign bodies
- For inserting cottonoids.

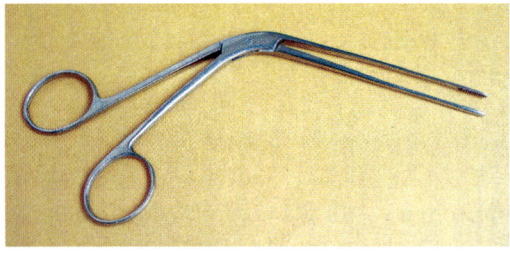

Fig. 99.9: Tilley's nasal dressing forceps

Hartmann's Nasal Dressing Forceps

- Shape of that tip is larger, oval and serrated

Uses: Similar to that of Tilley's nasal dressing forceps.

Tilley-Lichwitz Antral Trocar and Cannula
(Fig. 99.10)

Parts

- Handle with long pointed end and
- Cannula with a connecting end for irrigation syringe.

Uses: Diagnostic known as proof puncture to see pus in sinusitis, blood in hemoantrum, cytology for antral malignancy

Therapeutic

- Chronic maxillary sinusitis not responding to the conservative treatment.
- Instillation of medicine
- Aspiration of pus
- Oroantal fistula.

Method of Antral Puncture

It is done in the inferior meatus 1cm behind the anterior end of inferior turbinate, directing the trocar with the cannula, towards the outer canthus of ipsilateral eye, (under local / general anesthesia).

Complications

- Nasal mucosa laceration
- Soft tissue injury of the cheek
- Orbital injury
- Air embolism
- Hemorrhage

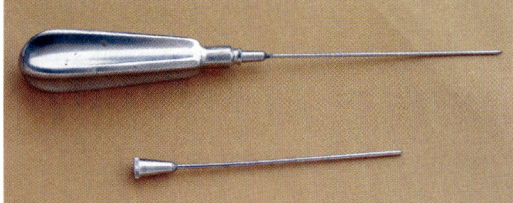

Fig. 99.10: Tilley-Lichwitz antral trocar and cannula

- Vasovagal attack
- Injury to the posterior wall of maxilla (pterygopalatine fossa).

Contraindications

- Acute infections and bleeding diathesis
(All instruments made of stainless steel unless otherwise stated).

Higginson's Syringe (Fig. 99.11)

Parts

It consists of rubber bulb of capacity around 30oz with tubes on either ends. One end has a valve to allow water into the bulb, other end fits to the antral puncture cannula.

Uses

- Antral wash.
  (Irrigation should be continued till clear washings come out).
- Nasal cavity irrigation in atrophic rhinitis.

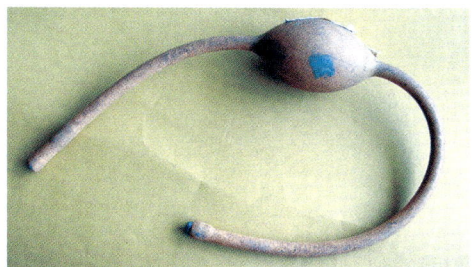

Fig. 99.11: Higginson's syringe

Tilley's Antral Harpoon (Fig. 99.12)

Uses

To perforate the maxillary antrum through the inferior meatus for inferior meatal antrostomy.

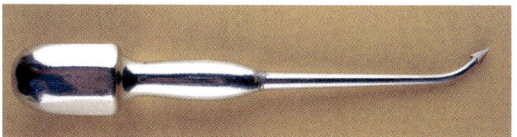

Fig. 99.12: Tilley's Antral Harpoon

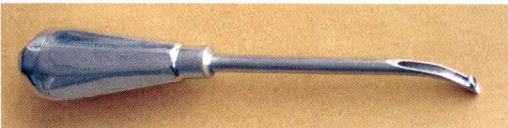

Fig. 99.13: Myle's nasoantral perforator

Myle's Nasoantral Perforator (99.13)

Uses

To perforate the maxillary antrum through the inferior meatus for inferior meatal antrostomy. It has a reverse cutting edge which helps to enlarge the antrostomy site after perforating the antrum.

Tilleys Antral Burr

Uses to make the antrostomy site smooth after perforating the antrum with antral harpoon.

Walsham's Forceps (Fig. 99.14)

Parts

Handle, blades with flat and blunt tips and a screw joint.

Uses

For disimpaction of fractured nasal bones. Rubber covering of the tip prevents injury to the skin.

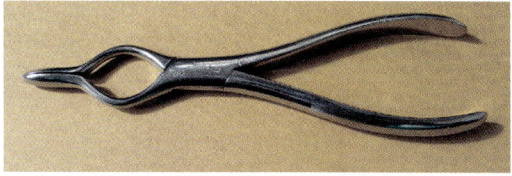

Fig. 99.14: Walsham's forceps

Asche's Septal Forceps (Fig. 99.15)

Parts

Similar to Walsham's forceps but both the blades are curved to enclose a space when blades are closed, so to prevent crush injury to septum.

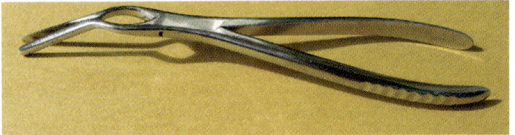

Fig. 99.15: Asche's septal forceps

Uses

To reposition the displaced septum following trauma. *Walsham* forceps. Used for disimpacting and reducing fractures of nasal bone.

Asche's septum forceps. Used for reducing fractures of nasal septum.

Freer's Elevator (Fig. 99.16)

It is a long slender instrument with central holding part and two curved flat ends. One end is sharp and the other is blunt.

Uses

For periosteal elevation

In septoplasty for mucoperichondrial and mucoperiosteal elevation.

In Functional Endoscopic Sinus Surgery (FESS) to identify uncinate process, middle meatal opening and bulla.

To separate temporalis fascia in myringoplasty operation.

Killian's Nasal Gouge (Fig. 99.17)

It is a bayonet shaped instrument with a grooved cutting edge at one end. Other end is flat.

The bend of the instrument offers better field of vision.

Uses

For reduction of spur, by engaging it in the groove of the cutting edge and gouging.

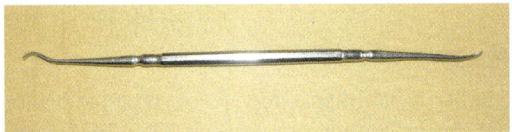

Fig. 99.16: Freer's elevator

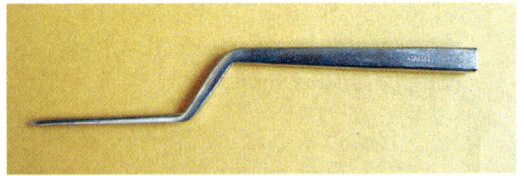

Fig. 99.17: Killian's nasal gouge

Mallet (Heermann) (Fig. 99.18)

Parts

Handle, shaft, and a non-reflecting head (light weight).

Uses

To give gentle blows on the gouge, during spur removal and osteotomy for rhinoplasty and other procedures.

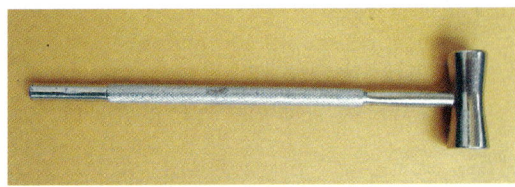

Fig. 99.18: Mallet (Heermann)

Ballenger's Swivel Knife (Fig. 99.19)

Parts

Handle, shaft, and a bipronged tip with cutting knife.

Knife can revolve through 360 degrees. So it can be positioned without rotating the instrument.

Uses

Submucous resection. To cut the cartilage, but not the bone.

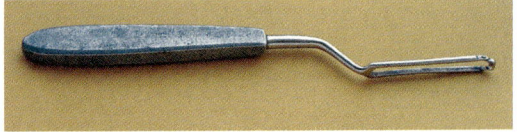

Fig. 99.19: Ballenger's swivel knife

Heymann's Turbinectomy Scissors (Fig. 99.20)

It has a bend at the center with narrow stout blades and blunt tip.

Uses

- For partial and total inferior turbinectomy
- For septal spurectomy (Endoscopic)

Advantages

The bend of the scissors, offers better field of vision.

Luc's Forceps (Fig. 99.21)

It has got a long arm and a short arm for better grip. The forceps has got a bend.

Uses

- Septoplasty for removal of bony septum

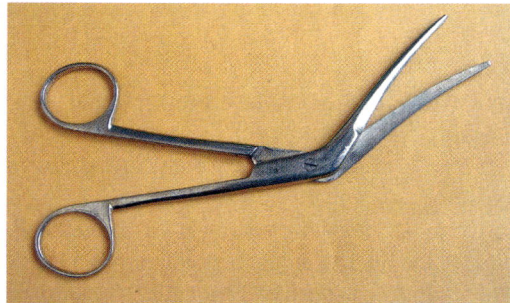

Fig. 99.20: Heymann's turbinectomy scissors

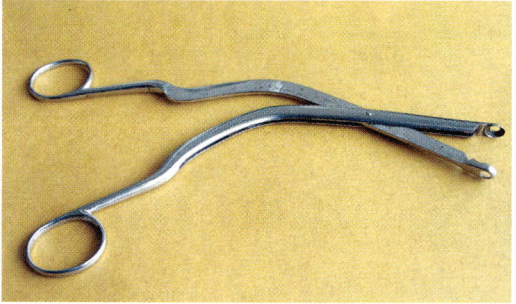

Fig. 99.21: Luc's forceps

- SMR for removal of cartilaginous and bony septum
- As a substitute for tonsil holding forceps
- To remove left over tags after adenoidectomy.
- To remove polyps
- Punch biopsy
- Punch biopsy
- Excision of angiofibroma and other benign tumor.

Irwin Moore's Forceps (Fig. 99.22)

Same as Luc's forceps, as it is fine and slender. It can be easily manipulated within the nasal cavity, for various surgical procedures.

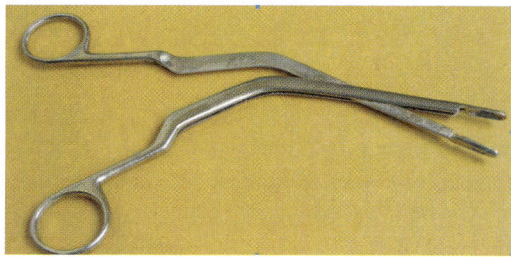

Fig. 99.22: Irwin Moore's forceps

Uses same as Luc's: Can be used for all kind of nasal surgery including angiofibroma excision.

Rhinoforce Takahashi Nasal Forceps (Fig. 99.23)

Working length of this straight forceps is 10 cm. Used for all types of endoscopic procedures like FESS, septoplasty and even endoscopic adenoidectomy.

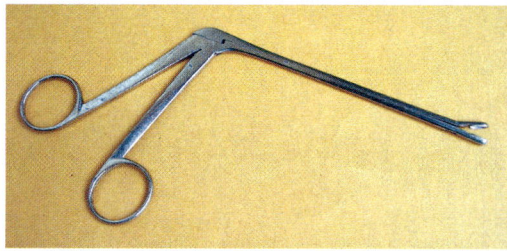

Fig. 99.23: Rhinoforce Takahashi nasal forceps

Blakesly Nasal Forceps Straight and 45 degrees Upturned (Fig. 99.24)

Various types of Blakesly forceps are cutting forceps available like straight, 30° upturn, 45° upturn, 70° upturn, 90° upturn in different sizes. They are used in endoscopic sinus surgeries for grasping and removal of tissue including polyps.

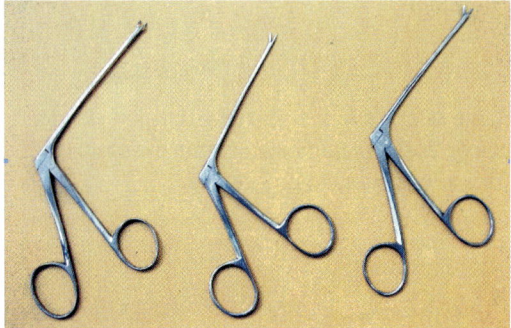

Fig. 99.24: Straight 45° upturned Blakesly nasal forceps are used for endoscopic sinus surgery specifically to excenterate the ethmoidal cells and to remove polyps

Stammbergers antrum punch forceps with backward cutting-right and left, upward and downward (Fig. 99.25)

It is used to enlarge the maxillary ostium while performing endoscopic middle meatal antrostomy.

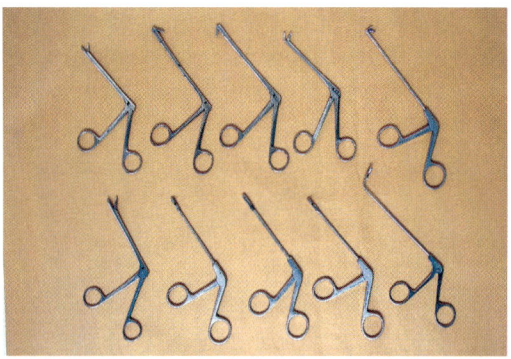

Fig. 99.25: Stammbergers antrum punch forceps with backward cutting-right and left, upward and downward

Hajek's Punch Forceps (Fig. 99.26)

It is used for removal of bone during antrostomy, Caldwell-Luc procedure, transpalatal approach, trans-sphenoidal approach, endoscopic Dacro Cysto Rhinostomy (DCR).

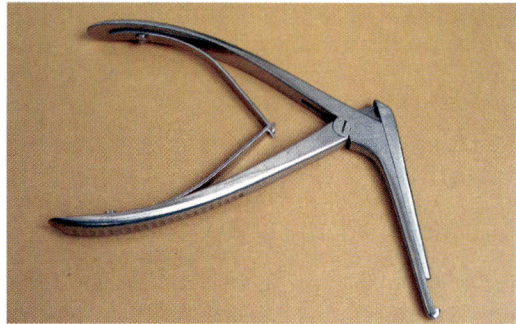

Fig. 99.26: Hajek's punch forceps

INSTRUMENTS IN ORAL CAVITY AND THROAT

Lack's Tongue Depressor (Fig. 99.27)

It's a plain variety of tongue depressor (other being Doughty type).

It's a 'L' shaped instrument with flat and curved ends.

Examiner holds the instrument at curved end, placing the flat end at junction anterior two thirds and posterior one third of the tongue (if anterior to this position a bulge will prevent proper visualization, if posterior it will initiate gag reflex).

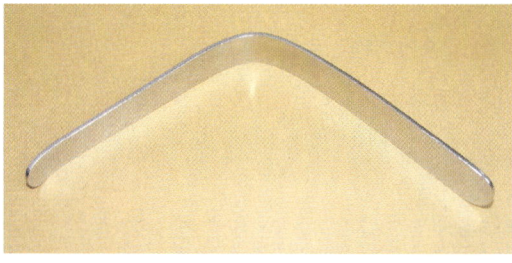

Fig. 99.27: Lack's tongue depressor

Uses

- Examination of oral cavity and oropharynx
- For posterior-rhinoscopy (as an adjunct)
- Cold spatula test.
- Check postnasal bleeding.
- Cheek retraction
- Checking out for loose-teeth
- During intraoral surgical procedures.
- Soft-palate retraction using curved end.

Other types

l Flat variety made of either steel or plastic.
l Glass tongue depressor.

Yankauer's Suction Cannula (Fig. 99.28)

Used to remove blood clot from the operating field during tonsillectomy adenoidectomy and oral and oropharyngeal surgeries.

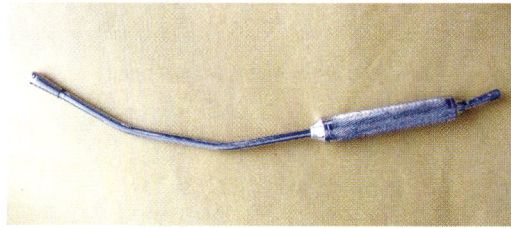

Fig. 99.28: Yankauer's suction cannula

Indirect-laryngoscopic Mirror
(Fig. 99.29)

Parts

Handle, shaft and a mirror, at an angle.

Method of Examination

Ask the patient to take mouth breathing, the mirror is warmed/dipped in savlon solution. Hold the instrument like a pen, pull the patient's tongue out and gently introduce into oral cavity, place it against soft palate and uvula without touching the posterior pharyngeal wall, to prevent gagging.

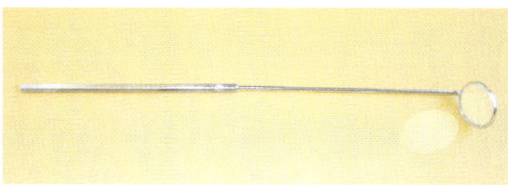

Fig. 99.29: Indirect-laryngoscopic mirror

Uses

Diagnostic

Examination of tongue base, valleculae, glossoepiglottic folds, pharyngoepiglottic folds, laryngeal inlet, vocal cords and pyriform fossae to rule out any foreign body, inflammatory and non inflammatory, neoplastic lesions.

Therapeutic

- To remove foreign body
- To give local anesthesia
- To take tissue from the growth for histo-pathological examination.

Prognostic

Post irradiated cases for evaluation of recurrences.

Rigid Telescope (70 Degree) (Fig. 99.30)

Parts: Light source
Fiberoptic cable.
Telescope: Eye-piece
Handle
Lens barrel.

Uses: Same as ILS examination

Extra advantages are:

- Better field of vision, magnification and illumination.
- Can be connected to a camera and monitor so that patient can see the images, which can be recorded for documentation and comparison.

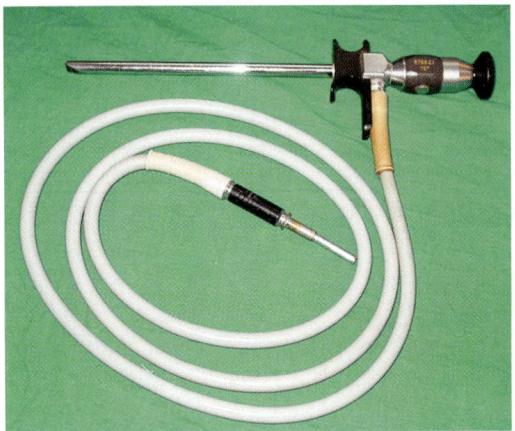

Fig. 99.30: Rigid Telescope (70 degree)

Doyen's Mouth Gag (Fig. 99.31)

Parts

Ring shaped finger grips with CROSS action joint and ratchet lock.

2 blades with curved tips. Covered with rubber caps.

Uses

To keep mouth open during intraoral procedures like glossectomy, soft-palate surgery, uvulopaltop-haryngoplasty, tongue-tie release, salivary gland calculi removal, dental surgeries, etc. Intraoral toilet in unconscious patients. To aid jaw movement in TMJ fibrosis/false ankylosis. To prevent tongue bite in epileptics.

Hajek's Cheek Retractor (Fig. 99.32)

It is an S-shaped instrument with smooth curved part-for cheek retraction and a right-angled part-for upper lip retraction.

The shape of the instrument confers the architecture of the face, so that assistant's hand does not obscure the view of surgeon.

Uses

Lip and cheek retraction during Caldwel-luc's and maxillectomy operations.

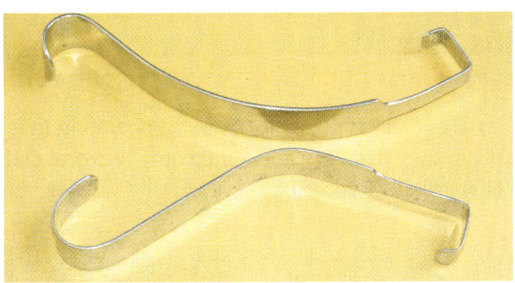

Fig. 99.32: Hajek's cheek retractor

INSTRUMENT USED IN TONSILLECTOMY AND ADENOIDECTOMY

I. Clar's; Head Light (Fig. 99.33)

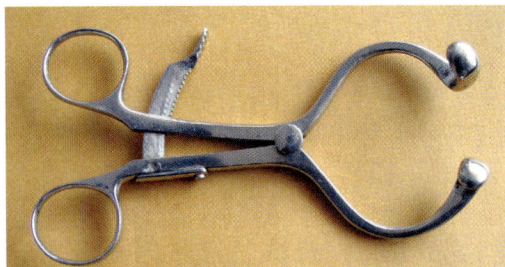

Fig. 99.31: Doyen's mouth gag

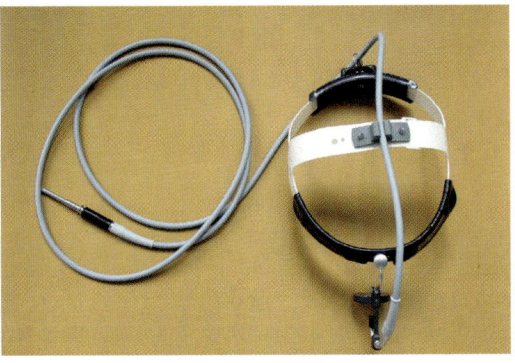

Fig. 99.33: Clar's; Head Light

II. Mouth Gag (Boyle-Davis)

Mouth gag consisting of two parts (Fig. 99.34):

1. Tongue bladem (by Boyle an anaesthesiology)
2. Jaw piece (Davis mouth gag)

Uses

(a) In dissection method of tonsillectomy
(c) Operations of the palate and the nasopharynx
(c) Operation in the pharynx
(d) Adenoidectomy
(e) Craniovertebral anomalies

Complications

Injury to the incisor tooth, injury to the lip and angle of mouth.

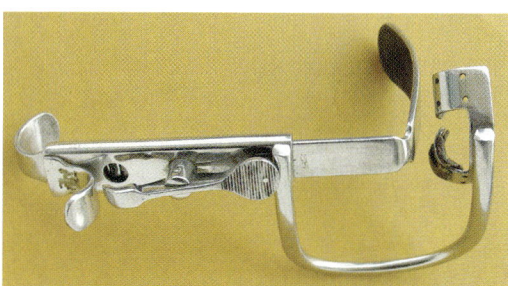

Fig. 99.34: Mouth gag

III. Draffin's Metallic Bipod Stand (Fig. 99.35)

Consists of two stands with ring to adjust the height.

Uses

To fix the Boyle-Davis Mouth gag to the operation table.

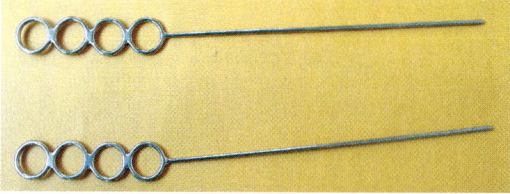

Fig. 99.35: Draffin's metallic Bipod stand

During tonsillectomy and other operations in the throat but not used in adenoidectomy operation to prevent excessive extension in the atlanto-occipital joint preventing atlanto-occipital joint dislocation.

IV. Denis Browne Tonsil Holding Forceps (Fig. 99.36)

- Has got a box joint, angular instrument
- Two sizes: Large and small
- Used to hold tonsil and pull inwardly during dissection method of tonsillectomy. Because of its special configuration less tissue trauma while holding the tonsil.

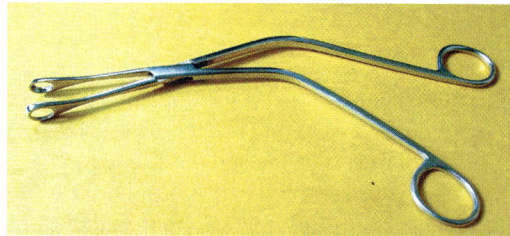

Fig. 99.36: Denis Browne Tonsil holding forceps

V. Waugh's Long Dissecting Forceps

Used during dissection of tonsils. It can also be used in catching bleeding points and putting swabs.

VI. Mollison's tonsil Dissector and Anterior Pillar Retractor (Fig. 99.37)

Double ended, one for retraction of anterior pillar, other for dissection.

Uses: In tonsillectomy (dissection method).

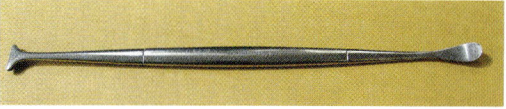

Fig. 99.37: Mollison's tonsil dissector and anterior pillar retractor

Pillar retractor used in the beginning of tonsillectomy to visualize the tonsil specially in fibrosed tonsil. Anterior pillar retractor will give a better view of the tonsil to grasp the tissue with tonsil holding forceps. Also same part of the instrument is used after tonsillectomy to retract the anterior pillar to visualize the bleeding point or to see the remnant of tonsillar tissue. The dissecting part is used to dissect the tonsil out of tonsillar fossa after the mucosal incision.

VII. Gwynne Evan's Tonsil Dissector

Double ended one side serrated the other side blunt, used in dissection tonsillectomy.

IX. Tonsillar Snare (Eve's) (Fig. 99.38)

A loop is attached at one end has Ratchet action where as other end has a thumb ring for better grip.

Uses: To snare out the lower pole of the tonsil at the end of dissection method. Advantage of using the snare to resect the tonsil is to minimize the bleeding by crushing the vascular pedicle not cutting unlike scissors. It also helps in coagulation by release of tissue thromboplastin a factor useful in pathway of coagulation cascade.

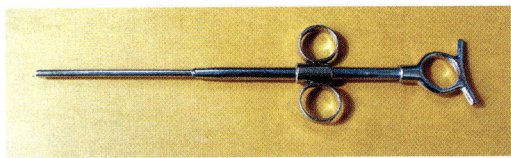

Fig. 99.38: Tonsillar snare (Eve's)

X. Tonsillar Knife (Fig. 99.39)

It is a sickle knife made of steel.

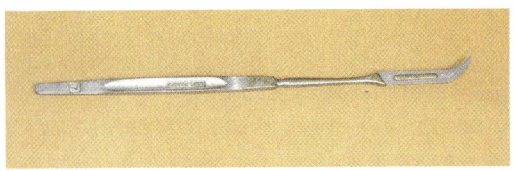

Fig. 99.39: Tonsillar Knife

Uses: For mucosal incision at the upper pole of tonsil during the beginning of tonsillectomy.

XI. Tonsillar Artery Forceps (Birkett's) (Fig. 99.40)

Long, slender straight artery forceps

Uses: To catch bleeding point along with a smaller tissue at the depth of tonsillar fossa. Because it is long and slender, provides a better view.

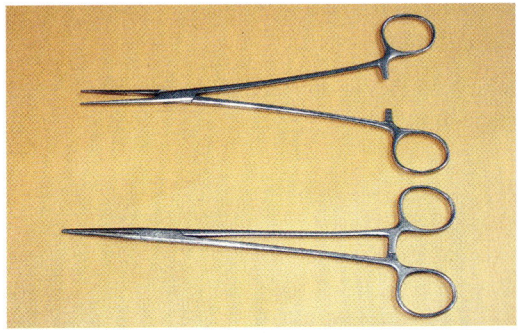

Fig. 99.40: Tonsillar artery forceps (Birkett's)

XII. Negus's Artery Forceps (replacement forceps) (Fig. 99.41)

It has a curved tip.

Uses: Use to replace the straight artery forceps after grasping the soft tissue around the tip of straight artery forceps. Because of curved tip, it is easier to slip the knot around it for ligating the bleeding vessel at a depth and ligature will not slip out during tying due to its curved tip.

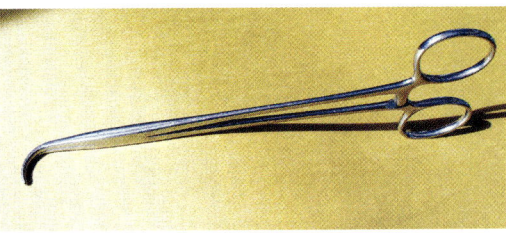

Fig. 99.41: Negus's artery forceps (replacement forceps)

XIII. Wilson's Artery Forceps (Fig. 99.42)

Long artery forceps with angulation in the middle and curved tip. Same as the Negus's artery forceps, not popular.

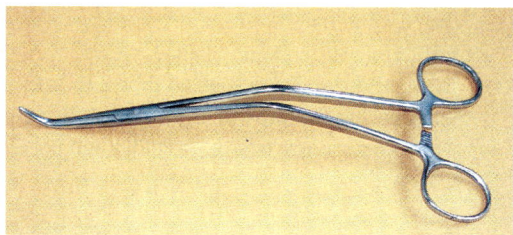

Fig. 99.42: Wilson's artery forceps

XIV. Negus's Ligature Slipper or Knot Tier (Fig. 99.43)

Uses: Helps to slip the ligature over the tip of Negus's forceps during ligation of vessels in the tonsillar bed.

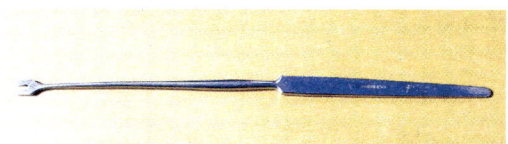

Fig. 99.43: Negus's ligature slipper or knot tier

XV. Peritonsillar Abscess (Quincy) Forceps (St. Clair Thompson) (Fig. 99.44)

It has a sharpened and angulated body.

Uses: Acts both as knife for incision and forceps to dilate the incision in peritonsillar abscess drainage.

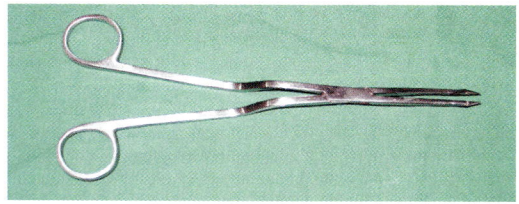

Fig. 99.44: Peritonsillar abscess forceps (St. Clair Thompson)

XVI. Adenoid Curette (St. Clair Thompson) (Fig. 99.45)

Two varieties: 1. With cage 2. Without cage

Available in 6 sizes approximately 8, 10, 12, 14, 16 and 18 mm blade.

Uses: It is used in adenoidectomy operation. The instrument is held in dagger holding fashion. The cage will prevent the tissue from slipping into the nasopharynx or larynx. The one without cage is used to remove tissue around the eustachian tube as the cage can injure the E-tube. While doing adenoidectomy neck of the patient should be flexed to avoid atlanto-occipital joint subluxation. Another precaution to avoid injury is to bring the adenoid tissue by a palpating finger from lateral wall to the midline at the onset of surgery and keeping line of dissection strictly in the midline.

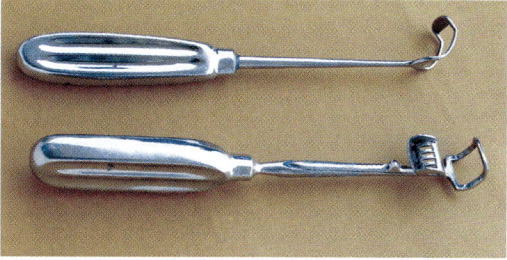

Fig. 99.45 Adenoid curette (St. Clair Thompson)

TRACHEOSTOMY INSTRUMENTS

1.Tracheal Hooks (Fig. 99.46)

Sharp and blunt

Parts

Handle and curved tip

Uses: Blunt hook is used to retract the isthmus of thyroid gland to expose tracheal wall

Sharp hook is used to retract cricoid cartilage by hooking at its lower border to stabilize trachea before making incision.

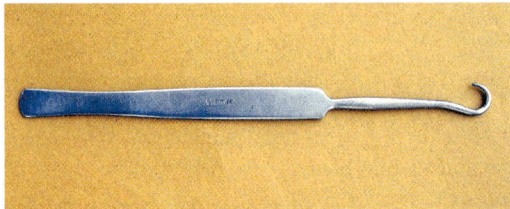

Fig. 99.46: Tracheal hooks

2. Trousseau's Tracheal Dilator
(Fig. 99.47)

Parts : It is similar to curved artery forceps, but Stout, cross action blades without lock mechanism (in case of an artery forceps while closing the handle the tip closes , but in dilator the tip opens , while closing the handle. Blades are curved with blunted tips (atraumatic).

Uses: For dilatation of tracheostomy opening at surgery to facilitate insertion of tracheostomy tube and also during tracheostomy tube changing.

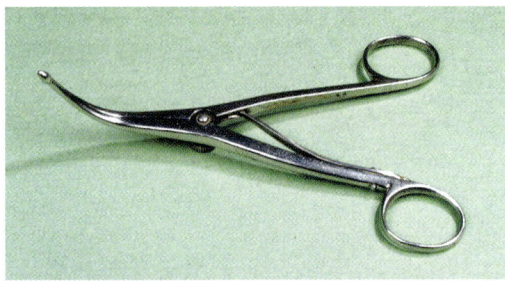

Fig. 99.47: Trousseau's tracheal dilator

3. Portex Tracheostomy Tube Cuffed/ Non-cuffed (Fig. 99.48)

Parts: Tube with shield

Flanges for strapping to secure the tube in position. Cuff, with Pilot bulb externally to know the cuff status. Obturator for guiding the tube insertion.

Advantages of Portex tracheostomy tube

- Cuff helps to prevent aspiration in conditions like vocal cord paralysis, comatose patients, etc.
- Cuff helps in positive pressure ventilation by preventing air leak around the tube
- For delivering inhalation anaesthesia
- Both cuffed and non-cuffed tube can safely used during radiotherapy as indicated
- This tube is more trachea friendly and better tolerated.

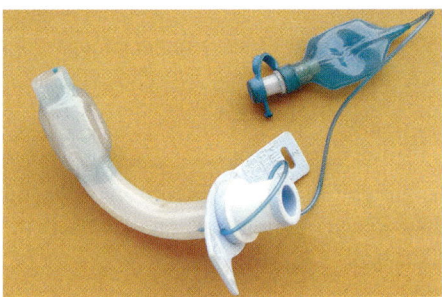

Fig. 99.48: Portex tracheostomy tube cuffed

4. Fuller's Tracheostomy Tube
(Fig. 99.49)

It is made of German silver.

Parts

Outer tube is bi-flanged and compressible. Inner tube is longer than outer tube with an opening in the back of the tube. This prevents obstruction of outer tube by the secretion and crusting. Inner tube can be easily taken out and cleaned and replaced.

Advantages

I. Acts as tracheal dilator as outer tube can be compressed. So tracheal dilator is not necessary while introducing this particular tube.

II. Opening in the back of the inner tube helps in
   - Phonation and re-education during decannulation

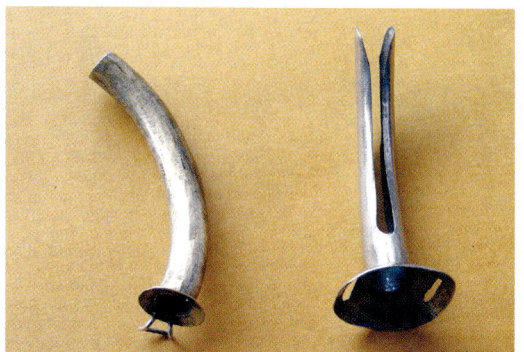

Fig. 99.49: Fuller's tracheostomy tube

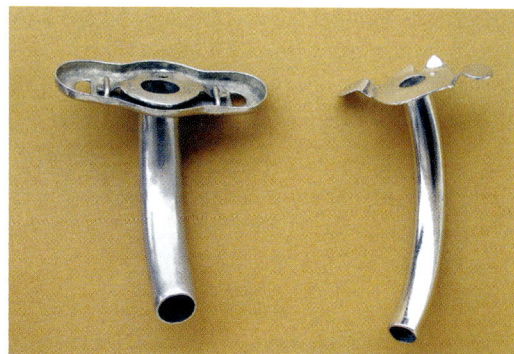

Fig. 99.50: Chevalier-Jackson's tracheostomy tube

- Patency of the airway above the tube can be checked by blocking the outer opening of tube
- Speaking valve can be used with the metal tube.

Disadvantages

- Flanges are weak and can break and become a foreign body in the bronchus.
- Flanges are sharp and can cause trauma to tracheal wall. (Tracheo innominate artery fistulas are reported following prolonged use of metal tubes)
- Cannot be used during radiotherapy.

5.Chevalier-Jackson's Tracheostomy Tube (Fig. 99.50)

Parts

It is made of German silver.

Outer tube	• Lock mechanism for inner tube • Holes on either side for straps • Shield for protection.
Inner tube	• Longer than outer tube to prevent outer tube blocking.
Obturator	• Guides the tube insertion.

Advantages

Speaking valve can be used with the metal tube.

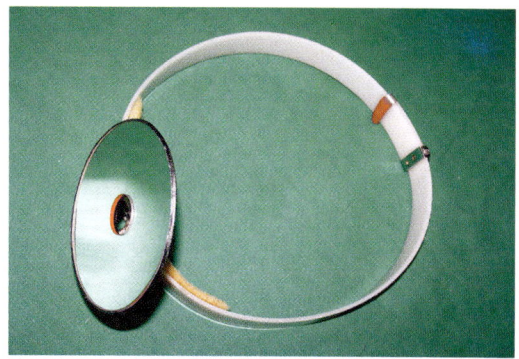

Fig. 99.51: Head mirror

Disadvantages

- Patient cannot phonate with tube in situ .
- Cannot be used during radiotherapy

INSTRUMENTS USED IN EXAMINATION AND SURGERY OF EAR

1. Head Mirror

Parts

Concave mirror
3 ½ inches in diameter
¾ inches in diameter round aperture
Fiber forehead band

Use: Has a focal length of 18 cm. Used to focus light from the bull's lamp. The distance between the bull's lamp and the examiner is about 30 cms.

2. The "Bull's Eye" Lamp (Fig. 99.52)

Gives an illumination of about 200 candle power without any image of the filament, and can be raised or lowered on the floor stand.

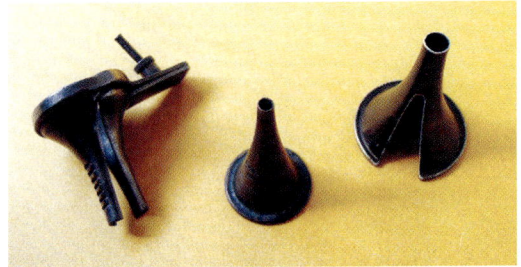

Fig. 99.53: Tonybee's ear speculum

Other varieties of Ear Speculum

1. Gruber
2. Heath
3. Yearsley's
4. Turner's
5. Tumarkins

4. Jobson Horne's Probe and Ring Curette (Fig. 99.54)

Parts: Has got a serrated end and ring curette at the other end.

Uses: Serrated probe end is used as cotton wool swab carrier to clean aural discharge. *To trace a sinus tract.* Curette is used to remove foreign body, wax, granulation tissue.

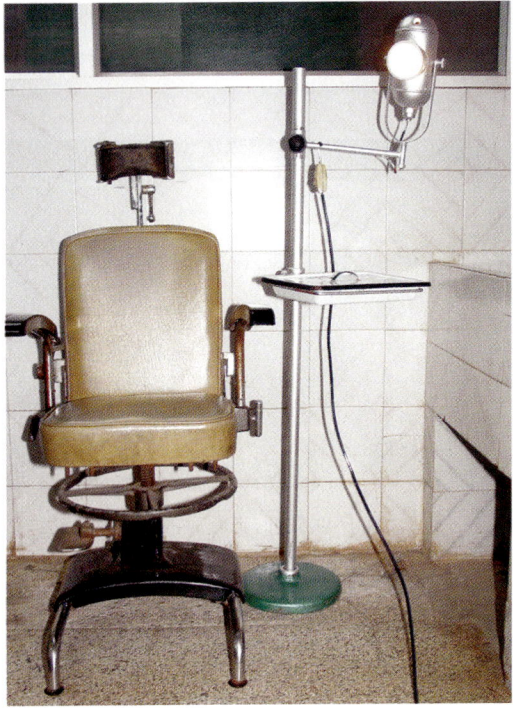

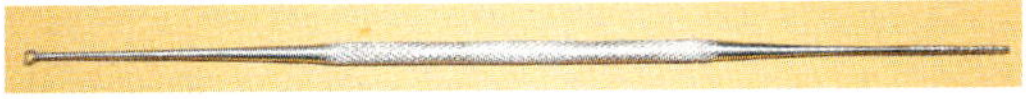

Fig. 99.52: The "Bull's Eye" lamp

Fig. 99.54 Jobson Horne's probe and ring curette

3. Toynbee's Ear Speculum (Fig. 99.53)

Comes in 3 sizes. Introduced by Sir William Wikk in 1844.

Uses

- In examination of ear
- In ear surgeries

5. Gardiner Browns Tuning Fork (Fig. 99.55)

History

In 1855 Heinrich Adolph Rinne (1819–1868) described the tuning fork test, which is still the best method for diagnosis of conductive versus sensori neural hearing loss.

Commonly used frequency in clinical examination: 256 Hz, 512 Hz, 1024 Hz

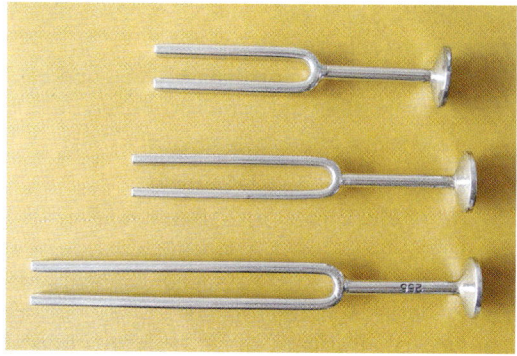

Fig. 99.55: Gardiner bBowns Tuning fork

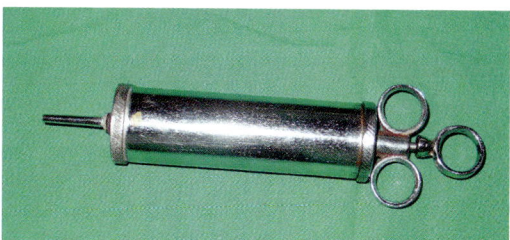

Fig. 99.56: Simpson's Aural Syringe

Parts

- Prongs
- Shoulder
  - l Base
  - l Stem
  - l Footplate

Uses: In tuning fork tests viz. Rinne's test, Weber's test, absolute bone conduction test.

Other types of Tuning Fork

- Hartman's
- Gradenigo's.

6. Simpson's Aural Syringe (Fig. 99.56)

- Is made up of metal (stainless steel)
- Has a capacity of 150 ml.
- Has two short pipes one bulbous and the other conical.

Uses

- Removal of FB
- Removal of wax
- In otitis externa to wash out fungal debris in case of otomycosis.
- What do you use for cleaning in syringing?
  Warm water at body temperature. Hot water causes burns, cold water causes caloric stimulation (vertigo).

Contraindication of Syringing.

- Perforated tympanic membrane
- Patients with history of head injury where there is possibility of temporal bone fracture / CSF otorrhea
- Hygroscopic foreign body

Technique

It is done in sitting position with the head bent to the side of the ear to be irrigated. A Macintosh drape has to be applied to the patient. To collect the irrigated fluid along with debris a kidney tray has to be placed over the shoulder. Pinna should be pulled upward outward and laterally and a jet of saline should be directed posterosuperiorly this is because posterosuperior meatal wall is shorter than anterior wall and floor.

Complications

- Vasovagal attack
- Injury to the external auditory canal and tympanic membrane
- The foreign body may get impacted.

Note

Suction and instrumentation under direct vision using an operating microscope is the safest method to remove foreign body or wax.

7. Rose Eustachian Tube Catheter (Fig. 99.57)

Metallic catheter with a curved proximal end and ring at its base. It is 12 to 15 cms in length.

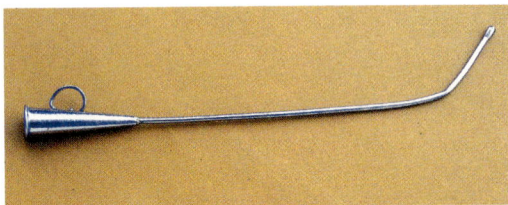

Fig. 99.57: Rose's Eustachian tube catheter

Uses

- To know the patency of the eustachian tube
- To inflate the middle ear
- To install medications to the middle ear
- Remove foreign body from the nose.
- Used as a suction cannula.

Note

Complications – Causes trauma to the Eustachian tube.

Other tests to evaluate Eustachian Tube Patency

- Valsalva maneuver
- Siegalization
- Politzerisation
- Toynbees maneuver
- Frenzels' maneuver
- Radiological evaluation–Basal or submento-Vertical view, salpingography, CT Scan, MRI
- Diagnostic nasal endoscopy.

Procedure of Catheterization

- Surface anesthesia by spraying 4 percent xylocaine.
- The catheter is passed with tip downward along the floor of nose till it reaches posterior wall of nasopharynx.
- Then tip is rotated 90 degree medially and withdrawn anteriorly till it touche's the posterior wall of nasal septum.
- Now catheter is rotated 180 degree laterally when tip of tube will be at the opening of Eustachian tube. By gentle manipulation of catheter at this stage will enable the examiner to enter the tube.

- Politzer bag is now attached to the catheter and air is insufflated.
- Sound heard in auscultation tube connected between patient and examiner, will give a clue to the status of Eustachian tube.

Inference

- Tubal block no insufflation sound can be heard.
- Partial block bubbling sound will be heard.
- Stenosis: Whistling sound.
- Normal insufflated air can be heard clearly.

Complication of the Procedure

- Excessive pain
- Epistaxis
- Syncope

8. Aural Dressing Forceps (Fig. 99.58)

- Hermann's aural forceps
- Tilleys aural forceps
- Henter tods aural forceps
- Heath's forceps

Uses

- In dressing and introduction of medicated pack in the external auditory canal
- Removal of foreign body and crust from EAC.

9. Agnew's Myringotome is also known as Politzer's myringotome

History

Named after Adam Potitzer (1835–1920) foremost teacher of otologic diagnosis, of Vienna School.

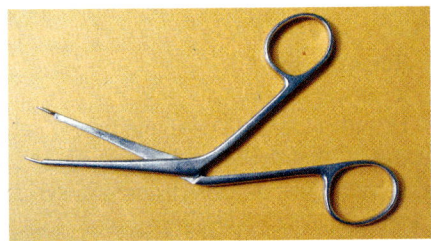

Fig. 99.58: Aural dressing forceps

Uses: To puncture tympanic membrane to place ventilation tubes in acute suppurative otitis media, secretary otitis media.

10. Mollisons Self Retaining Hemostatic Mastoid Retractor (Fig. 99.59)

Uses: In mastoid surgeries to retract soft tissues after incision and elevation of flaps.

Other retractors

Jansen's self retaining retractor.

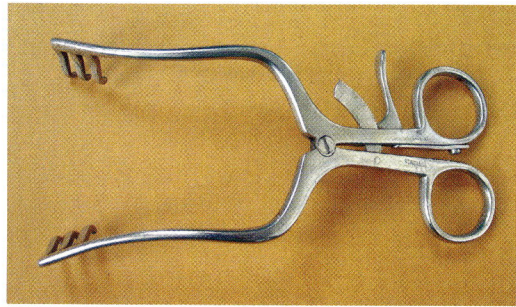

Fig. 99.59: Mollisons self retaining hemostatic mastoid retractor

11. Jenkins Gouges (Fig. 99.60)

Named after G.J.Jenkins (1874-1939) available in 10 widths

Uses: It is used in mastoidectomy to explore mastoid antrum and air cells.

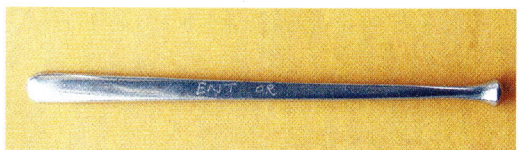

Fig. 99.60: Jenkins gouges

12. Farabeuf's Mastoid Elevator with Thumb Rest (Fig. 99.61)

- Made up of stainless steel
- Has a cutting edge

Use: To elevate the periosteum in mastoidectomy.

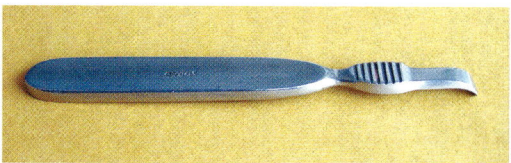

Fig. 99.61: Farabeuf's elevator with thumb rest

13. Lempert's Scoop (Fig. 99.62)

Named after Julius Lempert (1890-1968).

Uses: Used in different mastoid operations to curette diseased mastoid air cells and granulation tissue.

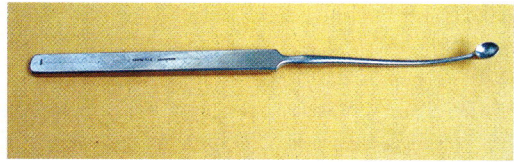

Fig. 99.62: Lempert's Scoop

14. Mac Ewen's curette; with cell seeker (Fig. 99.63)

History

Named after Sir William MacEwen (1848–1924) of Glasgow.

Parts: Has got two ends, one end curette and the other cell seeker.

Uses: Scoop is used to scoop out diseased air cells whereas cell seeker is used to seek the mastoid air cells and the antrum during mastoid operation. It is also used to identify the aditus. Maximum precaution should be taken to avoid incus dislocation while probing the aditus.

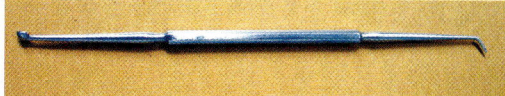

Fig. 99.63 Mac Ewen's curette; with cell seeker

Microsurgical Instruments

(Father of microsurgery of ear - Gunner Holmgren (1875-1954)

1. **Sickle knife:** For metal flap
2. **Ring curette**
3. House curette
4. **Knife for meatal skin incision**
5. Bayonet shaped elevators for meatal wall
6. Curette for tympanic ring
7. **Fine probe** to test the mobility of foot plate of stapes in stapedotomy
8. **Mobilizers** for severing adhesions involving stapes
9. **Oval scoops**
10. Oval window fenestrator
11. Straight needle
12. Perpendicular hook
13. **Wilson's Nibbling forceps:** For removal of superior rim during stapes mobilization
14. **Lempert's Nipper** (Fig. 99.64) for Head of Malleus
15. **Teflon Piston**
16. **Lempert's retractor:** Named after J. Lempert. Parts: 4 prongs and handle
    Uses: In various ear surgeries in retracting the skin by endaural route.
17. **Lempert's endaural speculum**
    Named after J.Lempert.

Uses: Used in endaural incisions.

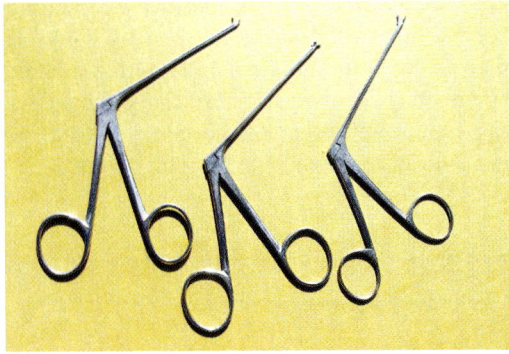

Fig. 99.64: Lempert's Nipper

STAPEDECTOMY

- Joseph Toynbee-demonstrated by anatomic dissections the common occurrence of stapes ankylosis as a cause of deafness.
- Fenestration operation was introduced in 1938 by Julius Lempert.
- In 1952 S.Rosen's – Endomeatal approach for stapes mobilization

Stapedotomy set (Figs 99.65a and b):

For stapedotomy operation

Contents: 10 instruments

(a) **Incision knife:** To make the transmeatal incision.
(b) **Metal flap elevator: To** elevate tympano-meatal flap.
(c) **House's Curette:** For curetting the postero-superior meatal wall for exposure of stapes.

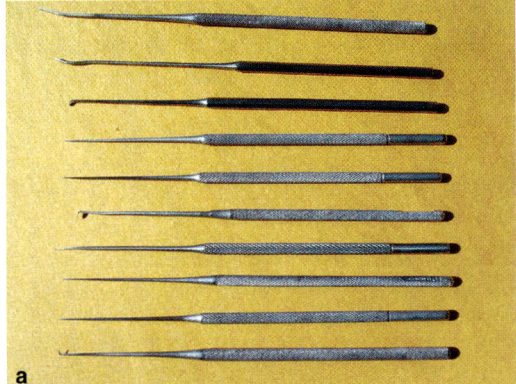

a

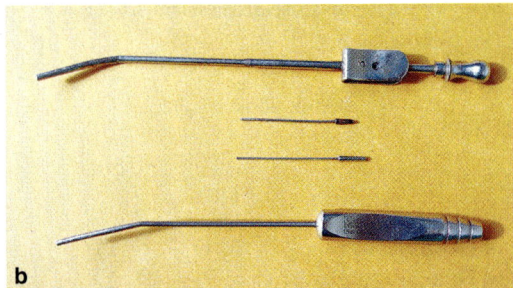

b

Figs 99.65a and b: Stapedotomy set

(d) **Sharp straight pick:** For making a puncture on the foot plate.

(e) **45 Degree and other angled pick (0.5mm):** To enlarge the puncture and enlarge the fenestra on the foot plate.

(f) **Crocodile aural scissors:** For cutting the stapedius tendon, fibrous adhesions, skin flaps, etc.

(g) **Crocodile aural forceps:** To insert the Teflon piston or other prosthesis, to remove bits of bone or soft tissue and to remove stapes superstructure.

(h) **Teflon Piston**
Diameter: 0.3 mm/0.6 mm/0.8 mm
Length: 3.5 mm to 6 mm
The measurement is made from the under surface of the lenticular process to the foot plate –usually 4 mm in length.

(i) **Zollner Suction tips.**

Uses: Microsuction tips used for suctioning blood during the procedure.

INSTRUMENTS TO PERFORM PER ORAL ENDOSCOPY

Direct Laryngoscope with Sliding Plate

Sliding part with proximal or Distal Illumination: Sliding part allows opening of the tube and thereby helping in guiding and directing the bronchoscope in case of children and difficult cases.

Anterior commissure direct laryngoscope (Fig. 99.66)

Types

1. Chevalier Jackson type
- Distal illumination of the laryngoscope

2. Negus type: **Proximal illumination**

Advantages
- Bright light and clear view
- Fogging unlikely
- Double illumination
- Broader so better view.

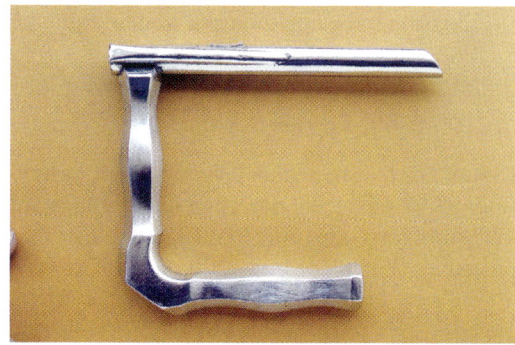

Fig. 99.66: Anterior commisure direct laryngoscope

Disadvantages
- Heavy and difficult to sterilize.

Distal Illumination

Advantages
- Lighter in weight.
- Completely sterilized.
- Narrow and easy to insert
- Unobstructed lumen for passage of instruments.

Disadvantages
- Less bright light
- Fogging due to secretions

Advantages of Anterior Commissure Direct Laryngoscope
- Anterior commissure can be visualized better.
- Vocal cord can be fixed in on position.
- Subglottis can be examined by manipulation of laryngoscope.

Uses

Diagnostic
- For detailed examination of the hypopharynx; and larynx
- For biopsy

Therapeutic
- Removal of foreign body

• Excision of benign tumor or nodule from the vocal cord.

Microlaryngoscope

Kleinssaur's suspension laryngoscope system (Figs 99.67 a to c) and operating microscope with 400 mm lens are commonly used for this procedure (Fig. 99.68).

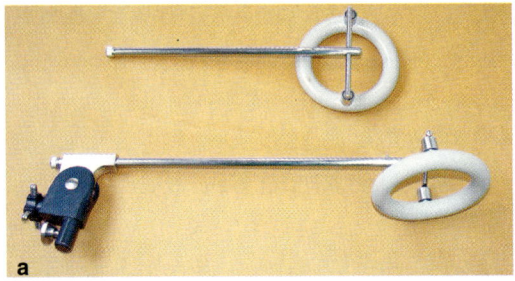

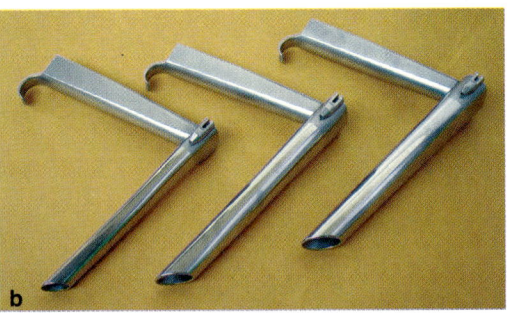

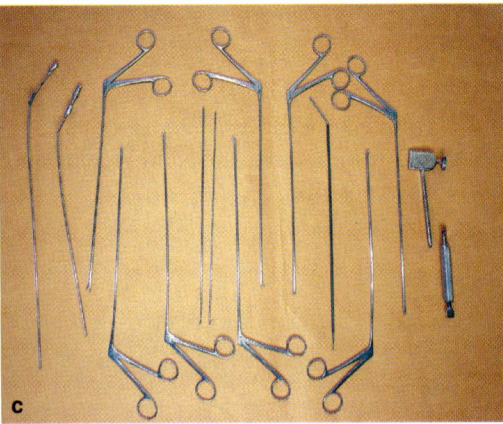

Figs 99.67a to c: Kleinssaur's suspension laryngoscope system

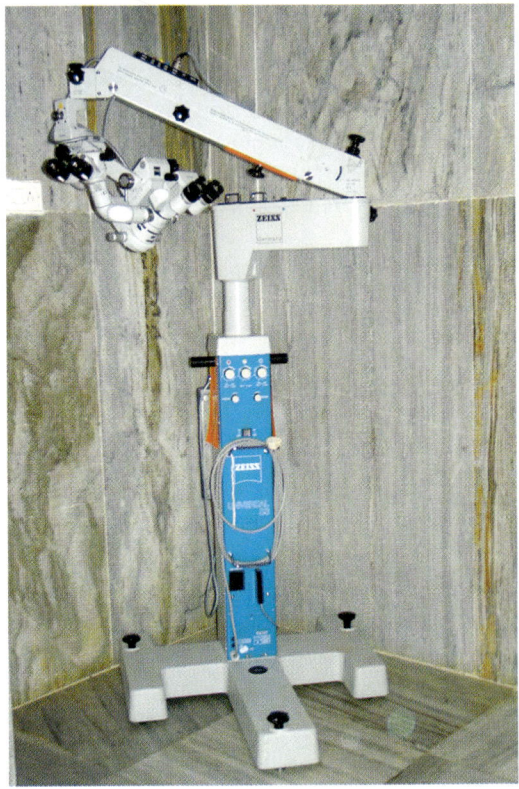

Fig. 99.68: Operating microscope for microlaryngeal and ear surgery

Advantages of microlaryngoscopy over direct laryngoscopy are

• Precision
• Better illumination and magnification
• Both hands of the surgeon will be free to perform precision surgery
• Laser laryngeal surgery can be performed with much ease.

Hypopharyngoscope (Fig. 99.69)

Diagnostic Indications

To examine and rule out growth in the pyriform fossa, postcricoid region and cervical esophagus and performing biopsy.

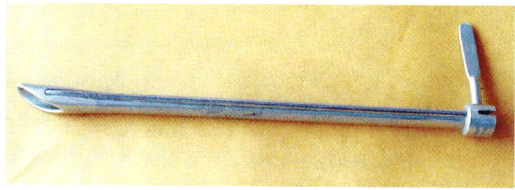

Fig. 99.69: Hypopharyngoscope

Therapeutic

- For removal of foreign body from pyriform fossa, postcricoid region and cervical esophagus
- Cricopharyngeal dilatation
- Use in cricopharyngeal myotomy
- Excision of cricopharyngeal web

Esophagoscope

Name: Chevalier Jackson's oesophagoscope (Fig. 99.70).

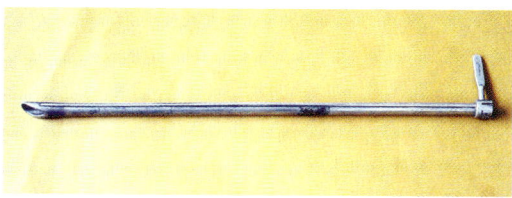

Fig. 99.70: Chevalier Jackson's esophagoscope

Uses

1. Diagnostic

- Malignancy of esophagus
- FB in oesophagus
- Cadiospasm
- Stricture of the esophagus
- Tracheoesophageal fistula
- Take biopsy from the esophageal lesion under direct vision

2. Therapeutic

- Removal of esophageal foreign body
- To guide bougies through the esophageal stricture

- To pass the M.B.tube
- Esophageal stenting to overcome obstruction and treatment of fistula
- Injection of sclerosing agent in esophageal varices

Prognostic

To follow up the patient after definitive therapy

Bronchoscope (Fig. 99.71)

Types

- Chevalier Jackson
- Negus type
- Fiberoptic

Negus type – Proximal illumination

C. Jackson type – Distal illumination

Sizes Available

Pediatric: 2.4 / 3.5 / 4.5

Adults: 6.5 / 7.5 / 8.5

Uses

Diagnostic

- To examine the bronchial tree for any pathological changes
- Take biopsy from a suspected site and collect bronchial secretions.

Therapeutic

- Removal of foreign bodies in bronchus
- Bronchial aspiration to remove viscid, purulent secretions.
- Tracheal and bronchial stenting

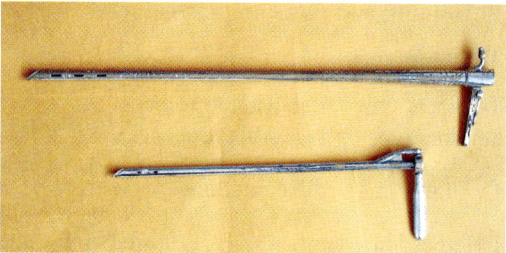

Fig. 99.71: Bronchoscope

SURGICAL INSTRUMENTS FOR NECK SURGERY

Classification

A. Cutting Instruments

I. Knives and blades (Fig. 99.72)

Eg:

Bard-Parker's
Beaver's
Fischer's tonsillar knife.

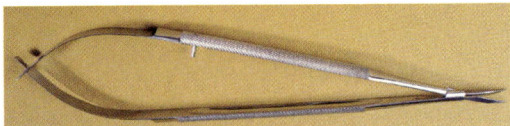

Fig. 99.73a: Iris cutting scissors

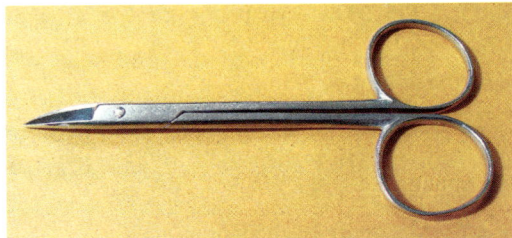

Fig. 99.73b: Metzenbaum's

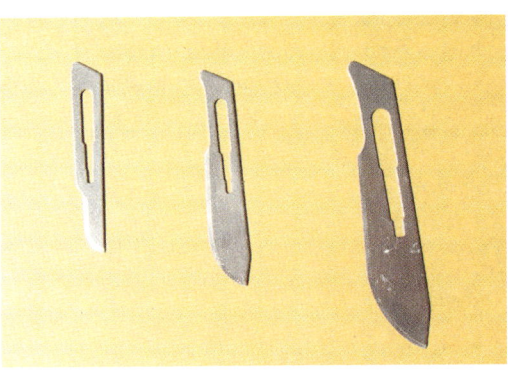

Fig. 99.72: Knives and blades

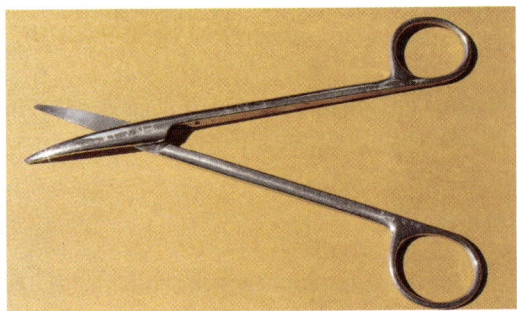

Fig. 99.74: Mayo's

II. Scissors

Small : E.g. Iris cutting scissors (Fig. 99.73a). Used in tympanoplsty procedures.
Medium : E.g. Metzenbaum's (Fig. 99.73b)
Large : E.g. Mayo's (Fig. 99.74)

B. Holding and Grasping instruments

Tissue forceps

Tweezers type   E.g. Thumb forceps
Scissors type   E.g. Allis, Babcock's

C. Clamping and Retraction

I. Hemostatic instruments. E.g. Halsted's mosquito Forceps

II. Retracting Instruments

- Plain e.g. Joseph's skin hook
- Self retaining, e.g. Jenson's and Mollison's

D. Suturing Instruments

Needle holders (Fig. 99.75)

- Ayer's and massion's—Long and narrow
- Johnson or Webster's—for delicate surgeries.

E. Accessory Instruments

 I. **Suction tubes**
       Frazier's — For minor surgeries
       Poole/Yankeur's — For major surgeries
 II. **Probes and directors,** e.g. Silver director
III. **Cautery tools**

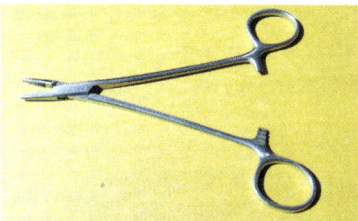

Fig. 99.75: Needle holders

BASIC SURGICAL INSTRUMENTS

- Sponge holding forceps:
- Towel clips:
  - Doyen's
  - Backhouse
- Bard-Parker's handle and knives:
- Dissecting forceps:
  - Thumb forceps
  - Adson's forceps
- Tissue forceps:
  - Allis'
  - Babcock's
  - Lane's
- Scissors:
  - Mayo's, Metzenbaum's
  - Lister's bandage cutting scissors
- Hemostatic (artery) forceps: Halsted's forceps
- Retractors:
  - Gigli's wire saw with handles
  - Chisel and Osteotomes
  - Cheatle's forceps
  - Magill's forceps
  - Ryle's tube

A small note on individual instruments is given below.

Sponge Holding Forceps (Foersters)
(Fig. 99.76)

Parts

- Long shaft
- Blades—are round and fenestrated, with serrations on inner aspect.
- Ratchet lock- helps to secure grip on to swab held

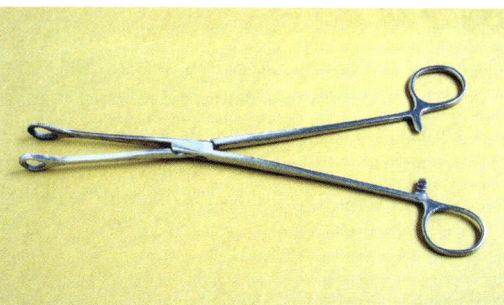

Fig. 99.76: Sponge holding forceps(foersters)

Uses

- For preparation of parts before surgery
- Hemostasis by pressure with swab
- In abdominal surgery to retract or to hold bowel or stomach
- For blunt gauge dissection.

Advantage

As the shafts are long, the hands of the surgeon are well away from cleaning area.

Towel Clips (Fig. 99.77)

- Doyen's towel clip
- Backhouse towel clip
  Short instruments with curved ends that end in sharp points.

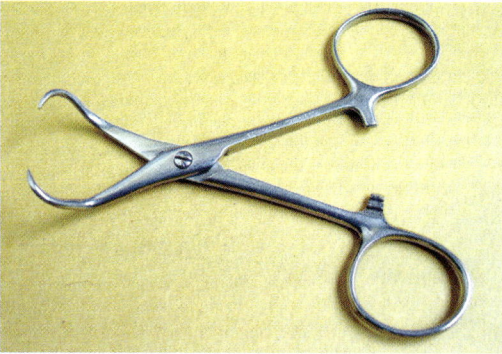

Fig. 99.77: Towel clips

Uses

- To fix the draping towels in position.
- To fix suction tubes/cautery cables to drapes
- To hold the sutured flaps in position.
- To hold the tongue in protruded position in intra-oral surgical procedures including partial glossectomies.

Bard-Parker Handle and Knives
(Fig. 99.78)

Advantage

- Light in weight, can be fixed to different blades.
- Short cutting edge and straight back.
- Good grip.
- Easy to sterilize.

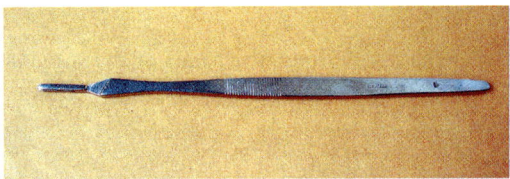

Fig. 99.78: Bard-parker handle and knives

Dissecting Forceps (Fig. 99.79)

Parts: Two blades joined at one end, the other end is narrow which may be:

- Plain with transverse serrations
  or
- Toothed for better grip

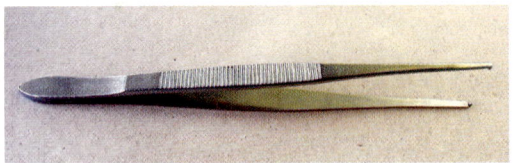

Fig. 99.79: Dissecting forceps

For delicate surgeries small light weighted **ADSON's** tissue forceps is used (Figs 99.80a and b).

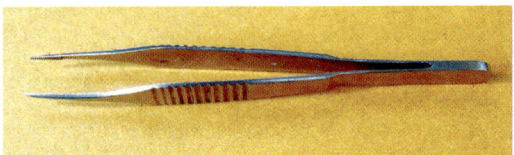

Fig. 99.80a: Plain with transverse serrations

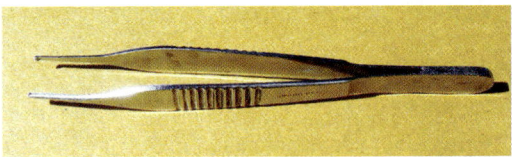

Fig. 99.80b: Toothed

Babcock's Tissue Forceps

Parts: It's a non-traumatic instrument with 2 ring shaped finger grips with a ratchet catch and fenestrated curved blades. Each blade has transverse bars with fine transverse serrations (Fig. 99.81).

Uses

- To hold soft tissues and delicate structures
- Available in long and short sizes.

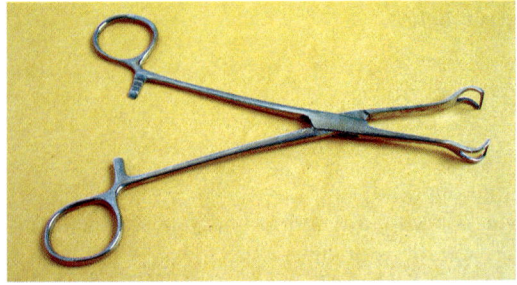

Fig. 99.81: Babcock's tissue forceps

Allis' Tissue Forceps (Fig. 99.82)

Parts

- 2 ring shaped finger grips, ratchet catch
- 2 tips which are flattened and curved inwards a little with fine teeth
- It offers better grip, but traumatic due to teeth

Uses

- To hold subcutaneous tissues
- To hold fascial flaps

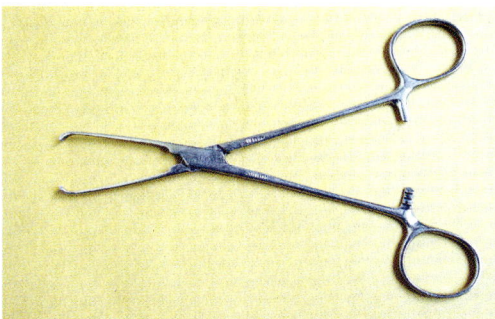

Fig. 99.82: Allis' tissue forceps

Lane's Tissue Forceps (Fig. 99.83)

Parts

- Ratchet catch
- 2 blades which are curved inwards and with 'one in two' fine teeth

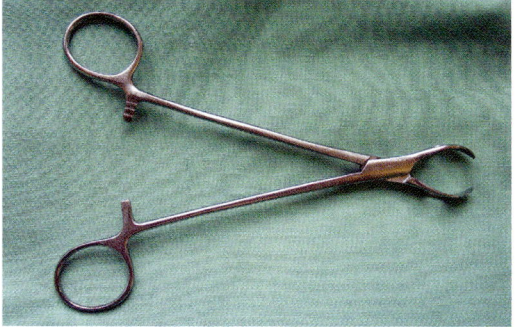

Fig. 99.83: Lane's tissue forceps

The curved and fenestrated blades allow the speculum to be held without crushing the tissues.

Uses

- To hold small tumors during dissection
- To hold and retract the edges of fascia

Moyinham's Tissue Forceps

It is similar to Allis' forceps except that blades are thinner and curved.

Scissors

These are sharp cutting instruments consisting of two blades each with ring shaped handle grips with screw joint.

Blades may be narrow or broad, tips may be blunt or pointed. Scissors may be

- Small/medium/large.
- Straight or curved.

Uses

- For tissue dissection
- To cut sutures and ligatures
- For suture removal.

Lister's Bandage Cutting Scissors
(Fig. 99.84)

Scissors is bent at an angle, to get below the bandage easily

The tip of the lower blade is flat and blunt (atraumatic)

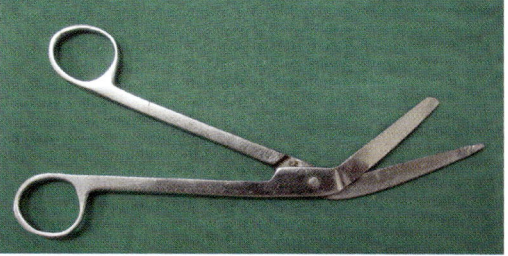

Fig. 99.84: Lister's bandage cutting scissors

Note: These scissors should not be boiled as it decrease the sharpness.

Sterilized by immersion in Lysol/ Cetrimide.

Hemostatic (artery) Forceps
(Figs 99.85a and b)

Parts: Designed for catching bleeding vessels and consists of ring shaped finger grip handles, blades with transverse serrations which can be long/short, straight/curved and with or without teeth at tip.

Pedicle clamp: Transverse serrations through out the extent of blades

Hemostat: Transverse serrations only at tip

Halsted's mosquito forceps is a fine short hemostat for fine vessels (Fig. 99.86).

Kocher's Artery Forceps (Fig. 99.87)

Is a pedicle clamp with teeth at tip

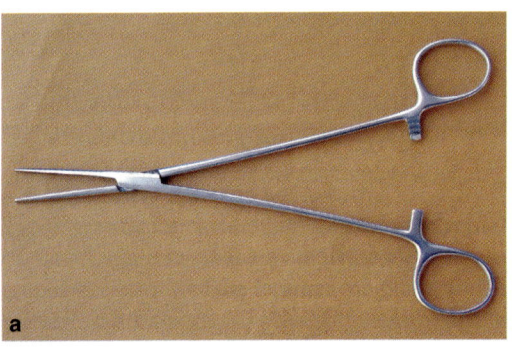

a

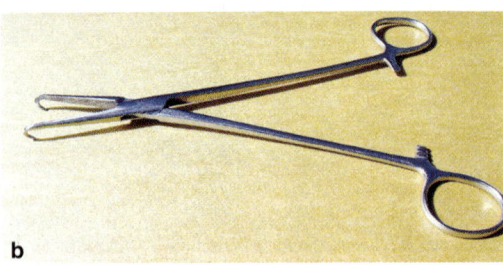

b

Figs 99.85a and b: Hemostatic (artery) forceps

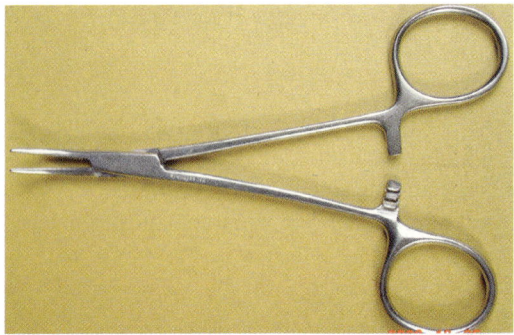

Fig. 99.86: Halsted's mosquito forceps

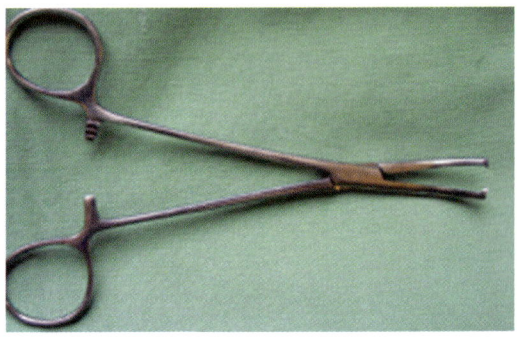

Fig. 99.87: Kocher's artery forceps

Bulldog Clamp (Fig. 99.88)

Atraumatic type of hemostat.

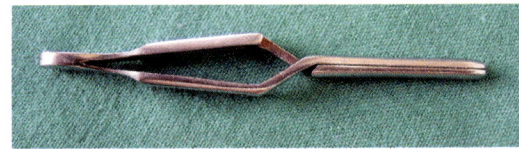

Fig. 99.88: Bulldog clamp

Mixter/Westphal Right Angled Forceps
(Fig. 99.89)

Uses

- To catch bleeding vessels
- As a pedicle clamp
- To hold cut edges of fascia, peritoneum, etc.
- As a sinus forceps/dressing forceps

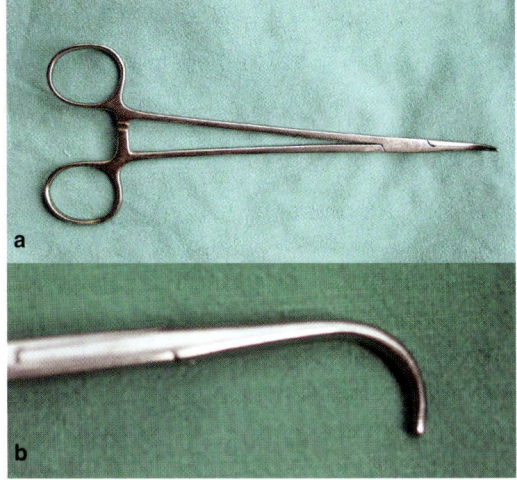

Figs 99.89a and b: Mixter/Westphal right angled forceps

- To hold the 'pea-nuts' for blunt dissection
- To feed the ligatures and to hold the ligature ends.
- To clamp catheters.

Retractors

Used to retract the structures away from operating field to provide adequate exposure.
Retractors may be

- Light/stout
- Broad and flat or hooked—single/double — e.g. Joseph skin hook
- Multiple, e.g. Cat's paw
- Plain/self-retaining.

Joseph's Skin Hooks
(Figs 99.90a and b)

Parts: Handle, shaft and hooked tip-single/double

Uses: To retract and lift skin margins while elevating the flaps.

Langenbeck's Retractor (Fig. 99.91)

Parts: Handle, shaft and a curved and flat retracting end.

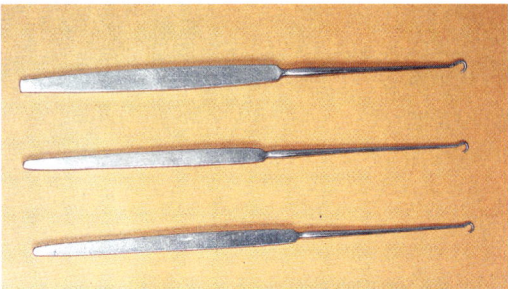

Fig. 99.90a: Joseph's skin hooks

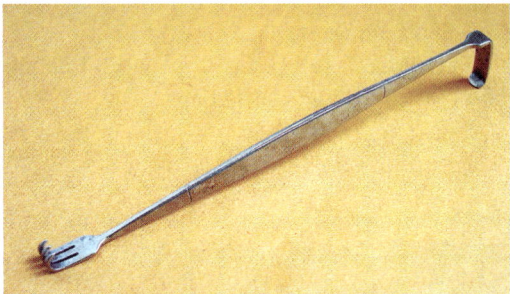

Fig. 99.90b: Cat's paw

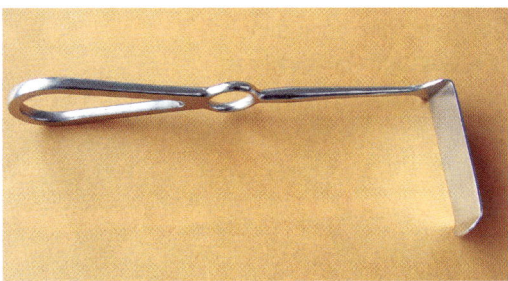

Fig. 99.91: Langenbeck's retractor

Czerney's Retractor

It is a double ended retractor, one is flat and the other is bipronged (U-shaped).

Gigli's Wire Saw with Handles
(Fig. 99.92)

Parts

- Two T-shaped handles, each with hook at vertical limb and
- Wire saw—acts as a cutting blade

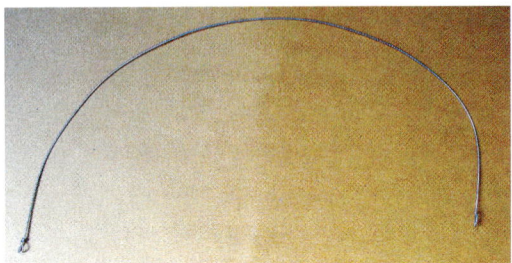

Fig. 99.92: Gigli's wire saw with handles

Uses: For cutting bone in maxillectomy and Mandibulectomy, etc.

For cutting skull bones in between trephine holes to reflect osteoplastic flaps

Chisel (Fig. 99.93)

Parts
- Head-to receive the mallet blows
- Shaft and a cutting edge which is bevelled on one side.

Uses
- To cut the bone tumors.
- Maxillofacial surgeries.

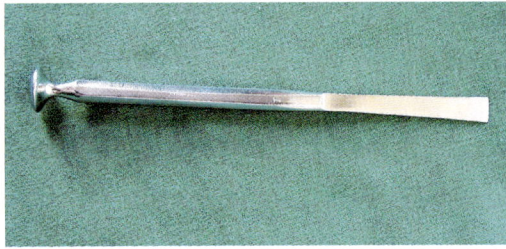

Fig. 99.93: Chisel

Osteotome (Fig. 99.94)

Designed similar to that of chisel except that the cutting edge is beveled on both sides.

Uses: Osteotomy and maxillectomy.

Cheatle's Forceps (Fig. 99.95)

It is a long instrument with ring shaped finger grip handle and two blades—flat and angled away from

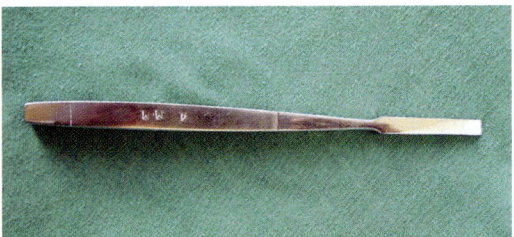

Fig. 99.94: Osteotome

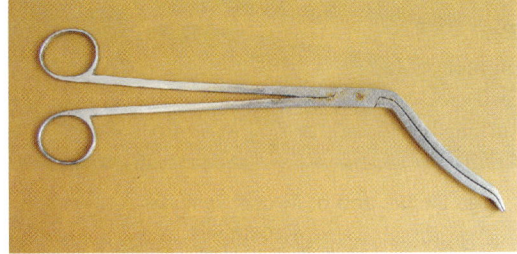

Fig. 99.95: Cheatle's forceps

handle. Blades are wavy for better gripping of objects. Available in large and small sizes.
Uses: To pick up the instruments from sterilizer and also to allow the transfer of instruments without contamination at surgery

The forceps is kept vertically with blades immersed down in antiseptic solution when not in use.

Magill's Forceps (Fig. 99.96)

It is a long and peculiarly angulated forceps with fenestrated and blunt blades, no locking mechanism.

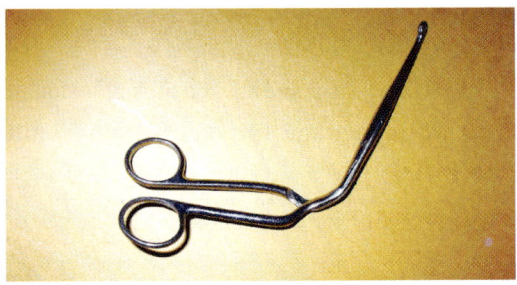

Fig. 99.96: Magill's forceps

Uses

- For endotracheal intubation
- For throat packing to prevent aspiration in anesthetized patient
- For passing nasogastric tube
- For removal of foreign bodies from pharynx in anesthetized patient

Nasogastric (Ryle's) Tube (Fig. 99.97)

Parts: It is a soft tube made of plastic, of length 30 inches. The tip is blunt and solid and contains lead shots subterminal openings on all sides. Outer surface has 3 markings to indicate the position of tip of nasogastric tube

- Cardiac orifice
- Body of stomach
- Pylorus

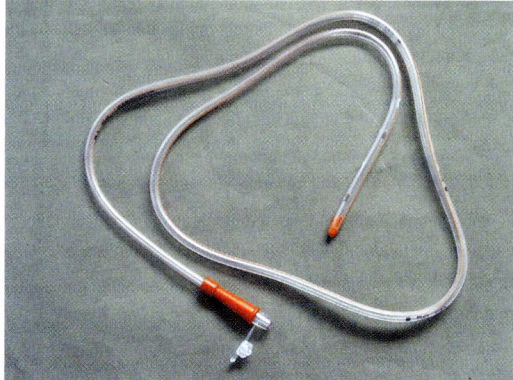

Fig. 99.97: Nasogastric (Ryle's) tube

Uses

Diagnostic
- To aspirate gastric/duodenal contents for evaluation
- For barium enema and duodenojejunography.

Therapeutic
- Nasogastric feeding
- To prevent aspiration in vocal cord palsy and other neurological lesions

- Gastric lavage
- Ice cold solution wash to control gastric hemorrhage
- Gastric decompression
- For administration of drugs

Contraindications

- Necrotic esophageal ulcer (Corrosive burns of esophagus is a relative contraindication)

Technique of Insertion
- Conscious patient- sitting position
- Unconscious-supine position
- Anesthetized patient- under direct laryngoscopy

Confirmation
- Aspiration of gastric contents
- Auscultation over epigastrium on insufflation air into tube.
- Outer end is placed under water to look for air bubble
- Direct laryngoscope
- Radiography

Complications
- Rhinitis and pharyngitis
- Esophageal ulcer
- Aspiration pneumonia and death
- Perforation and hemorrhage
- Coiling in pharynx leading to aspiration.

Montgomery T tube (Fig. 99.98)

Uses: For stenting of the trachea after releasing the tracheal stenosis. As it is made of silastic (inert material) it can be kept for long time inside the body.

Metallic (Nitilon) Stent: (Ultraflex Stent) (Figs 99.99 to 99.101)

Uses

- It can be both uncovered and covered as shown in the diagram.
- In tracheal stenosis after releasing the stenotic segment it can be used as a permanent stent.

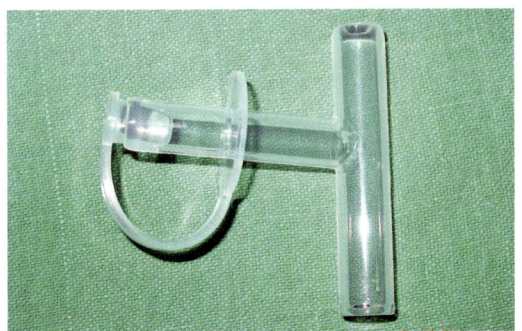

Fig. 99.98: Montogomery T tube

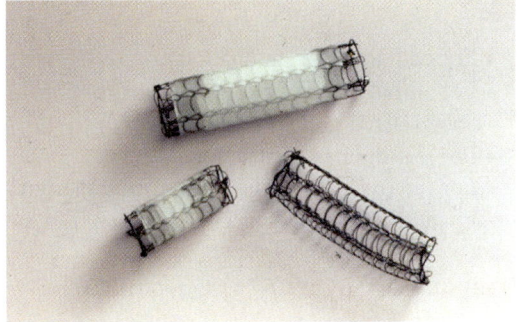

Fig. 99.99: Nitilon stent (Ultraflex stent)

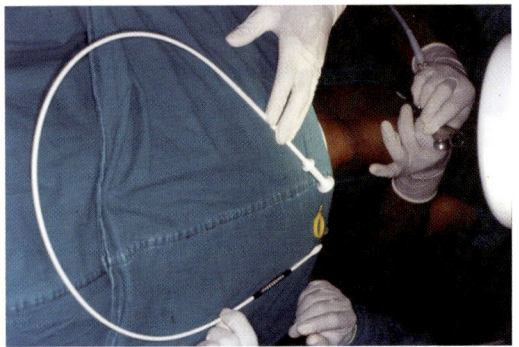

Fig. 99.100: Nitilon stent with applicator

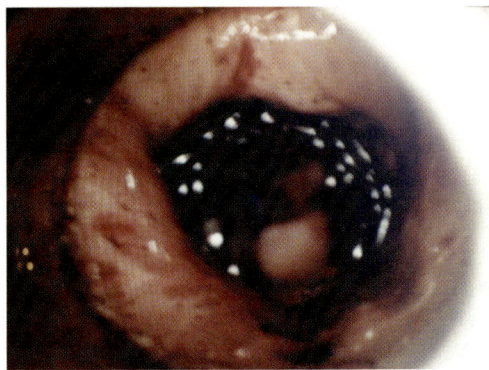

Fig. 99.101: Endoscopic view of nitilon stent

• No attempt should be made to stent the sub-glottis using this stent for fear of granulation tissue formation and re-stenosis. Photograph showing method of insertion of metallic stent.

100

Imaging Studies in ENT and Head and Neck

Imaging of Nose and Paranasal Sinuses

- Waters view
- Caldwell's view
- Base view
- Lateral view
- Optic canal view
- Pierr's view
- Nasal bone visualisation
- Mucocoele
- Malignancy of sinuses
- Juvenile nasopharyngeal angiofibroma
- CT Scan (Paranasal sinuses)
- Law's projection
- Schuller's view (Lateral oblique view).

IMAGING OF NOSE AND PARANASAL SINUSES

Radiological examination of the paranasal sinuses is complete only if all the sinuses are visualized. They include the frontal, the ethmoids, the maxillary and the sphenoid sinuses. Sinuses are generally visualized using four views:

- Caldwell view
- Waters view
- Lateral view
- Basal view

An additional view is the optic canal or Rhese view.

Waters View

(Occipitomental or inclined posteroanterior view)

Waters view, also known as occipitomental or inclined posteroanterior view, is the best view for visualizing the maxillary sinuses and the anterior ethmoidal air cells.

Structures visualized are:
- Floor of the orbit
- Frontal sinuses
- Anterior ethmoidal cells
- Maxillary sinus.

Caldwell's View

(Occipitofrontal view)

The frontal sinus and ethmoid sinus are best seen on Caldwells view (Fig. 100.1). In addition, the Caldwells view demonstrates the nasal floor to the best advantage.

Base View

(Submentovertical view or Jug handle view)

The Base view is used for visualization of

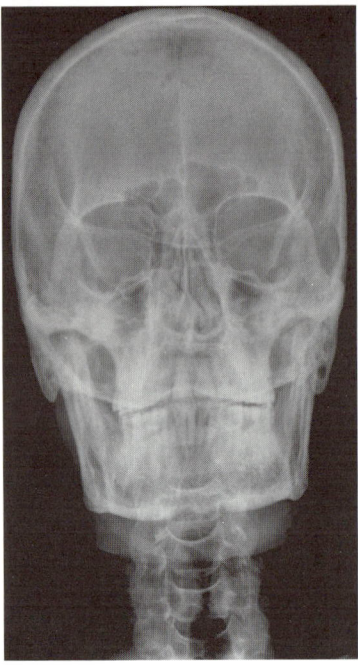

Fig. 100.1: Caldwell's view showing bilateral maxillary haziness with deviated nasal septum. Ethmoids are relatively clear

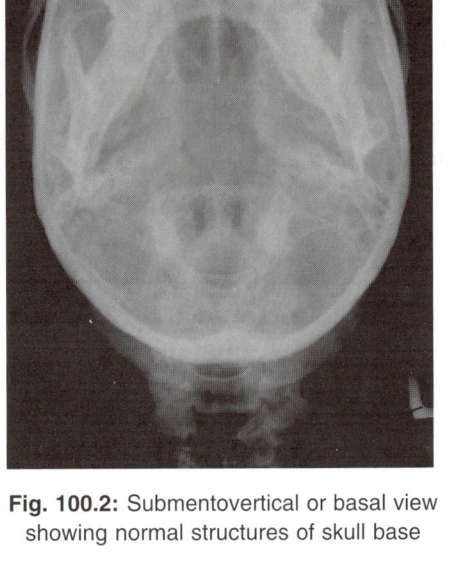

Fig. 100.2: Submentovertical or basal view showing normal structures of skull base

structures in the base of the skull and the structures of the skull (Fig. 100.2) which are oriented in a caudocephalad direction such as the anterior wall of the middle cranial fossa, lateral wall of the orbit and the lateral wall of the maxillary sinus.

Structures visualized are:

- *Medial and lateral pterygoid plates*, lateral represented by two lines posteromedially towards Foramen ovale. Absence of the lateral pterygoid plate due to bone destruction can be appreciated.
- *Foramen of the base of the skull,* oriented caudocephalically like Foramen ovale and foramen spinosum.
- *Pterygopalatine fossa* produces a short horizontal canal just posterior to the posterior wall of maxillary sinus and the anterior margin

of the junction of medial and lateral pterygoid plate. Enlargement of pterygopalatine fossa by a benign lesion such as JNA or destruction by a more aggressive tumor can be seen on base view.

- *Frontal sinus:* An overshot view can show the anterior and posterior walls of the frontal sinus.
- *Bony eustachian tube:* incus and malleus can be seen. Clouding of middle ear can be identified in the base view.
- *Triple lines of Baclesse* as mentioned by Barbosa (1961) in basal view is important to detect intracranial extension of tumor from nasopharynx. The S-shaped line represents the posterior wall of the maxillary sinus; erosion of this line indicates extension into the subtemporal fossa. The upper curvilinear line

represents the lateral wall of the orbit; erosion of this is evidence of invasion of tumor into the orbit. The lower curvilinear line, which is concave backward, represents the lesser wing of the sphenoid; erosion of this line is evidence of massive invasion of the base of the skull.

Lateral View

Lateral view can be used to visualize the pterygopalatine fossa, the hard palate and the posterior nasopharyngeal soft tissue shadow. It is the only view that shows the length and depth of sella turcica.

Optic Canal View-Rhese View

This view is useful to demonstrate the optic foramen or optic canal (Figs 100.3a and b). It gives a chance to visualize the frontal sinuses separately and also gives another view of the ethmoid air cells and the ipsilateral sphenoid sinus.

Pierr's View

Axial transoral projection. Also known as waters view with mouth open. Structures seen–axial projection of sphenoid sinus is projected through open mouth. The antra and nasal fossae are demonstrated.

Nasal Bone Visualization

Lateral Projection

Structures shown: Lateral projection of nasal bone is demonstrated and also the soft tissues of the nose. The figures (Fig. 100.4) show a fracture of nasal bones.

Tangential Projection

This projection is primarily used to demonstrate any medial or lateral displacement of fragments in fractures.

Waters View

Common questions asked are as follows:

1. **Name the X-ray:** plain X-ray paranasal sinus waters' view.
2. **Area of interest:** Maxillary and Frontal sinus
3. **Findings:** Maxillary sinus showing unilateral complete opacity of right maxillary

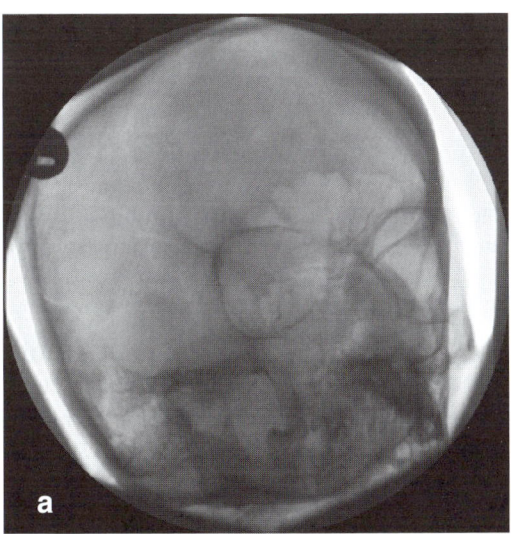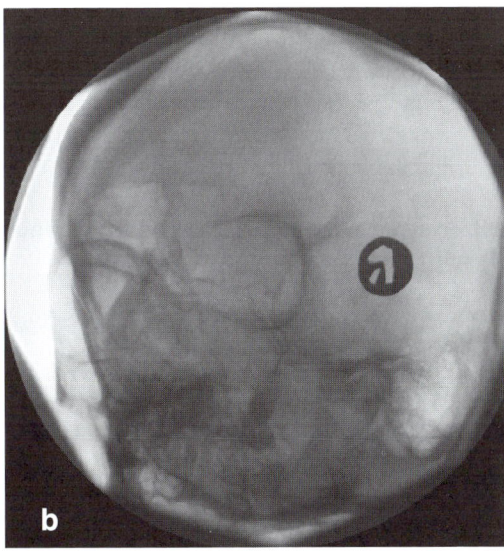

Figs 100.3a and b: Optic canal view showing optic foramen or optic canal

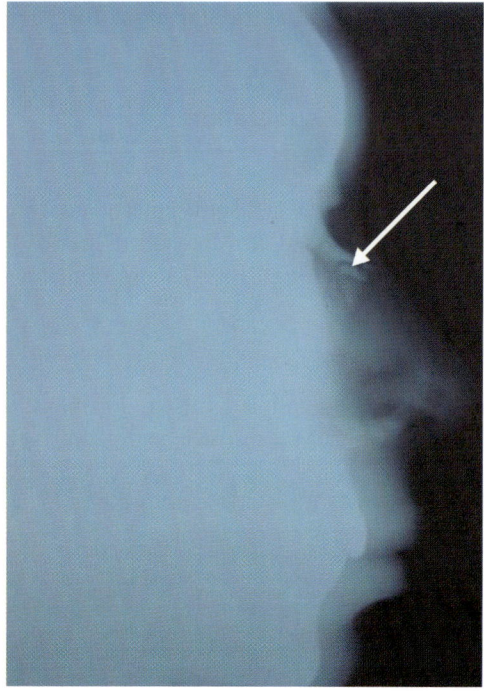

Fig. 100.4: Lateral projection showing fracture of nasal bone as pointed by arrow

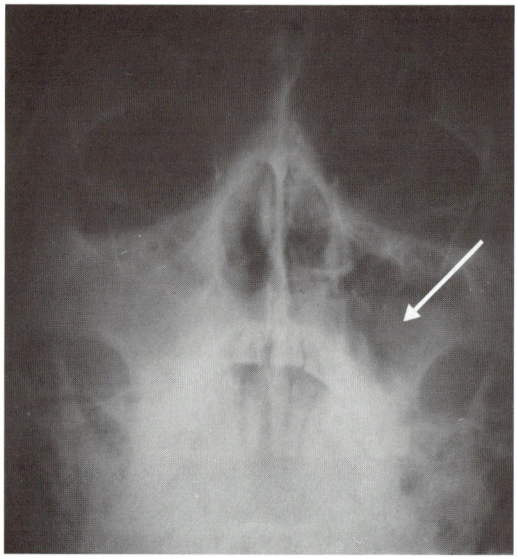

Fig. 100.5a: X-ray para nasal sinus waters' view showing unilateral opacity (right) with retension cyst (left)(✓)

sinus suggestive of maxillary sinusitis with smooth rounded opacity in left maxillary sinus suggestive of a mucous retention cyst (Fig. 100.5a). Opacity in both maxillary sinus can be seen in bilateral chronic maxillary sinusities (100.5c).

Differential Diagnosis of Maxillary Sinus Opacity

- Thickened maxillary bony wall
- Hemoantrum
- Thickened maxillary sinus wall
- Fibrous dysplasia
- Ossifying fibroma
- Dental cyst
- Dentigerous cyst
- Antral polyp/antrochoanal polyp
- Malignant growth of maxilla.

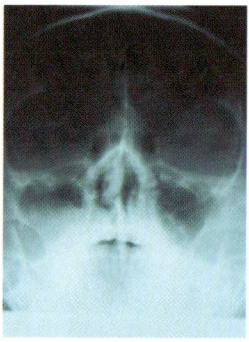 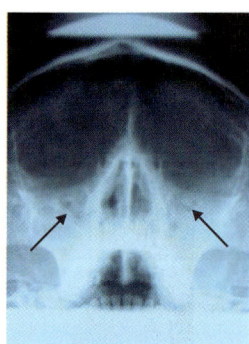

Fig. 100.5b: Fluid level in right maxillary sinus   **Fig. 100.5c:** Bilateral complete maxillary sinus opacity

4. **Whether acute or chronic sinusitis:** Chronic sinusitis invariably is associated with mucosal thickening which is missing in acute sinusitis whereas fluid level can be seen (Fig. 100.5b)

5. **How will you differentiate a polyp from mucosal cyst and fluid level:** X-ray PNS

should be taken in different position when fluid level will assume different positions which is absent in polyp and mucosal cyst.

MUCOCELE

Frontal Sinus

Cardinal findings are
1. Normal scalloped border of the frontal sinus becomes smoothened out to an even line.
2. Generally a diffused zone of sclerosis external to this smoothed anterior border.
3. There is bone destruction or displacement involving the superomedial border of the orbit adjacent to involved frontal sinus (Fig. 100.6).

Ethmoidal mucocele presents as round homogenous radiodensity in the ethmoid region. May cause lateral displacement of lamina papyracea and also cause destruction and lateral displacement of the superomedial wall of orbit or displacement downward of ethmomaxillary plate.

Sphenoid sinus mucocele generally balloon out all the walls of sphenoid sinus. Floor of sella turcica may be destroyed.

Retention Cyst

Most common site is the inferior portion of maxillary sinus (Fig. 100.5a). Smoothly marginated dome shaped mass of homogenous density. They have a thin calcific border similar to an egg shell. They do not cause bone destruction nor bone displacement.

Malignancy of Sinuses

Figure 100.7 shows X-ray paranasal sinus Waters view showing complete opacity of right maxillary sinus with evidence of bone destruction (antero-lateral wall).

Erosion of the roof of maxillary sinus will signify orbital involvement.

Medial wall of maxillary sinus destruction often signify maxilloethmoidal complex malignancy. Other conditions which can cause **bone destruction are as follows:**

Fungal sinusitis: Shows bone destruction of the sinus wall with evidence of inflammatory reaction on biopsy.

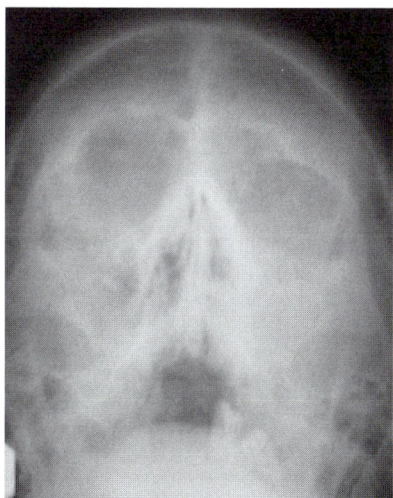

Fig. 100.6: X-ray PNS showing right frontal sinus mucocele with characteristic loss of scalloping

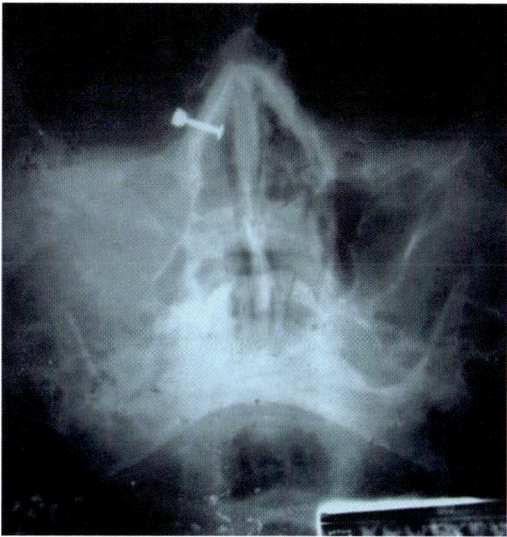

Fig. 100.7: Malignancy of right maxillary sinus (arrow showing destruction of anteromaxillary wall)

Wegeners granulomatosis: Opacification of sinuses with bone destruction.

Eosinophilic Granuloma

Brown's tumor (secondary deposit from parathyroid malignancy)

How do you confirm the diagnosis? Intranasal antrostomy and biopsy, Caldwell luc operation and biopsy, diagnostic nasal endoscopy and biopsy and antral lavage and cytology (Any one of the above).

What is the commonest malignancy in maxilla? - Squamous cell carcinoma.

What is the preferred line of manage- ment? Combined modality of treatment (either surgery with radiotherapy or radiotherapy with surgery with or without chemotherapy)

Ethmoid Sinus—malignancy

Opacification of sinus with bone destruction suggests presence of tumor. Bone destruction should be looked for in posterior part of lamina papyracea on Caldwells view.

What is the preferred surgical treatment for maxilloethmoidal complex malignancy?- Anterior craniofacial resection.

OSTEOMA (Figs 100.8 a and b)

X-ray PNS showing homogenous well localized dense opacity within the frontal sinus diagnosis is osteoma frontal sinus

JUVENILE NASOPHARYNGEAL ANGIOFIBROMA

It originates from sphenopalatine foramen and enlarges the foramen and erodes the bone locally at the base of medial pterygoid plates, the floor of sphenoid sinus and posterior wall of maxillary antrum. Extension leads to invasion of infratemporal fossa, orbit and middle cranial fossa. Indentation of posterior wall of maxilla in Plain X-ray skull (lateral view) called as **"antral sign or Holmann's sign"** indicates pterygopalatine fossa extension. Widening of space between

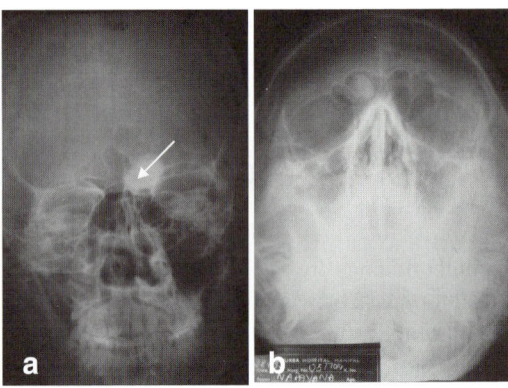

Figs 100.8a and b: Showing rounded homogenous dense opacity in the frontal sinus suggestive of osteoma (a) Caldwell's view, (b) Waters view

anterolateral wall and coronoid process which indicate sublabial extention of JNA (Fig. 100.9).

CT Scan of Paranasal Sinuses

CT Scan is currently the modality of choice in the evaluation of paranasal sinuses and the adjacent structures.

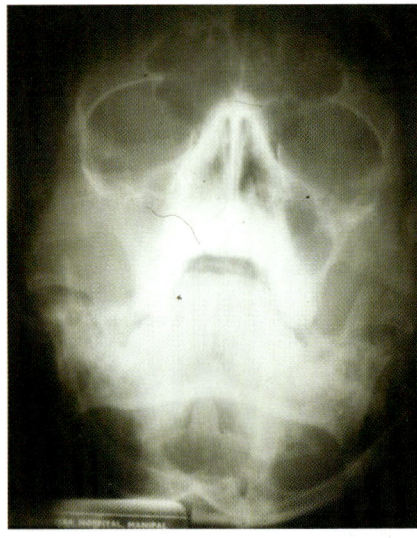

Fig. 100.9: X-ray showing increased distance between anterolateral wall of maxilla and coronoid process indicating extension of JNA through the pterygomaxillary fossa

ADVANTAGES OF CT OVER OTHER METHODS OF IMAGING

- CT can clearly show the fine bony anatomy of the osteomeatal complex
- Bony walls of the sinuses are better demonstrated
- Ability to optimally display bone, soft tissue and air facilitates accurate depiction of anatomy and extent of disease in and around the paranasal sinuses.
- Disease extending beyond the bony perimeters of sinuses into adjacent soft tissues of the orbit, brain and infratemporal fossa can be seen clearly.

Generally we take CT PNS in the coronal plane because

- It optimally shows the osteomeatal unit, relationship of the brain and the ethmoid roof and relationship of orbits to the paranasal sinuses.
- Coronal images correlate with the surgical approach and therefore should be obtained in all patients with inflammatory sinus disease, who are surgical candidates.

Coronal CT is not possible in:

- Intubated patients
- Young children
- In cases of cervical arthropathy
- Debilitated patients who will not tolerate the position. In such patients continuous axial images with coronal reconstruction are performed.

Scanning is performed from the anterior wall of the frontal sinus through the posterior wall of sphenoid sinus and contiguous 3 mm thick images are obtained.

A window level of 2000 Hounsefield - 200 Hounsefield is best. Figure 100.10 shows a normal CT scan of paranasal sinuses in axial sections.

Axial reconstruction can be helpful in displaying the position of internal carotid artery and optic nerves with respect to the bony margins of the posterior ethmoids and sphenoid sinuses (Fig. 100.10). MRI is not a reliable operative road map to guide the surgeon during FESS operation because of the following factor:

- It does not visualize the cortical bones resulting in an inability to discern the intricate anatomic relationships of the sinuses and their drainage portals.

MRI is most helpful in the following conditions:

- The evaluation of regional and intracranial complications of inflammatory sinus disease.
- In the detection of neoplastic processes.
- Improved display of anatomic relationship between intra and extraorbital compartment.
- Helpful in the evaluation of fungal sinusitis which show no signal on T2 image.
- Also useful in the evaluation of mucoceles and encephaloceles.

Anatomical Variations and Congenital Abnormalities

The significance of an anatomical variant is determined by its relationship with the osteomeatal channel and nasal air passages. The ability of the

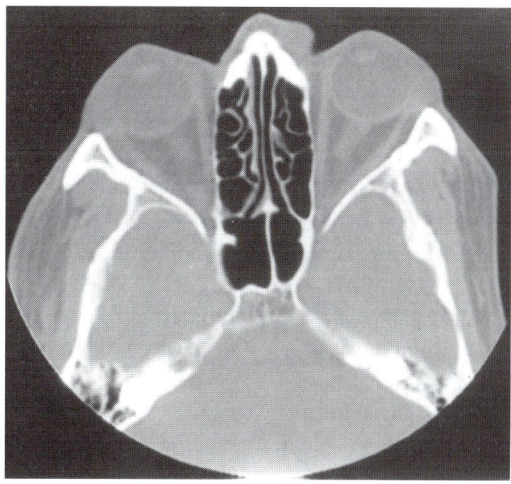

Fig. 100.10: Axial CT of paranasal sinuses and orbit

variations to obstruct air passages implies a role in the recurrence of sinusitis.

The common variations are:

- **Concha bullosa** which is an aeration in the middle turbinate which may enlarge to obstruct the middle meatus and the infundibulum.
- **Nasal septal deviation** which may compress the MT laterally narrowing the middle meatus.
- **Paradoxically curved middle turbinate**— Major curvature can project laterally and narrow the middle meatus and infundibulum.
- **Variations in uncinate process**—Atelectatic uncinate process-free edge of the uncinate process adheres to the orbital floor or inferior aspect of the lamina papyracea which may result in closure of infundibulum.
- **Haller cells**—The anterior ethmoid cells that extend along the medial roof of the maxillary sinus when enlarged they may cause narrowing of the infundibulum.
- **Onodi cells**—The lateral and posterior extensions of the posterior ethmoidal air cells, these cells may surround the optic nerve track and put the nerve at risk during surgery.
- **Giant ethmoidal bulla**—It may enlarge to narrow or obstruct the middle meatus and infundibulum.
- **Extensive pneumatization of sphenoid sinus** surrounding the optic nerve which can increase the risk of optic nerve damage during surgery.
- **Medial deviation or dehiscence of lamina papyracea**—Intraorbital contents are at increased risk during surgery
- **Aerated crista galli** may communicate with the frontal recess—This should be differentiated from ethmoid air cells to avoid extension of surgery into the cranial vault.
- **Cephaloceles** seen as an isolated soft tissue mass adjacent to ethmoidal or sphenoid roof
- **Asymmetry in ethmoid roof**—Incidence of intracranial penetration during FESS is higher when this variation exists.

Fungal Sinusitis

Maxillary and ethmoidal sinus involvement commonly points for suspicion of fungal sinusitis.

- Non-specific mucosal thickening.
- Sinus opacification with the central mycetoma and associated bone erosion.
- On MRI signal void on T2 weighted image as seen in the following MRI pictures (Figs 100.11a and b).
- Coronal postoperative CT Scan (Fig. 100.11c).
- Association of inflammatory sinus disease with involvement of adjacent nasal fossa and soft tissue of the cheek.

Allergic Fungal Sinusitis

Usually there will be unilateral involvement of the sinuses where there will be sinus opacity (Fig. 100.12). The following CT scan shows unilateral maxillary opacity on left side in a case of allergic fungal sinusitis.

Allergic sinusitis shows the following:

- Pan sinusitis with symmetrical involvement
- Nodular mucosal thickening with thickened turbinates
- Air fluid levels are rare unless there is secondary bacterial infection (Figs 100.13 and 100.14).

Mucous Retention Cyst

It is a small cyst commonly occurring in the maxillary sinus floor in patient with history of inflammatory disease. It appears as a homogenous well circumscribed hypo to isodense mass.

Mucocele

66 percent of mucocele are seen in frontal sinus. 25 percent in ethmoids, 10 percent in maxillary sinus. Appears as a hypodense non-enhancing mass that fills and expands a sinus cavity. An infected mucocele, a mucopyocele may show rim enhancement.

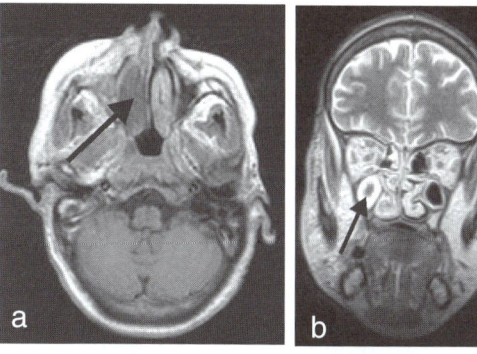

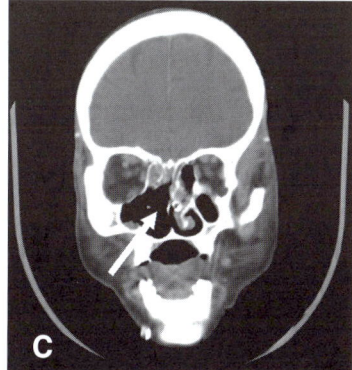

Figs 100.11a to c: (a) Axial, (b) Coronal, (c) Postoperative CT Scan

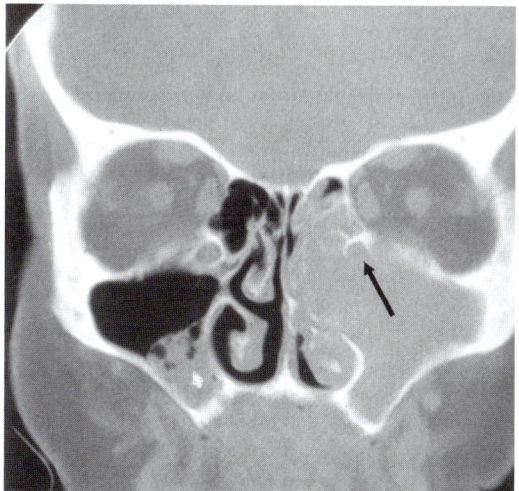

Fig. 100.12: Allergic fungal sinusitis involving left maxillary antrum and ethmoids

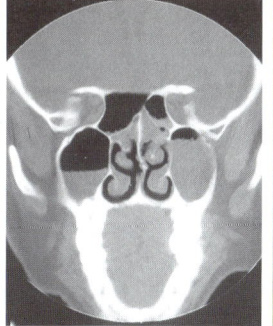

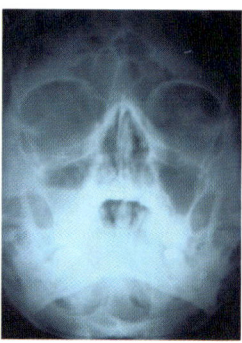

Fig. 100.13: Scan shows air fluid levels in both maxillary sinuses

Fig. 100.14: Fluid level is seen in right maxillary sinus

Inflammatory polyps seen in allergic sinusitis seen as smooth isodense to hypodense lesions

Malignancy of paranasal sinus or nasal cavity shows soft tissue mass within the antrum with bony erosion often obliterating the nasal cavity. The following scan shows a complete opacity with destruction of root of ethmoid and lamina papyracea, which is suggestive of malignant growth extending intracranially after destroying the bony barriers.

Another area of interest is **choanal atresia**. Shown here clearly are films depicting failure of canalization of choana leading to membranous and bony atresia (Figs 100.16 and 100.17).

Larynx Plain X-ray Neck Lateral View

Should be performed during quiet respiration to give maximum contrast of air filled passages and soft tissues. Structures seen are: air in upper respiratory passages outline the vallecula and cavities of larynx and trachea. Soft tissue structures like soft palate, base of tongue, epiglottis and aryepiglottic folds are seen against this air background.

Enlarged tonsils may be seen as oval densities and cartilagenous eustachian tube seen as narrow dark slit filled with air having a rim around it due to eustachian cushions.

Hyoid bone, thyroid and cricoid cartilages are seen. Increase in thickness of soft tissue in

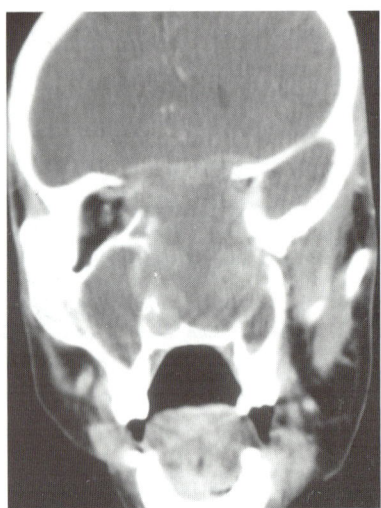

Fig. 100.15: Malignant growth of the maxillo-ethmoidal complex showing errosion of cribriform plate and lamina papyracea

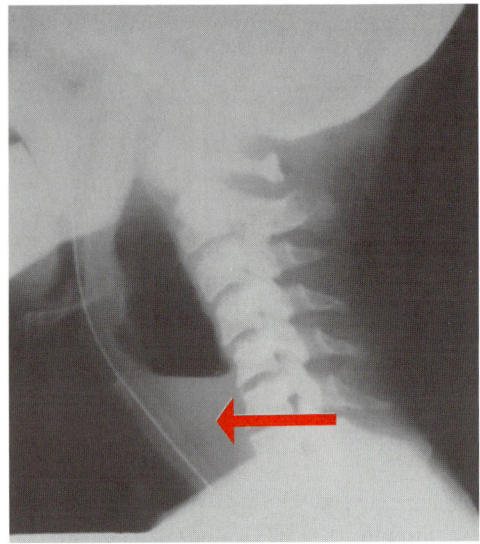

Fig. 100.18: X-ray lateral view neck showing acute retropharyngeal abscess

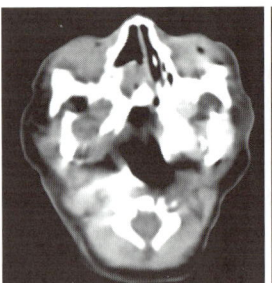

Fig 100.16: Membranous atresia

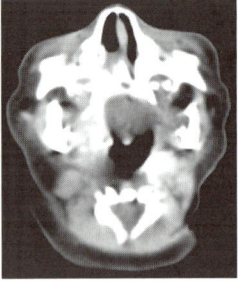

Fig. 100.17: Bony atresia

nasopharynx and prevertebral area may indicate edema, abscess, hematoma, cyst or tumor. Loss of normal spinal curvature noted in diseases, e.g. Retropharyngeal abscess (Fig. 100.18).

Common Questions Asked

Name the x-ray? (Fig. 100.18) This is a plain x-ray of soft tissue of neck, lower part of skull and upper part of mediastinum.

Area of interest—Prevertebral space- (as shown by an arrow) which is showing gross widening of prevertebral shadow with air fluid level with anterior displacement of trachea. Cervical spine has become straight loosing its normal curvature called as **'bamboo spine'** (Fig. 100.18).

Diagnosis—acute retropharyngeal abscess

Why it is not chronic retropharyngeal abscess? In chronic abscess there will be collapse of intervertebral space with erosion of body of vertebra, seen in caries spine. Chronic retropharyngeal abscess is seen in midline whereas acute initially will be seen in the side. Above x ray does not show any bone destruction so it is acute retropharyngeal abscess.

What are the complications of untreated retropharyngeal abscess?

- May rupture anteriorly leading to aspiration
- Tracheal wall may be eroded leading to tracheo esophageal fistula
- May involve parapharyngeal space leading to parapharyngeal abscess
- May burst inferiorly into posterior mediastinum via **Lincoln's highway** producing mediastinitis.
- May lead to general septicemia and death

What are the differences in modalities of drainage of acute from chronic retropharyngeal abscess?

Acute abscess is drained per orally where as **chronic** is drained externally for fear of fistula.

Surgical emphysema is seen as linear streaks of air in prevertebral plane.

Foreign bodies and growths in trachea and larynx are silhouetted against intraluminal air. Intraluminal air lies equidistant between anterior vertebral border and posterior profile of upper manubrium. This may be disturbed in kyphosis, scoliosis, etc. trachea displaced towards concavity of scoliosis and forwards with kyphosis.

This X-ray (Fig. 100.19) is a plain X-ray soft tissue neck with upper chest and lower skull, AP view showing smooth rounded radio-opaque shadow in the cricopharynx most probably a coin.

- **Why do you say it is in the cricopharynx but not in trachea?** Cricopharyngeal foreign body is seen in coronal plane in AP view where as tracheal foreign body is seen in sagittal plane in same view.

- **How will you confirm that foreign body is not in trachea?** By taking a lateral view which shows that tracheal air shadow is in front of the cricopharyngeal foreign body (Fig. 100.20).

- **How will you remove the foreign body from the cricopharynx?** By visualizing the foreign body with hypopharyngoscope and remove with foreign body removal forceps preferably under general anesthesia

- **What are the complications of untreated foreign body in the cricopharynx?**
  - Mucosal ulceration and perforation of hollow viscus
  - Retropharyngeal abscess
  - Laryngeal edema
  - Migration of foreign body from cricopharynx which may get stuck in the ileocecal junction, the 2nd narrowest part of GI tract
  - Mediastinitis and septicemia.

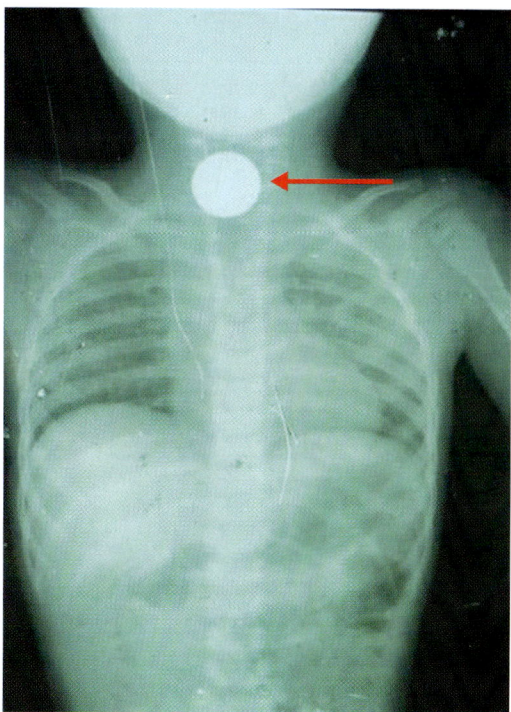

Fig. 100.19: AP view soft tissue neck showing foreign body (coin) at the level of cricopharynx

This is (Fig. 100.21) the lateral view X-ray **soft tissue** neck showing tracheal air column in front of a small linear radio opaque shadow at the level of C5, C6 probably a fish or chicken bone in the cricopharynx.

This X-ray (Fig. 100.22) lateral view neck soft tissue neck shows a linear long radio opaque foreign body showing an eye at the lower end occupying the air lucency of laryngotracheal region. It could be a stitching needle in the laryngopharynx.

CT Larynx

CT provides a non-invasive, quick and effective radiological investigations of the larynx and can be carried out in the face of respiratory obstruction or after suspected laryngeal injury. It gives an accurate assessment of laryngeal

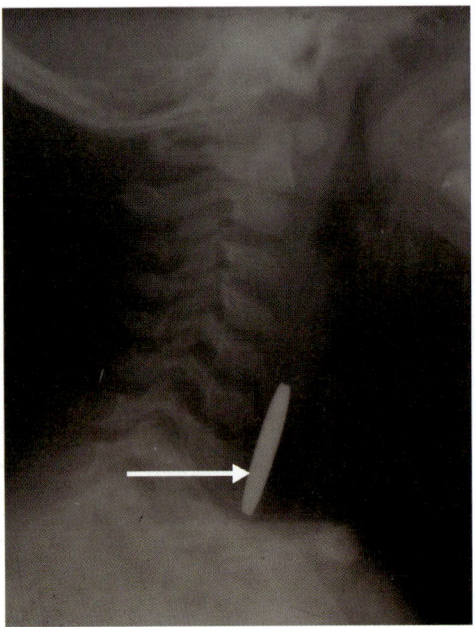

Fig. 100.20: lateral view X-ray neck soft tissue showing tracheal air column in front of cricopharyngeal foreign body

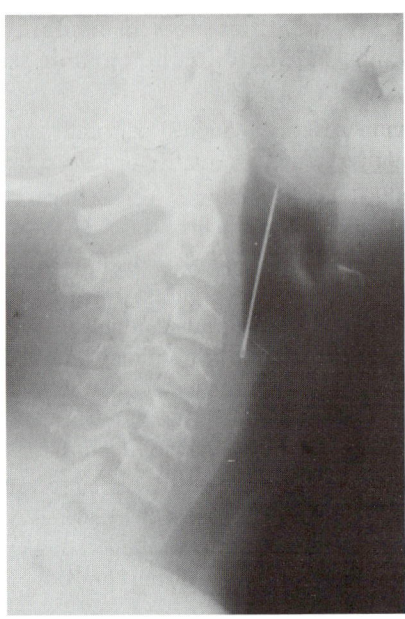

Fig. 100.22: Soft tissue X-ray neck lateral view showing linear long radio-opaque foreign body with an eye in the lower end (Needle)

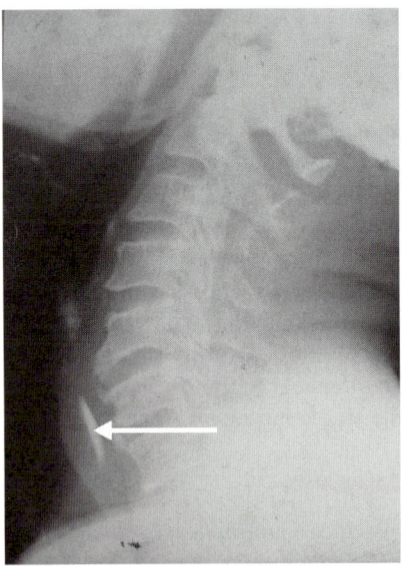

Fig. 100.21: Lateral view soft tissue neck showing small linear radio-opaque foreign body at the level of C5–C6

anatomy and involvement by tumor especially at the glottic level, especially important if a partial laryngectomy procedure is being contemplated

CT in larynx and hypopharynx is most useful in two areas

- Mass lesions benign and malignant
- Trauma – blunt or iatrogenic

Sections are made from the hyoid bone down to the lower margin of cricoid cartilage, contiguous 3 mm sections are necessary from the false cords to the subglottic area. Once beyond the confines of the larynx 5 mm sections are taken to evaluate lymph node bearing areas. IV contrast is used in all cases of laryngeal cancer as it improves visualization of the primary tumor and aids in evaluation of cervical metastatic disease.

CT is also useful in evaluating the spread of laryngeal cancer into the pre-epiglottic and paraepiglottic spaces. Minimum T1 glottic lesions may not be visible or may produce only slight thickening of cord on CT image. CT is useful to diagnose anterior commissure involvement for glottic tumors, posterior spread to the cricoarytenoid joints and inferiorly to the infraglottic region and cricoid. Evaluation of spread to the cricoid is extremely important since reconstruction of a functional glottis (in voice conservation surgery) is difficult once more than a small portion of cricoid is sacrificed at surgery. Fig. 100.23 is showing involvement of right paraglottic space (shown highlighted) which is well made out on CT scan.

Thyroid cartilage involvement can also be assessed by CT scan. Hemangiomas and paraganglionomas enhance intensely on CT scan.

Trauma to Larynx

CT scan is useful in detecting soft tissue injury to the larynx in conjunction with fractures. Fractures may be seen in the thyroid or cricoid cartilage. The following X-ray shows a fracture of thyroid cartilage as a result of trauma (Fig. 100.24).

Cricoid fracture is characteristically a double break, ring may be fractured in two or three places.

The cricoarytenoid joint maybe found to be dislocated with fairly minimal trauma to the lateral larynx.

Cricoarytenoid joint may be rarely dislocated in case of trauma and can be made out on CT scan (Figs. 100.25a and b) of the same patient.

Stenosis

Subglottic stenosis and tracheal stenosis can be evaluated by plain films, but imaging can give information about the cross sectional area of the remaining airway (Figs 100.26a and b).

MRI and CT imaging of Cervical Adenopathy and Neck Masses

CT and MRI are useful to demonstrate the precise location of a neck mass and its rela-tionship to adjacent vascular, muscular and neural structures.

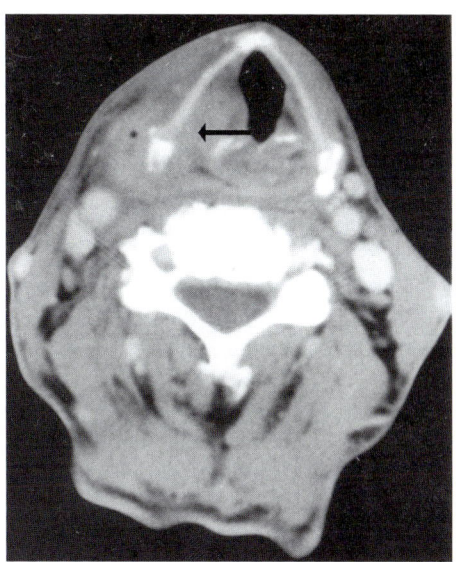

Fig. 100.23: Axial CT showing involvement of right paraglottic space by malignant growth

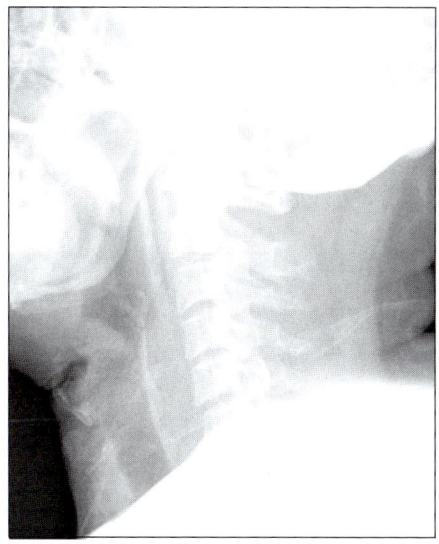

Fig. 100.24: Plain X-ray soft tissue neck showing fracture of thyroid and cricoid cartilage

Contiguous 5 mm thick axial images are taken from the level of superior orbital rim to the lung apex.

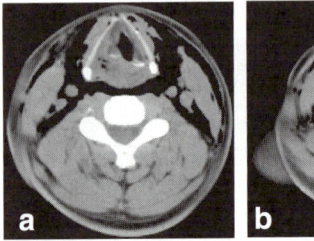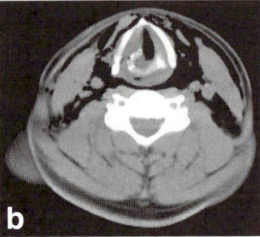

Figs 100.25a and b: CT scan showing fracture of cricoid and dislocation of cricoarytenoid joint associated with hematoma (right side)

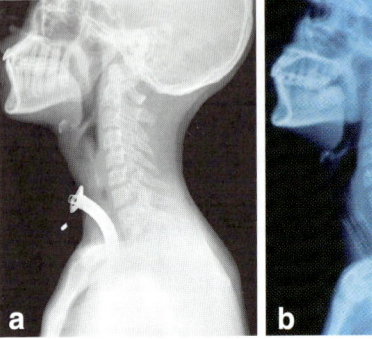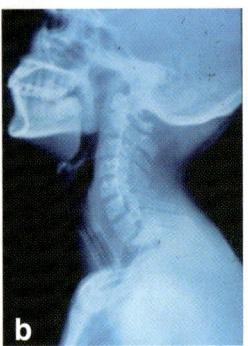

Figs. 100.26a and b: (a) Showing suprastomal stenosis with a metallic tracheostomy tube in situ. (b) Postoperative X-ray of the same patient after excision of stenosis. (a metallic distendable stent in situ after decannulation)

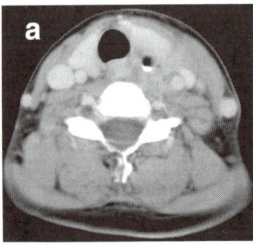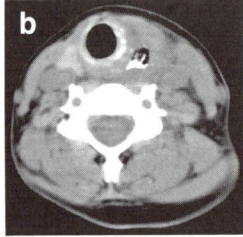

Figs 100.27a and b: CT scan showing pharyngeal pouch of 4th pharyngeal arch origin

MRI and CT imaging are considered complementary in case of imaging of neck masses. *Contrast enhanced CT is the imaging of choice in vascular mass lesion.*

Figs 100.27a and b depicting pharyngeal pouches of IV pharyngeal arch origin.

CT remains the gold standard for assessing palpable and non-palpable nodal metastasis in patient with head and neck tumors.

Based on the work of Mancuso and others following criteria have been adopted:

- Normal lymph nodes have an ovoid shape and are of homogenous soft tissue density and measure less than 1 cm in diameter
- Any node > 1.5 cm is abnormal which may be reactive or neoplastic
- Any node with a central lucency regardless of size is abnormal
- Obliteration of fascial planes surrounding a node is abnormal

Abscesses appear as single or multiloculated low density masses that conform to fascial planes. With contrast they show rim enhancement.

Essentially in the diagnosis of a neck abscess, clinical correlation is extremely important, because even a necrotic tumor, nodal disease with extension into adjacent soft tissues and a thrombosed vessel may all mimic an abscess on sectional images (Fig. 100.28)

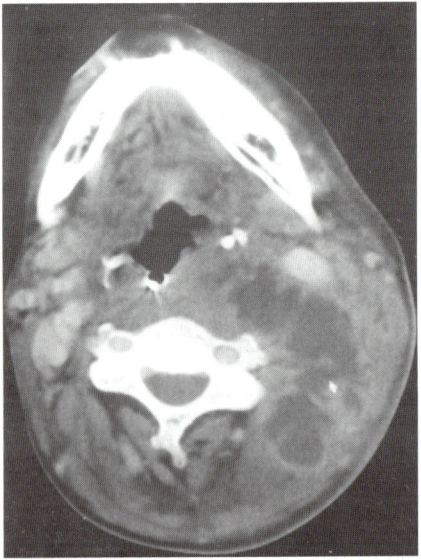

Fig. 100.28: Axial CT showing retropharyngeal abscess coming out to form multiple deep neck space abscesses

Masses of Vascular Origin

Glomus tumor presenting at the bifurcation of carotid is seen in CT as intense enhancement after IV contrast administration

Masses of Neural Origin

- **Schwannomas:** Most appear hypodense or isodense to skeletal muscle
- **Neurofibromas:** Enhancement pattern is variable
- **Lipomas:** Homogenous, non-enhancing mass isodense with subcutaneous fat
- **Larynogocele:** Internal larynogocele are limited to the paralaryngeal space while combined ones extend from paralaryngeal space into the anterior triangle and neck via fenestrations in the thyrohyoid membrane. On CT it shows as a thin rimmed fluid or air filled mass directly lateral to the thyrohyoid membrane.

Soft tissue imaging in the parapharyngeal, infratemporal fossa and pterygopalatine fossa

An axial CT scan with 5 mm contiguous sections form the basis of the examination . Contrast enhancement by bolus infusion is usual to show the position of vessel more clearly and is now the imaging investigation of choice.

The infratemporal fossa can be assessed by CT scan, so also the pterygopalatine fossa is well shown by axial CT.

Spread of tumors along the axis of pterygomaxillary fissure with expansion of walls is seen in JNA.

Intracranial extension can best be assessed with coronal scans.

Sagittal and coronal views are helpful in discerning the position of mass in relation to the carotid and jugular vessels.

The parapharyngeal mass in the anterior compartment in front of styloid is usually salivary in origin (Fig. 100.29). The important differentiation between a tumor of the deep lobe of parotid from a minor salivary gland tumors is the presence of a fat plane between them.

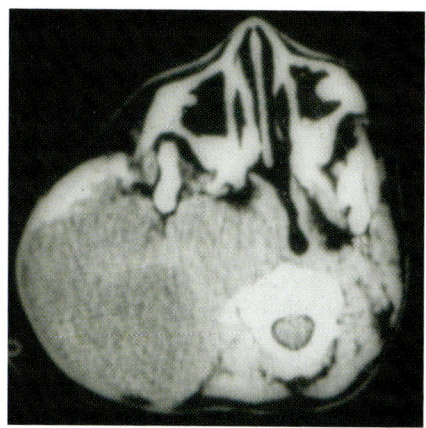

Fig. 100.29: CT sialogram depicting a small parotid being pushed laterally by a large parapharyngeal tumor

The internal carotid artery is usually (but not always) displaced anteromedially by neuromas and posteriorly by minor salivary gland tumors (Figs 100.30a and b).

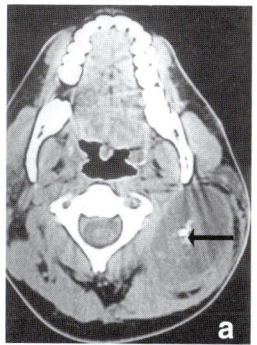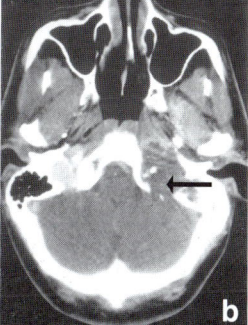

Figs 100.30a and b: These CT scans clearly show a parapharyngeal space tumor with central liquefaction and calcification extending above to destroy the jugular foramen

Imaging of Oropharynx and Tongue

Tumors of the oropharynx, particularly the tongue and the floor of the mouth, can be difficult to assess clinically and their extent hard to define (Fig. 100.31).

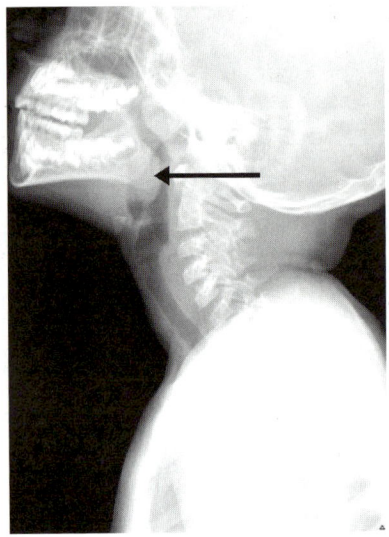

Fig. 100.31: X-ray soft tissue neck lateral view showing oropharyngeal mass (lingual thyroid)

Angiography

A sparsely vascular mass such as neurofibroma show puddling of contrast and anteromedial displacement of internal carotid artery. Paraganglionomas may also displace the internal carotid artery (Fig. 100.32). Carotid body tumors occur low in the neck and displace carotid artery laterally. Vascular masses such as glomus tumors and hemangioma in the neck, salivary gland and base of tongue are extremely difficult to excise and preoperative embolisation may be required.

Another tumor requiring a preoperative angiography and preoperative embolization is JNA. Shown here is an angiogram of a patient of Juvenile angiofibroma (JNA) which showed supply mainly from internal maxillary artery (Figs 100.33a and b).

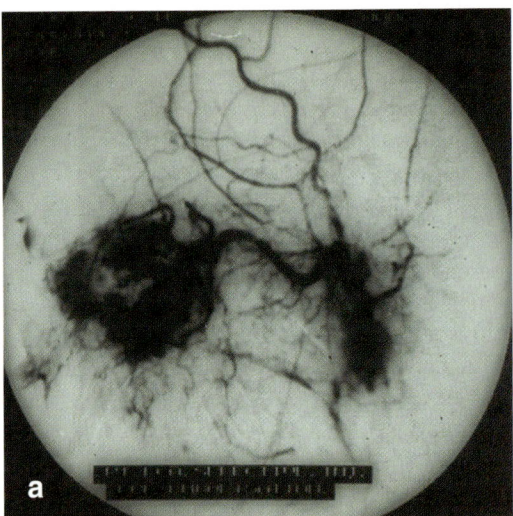

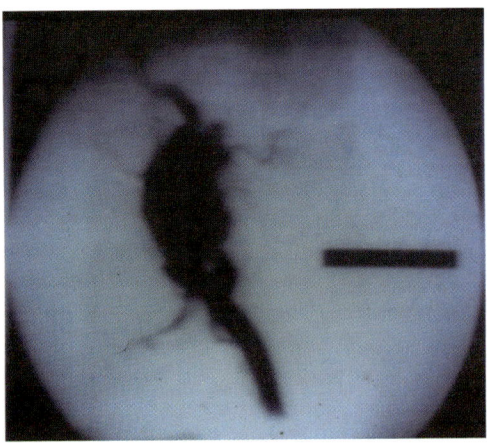

Fig. 100.32: Digital subtraction angiogram of a vagal body tumor with feeding tributaries from both internal and external carotid arteries

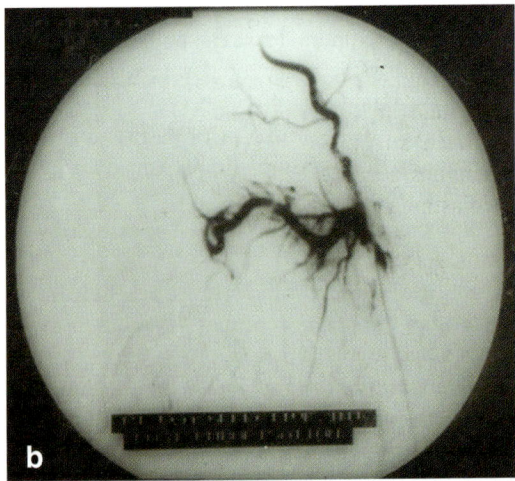

Figs 100.33a and b: (a) Pre-embolisation film (b) Post-embolization

Imaging of the Nasopharynx

CT and MRI give excellent visualization of the nasopharynx and can demonstrate the presence of tumor together with any spread to the skull bone.

In the case of malignancy of the nasopharynx. CT will show a mass in the nasopharynx extending into the soft tissues of the postnasal space and eroding the skull base. The fossa of Rosenmuller and eustachian recess are seen to be obliterated.

Thyroid Imaging

Thyroid may be imaged either with ultrasound or by nuclear medicine technique by giving an IV injection of technitium-99 pertechnate or iodine 131.

Thyroid imaging is useful in a patient with a suspected thyroid swelling to help determine its nature. Most solitary nodules do not take up radionuclide and are referred to as cold nodules, which may be a cyst, adenoma or carcinoma. Ultrasound will show whether it is cystic or solid.

A nodule may be functioning or hot nodules and takes up radionuclide and such nodules are invariably benign adenomas.

Thyroid masses may extend into the mediastinum and thyroid imaging using iodine-131 is the best method of detecting whether such a mass is arising from thyroid tissue.

The parathyroids are imaged using Thallium Technitium Subtraction scans. This is especially important in localizing a parathyroid adenoma prior to surgery since about 10 percent of adenomas occur in ectopic positions often in the mediastinum.

IMAGING STUDY OF THE EAR

Eight conventional views are used for evaluation of the temporal bones. The Laws, Schullers, Owens and Lateral or Modified Lateral views, Chause III and Towne's projection are modified frontal views, Transorbital, Stenvers and Basal view – are useful to expose the petrous pyramid, internal acoustic meatus and mastoid.

Law's Projection

Useful for study of pathological processes including the mastoid air cells and the sinus plate.

Structures Visualized

Extent of air cells in the mastoid process, temporal, squamous, zygomatic arch and the occipital bone.

In a well pneumatized mastoid cavity, the sinus plate separates the superficial air cells from the deeper air cells. Superior dural plate seen as a dense horizontal or oblique line merging with the sinus plate at a sharp angle forming the **angle of Citelli.**

Schuller's View (Lateral Oblique View)

To determine the extent and degree of pneumatization of the mastoids and the condition of the air cells. Also supplies information about the size of the external auditory canal and the relation of the external auditory canal to the sinus plate.

Structures visualized

Mastoids-extent of pneumatization and distribution and degree of aeration of air cells and the status of the trabecular pattern.

Internal auditory canal is seen below the external auditory canal.

It exposes the upper part of external auditory canal, epitypanum and when the middle ear is aerated portions of malleus and incus can also be seen.

Shown here (Figs 100.34a and b) are plain X-rays lateral oblique views of mastoid showing a smooth walled cavity involving the epitympanum and mastoid on left side probably a cholesteatoma cavity. Where as right side is showing secondary sclerosis in a patient having bilateral chronic suppurative otitis media, left atticoantral and right tubotympanic.

Temporomandibular joint and external auditory canal shadow should be identified before studying the details.

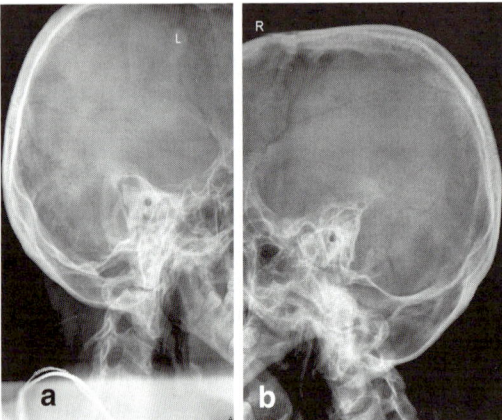

Figs 100.34a and b: (a) Smooth walled cavity involving the epitympanum and the mastoid on the left side (b) Right side showing secondary sclerosis of mastoid.

Differential diagnosis of a cavity on X-ray mastoid.

- Cholesteatoma cavity
- Postmastoidectomy
- Mega antrum
- Multiple myeloma
- Eosinophilic granuloma
- Gun shot injury
- Abnormal emissary vein
- Neoplastic lesions eroding the mastoid

How will you differentiate a postmastoid cavity from cholesteatoma cavity?

- Cholesteatoma cavity-wall will be smooth
- Cholesteatoma cavity will be localized to attic and antrum
- Its wall will be surrounded by a zone of sclerosis
- Cholestetoma mass will be seen in center of cavity with cotton wool appearance
- Postmastoidectomy cavity will appear as single cavity connecting attic antrum and canal in case of canal wall down mastoidec- tomy
- Wall of this will be irregular because of new bone formation.

Why should you take X-ray mastoid in chronic suppuartive otitis media?

- To know the normal and abnormal land marks like forward lying sinus plate and low lying dural plate
- To know the status of pneumatization , whether there is primary or secondary sclerosis
- To know the evidence of bone destruction or cavity formation

Owens View

The Owens projection is used to visualize the external auditory canal epitympanum, portions of the ossicles and the mastoid air cells.

Chause III View

The Chause III projection is the most reliable conventional projection for the study of middle ear. It is the best view to visualize the fistulas of horizontal semicircular canal.

Transorbital View

The transorbital view is mandatory in the study of possible acoustic neuroma, since it allows the study of the size and shape of internal auditory canal and the length of the posterior wall. This view also provides a general survey of the status of the cochlea, vestibule and semicircular canals.

Stenver's View

Stenver's view is useful in the study of all pathological process which involve the petrous pyramid and the apex such as petrositis and tumors of various types.

Town's view (Chamberlain Towne's, Worns and Bretton, Supraorbital Projection of Lysholen)

Useful for the study of inflammation of mastoid and petrous air cells. Internal auditory canal in acoustic neuroma, with large glomus jugulare tumor, erosion of jugular fossa and posteroinferior aspects of petrous pyramid may be recognized. Valvassori criteria are used to interpret the x ray to rule out acoustic neuroma. They are:

1. Shortening of posterior lip of the internal acoustic meatus
2. Difference of 1 cm diameter of internal acoustic meatus is significant
3. Distortion of the C shape of the meatus indicates intracanalicular tumor

20° Coronal Section CT of Middle Ear and Mastoid

This is a good view to study the abnormality of middle ear cavity (Fig. 100.35).

Lateral Sinus Thrombophlebitis

Sinus plate poorly defined and partially eroded (Fig. 100.36).

Jugular Venography

The jugular vein Venography is best to demonstrate a downward extension of glomus tumor into neck along the wall of jugular vein. It shows narrowing or obstruction of the vein extending inferiorly from the base of the skull.

Arteriography

Arteriography exposes the feeding vessels and their origin and this helps to plan the ligation of vessels during surgery. If embolization treatment is used arteriography will indicate which vessels must be selectively catheterized. Postembolization arteriographic studies are used to determine effectiveness of treatment.

CT Scan of Acoustic Neuroma

Coronal and axial sections of high definition CT are used to study these tumors. Examination may show indirect signs of tumor—such as displacement of 4th ventricle, narrowing of opposite cerebellopontine cistern by a displaced brainstem and in large lesion presence of

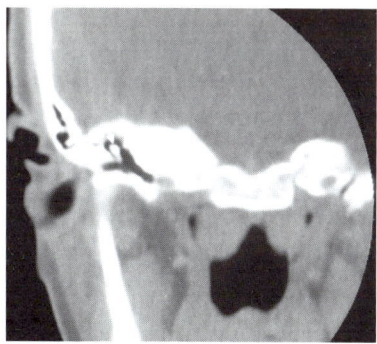

Fig. 100.35: 20° coronal section of middle ear and mastoid showing the malleus

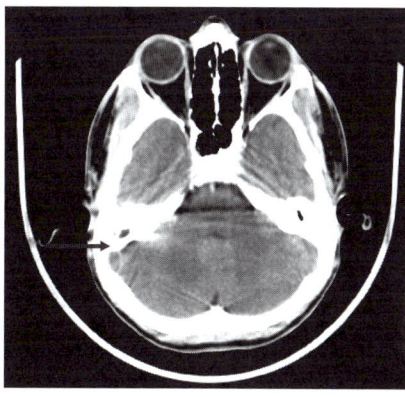

Fig. 100.36: Axial CT showing poorly defined and partially eroded sinus plate seen in lateral sinus thrombophlebitis

obstructive hydrocephalus. Postinfusion study demonstrates mass, because of enhancement of its density by the contrast material. In large lesions there is a central area of decreased absorption produced by cystic degeneration of the tumor.

Tumors under 2 cm are not well shown by CT and hence an air-contrast CT scan or MRI must be performed.

These are MRI and CT Scans of same patient showing an acoustic tumor (shown highlighted in Figs 100.37a and b).

Positron Emission Tomography (PET scan)

Newer functional radioisotopic scan, has been

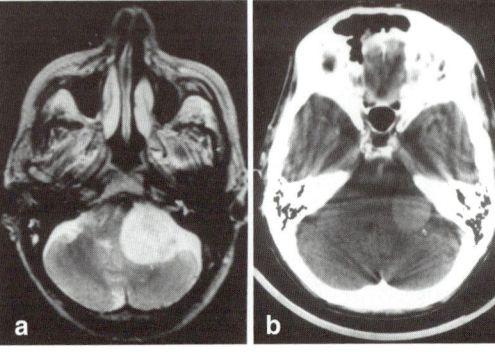

Figs 100.37a and b: (a) MRI and (b) CT scan, of same patient showing acoustic neuroma on the right side

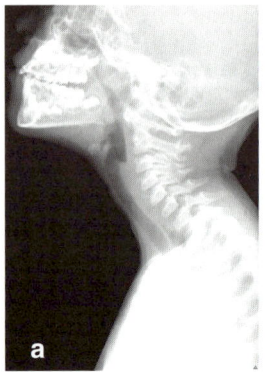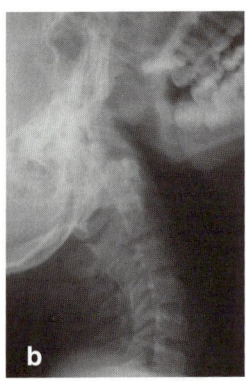

Figs 100.38a and b: Near total occlusion of naso-pharyngeal airway by hypertrophied adenoids

proposed for differentiation of malignant tumors from benign tumors on the basis of malignant tumors having higher metabolic rate and greater incorporation of radio-labeled deoxy glucose than benign lesions.

X-RAYS OF PHARYNX

NASOPHARYNX

Plain X-ray soft tissue nasopharynx : Lateral view.

Lateral projections are taken with patient quietly breathing through the nose. This maneuver will depress the soft palate against the tongue and causes the epiglottis to become more vertical thus opening up the laryngeal vestibule.

Structures Visualized

- Posterior margin of turbinates
- Adenoidal mass
- Salphingopharyngeal fold
- An increase in the midline soft tissues of the oropharynx greater than 4 mm is suspicious of an expansive process.
- In adults soft tissue in roof of nasopharynx should measure not more than 3 mm with regular outline and thickness.
- In children adenoid hypertrophy may be so pronounced as to obliterate the airspace

between posterosuperior wall of soft palate.

Both these X-rays show near total occlusion of airway by hypertrophied adenoids (Figs 100.38a and b).

These X-rays show preoperative and post operative views of chronic retropharyngeal abcess (Figs 100.39 and 100.40)

MRI of same patient (Figs 100.41a and b).

Showing destruction of vertebral body with encroachment onto spinal cord characteristic of chronic retropharyngeal abscess which resulted in quadriplegia in this patient.

- Below the cricoid the soft tissue thickness between the air filled trachea and spine should

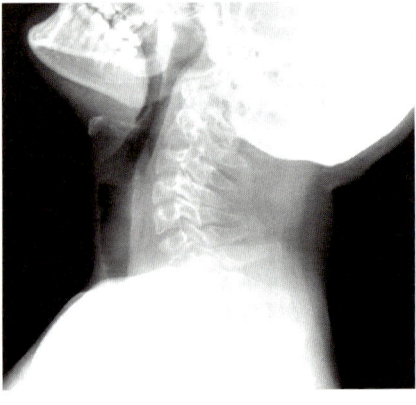

Fig. 100.39: Preoperative plain X-ray view of chronic retropharyngeal abscess

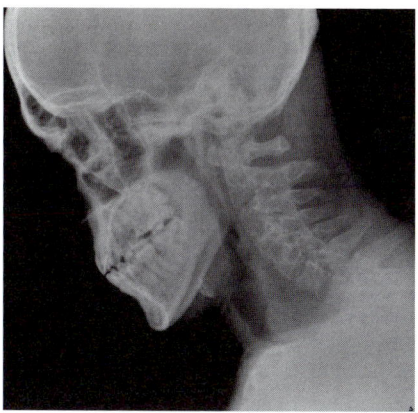

Fig. 100.40: Postoperative plain X-ray view of chronic retropharyngeal abcess

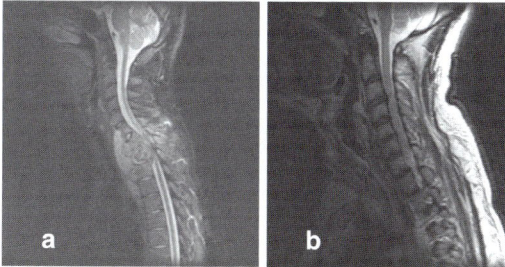

Figs 100.41a and b: MRI of the same patient showing destruction of the vertebral body with encroachment of spinal cord characteristic of chronic retropharyngeal abscess

not normally exceed three-fourth of diameter of corresponding cervical vertebra and if it is more it is suspicious of tumor, inflammation of postcricoid region or upper esophagus. The following X-ray shows a characteristic prevertebral soft tissue widening suggestive of a tumor (Fig. 100.42).

IMAGING OF SALIVARY GLANDS

Pathological changes in the salivary glands are investigated by

- Plain radiography.
- Contrast radiography.

Plain films are obtained to demonstrate any radiopaque calculi or calcification within the gland.

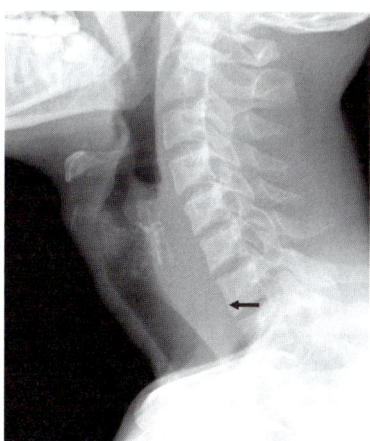

Fig. 100.42: Prevertebral soft tissue widening suggestive of tumor

Parotid gland: Lateral oblique view with open mouth position.

Submandibular gland: Lateral view with floor of mouth depressed with wooden spatula. Intraoral occlusal film is necessary to exclude a stone in Wharton's duct.

Opening of the Stensons and Whartons ducts are exposed and cannulated by a catheter or sialographic cannula and hand injection technique employed. Water soluble or an oily contrast medium (Ultrafluid Lipoidol) may be used.

Sialogresis considered in three phases.

- Ductal filling.
- Acinar filling.
- Evacuation.

Conventional sialography is still the best examination for duct architecture and diseases of duct system like sialectasis. These are sialograms of same patient which show sialectasis (Fig. 100.43).

Ultrasonography of Neck

Ultrasonography is non-invasive and inexpensive radiological examination. Used in ENT – head and neck surgery mainly for:

1. Identification of lymphadenopathy and other cervical masses.

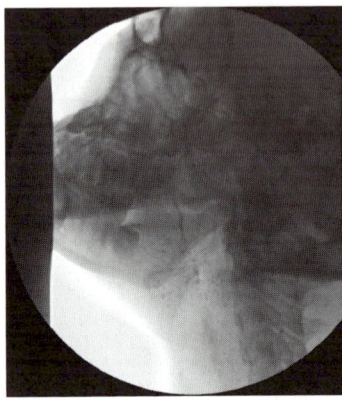

Fig. 100.43: Sialogram showing sialectasis

2. Differentiate between cysts and solid tumors.
3. In detecting venous thrombosis and carotid artery luminal involvement.
4. Relations of lesion to adjacent structures.
5. To aid in directing needle aspiration cytology in tumors that are difficult to localize clinically.
6. To differentiate between benign and malignant lesions.
7. To detect thyroid anomalies like agenesis, hypoplasia and ectopia and malignancy. Lymphadenopathy may be inflammatory and neoplastic

Normal lymph nodes in neck are usually 7 mm or less having typically smooth margins. They have homogenous echogenicity and are oval and elongated in shape.

Malignant lymph nodes are larger in size >1.5cm and rounded in shape. Most characteristic feature is presence of microcalcifications in an enlarged rounded mass. The architecture of metastatic lymph node is abnormal with intranodal cystic necrosis.

Lymphoma is a coalescence of individual nodes to form a large homogenous solid mass

Barium Swallow

Is a contrast study from oral cavity up to the fundus of stomach. Barium sulphate compound in different concentrations is being used. It is of more value for showing lesions of esophagus, pharyngeal pouches, fistula and for neurological swallowing problems, dysphagia, motility disorder like achalasia cardia, foreign body esophagus; perforation of esophagus (water soluble contrast medium—non-cardiac gastrograffin is used). Assessment of extrinsic compression of esophagus, to see for diverticula and webs.

Achalasia cardia: Plain radiograph show markedly dilated esophagus with air filled food levels. Single contrast barium examination with patient upright will show considerable residual solid material in a markedly dilated sigmoid shaped esophagus (Fig. 100.44).

Barium esophagogram showing a stricture in

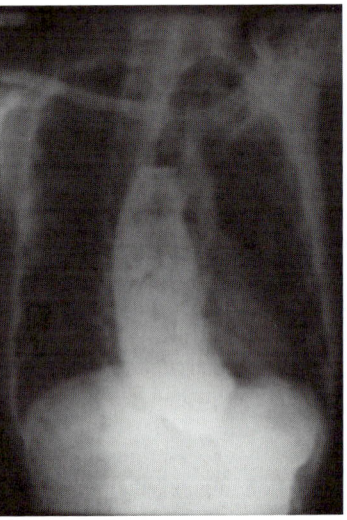

Fig. 100.44: Fusiform dilation of esophagus

the lower end of esophagus with fusiform dilatation of proximal portion suggestive of achalasia cardia or cardiospasm (Fig. 100.45).

How will you confirm your diagnosis?

Barium swallow and Upper GI endoscopy. (Chance of esophageal perforation is high in cardiac achalasia while doing rigid eso-phagoscopy).

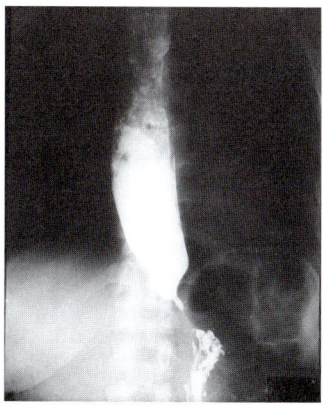

Fig. 100.45: Showing a smooth stricture with fusiform dilatation of esophagus

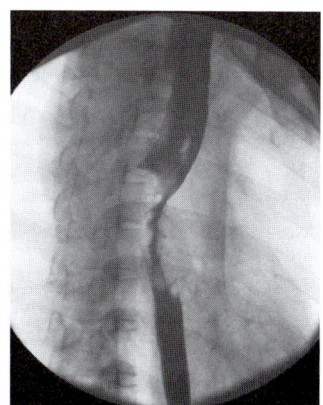

Fig. 100.46: Apple core appearance in malignancy middle third of esophagus

How will you treat this?

1. Medical management with amyl nitrate, anticholinergics like scopalamine
2. Minor surgical procedure like bougie / balloon dilatation
3. Heller's cardiomyotomy and laparoscopic procedures

Malignancy: Circumferential mass arising from esophageal mucosa produce an apple-core appearance (Fig.100.46).

Esophageal motility disturbance: Cork screw esophagus with multiple simultaneous non-peristaltic contractions.

This is (Fig.100.46) a barium swallow esophagogram showing irregular filling defect involving middle third of esophagus with minimal proximal dilatation. In the lower end of esophagus this filling defect is classically described as rat-tail appearance, suggestive of malignant growth.

What is the most common area of malignant change in esophagus?

Middle third.

What is the commonest malignancy seen in middle and lower third of esophagus?

Squamous cell carcinoma in middle third and adeno carcinoma in lower third.

How will you confirm the diagnosis?

Esophagoscopy and biopsy.

How will you differentiate benign stricture from malignant one?

- Benign strictures are multiple, preferably occurring at the normal constrictions of esophagus
- Benign strictures are more in posterior wall
- Benign ones are smooth
- Proximal dilatation is enormous in benign lesions classically called as fusiform dilatation
- Malignant strictures are usually solitary, irregular with minimal proximal dilatation with shouldering effect.

How will you treat squamous cell carcinoma of middle third esophagus?

- External radiation
- Laser excision with Stenting followed by radiation
- Mossou-Baubine tube stenting followed by radiation

How will you treat the malignancy of the lower third of esophagus?

Esophagogastrectomy.

The following barium swallow esophagograms show irregular filling defect in the lower end

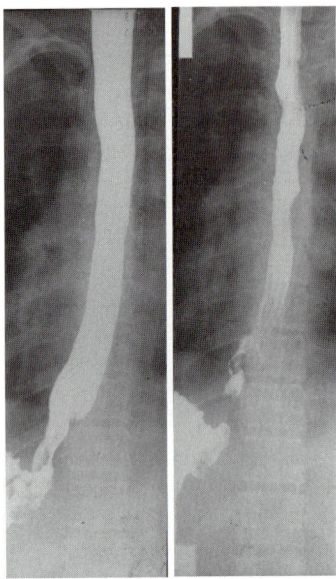

Fig. 100.47: Rat-tail appearance in malignancy lower third of esophagus

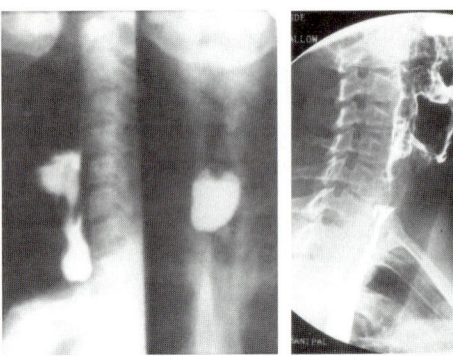

Fig. 100.48: Pre-and postoperative X-ray of pharyngeal pouch

suggestive of malignant growth (Figs 100.47a and b).

Barium swallow shows hypopharyngeal pouch (Fig. 100.48).

Postoperative contrast radiogram shows absence of pouch.

Practicals

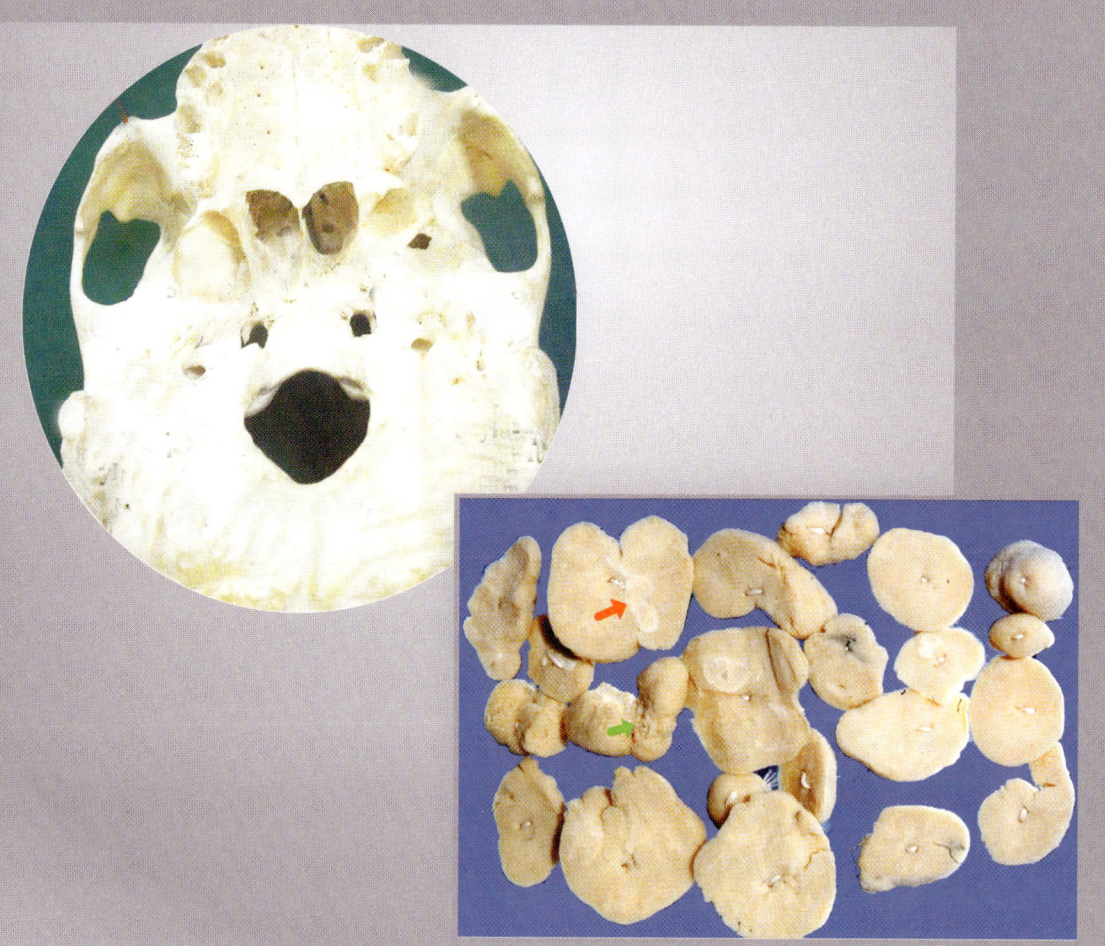

101

Osteology in ENT

Bones of the head and neck region including the skull is frequently given to the candidates appearing for the undergraduate and post-graduate examinations. The following are the points a candidate has to know:

1. Identification of the bone and its parts
2. Placing or holding it in the correct anatomical position
3. Various structures that may be attached to it or the structures that pass through the foramina and fissures.
4. Applied clinical and surgical importance
5. Attachments of the muscles and the ligaments have not been shown as it is understood that the candidate has adequate knowledge of that during the anatomy lectures. Salient points of applied and surgical importance have however been mentioned.

Floor of the Cranial Cavity (Anterior, Middle and Posterior Cranial Fossae) (Figs 101.1 and 101.2)

The floor of the anterior cranial fossa is formed by the roof of the orbits and the roof of the ethmoids (fovea ethmoidalis) and cribriform plates. It is limited posteriorly by posterior borders of the lesser wings of the sphenoid and by anterior margin of the chiasmatic groove.

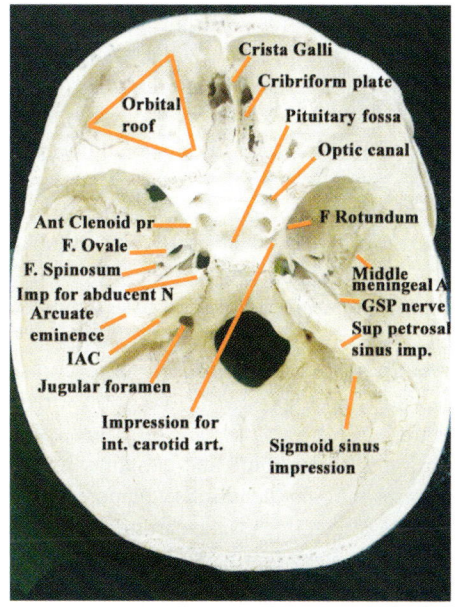

Fig. 101.1: Various features in the floor of the cranial cavity. GSP= greater superficial petrosal nerve, IAC= internal auditory canal

Cribriform plates are perforated by numerous nerve filaments of the olfactory nerve.

The middle cranial fossa is deeper than the anterior cranial fossa. It is narrow medially and wide laterally. It is bounded anteriorly by the lesser

885

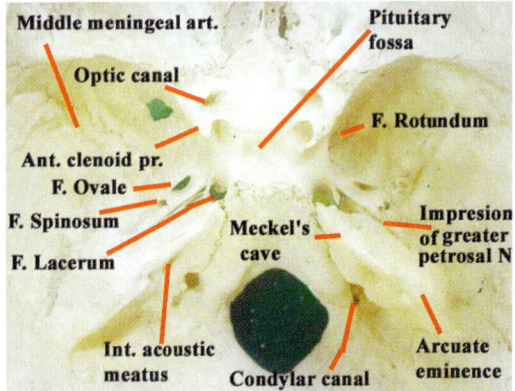

Middle meningeal art.
Pituitary fossa
Optic canal
F. Rotundum
Ant. clenoid pr.
F. Ovale
F. Spinosum
Meckel's cave
Impresion of greater petrosal N
F. Lacerum
Int. acoustic meatus
Condylar canal
Arcuate eminence

Fig. 101.2: A close-up view of the middle and part of the posterior cranial fossae

wing of the sphenoids, anterior clenoid process and anterior margins of the chiasmatic groove. Posteriorly it is limited by the superior angles of the petrous temporal bone and dorsum sellae. Lateral boundary is formed by squamous part of temporal, sphenoidal angles of the parietal bones and by the greater wings of the sphenoid. The middle cranial base has many foramina and fissures and the knowledge of these is essential to understand the spread of skull base tumors like nasopharyngeal carcinoma and angiofibroma. The chiasmatic groove contains the optic chiasma which ends on either side at the optic foramen containing the optic nerve. Sella turcica is a depression in the midline and contains the fossa hypophyses lodging the pituitary gland. On either sides of the sella turcica is the carotid groove. The foramina are seen in the middle cranial base including the foramina ovale, spinosum, rotundum and lacerum which are described later. Superior orbital fissure is bounded above by the lesser wing, below by the greater wing and medially, by the body of the sphenoid. It transmits the oculomotor, trochlear, ophthalmic division of the trigeminal and the abducent nerves. It also transmits the orbital branch of the middle meningeal artery and the ophthalmic veins.

The Dorello's canal is a bow-shaped canal through which courses the abducens nerve before reaching the cavernous sinus. It is located inside a venous confluence which occupies the space between the dural leaves of the petroclival area. The petrosphenoid ligament (Gruber's ligament), which forms the posteromedial wall of the canal, appears as a fibrous trabecula surrounded by venous blood. This is affected in petrositis causing abducent nerve palsy.

The superior angle of the petrous temporal bone contains the superior petrosal sinus. On the anterior surface of the petrous portion of the temporal bone are seen the arcuate eminence caused by the projection of the superior semicircular canal.

The posterior cranial fossa is the deepest of the three and is formed medially by the dorsum sellae, clivus of the sphenoid, occipital bone including the foramen magnum. Anterolaterally is the posterior surface of the petrous temporal bone. It features the internal acoustic meatus, jugular foramen, hypoglossal canal and the foramen magnum which are described later. The sigmoid and the transverse sinuses form sulci in the interior of this fossa.

Structures passing through Various Foramina at the Skull Base
(Figs 101.3 to 101.5)

1. Greater palatine foramen
   - Descending palatine vessels
   - Ascending palatine nerve
2. Foramen ovale (MALE structures)
   - Mandibular nerve
   - Accessory meningeal artery
   - Lesser petrosal nerve
   - Emissary vein
3. Foramen spinosum
   - Meningial artery
   - Recurrent branch from the mandibular nerve
4. Foramen rotundum
   - Maxillary nerve
5. Foramen lacerum
   - During life the foramen is closed by a fibro-cartilage in its lower part

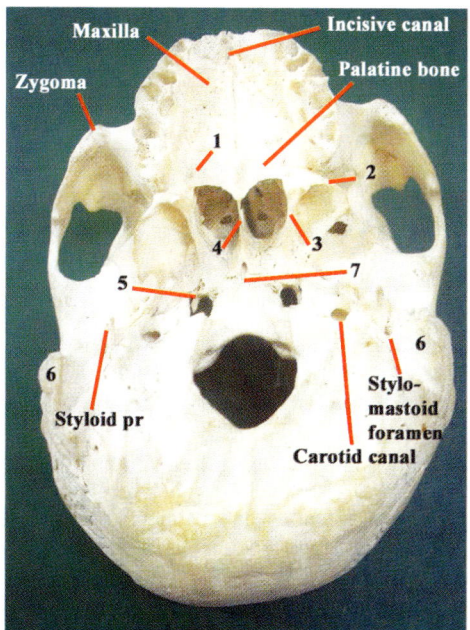

Fig. 101.3: Various features in the norma basalis of the skull. 1. Foramen for greater palatine artery, 2. Lateral pterygoid plate, 3. medial pterygoid plate, 4. Posterior end of the nasal septum formed by vomer, 5. Foramen lacerum, 6. Mastoid process and 7. Basisphenoid

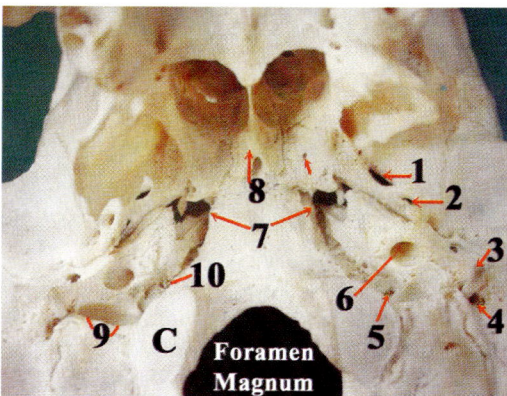

Fig. 101.4: Close-up view of the middle part of the norma basalis. 1. Foramen Ovale, 2. foramen spinosum, 3. Styloid process, 4. Stylo-mastoid foramen, 5. Jugular foramen, 6. Carotid canal, 7. Foramen Lacerum, 8. Vomer, 9. Jugular fossa and 10. Hypoglossal foramen

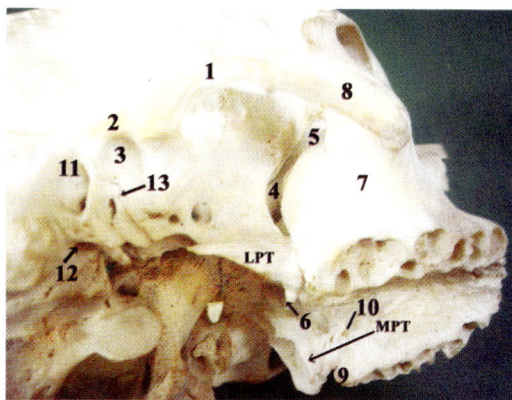

Fig. 101.5: Showing 1. Zygomatic arch, 2. Root of zygoma, 3. Glenoid fossa, 4. Pterygomalxillary fissure, 5. Inferior orbital fissure, 6. Pterygoid hamulus, 7. Right maxilla, 8. Zygoma, 9. Maxillary tuberosity, 10. Greater palatine foramen, 11. External auditory canal, 12. Stylomastoid foramen, 13. Petrotympanic fissure, MPT–Lateral pterygoid plate

- Upper and inner part is related to the internal carotid artery and the sympathetic plexus
6. Foramen magnum
   - Medulla oblongata that continues as spinal cord below the foramen magnum
   - Membranes covering the medulla and spinal cord
   - Cranial accessory nerves
   - Vertebral arteries
   - Anterior and posterior spinal arteries
   - Ligaments connecting the occipital bone with the axis
   - Vertebral veins.
7. Stylomastoid foramen
   - Facial nerve
   - Entrance of stylomastoid artery
8. Hypoglossal canal
   - Hypoglossal nerve
9. Jugular foramen
   It has three compartments:
   - Anterior
     - Inferior petrosal sinus
   - Intermediate

- Glossopharyngeal nerve
- Vagus nerve
- Spinal accessory nerve
- Posterior
  - Internal jugular vein which is the continuation of the sigmoid sinus at the jugular bulb just above the jugular foramen
  - Some meningeal branches from the occipital and ascending pharyngeal arteries
10. Carotid canal
  - Internal carotid artery and cortico sympathetic plexus around it

The details of osteology of the temporal bone and mandible are given in figure legend (101.6, 101.7 and 101.8). These descriptions are self-explanatory. The reader should refer and read along with respective bones to identify various structures by keeping in anatomical position.

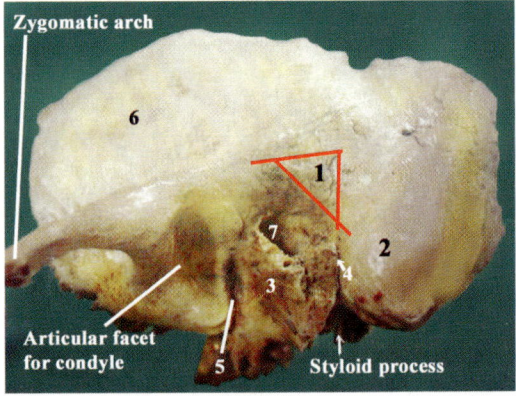

Fig. 101.6: Showing 1. Mac Even's supramastoid triangle, 2. Mastoid process, 3. Tympanic bone, 4. Tympanomastoid suture line, 5. Petrotympanic fissure, 6. Squamous part of the temporal bone, 7. External auditory canal

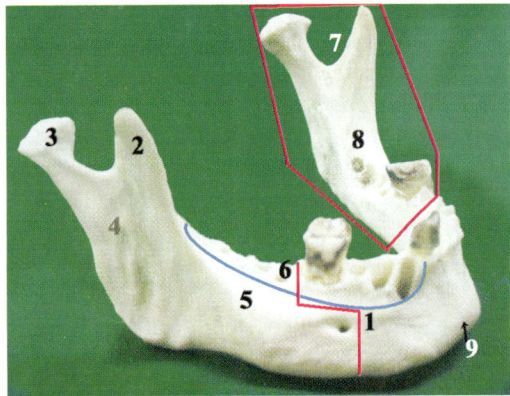

Fig. 101.7: Specimen of the mandible showing 1. Mental foramen, 2. Coronoid process, 3. Condyle of the mandible, 4. Ascending ramus of the mandible, 5. Body of the mandible, 6. Alveolar process with tooth sockets, 7. Coronoid notch and 8. Retromolar trigone. Pink line on the right side shows paramedian mandibulotomy, on the lofe side, area lined with pink boundary shows area of resection for hemimandibulectomy. Blue line shows area to be removed in marginal mandibulectomy

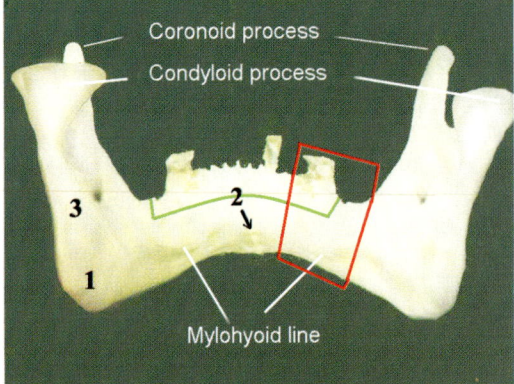

Fig. 101.8: Specimen of the mandible viewed from behind depicting the internal surface. Red square area shown extent of resection in segmental mandibulectomy. Green line shows ara of resection in marginal mandibulectomy in floor of the mouth cancer. Genial tuberosities should be spared to prevent falling back of tongue as genio-glossus muscle gets detached. Various areas shown are 1. Angle of mandible, 2. Genial tuberosity 3. Mandibular foramen for inferior alveolar nerve

102

Operative Specimens of ENT—Head and Neck

The following operative specimens are discussed here:

1. Total laryngectomy specimen
2. Total laryngectomy with partial pharyngectomy
3. Total Laryngo-pharyngo-esopharyngectomy (TLPE)
4. Total maxillectomy specimen
5. Composite wide resection of the oral malignancy with hemimandibulectomy
6. Tubercular lymphadenitis
7. Antrochoanal polyp
8. Rhinosporidiosis

Any operative specimen should be studied under the following parameters:

- Identification of the specimen and reasons for the same. We should be able to identify the normal and the abnormal structures in the specimen.
- Specific findings in the specimen
- Extent of resection
- Indications/differential diagnosis for such surgical resection
- Preoperative work-up that would be necessary
- Anesthetic considerations, if any
- Operative procedure and variants if any

- Reconstruction options
- Postoperative management
- Complications of the procedure

The details of the surgical procedures are discussed in the respective chapters. Hence the theoretical aspects of the surgical procedures are not discussed here.

Specimen 1

The Fig. 102.1 shows a resected specimen after total laryngectomy. The specimen has been split open to visualize the following structures:

- Epiglottis
- Arytenoid cartilage
- Aryepiglottic folds
- Thyroid cartilage
- Cricoid cartilage
- Vocal cord (VC)
- Ventricular band (VB)
- Anterior commisure
- Subglottis.

A proliferative growth (T) is seen involving the posterior two third of the left vocal cord. Fullness of the left ventricular band is seen which is well appreciated when compared to that of the right side. There is prolapse of the ventricular mucosa

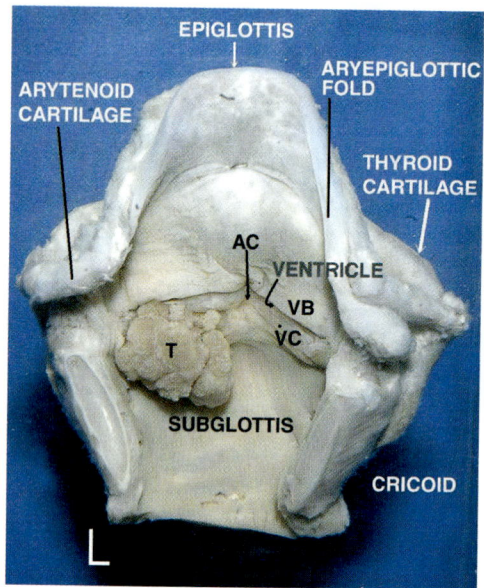

Fig. 102.1: Resected specimen after total laryngectomy

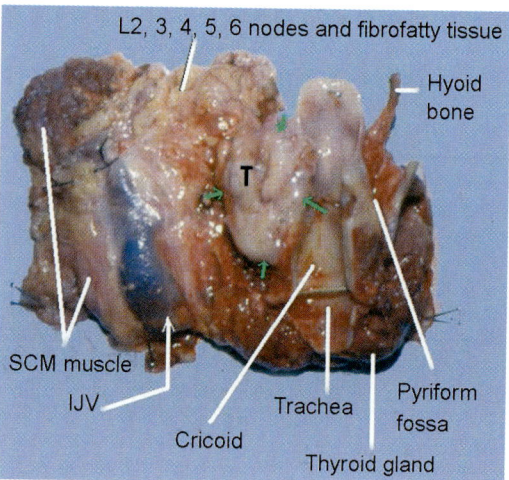

Fig. 102.2: Resected specimen after total laryngectomy with partial pharyngectomy and left radical neck dissection

on the left side. The left vocal process of the arytenoid cartilage is involved. The growth is extending about 10 mm to the subglottis. The anterior commisure appears to be normal. The resected margins are grossly free from the lesion. The lesion has a characteristic 'cauliflower' appearance and is grossly suggestive of malignancy of the left glottis. However possibility of other conditions likes verrucous carcinoma, tuberculosis of the larynx, etc should be kept in mind. The indications for total laryngectomy are

1. Transglottic growth causing cord fixation (T3)
2. Cartilage involvement (T4).

A conservation surgery or near-total laryngectomy may be done if the cricoid cartilage is free and one cricoarytenoid joint is free of disease.

Specimen 2

This is a resected specimen (Fig. 102.2) of total laryngectomy with partial pharyngectomy and left

radical neck dissection for an ulceroproliferative growth (T) involving the left pyriform fossa (medial, anterior and lateral walls) extending up to the left pharyngoepiglottic fold and not involving the apex of the pyriform fossa. The larynx has been split open by cutting the cricoid cartilage in the midline between the two arytenoid cartilages. The hyoid and the thyroid cartilages are well visualized and so is the proximal trachea. The left radical neck dissection specimen contains the resected part of the sternocleidomastoid muscle, internal jugular vein, lymph nodes and the cervical fascia with fatty-alveolar tissue from the anterior and posterior triangles. The thyroid gland also has been resected in total. Following the resection the pharyngeal defect is closed primarily and a permanent tracheostomy is done.

Specimen 3 (Fig. 102.3)

This is resected specimen following total laryngo-pharyngo-esophagectomy (TLPE) for postcricoid carcinoma. Entire esophagus is resected but entire esophagus is not shown in the above picture. The ulceroproliferative growth involves the postcricoid area and right pyriform fossa. Inferiorly it is

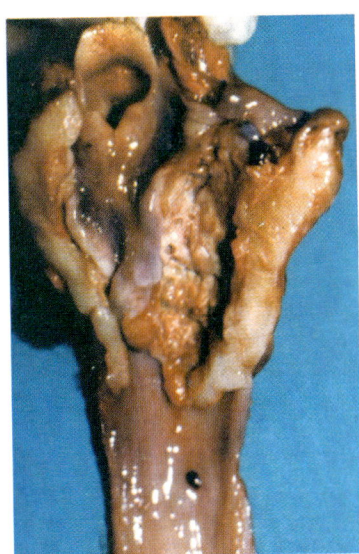

Fig. 102.3: Total laryngo-pharyngo-esophagectomy (TLPE)

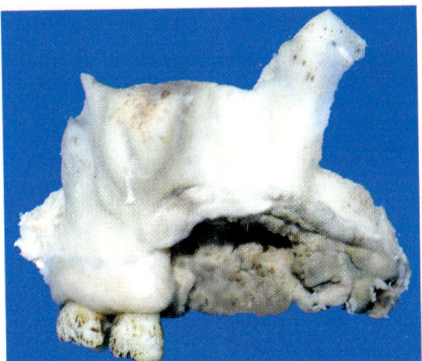

Fig. 102.4: Operated specimen of partial maxillectomy

extending beyond the lower end of the cricoid cartilage and is thus involving about one cm of the proximal esophagus. Superiorly it is extending till the right pharyngoepiglottic fold. The pharynx has been split open to show the entire lesion. Following the resection, reconstruction of the proximal gut is done by gastric pull-up and pharyngogastric anastomosis or by colonic transposition and pharyngocolonic anastomosis.

Specimen 4

This is an operated specimen of partial maxillectomy showing the growth in the alveolar process extending to the interior of the maxillary sinus. The specimen should be examined on both medial and lateral aspects to know the extent of the growth. The indications for partial maxillectomy are growth confined to the infrastructure of the maxilla, malignancy of the upper alveolus, etc.

Specimen 5

The Figure 102.5 shows a specimen following right hemimandibulectomy, with wide excision of

the growth involving buccal mucosa with extension to retromolar trigone (arrow). Entire half of the mandible till the mental foramen is resected in this case. The mylohyoid line and the mandibular foramen with the inferior alveolar nerve passing into it may be appreciated. An ulcero-proliferative growth (T) is seen in the buccal mucosa extending from the level of canine tooth anteriorly to the retromolar trigone posteriorly. Involvement of the mandible clinically or radiologically is an indication for hemi or segmental mandibulectomy. Involvement of the mandibular canal for the inferior alveolar nerve necessitates a hemimandibulectomy for complete resection. The mandibular defect may be reconstructed by various procedures like osteomyocutaneous pedicle flap like pectoralis major myocutaneous flap with the rib or trapezius flap with scapular

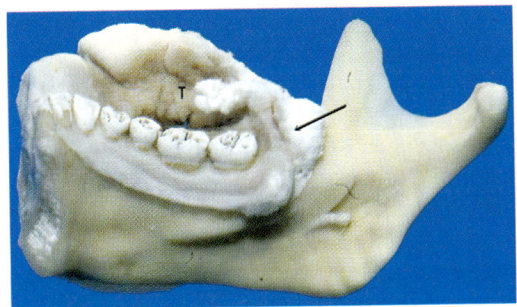

Fig. 102.5: Right hemimandibulectomy

crest or free flaps like fibular free flap or osteointegrated fibular free flaps which are more popular these days.

Specimen 6

The Figure 102.6 shows multiple resected cervical lymph nodes in a case of suspected tubercular lymphadenitis. Cut lymph nodes show areas of caceation as shown by red arrow. Also shown are areas of matting (green arrow) characteristic of tubercular lymphadenitis.

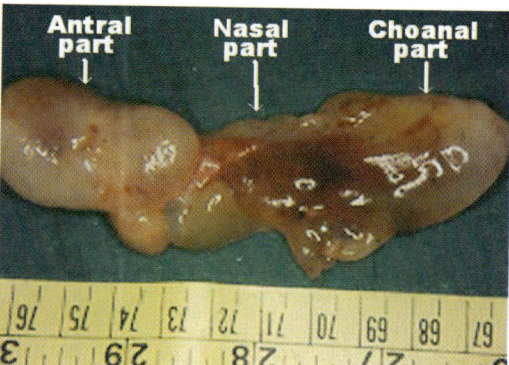

Fig. 102.7: Antrochoanal polyp

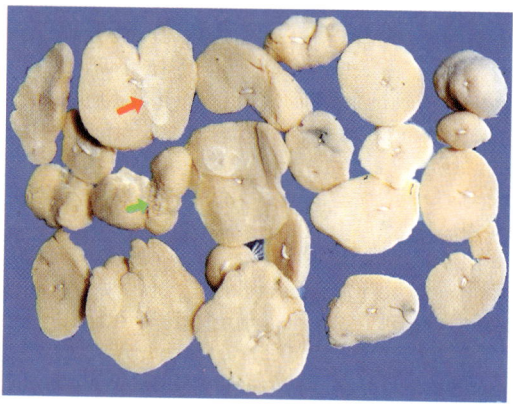

Fig. 102.6: Multiple lymph nodes in tubercular cervical lymphadenitis. Red arrow shows the site of central necrosis within the lymph node

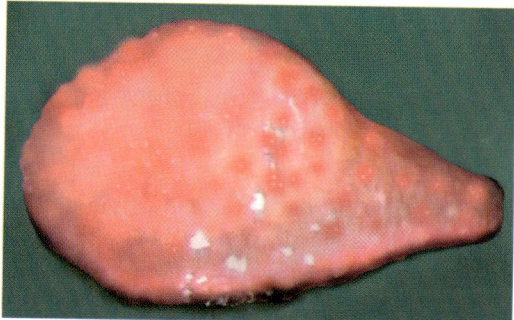

Fig. 102.8: Rhinosporidiosis

Specimen 7

This is a resected specimen of an antrochoanal polyp. The polyp is a prolapsed edematous mucosa of the sinuses or the nasal cavity and has a characteristic pale grape like appearance with smooth glossy surface and is soft in consistency. This specimen of antrochoanal polyp has three parts as shown in the Fig. 102.7. Complete removal of the polyp is ascertained by the presence of these three parts as it has two constrictions, one at the maxillary ostium and the other at the choana. Differential diagnosis of unilateral polypoidal nasal mass includes meningocele/

meningoencephalocele, intranasal dermoid, intranasal glioma, inverted papilloma, rhinosporidiosis, hemangioma, angioma of the septum, choristoma, olfactory neuroblastoma, etc.

Specimen 8

This is a resected specimen of rhinosporidiosis. The gross specimen is a pedunculated mass and has the characteristic pinkish-red color with granular surface studded with white spots (sporangia) giving it a classical 'Strawberry appearance'. It often has a pedicle and the mass is surgically excised by cutting the pedicle using cautery or laser. The base of the pedicle is then cauterized to destroy the submucosal sponangia (Fig. 102.8).

Case Studies

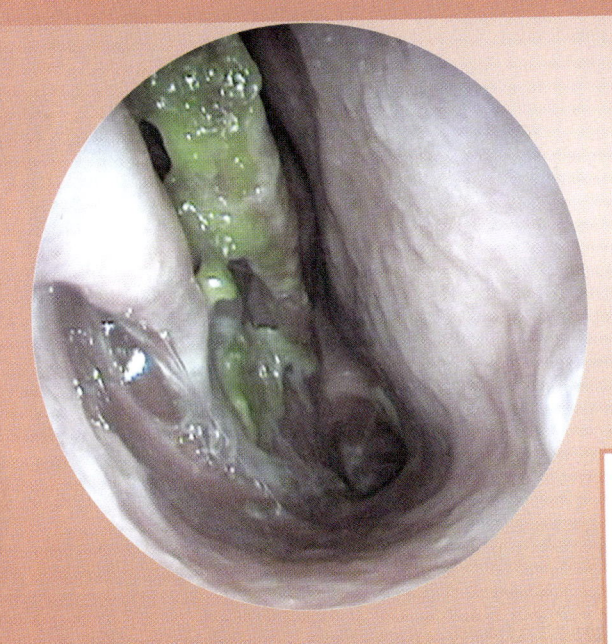

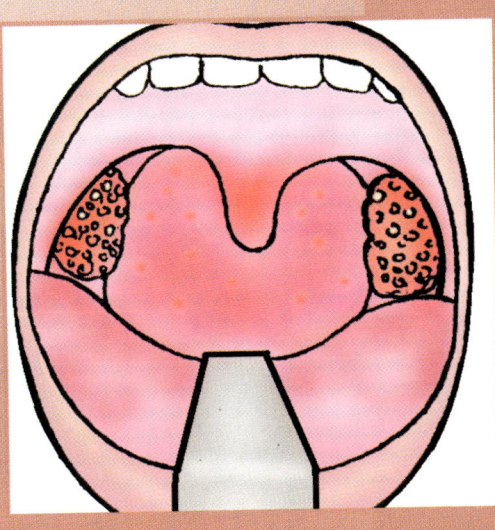

103

Clinical Case Discussion

SAMPLE CASES

- Case-I CSOM (TTD)
- Case-II Recurrent rhinosporidiosis
- Case-III B/L ethmoidal polyps
- Case-IV CSOM (AAD)
- Case-V Primary atrophic rhinitis
- Case-VI Chronic tonsillitis with adenoid hypertrophy

Following are model clinical presentations given for the sake of helping the students. It is imperative that students take a thorough clinical history before proceeding on to examination proper. Detailed history is taken which includes:

(a) Basic data regarding patient's name, age, sex, occupation, address, etc.
(b) Chief complaints with duration of each complaint
(c) History of presenting illness
(d) Treatment history
(e) Past history
(f) Family history.

(Full forms of abbreviations are given on page 905 of this chapter)

CASE - 1

Name	-	K
Age	-	30 years
Sex	-	Female
Address	-	Mapusa, Goa.

Chief complaints

- Right ear discharge since childhood
- Decreased hearing in right ear - 5 years
- Headache since 8 months

History of Presenting Illness

Right ear discharge started since childhood, which was insidious in onset, intermittent, profuse, mucoid to mucopurulent, non-foul smelling, non bloodstained, more during episodes of upper respiratory tract infection, relieved on putting ear drops. Last ear discharge was three months back. Decreased hearing in the right ear started five years back, insidious in onset, and slowly progressive. No history of giddiness or tinnitus.

Headache: Eight months duration, insidious in onset, gradually progressive, intermittent, mainly bi-frontal, more on bending forward, more in the morning and more during episodes of URI. History of recurrent hawking sensation is present. No history of visual aura, vomiting or decreased vision, recurrent nose block/mouth breathing, allergy to dust or excessive sneezing, bloodstained nasal discharge.

Past History

No history of diabetes mellitus, hypertension, bronchial asthma, ischemic heart disease, pulmonary tuberculosis or drug allergy.

Treatment History

Patient had consulted local doctor for ear discharge and was given ear drops, after which ear discharge subsided. Patient had taken ayurvedic treatment for headache and was given treatment in the form of ointment.

Family History

Married and has one child. No significant illness in the family.

Personal History

- Sleep and appetite are normal.
- Bowel and bladder habits are normal.

Menstrual History

- Patient is having regular menstrual cycles.
- Last menstrual period—Feb 21.

General Physical Examination

- Moderately built and nourished
- No pallor, cyanosis, icterus, koilonychia, clubbing, lymphadenopathy or pedal edema.
- *Pulse rate:* 80/min, regular
- *BP:* 120/80 mm Hg in right arm supine position.
- *Temperature:* Normal
- *Respiratory rate:* 15/min

Examination of the Ear

	Right	Left
• Preauricular region	Normal	Normal
• Pinna	Normal	Normal
• Postauricular region	Normal	Normal
• Tragal tenderness	Absent	Absent
• Mastoid tenderness	Absent	Absent
• External auditory canal	Normal	Normal
• Tympanic membrane (Fig. 103.1a)	Large central perforation	Retracted
• Mobility present on valsalva maneuver	-	Present
• MEM	Dry	Not seen
• HOM	Foreshortened	
• ETO	Visible	Not seen
• TM Joint	Normal	Normal
• Fistula sign	Negative	Negative
• Facial nerve	Normal	Normal

Tuning fork test:

Rinne 256	Negative	Positive
512	Negative	Positive
1024	Positive	Positive
Weber	Lateralized toright	
ABC	N	N

Examination of the Nose and PNS

- Paranasal sinus tenderness absent.
- *Cold spatula test:* Decreased fogging on the left side.
- *External osseocartilaginous framework:* Normal.
- *Vestibule, columella:* Normal
- *Anterior rhinoscopy:* S-shaped DNS to left to post deviation with spur with right-sided inferior turbinate hypertrophy. Discharge is seen left middle meatus. Right side middle meatus could not be visualized due to spur (Fig.103.1b).
- *Nasal mucosa:* Congested.

Postnasal Examination

- *Posterior end of septum:* Normal
- *Choana:* Normal
- *B/L posterior end of inferior and middle turbinates:* Normal

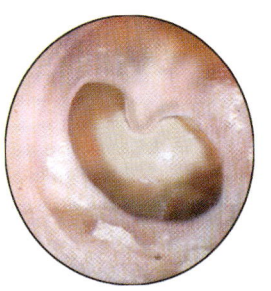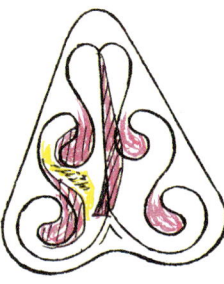

Figs 103.1a and b: (a) Large central perforation (right tympanic membrane). (b) 'S' shaped DNS to left

- Discharge seen in both middle meatus.
- Bilateral ETO congested, discharge seen.

Oral Cavity and Oropharynx

- Mouth opening adequate
- *Lips:* Normal
- *Gingivobuccal sulcus:* Normal
- *Gums, teeth:* Normal
- *Orodental hygiene:* Normal
- *Floor of mouth:* Normal
- *Tongue:* Normal
- *Retromolar trigone:* Normal
- *Palate:* Normal
- *Anterior pillars:* Normal
- *Uvula:* Normal
- *Posterior pillars:* Normal
- *Posterior pharyngeal wall:* Congested and granular.
- *Postnasal discharge:* ++

Indirect Laryngoscopy

- *Base of tongue:* Normal
- *Glossoepiglottic fold:* Normal
- *Valleculae:* Normal
- *Epiglottis:* Normal
- *Pharyngoepiglottic fold:* Normal
- *Bilateral pyriform fossae:* Normal
- *Bilateral arytenoids:* Normal
- *Bilateral aryepiglottic fold:* Normal
- *Ventricular bands:* Normal
- *Bilateral vocal cords:* Normal

Head and Neck Examination

Trachea appears central

- Laryngeal crepitus+
- No dilated veins, scars or sinuses
- No palpable lymph nodes
- Cranial nerve examination—Normal

Systemic Examination

- *Respiratory system:* Bilateral vesicular sounds heard
- *CVS S1S2:* Normal
- *Per abdominal examination:* Abdomen soft, no organomegaly
- *CNS:* Higher mental functions—Normal
- Cranial nerves appear intact

Summary

The whole history has to be summarized, only positive findings both in the clinical history and ENT examination should be mentioned. Negative clinical history and findings to be completely omitted.

Provisional Diagnosis

Right CSOM, TTD, inactive stage, with moderate CHL with S-shaped DNS with right sided inferior and left middle turbinate hypertrophy with chronic sinusitis.

Commonly asked questions

- Why do you say it is tubo-tympanic disease (safe type) of Chronic Suppurative Otitis Media?
- What are the different types of discharges that can be associated with otitis media?
- What could be the cause of otitis media in this case?
- Can you mention the stages of tubotympanic disease (safe type) of Chronic Suppurative Otitis Media?
- Why do you say the patient suffers from moderate conductive hearing loss in this case?

- What are the investigations you would ask for in this case and why?
- What is the role of operating microscope in examination of this case?
- What do you mean by air-bone gap?
- How will you perform Patch test?
- Is it necessary to treat chronic sinusitis before treating Chronic Suppurative Otitis Media?
- What is the aim of your treatment in this case?
- How will you manage this case?

CASE - 2

Name - C
Age - 37 years
Sex - Male
Occupation - Tailor
Address - Madhurai Dt., Tamil Nadu

Chief complaints

- Left sided nasal obstruction -20 years
- Recurrent bouts of bleeding from left nostril - 20 years

History of Presenting Illness

Patient with history of bathing in public ponds since childhood comes with history of left sided nasal obstruction, which was insidious in onset and gradually progressive. This was associated with a reddish mass protruding from the left nostril.

Patient also gives history of recurrent bouts of bleeding (epistaxis) from the left nostril, which was provoked by sneezing and coughing. Patient lost about 10 to 15 ml of blood in each episode. It was relieved by application of cold compresses to the nose. Initially patient had 1 to 2 episodes per week, but as the mass started growing out of the nasal cavity the frequency increased. The patient consulted a local doctor for the same and was advised surgery.

Patient also gives history of bitemporal headache, which is more towards the evening. It is associated with hawking sensation. Headache increases during episodes of URTI.

Treatment History

Patient gives history of undergoing multiple nasal surgeries in the past for the above complaints in 1985, 86, 87, 88, 93 and 2002. Presently patient is on tab dapsone100 mg O.D and nasal douches.

Examination of the Nose and PNS

- Right maxillary sinus tenderness is present.
- *Cold spatula test*: Decreased fogging on the left side.
- *External framework:* Normal
- *Columella and vestibule:* Normal

Anterior Rhinoscopy

Pinkish pedunculated granular sessile mass studded with greyish white specks resembling a ripe strawberry attached to the septum which is confirmed by probing. The mass is seen protruding from left nostril (Figs 103.2a and b).

On the right side anterior DNS to the right with synechiae between septum and inferior turbinate is seen. Mucoid discharge was present in middle meatus (Fig. 103.3).

Postnasal Examination

- *Posterior end of septum:* Normal
- *Posterior end of middle and inferior turbinates:* Normal
- *Nasopharynx:* Normal

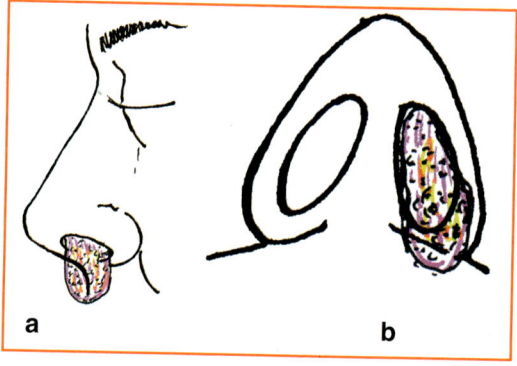

Figs 103.2a and b: Mass is seen protruding from left nostril

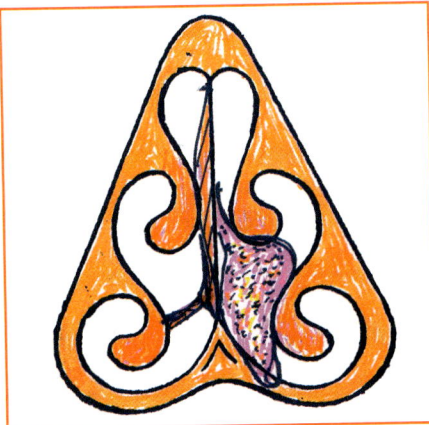

Fig. 103.3: Anterior rhinoscopy showing synechia nasal cavity between septum and inferior turbinate left and pinkish granular pedunculated mass right nasal cavity, surface of which is studded with yellowish white spots

- No similar strawberry like mass seen.
- *Left ETO:* Normal
- *Right ETO:* Mucoid discharge seen.
- *Oral cavity and oropharynx:* Normal
- *Indirect laryngoscopy:* WNL
- *Head and neck examination:* Normal

Examination of Ear

Pinna, external auditory canal, tympanic membranes are bilaterally normal

Summary

The whole history has to be summarized, only positive findings both in the clinical history and ENT examination should be mentioned. Negative clinical history and findings to be completely omitted.

Provisional Diagnosis

Recurrent rhinosporidiosis of left nasal cavity with DNS to the right, with synechiae between septum and right inferior turbinate, associated with chronic sinusitis on right side.

Commonly asked questions

- Why do you give a provisional diagnosis of recurrent rhinosporidiosis?
- What are the differential diagnosis you will keep in mind?
- What do you mean by synechiae and how will you prevent it?
- What could be the cause of chronic sinusitis on the right side?
- Can you give the life cycle of rhinosporidiosis?
- What is the latest organism thought to be the cause of rhinosporidiosis?
- What do you mean by malignant rhinosporidiosis?
- How will you investigate this case? What is the line of management you will adopt?
- How will you prevent recurrence?

CASE - 3

Name	- A
Age	- 60 years
Sex	- Female
Occupation	- Housewife
Address	- Manderi, Kannur, Kerala.

Chief complaints

- *Recurrent attacks of URTI:* 15 years duration
- *Hawking:* 15 years
- *Nose block:* 3 months

History of Presenting Illness

Patient was apparently normal till 15 years back when she developed recurrent attacks of URTI. This was associated with sneezing, itching and watering of the eyes on exposure to dust patient also case of watery nasal discharge. History of dust allergy was present. Patient also complains of left sided headache during attacks of URTI, which aggravates on bending forward. No diurnal variation, mainly in frontal region, does not radiate, not associated with nausea/vomiting/blurring of vision. Headache is associated with mucopurulent nasal discharge and hawking.

Nose block started three months back which was insidious in onset and gradually progressive bilaterally but more on the left side, present throughout the day, increased during attacks of URTI. History of mouth breathing present during attacks of URTI, no other ENT complaints.

Past History

- Patient is a known bronchial asthmatic on bronchodilator therapy since 5 years.
- History of diabetes mellitus present, on oral hypoglycemic drugs since 2 years.
- No history of ischemic heart disease, pulmonary tuberculosis, hypertension.

Treatment History

- Consulted a local doctor who referred him to this hospital.

Menstrual History

- Attained menopause 6 years back

Family History

- Patients mother and father both suffer from bronchial asthma.
- Married and has three children. No one has similar complaints.

Personal History

- *Sleep, bowel and bladder habits:* Normal.
- No history of loss of weight /loss of appetite.

General Examination

- Conscious and cooperative.
- Moderately built and nourished.
- Bilateral allergic shiner's present.
- No pallor, icterus, cyanosis, koilonychia, lymphadenopathy, clubbing or pedal edema.
- *Pulse rate:* 82/min., regular rhythm and good volume.
- *BP:* 140/90 mm Hg in right arm supine position.
- *RR:* 18/min
- *Temperature:* 98.4° F

Examination of the Nose and PNS

- *External framework:* Normal
- Transverse crease seen above the tip of the nose.
- No PNS tenderness.
- *Cold spatula test:* Bilateral decreased fogging, more decreased on the left side.
- *Columella:* Caudal dislocation of septum to left.

Anterior Rhinoscopy

- DNS with spur on the left side.
- Bilateral inferior turbinate is hypertrophied and pale.
- Multiple glistening greyish white, smooth pedunculated polypoidal masses, appear like a bunch of grapes seen in both middle meatus (Figs 103.4 and 103.5).

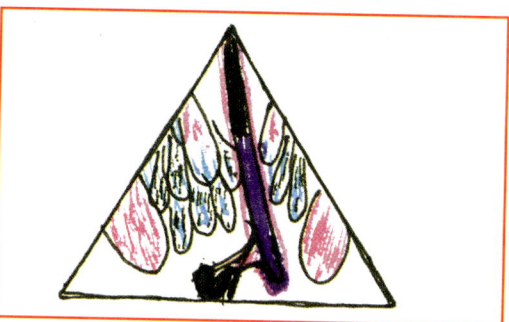

Fig. 103.4: DNS with spur on the left side with bilateral ethmoidal polyposis

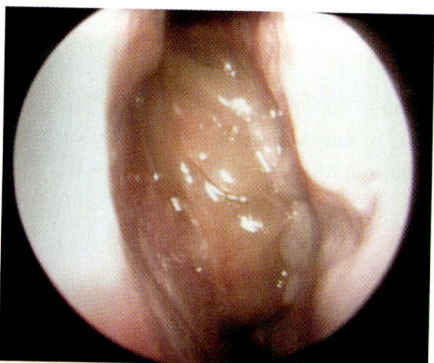

Fig. 103.5: Endoscopic photograph showing typical appearance of ethmoidal polyp

- *On probing:* Each mass can be probed all around .
- They are insensitive to touch, consistency, does not bleed.

Postnasal Examination

- *Posterior end of septum:* Normal
- *Posterior end of inferior and middle turbinate:* Normal
- Mucopurulent discharge seen around bilateral ETO.

Oral Cavity and Oropharynx	
Orodental hygiene	– Fair
Lips, angle of mouth	– Normal
Mouth opening	– Adequate
Glossolingual sulcus	– Normal
Glossobuccal sulcus	– Normal
Gums, teeth	– Normal
Tongue	– Normal
Palate	– Normal
Anterior and posterior pillars	– Normal
Uvula	– Normal
Tonsils	– Normal
PPW	– Granular
PND	– +

Indirect laryngoscopy (ILS)

Base of tongue	– Normal
Glossoepiglottic fold	– Normal
Bilateral valleculae	– Normal
Epiglottis	– Normal
Bilateral pharyngoepiglottic folds	– Normal
Bilateral pyriform fossae	– Normal
Bilateral arytenoids	– Normal
Bilateral aryepiglottic folds	– Normal
Bilateral ventricular bands	– Normal
Bilateral vocal cords	– Normal

Head and Neck Examination

- *Laryngeal framework:* Normal
- *Laryngeal crepitus:* +
- Trachea central
- Bilateral carotid pulsations felt.

Examination of the Ear

	Right	Left
• Preauricular region	Normal	Normal
• Pinna	Normal	Normal
• Postauricular region	Normal	Normal
• EAC	Normal	Normal
• TM	Intact	Intact
• Fistula sign negative bilateral		
• No mastoid or tragal tenderness seen bilateral		
• Facial nerve intact bilateral		

Tuning fork test (TFT)

• Rinne	256	+	+
	512	+	+
	1024	+	+
• Weber		Central	
• ABC		N Bilaterally	

Systemic Examination

- *CVS:* S1, S2 heard, no murmurs
- *RS:* No adventitious sounds heard. Vesicular sounds heard bilaterally.
- *CNS:* Higher mental functions—Normal.
- *PA:* Abdomen soft, no organomegaly.

Summary

The whole history has to be summarized, only positive findings both in the clinical history and ENT examination should be mentioned. Negative clinical history and findings to be completely omitted.

Provisional Diagnosis

Bilateral ethmoidal polyposis with allergic rhinosinusitis with 'S' shaped DNS with caudal dislocation to the left with granular pharyngitis associated with bronchial asthma and diabetes mellitus.

Commonly asked questions

- What do you mean by 'polyp'?
- Why do you give a diagnosis of bilateral ethmoidal polyps?
- What are the differences between ethmoidal and antrochoanal polyp?
- What is the pathogenesis for polyp formation?
- What is the differential diagnosis for polypoidal masses?
- What do you mean by allergic fungal sinusitis?
- How often do you find ethmoidal polyps being associated with bronchial asthma?
- What is Sampter's triad?
- How will you investigate this case? How important is CT Scan in this case?
- What are the various tests done to diagnose allergic rhinitis?
- What is allergic salute?
- Do you think FESS is required in this case?
- What is the principle behind FESS?

CASE - 4

Name   - H
Age   - 40 years
Sex   - Male
Occupation - Factory worker
Address   - Kannur, Kerala
Chief complaints

- Left ear discharge since 15 years.
- Decreased hearing in the left ear since 10 years.

History of Presenting Complaints

Patient was apparently normal since 15 years when he developed left ear discharge. Discharge was continuous, scanty, purulent, foul smelling, occasionally blood stained, does not subside with ear drops and not associated with URTI.

- History of decreased hearing since 10 years, insidious onset and gradually progressive.
- No history of tinnitus, giddiness, ear block or pain.
- No history of facial weakness or asymmetry.
- No other ENT complaints.

Past History

- History of Diabetes mellitus and Hypertension present, on medication since two months
- No history of bronchial asthma, pulmonary tuberculosis, ischemic heart disease.
- No history of previous surgeries

Treatment History

Patient had consulted a local doctor for the same complaints who had prescribed ear drops. Patient had no improvement with the treatment.

Family History

- Married and has two children (boys).

Personal History

- Mixed diet
- Sleep, bowel and bladder habits are normal.
- No history of loss of weight or appetite.
- Smokes 9 to 10 beedis /day for last 10 to 15 years.
- Consumes alcohol occasionally.

General Examination

- Moderately built and nourished
- No pallor, cyanosis, icterus, clubbing, koilonychia, lymphadenopathy, pedal edema.
- *Pulse rate:* 86/min, regular rhythm and good volume.
- *BP:* 140/90 in right arm supine position
- *Temperature:* Normal
- *RR:* 20 breathes/min.

Examination of the Ear

	Right	*Left*
• Preauricular region	Normal	Normal
• Pinna	Normal	Normal
• Postauricular region	Normal	Normal
• No mastoid/tragal tenderness b/l		
• EAC	Normal	Normal
• TM	Retracted	Marginal perforation involving foreshortened. Granulations at the posteror margin. Posterior margin:ill-defined (Fig. 10.3.6).
• TMJ	Normal	Normal

- *Fistula sign negative:* Bilaterally.
- *Facial nerve clinically intact:* Bilaterally.

Tuning fork tests (TFT)

Rinne		
256	+	-
512	+	-
1024	+	+
Weber	Lateralized to left	
ABC	Normal bilaterally	

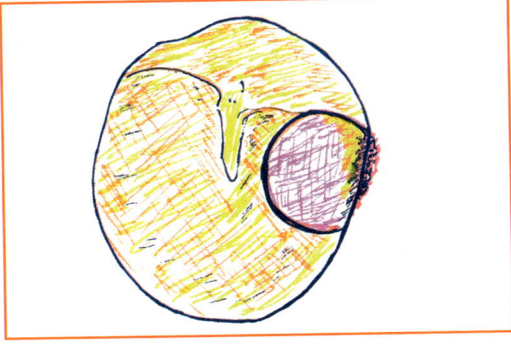

Fig. 103.6: Marginal perforation involving PSQ of left tympamic membrane associated with granulations

Examination of the Nose and PNS

- No PNS tenderness
- *Cold spatula test:* Equal fogging bilaterally.
- *External osseocartilaginous framework:* Normal
- *Columella, vestibule:* Normal
- *Anterior rhinoscopy:* DNS to left bilateral inferior turbinate hypertrophied, left middle turbinate hypertrophied.

Postnasal Examination

- *Posterior end of septum and turbinates:* Normal
- *Bilateral eustachian tube orifice:* Normal
- *Nasopharynx:* Normal

Oral Cavity and Oropharynx

- Mouth opening adequate
- Orodental hygiene fair
- Lips, gums are normal
- Gingivobuccal sulcus is normal
- Gingivolabial sulcus is normal
- *Buccal mucosa:* Normal
- *Tongue:* Normal
- *Palate:* Normal
- *Anterior pillar:* Normal
- *Tonsils:* Normal
- *Posterior pillars:* Normal
- *Uvula:* Normal
- *Posterior pharyngeal wall:* Normal
- *ILS:* WNL
- *Neck:* WNL

Summary

The whole history has to be summarized, only positive findings both in the clinical history and ENT examination should be mentioned. Negative clinical history and findings to be completely omitted.

Provisional Diagnosis

Left CSOM-AAD-secondary acquired cholesteatoma with moderate conductive hearing loss with DNS to right with DM and HTN.

Commonly asked questions

- Why do you diagnose this case as Chronic Suppurative Otitis Media (Attico-antral disease)- Unsafe Type?
- What is the definition of Attico-antral disease/ cholesteatoma/?
- What do you mean by secondary acquired cholesteatoma?
- How will you differentiate primary acquired cholesteatoma?
- How will you classify cholesteatoma, explain its genesis?
- How will you differentiate simple retraction pocket from cholesteatoma?
- What could be the cause in this case?
- How the disease spreads (pathways)?
- What is congenital cholesteatoma?
- What are the investigations you will do to confirm your diagnosis?
- Do you think that deviated nasal septum could be the causative factor of the disease of the ear?
- What radiological findings do you expect in this case?
- What is the differential diagnosis of cavity in the mastoid?
- What is the aim of your treatment?
- How will you decide about when the patient requires canal wall down or intact wall mastoidectomy?
- What are the problems encountered following postmastoidectomy cavity?

CASE - 5

Name - R
Age - 15 years
Sex - Female
Occupation - Student

Chief complaints

- Nasal discharge with crusts since three years
- Hyposmia since three years
- Occasional epistaxis while removal of crusts

History of Presenting Illness

Patient was apparently normal three years back when she started complaining of insidious onset of nasal discharge from both nostrils, gradually progressive, greenish associated with crusting of the nasal cavities and foul smell appreciated by the bystanders.

Patient also gives history of scanty bleeding whenever she attempts to remove these crusts.

There is also associated hyposmia of three years duration, which is continuous.

Examination of the Nose and PNS

- No PNS tenderness present.
- Cold spatula test—there is decreased fogging on the left side
- External osseocartilaginous framework - Normal
- Vestibule, columella—Normal
- Anterior rhinoscopy
- Both nasal cavities appear roomier right > left
- Nasal mucosa appears congested
- Mucoid discharge is seen in floor of both nasal cavity.
- Bilateral inferior and middle turbinate atrophic (Figs 103.7a and b).
- Mucopurulent discharge is seen in both middle meatus.

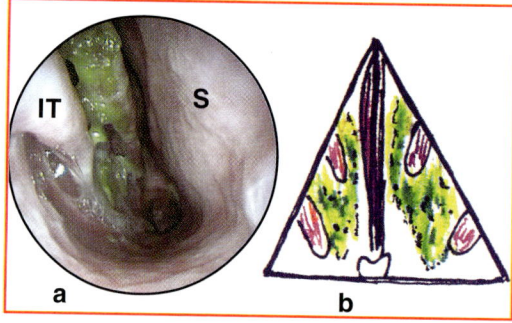

Figs 103.7a and b: (a) Endoscopic picture showing classical features like greenish crusts present on the IT, MT and atrophy of the inferior turbinate and roomy nasal cavity as seen in atrophic rhinitis, (b) Showing diagrammatic depiction of the nasal cavity in the present case

- Greenish crusts present on the inferior turbinate, middle turbinate, septum on both sides which bleeds on removal.
- Posterior DNS to the left

Postnasal Examination

- Greenish crusts seen on the posterior ends of inferior and middle turbinate and choana.
- *Bilateral eustachian tube orifice:* Normal.

Examination of the Ear

- EAC-wax present on the right side.
- Tympanic membrane not seen on the right side due to wax and is intact and mildly retracted on the left side.

Summary

The whole history has to be summarized, only positive findings both in the clinical history and ENT examination should be mentioned. Negative clinical history and findings to be completely omitted.

Provisional Diagnosis

Primary atrophic rhinitis with posterior DNS to the left.

Commonly asked questions

- Why do you say this is a case of primary atrophic rhinitis?
- What are the types of atrophic rhinitis?
- What are the types of primary atrophic rhinitis?
- What do you mean by secondary atrophic rhinitis? What are the causes?
- What do you mean by ozaena and merciful anosmia?
- What are the investigations you would like to do in this case?
- What are the histopathological features seen in the biopsy specimen of an atrophic rhinitis patients?
- What is the differential diagnosis?

- What is rhinitis sicca?
- How will you treat a case of atrophic rhinitis?
- When should you do recanalization in Young's/Modified Young's operation?

CASE - 6

Name - S
Age - 6 years
Sex - Male
Occupation - Student
Address - Kerala

Chief complaints

- Recurrent attacks of URTI since three years.
- Throat pain since one year.
- Mouth breathing and snoring since six months.

History of Presenting illness

Patient was apparently normal three years back when he started developing insidious onset of recurrent episodes of URTI, accompanied by mucoid to mucopurulent nasal discharge, low grade fever and nasal obstruction

There was also associated throat pain with difficulty in swallowing food during the attacks. History of mouth breathing and snoring present since last 6 months.

Examination of the Nose

- No PNS tenderness present
- Cold spatula test shows decreased fogging bilaterally
- *External osseocartilaginous framework:* Normal
- *Vestibule, columella:* Normal
- Anterior rhinoscopy
- Anterior DNS to the left
- Nasal mucosa appears pale
- Right inferior and middle turbinate appears hypertrophied
- Mucoid discharge in bilateral middle meatus.

Postnasal Examination

- Enlarged adenoids seen in the upper part of nasopharynx partly obscuring the choanae.
- Mucoid discharge in bilateral eustachian tube orifice.

Oral Cavity and Oropharynx

- Mouth opening adequate
- Orodental hygiene fair
- *Lips, gums:* Normal
- Overcrowding of teeth present
- *Floor of mouth:* Normal
- *Tongue:* Normal
- *Retromolar trigone:* Normal
- High arched palate
- Anterior pillar congested bilaterally.
- Hypertrophied tonsils congested bilateral grade 2 (Fig. 103.8)
- Septic squeeze negative bilateral
- *Posterior pillars:* Normal
- PND ±
- Indirect laryngoscopy
- *Base of tongue:* Normal

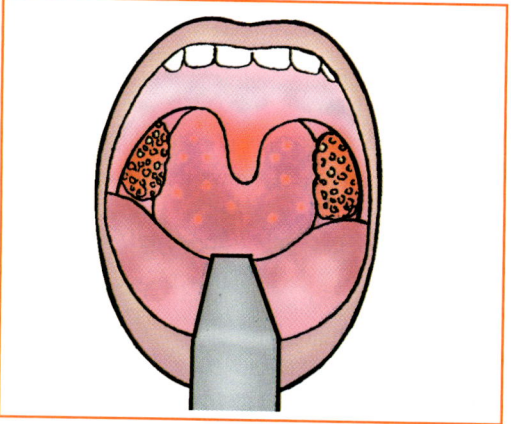

Fig. 103.8: Hypertrophied tonsils congested bilaterally (grade 2) with congestion of anterior pillar

- *Bilateral glossoepiglottic fold:* Normal
- *Bilateral valleculae:* Normal
- *Epiglottis:* Normal
- *Bilateral pharyngoepiglottic fold:* Normal
- *Bilateral pyriform fossae:* Normal
- *Bilateral aryepiglottic fold:* Normal
- *Bilateral arytenoids:* Normal
- *Bilateral ventricular bands:* Normal
- *Bilateral vocal cords mobile:* Normal

Head and Neck Examination

Bilateral jugulodigastric lymph nodes 2 × 2 cms palpable, firm, non-tender and mobile.

Provisional Diagnosis

Chronic parenchymatous tonsillitis with adenoid hypertrophy.

Commonly asked questions

- Why do you say that the patient is having chronic tonsillitis with adenoiditis?
- What are the cardinal signs of chronic tonsillitis?
- What are the features of adenoid facies?
- How will you differentiate tonsil from adenoid?
- How will you grade tonsillar and adenoid hypertrophy?
- Can you briefly mention their immunological role?
- What is the differential diagnosis of white patch on tonsil?
- How will you investigate this case?
- What treatment will you offer to the patient?
- What are the indications of tonsillectomy?
- What are the complication involved in tonsillectomy and adenoidectomy?
- When is tonsillectomy and adenoidectomy contraindicated?

Index